CURRENT PEDIATRIC THERAPY
13

SYDNEY S. GELLIS, M.D.

Professor and Emeritus Chairman, Department of Pediatrics,
Tufts University School of Medicine;
Pediatrician-in-Chief Emeritus, Boston Floating Hospital
for Infants and Children,
New England Medical Center, Inc., Boston, Massachusetts

BENJAMIN M. KAGAN, M.D.

Senior Consultant and Director Emeritus, Department of Pediatrics,
Cedars-Sinai Medical Center;
Professor of Pediatrics Emeritus, University of California at Los Angeles,
Los Angeles, California

1990
W.B. SAUNDERS COMPANY

Harcourt Brace Jovanovich, Inc.

Philadelphia   London   Toronto   Montreal   Sydney   Tokyo

W. B. SAUNDERS COMPANY
Harcourt Brace Jovanovich, Inc.

The Curtis Center
Independence Square West
Philadelphia, PA 19106

The Library of Congress Catalogued the First Issue of This Serial As Follows:

RJ52   Current pediatric therapy.   1964–
C8   Philadelphia, Saunders.

      v. 28 cm. biennial.

      Editors: 1964–   S. S. Gellis and B. M. Kagan.

      1. Pediatrics—Collected works.   2. Therapeutics—Collected works.   I. Gellis, Sydney S., ed.   II. Kagan, Benjamin M., ed.

      RJ52.C8   618.9/2006   64–10484 rev

      Library of Congress   [r66i3]

Editor: Lisette Bralow

Developmental Editor: Hazel Hacker

Manuscript Editor: Donna Walker

Production Manager: Frank Polizzano

Indexer: Dennis Dolan

CURRENT PEDIATRIC THERAPY—13   ISBN   0–7216–2334–4

Printed in the United States of America.

Last digit is the print number: 9   8   7   6   5   4   3   2   1

Contributors

James M. Adams, M.D.
Associate Professor of Clinical Pediatrics, Baylor College of Medicine; Director, Neonatal Intensive Care Unit and Transport System, Texas Children's Hospital and The Woman's Hospital of Texas, Houston, Texas
Tetanus Neonatorum

Raymond D. Adelman, M.D.
Professor and Chairman, Department of Pediatrics, Eastern Virginia Medical School; Vice President for Medical Affairs and Consultant in Pediatric Nephrology, Children's Hospital of the King's Daughters, Norfolk, Virginia
Perinephric and Intranephric Abscess

Laurie S. Ahlgren, M.D.
Assistant Professor of Surgery, Tufts University School of Medicine; Lecturer in Surgery, Boston University School of Medicine; Attending Pediatric Surgeon, Boston Floating Hospital for Infants and Children/New England Medical Center; Chief of Pediatric Surgery, Boston City Hospital, Boston, Massachusetts
Burns

D. A. Allen, Ed.D.
Associate Professor in Child Psychiatry, Albert Einstein College of Medicine; Director of Infant and Preschool Therapeutic Nurseries, Albert Einstein and Bronx Municipal Hospital Center, Bronx, New York
Autism

A. Loren Amacher, M.D., F.R.C.S.(C)
Department of Neurosurgery, Geisinger Medical Center, Danville, Pennsylvania
Brain Tumors

Mary G. Ampola, M.D.
Associate Professor of Pediatrics, Tufts University School of Medicine; Acting Chief, Clinical Genetics Division, and Director, Pediatric Amino Acid Laboratory and PKU-IEM Clinic, New England Medical Center, Boston, Massachusetts
Disorders of Amino Acid Metabolism

John A. Anderson, M.D.
Clinical Professor of Pediatrics, University of Michigan Medical School, Ann Arbor; Head, Division of Allergy and Clinical Immunology, Department of Medicine, Henry Ford Hospital, Detroit, Michigan
Physical Allergy

Bascom F. Anthony, M.D.
Professor of Pediatrics, University of California, Los Angeles School of Medicine, Los Angeles; Chief, Division of Infectious Diseases and Associate Chair, Department of Pediatrics, Harbor-UCLA Medical Center, Torrance, California
Group A Streptococcal Infections

Leonard Apt, M.D.
Professor of Ophthalmology, Director Emeritus of the Division of Pediatric Ophthalmology, Jules Stein Eye Institute, Los Angeles School of Medicine; Special Consultant in Pediatric Ophthalmology for the Los Angeles City Health Department and the Bureau of Maternal and Child Health, Department of Public Health, State of California, Los Angeles, California
The Eye

Kenneth A. Arndt, M.D.
Professor of Dermatology, Harvard Medical School; Dermatologist-in-Chief, Beth Israel Hospital, Boston, Massachusetts
Topical Therapy: A Dermatologic Formulary for Pediatric Practice

Stephen C. Aronoff, M.D.
Associate Professor of Pediatrics, Case Western Reserve University School of Medicine; Acting Chief, Division of Pediatric Infectious Diseases, Rainbow Babies and Children's Hospital, Cleveland, Ohio
Management of Septic Shock

Felicia B. Axelrod, M.D.
Professor of Pediatrics, New York University School of Medicine; Attending in Pediatrics, New York University Medical Center, New York, New York
Familial Dysautonomia

George E. Bacon, M.D.
Professor and Chairman, Department of Pediatrics, Texas Tech University School of Medicine; Chief, Pediatric Service, Lubbock General Hospital, Lubbock, Texas
Disorders of the Adrenal Gland

Robert L. Baehner, M.D.
Professor and Executive Chairman of Pediatrics, University of Southern California School of Medicine; Chairman of Academic Affairs and Physician-in-Chief, Children's Hospital of Los Angeles, Los Angeles, California
Aplastic Anemia

Carol J. Baker, M.D.

Professor of Pediatrics, Microbiology and Immunology, Baylor College of Medicine; Active Staff, Texas Children's Hospital, Harris County Hospital District and Woman's Hospital of Texas, Houston, Texas

Group B Streptococcal Infections

Anthony H. Balcom, M.D.

Clinical Fellow, Hospital For Sick Children, Toronto, Ontario

Penis, Spermatic Cord, and Testes

William F. Balistreri, M.D.

Fellow, Pediatric Gastroenterology and Nutrition, Children's Hospital Medical Center, Cincinnati, Ohio

Cirrhosis

Giulio J. Barbero, M.D.

Professor of Child Health, University of Missouri School of Medicine; University of Missouri Hospital, Colombia, Missouri

Pylorospasm, Pyloric Stenosis

Gabor Barabas, M.D.

Associate Clinical Professor of Pediatrics, University of Medicine and Dentistry of New Jersey—Robert Wood Johnson Medical School, New Brunswick; Consulting Pediatric Neurologist, Monmouth Medical Center, Red Bank; and Robert Wood Johnson—University Hospital, New Brunswick, New Jersey

Childhood Sleep Disturbances and Disorders of Arousal

Dorsey M. Bass, M.D.

Research Fellow in Medicine, Stanford University; Assistant Clinical Professor of Pediatric Gastroenterology, Stanford University Hospital, Stanford, California

Acute and Chronic Nonspecific Diarrhea Syndromes

James W. Bass, M.D., M.P.H.

Professor of Pediatrics, Uniformed Services University of the Health Sciences, Bethesda, Maryland; Clinical Professor of Pediatrics, University of Hawaii School of Medicine, and Chairman, Department of Pediatrics, Tripler Army Medical Center, Honolulu, Hawaii

Toxoplasmosis

Maha K. Bassila, M.D.

Assistant Professor of Otorhinolaryngology, Albert Einstein College of Medicine; Full-time Attending Physician in Otorhinolaryngology, Montefiore Medical Center, Albert Einstein Weiler Hospital, Bronx Municipal Hospital, and North Central Bronx Hospital, Bronx, New York

Malformations of the Nose; Tumors and Polyps of the Nose; Nasal Injuries

Mark L. Batshaw, M.D.

Professor of Pediatrics and Neurology, University of Pennsylvania School of Medicine; Physician-in-Chief, Children's Seashore House, Atlantic City, New Jersey; Chief, Division of Child Development and Rehabilitation, Children's Hospital of Philadelphia, Philadelphia, Pennsylvania

Mental Retardation

David Baum, M.D.

Professor of Pediatrics and Chief, Division of Pediatric Cardiology, Stanford University School of Medicine; Pediatric Cardiologist, Stanford Medical Center and Children's Hospital at Stanford; Consultant in Pediatric Cardiology for the U.S. Army, Silas B. Hayes Hospital, Fort Ord, California

Acute Rheumatic Fever

Arthur L. Beaudet, M.D.

Investigator, Howard Hughes Medical Institute and Professor, Institute for Molecular Genetics, Baylor College of Medicine; Chief, Genetic Service, Texas Children's Hospital, Houston, Texas

Lysosomal Storage Disease

Robert C. Beckerman, M.D.

Professor of Pediatrics and Physiology and Section Chief, Pediatric Pulmonary Medicine; Tulane University School of Medicine, Tulane University Medical Center and Charity Hospital of New Orleans, New Orleans, Louisiana

Primary Pulmonary Hemosiderosis

Douglas W. Bell, M.D.

Clinical Instructor of Otolaryngology, Harvard Medical School; Associate in Otolaryngology, Children's Hospital, Boston, Massachusetts

Salivary Gland Tumors; Thyroglossal Duct Cysts; Branchial Arch Cysts and Sinuses

Bruce O. Berg, M.D.

University of California, San Francisco; Professor of Neurology and Pediatrics, Director of Child Neurology, University of California Medical Center, San Francisco, California

Congenital Muscular Defects

Abraham B. Bergman, M.D.

Professor of Pediatrics, University of Washington School of Medicine; Director, Department of Pediatrics, Harborview Medical Center, Seattle, Washington

Sudden Infant Death Syndrome and Recurrent Apnea

Stanley Berlow, M.D.

Madison, Wisconsin

Hyperphenylalaninemias

Bernard A. Berman, M.D.

Associate Clinical Professor of Pediatrics, Tufts University School of Medicine; Director, Pediatric Allergy, St. Elizabeth Hospital, Boston, Massachusetts

Treatment of Allergic Rhinitis

Shelly C. Bernstein, M.D., Ph.D.

Associate in Pediatrics, University of Massachusetts Medical School; Associate in Pediatrics, University of Massachusetts Hospital, Worcester, Massachusetts

Polycythemia

Leonard Bielory, M.D., F.A.C.P., F.A.A.A.I.

Director, Division of Allergy and Immunology and Assistant Professor of Medicine, University of Medicine and Dentistry of New Jersey-Rutgers Medical School, Newark; Director, Division of Allergy and Immunology and Attending Staff, University of Medicine and Dentistry of New Jersey-University Hospi-

tal, Newark; Attending Staff, Saint Barnabas Medical Center, Livingston, New Jersey
Serum Sickness

Jeffrey A. Biller, M.D.

Assistant Clinical Professor of Pediatrics, Tufts University School of Medicine; Assistant in Pediatrics, New England Medical Center, Boston, Massachusetts
Recurrent Abdominal Pain

Cynthia Black-Payne, M.D.

Assistant Professor of Pediatrics, Section of Pediatric Infectious Diseases, Louisiana State University School of Medicine; Attending Physician and Consultant, Louisiana State University Hospital, Shreveport, Louisiana
Histoplasmosis

Joseph A. Bocchini, Jr., M.D.

Associate Professor of Pediatrics and Chief, Section of Pediatric Infectious Diseases, Louisiana State University School of Medicine; Attending Physician and Consultant, Louisiana State University Medical Center, Shreveport, Louisiana
Histoplasmosis

E. Thomas Boles, Jr., M.D.

Professor of Surgery, Ohio State University College of Medicine; Chief, Department of Pediatric Surgery, Children's Hospital; Director, Division of Pediatric Surgery, University Hospital; Attending Staff, Children's and University Hospitals, Columbus, Ohio
Foreign Bodies in the Alimentary Tract

Bruce R. Boynton, M.D., M.P.H.

Associate Professor of Pediatrics, University of Kentucky College of Medicine; Chief, Division of Neonatology, A. B. Chandler Medical Center, Lexington, Kentucky
Meconium Aspiration Syndrome

Murray Braun, M.D.

Clinical Assistant Professor of Pediatric Neurology, Boston University School of Medicine, Boston, Massachusetts
Injuries to the Brachial Plexus

Itzhak Brook, M.D.

Professor of Pediatrics and Surgery, Uniformed Services University for the Health Sciences, Attending Physician and Consultant in Infectious Diseases, National Naval Medical Center, Bethesda, Maryland, and Walter Reed Army Medical Center, Washington, D.C.
Infections Due to Anaerobic Cocci and Gram-Negative Bacilli

John G. Brooks, M.D.

Professor of Pediatrics, University of Rochester School of Medicine; Director, Pediatric Pulmonology, Strong Memorial Hospital, Rochester, New York
Pleural Effusion

John F. Brown, Jr., M.D. (deceased)

Assistant Professor Emeritus of Medicine, University of Southern California School of Medicine; Attending Staff, Pulmonary Disease Service, Los Angeles County-University of Southern California Medical

Center; Consultant, Barlow Hospital, Los Angeles, California
Mucormycosis

Philip A. Brunell, M.D.

Professor of Pediatrics, University of California, Los Angeles, School of Medicine; Associate Director, Ahmanson Pediatric Center; Director, Pediatric Infectious Diseases, Cedars-Sinai Medical Center, Los Angeles, California
Varicella and Herpes Zoster; Immunization

Philip J. Brunquell, M.D.

Assistant Professor of Pediatrics and Neurology, University of Connecticut School of Medicine, Farmington; Director, Clinical Neurophysiology Laboratories, Newington Children's Hospital, Newington, Connecticut
Degenerative Diseases of the Central Nervous System

Ruth D. Bruun, M.D.

Clinical Associate Professor of Psychiatry, Cornell University Medical College; Attending Psychiatrist, New York Hospital-Cornell Medical Center, New York, New York
Tourette Syndrome

Kevin A. Burbige, M.D., F.A.A.P., F.A.C.S.

Assistant Professor of Urology, College of Physicians and Surgeons of Columbia University; Attending Urologist, St. Luke-Roosevelt Medical Center, New York, New York
Neurogenic Bladder

Victor E. Calcaterra, M.D.

Assistant Professor of Otolaryngology, Tufts University School of Medicine; Senior Surgeon, Department of Otolaryngology, New England Medical Center, Boston, Massachusetts
Foreign Bodies in the Ear; Injuries of the Middle Ear

Thomas R. Caraccio, Pharm. D., D.A.B.A.T.

Adjunct Assistant Clinical Professor of Pharmacy, St. John's University College of Pharmacy, Jamaica; Visiting Assistant Clinical Professor of Pharmacology and Toxicology, New York College of Osteopathic Medicine, Old Westbury; Clinical Coordinator, Nassau County Medical Center, Long Island Regional Poison Control Center, East Meadow, New York
Salicylate Poisoning; Acetaminophen Poisoning

Hugh A. Carithers, M.D.

Clinical Professor of Pediatrics, University of Florida School of Medicine; Consulting Pediatrician, St. Vincent's and University Hospitals, Jacksonville, Florida
Cat Scratch Disease

Kathleen S. Carlson, M.D.

Clinical Assistant Professor of Pediatrics, Medical College of Ohio; Neonatologist, The Toledo Hospital, Toledo, Ohio
Management of the Newborn at Delivery

Gail H. Cassell, M.S., Ph.D

Professor and Chairman, Department of Microbiology, School of Medicine and Dentistry, University of Alabama at Birmingham, Birmingham, Alabama
Mycoplasma Infections

Edmund Cataldo, D.D.S., M.S.

Professor and Chairman, Department of Oral Pathology, Oral Diagnosis and Oral Radiology, Tufts University School of Dental Medicine; Chief, Oral Pathology, New England Medical Center Hospital, Boston, Massachusetts

Congenital Epulis of the Neonate

J. Julian Chisolm, Jr., M.D.

Associate Professor of Pediatrics, Johns Hopkins University School of Medicine; Director, Lead Poisoning Program, Kennedy Institute; Staff Pediatrician, Johns Hopkins Hospital; Staff Pediatrician, Francis Scott Key Medical Center, Baltimore, Maryland

Increased Lead Absorption and Acute Lead Poisoning

Sterling K. Clarren, M.D.

Aldrich Professor of Pediatrics and Head, Division of Embryology, Teratology, and Congenital Defects, Department of Pediatrics, University of Washington School of Medicine; Head, Department of Congenital Defects, Children's Hospital and Medical Center, Seattle, Washington

Maternal Alcohol Ingestion: Effects on the Developing Fetus

Luis A. Clavell, M.D.

Associate Professor of Pediatrics, University of Puerto Rico; Director, Pediatric Oncology, University Pediatric Hospital, San Juan, Puerto Rico

Lymphangioma

T. G. Cleary, M.D.

Associate Professor of Pediatrics, University of Texas Medical School at Houston; M. D. Anderson Tumor Institute, and Hermann Hospital, Houston, Texas

Endocarditis

William W. Cleveland, M.D.

Professor of Pediatrics, University of Miami School of Medicine; Pediatric Staff, Jackson Memorial Hospital, Miami Children's Hospital, and Baptist Hospital, Miami, Florida

Gynecomastia

John P. Cloherty, M.D.

Assistant Clinical Professor of Pediatrics, Harvard Medical School; Associate in Neonatology, Joint Programs in Neonatology, Brigham and Women's Hospital, Children's Hospital, and Beth Israel Hospital, Boston, Massachusetts

Infants Born to Diabetic Mothers

William D. Cochran, M.D.

Associate Clinical Professor of Pediatrics, Harvard Medical School; Pediatrician in Charge, Beth Israel Hospital; Senior Associate in Medicine, The Children's Hospital; Senior Member, Newborn Medicine, Brigham and Women's Hospital; Senior Member, Joint Program in Neonatology, Beth Israel Hospital, The Children's Hospital, and Brigham and Women's Hospital, Boston, Massachusetts

Birth Injuries

Bernard A. Cohen, M.D.

Assistant Professor of Pediatrics and Dermatology, University of Pittsburgh School of Medicine; Director of Pediatric Dermatology, Children's Hospital of Pittsburgh, Pittsburgh, Pennsylvania

Arthropod Bites and Stings

Dale Coln, M.D.

Associate Professor of Surgery, University of Texas Southwestern Medical Center; Director of Pediatric Surgery, Baylor University Medical Center, Dallas, Texas

Chylothorax

Paul M. Colombani, M.D.

Associate Professor of Surgery, Pediatrics and Oncology, Johns Hopkins University School of Medicine; Attending Surgeon, Johns Hopkins Hospital, Baltimore, Maryland

Neonatal Pneumothorax and Pneumomediastinum

Kenneth L. Cox, M.D.

Director of Pediatric Gastroenterology, Pacific Presbyterian Medical Center, San Francisco, California

Pancreatic Diseases

Donald B. Darling, M.D.

Professor of Pediatrics and Radiology, Tufts University School of Medicine; Senior Radiologist, New England Medical Center Hospitals, Boston, Massachusetts

Infantile Cortical Hyperostosis

J. Michael Dean, M.D.

Chief, Division of Pediatric Critical Care, Associate Professor of Pediatrics, University of Utah School of Medicine; Director, Pediatric Intensive Care Unit, Primary Children's Medical Center, Salt Lake City, Utah

Near-Drowning

Steven Demeter, M.D.

Clinical Assistant Professor of Neurology and Psychiatry, University of Rochester School of Medicine; Attending Neurologist and Associate Attending Psychiatrist, Strong Memorial Hospital; Neurology Consultant, Rochester Psychiatric Center, Rochester, New York

Tourette Syndrome

Darryl C. De Vivo, M.D.

Sydney Carter Professor of Neurology, Professor of Pediatrics, and Director of Pediatric Neurology, College of Physicians and Surgeons of Columbia University; Attending Neurologist and Attending Pediatrician, Presbyterian Hospital, New York, New York

Cerebral Edema

William H. Dietz, M.D., Ph.D.

Associate Professor of Pediatrics, Tufts University School of Medicine; Director of Clinical Nutrition, The Floating Hospital for Infants and Children/New England Medical Center, Boston, Massachusetts

Nutrition

Donna DiMichele, M.D.

Instructor, New England Medical Center, Tufts University; Instructor, The Floating Hospital for Infants and Children/New England Medical Center, Boston, Massachusetts

Pediatric Hemostasis and Thrombosis

Joan DiPalma, M.D.
Assistant Professor of Pediatrics, Georgetown University's Children's Medical Center; Georgetown University Hospital, Washington, D.C.
Pylorospasm; Pyloric Stenosis

Andrea M. Dominey, M.D.
Fellow, Pediatric Dermatology, Baylor College of Medicine, Houston, Texas
Nevi and Nevoid Tumors

George N. Donnell, M.D.
Professor of Pediatrics, University of Southern California, Los Angeles, School of Medicine; Professor of Pediatrics, Department of Pediatrics, Children's Hospital of Los Angeles, Los Angeles, California
Galactosemias

Henry L. Dorkin, M.D.
Associate Professor of Pediatrics, Tufts University School of Medicine; Chief, Pediatric Pulmonology and Allergy Division, New England Medical Center, Boston, Massachusetts
Lobar Emphysema

James M. Drake, M.D.
Lecturer, University of Toronto; Staff Neurosurgeon, Hospital for Sick Children, Toronto, Ontario
Extradural and Subdural Hematoma

John W. Duckett, M.D.
Professor of Urology in Surgery, University of Pennsylvania School of Medicine; Director, Division of Urology, Children's Hospital of Philadelphia, Philadelphia, Pennsylvania
Disorders of the Bladder and Urethra

Joseph Y. Dwoskin, M.D.
Clinical Assistant Professor of Urology, State University of New York at Buffalo Medical School; Attending Physician, Buffalo Children's Hospital; Chairman, Department of Urology, Mercy Hospital of Buffalo, Buffalo, New York
Vesicoureteral Reflux

Heinz F. Eichenwald, M.D.
William Buchanan Professor, Department of Pediatrics, University of Texas Southwestern Medical Center at Dallas; Attending Physician, Children's Medical Center of Dallas and Parkland Memorial Hospital, Dallas, Texas
Plague

Arnold H. Einhorn, M.D.
Professor and Associate Chairman of Pediatrics, Director of Pediatric Residency Training Program, George Washington University School of Medicine; Chairman, Department of Pediatric Medicine, Children's National Medical Center, Washington, D.C.
Iron Poisoning

Arthur R. Euler, M.D.
Associate Clinical Professor of Pediatrics, University of Michigan, Ann Arbor, Michigan
Disorders of the Esophagus

Hugh E. Evans, M.D.
Chairman, Department of Pediatrics, University of Medicine and Dentistry of New Jersey, Newark; Director, Department of Pediatrics, University Hospital, Newark, New Jersey
Syphilis

Ralph D. Feigin, M.D.
J. S. Abercrombie Professor of Pediatrics and Chairman, Department of Pediatrics, Baylor College of Medicine; Physician-in-Chief, Texas Children's Hospital; Physician-in-Chief, Pediatric Services, Harris County Hospital District (Ben Taub General Hospital); Chief, Pediatric Service, The Methodist Hospital, Houston, Texas
Leptospirosis

Sandor Feldman, M.D.
Professor of Pediatrics, University of Mississippi Medical Center; Infection Control Officer, Children's Hospital; Chief, Division of Pediatric Infectious Diseases, Department of Pediatrics, University of Mississippi Medical Center, Jackson, Mississippi
Typhoid Fever, Salmonellosis

Robert H. Feldt, M.D.
Professor of Pediatrics, Mayo Medical School; Consultant in Pediatric Cardiology, Mayo Clinic and Hospitals, Rochester, Minnesota
Cardiomyopathies and Related Diseases

James Feusner, M.D.
Associate Clinical Professor of Pediatrics, University of California School of Medicine, San Francisco; Director of Oncology, Children's Hospital of Oakland; Assistant Clinical Professor, Department of Pediatrics, UCSF Medical Center, San Francisco, California
Neuroblastoma

Robert M. Filler, M.D., F.R.C.S.(C)
Professor of Surgery, University of Toronto Faculty of Medicine; Surgeon-in-Chief, The Hospital for Sick Children, Toronto, Ontario
Intrathoracic Cysts; Tumors of the Chest; Neonatal Intestinal Obstruction

Laurence Finberg, M.D.
Professor of Pediatrics, State University of New York, Brooklyn; Department Chairman, University Hospital of Brooklyn; Attending Pediatrician, Kings County Hospital, Brooklyn, New York
Parenteral Fluid and Electrolyte Therapy

Jo-David Fine, M.D.
Associate Professor of Dermatology and Director of Dermatologic Research, University of Alabama School of Medicine; Attending in Dermatology, University of Alabama Hospitals; Chief, Dermatology Section, Medical Service, Birmingham Veterans Administration Medical Center, Birmingham, Alabama
Topical Therapy: A Dermatologic Formulary for Pediatric Practice

Richard N. Fine, M.D.
Professor of Pediatrics, University of California, Los Angeles Center for the Health Sciences; Head, Division of Pediatric Nephrology, UCLA Medical Center, Los Angeles, California
Peritoneal Dialysis

Adam Finn, B.M., B.Ch., M.R.C.P.
Lecturer in Immunology, Institute of Child Health; Honorary Senior Registrar, Hospital For Sick Children, London, England
Rabies; Infectious Mononucleosis and Epstein-Barr Virus–Related Syndromes

Nathan Fischel-Ghodsian, M.D.
Assistant Professor of Pediatrics, University of California, Los Angeles, School of Medicine; Director, Molecular Hematology, and Pediatric Hematology/Oncology, Ahmanson Pediatric Center, Cedars-Sinai Medical Center, Los Angeles, California
Anemia of Iron Deficiency and Chronic Disease

Alfred J. Fish, M.D.
Professor of Pediatrics, University of Minnesota Medical School; University of Minnesota Hospitals, Minneapolis Children's Medical Center, Minneapolis; St. Paul Ramsay Hospital, St. Paul, Minnesota
Glomerulonephritis

Joseph F. Fitzgerald, M.D.
Professor of Pediatrics, Indiana University School of Medicine; Director, Division of Gastroenterology and Nutrition, James Whitcomb Riley Hospital for Children, Indianapolis, Indiana
Chronic Active Hepatitis

David R. Fleisher, M.D.
Clinical Professor of Pediatrics, University of California, Los Angeles, School of Medicine; Attending Pediatrician and Associate Director, Division of Pediatric Gastroenterology, Cedars-Sinai Medical Center, Los Angeles, California
Nausea and Vomiting

Laurie S. Fouser, M.D.
Acting Assistant Professor of Pediatrics, University of Washington School of Medicine; Staff Neurologist, Children's Hosptial and Medical Center, Seattle, Washington
Glomerulonephritis

Ivan D. Frantz, III, M.D.
Professor of Pediatrics, Tufts University School of Medicine; Chief, Division of Newborn Medicine, Floating Hospital for Infants and Children/New England Medical Center; Director, Boston Perinatal Center, Boston, Massachusetts
Necrotizing Enterocolitis; Respiratory Distress Syndrome

Robert M. Freedom, M.D., F.R.C.P.(C), F.A.C.C.
Professor of Pediatrics (Cardiology and Pathology), University of Toronto Faculty of Medicine; Director, Division of Cardiology, The Hospital for Sick Children, Toronto, Ontario
Primary Cardiac Neoplasms

Louis Friedlander, M.D.
Clinical Professor of Pediatrics, University of Southern California School of Medicine and Los Angeles County University of Southern California Medical Center, Los Angeles, California
Vulva and Vagina

Emily D. Friedman, M.D.
Assistant Professor of Neurosurgery, University of Pennsylvania School of Medicine; Hospital of The University of Pennsylvania, Philadelphia, Pennsylvania
Cerebral Edema

David R. Fulton, M.D.
Associate Professor of Pediatrics, Tufts University School of Medicine; Cardiologist, The Floating Hospital for Infants and Children, Boston, Massachusetts
Congestive Heart Failure

Bruce Furie, M.D.
Professor of Medicine, Tufts University School of Medicine; New England Medical Center, Boston, Massachusetts
Pediatric Hemostasis and Thrombosis

Toni M. Ganzel, M.D.
Associate Professor of Surgery, Division of Otolaryngology, Department of Surgery, University of Louisville, Chief of Otolaryngology, Kosair Children's Hospital, Louisville, Kentucky
Recurrent Acute Parotitis

Margaret P. Gean, M.D.
Assistant Professor of Psychiatry, Tufts University School of Medicine; Psychiatrist and Deputy Chief, Division of Child and Adolescent Psychiatry; Director, Outpatient Child and Adolescent Psychiatry, and Director, Infant and Toddler Program, New England Medical Center, Boston, Massachusetts
Psychiatric Disorders of Infants and Toddlers

Mitchell E. Geffner, M.D.
Associate Professor of Pediatrics, University of California School of Medicine, Los Angeles, Los Angeles, California
Short Stature; Tall Stature

Robert H. Gelber, M.D.
Associate Clinical Professor, Department of Epidemiology and Biostatistics and Dermatology, University of California, San Francisco; Associate Clinical Professor, Department of Dermatology, Stanford University, Palo Alto; Medical Director, Northern California Regional Hansen's Disease Program, Kuzell Institute, San Francisco, California
Leprosy

Stephen E. Gellis, M.D.
Assistant Professor of Dermatology (Pediatrics), Harvard Medical School; Associate Physician, Chief of Dermatology Program, Children's Hospital, Boston, Massachusetts
Miscellaneous Dermatoses

Welton M. Gersony, M.D.
Professor of Pediatrics and Director, Division of Pediatric Cardiology, College of Physicians and Surgeons of Columbia University; Attending Pediatrician, Babies Hospital, Columbia-Presbyterian Medical Center, New York, New York
Cardiac Arrhythmias

Hubert L. Gerstman, D.Ed.
Clinical Assistant Professor of Otolaryngology, Department of Surgery, State University of New York at Stonybrook; Chief, Speech, Language and Hearing Program, University Hospital, Stonybrook, New York
Hearing Loss

Frances M. Gill, M.D.
Associate Professor of Pediatrics, University of Pennsylvania School of Medicine; Senior Physician, The Children's Hospital of Philadelphia, Philadelphia, Pennsylvania
Hemolytic Anemia

Herbert E. Gilmore, M.D.
Assistant Professor of Pediatrics (Neurology), Tufts University School of Medicine; Pediatric Neurologist, Boston Floating Hospital for Infants and Children/New England Medical Center, Boston, Massachusetts
Congenital Hypotonia

Janet R. Gilsdorf, M.D.
Associate Professor, University of Michigan Medical School; Director, Pediatric Infectious Diseases, C.S. Mott Children's Hospital, University of Michigan Medical Center, Ann Arbor, Michigan
Haemophilus Influenzae Infections

Eli Gold, M.D.
Clinical Professor of Pediatrics, University of Washington School of Medicine; Attending Pediatrician, Children's Hospital and Medical Center, Harborview Medical Center, Seattle, Washington
Meningococcal Disease

Richard B. Goldbloom, M.D., F.R.C.P.(C)
Professor of Pediatrics, Dalhousie University; Attending Physician, The Izaak Walton Killam Children's Hospital, Halifax, Nova Scotia
Pica; The Tonsil and Adenoid Problem

Dennis Goldfinger, M.D.
Director, Division of Transfusion Medicine, Department of Pathology and Laboratory Medicine, Cedars-Sinai Medical Center, Los Angeles, California
Adverse Reactions to Blood Transfusion

David Goldring, M.D.
Professor Emeritus and Lecturer in Pediatrics, Director Emeritus of Pediatric Cardiology, Washington University Medical School, St. Louis, Missouri
Systemic Hypertension

Manuel R. Gomez, M.D.
Professor of Pediatric Neurology, Mayo Medical School; St. Mary's Hospital, Methodist Hospital, Rochester, Minnesota
Neurocutaneous Syndromes

Gary M. Gorlick, M.D., M.P.H., F.A.A.P.
Assistant Clinical Professor of Pediatrics, University of California, Los Angeles, School of Medicine; Attending Pediatrician, Cedars-Sinai Medical Center, Los Angeles, California
Eruptions in the Diaper Region

Jeffrey B. Gould, M.D., M.P.H.
Professor and Chairman, Maternal and Child Health Program, University of California School of Public Health, Berkeley; Neonatologist, Highland Hospital, Oakland, California
Preparation of the Neonate for Transfer

David F. Graft, M.D.
Clinical Assistant Professor of Pediatrics, University of Minnesota School of Medicine; Active Staff, Methodist Hospital; Courtesy Staff, Minneapolis Children's Hospital, Minneapolis, Minnesota
Insect Stings

H. Gordon Green, M.D.
Clinical Associate Professor of Pediatrics, University of Texas Southwestern Medical Center; Medical Staff, Children's Medical Center, Dallas, Texas
Chylothorax

Morris Green, M.D.
Perry W. Lesh Professor of Pediatrics, Indiana University School of Medicine; Attending Pediatrician, James Whitcomb Riley Hospital for Children, Indianapolis, Indiana
The Child and the Death of a Loved One

Neil E. Green, M.D.
Professor and Vice Chairman, Department of Orthopaedics and Rehabilitation, Vanderbilt University School of Medicine; Chief of Pediatric Orthopaedics, Vanderbilt University Medical Center, Nashville, Tennessee
Bone and Joint Infections

Melvin Greer, M.D.
Professor and Chairman, Department of Neurology, University of Florida College of Medicine; Chief Neurologist, Shands Hospital, Gainesville, Florida
Benign Intracranial Hypertension

Robert C. Griggs, M.D.
Chairman of Neurology and Professor of Neurology and Pediatrics, University of Rochester School of Medicine and Dentistry; Neurologist-in-Chief, Strong Memorial Hospital, Rochester, New York
Periodic Paralysis

Moses Grossman, M.D.
Professor and Vice Chairman of Pediatrics, University of California, San Francisco, School of Medicine; Chief of Pediatrics, San Francisco General Hospital, San Francisco, California
Brucellosis; Rat Bite Fever

Kenneth M. Grundfast, M.D.
Associate Professor, Division of Otolaryngology, Department of Surgery, George Washington University School of Medicine; Chairman, Department of Otolaryngology, Children's Hospital National Medical Center, Washington, D.C.
Disorders of the Larynx

Joyce D. Gryboski, M.D.
Professor of Pediatrics, Yale University School of Medicine, New Haven, Connecticut
Irritable Bowel Syndrome

Warren G. Guntheroth, M.D.
Professor of Pediatrics and Head, Division of Pediatric Cardiology; University of Washington School of

Medicine; University of Washington Medical Center, Seattle, Washington
Peripheral Vascular Disease

Kevin E. Halbert, M.D.
Fellow in Neonatology, University of Cincinnati College of Medicine, University of Cincinnati Medical Center and Children's Hospital Medical Center, Cincinnati, Ohio
Parathyroid Disease

J. Alex Haller, Jr., M.D.
Professor of Pediatrics, Professor of Emergency Medicine, and Robert Garrett Professor of Pediatric Surgery, Johns Hopkins University School of Medicine; Professor of Surgery and Pediatric Surgery, University of Maryland Hospital; Children's Surgeon-in-Charge, Johns Hopkins Hospital, Baltimore, Maryland
Intussusception, Neonatal Pneumothorax and Pseudomediastinum

Jerome S. Haller, M.D.
Professor of Neurology and Pediatrics, Albany Medical College; Full-time Staff, Albany Medical Center, Albany, New York
Reye Syndrome

K. Michael Hambidge, M.D., F.R.C.P., Sc.D.
Professor of Pediatrics, University of Colorado Health Sciences Center; University Hospital, Denver, Colorado
Zinc Deficiency; Breast Feeding

Brian L. Hamilton, M.D., Ph.D.
Associate Professor of Clinical Pediatrics, Department of Pediatrics, Associate Professor, Department of Microbiology and Immunology, University of Miami School of Medicine; Attending Pediatrician, Jackson Memorial Hospital, Miami, Florida
The Immunodeficiencies, Including HIV-1 Infection

Steven D. Handler, M.D.
Associate Professor, Otolaryngology and Human Communication, University of Pennsylvania School of Medicine; Associate Director, Otolaryngology, Children's Hospital of Philadelphia, Philadelphia, Pennsylvania
Epistaxis, Foreign Bodies in the Nose and Pharynx; Labyrinthitis

Ronald C. Hansen, M.D.
Associate Professor of Internal Medicine (Dermatology) and Pediatrics, University of Arizona College of Medicine, Tucson; Staff Dermatologist, University Medical Center, Tucson; Consultant, Dermatology, Tucson Medical Center, Tucson, Phoenix Children's Hospital, St. Joseph's Medical Center, Maricopa Medical Center, Phoenix, Arizona
Discoid Lupus Erythematosus

James Barry Hanshaw, M.D.
Professor of Pediatrics, Dean Emeritus, University of Massachusetts Medical School; Active Staff, University of Massachusetts Hospital; Consultant, St. Vincent Hospital, Worcester, Massachusetts
Cytomegalovirus Infections

Herbert S. Harned, Jr., M.D.
Professor Emeritus of Pediatrics, University of North Carolina School of Medicine; Attending Physician, University of North Carolina Hospitals, Chapel Hill, North Carolina
Hypotension

H. Robert Harrison, D. Phil., M.D., M.P.H.
Associate Chief, Pediatric Infectious Diseases, Scottish Rite Children's Medical Center, Atlanta, Georgia
Coccidioidomycosis

Gregory F. Hayden, M.D.
Associate Professor of Pediatrics, University of Virginia School of Medicine; Attending Pediatrician, Children's Medical Center of The University of Virginia, Charlottesville, Virginia
Mumps

Felix P. Heald, M.D.
Professor of Pediatrics, University of Maryland School of Medicine; Director, Division of Adolescent Medicine, University of Maryland Medical System, Baltimore, Maryland
Obesity

Douglas C. Heiner, M.D., Ph.D.
Professor of Pediatrics, University of California, Los Angeles; Chief, Division of Immunology and Allergy, Harbor-UCLA Medical Center; Staff Physician, Harbor-UCLA Medical Center, Los Angeles, California
Toxocara Canis Infections, Including Visceral Larva Migrans; Anaphylaxis

Terry W. Hensle, M.D.
Professor of Clinical Urology, Columbia University College of Physicians and Surgeons; Director, Pediatric Urology, Babies Hospital and Columbia Presbyterian Medical Center, New York, New York
Neurogenic Bladder

John J. Herbst, M.D.
Professor and Chairman, Department of Pediatrics, Louisiana State University School of Medicine at Shreveport; Attending Physician, University Hospital, Louisiana State University Medical Center, Shreveport, Louisiana
Gastroesophageal Reflux

John T. Herrin, M.B.B.S., F.R.A.C.P.
Associate Clinical Professor of Pediatrics, Harvard Medical School; Chief of Pediatric Nephrology, Massachusetts General Hospital; Chief of Pediatrics, Shriners Burns Institute, Boston, Massachusetts
Chronic Renal Failure

Layne Hersh, M.D.
Consultant, Woodland Memorial Hospital, Carmichael, California
Warts and Molluscum Contagiosum

Fred S. Herzon, M.D.
Professor of Otolaryngology-Head and Neck Surgery, University of New Mexico School of Medicine; Attending in Otolaryngology, University Hospital, Albuquerque, New Mexico
Retropharyngeal and Peritonsillar Abscesses

Joan E. Hodgman, M.D.

Professor of Pediatrics, University of Southern California School of Medicine; Director, Newborn Division, Los Angeles County/University of Southern California Medical Center, Los Angeles, California

Bronchopulmonary Dysplasia

Norman B. Hodgson, M.D.

Clinical Professor of Urology, Medical College of Wisconsin, Madison; Staff, Children's Hospital of Wisconsin, Columbia Hospital, Good Samaritan Medical Center, Veterans Administration Medical Center, St. Joseph's Hospital, West Allis Memorial Hospital, and Froedtert Memorial Lutheran Hospital, Milwaukee, Wisconsin

Penis, Spermatic Cord, and Testes

Gregory L. Holmes, M.D.

Associate Professor of Neurology, Harvard Medical School; Director, Clinical Neurophysiology Laboratory, and Director, Epilepsy Unit, The Children's Hospital, Boston, Massachusetts

Seizure Disorders

Paul J. Honig, M.D.

Professor of Pediatrics and Dermatology, University of Pennsylvania School of Medicine; Children's Hospital of Philadelphia, Philadelphia, Pennsylvania

Rickettsial Diseases

Debra A. Horney, M.D.

Clinical Assistant Professor, University of California, Davis, Medical School, Davis, California

Papulosquamous Disorders

Walter T. Hughes, M.D.

Professor of Pediatrics, University of Tennessee College of Medicine; Chairman, Department of Infectious Diseases, St. Jude Children's Research Hospital, Memphis, Tennessee

Tularemia; Pneumocystis Carinii *Pneumonitis*

Sidney Hurwitz, M.D.

Clinical Professor of Pediatrics and Dermatology, Yale University School of Medicine; Attending Physician in Pediatrics and Dermatology, Yale-New Haven Medical Center and Hospital of St. Raphael, New Haven, Connecticut

Scabies and Pediculosis; The Genodermatoses

Carol B. Hyman, M.D.

Associate Professor of Clinical Pediatrics, University of Southern California School of Medicine; Attending in Pediatric Hematology/Oncology, Department of Pediatrics, Cedars-Sinai Medical Center, Los Angeles, California

Thalassemia

Susan T. Iannaccone, M.D.

Associate Professor of Neurology, University of Cincinnati Medical Center; Associate Professor of Neurology, Children's Hospital Medical Center and University Hospital, Cincinnati, Ohio

Myasthenia Gravis

Laura S. Inselman, M.D.

Assistant Professor of Pediatrics, University of Connecticut Health Center, Farmington, and Assistant Clinical Professor of Pediatrics, Yale University School of Medicine, New Haven; Clinical Director, Pediatric Pulmonology, Newington Children's Hospital, Newington, Connecticut

Tuberculosis

Silvia Iosub, M.D.

Professor of Pediatrics, New York Medical College, Valhalla; Attending Physician, Metropolitan Hospital Center, New York, and Lincoln Medical and Mental Health Center, Bronx, New York

Gianotti Disease

Shunzaburo Iwatsuki, M.D.

Professor of Surgery, University of Pittsburgh School of Medicine; Presbyterian-University Hospital, Children's Hospital of Pittsburgh, and Veterans Administration Hospital, Oakland, Pittsburgh, Pennsylvania

Tumors of the Liver

Ian T. Jackson, M.D., F.R.C.S., F.A.C.S., F.R.A.C.S.(Hon)

Director, Institute of Craniofacial, Plastic, and Reconstructive Surgery, Providence Hospital, Southfield, Michigan

Craniofacial Malformations

Alvin H. Jacobs, M.D.

Professor Emeritus of Dermatology and Pediatrics, Stanford University Medical Center, Stanford, California

Atopic Dermatitis

Norman Jaffe, M.D., D.Sc.

Professor of Pediatrics, University of Texas Medical School at Houston; Chief, Section of Solid Tumors, Division of Pediatrics, M.D. Anderson Cancer Center, Houston, Texas

Langerhans Cell Histiocytosis (The Histiocytosis Syndromes)

Joseph J. Jankowski, M.D.

Associate Clinical Professor of Psychiatry, Tufts University School of Medicine; Director, Consultation/Liaison and Emergency Services, Division of Child Psychiatry, New England Medical Center Hospital, Boston, Massachusetts

Psychiatric Disorders

Michael Jellinek, M.D.

Associate Professor of Psychiatry (Pediatrics), Harvard Medical School; Chief, Child Psychiatry Service; Director, Outpatient Psychiatry, Massachusetts General Hospital, Boston, Massachusetts

Children of Divorcing Parents

Venusto H. San Joaquin, M.D.

Associate Professor of Pediatrics, University of Oklahoma Health Sciences Center; Staff, Pediatric Infectious Disease Service, Children's Hospital of Oklahoma, Oklahoma City, Oklahoma

Cholera

Carey L. Johnson, M.D.

Clinical Instructor, University of California, Los Angeles, School of Medicine; Medical Genetics Fellow, Cedars-Sinai Medical Center, Los Angeles, California

Genetic Diseases

Hassan Hesham A-Kader, M.D., M.Sc.
Fellow, Pediatric Gastroenterology and Nutrition, Children's Hospital Medical Center, Cincinnati, Ohio
Cirrhosis

George W. Kaplan, M.D.
Clinical Professor of Surgery/Urology and Pediatrics; Chief of Pediatric Urology, University of California, San Diego School of Medicine; Chief of Urology, Children's Hospital; Attending Staff, University Hospital, San Diego, California
Urolithiasis

Sheldon L. Kaplan, M.D.
Professor, Department of Pediatrics, Baylor College of Medicine; Chief, Infectious Disease Service, Texas Children's Hospital, Houston, Texas
Pneumonia; Aseptic Meningitis

Evan J. Kass, M.D., F.A.C.S., F.A.A.P.
Chief, Division of Pediatric Urology, William Beaumont Hospital, Royal Oak, Michigan
Hydronephrosis and Disorders of the Ureter

Arnold E. Katz, M.D., M.S.
Professor of Surgery and Chief, Divisions of Otolaryngology and Head and Neck Surgery, State University of New York, Stonybrook, New York
Hearing Loss

Panayotis P. Kelalis, M.D.
Dr. Anson L. Clark Professor of Pediatric Urology, Mayo Medical School; Chairman, Department of Urology, Mayo Clinic and Mayo Foundation, Rochester, Minnesota
Extrophy of the Bladder

Edwin L. Kendig, Jr., M.D.
Professor of Pediatrics, Medical College of Virginia, Health Sciences Division, Virginia Commonwealth University; Director, Child Chest Clinic, Medical College of Virginia Hospitals; Coordinator, Hospital Affiliations, St. Mary's Hospital, Richmond, Virginia
Sarcoidosis

Joseph L. Kennedy, Jr., M.D.
Associate Professor of Pediatrics, Tufts University School of Medicine; Director of Neonatology, St. Margaret's Hospital, Boston, Massachusetts
Disturbances of Intrauterine Growth; Disorders of the Umbilicus

Thomas L. Kennedy, III, M.D.
Associate Clinical Professor of Pediatrics, Yale School of Medicine, New Haven; Chairman, Department of Pediatrics, Bridgeport Hospital, Bridgeport, Connecticut
Renal Venous Thrombosis

Keith J. Kimble, M.D.
Assistant Clinical Professor of Anesthesiology and Pediatrics, University of California, Los Angeles, School of Medicine; Coordinator, Section of Pediatric Anesthesia, Department of Anesthesia; Attending Intensivist, Pediatric Intensive Care Unit, Department of Pediatrics, Cedars-Sinai Medical Center, Los Angeles, California
Malignant Hyperthermia

George T. Klauber, M.D.
Professor of Urology and Pediatrics and Chief of Pediatric Urology, Tufts University School of Medicine; Chief of Pediatric Urology, Floating Hospital for Infants and Children/New England Medical Center, Boston, Massachusetts
Malignant Tumors of the Kidney

Jerome O. Klein, M.D.
Professor of Pediatrics, Boston University School of Medicine; Director, Division of Pediatric Infectious Diseases, Boston City Hospital, Boston, Massachusetts
Otitis Media

Stanley J. Kogan, M.D.
Professor of Urology, New York Medical College, Visiting Associate Professor of Pediatrics, Albert Einstein College of Medicine, Bronx; Co-Director, Section of Pediatric Urology, Westchester County Medical Center, Valhalla; Attending Pediatric Urologist, Weiler Hospital of Albert Einstein College of Medicine, Montefiore Medical Center, Bronx, New York
Ambiguous Genitalia

Anne Kolbe, M.B., B.S.
Department of Pediatric Surgery, Grafton Medical Center, Auckland, New Zealand
Peritonitis

Peter K. Kottmeier, M.D.
Professor and Chief, Pediatric Surgery, Health Science Center at Brooklyn, State University of New York, Brooklyn, New York
Peptic Ulcers; Gastritis

Martin A. Koyle, M.D., F.A.A.P., F.A.C.S.
Associate Professor of Surgery/Pediatric Urology, University of Colorado School of Medicine and the Children's Hospital; Consulting Pediatric Urologist, Rose Medical Center, Denver, Colorado
Undescended Testes

Adriane S. Kozlovsky, M.S., R.D., L.D.
Instructor in Nutrition, University of Maryland School of Medicine, Baltimore, Maryland
Obesity

Bernice R. Krafchik, M.D.
Associate Professor, Department of Dermatology, University of Toronto; Active Staff, Hospital for Sick Children, Toronto, Ontario
Urticaria

Stephen A. Kramer, M.D.
Associate Professor of Urology, Mayo Medical School; Consultant, Department of Urology, Mayo Clinic and Mayo Foundation, Rochester, Minnesota
Exstrophy of the Bladder

Richard E. Kravath, M.D.
Professor of Clinical Pediatrics, State University of New York Health Science Center at Brooklyn College of Medicine; Director of Pediatric In-Patient Service, Kings County Medical Center; University Hospital of Brooklyn, Brooklyn, New York
Parenteral Fluid and Electrolyte Therapy

Saul Krugman, M.D.
Professor of Pediatrics, New York University School of Medicine; Attending Physician, Bellevue and University Hospitals, New York, New York
Viral Hepatitis

John W. Kulig, M.D.
Assistant Professor of Pediatrics, Tufts University School of Medicine; Director, Adolescent Medicine, Floating Hospital for Infants and Children/New England Medical Center, Boston, Massachusetts
Sex Education; Adolescent Sexuality, Contraception, Pregnancy, and Abortion

Nancy L. Kuntz, M.D.
Clinical Assistant Professor, John Burns School of Medicine, University of Hawaii, Consultant Neurologist, Kapiolani Medical Center for Women and Children, Honolulu, Hawaii
Chronic Inflammatory Demyelinating Polyradiculoneuropathy

Cheryl C. Kürer, M.D.
Assistant Professor of Pediatrics, University of Pennsylvania School of Medicine and Children's Hospital of Philadelphia, Philadelphia, Pennsylvania; Assistant Professor of Pediatrics, Albert Einstein College of Medicine, Schneider Children's Hospital, and Long Island Jewish Medical Center, New Hyde Park, New York
Mitral Valve Prolapse

Paul S. Kurtin, M.D.
Assistant Professor of Pediatrics and Medicine, Tufts University School of Medicine; Chief, Division of Pediatric Nephrology, New England Medical Center, Boston, Massachusetts
The Nephrotic Syndrome; Hemolytic-Uremic Syndrome

Peter O. Kwiterovich, Jr., M.D.
Chief, Lipid Research Atherosclerosis Unit, Professor of Pediatrics, and Professor of Medicine, Johns Hopkins University School of Medicine; Active Staff, Pediatrics, and Director, Lipid Clinic, Johns Hopkins Hospital, Baltimore; Chairman, National Cholesterol Education Program, National Heart, Lungs, and Blood Institute, Bethesda, Maryland
Hyperlipoproteinemia

Daniel J. Lacey, M.D., Ph.D.
Associate Professor of Neurology and Pediatrics, Wright State University; Director of Child Neurology, Children's Medical Center, Dayton, Ohio
Infantile Spasms

Philip Lanzkowsky, M.D., F.R.C.P., D.C.H., F.A.A.P.
Professor of Pediatrics, Albert Einstein College of Medicine; Chief of Pediatric Hematology and Oncology, Chairman of Pediatrics, Chief of Staff, Schneider Children's Hospital, Long Island Jewish Medical Center, New Hyde Park, New York
Megaloblastic Anemia

Eric Larsen, M.D.
Instructor, Department of Pediatrics, Harvard Medical School; Instructor in Pediatrics, Dana Farber Cancer Institute; Associate in Hematology, The Children's Hospital, Boston, Massachusetts
Pediatric Hemostasis and Thrombosis

Laurie A. Latchaw, M.D.
Assistant Professor of Surgery, Tufts University School of Medicine; Staff Surgeon, New England Medical Center, Boston, Massachusetts
Preoperative and Postoperative Care of Patients Undergoing Gastrointestinal Surgery

Mark C. Leeson, M.D., F.A.C.S.
Assistant Professor of Orthopaedic Surgery, Northeast Ohio Universities College of Medicine; Director, Orthopaedic Resident Education and Research, Akron General Medical Center, Akron, Ohio
Malignant Bone Tumors

Thomas J. A. Lehman, M.D.
Chief, Division of Pediatric Rheumatology, Hospital for Special Surgery; Associate Professor of Pediatrics, Cornell University Medical Center; Chief, Division of Pediatric Rheumatology, Hospital for Special Surgery, New York, New York
Familial Mediterranean Fever

Carl Lenarsky, M.D.
Assistant Professor of Pediatrics, University of Southern California School of Medicine; Clinical Director, Division of Research Immunology and Bone Marrow Transplantation, Children's Hospital of Los Angeles, Los Angeles, California
Aplastic Anemia

Lucille A. Lester, M.D.
Associate Professor, Department of Pediatrics, University of Chicago Pritzker School of Medicine; Associate Professor of Allergy, Immunology and Pulmonary, and Director of Cystic Fibrosis Center, Wyler Children's Hospital, University of Chicago, Chicago, Illinois
Cystic Fibrosis

Melvin D. Levine, M.D.
Professor of Pediatrics, University of North Carolina School of Medicine; Director, Center for Development and Learning, University of North Carolina, Chapel Hill, North Carolina
Constipation and Encopresis

Selwyn B. Levitt, M.D.
Clinical Professor of Urology, New York Medical College; Visiting Clinical Professor of Pediatrics, Albert Einstein College of Medicine, Bronx; Co-Director, Division of Pediatric Urology, Westchester Medical Center, Valhalla; Attending Pediatric Urologist, Albert Einstein College Hospital and Montefiore Hospital and Medical Center, Bronx, New York
Ambiguous Genitalia

Moise L. Levy, M.D.
Assistant Professor of Dermatology and Pediatrics and Chief of Pediatric Dermatology, Baylor College of Medicine; Chief, Dermatology Service, and Active Staff, Texas Children's Hospital; Active Staff, The Methodist Hospital, Harris County Hospital District, Houston, Texas
Photodermatoses; Nevi and Nevoid Tumors

Nancy C. Lewis, M.D.

Pediatric Pulmonologist; Director, Cystic Fibrosis Center, Children's Hospital, Oakland, Oakland, California

Right Middle Lobe Syndrome; Viral Pneumonia

Gerald M. Loughlin, M.D.

Director, Eudowood Division of Pediatric Respiratory Sciences; Associate Professor of Pediatrics; Johns Hopkins Medical Institutions; Johns Hopkins Hospital, Baltimore, Maryland

Pulmonary Edema

Anne W. Lucky, M.D.

Adjunct Associate Professor of Dermatology and Pediatrics, University of Cincinnati College of Medicine; Director, Dermatology Clinic, The Children's Hospital Medical Center, Cincinnati, Ohio

Disorders of the Hair and Scalp; Disorders of Sebaceous Glands and Sweat Glands

E. Dennis Lyne, M.D.

Head, Division of Pediatric Orthopedic Surgery, and Division of Rehabilitation in The Bone and Joint Institute, Henry Ford Hospital, Detroit; Staff, St. Joseph's Hospital, Pontiac, Michigan

Orthopedic Disorders of the Upper Extremity

Max Maizels, M.D.

Associate Professor of Urology, Northwestern University Medical School; Active Attending, Children's Memorial Hospital; Associate Attending, McGaw Medical Center, Chicago, Illinois

Renal Hypoplasia and Dysplasia

Eric S. Maller, M.D.

Instructor of Pediatrics, Harvard Medical School; Assistant in Medicine (Gastroenterology and Nutrition), The Children's Hospital, Boston, Massachusetts

Disorders of the Hepatobiliary Tree

Eberhard M. Mann, M.D.

Associate Professor, University of Hawaii, John A. Burns School of Medicine; Medical Consultant, Sex Abuse Treatment Center, Kapiolani Medical Center for Women and Children, Honolulu, Hawaii

Sexual Abuse and Rape

Catherine S. Manno, M.D.

Assistant Professor of Pediatrics, University of Pennsylvania School of Medicine; Assistant Physician, Children's Hospital of Philadelphia, Philadelphia, Pennsylvania

Hemolytic Anemia

Andrew M. Margileth, M.D.

Professor, Department of Pediatrics, F. Edward Hébert School of Medicine, Uniformed Services University of the Health Sciences; Consultant in Pediatrics and Pediatric Dermatology, Bethesda Naval Hospital, Bethesda, Maryland; Consultant in Pediatrics and Pediatric Dermatology, Walter Reed Army Medical Center, Washington, D.C.

Nontuberculous (Atypical) Mycobacterial Diseases

Melvin I. Marks, M.D.

Professor and Vice-Chairman, Department of Pediatrics, University of California, Irvine College of Medicine; Medical Director, Memorial Miller Children's Hospital, Long Beach, California

Pertussis; **Campylobacter** *Infections;* **Yersinia Enterocolitica** *Infections*

Richard J. Martin, M.D.

Professor of Pediatrics, Case Western Reserve University School of Medicine; Co-director of Neonatology, Rainbow Babies and Children's Hospital, Cleveland, Ohio

Neonatal Atelectasis

John T. McBride, M.D.

Associate Professor of Pediatrics, University of Rochester School of Medicine and Dentistry; Attending Pediatrician, Strong Memorial Hospital, Rochester, New York

Aspiration Pneumonia

John C. McQuitty, M.D.

Associate Clinical Professor, University of California, San Francisco; Director of Pulmonary Medicine, Children's Hospital Oakland, Oakland, California

Congenital Deformities of the Anterior Chest Wall

Marian E. Melish, M.D.

Professor of Pediatrics, Tropical Medicine and Microbiology, John A. Burns School of Medicine, University of Hawaii; Consultant, Infectious Diseases, Kapiolani Medical Center for Women and Children, Honolulu, Hawaii

Kawasaki Syndrome

Lee Todd Miller, M.D.

Assistant Professor of Clinical Pediatrics, University of California, Los Angeles, School of Medicine; Director, Pediatric Residency Training Program, Cedars-Sinai Medical Center, Los Angeles, California

Lyme Disease

Howard C. Mofenson, M.D., F.A.A.P., F.A.C.I.

Professor of Clinical Pediatrics, State University of New York at Stonybrook; Professor of Pharmacology and Toxicology, New York College of Osteopathy, Old Westbury; Professor of Clinical Pharmacy, St. John's University College of Pharmacy, Jamaica; Director, Long Island Regional Poison Control Center; Director, Pediatric Pharmacology, Nassau County Medical Center, East Meadow; Attending Staff, Winthrop University Hospital, Mineola, New York

Acute Poisoning; Salicylate Poisoning; Acetaminophen Poisoning

Edward A. Mortimer, Jr., M.D.

Professor and Vice Chairman, Department of Epidemiology and Biostatistics, and Professor of Pediatrics, Case Western Reserve University School of Medicine, Cleveland, Ohio

Measles

Michael J. Muszynski, M.D.

Assistant Director of Medical Education; Director, Pediatric Infectious Disease Program, Arnold Palmer Hospital for Children and Women, Orlando Regional Medical Center, Orlando, Florida

Infections due to **Escherichia Coli,** *Proteus, Klebsiella,* **Enterobacter-Serratia,** *Pseudomonas, and other Gram-Negative Bacilli*

Gary J. Myers, M.D.

Professor, Department of Pediatrics and Neurology, University of Alabama School of Medicine, The University of Alabama at Birmingham, Birmingham, Alabama

Myelodysplasia

Alexander S. Nadas, M.D.

Professor of Pediatrics, Emeritus, Harvard Medical School; Chief, Emeritus, Department of Cardiology, and Senior Associate in Cardiology, Children's Hospital, Boston, Massachusetts

Congenital Heart Disease

Lawrence S. Neinstein, M.D.

Associate Professor of Medicine and Pediatrics, University of Southern California School of Medicine; Associate Director, Division of Adolescent Medicine, Children's Hospital of Los Angeles, Los Angeles, California

Homosexual Behavior

Marianne R. Neifert, M.D.

Associate Clinical Professor of Pediatrics, University of Colorado School of Medicine, University of Colorado Health Sciences Center; Medical Director, Lactation Program, AMI Saint Luke's Hospital, Denver, Colorado

Breast Feeding

David B. Nelson, M.D., M.Sc.

Associate Professor of Pediatrics and Director, Medical Education, Medical College of Wisconsin; Attending Physician, Children's Hospital of Wisconsin, Milwaukee, Wisconsin

Bronchitis and Bronchiolitis

Heber C. Nielsen, M.D.

Associate Professor of Pediatrics, Tufts University School of Medicine; Associate Professor of Pediatrics, Division of Newborn Medicine, Floating Hospital for Infants and Children/New England Medical Center, Boston, Massachusetts

Hemolytic Disease of the Newborn

Michael J. Noetzel, M.D.

Assistant Professor, Edward Mallinckrodt Department of Pediatrics and Department of Neurology and Neurological Surgery, Washington University School of Medicine; Director, Down's Syndrome Medical Clinic, St. Louis Children's Hospital; Assistant Pediatrician and Neurologist, Barnes and Allied Hospitals; Consultant in Child Neurology, Irene Walter Johnson Institute of Rehabilitation, St. Louis, Missouri

Intracranial Hemorrhage; Hydrocephalus

James J. Nora, M.D., M.P.H.

Professor of Pediatrics, Genetics, and Preventive Medicine, University of Colorado School of Medicine; Director of Preventive Cardiology, University Hospital; Director of Genetics, Rose Medical Center, Denver, Colorado

The Child at Risk of Coronary Disease as an Adult

Antonia C. Novello, M.D., M.P.H.

Deputy Director for the National Institute of Child Health and Human Development, Washington, D.C.

Hemodialysis, Renal Transplantation

Sharon E. Oberfield, M.D.

Assistant Professor of Pediatrics, College of Physicians and Surgeons of Columbia University; Associate Attending Physician, St. Luke's–Roosevelt Hospital Center, New York, New York

Diabetes Insipidus

William Oh, M.D.

Professor and Chairman, Department of Pediatrics, Brown University Program in Medicine; Pediatrician-in-Chief, Woman and Infant Hospital and Rhode Island Hospital, Providence, Rhode Island

Neonatal Polycythemia and Hyperviscosity

Gary D. Overturf, M.D.

Professor of Pediatrics, University of California, Los Angeles, School of Medicine; Associate Chief of Pediatrics, Olive View Medical Center, Los Angeles, California

Systemic Mycoses

Charles N. Paidas, M.D.

Instructor, ATLS (Advanced Trauma Life Support) 1988; Instructor, APLS (Advanced Pediatric Life Support), The Johns Hopkins Hospital, Baltimore, Maryland

Intussusception

Dachling Pang, M.D., F.R.C.S.(C)

Associate Professor of Neurosurgery, University of Pittsburgh School of Medicine: Chief of Pediatric Neurosurgery, Children's Hospital, Pittsburgh, Pennsylvania

Rhinitis and Sinusitis

Frederick M. Parkins, D.D.S., M.S.D., Ph.D.

Professor of Pediatric Dentistry, Department of Growth and Special Care, School of Dentistry, University of Louisville; Medical Staff, Kosair Children's Hospital, Louisville, Kentucky

Recurrent Acute Parotitis

Umesh B. Patil, M.D.

Professor of Urology and Paediatrics, Health Science Center, State University of New York; Attending Staff, University Hospital, Crouse-Irving Memorial Hospital, St. Joseph's Hospital, Syracuse, New York

Patent Urachus and Urachal Cysts

Nicholas A. Patrone, M.D., F.A.C.P.

Associate Professor of Medicine and Pediatrics and Section Head, Pediatric Rheumatology, East Carolina University School of Medicine; Consulting Assistant Professor of Pediatrics, Duke University School of Medicine, Durham; Attending Staff, Pitt County Memorial Hospital, Greenville, North Carolina

Eosinophilic Fasciitis

Jerome A. Paulson, M.D.

Associate Clinical Professor of Pediatrics, Georgetown University School of Medicine, Washington, D.C.

Animal and Human Bites and Bite-Related Infections

Samuel H. Pepkowitz, M.D.

Associate Director, Division of Transfusion Medicine, Department of Pathology and Laboratory Medicine, Cedars-Sinai Medical Center, Los Angeles, California

Adverse Reactions to Blood Transfusion

Michael J. Pettei, M.D., Ph.D.
Assistant Professor of Pediatrics, Albert Einstein College of Medicine; Co-Chief, Division of Gastroenterology and Nutrition, Schneider Children's Hospital of the Long Island Jewish Medical Center, New Hyde Park, New York
Early Childhood Obesity

Carol F. Phillips, M.D.
Professor and Chairman, Department of Pediatrics, University of Vermont College of Medicine; Chief of Pediatric Service, Medical Center Hospital of Vermont, Burlington, Vermont
Psittacosis; Chlamydia Infections

Larry K. Pickering, M.D.
Professor of Pediatrics, Director of Pediatric Infectious Diseases, University of Texas Medical School at Houston, Houston, Texas
Shigellosis

Rosita S. Pildes, M.D.
Professor of Pediatrics, University of Illinois College of Medicine; Chairman, Division of Neonatology, Cook County Children's Hospital, Chicago, Illinois
Infants of Drug-Dependent Mothers

Donald Pinkel, M.D.
Professor of Pediatrics, University of Texas M.D. Anderson Cancer Center; Pediatrician and Director, Pediatric Leukemia Research Program; Mansfield and Levine Chair in Cancer Research, University of Texas M.D. Anderson Cancer Center, Houston, Texas
Acute Leukemia

Philip A. Pizzo, M.D.
Professor of Pediatrics, Uniformed Services University for the Health Sciences; Chief of Pediatrics, Head of Infectious Diseases, National Cancer Institute, National Institutes of Health, Bethesda, Maryland
Leukopenia, Neutropenia, and Agranulocytosis

Stanley A. Plotkin, M.D.
Professor of Pediatrics and Microbiology, University of Pennsylvania; Professor, The Wistar Institute; Senior Physician, Children's Hospital of Philadelphia, Philadelphia, Pennsylvania
Rabies; Infectious Mononucleosis and Epstein-Barr Virus–Related Syndromes

Richard A. Polin, M.D.
Professor of Pediatrics, University of Pennsylvania School of Medicine; Associate Chairman, Department of Pediatrics, Children's Hospital of Philadelphia, Philadelphia, Pennsylvania
Neonatal Septicemia, Meningitis, and Pneumonia

Paul G. Quie, M.D.
Professor of Pediatrics, University of Minnesota Medical School; Chief, Pediatric Infectious Diseases, University of Minnesota Hospital, Minneapolis, Minnesota
Staphylococcal Infections

Sharon S. Raimer, M.D.
Professor of Dermatology and Pediatrics, University of Texas Medical Branch, Galveston, Texas
Skin Diseases of the Neonate

Max L. Ramenofsky, M.D.
Professor of Surgery and Pediatrics, University of Pittsburgh School of Medicine; Children's Hospital of Pittsburgh, Pittsburgh, Pennsylvania
Lymphangitis; Lymph Node Infections (Lymphadenitis)

I. Rapin, M.D.
Professor of Neurology and Pediatrics (Neurology), Albert Einstein College of Medicine; Attending Neurologist and Child Neurologist, Einstein Affiliated Hospitals, Bronx, New York
Autism

James E. Rasmussen, M.D.
Professor of Dermatology and Pediatrics, University of Michigan Medical School; Chief of Clinic in Dermatology and Chief of Pediatric Inpatient and Dermatology Outpatient Services, University of Michigan Hospitals, Ann Arbor, Michigan
Erythema Multiforme

C. George Ray, M.D.
Professor, Pathology and Pediatrics, University of Arizona College of Medicine; Active Medical Staff, University Medical Center, Tucson, Arizona
Diphtheria

Edward F. Reda, M.D.
Assistant Professor of Urology, New York Medical College, Valhalla; Chief of Pediatric Urology, Lincoln Hospital; Voluntary Attending in Pediatric Urology, Montefiore Medical Center, Bronx, Flushing Hospital, Flushing, and Nyack Hospital, Nyack, New York
Ambiguous Genitalia

Owen M. Rennert, M.D.
Professor and Chairman, Department of Pediatrics, Georgetown University School of Medicine; Pediatrician in Chief, Georgetown University Hospital, Washington, D.C.
Hepatolenticular Degeneration (Wilson's Disease)

Thomas S. Renshaw, M.D.
Professor of Orthopaedic Surgery, University of Connecticut School of Medicine, Farmington; Director of Orthopaedic Surgery, Newington Children's Hospital, Newington, Connecticut
Torticollis

Warren Richards, M.D.
Professor of Pediatrics, University of Southern California School of Medicine; Head, Division of Allergy and Clinical Immunology, Children's Hospital of Los Angeles, Los Angeles, California
Allergic Gastrointestinal Disorders

Sylvia Onesti Richardson, M.D.
Distinguished Professor, Communication Sciences and Disorders, and Clinical Professor of Pediatrics, University of South Florida, Tampa, Florida
Voice, Speech, and Language Disorders

Harris D. Riley, Jr., M.D.
Distinguished Professor of Pediatrics, University of Oklahoma College of Medicine; Attending Physician, Children's Hospital of Oklahoma, University of Oklahoma Health Sciences Center, Oklahoma City, Oklahoma

Infections due to **Escherichia Coli,** *Proteus, Klebsiella,* **Enterobacter-Serratia,** *Pseudomonas, and other Gram-Negative Bacilli*

David L. Rimoin, M.D., Ph.D.

Professor of Pediatrics and Medicine, University of California, Los Angeles, School of Medicine; Steven Spielberg Chairman of Pediatrics, Director, Ahmanson Pediatrics Center; Director, Medical Genetics-Birth Defects Center, Cedars-Sinai Medical Center, Los Angeles, California

Genetic Diseases

Judith E. Robinson, M.D.

Assistant Professor of Psychiatry, Tufts Medical School; Director of Inpatient Child Psychiatry, New England Medical Center, Boston, Massachusetts

Psychosomatic Illness

Alan M. Robson, M.D., F.R.C.P.

Professor of Pediatrics, Tulane University School of Medicine, and Louisiana State University School of Medicine; Medical Director, Children's Hospital, New Orleans, Louisiana

Systemic Hypertension

Robert L. Rosenfield, M.D.

Professor of Pediatrics and Medicine, University of Chicago Pritzker School of Medicine; Head, Section of Pediatric Endocrinology, Wyler Children's Hospital, Chicago, Illinois

Endocrine Disorders of the Testis

Philip Rosenthal, M.D.

Visiting Associate Professor of Pediatrics, University of California, Los Angeles, School of Medicine; Director, Pediatric Gastroenterology and Nutrition; Medical Director, Pediatric Liver Transplantation Program, Cedars-Sinai Medical Center, Los Angeles, California

Disorders of Porphyrin, Purine, and Pyrimidine Metabolism

N. Paul Rosman, M.D.

Professor of Pediatrics and Neurology, Tufts University School of Medicine; Chief, Division of Pediatric Neurology, Floating Hospital for Infants and Children; Director, Center for Children with Special Needs, New England Medical Center Hospital, Boston, Massachusetts

Febrile Convulsions; Headache

Barry H. Rumack, M.D.

Professor of Pediatrics, University of Colorado Health Sciences Center; Director, Rocky Mountain Poison and Drug Center; Denver General Hospital, The Children's Hospital, St. Anthony's Hospital, and University of Colorado Health Sciences Center, Denver, Colorado

Botulinal Food Poisoning

Michael E. Ryan, D.O.

Clinical Associate Professor, Jefferson Medical College, Philadelphia; Director, Pediatric Subspecialties, Geisinger Clinic, Danville, Pennsylvania

Legionella *Infections*

Joseph W. St. Geme, III, M.D.

Postdoctoral Fellow, Department of Microbiology and Immunology, Stanford University School of Medicine, Stanford, California

Neonatal Septicemia, Meningitis, and Pneumonia

Joy H. Samuels-Reid, M.D.

Department of Pediatrics, Howard University Hospital, Washington, D.C.

Sickle Cell Disease

Julio V. Santiago, M.D.

Professor of Pediatrics and Co-Director of Pediatric Endocrinology, Washington University School of Medicine; Division of Endocrinology and Metabolism, St. Louis Children's Hospital, St. Louis, Missouri

Systemic Hypertension

Lawrence Schachne, M.D.

Professor of Pediatrics and Professor of Dermatology, and Director, Division of Pediatric Dermatology, University of Miami School of Medicine, Miami, Florida

Erythema Nodosum; Drug Reactions and the Skin; Fungal Infections

Hal C. Scherz, M.D.

Clinical Assistant Professor of Surgery/Urology, University of California, San Diego, School of Medicine; Associate Staff, Children's Hospital, Attending Staff, University Hospital, San Diego, California

Urolithiasis

Gilbert M. Schiff, M.D.

President, James N. Gamble Institute of Medical Research, Professor of Medicine, University of Cincinnati College of Medicine, Attending Physician, The Christ Hospital, Cincinnati Children's Hospital, and University Hospital, Cincinnati, Ohio

Enteroviruses

Virginia E. Schuett, M.S.

Seattle, Washington

Hyperphenylalaninemias

James F. Schwartz, M.D.

Professor of Pediatrics and Neurology, Emory University School of Medicine; Chief of Pediatrics, Henrietta Egleston Hospital for Children, Emory University Hospital, Grady Memorial Hospital, Atlanta, Georgia

Acute Ataxia

Richard H. Schwartz, M.D.

Clinical Professor of Pediatrics, Georgetown University School of Medicine and George Washington University School of Medicine, Washington, D.C.; Clinical Professor of Family Practice, Medical College of Virginia, Richmond; Attending Pediatrician, Fairfax Hospital, Falls Church, Virginia

Nasopharyngitis

Molly R. Schwenn, M.D.

Assistant Professor, Tufts University School of Medicine; Assistant Pediatrician and Clinical Director, Pediatric Hematology/Oncology, Floating Hospital for Infants and Children/New England Medical Center Hospital, Boston, Massachusetts

Burkitt's Lymphoma

Gwendolyn B. Scott, M.D.
Director, Division of Immunology and Infectious Disease, Department of Pediatrics, University of Miami School of Medicine; Head, Pediatric Immunology and Infectious Disease, Jackson Memorial Hospital, Miami, Florida
The Immunodeficiencies, Including HIV-1 Infection

Roland B. Scott, M.D.
Washington, D.C.
Sickle Cell Disease

Susan M. Scott, M.D.
Assistant Professor of Pediatrics, University of New Mexico School of Medicine; University of New Mexico Hospital, Albuquerque, New Mexico
Rickets; Tetany

John H. Seashore, M.D.
Professor of Surgery and Pediatrics, Yale University School of Medicine; Attending Physician, Yale-New Haven Hospital, New Haven, Connecticut
Disorders of the Anus and Rectum

Boris Senior, M.D.
Professor of Pediatrics, Tufts University School of Medicine; Chief, Pediatric-Endocrine-Metabolic Service, Floating Hospital For Infants and Children, Boston, Massachusetts
Hypoglycemia

D. H. Shaffner, Jr., M.D.
Instructor, Johns Hopkins University School of Medicine; Instructor, Department of Anesthesiology and Critical Care Medicine, Johns Hopkins Hospital, Baltimore, Maryland
Management of Septic Shock

Bruce K. Shapiro, M.D.
Associate Professor of Pediatrics, Johns Hopkins University School of Medicine; Kennedy Institute for Handicapped Children, Johns Hopkins Hospital, Baltimore, Maryland
Mental Retardation

Stephen R. Shapiro, M.D.
Assistant Clinical Professor of Pediatrics, University of California, Davis; Sutter Community Hospitals, and Mercy General Hospital, Sacramento, California
Perinephric and Intranephric Abscess

Bennett A. Shaywitz, M.D.
Professor of Pediatrics, Neurology and Child Study Center, Yale University School of Medicine; Director of Pediatric Neurology, Yale-New Haven Hospital, New Haven, Connecticut
Hypoxic Encephalopathy

Nancy F. Sheard, Sc.D., R.D.
Assistant Professor, Department of Nutrition, University of Massachusetts, Amherst, Massachusetts
Total Parenteral Nutrition in Infants

I. Ronald Shenker, M.D.
Associate Professor of Pediatrics, Albert Einstein College of Medicine; Chief, Adolescent Medicine, Schneider Children's Hospital of the Long Island Jewish Medical Center, New Hyde Park, New York
Later Childhood and Adolescent Obesity

Sheila Sherlock, D.B.E., M.D.
Professor of Medicine, School of Medicine, University of London; Consulting Physician, Royal Free Hospital, London, England
Portal Hypertension

Mitchell D. Shub, M.D.
Director of Medical Education and Assistant Lecturer, University of Arizona College of Medicine; Attending Pediatrician, Children's Hospital, Phoenix, Arizona
Protracted Diarrhea of Infancy; Chronic Diarrhea and Malabsorption Syndromes

William K. Sieber, M.D.
Clinical Professor of Surgery, University of Pittsburgh School of Medicine; Senior Staff in Surgery, Children's Hospital of Pittsburgh; Active Staff, Department of Surgery, Presbyterian University Hospital of Pittsburgh; Active Staff, Pediatric Surgery, Western Pennsylvania Hospital, and Forbes Regional Health Center, Pittsburgh, Pennsylvania
Hirschsprung's Disease

Irwin M. Siegel, M.D.
Associate Professor, Departments of Orthopaedic Surgery and Neurological Sciences, Rush-Presbyterian-St. Luke's Medical Center; Attending Orthopaedic Surgeon, Louis A. Weiss Memorial Hospital, Chicago, Illinois
Muscular Dystrophy and Related Myopathies

Richard H. Sills, M.D.
Director of Pediatric Hematology/Oncology, Children's Hospital of New Jersey, Newark; Associate Professor of Pediatrics, University of Medicine and Dentistry of New Jersey, Newark; Specialist in Pediatric Hematology/Oncology, St. Barnabas Medical Center, Livingston, New Jersey
Disseminated Intravascular Coagulation and Purpura Fulminans

Robert A. Silverman, M.D.
Clinical Associate Professor of Pediatrics, Georgetown University School of Medicine; Georgetown University Medical Center, Washington, D.C.
Disorders of Pigmentation

William D. Singer, M.D.
Assistant Professor of Pediatrics, Harvard Medical School, Boston; Associate Chief of Pediatrics, Cambridge Hospital, Cambridge, Massachusetts
Spasmus Nutans

Fady A. Sinno, M.D.
General Surgery Resident, St. Agnes Hospital, Baltimore, Maryland
Peritonitis

R. Michael Sly, M.D.
Professor of Pediatrics, George Washington University School of Medicine and Health Sciences; Chairman of Allergy and Immunology, Children's National Medical Center, Washington, D.C.
Asthma

Jeffrey F. Smallhorn, M.D., F.R.C.P.(C), F.A.C.C.
Associate Professor, University of Toronto Faculty of

Medicine; Director, Section of Echocardiography, Division of Cardiology, Department of Pediatrics, The Hospital for Sick Children, Toronto, Ontario
Primary Cardiac Neoplasms

Peter S. Smith, M.D.
Associate Professor of Pediatrics, Brown University; Associate Director, Pediatric Hematology–Oncology, Rhode Island Hospital, Providence, Rhode Island
Lymphedema

Russell D. Snyder, M.D.
Professor of Neurology and Pediatrics, University of New Mexico School of Medicine; Director, Division of Pediatric Neurology; Active Staff at University of New Mexico Hospital and Albuquerque Veterans Administration Hospital; Consulting Staff at Gallup Indian Medical Center, Presbyterian Hospital, St. Joseph's Hospital, and Heights Psychiatric Hospital, Albuquerque, New Mexico
Disorders of Learning; Attention Deficit Disorder

Gail E. Solomon, M.D.
Associate Professor of Clinical Neurology in Pediatrics, New York Hospital-Cornell University Medical Center; Associate Attending in Neurology and Pediatrics, New York Hospital-Cornell University Medical Center, New York, New York
Cerebrovascular Disease in Infancy and Childhood

William Spivak, M.D.
Associate Clinical Professor of Pediatrics, Albert Einstein College of Medicine; Assistant Attending Pediatrician, Montefiore Medical Center, Bronx, New York
Nonhemolytic Unconjugated Hyperbilirubinemia

Mary K. Spraker, M.D.
Associate Professor of Dermatology and Pediatrics, Emory University School of Medicine; Chief of Dermatology, Henrietta Egleston Hospital for Children, Atlanta, Georgia
Chronic Nonhereditary Vesiculobullous Disorders of Childhood; Other Skin Tumors

Gopal Srinivasan, M.D.
Professor of Pediatrics, University of Health Sciences/ Chicago Medical School; Attending Physician, Cook County Children's Hospital, Chicago, Illinois
Infants of Drug-Dependent Mothers

Lynn T. Staheli, M.D.
Professor of Orthopedic Surgery, University of Washington School of Medicine; Director, Department of Orthopedics, Children's Orthopedic Hospital and Medical Center, Seattle, Washington
The Hip

F. Bruder Stapleton, M.D.
A. Conger Goodyear Professor and Chairman, Department of Pediatrics, State University of New York at Buffalo; Pediatrician-in-Chief, Children's Hospital of Buffalo, Buffalo, New York
Idiopathic Hypercalcemia

Thomas E. Starzl, M.D., Ph.D.
Distinguished Service Professor of Surgery, University of Pittsburgh School of Medicine; Presbyterian-University Hospital, Children's Hospital of Pittsburgh, and Veterans Administration Hospital, Oak-

land, Pittsburgh, Pennsylvania
Tumors of the Liver

Robert C. Stern, M.D.
Professor of Pediatrics, Case Western Reserve University School of Medicine; Associate Pediatrician, Rainbow Babies and Children's Hospital, Cleveland, Ohio
Pulmonary Thromboembolism; Bronchiectasis; Pulmonary Thromboembolism

Dennis C. Stokes, M.D.
Associate Professor of Pediatrics, University of Tennessee, Memphis; Director, Cardiopulmonary-Critical Care Division, St. Jude Children's Research Hospital, Memphis, Tennessee
The Croup Syndrome

D. Eugene Strandness, Jr., M.D.
Professor of Surgery, University of Washington School of Medicine; University Hospital, Seattle, Washington
Peripheral Vascular Disease

Victor C. Strasburger, M.D.
Associate Professor of Pediatrics, Chief, Division of Adolescent Medicine, Department of Pediatrics, University of New Mexico School of Medicine; Attending Physician, University Hospital and New Mexico Children's Hospital, Albuquerque, New Mexico
Uterus, Tubes, and Ovaries

Richard H. Strauss, M.D.
Assistant Clinical Professor of Pediatrics, University of Wisconsin Medical School, Madison; Director, Pediatric Intensive Care Unit, Gundersen Clinic/Lutheran Hospital, La Crosse, Wisconsin
Head Injury

Denise J. Strieder, M.D.
Associate Professor of Pediatrics, Harvard Medical School; Pediatrician, Massachusetts General Hospital, Boston, Massachusetts
Atelectasis

Donald K. Stritzke, M.D.
Tacoma, Washington
Penis, Spermatic Cord, and Testes

Dennis M. Styne, M.D.
Associate Professor of Pediatrics, University of California, Davis, School of Medicine; Chairman, Department of Pediatrics, University of California, Davis, Medical Center, Sacramento, California
Thyroid Disease

Se Mo Suh, M.D., Ph.D.
Professor of Pediatrics, John A. Burns School of Medicine, University of Hawaii; Chief of Pediatric Endocrinology, Kapiolani Medical Center for Women and Children, Honolulu, Hawaii
Magnesium Deficiency

Michael D. Sussman, M.D.
Professor and Head, Division of Pediatric Orthopedic Surgery, and Professor of Pediatrics, University of Virginia School of Medicine, Charlottesville, Virginia
Disorders of the Spine and Shoulder Girdle

Ilona S. Szer, M.D.
Assistant Professor in Pediatrics, Tufts University School of Medicine; Associate Director, Division of

Pediatric Rheumatology, Floating Hospital for Infants and Children, Boston, Massachusetts
Rheumatic Diseases of Childhood

Lawrence T. Taft, M.D.
Professor of Pediatrics, University of Medicine and Dentistry of New Jersey Robert Wood-Johnson Medical School; Attending, Robert Wood-Johnson University Hospital; Consultant, St. Peter's Medical Center, New Brunswick, New Jersey
Cerebral Palsy

Anabel J. Teberg, M.D.
Upland, California
Listeria Monocytogenes *Infection*

M. Michael Thaler, M.D.
Professor of Pediatrics, University of California, San Francisco, School of Medicine; Attending Physician, University of California, San Francisco, School of Medicine, Moffitt-Lang Hospital, San Francisco, California
Disorders of Porphyrin, Purine, and Pyrimidine Metabolism

Joel A. Thompson, M.D.
Associate Professor of Pediatrics and Neurology and Chief, Division of Pediatric Neurology, University of Utah Medical Center and Primary Children's Medical Center, Salt Lake City, Utah
Infant Botulism

James K. Todd, M.D.
Professor of Pediatrics and Microbiology/Immunology, University of Colorado School of Medicine; Director of Infectious Diseases, The Children's Hospital, Denver, Colorado
Bacterial Meningitis and Septicemia Beyond the Neonatal Period

William E. Truog, M.D.
Professor of Pediatrics, University of Washington School of Medicine; Medical Director, Infant Intensive Care Unit, Children's Hospital and Medical Center, Seattle, Washington
Pneumothorax and Pneumomediastinum

Reginald C. Tsang, M.B.B.S.
Professor of Pediatrics and of Obstetrics and Gynecology, University of Cincinnati College of Medicine; Attending Physician, University of Cincinnati Medical Center and Children's Hospital Medical Center, Cincinnati, Ohio
Parathyroid Disease

John N. Udall, Jr., M.D., Ph.D.
Associate Professor of Pediatrics, Chief of Pediatric Gastroenterology, University of Arizona School of Medicine; Chief, Pediatric Gastroenterology, University Medical Center, Tucson, Arizona
Vitamin Deficiencies and Excesses

David T. Uehling, M.D.
Professor and Chairman, Division of Urology, University of Wisconsin Medical School; University of Wisconsin Hospital, Madison, Wisconsin
Urinary Tract Infections

Martin H. Ulshen, M.D.
Associate Professor of Pediatrics, University of North Carolina School of Medicine; Attending Pediatric Gastroenterologist, Children's Hospital; University of North Carolina Hospital, Chapel Hill, North Carolina
Protracted Diarrhea of Infancy; Chronic Diarrhea and Malabsorption Syndromes

Louis E. Underwood, M.D.
Professor of Pediatrics, University of North Carolina School of Medicine, Chapel Hill, North Carolina
Hypopituitarism and Growth Hormone Therapy

Paul T. Urea, M.D., M.P.H.
Clinical Instructor, Department of Ophthalmology, University of Southern California School of Medicine, Los Angeles; Practicing Ophthalmologist, Monterey Park, California
The Eye

Timos Valaes, M.D.
Professor of Pediatrics, Tufts University School of Medicine; Neonatologist, Floating Hospital for Infants and Children/New England Medical Center Hospital, Boston, Massachusetts
Neonatal Ascites

Victoria L. Vetter, M.D.
Associate Professor of Pediatrics, University of Pennsylvania School of Medicine; Senior Cardiologist and Director, Electrophysiology and Electrocardiography Laboratories, Children's Hospital of Philadelphia, Philadelphia, Pennsylvania
Mitral Valve Prolapse

Nancy E. Vinton, M.D.
Assistant Professor in Pediatrics, Tufts University School of Medicine; Assistant Pediatrician, Floating Hospital for Infants and Children/New England Medical Center Hospital, Boston, Massachusetts
Nutrition; Malformations of the Intestine; Inflammatory Bowel Disease

Jeffrey Wacksman, M.D., F.A.A.P
Assistant Professor of Surgery, Division of Urology, University of Cincinnati College of Medicine; Associate Director, Division of Pediatric Urology, Children's Hospital Medical Center, Cincinnati, Ohio
Hernias and Hydroceles

Ken B. Waites, M.D.
Research Assistant Professor, Department of Microbiology, University of Alabama at Birmingham Schools of Medicine and Dentistry, Birmingham, Alabama
Mycoplasma Infections

Ellen R. Wald, M.D.
Professor of Pediatrics, University of Pittsburgh School of Medicine; Associate Medical Director, Ambulatory Care Division; Member, Division of Infectious Diseases, Children's Hospital of Pittsburgh, Pittsburgh, Pennsylvania
Rhinitis and Sinusitis

W. Allan Walker, M.D.
Professor of Pediatrics, Harvard Medical School;

Chief, Combined Program in Pediatric Gastroenterology and Nutrition, Children's Hospital, Boston, Massachusetts
Acute and Chronic Nonspecific Diarrhea Syndromes; Disorders of the Hepatobiliary Tree

Michael A. Wall, M.D.
Associate Professor of Pediatrics and Chief, Pediatric Pulmonary Section, Oregon Health Sciences University, Portland, Oregon
Emphysema

Michele C. Walsh-Sukys, M.D.
Assistant Professor of Pediatrics, Case Western Reserve University School of Medicine; Attending Neonatologist, Rainbow Babies and Children's Hospital, Cleveland, Ohio
Neonatal Atelectasis

Eli R. Wayne, M.D.
Associate Professor of Pediatric Surgery, University of Colorado School of Medicine; Attending Pediatric Surgeon, Children's Hospital, Denver, Denver, Colorado
Congenital Diaphragmatic Hernia

H. James Wedner, M.D.
Associate Professor of Medicine, Washington University School of Medicine; Associate Physician, Barnes Hospital, St. Louis, Missouri
Adverse Reactions to Drugs

Paul F. Wehrle, M.D.
Professor of Pediatrics, University of California, Irvine, School of Medicine; Los Angeles County-USC Medical Center; University of California, Irvine Medical Center, Irvine, California
Influenza

Marvin L. Weil, M.D.
Professor Emeritus of Pediatrics and Neurology, University of California, Los Angeles, School of Medicine, Los Angeles, California; Visiting Scholar, University of Oxford, Oxford, England
Brain Abscess; Spinal Epidural Abscesses; Myositis Ossificans; Encephalitic Infections—Postinfectious and Postvaccinal

Louis M. Weiss, M.D., M.P.H.
Assistant Professor of Medicine, Division of Infectious Diseases and Assistant Professor of Pathology, Division of Parisitology and Tropical Medicine, Albert Einstein College of Medicine; Assistant Attending Staff, Bronx Municipal Hospital; Assistant Attending Staff, Albert Einstein Hospital-Waecom Division of Montefiore Hospital; Attending Staff, Westchester Square Hospital; Bronx, New York
Malaria; Cysticercosis; Babesiosis

Marc Weissbluth, M.D.
Associate Professor, Department of Pediatrics, Northwestern University School of Medicine; Active Attending Pediatrician, The Children's Memorial Hospital, Chicago, Illinois
Colic

William L. Weston, M.D.
Professor of Dermatology and Pediatrics, Chairman,

Department of Dermatology, University of Colorado School of Medicine; Chief of Dermatology, University Hospital; The Children's Hospital, Denver, Colorado
Contact Dermatitis

George E. White, A.B., D.D.S., Ph.D., D.B.A., F.A.G.D., F.I.C.D.
Chairman and Associate Professor, Department of Pediatric Dentistry, Tufts University School of Dental Medicine; New England Medical Center Hospital, Boston, Massachusetts
Nursing Caries

Jerry A. Winkelstein, M.D.
Eudowood Professor of Pediatrics, Johns Hopkins University School of Medicine; Director, Division of Allergy and Immunology, Department of Pediatrics, Johns Hopkins Hospital, Baltimore, Maryland
Postsplenectomy Syndrome

Murray Wittner, M.D., Ph.D.
Professor of Pathology and Parasitology, Albert Einstein College of Medicine; Attending Physician and Director, Parasitology and Tropical Disease Clinic and Laboratory, Bronx Municipal Hospital Center, Weiler Hospital, Bronx, New York
Cysticercosis; Malaria; Babesiosis

Joseph I. Wolfsdorf, M.D.
Assistant Professor of Pediatrics, Harvard Medical School; Associate in Endocrinology, The Children's Hospital of Boston; Chief of Pediatrics, Joslin Diabetes Center; Physician, New England Deaconess Hospital, Boston, Massachusetts
Diabetes Mellitus

Shiao Y. Woo, M.D.
Assistant Professor, Radiotherapy and Pediatrics, University of Texas; Assistant Radiotherapist and Pediatrician, University of Texas M. D. Anderson Cancer Center, Houston, Texas
Malignant Lymphoma

Francis S. Wright, M.D.
Professor of Pediatrics, Ohio State University College of Medicine; Chief, Division of Neurology, Columbus Children's Hospital, Columbus, Ohio
Spinal Diseases; Guillain-Barré Syndrome

Terry Yamauchi, M.D.
Professor of Pediatrics, Vice-Chairman of Pediatrics and Associate Dean, College of Medicine, University of Arkansas for Medical Sciences, Arkansas Children's Hospital, Little Rock, Arkansas
Herpes Simplex Virus Infection

George H. Zalzal, M.D.
Assistant Professor of Otolaryngology and Pediatrics, George Washington University; Attending Staff, Children's National Medical Center, Washington, D.C.
Disorders of the Larynx

Harvey A. Zarem, M.D.
Professor Emeritus and Clinical Professor of Surgery, Division of Plastic Surgery, University of California, Los Angeles School of Medicine; UCLA Medical Center, Los Angeles, and St. John's Hospital, Santa Monica, California
Diseases and Injuries of the Oral Region

Ekhard E. Ziegler, M.D.
Professor of Pediatrics, University of Iowa College of Medicine; Staff Physician, University of Iowa Hospitals and Clinics, Iowa City, Iowa
Feeding the Low Birth Weight Infant

William H. Zinkham, M.D.
Distinguished Service Professor of Pediatrics and Professor of Oncology, Johns Hopkins University School of Medicine; Director of Pediatric Hematology, Johns Hopkins Hospital, Baltimore, Maryland
Indications for Splenectomy

Philip R. Ziring, M.D.
Associate Clinical Professor of Pediatrics, University of California, San Francisco; Chairman, Department of Pediatrics, Pacific Presbyterian Medical Center, San Francisco, California
Rubella and Congenital Rubella

Preface

Since *Current Pediatric Therapy* was first published in 1964, its goal has been to provide information on the therapeutic needs of infants and children in terms of dosages, prescriptions, modified regimens, immunization schedules, and rehabilitation measures. In every one of the past 12 editions, as well as in this current volume, some of the treatments described are new and some are traditional. The single, inflexible requirement has been that all be proven effective in clinical practice.

In the course of some 27 years, the issues of major concern in the care of infants and children have altered somewhat. Smallpox has been eradicated throughout the world, for example, and wide use of highly effective vaccines has drastically decreased the number of cases of such diseases as pertussis, whooping cough, and polio seen by the average practitioner. Conversely, new problems such as AIDS, substance abuse, and toxic shock have become more prevalent, requiring those who care for children to learn about these problems and how to manage them.

It is partly because fewer cases of some disorders are seen today that we continue to include them in this work—so there is still a resource available for management of these problems. In addition, we have expanded other sections to deal with "new" problems seen in the pediatrician's office. This volume includes more information on treatment of newborn infants and on management of teenage ailments such as sexually transmitted disorders and drug abuse.

As from the beginning, it is assumed that a correct diagnosis has been made previously and that the information sought relates solely to management. The reader will also note that the book contains few, if any, references. Each writer has been asked to describe the treatment that has worked for him or her rather than to give a review of the studies of others.

The editors are indebted to the many contributors who have generously taken the time to share their modes of treatment. Each one presents a workable solution to a problem that will ease the life of a child and calm a worried parent. It is our hope that the use of this body of knowledge will provide answers for the practitioner and an ultimate benefit to each patient.

Sydney S. Gellis, M.D.
Benjamin M. Kagan, M.D.

Contents

4   RESPIRATORY TRACT

7   BLOOD

8   SPLEEN AND LYMPHATIC SYSTEM

15 SKIN

16 THE EYE

17 THE EAR

18 INFECTIOUS DISEASES

24   MISCELLANEOUS

1

Nutrition

UNDERNUTRITION

NANCY E. VINTON, M.D.,
and WILLIAM H. DIETZ, Jr., M.D., Ph.D.

In the United States, "failure to thrive" has become the euphemism for undernutrition. In this section, we will use the term *undernutrition* to describe states of protein and energy deficiency, rather than *malnutrition,* which is a more general term that encompasses obesity, undernutrition, and nutrient imbalance. Undernutrition occurs frequently in pediatric hospitals. Failure to thrive accounts for 1 to 5 per cent of all pediatric hospital admissions, and up to 30 per cent of all hospitalized children may have one or more signs of undernutrition.

The treatment of undernutrition begins with an assessment of the child's overall nutritional status (Table 1). Classifications of the degree of undernutrition begin with the measurement of height and weight and comparison with the standard growth charts published by the National Center for Health Statistics (NCHS) to determine whether the child is acutely or chronically undernourished. Growth of upper socioeconomic class populations in developing countries shows a distribution similar to that of the NCHS, indicating that the NCHS standards are a valid standard against which the growth of children in the third world or immigrants to the United States should be compared.

Acute malnutrition, or wasting, is characterized by a weight for height that is less than the fifth percentile. Chronic undernutrition, or stunting, is characterized by a height for age that is less than the fifth percentile,

TABLE 1. Clinical and Laboratory Assessment of Undernutrition

History—time of onset, family growth patterns, parental height
Dietary—usual intake, eating behavior, swallowing abnormalities
Development—delayed, comparison of social and motor
Physical—signs of organic disease, edema, hair texture and pluckability
Anthropometry—height, weight, weight for height, mid-arm circumference, triceps skinfold
Laboratory—lymphocyte count, albumin, transferrin

but a normal weight for height. Some children may be both wasted and stunted, as seen with marasmus, a severe form of energy deficiency in which both height for age and weight for height are less than the fifth percentile. Children with severe protein deficiency, or kwashiorkor, may present with a normal weight for height secondary to hypoalbuminemia and edema. Recognition of kwashiorkor affects therapy because children with kwashiorkor are frequently anergic, incapable of inflammatory responses, and must be treated as if they were immunodeficient.

Anthropometric assessment also provides clear expectations for the course of recovery. Children with acute undernutrition demonstrate rapid weight gain in the early stages of recovery, whereas children with chronic undernutrition do not. In cases in which height velocity has been affected, catch-up growth, defined as a height velocity two to three times that observed in normal children of the same age and sex, may require several months to become apparent. The formula for estimating the calorie requirements for catch-up growth is ideal weight times requirement for weight for age divided by actual weight (Table 2).

The second determination that directly affects therapy is whether the undernutrition is organic or psychosocial in origin. Together, neurologic and gastrointestinal diseases account for 60 to 80 per cent of all organic causes of undernutrition. Clearly, resolution of undernutrition that accompanies another illness requires successful therapy for the illness before the nutritional problems will resolve. Underlying diseases, such as occult carcinoma or inflammatory bowel disease, or intercurrent infections, such as pneumonia or measles, frequently accompany undernutrition. Parental guilt at having a malnourished child or strenuous efforts to nourish a child with a primary illness who will not eat may promote the development of a secondary eating disorder that may persist after the original illness has resolved. The diagnosis and treatment of both primary and secondary psychosocial components of undernutrition usually require the assistance of a social worker or psychologist.

Initial intervention in the treatment of undernutrition

1

TABLE 2. Calculation of Catch-Up Requirements

1. Determine weight-age by extrapolation to the 50th percentile
2. Determine ideal weight for actual height

$$\frac{(\text{kcal or gm protein for weight age} \times \text{ideal body weight})}{\text{actual weight}}$$

age	kcal/kg	gm prot/kg
0–6 months	115	2.2
6–12 months	105	2.0
1–3 years	100	1.8
4–6 years	85	1.5

may require acute management of dehydration and electrolyte imbalance. Fluid resuscitation may be particularly important if diarrhea accompanies undernutrition. A danger of acute phase therapy is that overly vigorous hydration or calorie supplementation may precipitate congestive heart failure. Children with a kwashiorkor-like syndrome who have severe hypoalbuminemia and anemia are at particular risk. Hypoglycemia and hypothermia may also be present initially. During this early phase of nutritional rehabilitation, the child may have increased requirements for potassium (as much as twice maintenance requirements—6 to 8 mEq/day), as well as for calcium, magnesium, and phosphorus. These metabolic imbalances may be exacerbated if hypercaloric, hypertonic parenteral nutrition solutions are used in the acute phase of management. Sudden death from hypophosphatemia has been reported with overzealous hypercaloric repletion started within the first 24 hours of intervention. The coincident vitamin and trace element deficiencies seen with malnutrition are reviewed in a later chapter.

The following algorithm presents a useful approach to the treatment of undernutrition after fluid and metabolite imbalances are corrected. The principal decisions depend on the degree to which intestinal absorption is impaired and the length of time that nutritional support is required. If the gut is functional, it should be used. If it is not, and nutritional support is required for less than 5 days, peripheral parenteral nutritional support is warranted. If nutritional support is required for more than 5 days, use of a central line must be considered.

To institute parenteral nutrition, initial volumes to be infused should be based on the child's maintenance fluid requirements (usually 100 ml/kg/day). Fluid intake at this level generally provides adequate protein intake of 2 gm/kg/day if a 2 per cent amino acid mixture is utilized. Dextrose concentrations may be increased by 5 per cent per day as long as glucose intolerance does not arise. Serum glucose should be monitored on a regular basis (every 6 hours). Concurrent sepsis or infection increases the likelihood of hyperglycemia. Only 10 per cent dextrose solutions may be used with peripheral parenteral nutrition. Intravenous fats are calorically dense and are often essential in the care of the fluid-restricted patient. Up to 60 per cent of total calories, or 4 gm/kg/day, may be given as lipid provided that hyperlipidemia (triglyceride level greater than 200 more than 4 hours after infusion is completed) does not result. Weekly monitoring of liver function tests is

necessary to screen for total parenteral nutrition–associated liver disease.

If the gut is functional, the decision regarding the mode of nutritional support depends on whether the patient can increase oral intake or consume an additional dietary supplement. If the patient cannot increase oral intake, bolus or continuous nasogastric tube feedings must be considered. However, in patients with gastroesophageal reflux, coma, or other neurologic impairment, a nasojejunal tube may be required to minimize the likelihood of aspiration. If tube feedings are required for periods greater than 2 months, and if tube feedings constitute the major route of nutrient delivery, a feeding gastrostomy should be considered. Continuous drip tube feedings have an increased risk of bacteria overgrowth. These solutions should be changed every 12 hours.

The nutrient solution used depends on the gastrointestinal function of the patient. If intestinal function is intact, whole proteins, long-chain fats, and complex carbohydrates may be used. However, a sufficient diversity of enteral products now exists that the nutrient solution can be specifically tailored to the patient's intestinal absorptive capacity and nutritional requirements. The choice of full-strength versus half-strength and lactose-free versus milk formula must be based on the response of stool output and presence of reducing substances. However, trophic stimulation (e.g., from pancreatic secretions, polyamines, glutamine) is necessary for the recuperation of gut impairment due to undernutrition and may be accomplished using continuous drip feedings at 1 cc/hr for 4 days. Thereafter, feedings may be increased as tolerated.

The nutritional rehabilitation of both protein and energy deficiency is similar and depends on calorie intake and protein quality. In kwashiorkor, resolution of edema occurs with increased calorie intake, not increased protein intake, and often precedes changes in serum albumin. Adequate protein intake may be as low as 8 per cent of total calories, as long as the protein is of high quality. After a period of 2 to 4 days for stabilization during the acute phase, calorie intakes of 150 kcal/kg/day usually result in weight increases of 10 gm/kg/day, and 200 to 250 kcal/kg/day will accelerate weight gains to 15 to 20 gm/kg/day. This rapid accretion of body weight appears to occur within normal body composition.

In the absence of other illness, good evidence of recovery may be anticipated in most children after the first 10 to 12 days of therapy. At this time the consolidation phase of renutrition must be instituted. Protracted caloric supplementation is usually required to achieve full recovery. Enrollment in WIC or Food Stamps may be essential to provide the child with sufficient calorie support. Early intervention programs may be helpful to reverse the impaired cognitive development that may accompany undernutrition. Additional counseling may foster parental nurturance that may have diminished in the absence of the infant's ability to elicit parenting responses. Education of caretakers regarding the child's nutritional needs is most important. However, these educational goals may not be achieved without securing social and financial support for these often long-term nutritional interventions.

EARLY CHILDHOOD OBESITY

MICHAEL J. PETTEI, M.D., Ph.D.

Obesity is estimated to be the most common form of pediatric malnutrition in the United States, occurring in 5 to 20 per cent of children. Although there is no uniformly accepted definition of obesity, the most useful pediatric assessment is obtained by the standard plot of weight and height on growth charts. In general, it is necessary to relate weight to height; otherwise, children who are simply tall with proportionately high weights may be labeled obese. Weight for height, or per cent of ideal body weight, may be calculated by dividing actual weight by the child's ideal weight for height. Obesity may then be defined as 20 per cent over ideal weight for height (120 per cent IBW). The treatment of obesity in childhood is important for two reasons: First, the psychosocial consequences of obesity are often severe. It has been well demonstrated that even young children discriminate against their obese peers. Many subsequently suffer from low self-esteem, social isolation, rejection, and depression. Secondly, obesity during childhood is associated with an increased risk of becoming an obese adult. The mildly obese school-age child is four times more likely to become an obese adult than his nonobese counterpart. This risk ratio increases with greater degrees of obesity and age. Since adult obesity is one of the leading causes of morbidity and mortality in the adult population, the treatment of childhood obesity becomes a significant public health measure.

The treatment of obesity can be a frustrating, difficult, and often unsuccessful endeavor. In theory, since obesity is simply the long-term accumulation of a positive net energy balance in the form of fat, treatment should be quite straightforward. Reduction of caloric intake and/or increased caloric expenditure (activity) should result in a caloric deficit requiring the mobilization of fat stores. Because of complex cultural and family factors that affect how an individual eats and acts, alteration of these behaviors is exceedingly difficult to achieve. Since many parents are concerned about a metabolic cause for their child's obesity, it should be explained initially that while there may be genetic susceptibility to obesity, environmental factors affecting food intake and activity seem critical. The rare endocrinopathy or genetic syndrome can usually be excluded by a thorough history and physical examination. Since overweight children tend to be tall, the short obese child should raise the possibility of an associated disorder. Therapy should be appropriate to the child's age and degree of obesity.

During infancy, only correct feeding practices should be outlined. Specific recommendations regarding the volume of formula and portion sizes appropriate for age should be provided. Solids should not be introduced before 4 months of age. Cereal should not be placed in the bottle, and excessive juice intake can be controlled by offering it in a cup to the older infant. Overfeeding by forcing the last ounce or finishing the jar must be avoided. Infants need not have "desserts" such as ice cream and cake. Finally, all infant crying should not be mistaken for hunger. When an infant cries despite a recent feeding, other comforting methods (such as holding) should be tried first.

For preschool children, management begins with a careful dietary history and, if possible, a 72-hour intake record. This allows an estimate of the caloric intake as well as the family food preferences. Weight reduction is usually not appropriate during infancy and early childhood. Instead, cessation or reduction of weight gain should be the goal. In this way, the child will slowly outgrow the obesity. Initially, modest reductions in caloric intake of 10 to 15 per cent (based on initial intake records) should be devised and modified gradually until cessation of weight gain occurs. A nutritionist can be invaluable in devising a diet that is balanced yet takes into account the family's eating habits. Elimination of high caloric density foods (regular fat milk, mayonnaise, ice cream, etc.) and emphasis on low energy density foods that are known to be liked by the family are preferable. Some general recommendations for this age group include not using food as a reward, substituting water for soda or juices, limiting milk intake to 24 ounces/day, and establishing meal or snack times as the only times for food.

In the older school-age child, a weight reduction program is not unreasonable. A comprehensive program should include three factors: exercise, diet, and behavior modification. An exercise program that provides energy expenditures should be followed. A common approach is to enroll the child in extracurricular physical activity programs in his or her school or community. Second, a diet should be provided that will produce a weight loss yet is relatively easy to adhere to and promotes growth. Gradual weight reduction (depending on age) is desirable. The diet should be balanced in nutrients but reduce energy intake by about 25 to 30 per cent. Again, the aid of a nutritionist utilizing the principles outlined above should be enlisted for the individualized diet prescription. Particular care needs to be taken to incorporate sufficient calcium and iron into these diets, which may require supplementation. More restrictive diets and protein-sparing modified fasts should be used only in specialized centers with close monitoring. Third, *behavior modification* therapy involving both parent and child ensures that the diet and exercise information will be utilized. Self-monitoring of food intake (recording what, when, why, and where food is eaten) is the mainstay of behavior modification. Careful examination of the self-monitoring records usually reveals the nature of the child's eating problems and where intervention is needed. Stimulus control methods are used to control the circumstances that evoke eating. Such factors include limiting the availability of high-calorie foods in the home, eating only in the kitchen or dining room at scheduled times, avoiding other activities (e.g., watching television) while eating, and discarding "leftovers" rapidly. Serving dishes should be removed from the table after the initial serving and "seconds" should be given only after a short wait to allow satiety to occur. Reinforcement is the principal technique used to modify childhood behavior. Since weight loss may not be very important to the child, it is crucial to use external reinforcement with most children to increase their acquisition of new eating behaviors. The most effective rewards are usually immediate, consistent, and appropriate to the behavior. Rewards should not be so expensive that they are impossible to give on a routine basis. Larger rewards can also be contracted between parents and child.

Finally, it must be recognized that parents exert a powerful influence over the eating and exercise behaviors of their children. A successful pediatric weight reduction program is unlikely without changes within the family. Parents usually determine the amount and kind of food in the home, promote specific patterns of eating and activity, and exert pressures (sometimes subconsciously) for a child to maintain a given appearance. A program directed at the entire family unit, utilizing family therapists if necessary, probably stands the greater chance of success.

LATER CHILDHOOD AND ADOLESCENT OBESITY

I. RONALD SHENKER, M.D.

The treatment of obesity in children and adolescents is not easy. It is time-consuming, frustrating, and not infrequently unsuccessful. Obesity prevention and management remain an enigma for the physician. The basic tenets of therapy—reduced caloric intake and/or increased caloric utilization—are particularly difficult to achieve except in the most highly motivated patients. During childhood one must direct the bulk of attention to the parent, whereas by the time of adolescence most management programs must deal in an intimate fashion with the patient.

Exogenous obesity is an eating disorder, and as such therapy must be directed to reducing excessive intake. Psychological factors are undoubtedly important in the vast majority of patients, but dealing with these underlying factors alone does not control the symptomatology or outcome of the eating behavior. An active directive approach is needed.

Patient motivation is the key to success and must be assessed during the initial consultation. Although it has been demonstrated that self-image and self-assessment are more realistic in adolescent boys with obesity than in girls, the latter are often more motivated to reduce body fat and are more prone to follow a planned dietary and exercise regimen. Early adolescent boys are the least motivated or successful in adherence to a therapeutic plan.

The physician and patient must form an alliance for therapy. A transference undoubtedly occurs but is less obvious than in conventional (psycho)therapy. Female adolescents may wish to please their (male) physicians.

Although this is a poor long-term motivation for weight reduction, any reasonable method of getting the patient on the right program for weight reduction should be utilized.

Preparation for new school entrance, such as high school or college, may be an important motivator. The physician should explore why the patient comes for treatment at a specific time, especially in the face of long-term obesity. Motivation should be explored, exploited, and encouraged.

The goal of treatment is long-term. An appropriate assessment of ideal body weight based on standard growth charts is determined. An individual who is 20 per cent over ideal weight for height may be considered obese. In many instances "eyeball" diagnosis may not always be easy. Body weight does not necessarily indicate the degree of body fatness and may result in a diagnosis of obesity in those individuals whose excess weight for height is due to lean tissue. This may be more true for adolescent males than for females. Measurement of the triceps skinfold and mid-arm circumference, with calculation of the mid-arm muscle circumference, is helpful in assessing the contribution of fat and lean tissue to body weight. Age-adjusted standards are available for the adolescent population. The use of the body mass index (BMI = weight in kilograms/the square of the height in meters) can also be helpful in the diagnosis of obesity. A BMI of 25 to 30 is associated with overweight, and a BMI greater than 30 suggests obesity.

The patient should be examined undressed at the initial visit. Naturally, causes for obesity other than overeating are to be excluded, such as genetic conditions, hypothalamic disorders, and endocrine causes. These are rare. However, the objectives of dietary control apply to all forms of obesity.

The patient's body build should be noted and discussed with the patient. Realistic outcomes are to be agreed upon by patient, physician, and parent. "The apple doesn't fall far from the tree" is a worthwhile axiom to discuss with the patient and family. The role of genetic and environmental factors should be mentioned. An important goal of successful treatment is patient acceptance of self as he or she will be. Even if the ultimate weight loss is modest, the goal of self-acceptance is to be strived for.

Although many patients have short-term motivation, no therapeutic program should have short-term goals. Discuss the patient's goal in terms of 3, 6, or even 12 months from the initial visit. One pound of fat is equal to 3500 calories. Therefore, a program of caloric deprivation and exercise in which a deficit of 3500 calories per week is achieved results in weight loss of 1 pound per week, or about 12 pounds in 3 months. This weight will not be reduced in an even manner. Typically weight loss is fastest in the first few weeks and then becomes more resistant. But an appreciation of a weight loss potential of 25 pounds in 6 months may be realistic and achievable for some adolescents with above-average motivation.

The diet prescribed should be nutritionally sound and easy to follow. Examples are given in Tables 1 and

TABLE 1. 1200-Calorie Meal Plan

Breakfast		Lunch		Dinner	
Select 1 of the following:		Select 1 of the following:		Select 1 of the following:	
Orange juice	—4 fl oz	Chicken (skinless)	—3 oz wt cooked	Beef, lean	—3 oz wt cooked
Grapefruit juice	—4 fl oz	Turkey (skinless)	—3 oz wt cooked	Lamb, lean	—3 oz wt cooked
Apple juice	—4 fl oz	Beef, lean	—2 oz wt cooked	Veal, lean	—4 oz wt cooked
Banana	—½ small	Tuna (7 oz wt can)	—½ can drained	Pork, lean	—4 oz wt cooked
Grapefruit	—½	Cottage cheese	—½ cup	Chicken, skinless	—4 oz wt cooked
Strawberries	—¾ cup	Hard cheese	—2 oz wt (limit to 1 × week)	Turkey, skinless	—4 oz wt cooked
		Peanut butter	—2 level tbs (limit to 1 × week)	Fish	—4 oz wt cooked
Select 1 of the following:		Select 1 of the following:		Select 1 of the following:	
Bagel (frozen type)	—1	Bagel (frozen type)	—½	Potato, white	—1 small
Bread—regular	—1 sl	Bread—regular	—1 sl	Potato, sweet	—¼ small
Bread—low calorie	—2 sl	Bread—low calorie	—2 sl	Pasta, cooked	—½ cup
Cold cereal	—¾ cup	Sandwich roll	—½	Rice, cooked	—½ cup
Cooked cereal	—½ cup	Pita pocket	—1 small	Bread, regular	—1 sl
English muffin	—½	English muffin	—½	Bread, diet	—2 sl
				Corn, niblets	—⅓ cup
				Corn on the cob	—½ ear
Select 1 of the following:		Select a minimum of 1 serving:		Select 2 of the following:	
Low fat milk (1%)	—8 fl oz	Tossed green salad	—1 cup	½ cup cooked vegetable:	1 portion raw vegetable:
Skim milk	—8 fl oz	Carrot	—1	Asparagus	Tossed salad—1 cup
Plain low-fat yogurt	—½ cup	Celery	—2 stalks	Beets	Carrot—1
Cottage cheese	—¼ cup	Dill pickle	—1	Broccoli	Celery—2 stalks
Egg	—1 (limit to 2 × week)	Tomato	—½ whole	Carrots	Lettuce—1 cup
		Cherry tomato	—½ cup	Cauliflower	Tomato—½ whole
		Green pepper	—½	Collard greens	Green pepper—1
				Endive	
				Green beans	
				Spinach, kale	
*Select 1 of the following:		*Select 1 of the following:		Select 1 of the following:	
Cream cheese	—1 tbs	Apple	—1	Apple	—1
Margarine	—1 tsp	Banana	—½	Banana	—½ small
Diet margarine	—2 tsp	Blueberries	—¾ cup	Blueberries	—¾ cup
Butter	—1 tsp	Orange	—1	Orange	—1
*The allowance from this group only may be saved and used at other meals.		Peach	—1	Peach	—1
		Pear	—1	Pear	—1
		Strawberries	—1 cup	Strawberries	—1 cup
		Tangerine	—2	Tangerine	—2
		Watermelon, pieces	—1 cup	Watermelon, pieces	—1 cup
		*This may be saved for a between-meal snack.			
		Select 1 of the following:		Select 1 of the following:	
		Butter	—1 tsp	Butter	—1 tsp
		Margarine	—1 tsp	Margarine	—1 tsp
		Diet margarine	—2 tsp	Diet margarine	—2 tsp
		Mayonnaise	—1 tsp	Mayonnaise	—1 tsp
		Diet mayonnaise	—2 tsp	Diet mayonnaise	—2 tsp
		Salad dressing	—1 tbs	Salad dressing	—1 tbs
		Select 1 of the following:		Select 1 of the following:	
		Low fat milk (1%)	—8 fl oz	Low fat milk (1%)	—8 fl oz
		Skim milk	—8 fl oz	Skim milk	—8 fl oz

2 for nutritionally balanced diets of 1200 and 1500 calories per day. Intake of calories only during prescribed meals and snacks should be stressed. Dietary education should be occurring during weekly physician visits so that a newly learned eating behavior is maintained. Modification and individualization of the diet require time and detailed explanations. A nutritionist is particularly helpful in this regard. The pediatrician would be wise to seek out such a consultant. Being given a specific diet is an important tangible aid to the patient. Give duplicate copies to the patient and parent.

Frequent physician visits are essential to a successful weight reduction program. If follow-up visits are less than weekly for the first weeks, treatment is doomed to failure. Physician-patient rapport and trust are built during these visits, which always include a weight check under uniform conditions. Since enthusiasm is often high for both patient and physician at the outset, the first few weeks often have a successful outcome, especially for the adolescent girl. Although intake of food is stressed in the earliest visits, weight maintenance with increased exercise and modestly increased calories if they have been severely restricted (i.e., 1000 or below) should be discussed in detail as follow-up proceeds

TABLE 2. 1500-Calorie Meal Plan

Breakfast	Lunch	Dinner
Select 1 of the following: Orange juice —4 fl oz Grapefruit juice —4 fl oz Apple juice —4 fl oz Banana —½ small Grapefruit —½ Strawberries —¾ cup	Select 1 of the following: Chicken (skinless) —3 oz wt cooked Turkey (skinless) —3 oz wt cooked Beef, lean —2 oz wt cooked Tuna (7 oz wt can) —½ can drained Cottage cheese —½ cup Hard cheese —2 oz wt (limit to 1× week) Peanut butter —2 level tbs (limit to 1× week)	Select 1 of the following: Beef, lean —3 oz wt cooked Lamb, lean —3 oz wt cooked Veal, lean —4 oz wt cooked Pork, lean —4 oz wt cooked Chicken, skinless —4 oz wt cooked Turkey, skinless —4 oz wt cooked Fish —4 oz wt cooked
Select 1 of the following: Bagel (frozen type) —1 Bread —2 slices Cold cereal —1½ cups Cooked cereal —1 cup English muffin —1	Select 1 of the following: Bread —2 slices Bagel (frozen type) —1 Sandwich roll —1 Pita pocket —1 large (160 calories) English muffin —1	Select 1 of the following: Potato, white —1 average Potato, sweet —½ small Pasta —1 cup cooked Rice —1 cup cooked Bread —2 slices Sandwich roll —1 Corn, niblets —⅔ cup
Select 1 of the following: Low fat milk (1%) —8 fl oz Skim milk —8 fl oz Plain low-fat yogurt —½ cup Cottage cheese —¼ cup Egg —1 (limit to 2× week)	Select a minimum of 1 serving: Tossed green salad —1 cup Carrot —1 Celery —2 stalks Dill pickle —1 Tomato —½ whole Cherry tomato —½ cup Green pepper —½	Select 2 of the following: ½ cup cooked vegetable: 1 portion raw vegetable: Asparagus / Tossed salad—1 cup Beets / Carrot—1 Broccoli / Celery—2 stalks Carrots / Lettuce—1 cup Cauliflower / Tomato—½ whole Collard greens / Green pepper—1 Endive Green beans Spinach, kale
*Select 1 of the following: Cream cheese —1 tbs Margarine —1 tsp Diet margarine —2 tsp Butter —1 tsp *The allowance from this group only may be saved and used at other meals.	*Select 1 of the following: Apple —1 Banana —½ small Blueberries —¾ cup Orange —1 Peach —1 Pear —1 Strawberries —1 cup Tangerine —2 Watermelon, pieces —1 cup *This may be saved for a between-meal snack.	Select 1 of the following: Apple —1 Banana —½ small Blueberries —¾ cup Orange —1 Peach —1 Pear —1 Strawberries —1 cup Tangerine —2 Watermelon, pieces —1 cup
	Select 1 of the following: Butter —1 tsp Margarine —1 tsp Diet margarine —2 tsp Mayonnaise —1 tsp Diet mayonnaise —2 tsp Salad dressing —1 tbs	Select 1 of the following: Butter —1 tsp Margarine —1 tsp Diet margarine —2 tsp Mayonnaise —1 tsp Diet mayonnaise —2 tsp Salad dressing —1 tbs
	Select 1 of the following: Low fat milk (1%) —8 fl oz Skim milk —8 fl oz	Select 1 of the following: Low fat milk (1%) —8 fl oz Skim milk —8 fl oz

beyond the first few weeks. Examples of 10 activities with caloric energy utilization as seen in Table 3 should be discussed.

Some patients respond to specific behavior techniques to reduce intake. These may be used in combination with prescribed meal plans, although some behavior modification programs omit prescribed diets. There are behavior modification programs targeted specifically for the adolescent population. Behavior modification techniques utilized to reduce intake may include attempts to prolong the duration of meals, the use of smaller plates and eating utensils, and recording of foods consumed in a food diary. Parental rewards are a form of behavior modification and are helpful in some children and adolescents.

The role of the family is often the key to outcome. If youngsters are in the center of family strife, they will be unable to co-operate with a successful weight reduction program. The concept of the vulnerable child, a pathologic mechanism seen in the anorexic patient and in other psychosomatic conditions, is also applicable to the obese. Ancillary psychological and psychiatric evaluation may be needed in some obese youngsters.

Dietary modification is best implemented when the entire family participates. Parents control the food purchased for the household. Thus, access to high-calorie

TABLE 3. Burning Off Calories by the Hour

Activity	Calories Utilized Per Hour If Body Weight Is		
	117 Pounds	*152 Pounds*	*196 Pounds*
Resting in bed or sleeping	55	72	93
Dancing, vigorous	264	344	444
Walking, 4 mph	307	400	518
Volleyball	265	345	445
Basketball, moderate	327	426	550
Bicycling, level 5.5 mph	233	304	392
Ping pong	180	235	302
Tennis, moderate	322	420	541
Bowling	310	404	520
Skiing downhill	449	585	755

or low-calorie foods at home and snacks is often parent-dependent. Children and adolescents who are expected to forgo their favorite foods and desserts while other family members are enjoying them soon become resentful. This undoubtedly results in greater dietary indiscretion outside the household. A well-balanced, calorically controlled diet is beneficial to others in the family, and the adolescent will not feel singled-out. Here again, the intact nonpathologic family can be of great support.

Since peer support and struggles for independence are so developmentally important for the adolescent, adjuncts to obesity therapy are group meetings, therapy, and counseling, which may be the primary appropriate treatment for some. Youngsters do best in peer groups. They generally should not become part of an adult obesity group. In the peer group, patients are able to see, identify with, and help themselves and others in the struggle to maintain an appropriate weight.

Drug treatment has no place in the treatment of childhood or adolescent obesity.

Finally, obesity prevention is obviously preferable to obesity treatment. It should begin in childhood. However, the major therapeutic tool available, dietary restriction, cannot be prescribed without regard to nutritional needs and growth requirements. Allowing the child to "grow into his weight" is often indicated, as opposed to weight reduction. The results here are often less obvious and more frustrating to supervise. Natural periods of decreased intake after the rapid growth of the first 2 years of life should be appreciated. Parental guidance is essential to prevent obesity. Social and cultural factors must also be considered.

The final recommendation for the physician who treats the obese patient is to approach the patient with enthusiasm for potential success. An "upbeat" attitude may help patient motivation, which remains the single most important factor for a successful treatment outcome.

VITAMIN DEFICIENCIES AND EXCESSES

JOHN N. UDALL, Jr., M.D., Ph.D.

Health professionals who deal with children should be aware of the recommended daily allowances for vitamins (Table 1). A knowledge of the signs/symptoms of vitamin deficiencies and excesses is also important so treatment may be instituted before severe and permanent functional impairment of vital organs occurs.

FAT-SOLUBLE VITAMINS

The fat-soluble vitamins A, D, E, and K are insoluble in water and therefore must circulate in association with lipid-solubilizing carrier systems. Diseases of the pancreas (cystic fibrosis), liver (biliary atresia), or intestine (celiac disease) that impair fat digestion and/or fat absorption may result in a deficiency of one or more of these vitamins.

Vitamin A (Retinol). This vitamin is important for growth, healthy skin, and vision. Deficiency of vitamin A results in growth failure, apathy, mental retardation, skin and corneal changes, and occasionally intracranial hypertension. Xerophthalmia, the term in general use to cover all the ocular manifestations of vitamin A deficiency, is the most common cause of blindness in young children throughout the world.

The treatment of xerophthalmia may be divided into emergency treatment and maintenance therapy. Emergency treatment consists of the oral administration of 100,000 IU of vitamin A (retinyl palmitate in oil) given immediately and repeated on the second day. The response may take several days to appear, but this regimen is adequate to obtain maximal effect. If there is vomiting or severe diarrhea, the dose should be administered intramuscularly, but the preparation must be water dispersible because oily preparations are not absorbed from the injection site. A final dose of 200,000 IU should be given before discharge to boost liver storage. Maintenance therapy consists of administration of the recommended dietary allowance of the vitamin.

Vitamin A intoxication, with resultant intracranial hypertension (vomiting, headache, stupor), skeletal changes, and skin rash, has been reported in infants, from an excessive number of vitamin A tablets or from dietary excesses. Regular daily ingestion of retinol supplements exceeding 3000 retinol equivalents (RE) (10,000 IU) by infants and children is recommended only under the direction of a physician. Toxicity in adults is seen with daily intakes of more than 15,000 RE for long periods. The goal of treatment of vitamin A toxicity is obviously to eliminate the dietary source of the excessive vitamin A. Symptoms rapidly subside on withdrawal of the vitamin, and complete recovery always results.

A comment should be made in regard to vitamin A analogs such as isotretinoin and 13-cis-retinoic acid. The use of these analogs for the treatment of acne has been accepted enthusiastically by teenagers because of their effectiveness. However, there is concern regarding the use of large doses of these analogs in teenagers who could become pregnant. Recently it has been recognized that there is a relationship between maternal consumption of large doses of vitamin A and multiple congenital abnormalities in offspring.

Vitamin D. Rickets in children results when vitamin D deficiency occurs before the epiphyses of bones have closed. Rickets has been found in premature infants consuming formulas containing 400 IU vitamin D/liter,

TABLE 1. 1989 Recommended Daily Dietary Allowances

Age (Years) and Sex Group	Weight		Height		Protein (gm)	Fat-Soluble Vitamins				Water-Soluble Vitamins							Minerals						
	kg	lb	cm	in		Vita-min A (µg RE*)	Vita-min D (µg†)	Vita-min E (µg α-TE‡)	Vita-min K	Vita-min C	Thia-min	Ribo-flavin	Niacin	Vita-min B$_6$	Fo-late	Vita-min B$_{12}$	Cal-cium	Phos-pho-rus	Mag-nes-ium	Iron	Zinc	Iodine	Sele-nium
Infants																							
0.0–0.5	6	13	60	24	13	375	7.5	3	5	30	0.3	0.4	5	0.3	25	0.3	400	300	40	6	5	40	10
0.5–1.0	9	20	71	28	14	375	10	4	10	35	0.4	0.5	6	0.6	35	0.5	600	500	60	10	5	50	15
Children																							
1–3	13	29	90	35	16	400	10	6	15	40	0.7	0.8	9	1.0	50	0.7	800	800	80	10	10	70	20
4–6	20	44	112	44	24	500	10	7	20	45	0.9	1.1	12	1.1	75	1.0	800	800	120	10	10	90	20
7–10	28	62	132	52	28	700	10	7	30	45	1.0	1.2	13	1.4	100	1.4	800	800	170	10	10	120	30
Males																							
11–14	45	99	157	62	45	1,000	10	10	45	50	1.3	1.5	17	1.7	150	2.0	1,200	1,200	270	12	15	150	40
15–18	66	145	176	69	59	1,000	10	10	65	60	1.5	1.8	20	2.0	200	2.0	1,200	1,200	400	12	15	150	50
19–24	72	160	177	70	58	1,000	10	10	70	60	1.5	1.7	19	2.0	200	2.0	1,200	1,200	350	10	15	150	70
Females																							
11–14	46	101	157	62	46	800	10	8	45	50	1.1	1.3	15	1.4	150	2.0	1,200	1,200	280	15	12	150	45
15–18	55	120	163	64	44	800	10	8	55	60	1.1	1.3	15	1.5	180	2.0	1,200	1,200	300	15	12	150	50

Adapted from the National Academy of Sciences—National Research Council. The allowances, expressed as average daily intakes over time, are intended to provide for individual variations among most normal persons as they live in the United States under usual environmental stresses. Diets should be based on a variety of common foods in order to provide other nutrients for which human requirements have been less well defined.

*Retinol equivalents. 1 retinol equivalent = 1 µg retinol or 6 µg β-carotene. See text for calculation of vitamin A activity of diets as retinol equivalents.

†As cholecalciferol. 10 µg cholecalciferol = 400 IU of vitamin D.

‡α-Tocopherol equivalents. 1 mg d-α tocopherol = 1 α-TE.

probably because of low intake of nutrients in general. Black infants who are infrequently exposed to the sun and who are breast-fed by mothers with impaired vitamin D intake may be at risk for the development of rickets, especially during the winter months. Some patients with nephrotic syndrome may also develop vitamin D deficiency. Vitamin D–dependent rickets may be due to a recessively inherited deficiency of the renal 1α-hydroxylase enzyme or a receptor defect. In mild cases of vitamin D deficiency, 1600 IU/day of vitamin D is the recommended therapy; in advanced cases 5000 IU/day should be administered. Treatment of vitamin D–dependent rickets consists of pharmacologic amounts of vitamin D or physiologic amounts of 1,25-(OH)$_2$D$_3$.

Excessive doses of vitamin D result in the mobilization of calcium and phosphorus from bony tissues and their redeposition in soft tissues. This occurs principally in the walls of blood vessels but also in kidney tubules, bronchi, and the heart. Vitamin D intoxication may be fatal. Preliminary symptoms of toxicity include anorexia, thirst, urinary urgency, vomiting, and diarrhea. When hypervitaminosis is present, the first step in management is to stop administration of all forms of vitamin D immediately and restrict dietary calcium intake. It is also important to maintain good hydration and urine output and correct any deficiency in serum sodium or potassium. Furosemide may be required (0.5–1.0 mg/kg initially, given orally or parenterally). This may be repeated at 6 to 12 hours if necessary. Prednisone (2 mg/kg/24 hr) may also be used in refractory cases.

Vitamin E (Tocopherol). Vitamin E deficiency has been implicated in hemolytic anemia of preterm infants and glutathionine synthetase deficiency. A dietary intake of 3 to 5 mg α-TE (tocopherol equivalents) should avoid deficiency states during infancy. Data concerning toxicity are confusing. However, recently the use of a commercially available parenteral vitamin E preparation was associated with several infant deaths. The reason for the toxicity of this preparation has not yet been fully established. However, preliminary data from toxicologic studies suggest that the emulsifier polysorbate used in the vitamin E preparation may have exerted the major toxicologic effect.

Vitamin K. Newborn infants represent a special case when considering vitamin K nutrition because the placenta is a relatively poor organ for the transmission of lipids, and the gut flora important for vitamin K production is meager during the first few days of life. Therefore, vitamin K–dependent factors (plasma prothrombin concentration) may be only 30 per cent of normal on the second and third days of life. Premature infants are even more susceptible than full-term infants to vitamin K deficiency. If prothrombin values fall below 10 per cent, hemorrhagic disease of the newborn may occur. It is for this reason that 0.5 to 1.0 mg of phylloquinone is administered intramuscularly on the first day of life. This is an effective way of preventing hemorrhagic disease. It should also be noted that broad-spectrum antibiotics that dramatically suppress or alter intestinal flora may put an infant or child at an increased risk for vitamin K deficiency.

WATER-SOLUBLE VITAMINS

The water-soluble vitamins include thiamine (B$_1$), riboflavin (B$_2$), niacin (B$_3$), pyridoxine (B$_6$), folic acid, cyanocobalamin (B$_{12}$), and several others. These vitamins act primarily as cofactors in biochemical reactions. The entire group is widely distributed in plants and animals. Because they are found so extensively in nature, a vitamin deficiency of any one of them is unusual. When deficiencies occur in industrial nations, they are commonly associated with chronic illness, food faddism, or the chronic use of alcohol or drugs that interfere with the normal absorption or metabolism of a specific vitamin. In contrast, deficiencies of water-soluble vitamins in underdeveloped countries usually coexist with protein-calorie malnutrition.

Thiamine (B$_1$). Patients with simple thiamine deficiency can be treated orally with 5 mg of thiamine daily. Severely ill children should receive 10 mg intravenously twice a day. In the management of fulminant heart disease, 100 mg thiamine hydrochloride plus vigorous treatment of congestive heart failure is necessary. No toxic effects of thiamine administered by mouth have been reported. However, there have been reports of hypersensitivity to thiamine given parenterally.

Riboflavin (B$_2$). Riboflavin-deficient infants respond to 0.5 mg twice daily. Children who are deficient should be treated with 1.0 mg given orally three times a day for several weeks. Since dietary protein influences riboflavin status, it is important that protein and calories in the diet be adequate. Riboflavin toxicity has not been demonstrated in man or animals.

Niacin (B$_3$). Pellagra, the disease of niacin deficiency, is characterized by the classic "three D's": *d*ermatitis, *d*iarrhea, and *d*ementia. Early symptoms include glossitis, stomatitis, insomnia, anorexia, weakness, irritability, abdominal pain, forgetfulness, morbid fear, and vertigo. Treatment of the deficiency is usually more effective with oral rather than parenteral niacin, since blood levels remain elevated longer following oral treatment. The usual daily dose is about 10 times the RDA, or 100 mg in an adult. Additionally, a high-calorie, high-protein diet supplemented by the administration of the entire B vitamin group should be instituted. Ingestion of large amounts of nicotinic acid but not nicotinamide may produce vascular dilation. This is associated with "flushing" and headaches. The effect comes on within 7 to 10 minutes of nicotinic acid administration and lasts about 30 minutes.

Pyridoxine (B$_6$). Inborn errors in pyridoxine metabolism require a dose of pyridoxine several times the usual requirement, in some instances as much as 200 to 600 mg of pyridoxine/day to effect a clinical response. Pyridoxine-dependent convulsions in the neonate usually respond to 5 to 10 mg of pyridoxine intravenously. These infants can then be maintained on 10 to 25 mg daily. Toxicity from excessive amounts has not been reported until recently. This has been noted in adults who have been shown to develop severe sensory nervous system dysfunction after chronic daily megadoses of pyridoxine.

Cyanocobalamin (B$_{12}$). Vitamin B$_{12}$ deficiency (megaloblastic anemia) is rare in infants because amounts acquired from the mother during fetal life are usually sufficient to carry the infant through the first year of life, especially since those amounts are generally supplemented by additional supplies from mother's (or other) milk. The RDA for children 1 to 3 years old is 0.7 μg/day, for 4- to 6-year olds it is 1.0 μg/day, for 7- to 10-year olds it is 1.4 μg/day, and for adolescents and nonpregnant adults it is 2.0 μg/day.

Deficiency occurs in pernicious anemia. Although congenital and juvenile pernicious anemias are rare, both require treatment for life. The use of vitamin B$_{12}$ in megatherapy for various conditions is not valid. The only legitimate need for megatherapy with vitamin B$_{12}$ is for the rare patient with a congenital defect in vitamin B$_{12}$ metabolism, such as vitamin B$_{12}$–responsive methylmalonic acidemia.

Folacin. Folacin is the generic term for compounds having nutritional properties and a chemical structure similar to folic acid. Folic acid deficiency is the most common cause of megaloblastic anemia in infants and children. An appropriate maintenance dose to prevent folate deficiency in a premature infant is 0.05 to 0.1 mg/day. The RDA for infants up to 6 months of age is 25 μg/day; for infants 6 to 12 months it is 35 μg/day; for 1- to 3-year olds it is 50 μg/day; for 4- to 6-year olds it is 75 μg/day; for 7- to 10-year olds it is 100 μg/day; and for older children and adults it is 200 μg/day. Less than 5 μg of folacin/kg body weight produces hematologic response in children with vitamin B$_{12}$ deficiency. However, 1 to 5 mg orally given daily is recommended for children with folacin deficiency.

Vitamin C. Deficiency of vitamin C causes scurvy, which is characterized by weakness, petechial hemorrhages in the skin, ecchymosis, gingival and subperiosteal hemorrhage, and defects in bone development in children. It is prevented by 10 mg/day of ascorbic acid. In order to attain better tissue saturation, however, the RDA is 40 to 50 mg/day in children and 60 mg/day in adults. The usual treatment of infantile scurvy is 25 mg four times a day for 4 to 5 days and then 25 mg twice a day until healing occurs.

Excessive quantities of ascorbic acid, 2.0 to 5.0 gm/day,* have been suggested for prophylaxis or treatment of upper respiratory tract infections. There is no substantial evidence that these large amounts consistently affect the incidence and severity of this illness. These amounts will acidify the urine and may lead to nephrolithiasis.

---

*Two to 5 gm exceeds the manufacturer's recommended dose.

TOTAL PARENTERAL NUTRITION IN INFANTS
NANCY F. SHEARD, Sc.D., R.D.,
and W. ALLAN WALKER, M.D.

INDICATIONS

The optimal route for the provision of nutritional support is the gastrointestinal tract. This mode is safer, more physiologic, and considerably less expensive than parenteral nutrition. However, in our experience, 5 to 10 per cent of hospitalized children require some form of parenteral nutritional (PN) support. At our institution, nearly 60 per cent of these children are under 1 year of age (exclusive of premature infants). Infants and children suffering from congenital heart disease, gastrointestinal disease, and neoplastic disease are most likely to require PN support. In general, PN is indicated in a full-term infant who will be unable to feed enterally for at least 5 to 7 days.

NUTRIENT REQUIREMENTS

Intravenous nutrient requirements have not been well-characterized. Also, the nutritional needs of hospitalized infants are dependent on disease state (i.e., febrile, stressed), activity level, and nutrient losses. During acute illnesses, we estimate caloric requirements using the basal metabolic rate (based on weight) with additional calories provided pursuant to the medical and metabolic status of the patient. We routinely use the Recommended Dietary Allowances for calories in infants who are in the convalescent stage of their illness (Table 1).

Protein needs are estimated using the RDA and are increased depending on losses and level of catabolic stress. Protein restriction, which may be required in renal or liver disease, is determined by the clinical status of the patient. Protein overload is monitored using blood urea nitrogen and ammonia levels.

Guidelines for intravenous electrolytes, minerals, and trace elements are provided in Table 1.

COMPONENTS

PN solutions contain specified amounts of dextrose, amino acids, minerals, electrolytes, and vitamins. We have found that the majority of the needs of our patients can be met with one of the standard PN solutions shown in Table 2. Intravenous (IV) fat emulsions are used as a source of both calories and essential fatty acids. Approximately 20 to 30 per cent of calories are derived from IV lipids. Both 10 per cent and 20 per cent lipid emulsions are used.

The concentration of electrolytes and minerals in our standard solutions has been calculated to meet intravenous requirements when the patient receives the solution at maintenance fluid rates. Transient increases in electrolyte requirements due to increased losses are met using a separate IV solution that more closely matches the fluid being lost. A pediatric trace element mixture which includes zinc, copper, manganese, and chromium is added to each bag of PN solution that the patient receives. Pediatric multivitamins are also placed in the first bag of the day to ensure that the patient receives the full recommended dose.

ADMINISTRATION

PN can be administered either peripherally or centrally. If therapy is expected to be short-term (less than 1 week) and the child's nutritional status is adequate, peripheral PN is an appropriate method of supplying nutrients. It is our policy to administer no more than 10 per cent dextrose and 2 per cent amino acids via a peripheral vein. Because the caloric density of peripheral PN is low (0.4 kcal/cc), it is usually necessary to administer this solution at 1.5 times the maintenance fluid rate as well as to provide approximately 50 per cent of total calories as lipid (3 to 4 gm fat/kg/day).

TABLE 1. Daily Intravenous Nutrient Requirements

Calories	95–110	kcal/kg
Protein	2–3	gm/kg
Sodium	2–4	mEq/kg
Potassium	2–3	mEq/kg
Chloride	2–3	mEq/kg
Magnesium	0.25–0.5	mEq/kg
Calcium	1–2.5	mEq/kg
Phosphorus	1–2	mmol/kg
Zinc	100–300	µg/kg
Copper	20	µg/kg
Chromium	0.14–0.2	µg/kg
Manganese	2–10	µg/kg

From Nelson N (ed): Current Therapy in Neonatal-Perinatal Medicine, 2nd ed. Philadelphia, B.C. Decker, 1990.

TABLE 2. Standard Parenteral Nutrition Solutions

Per 1000 ml	PN-10	PN-20	PN-25	PN-30
Amino acids	20 gm	20 gm	40 gm	30 gm
Dextrose	100 gm	200 gm	250 gm	300 gm
Potassium	20 mEq	20 mEq	20 mEq	20 mEq
Sodium	30 mEq	30 mEq	30 mEq	30 mEq
Calcium	15 mEq	15 mEq	15 mEq	15 mEq
Magnesium	10 mEq	10 mEq	10 mEq	10 mEq
Phosphorus	10 mM	10 mM	10 mM	10 mM
Chloride	30 mEq	30 mEq	30 mEq	30 mEq
Acetate	35 mEq	35 mEq	65 mEq	50 mEq
Zinc	1.0 mg	1.0 mg	1.0 mg	1.0 mg
Copper	0.2 mg	0.2 mg	0.2 mg	0.2 mg
Chromium	2 µg	2 µg	2 µg	2 µg
Manganese	60 µg	60 µg	60 µg	60 µg
Vitamins*	yes	yes	yes	yes
Calories	410	750	990	1120

*Pediatric multivitamins are added to the first bottle of the day.
From Nelson N (ed): Current Therapy in Neonatal-Perinatal Medicine, 2nd ed. Philadelphia, B.C. Decker, 1990.

Placement of a central venous catheter is indicated when the duration of therapy is expected to be greater than 1 week, when fluid restriction prohibits use of peripheral PN, or when nutritional status is compromised and nutrient requirements cannot be adequately met via the gastrointestinal tract. Central lines are most often placed in the operating room by a skilled pediatric surgeon. A Silastic catheter is threaded into the superior vena cava via the subclavian vein. The exterior end is then tunneled under the skin, exiting from the chest. A Dacron cuff is situated midway in the tunnel to aid in infection control and to prevent catheter dislodgement.

INITIATING CENTRAL PN

A 10 per cent dextrose solution is initiated at maintenance fluid rates. Over 8 to 12 hours, this rate can be increased to 1.5 times maintenance rate. On the second day of therapy, PN 20/2 (infused at maintenance rates) is ordered. As necessary, either the rate of infusion or the glucose concentration is increased over the next 24 hours. Intravenous lipid emulsions are generally begun on the second day at a rate of 0.5 gm/kg/day. Lipids are infused over 24 hours. The rate is doubled every 12 to 24 hours until the desired lipid rate is reached (3 to 4 gm/kg/day).

MONITORING

The Nutrition Support Service monitors patients receiving parenteral nutrition on a daily basis. Weight, vital signs, and nutrient intake are recorded on a daily flow sheet. Glucose tolerance is assessed by checking urine glucose with each voiding. A blood glucose level is determined if glucosuria is 2+ or greater.

A panel of laboratory tests, which includes electrolytes, renal function tests, and liver function tests, is ordered prior to the initiation of PN and weekly thereafter (Table 3). Serum electrolyte, glucose, and triglyceride levels are checked more often depending on the clinical course.

COMPLICATIONS

There are three general types of complications associated with the use of PN. These include mechanical,

TABLE 3. Monitoring Parenteral Nutrition

Parameter	Daily	Weekly*
Weight	x	
Fluid balance	x	
Vital signs	x	
Urine sugar/acetone	x	
Catheter site/function	x	
Laboratory functions		
Sodium		x
Potassium		x
Chloride		x
Tco₂		x
Glucose		x
BUN		x
Creatinine		x
Triglycerides		x
Calcium		x
Magnesium		x
Phosphorus		x
Albumin		x
T. protein		x
SGPT		x
Alkaline phosphatase		x
Bilirubin (direct/total)		x

*More frequently if clinical condition indicates.

infectious, and metabolic problems. The most serious mechanical complications usually take place during placement of the line and are rare. Catheter-related problems that occur more commonly include occlusion of the line and catheter breakage. Through proper line management these problems are preventable.

Infectious complications associated with central venous lines occur in 5 to 10 per cent of pediatric patients. *Staphylococcus aureus* and *S. epidermidis* are the most common organisms. Exit site or tunnel infections can be treated with topical and/or intravenous antibiotics, respectively. Systemic infections are managed initially with broad-spectrum antibiotics. After the organism is cultured, specific antibiotic coverage is begun. Treatment through the line is continued for 14 to 21 days.

The catheter is removed if fever persists or if the patient's clinical condition worsens.

Metabolic complications associated with PN can occur in both the short term and the long term. Short-term complications such as glucose or lipid intolerance, fluid and electrolyte imbalance, and vitamin/mineral deficiencies are generally prevented by appropriate administration of PN solutions and careful monitoring of clinical and laboratory findings. The most frequent and serious long-term complication of PN is cholestatic liver disease. The etiology of this disorder is unknown and is most likely multifactorial. Recent evidence suggests that the administration of at least small amounts of enteral feedings can aid in the management of this disease.

SPECIAL CONSIDERATIONS

In specific cases, PN solutions can be cycled to allow patients freedom from infusion equipment. In addition, recent preliminary data suggest that cycling can decrease the incidence of PN-related cholestasis. In our experience, infants tend to require a longer period to wean from solutions and can be infusion-free for less time (usually 6 to 8 hours). Home PN has been successfully used in infants under 1 year of age.

Specialized amino acid solutions that have been designed for use in specific disease states (i.e., renal, hepatic, trauma) have not been sufficiently tested in pediatric patients. We routinely use standard amino acid solutions in infants with renal or hepatic disease, initially restricting the total protein load to 0.5 to 1.0 gm protein/kg/day. Protein intake is advanced as tolerated.

Newer amino acid formulations which contain taurine and cysteine are currently in use at our institution for children less than 1 year of age. The efficacy of these solutions over older formulations is still undetermined. Although these solutions are more costly, the theoretical advantage of providing a more complete amino acid mixture deserves consideration.

2

Mental and Emotional Disturbances

MENTAL RETARDATION

BRUCE K. SHAPIRO, M.D.
and MARK L. BATSHAW, M.D.

Mental retardation is defined as significant subaverage general intellectual functioning associated with impairment of adaptive behavior and manifested during the developmental period. Treatment is palliative, as the underlying defect cannot be corrected. However, there are many ways pediatricians can help the mentally retarded child reach his potential, aid the family in coping, and, in some cases, prevent the occurrence of mental retardation in future children. The first step is correct and early diagnosis to provide genetic counseling. Next, the pediatrician needs to advise the parents about appropriate expectations. Then, therapy must be directed at the child's educational needs, behavioral problems, and other associated deficits. Finally, there needs to be a periodic review of progress.

Early Diagnosis. Early diagnosis allows for the easing of parental anxiety, realistic goal setting, and greater acceptance of the child. Severely retarded children demonstrate major developmental delays at an early age, making the diagnosis straightforward. However, many mildly retarded children will not have significant developmental delays during the first year of life. Certain groups of children are at increased risk: premature infants, children who are small for gestational age, and infants who have suffered perinatal insults. However, most retarded children do not fall into an identifiable "at risk" group. Thus, taking a complete developmental history is important for all children with developmental delays.

The parents will usually bring the retarded child to a pediatrician because the child is failing to fulfill developmental expectations. In early infancy, these include questions about hearing or vision and problems in feeding or swallowing. After 6 months of age, motor delay is the most common complaint. Language and

behavior problems become prominent between 2 and 4 years, and school failure becomes evident in nursery school or in the early primary grades. Once identified, the child should be referred to an interdisciplinary evaluation center—e.g., school, university-affiliated facility (UAF), or state diagnostic and evaluation center. Evaluation should include an examination by a developmental pediatrician and formal psychological testing. In addition to medical consultations, evaluations may be required from experts in behavioral psychology, special education, social work, speech, language and audiology, nursing, and physical and occupational therapies.

Etiology. Most cases of mental retardation remain idiopathic, especially in the mildly retarded group, which composes over 85 per cent of the total mental retardation population. However, among retarded individuals with IQ less than 50, determination of etiology is often possible. A diagnosis allows the parents to know why their child is retarded. It helps to reduce the guilt of "what could I have done differently to prevent this child's handicap" and allows association with other parents who have children with a similar diagnosis. It also permits prediction of future outcome based on reported experience with other children having similar diagnoses. Finally, it is important for genetic counseling. Among idiopathic cases of severe-profound mental retardation, the empiric recurrence risk is 3 to 5 per cent. However, in chromosomal or single gene defects, recurrence risks can be as high as 25 to 50 per cent. Because of the diversity of conditions leading to mental retardation, there is no screening evaluation possible. A complete history and physical may give leads which should then be fully investigated, but fishing expeditions should be avoided. For example, skull x-rays, metabolic screens, and CT scans have not proved useful as diagnostic screening techniques in children with mental retardation.

Genetic Counseling. Various techniques of prenatal diagnosis are available for families with children having mental retardation of genetic origin. For prenatal diagnosis to be successful, three conditions must be met. First, a correct diagnosis must be established. Second, the mother must be known to be at an increased risk for having a handicapped child—e.g., the increased risk of Down's syndrome in a mother over 35 years old, the recurrence risk in a mother who has borne a Down's child or a child with fragile X syndrome, or a mother who is a translocation carrier. Third, the disorder must be identifiable by amniocentesis or other prenatal diagnostic techniques.

The most common form of prenatal diagnosis involves amniocentesis. The amniotic fluid can be used for alpha-fetoprotein determination of neural tube defects. The amniocytes are cultured for karyotyping, to determine the sex of the fetus or to detect chromosomal anomalies. Enzyme assays for inborn errors of metabolism can also be performed on the amniocytes. Fetal cells can be obtained for molecular genetic studies. Chorionic villus sampling is being investigated as an alternative to amniocentesis. This procedure permits the same types of analyses as amniocentesis but can be performed at an earlier stage of gestation (9 to 11 weeks gestation). However, the safety and accuracy of this procedure are still being investigated. A second technique of prenatal diagnosis involves fetoscopy, which allows direct visualization of body parts so that syndromes associated with absent or deformed limbs can be identified. Fetal skin and liver biopsy have also been performed during fetoscopy. Fetal ultrasonography, a method of indirect visualization, is now being used for definition of neural tube defects, microcephaly, and congenital heart defects.

The primary purpose of prenatal diagnosis has been to identify an affected fetus and offer therapeutic abortion. However, it may also influence the timing and mode of delivery or the perinatal care of the infant. For instance, a child with a complete urea cycle enzyme deficiency, organic acidemia, or maple syrup urine disease will become comatose during the first week of life. If diagnosed prenatally or at birth, the child can be started on appropriate therapy, and coma can be avoided. We are even approaching a time when fetal therapy may be possible. The classic example is the use of intrauterine transfusion for erythroblastosis fetalis. However, recently ventricular shunts have been placed in hydrocephalic fetuses, thyroxine has been injected into a hypothyroid fetus, and vitamin B_{12} has been given to a fetus with methylmalonic acidemia.

TREATMENT

General Pediatric Care. Besides these special services, the mentally retarded child requires the same basic pediatric supervision as the child with normal intelligence. This includes following immunization schedules, growth parameters, and treating intercurrent infections. However, there may be additional concerns under certain circumstances. Mentally retarded children in classes or institutions where hepatitis B antigen has been identified may require the hepatitis B vaccine. Multiply handicapped children with recurrent respiratory infections may benefit from influenza vaccine.

Weight gain may be deficient or excessive and requires nutritional intervention. Counseling of parents concerning reduced growth potential is also necessary. Dental hygiene needs to be addressed, especially for children who are receiving phenytoin or who are incapable of self-brushing. Preventive dental measures include decreasing the intake of sucrose-containing sweets by substituting noncariogenic snacks such as fruits and potato chips for candy and sugar-laden cereals. Toothbrushing and the use of fluoride should also be emphasized.

Consideration of Associated Dysfunctions. Mental retardation is often accompanied by associated deficits that further limit the child's adaptive abilities. In their most obvious forms, associated dysfunctions can be considered additional diagnoses—cerebral palsy, visual deficits, seizure disorders, speech disorders, autism, and other disorders of language, behavior, and perception. *Formes frustes* of these disorders have also been recognized—clumsiness, attentional peculiarities, articulation disorders, hyperactivity, and school underachievement. The severity and frequency of the associated dysfunctions tend to be proportional to the degree of mental retardation but may be more incapacitating than the mental retardation itself. Failure to appreciate the effects of associated deficits usually results in unsuccessful habilitation and may heighten behavioral problems.

Early Intervention. Early intervention is based on the assumption that children who receive remedial services at an earlier age will have a better outcome. While the value of early intervention is unproved, The Early Intervention Amendments to Education of the Handicapped Act of 1986 (Public Law 99–457) have mandated services to children who demonstrate developmental delays or are at risk for such disorders. Under this law early intervention services must include, for each eligible child, a multidisciplinary assessment and a written Individualized Family Service Plan (IFSP) developed by a multidisciplinary team and the parents. The IFSP must contain: (1) a statement of the child's present level of development; (2) a statement of the family's strengths and needs related to enhancing the child's development; (3) a statement of major outcomes expected to be achieved for the child and family and the criteria, procedures, and timelines for determining progress; (4) the specific early intervention services required to meet the needs of the child and family, including the projected dates for the initiation of services, frequency, intensity and expected duration; (5) the name of the case manager responsible for implementing the plan; and (6) the procedures for transition from early intervention to preschool services. The initial assessment and plan will be reviewed at least semiannually. This program targets children between 3 and 5 years old and will be implemented in the 1990–91 school year. It also creates a discretionary program to address the special needs of handicapped infants from birth through age 2.

Educational Placement. If a mentally retarded child is placed in an inappropriate educational setting, his progress will be slowed, and behavioral problems are likely to increase. In 1975, Public Law 94-142, the

Education for all Handicapped Children's Act, came into force to ensure education for the retarded. The provisions of this law include identification, location, and evaluation of all handicapped children; provision of a full appropriate public education for all handicapped children; and preparation and implementation of an individualized educational plan (IEP).

The goals for education should be based on the child's developmental level and the future goals for independence. If the child is mildly retarded (IQ 55 to 69), his prognosis for independence is good. Most of these individuals marry and hold jobs, although they are generally the last hired and first fired. Social-adaptive skills are also impaired, and this results in greater risks of deviant behavior and the need for assistance from social agencies. In school, these children need to gain basic academic and vocational skills and training in social interactions. Some may attain functional literacy (defined as a fourth grade education). The moderately retarded child (IQ 40 to 54) can look toward independence in self-care skills and partial social independence in a sheltered environment. Education needs to stress "survival" vocabulary and arithmetic and self-care skills. These children will not read for information. The severely-profoundly retarded child (I.Q. less than 40) may develop some language and self-help skills; however, he will remain basically dependent throughout life. If the child has associated deficits such as cerebral palsy or seizures, his function will be further impaired.

The appropriate placement for each of these groups of children should be guided primarily by their developmental level rather than by their chronological age. Although mainstreaming into homeroom, art, music, and physical education may be appropriate for the mildly retarded child, it has little benefit for children with more severe handicaps. The pediatrician should examine the individual educational program (IEP) to see if it appears appropriate in relation to the child's developmental level, especially if behavioral problems or poor school performance become evident.

Recreation is important to the mentally retarded child. Athletics should be encouraged. In general, retarded children do better in individual or small group activities than in the more complicated team sports. Activities requiring gross motor skills rather than fine motor coordination are most appropriate. Examples include track and field, swimming, and hiking. Although some physical limitations may be medically necessary, they should be as few as possible.

Behavior Management. Behavioral problems occur with greater frequency in retarded children than in normal children. The causes are complex and may result from the interaction of a variety of factors, including (1) inappropriate expectations of the child's developmental level; (2) organic behaviors: hyperactivity, short attention span, lack of perseverance, self-injurious or self-directed behaviors; and (3) family problems.

These factors are not mutually exclusive and multiple causes are the rule. The majority of behavioral problems can be ameliorated by altering the child's environment, e.g., changing him to a more appropriate classroom

setting and helping the parents understand that although he is 15 years old, he may not have the judgment to cross the street unsupervised. However, behaviors arising from organic deficits are less amenable to treatment by simple means. Two additional methodologies are employed to treat behavioral problems: behavior modification and/or psychotropic drugs.

Behavior modification has proved effective in the control of various behavioral problems: hyperactivity and self-stimulatory, self-injurious, aggressive, and noncompliant behaviors. The basic premise in behavior modification is that behavior is controlled by its consequences. Thus, if a behavior is reinforced, it will occur with greater frequency in the future. If it is not reinforced, it will be less likely to recur. This theory leads to three basic methods of controlling behavior: reinforcement, punishment, and extinction.

Reinforcement leads to an increase in the frequency of a desired behavior. In positive reinforcement, food or social reinforcers, such as hugs, food, or money, are given contingent on compliant behavior. Punishment differs from reinforcement in that it reduces the frequency of a behavior by use of aversive consequences or by the withdrawal of positive reinforcement. Aversive approaches are infrequently used to control noncompliant or self-injurious behaviors. The other form of punishment, "timing out," involves placing the child in a situation or room that lacks anything of interest to him. This isolates him for 1 to 10 minutes from any social activity that would provide positive reinforcement.

Extinction involves the removal of positive reinforcement from a situation that was previously rewarding. In effect, the prior relationship between the behavior and the consequence is disconnected. An example is ignoring self-stimulatory behavior while providing positive reinforcement as soon as the child stops. Usually, the targeted behavior will increase initially and then gradually diminish. Often extinction is paired with a procedure called differential reinforcement of other behaviors (DRO). While the self-stimulatory behavior is being extinguished, an incompatible behavior such as stringing beads is being reinforced. As a group, these behavioral approaches appear to be as effective as psychotropic drugs, although they obviously take more time and effort and long-term outcome studies have not been performed.

Mental retardation does not usually mandate the use of *psychotropic agents*. Drugs should not be used as a substitute for programming but rather to facilitate learning and social interactions or to suppress behaviors that are harmful to the patient or others. The drugs most commonly used to control behavior fall into the groups of phenothiazines, butyrophenones, and amphetamines. Phenothiazines include chlorpromazine (Thorazine), thioridazine (Mellaril), and trifluoperazine (Stelazine). These drugs act as dopamine antagonists. They result in sedation and decreased levels of motor activity, anxiety, combativeness, and hyperactivity. They also impair attention span. The usual dose in childhood for chlorpromazine or thioridazine is 25 to 200 mg/day, but this dosage needs to be individually titrated. The peak drug levels following oral intake occur in 2 to 3 hours. The half-life varies from 2 to 5 days. Common side effects include hyperphagia and lethargy. Uncommon toxic effects include blood dyscrasias, cholestatic jaundice, dermatitis, and increased seizure frequency. After long-term therapy, tardive dyskinesia and akathisia may occur. These symptoms do not always disappear following termination of drug therapy. Haloperidol (Haldol), a butyrophenone, has similar therapeutic effects. However, it produces more frequent extrapyramidal side effects. The usual dosage range is 0.5 to 7.5 mg/day.

Stimulants such as methylphenidate (Ritalin) or dextroamphetamine (Dexedrine) have been shown to be effective in the short-term control of hyperactivity and attentional problems in children with normal intellectual functioning. However, they are much less effective in controlling hyperactivity in mentally retarded children. Because they have fewer or less severe side effects than phenolthiazines, stimulants are still worth trying in the mentally retarded child. Dosage ranges from 0.5 to 2.0 mg/kg/day for methylphenidate* and 0.25 to 1.0 mg/kg/day for dextroamphetamine.† Peak levels occur in 2 hours, and the half-life is 2 to 4 hours. Antidepressants may be used for affective symptoms; lithium or propranolol are used for aggression.

A 1- to 2-week trial should be sufficient to evaluate the effectiveness of a medication in controlling behavior. Preferably, the study should be done with the teacher remaining unaware of the drug condition and keeping records of attention, behavior, and hyperactivity. Drug holidays should be attempted at least yearly to evaluate the need for continued medication. Psychotropic approaches using antihistamines, megavitamin therapy, and caffeine have been found to be ineffective.

Thus, the benefits of psychotropic drugs in mentally retarded children are modest and the risks, especially of phenothiazines and butyrophenones, are not inconsiderable. The risk-benefit ratio is not clearly positive in many children. Psychotropic drugs should then be used as a last resort, on a short-term basis, and only in combination with an appropriate behavior modification and educational program.

Family Counseling. The emotional impact of having a mentally retarded child is enormous. The stages of grief the family passes through are similar to those of parents who have lost a child. The initial response is one of disbelief. The parents will rarely hear what you say after the words mental retardation are mentioned. Thus, the parents may find it difficult to absorb medical information about their child at this time.

After the initial shock and denial, the parents start to feel guilty. The mother especially may feel that she could have done something during her pregnancy to prevent the handicap or could have given better care to the child or sought medical attention sooner. Accompanying these are feelings of anger, "Why us?" The

parents may direct their anger at each other, at God, at the pediatrician, or even at their child. The risk of child abuse is increased. The parents also feel isolated. They may feel they are the only ones with this problem. They need reassurance from the pediatrician and may also benefit from a parents' support group.*

The next step in coping involves bargaining: "If only we try harder, perhaps he will be normal." The pediatrician needs to help the parents maintain realistic expectations during this time. Some parents may intellectualize, accumulating a great deal of medical information about the child instead of confronting their own feelings. Some parents remain in this stage forever. Others move on eventually to a stage of acceptance.

Having a mentally retarded child also affects the stability of a marriage and the emotional health of the siblings. It is not uncommon for parents to be at different stages of coping. Further, one parent may want to talk about his or her feelings while the other does not; this leads to feelings of frustration and isolation. The siblings may share this anxiety. They are stigmatized as being the brother or sister of the "mental kid," and they may worry that they can "catch" the mental retardation. While feeling relieved that they are not retarded themselves, the siblings may also feel guilty about being normal. They may also feel resentful that the parents spend more time with the mentally retarded child than with them. They may even be worried that they will have to care for their handicapped sibling when they grow up. The grandparents need also to be considered, as they may assume some of the care of the child and will certainly influence the attitudes of the parents. Thus, counseling of the entire family is needed.

Re-evaluations. Although mental retardation is considered a static encephalopathy, there is a need for periodic review. As the child and family grow, new information must be imparted, goals readjusted, and habilitation programming altered. A review requires information about health status, family functioning, child functioning at home and at school, and the nature of the school programs. Other information, such as formal psychological or educational testing, may be needed. Annual reviews are generally necessary until school age. These reviews should also be undertaken any time the child is not meeting previous expectations.

Life Cycle Issues. As the child grows, he moves from one service provision system to another. This also marks the time for a review. Re-evaluation is necessary with the move from preschool to primary grades, from primary to intermediate grades, from intermediate to senior programming, and at the conclusion of school. By this time, the child has been abandoned by other adolescents. The disparity between cognitive abilities and chronological age prevents the retarded adolescent from fitting in. This isolation promotes social awkwardness and diminishes the adolescent's self-esteem. Many parents feel incompetent to deal with issues of emerging sexuality in their retarded children.

The teaching of sexuality, dealing with menses, mas-

---

*Manufacturer's warning: Safety and efficacy in children under 6 years of age have not been established.

†Dextroamphetamine is not recommended for children under 3 years of age with attention deficit disorder with hyperactivity.

---

*Batshaw M, Perret Y: *Children with Handicaps*, Brookes Publishing Co., 1986.

turbation, and inappropriate closeness are some of the more common issues brought up by parents of retarded adolescents. In the severely retarded patients, sexual drive is limited, and few problems other than masturbation develop. These youngsters should be taught that masturbation is acceptable behavior in the privacy of their room but not in public. In the moderately retarded patient, sexual drive may be normal, although late in developing. As judgment is limited, close parental supervision is essential. Contraception should be afforded to all retarded individuals who are sexually active. Although controversy regarding reversible versus irreversible methods of contraception continues to exist, the present legal climate precludes irreversible contraception in most cases.

Late adolescence coincides with the transition from intermediate to senior programs. School will be ending, and long-term planning concerning vocation, living situation, and independence should be in progress. Such planning needs to be based more on achievement than on potential. It is not uncommon to see a leveling off of academic abilities, and this should not be confused with a progressive neurologic disorder. Heterosexual activities, marriage, contraception, and social integration are all common concerns at this age. With the completion of school, there is no clearly identified service system for the retarded person. Plans for living arrangements and vocational pursuits should be in place and able to be activated when school is completed.

In the past, the answer to placement for the retarded patient was institutionalization. Many of those individuals are now being de-institutionalized and placed into group homes or smaller institutions or returned to their families. In general, the only patient who will be institutionalized in the foreseeable future is the multiply handicapped child whose parents cannot cope with the combined medical, behavioral, and intellectual problems. Many moderately severely retarded individuals still remain at home and attend activity centers or sheltered workshops. However, supportive employment programs have begun to extend to young adults with moderate-severe mental retardation. Rather than teach "prerequisite" skills, job "coaches" train people to perform specific tasks (e.g., dish washing) in the actual work setting and work to facilitate the acceptance of the new worker. As a result, people with mental retardation are successfully moving into competitive employment. Alternate living situations such as group homes and supervised apartments continue to expand, but the numbers are insufficient to meet the demand and issues of community acceptance and supervision remain controversial.

PSYCHIATRIC DISORDERS

JOSEPH J. JANKOWSKI, M.D.

Diagnostic assessment in child psychiatry has assumed increasing importance as its knowledge base has expanded. Such an assessment must be available to develop a treatment plan.

The child psychiatric diagnostic assessment usually consists of four to six interviews with the child and two to three with the parents. The components of such an assessment are as follows below:

Components of Assessment

1. *Chief complaint*—A clear statement of the presenting complaint that led the child to be referred for assessment.

2. *Present illness*—A clarification and expansion of those issues related to the presenting problem.

3. *Past history*—A review of the child's development, behavior, and past medical and psychiatric history.

4. *Family history*—An inclusion of family variables to help assess the child further, e.g., psychosocial, genetic, psychiatric and medical aspects of first- and second-degree family members.

5. *Ancillary history*—Information obtained from other human service providers, e.g., pediatricians, schools, therapists.

6. *Clinical interviews with child*—Interviews utilized to conduct a mental status examination and to assess levels of emotional, cognitive, and motor functioning.

7. *Parent interviews*—Utilized to determine if the parent(s) themselves have a psychiatric problem; also used to help determine the parent's capacity to aid the child and be involved in an intervention plan.

8. *Psychological testing*—Used to assess levels of cognitive and emotional functioning. At times formal assessment of cognitive level can be helpful with learning-disabled youngsters who appear bright but have difficulty in learning. Projective tests provide an opportunity to further evaluate anxiety, affective, or psychotic disorders.

9. *Physical evaluation of child*—The pediatric examination is helpful to rule out potential organic causes of the behavior.

10. *Laboratory tests*—Screening tests of urine and blood are performed by pediatricians. Special tests such as EEG, CAT scan, MRI, liver, renal and thyroid function studies, ECG, and antinuclear antibody tests are ordered when needed to help further establish the diagnosis or be helpful in selecting a treatment modality.

11. *Formulation*—Develop a summary of the child's problem in terms of internal and external forces that impinge on the child and might be causing his or her psychiatric problem. A biopsychosocial model is currently most often used in such a formulation.

12. *Diagnosis*—Psychiatry currently uses the DSM III-R diagnostic/classification format, which utilizes five axes as follows:

Axis I—All clinical psychiatric syndromes
Axis II—Specific developmental and personality syndromes
Axis III—Physical disorders
Axis IV—Severity of psychosocial stressors
Axis V—Highest level of adaptive functioning

The results of the diagnostic assessment are used to develop a treatment plan. In fashioning such a plan, the clinician must keep in mind a variety of factors. It is rare that the treatment plan would only involve the child. Most likely there are aspects of the plan to include the child, family, and community.

The types of psychiatric treatment available are numerous. Often the clinician selects that type with which he or she is most familiar or competent. However, the clinical demands of the case usually dictate the type of treatment to be used. Types of psychiatric treatment are listed below.

Types of Psychiatric Treatment

Psychotherapy

1. *Psychoanalysis*—Uses analysis to uncover unconscious internalized conflicts. By making these more available to consciousness, resistances to treatment are overcome and the patient is freed to proceed more effectively with his or her development and life.

2. *Psychodynamically oriented psychotherapy*—Utilizes the special relationship between therapist and patient to help the patient gain a better understanding of himself or herself and to use more acceptable avenues of expressing feelings and affect.

3. *Behavior therapy*—Incorporates a learning-reinforcement model to obtain modification of behavior.

4. *Cognitive therapy*—Helps patients to cognitively correct misperceptions of their own and others' behavior as they interact with them.

5. *Supportive therapy*—Provides support and nurturance to those in need, e.g., a patient dealing with a chronic medical illness.

6. *Relationship therapy*—Uses the patient/therapist therapeutic alliance to affect change through suggestion and clarification.

7. *Nontraditional psychotherapy*—Includes the use of a variety of treatment techniques for patients who do not respond to more traditional methods listed above, e.g., includes outreach, home visits, environmental changes, and assistance with reality problems.

8. *Group therapy*—Provides a group of similar-aged children the opportunity of reliving experiences in relating to peers or family members in a controlled setting.

9. *Family therapy*—Family members in any combination meet to discuss the patient and their own mutual problems. The family is viewed as a small psychobiologic system in which the patient lives, experiences daily life, and deals with hierarchical social constructs, generational boundaries, and group phenomena. The treatment focuses on helping the patient and family understand the patient's problem and to institute appropriate intervention.

10. *Marital therapy*—Parents are engaged in couple's treatment for themselves to work on issues related to their marriage and how they effect their child.

Biologic Therapy

1. *Medications*—A number of medications are now used for a variety of child psychiatric problems. They include neuroleptics, stimulants, salts, antidepressants, minor tranquilizers, and anti-anxiety agents. Before these medications are used, the child should be properly evaluated medically, including laboratory studies. These medications should be administered by a child psychiatrist and the child monitored carefully for response and side effects. Dose responses are highly individualized.

2. *Biofeedback*—Psychophysiologic states are altered by using feedback of visceral states to patients.

3. *Vitamin therapy*—Has been advocated in the past for patients with attention deficit disorder with hyperactivity and schizophrenia. However, it has not been found to be helpful in controlled clinical trials for either of these conditions.

4. *Electroconvulsive therapy*—Used only rarely for children or adolescents, e.g., for critically ill children who are suicidal but for whom medications such as antidepressants are medically contraindicated.

Social Therapy

1. *Milieu therapy*—Takes place within a therapeutic community such as a child psychiatry inpatient setting. The organization and functioning of the setting itself promote healthy responses and discourage deviant or pathologic behavior.

2. *Therapeutic recreational program*—A group therapeutic experience provided within a recreational format.

Adjunctive Therapy

1. *Parental guidance/counseling*—Helps the parent with child/parent problems through suggestion, planning, and environmental changes. There is an effort with this therapy to improve or optimize the child's normal development.

2. *Psychiatric treatment of parents*—If a parent is psychiatrically troubled, he or she is referred for treatment intervention. This is needed when the parent's psychiatric illness is either causing or impeding the treatment of the child's problem.

3. *Case consultation*—This can be provided to schools, health providers, courts, or other community agencies that are involved in the care of the child. Such intervention helps the other human service provider to understand the extent of the child's problem and what can be done to remedy it. The human service provider may be asked to take an active part in the child's intervention.

4. *Psychoeducational therapy*—Includes a special therapeutic program developed in the context of learning and the school.

5. *Hypnosis*—Involves the induction of a trance state or period of dissociation by using a heightened degree of concentration. This is short-lived and used for treatments that are uncomfortable or cause severe side effects, e.g., antimetabolic treatment for oncologic illnesses.

6. *Guided imagery*—Focuses on a topic of pleasure in helping the patient dissociate from an unpleasurable experience. This is used for patients who are about to undergo or are recovering from severe medical or surgical procedures.

The length of treatment varies with the patient and clinical condition. Treatment can be provided in outpatient, inpatient, day treatment, or residential settings. Psychiatric patients who develop medical problems often have their psychiatric illnesses reawakened or made worse by the medical treatment, e.g., medications, hospitalization, or confinement.

Play therapy is a type of therapy using play as the major form of communication. With play, the therapist can use a number of different theoretical treatment approaches, e.g., psychodynamic, behavioral, or cognitive. Play therapy is used commonly for younger children, especially preschoolers and early school-age children, perhaps up to the junior high level. Beyond junior high, the children begin to prefer sitting and talking about their problems, playing games, and drawing. In effect, a modification of play therapy to suit the maturing child is often used.

INFANTS AND TODDLERS (BIRTH TO 3 YEARS)

See chapter by Gean.

THE PRESCHOOL YEARS (3 TO 5 YEARS)

Behavioral disorders in this age group are difficult to contrast from normal behavior because there is a natural confluence between the vicissitudes of normal development and pathology at this age. In many instances, phobias, problems with bowel training, lack of co-operativeness, and oppositional features are short-lived and change over time with environmental supports and/or intervention. The parents usually need encouragement to be patient and observe the child further while at the same time examining their own behaviors or issues within the environment that could cause these symptoms. Careful scrutiny is required by the clinician to determine the multiple factors that might influence development and contribute to the establishment of a correct diagnosis.

As the child progresses from ages 3 to 5, the diagnostic task becomes more clear because psychological and maladaptive problems begin to manifest themselves by symptoms of anxiety, depression, and more clearly defined behavioral disorders. Organic brain syndromes must always be ruled out.

The most common DSM III-R diagnosable disorders seen in this age group are pervasive developmental disorder, mental retardation, language disorder, anxiety disorder, oppositional disorder, and parent/child problems. The first three are dealt with elsewhere in this book. Anxiety disorders are presented in the school-aged section of this chapter. Oppositional disorders and parent/child problems are reviewed here.

Oppositional Disorder

This disorder is characterized by a pattern of negative, provocative, disobedient behavior often directed at an authority figure such as a parent and/or teacher. Important features are its persistence and self-defeating nature. Rules are violated, suggestions are negated, and refusals to do things are common. Such behavior eventually robs the child of constructive and pleasurable experiences, leading to sadness, withdrawal, and anger.

If the child experiences an act as aggression, e.g., limit setting, the results likely will be tantrum behavior, withdrawal, anger, and/or further opposition. Such children often present with sleep difficulties, poor eating patterns, and excessive aggression toward others such as hitting, kicking, biting, and spitting. These children commonly reveal developmental delays, deficits in language, poor communication, and learning problems.

It is important to intervene early with such children because they rapidly become persona non grata in educational settings and are rejected by their peer group. A thorough diagnostic evaluation should include family evaluation as well as developmental and learning disability testing.

Since such children have difficulty in communicating verbally, play therapy is the approach of choice. By using play materials and themes, the clinician can engage the child in a therapeutic alliance and express important affectively laden material. These children commonly have experienced either real or perceived losses such as an ill parent, the recent birth of a sibling, or the withdrawal of the primary caretaker for any reason.

If the symptoms result in the patient being unmanageable at home or school, behavioral techniques—especially positive reinforcement—are helpful. In the event that neither individual psychotherapy using play therapy nor behavioral management is successful, the patient will need to be referred to a day treatment program. In such a setting, milieu treatment can be used as a major intervention and can be very helpful.

When cognitive or learning disabilities are noted, these need to receive remediation through the educational system. If the family is experiencing problems, intervention with the family or with a family member may be needed.

Parent/Child Problems

Although this is a V-code in DSM III-R, indicating that it is considered to be of less importance than other primary psychiatric disorders, the parent/child problems observed within this age group are common and result in developmental delays and behavior problems. When this is ascertained by diagnostic assessment, intervention is needed with the parent and/or family. Parents may require parental guidance, counseling, or psychotherapy for themselves.

In some cases, the environmental issues predominate such as constant upheaval or chaotic family life, homelessness, parental medical illness, or significant psychiatric disturbance in the parent(s). In such cases nontraditional therapeutic techniques are needed such as home visiting, outreach, and consultation with other human service providers in the community.

SCHOOL-AGE CHILDREN (AGES 5 TO 12)

This developmental period of primary school age has been variously described. Freud described it as the period of latency. Erickson named it the period of industry, and Piaget referred to it as the stage of concrete operations. It is an interesting age of development which carries the child on the one hand through a progressively sophisticated cognitive development while on the other hand a period of diminished libidinal (sexual) intensity. Most of the children who develop problems at this age do not show the normal characteristics of latency. Instead they present with symptoms or behavior that indicates problems internal to themselves or with their families or environment.

The disorders seen most commonly during this stage are anxiety disorders, obsessive-compulsive disorder, conduct disorders, enuresis, encopresis, Gilles de la Tourette's syndrome, somatoform disorders, and elective mutism. They are presented in this section.

Anxiety Disorders

The main characteristic of the three subgroups of anxiety disorders of childhood and adolescence is excessive anxiety manifested by abnormal worry, social avoidance, and fear of separation. The three subgroups include overanxious disorder, avoidant disorder, and separation anxiety.

Overanxious Disorder. This is manifested by excessive worrying and fearful behavior not focused on a special situation or object and not due to an identified psychosocial stressor. These children are chronic worriers. They worry about impending issues or events in their life, e.g., upcoming school examinations. These worries appear to be obsessive and ruminative. The children often feel inadequate and shy despite statements of support.

Individual and family therapy are used for this problem. The length of treatment is usually 1 to 1.5 years and the child is seen once per week while the family is also seen. The type of treatment may vary from psychoanalytic to psychodynamic to behavior treatment, depending on the available skill and interest of the therapist. Minor tranquilizers and beta-adrenergic blocking agents have been tried with inconclusive results.

Avoidant Disorder. This disorder is characterized by persistent and excessive avoidance of social contact with strangers. The avoidance is severe enough to interfere with relationships with peers, family, and school. These children tend to cling and whisper to their parents and become overly anxious and panicky when meeting strangers or being exposed to strange situations. These children appear withdrawn and inarticulate or even mute when their social anxiety is severe. They are often teased by peers and appear socially immature.

Treatment includes individual psychotherapy with the child. If the child can form a therapeutic alliance with the therapist, he or she can expand that to include others in the environment. Often family therapy needs to be provided concurrently. Medications and behavior therapy have been used with mixed results.

Separation Anxiety. The major feature of this disorder is excessive anxiety with separation from the major attachment figure. Sometimes the attachment itself may be to home or other familiar surroundings. The anxiety in these children can reach the level of panic or a phobic response. The most common example is school phobia, in which the child avoids going to school and cannot leave the primary attachment object. This is often preceded by headaches or other somatic complaints that are viewed as avoiding school but are actually prodromal to the syndrome of school phobia itself.

A follow-up study of adults who had school phobia as children found that a large percentage continued to have symptoms of separation anxiety as adults, manifested by inability to move from home or community, avoidance of new situations, and inhibition in social relationships.

The treatment of school phobia includes having the primary attachment object take the child bodily to school and remain in the class if needed. Gradually the attachment object can move away from the class by first sitting outside the door, then in the hall or principal's office, and eventually going home but being "on call."

If the diagnostic assessment points out that the child is depressed, antidepressant medication can be used. Recently antidepressant medication has been used successfully even when depression was not observed during interview or psychological testing. Imipramine (5 mg/kg) is used for this disorder. If a thought disorder is additionally found, a neuroleptic can be used.

Obsessive-Compulsive Disorder

The features of this disorder consist of obsessions such as recurrent and persistent thoughts, ideas, fears, and concerns that are senseless. Additionally, these children suffer from compulsions to perform repetitive, stereotyped acts. The compulsive behavior is not an end in itself but is expected to produce or prevent some future event or situation. Both of these aspects—the obsessions and compulsions—are not related to reality. The child usually realizes the uselessness of the behavior but cannot voluntarily stop it.

Obsessive-compulsive symptoms are found in other psychiatric disorders such as schizophrenia, major depression, organic mental disorder, and Tourette's syndrome. These must be ruled out during the diagnostic assessment.

The treatment of such children has met with mixed results. Individual and family therapies have been used with moderate success. Carbamazepine has been used with some success and clonazepam with increasing success.

Conduct Disorder

These disorders include children with a repetitive pattern of violating the basic rights of others and breaking the rules of societal norms. The specific types included in DSM III-R are group, solitary aggressive, and undifferentiated.

The etiology of this disorder is not known. Parental, societal, intrapsychic, environmental, and organic factors have been involved. It is important to note that there is a high incidence of neurologic abnormalities, e.g., seizures, abnormal EEGs, and learning disabilities, in this group of disorders. These children should therefore have a thorough medical/neurologic evaluation as well as neuropsychiatric testing during the diagnostic assessment.

Many types of psychiatric treatment have been used to help these patients, but none has distinguished itself as being consistently effective except for residential treatment. Often these children require multiple modalities of treatment, including help with a learning disability, medical treatment for a seizure disorder, and family and individual treatment. The families of these children often contain members with serious psychiatric disorders, substance abuse, and criminality. This makes it difficult to treat them as outpatients because their families are often resistant to conventional treatment approaches. Nontraditional methods of outreach, home visits, and intervention at the school and court have been more successful. Also, after their residential treatment is completed, they are often sent back to families who cannot care for them properly and recidivism is high. Psychoactive medications have not been helpful unless the patients have a concomitant depression, attention deficit disorder, or thought disorder that responds to the medications.

Attention Deficit Hyperactivity Disorder

See chapter by Snyder.

Functional Enuresis

This entity is defined by repeated involuntary voiding of urine during the day or night. This voiding is involuntary and not the result of an organic problem. Primary enuresis *has not been* preceded by a period of urinary continence for at least 1 year. Secondary enuresis *has been* preceded by urinary continence for 1 year. Enuresis may be nocturnal (during sleep) or diurnal (during waking hours) or both (diurnal and nocturnal). By definition, primary enuresis begins by 5 years of age. Before 5, enuresis is often considered to be a maturational problem unless there is an organic cause. By age 5 75 per cent of normal children are dry, and by age 10 95 per cent are dry. By age 18, only 2 per cent of adolescents are enuretic. Males are involved twice as often as females.

Psychological issues play a role in this problem but are probably not causative. It is well known that enuretic children develop poor self-esteem and have problems with family and peers because of their persistent wetting and its consequences. Also, patients with secondary enuresis have episodes of enuresis during periods of stress or emotional turmoil.

Family history plays an important role. It is known that 75 per cent of all children with functional enuresis have a first-degree relative who has had the same disorder.

Continence is the result of voluntary control over the levator ani muscles to inhibit the micturition reflex and fill the bladder with urine. To micturate, the abdominal muscles must contract and the levator ani relax voluntarily. In some enuretic patients these abilities do not mature developmentally, and the patient fails to attain proper bladder enlargement.

Sleep stage data regarding enuresis have been conflicting. Sleep states—REM, Stage 2, and arousal from Stage 4—have been incriminated but have not been found consistently in all patients.

Patients with enuresis often require a medical evaluation to rule out obstructive uropathy, epilepsy, diabetes mellitus, spinal tumors, diabetes insipidus, foreign body, paraphimosis, vaginitis, and intestinal parasites.

Treatment procedures include the following:

1. *Conditioning devices*—These are very successful, but their efficacy is often short-lived. They include the use of a pad on which the child sleeps. This pad has a wire embedded in it which when wet triggers a bell or buzzer to wake the child and interrupt the enuretic phase.

2. *Psychotherapy*—Supportive approaches are helpful to promote feelings of confidence and hope in the patient and family. This is especially helpful when coupled with the conditioning devices. The patient can also be helped with peer problems and the enlistment of the family to aid in the problem rather than to be negative about it.

3. *Medication*—Anticholinergics can be used to help bladder retention. The most commonly used is imipramine, a tricyclic antidepressant. The usual dosage for a 6- to 12-year-old child is 25 to 75 mg/day. If the enuresis is nocturnal, the medication should be given 2 hours before bedtime. If it is diurnal, the medication should be given in three divided doses.

4. *Bladder training*—Since many enuretics have smaller than normal functional bladder capacities, bladder training to increase the size of the bladder has been successful. This method is often used in conjunction with other treatments mentioned above.

5. *Sleep awakening*—To aid in voiding, this approach has had marginal success. Parents feel they are doing something constructive and are helped psychologically by being part of the treatment process. This procedure is best used with other treatment modalities listed above.

6. *Hypnosis*—It is unclear whether this modality is helpful. Some report good success, whereas others report difficulty in hypnotizing the child or complain about recidivism. It is not considered a primary treatment approach.

Encopresis

See chapter by Barabas.

Tourette's Syndrome

See chapter by Demeter and Bruun.

Somatoform Disorders

This group of disorders includes those in which somatic symptoms are present and suggest a physical disorder for which there are no organic findings. Interestingly, real physical symptoms are often exaggerated by existing psychological issues. The disorders include somatization disorder, conversion disorder, hypochondriasis, and psychogenic pain disorder.

Somatization Disorder. This entity includes recurrent and multiple somatic complaints of several years duration for which no organic basis has been found.

The disorder is less commonly diagnosed in males. It tends to be chronic but has periods of remission. Often the patients are anxious or depressed, and suicide threats and attempts can occur.

A striking aspect of these patients is how they present clinically, i.e., in a dramatic, exaggerated, and emotionally laden fashion. They describe their symptoms in colorful language and attend more to how the symptoms have affected them and their lives than to the symptoms themselves.

These patients tend to have a poor prognosis unless

they receive intensive intervention. They move from physician to physician and do not remain with one long enough to be treated. If they appear depressed or complain of suicidal thoughts or ideation, they may be candidates for a trial on antidepressant medication. These patients, unfortunately, often incorporate the side effects of the antidepressant medication into their medical complaints and stop taking the medications.

The medical physician and psychiatric clinician must be careful not to discount their medical complaints entirely, because they have been known to develop serious medical or surgical illnesses concurrently with their somatiform disorder.

Conversion Disorder. This disorder includes the loss of or alteration in physical functioning that mimics an organic disorder but is basically the expression of a psychological conflict. Most obvious conversion disorders appear as neurologic disease, e.g., paralysis, seizures, blindness, anesthesia, and aphonia. It is hypothesized that such symptoms help the patient keep an internal conflict out of consciousness and/or allow for secondary gain, e.g., avoiding unpleasant, upsetting, or unwanted activities.

Frequently the symptoms are related to stressful events, including losses and family disruption. Children and adolescents often do not show "la belle indifférence," i.e., an attitude of detachment or lack of concern for the symptoms. Also a histrionic personality pattern is not usually found, and males are seen with this disorder as often as females.

Organic disease is difficult to distinguish from conversion disorder. For example, it would be common for a patient with multiple sclerosis to present with vague, remitting signs, including transient loss of function.

Symptom removal does not result in symptom substitution. The symptoms may recur with time, after a period of intervention. Many types of psychiatric intervention have been utilized, including reassurance, suggestion, behavioral modification, placebo, rehabilitation treatment, hypnosis, minor tranquilizers (e.g., anti-anxiety agents or beta-adrenergic blocking agents), biofeedback, and relaxation techniques. Not one of these treatment modalities stands out as being better than another.

It is important that all medical providers agree that the child does not have an organic illness and that the child be given a way out of his or her symptoms.

Individual and family psychotherapy are often prescribed to help the child and family deal with the symptoms. The referral for care must be done in terms of the detrimental effect the symptoms have on the child and how the child can overcome them.

Not uncommonly these children require inpatient child psychiatric hospitalization to make a large enough impact on the child and family, especially if their symptoms severely compromise functioning, e.g., paralysis, inability to go to school.

Hypochondriasis. This disorder includes an unrealistic interpretation of physical signs as being abnormal, thereby leading to a preoccupation with having a serious medical illness despite reassurance. Medical evaluations do not support the diagnosis of an organic illness. The

preoccupations of these patients may be with all sorts of bodily functions. Normal sensations are often interpreted as disease states by these patients.

In this illness the patient is taken from doctor to doctor trying to get treatment for his or her recurring medical complaints. The patient often is depressed and/or anxious and has obsessive-compulsive personality traits. Sometimes these symptoms are secondary to a more serious psychiatric disturbance, e.g., major affective disorder or psychosis.

Very often these children miss a great deal of school and become withdrawn, remaining away from peers. In some cases, the parents are very troubled and take the child from doctor to doctor, insisting that the child has a medical/surgical problem.

As with other disorders in this group, it is important to rule out a medical illness. Once that is done, the patient needs to be supported and not abandoned by the medical doctor. At the same time the child should be referred to a child psychiatric clinician for a diagnostic assessment.

Individual and family psychotherapy have been used with success. However, most success has been reported with group psychotherapy which includes patients with the same type of problem.

Psychogenic Pain Disorder. In this disorder, pain in the absence of physical findings is the major finding. The pain symptoms may either be dissimilar to any known anatomic distribution or may be similar to a known disease entity. Psychological factors are usually related temporally to the onset or exacerbation of the pain. Such pain may be accompanied by spasms or paresthesias.

These patients are at great risk of becoming abusers of pain medications. They seek out physicians who will give them continuous pain medications to which they can potentially become addicted.

Often the pain allows the child to avoid an unpleasant or unwanted activity. It also enables the patient to receive support from his parents or family when otherwise he would not.

Abdominal pain, limb pain, and recurrent headaches are frequently seen in these children. Pediatric oncology services commonly treat patients for pain that is exacerbated psychologically but related to chemotherapeutic side effects.

Before treatment is instituted, each case deserves a complete psychiatric evaluation. Many of these children suffer from other underlying psychiatric problems, e.g., affective, anxiety, or adjustment disorders. In those cases, individual, family, and group psychotherapies are helpful.

In oncology pain patients, pain is based in real illness and the clinician needs to decrease the psychological concerns regarding their oncologic illness or the side effects of medication to reduce or alleviate their pain symptoms.

Psychogenic pain patients respond best to relaxation, hypnotic, and guided imagery techniques. Such treatment helps to alter the perception of pain itself and decreases the anxious and exaggerated reactions to the illness, pain, or medication side effects.

Antidepressant medication (amitriptyline) has been used to help patients with chronic pain (lasting greater than 6 months) deal with their symptoms.

Most often parents and families also need to be involved in the patient's treatment. They live with and respond to the patient daily and need respite as well as a technique to deal with the patient's continuing complaints of pain.

Elective Mutism

This disorder is characterized by a refusal of the child to speak in almost all social situations. He or she understood language and communicated well before the onset of mutism. In some cases, the child continues to communicate with facial gestures, head nodding, and arm or body movements.

This problem develops without apparent reason. It differs from traumatic mutism, which occurs immediately after a shocking experience, either psychological, physical, or both. During the period of elective mutism, the child selects one or several family members or friends to whom he or she speaks exclusively; otherwise, verbal communication ceases entirely.

It is strongly believed that elective mutism is due to a psychological problem that reflects intrapsychic or environmental stress or both. The children who are vulnerable to developing elective mutism are shy, inhibited, and withdrawn. Whatever precipitates the mutism results in an exaggeration of these pre-existing personality traits.

Four types of elective mutism have been described as follows: symbiotic, speech phobic, reactive, and passive-aggressive.

In evaluating these children, issues to be ruled out include mental retardation, deafness, akinetic mutism secondary to disease of the reticular activating system, pervasive developmental disorder, autism, childhood psychosis, hysteria, and conversion reaction.

Individual and family psychotherapy have been used with good results. Speech therapy and behavior modification are usually added to the treatment regimen. Hypnosis has been reported to be helpful, but recidivism remains a major problem of this intervention.

ADOLESCENCE (AGES 12 TO 19)

This stage of development encompasses a wide range of physical, cognitive, and emotional aspects of development. As contrasted with the school-aged child, the adolescent has a greatly expanded mental ability and an increased capacity for introspection and abstract thought.

Adolescence is divided into three phases—early, middle, and late. Early adolescence (ages 12 to 15) includes entry into junior high school. Developmental tasks are obvious, including a full range of Tanner's biologic stages. There is, however, great biologic variability from child to child. Concerns about body image, normality, attractiveness, and physical vulnerability are obvious. Peer pressure is intense and rebelliousness common. Formal operations (Piaget) begin cognitively at this stage and continue developing throughout adolescence.

Middle adolescence (ages 15 to 17) begins with entry into high school. Most have achieved Tanner's five biologic stages by this time. This group begins to use generalizations and abstract thinking for their own gain. Their cognitive and emotional responses are more sophisticated and differentiated. Identity concerns first appear, and heterosexual interests become more normative. Also, there is an increased orientation to society at large.

Late adolescence (ages 17 to 20) includes that period when the integration of body image, autonomy, and self into an identity occurs. Educational and vocational choices are made. Also there is movement toward commitment and intimacy. During this stage, there is a preparation to move from adolescence to adulthood, a difficult step for many persons.

During adolescence, certain psychiatric disorders are more common than others. Those included in this section are adjustment disorders, brief reactive psychosis, identity disorder, affective disorders, and eating disorders. Conduct disorders, reported earlier, are also expressed commonly in this age group.

Adjustment Disorders

These disorders are defined as "maladaptive reactions to psychosocial stressors which occur within a three month period after the onset of the stressor and are indicated by impairment in occupational (including school) functioning or usual social relationships with others." Stressors may include physical illness, family discord, losses, abuse, or neglect. The specific symptomatology depends on the child's specific psychological defenses, the type and intensity of stressor, and the stage of development of the child.

Adolescent turmoil can be on the one hand normal and on the other pathologic. Regressive behavior in adolescents can easily be elicited by environmental stressors because of developmental stage-specific vulnerabilities.

Adjustment disorders in adolescence may be manifested by acting out behavior, depression, eating problems, sleep disorders, psychosomatic difficulties, and delinquency.

The types of this disorder are varied but include responses to stressors revealing anxious or depressed mood, disturbance in conduct or emotions, physical complaints, withdrawal, and work or academic inhibition.

With some children, the disorder improves when the stressor is removed. However, with many others, this does not happen. Pathologic responses may continue long after the stressor is removed. Also, certain stressors such as divorce, family upheaval, sexual abuse, and death of a parent may have a long-lasting effect on the child.

Various treatment options include short-term individual psychotherapy, family therapy, and group therapy. Each case must be evaluated individually to assess the child's defenses, the nature of the stressor, and how amenable the child and family are to environmental intervention, if that is needed.

Brief Reactive Psychosis

This is indicated by "the sudden onset of psychotic symptoms of at least a few hours, but not more than one month's duration with eventual full return to premorbid level of functioning." Emotional turmoil includes incoherence, delusions, hallucinations, and aberrant behavior. These symptoms are usually preceded by stressful life events to which the patient reacts strongly. This disorder is characterized by acute, florid symptoms, brief duration, and a good prognosis.

At the time the symptoms occur, the patient presents as severely disturbed and can be self-destructive and dangerous. Unstable personalities are more vulnerable to this disorder. It is not considered one of the spectrum disorders of schizophrenia even though in the past these patients had been diagnosed as having acute schizophrenic disorder, schizoaffective disorder, or catatonic or paranoid schizophrenia.

The psychotic symptoms generally remit in several days to 1 week. Such patients often need *brief inpatient* hospitalization with neuroleptic medication and supervision. Individual psychotherapy is helpful after discharge to deal with underlying stressors, whether intrapsychic or environmental.

For the pediatrician, it is important to rule out drug-induced states, epilepsy, head injury, and brain tumor.

If the symptoms persist beyond several weeks, the diagnosis must be revised to a schizophrenia spectrum illness.

Identity Disorder

This is described as "severe subjective distress regarding the inability to integrate aspects of the self into a relatively coherent and acceptable sense of self. There is uncertainty about long term goals, career choices, friendship patterns, sexual orientation and behavior, religious identification, moral value systems and group loyalties."

The symptoms of the illness show a marked discrepancy in how the patient sees him- or herself as contrasted to how others see him or her. The patient manifests moderate anxiety, depression, self-doubt, overconcern about the future, and an inability to make choices and tends to establish a negative pattern of identity.

The conflict is often expressed when the youth is expected to be more independent of the parents. The onset may be rapid but more likely gradual over several weeks to months. These patients commonly show a loss of interest and withdrawal from school, friends, and formerly pleasurable activities. Sleep and eating difficulties are common.

The course of the illness is brief, not lasting more than 1 year. If it lasts longer, further psychiatric evaluation should be undertaken.

Supportive and individual psychotherapy are most helpful. Continued growth and development should be encouraged in the process. These patients respond well to the empathic intervention of the therapist. It is expected that these patients will use the therapeutic relationship to separate from their parents and begin differentiating themselves with a separate identity.

Affective Disorders

These disorders, as described in adult patients, are also found in children and adolescents. They are referred to as "Mood Disorders" in DSM III-R and include the moods of depression and mania with variations of each. The disorders are called major depressive disorder, bipolar disorder, cyclothymia, and dysthymia (depressive neurosis).

Major Depressive Disorder. This includes one or more major depressive episodes without a history of mania. This includes a depressed mood, irritability, and loss of interest or pleasure in activities for a period of at least 2 weeks. Associated symptoms include appetite disturbance, change in weight, sleep disturbance, psychomotor agitation or retardation, decreased energy, feelings of worthlessness, excessive or inappropriate guilt, difficulty thinking or concentrating, recurrent thoughts of death, or suicidal ideation/attempts.

Although adult symptoms are used to classify major depressive illness, the child's changing developmental state and cognitive level often influence the presentation of symptoms. Children have difficulty in verbalizing depressive symptoms, but adolescents are quite vocal about them. Parents often do not recognize depressive signs in their children or adolescents. However, teachers and other human service providers are more reliable in such reporting.

Often there is a tendency to feel that unhappiness or sadness is merely a fleeting symptom in children and adolescents. However, it has been shown that depressive symptoms in children and adolescents actually remain stable over time. The diagnosis is made principally by interview, observation, and history. Laboratory tests such as the dexamethasone suppression test (DSI), serum MHPG, CNS 5-HIAA levels, and thyrotropin-releasing hormone test are not consistently reliable in children and adolescents.

These disorders are treated with tricyclic antidepressants or monoamine oxidase (MAO) inhibitors coupled with psychotherapy. The dose of imipramine is 6 mg/kg/day. It has been shown that most children/adolescents show the greatest improvement with a combination of medication and psychotherapy. Individual and family psychotherapy are those used most frequently with medication.

Before antidepressant medication is started, the patient should have a CBC, urinalysis, BUN, creatinine, electrolytes, liver and thyroid function studies, and an ECG. The antidepressant medications should be given for a period of 4 months, after which a drug-free trial can be attempted. If the symptoms recur, the medication should be restarted.

A major problem encountered with patients who have this disorder is suicidality. This topic will be discussed later in the chapter.

Bipolar Disorder. This includes one or more manic episodes, usually accompanied by one or several depressive episodes. Manic episodes are described as a distinct period during which the predominant mood is either elevated, expansive, or irritable with associated symptoms such as inflated self-esteem or grandiosity, decreased need for sleep, pressured speech, flight of ideas, distractibility, increased involvement in goal-directed activity, psychomotor agitation, and an excessive involvement in pleasurable activities that have a high potential for painful consequences.

Bipolar disorders can occur in children and adolescents. The symptoms generally reflect the specific developmental level of the child/adolescent and the predominant environmental influences, e.g., school and family.

These patients are best treated with lithium and/or carbamazepine in addition to individual and/or family psychotherapy. Lithium should be given at a dosage to reach a blood level of 0.5 to 1.5 mEq/L. Afterwards the medication needs to be maintained at that level. Laboratory studies to be done before instituting medication include CBC, urinalysis, BUN, creatinine, electrolytes, liver and thyroid function studies, and ECG. After 6 months of treatment, the medication can be tapered and a drug-free trial attempted. If the symptoms recur, the medication can be restarted.

Cyclothymia. The basic feature of this disorder is a chronic mood disturbance of at least 1 year's duration involving numerous hypomanic episodes and periods of depressed mood. The boundaries between cyclothymia and bipolar disorder are not well defined. Some feel that cyclothymia is a mild form of a bipolar disorder. A feature to help differentiate it from a bipolar disorder includes manic-like behavior without marked impairment in social or occupational functioning.

Many patients with this disorder treat themselves and become substance abusers. Major depression and bipolar disorders are more common within the first-degree biologic relatives of individuals with this disorder. Significant numbers of adolescents with this disorder go on to develop a full-fledged bipolar disorder in later years.

Most of these patients refuse treatment because their level of impairment is small to nonexistent. If impairment or concern appears, they are referred for a psychiatric evaluation and usually placed in individual and/or family psychotherapy.

Dysthymia. This disorder is a chronic disturbance of mood involving a depressed or irritable mood for a majority of days during a period of 1 year. Associated symptoms include poor appetite or overeating, insomnia or hypersomnia, low energy or fatigue, low self-esteem, poor concentration or difficulty making decisions, and feelings of hopelessness. The disorder begins without a clear onset and has a chronic course. Impairment is mild in school and family settings. These children/adolescents do not quite meet the criteria for major depression.

This disorder in children and adolescents often leads to a chronic, recurrent course with a high likelihood of developing major depressive disorder in the future.

Families need to be educated about potential symptoms to be aware of progressively more serious depressive symptoms that may express themselves. As impairment begins, these patients are referred for psychiatric evaluation and are initially treated with individual and/or family psychotherapy.

Eating Disorders

Anorexia Nervosa

This disorder is defined as an "inability to maintain body weight over a minimal weight range for age and height, e.g., weight loss leading to maintenance of body weight 15% below that expected; or failure to make expected weight gain during period of growth, leading to body weight 15% below that expected. Other essential features include an intense fear of gaining weight or becoming fat even though underweight, a distorted body image, and amenorrhea." The major age distribution is from 14 to 18 years of age, and 90 per cent are female. The skewed sex distribution is perhaps related to psychosocial issues within the female subculture of this age group. Psychological theories abound but remain unproven. Recent studies indicate that affective disorders are more common among first-degree relatives. Many predisposing factors have been considered, e.g., puberty, separation from family, and significant losses, but these remain unproven.

The above symptoms can occur in several psychiatric disorders, e.g., major depressive disorders, obsessive-compulsive disorder, and psychotic disorders. In addition, medical causes need to be ruled out. Once the psychiatric clinician is secure in the diagnosis, treatment can begin.

Outpatient psychiatric treatment is helpful only during the early phases of the illness when the weight losses are between 10 and 15 per cent of ideal body weight. In such cases, a contract needs to be made for appropriate rewards for weight gain and with the goal of avoiding hospitalization. Family therapy must accompany individual sessions.

Inpatient psychiatric hospitalization is needed for patients who have lost 15 to 20 per cent of their ideal body weight. Specialized facilities are used to treat these patients because of their manipulation, deviousness, and resistance to treatment. Efforts are made to institute a behavior therapy program (e.g., operant conditioning) with positive reinforcement, including visiting privileges with family and friends, social activities, and increased physical activity based on appropriate weight gain. It is expected that these patients will gain 0.10 kg (0.25 lb) per day. A weight gain plan includes (a) restricting the patient to bed until normal weight has been achieved; (b) close supervision of all eating by staff; (c) serving an adequate amount of appetizing food consisting of 3000 calories per day.

Tube feedings and total parenteral nutrition (TPN) are used in severe cases in which patients have lost greater that 25 per cent of ideal body weight and are not responsive to the weight gain plan mentioned above. It is best to avoid these procedures if possible, since they both carry risks.

Medications are helpful if the patient reveals psychotic, depressive, or anxiety symptoms. In such cases, a neuroleptic (chlorpromazine), antidepressants (amitriptyline, clomipramine), and antianxiety agents (alprazolam) have been used with mixed results.

It is important to keep in mind that many of the psychological symptoms seen in these patients may be related to their semistarvation status. With an increase in food intake and weight gain, the aberrant psychological concentration, obsessiveness about weight gain, and lack of sexual interest improve. Menses also generally recur after restoration of normal body weight.

Individual and family psychotherapies are often provided while the patient is on the inpatient service and following discharge. Psychotherapy should focus on the patient's being made aware of her behavior, fear of failure, and concerns about being independent from the family and moving on into adulthood.

Prognosis is difficult to predict, since the illness ranges from mild to severe. Those who are able to maintain normal weight for lengthy periods do best.

Bulimia

Important aspects of this disorder include "recurrent episodes of binge eating (rapid consumption of a large amount of food in a discrete period of time); a feeling of lack of control over eating behavior during binges; self-induced vomiting, use of laxatives or diuretics, strict dieting or fasting, or vigorous exercise in order to prevent weight gain, and persistent overconcern with body shape and weight." Most individuals with this disorder are within a normal weight range but many fluctuate with weight gains or losses equal to 10 to 15 per cent either above or below ideal body weight. In some patients, bulimia and anorexia nervosa symptomatology coexists. In those cases more psychopathology exists, usually an affective disorder. The age range is from 15 to 30 years, and females are primarily involved. First-degree relatives are often obese.

Persistent self-induced vomiting seen in this disorder often leads to dental caries, erosion of enamel and gums, parotid enlargement, esophageal tears, and acute gastric dilatation. Menstrual problems are seen commonly.

These patients are generally treated initially as outpatients unless their symptoms escalate to losing considerable weight (i.e., 15 to 20 per cent weight loss from ideal) with concurrent anorexic symptoms or serious medical complications. As an outpatient, he or she is treated commonly with a cognitive behavioral modality incorporating three stages. These include the following:

STAGE 1. Maintain a record of all meals and binging episodes. Afterwards a contract is developed to restrict eating to three or four specific meals. Development of self-control is important in this stage.

STAGE 2. The patient begins to identify issues that lead to loss of control regarding eating and binging.

STAGE 3. The patient is helped to assume and maintain control over those periods that lead to the binging.

This therapeutic modality often includes individual and group therapy sessions. If this approach is not helpful, the patient will need an inpatient hospitalization to utilize a more controlled setting to control the binging.

Recently, antidepressant medications, both tricyclic and MAO inhibitors, have been used with success in those patients who either exhibit major affective symptoms themselves or whose first-degree relatives do. Such medication is often coupled to the cognitive behavioral therapy program mentioned above.

PSYCHOLOGICAL REACTIONS TO CHRONIC ILLNESS AND HANDICAP

When a child is noted to have a chronic illness, it affects the child's entire environment and those within it. Following the diagnosis of the chronic illness, the child, parents, and siblings must adjust and readjust over a period of years as development occurs. In attempting to discuss this topic I decided to separately outline the problems of the child, parents, and siblings and to offer intervention strategies for each.

Problems

Child

Given the diagnosis itself, the child is not immediately aware of the course of the illness or its repercussions for the future. However, over time, the child undergoes a phase of mourning the loss of his or her own normal physical state. This is demonstrated by feelings of denial, anger, sadness, and withdrawal/depression. It may take several years before a child can come to terms with and accept his or her own chronic illness.

Since chronic illnesses do not improve linearly with medications, but instead exhibit remissions and exacerbations, the clinical course is frustrating for the child. The child does not understand why the illness does not get better and remain that way. He or she also hopes that the current remission will last forever and becomes angry that the latest exacerbation has occurred at an inopportune and unexpected time.

A patient with a chronic illness must reorient his or her life and develop a new identity as a person. Children typically resist this, hoping that they can return to their formerly healthy state.

Despair evolves as they realize that the medications have only an ameliorative and not a curative function.

They have less contact with peers if their illness requires multiple modalities of medical treatment. Such treatments, e.g., pulmonary toilet or physical therapy, usually result in their not being as available for peer activities.

Special arrangements for school are often needed. Loss of school days necessitates special educational programming, e.g., tutorial services at home. Physical disabilities often require alternate approaches to help with loss of strength or capabilities, e.g., use of computers, special transportation.

Medication can have disfiguring side effects, e.g., moon facies secondary to use of steroids.

Restricted mobility, need for special procedures, and physical side effects of a chronic illness can result in the child's not being accepted by his or her peer group, e.g., need to use a wheelchair, peritoneal dialysis, or extreme physical weakness.

Inability to either perform or maintain muscular activities results in curtailment of sports programs.

Parents

Parents themselves undergo a mourning phase as they learn about and integrate the fact that their child has a chronic illness. This is demonstrated by a period of denial, anger, depression, or withdrawal. Sometimes the parent, instead of becoming depressed or withdrawn, may become overinvolved in the physical or medical care of his or her child as a reaction to the mourning process.

The needs of the child place enormous stress on each parent individually as well as on the couple and the role of each as parent. Marriages are often strained by the demands of caring for a child with a chronic illness. They can be disrupted if one or the other parent leaves the marriage or family psychologically either to care for the ill child or to escape the reality of the child's chronic illness. Also, parents commonly leave the family by spending increasingly more time away from home in order to avoid dealing with the problems created by the child's chronic illness.

During times of stress generated by the chronic illness of a child, parents often try to maintain control of their child's fate. They want to know about laboratory tests and the expected course of the illness and often develop a questioning attitude about the medications being used. Such parents usually carry all of their child's medical records with them to gain control over the child's medical issues. They become fearful that if they do not, their child will be treated less than optimally and might not get better.

Financial demands are heightened on families because of costly medical treatments, including medication and outpatient and inpatient visits as well as loss of work, travel, and need for babysitters to help with other siblings left at home.

As with their children, the variable course of the chronic illness places uncommon stress on the parents. With remissions their hopes are raised, and with exacerbations they are dashed.

Underlying problems in the marriage or personal psychological vulnerabilities of the parents tend to be exposed during the care of a child with a chronic illness.

Siblings

Siblings of children with a chronic illness often feel deprived of their parent's attention/nurturance. The parents are usually too involved with the ill child and unintentionally exclude the healthy siblings.

To overcome these feelings of unintentional parental deprivation, siblings may begin to exhibit physical or hypochondriacal symptoms to recapture the parent's attention/nurturance.

As a result of this deprivation, siblings begin to reveal developmentally related symptomatology. Under age 7 years they may reveal developmental lags or symptoms of crying, eating or bowel problems, whining, clinging, withdrawal, or overaggressiveness. Those from 7 to 12 may present problems with school, learning, and peer relationships. Adolescents often show problems with affect—depression, peer withdrawal, overinvolvement, or antisocial behavior—and commonly reveal academic problems.

Intervention

Child

1. Explain the nature of their illness and medication side effects in developmentally acceptable terms and concepts.

2. Prepare for visits to the physician, hospital, laboratory, or rehabilitation service, especially if procedures are to be carried out.

3. Normalize the child's life at all costs even if it means taking appropriate risks. Such risks need to be discussed with the child beforehand and supported by parents and pediatrician, especially if the child wants to try doing something that may exacerbate the illness.

4. Develop special arrangements with the school as needed, e.g., bus pick-up, special classes, alternative to gym class, medications administered by school nurse.

5. Encourage peers to visit and be involved with the patient. Opportunities for peer contact must be arranged through schools, playgrounds, camps, and other organized activities.

6. Realistically assess the child's strengths and encourage their development and use. For example, a patient with rheumatoid arthritis who no longer can play soccer should be supported to develop his fine artistic abilities.

7. If the child becomes depressed or withdrawn, a formal child psychiatric evaluation may be indicated.

Parents

1. Encourage parents to join a parent support group to share common experiences and provide support to each other.

2. Provide parents with available resource material regarding the chronic illness of their child. This will help them gain a feeling of control through mastery of information.

3. Make available supportive psychotherapy to help the parents accept and adjust to their child's chronic illness as needed.

4. Support parents to establish and maintain an interest of their own separate from their child's chronic illness. This will help them continue developing as individuals and avoid overinvolvement with the chronically ill child.

5. Help parents plan for a respite from caring constantly for their ill child. Such care is often emotionally taxing and physically exhausting. They often need a rest from it intermittently to maintain their own emotional and physical well-being to carry on as parents and individuals.

6. Anticipate babysitting needs for siblings when the ill child is hospitalized.

7. Optimize family function by including the chronically ill child as much as possible while maintaining the needs of the family. If the family wishes to take a trip, arrangements could be made either to take the patient or to have the patient cared for while the other family members are away.

Siblings

1. Involve siblings separately with each parent independent of the chronically ill patient.

2. Arrange a regular basis for siblings to have a special designated time to be with one or both parents, without the ill patient present.

3. Encourage the parents to view each sibling as a separate person who has his or her own life and needs. Siblings should not be fused as a group within the family. They need to be seen and treated as individuals.

4. Remind parents to be involved in the specific

TABLE 1. Suicide Risk Factors in Adolescents: Attempted vs Completed

	Suicides Completed	Suicides Attempted
Sex	Male	Female
Stressors	Losses, failure	Losses, changes in social relationship
School attendance	Stable	Stable
Desire environmental changes	Not necessarily	Yes
Psychiatric status	Depressed	Depressed
	Substance abuse	Personality disorder
	Schizophrenic	Borderline
	Spectrum disorder	Histrionic
		Antisocial
Methods used	Firearms	Overdose of medication
	Jump off high places	Wrist slashing
	Hanging	
	Auto exhaust	

activities of the siblings at school, in the community, and with their peers. At times, these activities may need to supersede the needs of the chronically ill child.

5. Refer the siblings for a psychiatric evaluation if they begin showing signs of depression, anger, withdrawal, or other psychological symptoms. All too often they are expected to be the perfect, normal child because they do not have a chronic illness.

SUICIDE RISK—EVALUATION AND TREATMENT

Suicide is the second leading cause of death among adolescents, the first being accidents. This does not mean, however, that young children do not commit suicide. Suicides have been reported in preschool children, and most children 7 years and older have heard the word *suicide* and know what it means.

Suicidal ideation is frequently expressed by younger children when angry at an authority figure. However, this is less of a concern than the child who is depressed and denies suicidal thoughts. Those who are serious about suicide think about it quietly, deny the thoughts to others, and often plan detailed ways to end their lives.

Since children cannot understand the abstractness or finality of life with suicide, it was thought previously that they did not understand what they were doing and perhaps this was related to the lesser incidence of suicide at this age. Such thinking has been challenged, since suicide and the abstract thinking of death are dissimilar and probably not related to each other. It is true, however, that most young children, i.e., under age 12, who attempt or commit suicide are depressed. This depression is frequently not recognized by their family or human service providers. Looking back on the child's life after the attempt, clues were given but not pieced together as important because it was generally inconceivable to the adults in the child's environment that such an event could happen. In fact, even after overt attempts and gestures have occurred, the parents and involved human service providers, e.g., school and pediatricians, often do not take them seriously because they think the child is too young to commit suicide.

Adolescents, given normal developmental losses, such as changes in dependency of childhood, loss or sepa-

ration from parents, changes in interpersonal relationships with peers, and a sense of failure in fulfilling personal expectations, can develop serious depressed feelings. Rapid and extreme mood swings, coupled with the adolescent's difficulty in seeing beyond the intensity of the event, can lead the depressed adolescent to make an impulsive suicide gesture or attempt. Adolescents at highest risk have (a) history of parental suicide; (b) thought about the means of killing themselves previously; (c) experienced severe mood swings, especially depression; (d) talked about suicide with peers or family; (e) history of impulsivity; and (f) tended to be accident prone.

There are differences, however, between those who attempt and those who complete suicides (Table 1).

The principal role of the pediatrician in assessing suicidal risk is to listen carefully to what is being told in the history, whether a child or adolescent. Given the fact that depression is greatly underreported by parents, the pediatric clinician himself must assess the affect of the child. Where suspicion or concern exists, questions must be utilized to elicit prior suicidal thoughts, plans, and past attempts. If such information is obtained, the pediatrician should contact a child psychiatrist immediately on an emergency basis. The child psychiatrist will try to assess the level of seriousness of the ideation or plan and treat the child/adolescent accordingly.

If there is a heightened concern on the part of the pediatrician, the child should not be allowed to go home, even if the parents give assurance that they will observe the child on a 24-hour basis. Most parents and families are not trained to provide such safety for suicidal patients. Such safety, in fact, can be provided only within an environment where precautions are provided by 24-hour professional staff and the patient is not allowed out of the staff's view at any time. Such concerns of suicide are considered a psychiatric emergency.

Such children and adolescents will most likely require inpatient psychiatric hospitalization. There are few cases in which the child or adolescent can be discharged home immediately following a suicide attempt regardless of magnitude. Such a patient should be seen by a child psychiatrist before disposition is made.

PSYCHIATRIC DISORDERS OF INFANTS AND TODDLERS

MARGARET P. GEAN, M.D.

Extensive research and clinical work have established the existence of psychiatric disorders in children under 3 years of age. They may result from external stressors such as trauma, inadequate or distorted caretaking, and medical illness, as well as developmental difficulties, temperament, and genetically transmitted psychiatric illnesses. Additionally, psychiatric interventions are sometimes warranted even in this young age range to prevent iatrogenic difficulties and manage the responses to traumatic circumstances. Early detection and treatment of psychosocial difficulties can optimize development in children with impairments ranging from prematurity and mental retardation to the consequences of hospitalization and repetitive, painful medical procedures that distort the normal developmental progression of the first years of life.

The relationship between etiology, signs and symptoms, and diagnosis of psychiatric disorders in this age range is unique to a given situation. Multiple etiologies may contribute to the maintenance of one symptom, and multiple symptoms may arise in response to one etiology. Additionally, the presenting symptoms are of little guidance in determining either etiology or treatment plans. This is in part due to the psychoneurophysiologic immaturity of the young child. Boundaries between physical and emotional reactions are much less rigid than at later developmental phases.

As the following comments are directed toward treatment of particular psychiatric disorders in this very young population, a word of caution is in order. Treatment may fail or cause iatrogenic disorders if an inaccurate diagnosis and/or etiology is assumed. That caution established, helping parents adjust their care-taking to the specific needs of their infants and toddlers as well as to their own parenting limitations may prevent chronic dysfunction for many years to come. Even in geographic areas where optimal treatment is not available, an accurate diagnosis and understanding of the cause(s) of these disorders may be quite therapeutic. Knowing what is wrong affords parents an opportunity to use resources and even carry out their own therapeutic interventions. Telling parents to "wait and see" or that "the child will grow out of it" is no longer the only intervention for behavioral, developmental, and emotional problems of the first 3 years of life.

The following categories were chosen to reflect the presenting concerns of parents; however, the various DSM III-R diagnoses are noted for cross-referencing purposes. The term *parents* should not be abbreviated to mean "mother" or "father" only, unless it is a single-parent family. An effective treatment can be planned only with knowledge of the attitudes and information about the disorder from both parents. Implementation of the treatment requires agreement by both parents. In life-threatening, abusive, or neglectful circumstances, parents' unwillingness to cooperate may entail the in-

volvement of protective service agencies. It will be assumed that the physician or other staff and consultants have been able to arrive at an accurate description of the symptomatology as well as an accurate conclusion as to the etiology.

DEVELOPMENTAL PROBLEMS

In establishing which areas of mental, language, social, emotional, and physical development are disordered, it is important to distinguish between the areas that are age-appropriate and those that are delayed. Additionally, areas that are deviant and not appropriate for any particular developmental stage must be described. One should take into account the rate at which one expects a child to progress considering such issues as prematurity and mental retardation.

Children with developmental difficulties secondary to prematurity without neurologic damage and without environmental deprivation can generally be expected to make substantial developmental gains and reach chronologically equivalent developmental levels over a period of months to a few years. Children who have marked deviations in their developmental patterns (i.e., mental retardations and pervasive developmental disorders) may never approximate overall age-appropriate developmental status. They should, however, be given the opportunity to establish their own optimal rate of progress and are in need of programs that will ensure that they attain maximum levels of development. These children can easily and inadvertently be further impaired by inadequate or inappropriate treatment and environmental deprivation.

The following are suggested therapeutic interventions for children with developmental disorders.

1. Consult with the Parents

Parents should be given a summary of the evaluation and tests, including a description of the child's different developmental areas of strength and weakness, the age-equivalence of the developmental delays (e.g., a 24-month-old child chronologically is functioning at a 15-month level), and the working diagnosis or differential diagnosis and prognosis. Types of treatment, organizations for parents of children with similar disorders, and referral to resources to further treat the problem are needed. An outline of how the disorder will be monitored and further medical evaluations to refine the diagnosis and treatment are invaluable.

2. Early Intervention Programs

Referral to an early intervention program allows specialists in specific developmental areas to address detailed therapeutic needs. Working directly with the child can be facilitated by teaching the parents to meet the child at his developmental level rather than his chronological level. Reinforcement of skills taught by the program can also be implemented at home. The age of the child and severity and pervasiveness of the developmental disorder will help determine frequency and location of the treatment. Many areas have therapeutic nursery schools and as children approach 3 years of age, public school systems provide services for special-needs children.

3. Frequent Periodic Re-evaluation

Over at least the first 3 to 4 years of life, the rate of developmental progress and adjustment of the therapeutic interventions necessitate many check-ups per year. These also assist the parents with their frustrations and increase the likelihood of compliance with treatment. Revision of the diagnosis and prognosis, prevention of fixation of dysfunctional parent-child relationships, and early identification of emotional disorders in the children are more likely with close continuity of care.

4. Parent Guidance and Education

Education about the emotional and social expectations of a child with a developmental disorder is essential to prevent externally induced behavioral problems. For example, the slower rate of developing sustained eye contact and reciprocal interactions of the premature infant, the need for firm behavioral training for communication and social skills of the autistic child, and the slower, less intense emotional attachments of some retarded children should not be misinterpreted by the parents as "bad" behaviors of the child. They are best considered as part of the particular disability, which should be met with education of the parents and guidance about how best to assist the child in developing healthfully in all areas.

5. Parent Support

Although implementation of the four preceding areas of intervention provides parent support, the intensity of the emotional reaction of parents to their children's disabilities frequently leads to sleeplessness, depression, marital discord and disruption, and dysfunction in all areas of life. Questions by the physician about the parents' responses and how they are managing the stress of a child's problems may be met with denial. Offers to be of assistance, referrals to groups or individuals with similarly diagnosed children, referrals for individual counseling, psychiatric evaluation and treatment, and marital counseling may be utilized even if not overtly accepted. Financial resources are often depleted and information about state, federal, and local funding for medical and educational treatment should be made available.

6. Problems of Behavior, Emotions, and Parent-Child Interaction

Direct observations and parent's information to the physician should be elicited to prevent a worsening of the situation. In general, parents should be helped to provide structure and consistency in the child's day-to-day activities and schedule and should be encouraged to give positive praise and reinforcement for behaviors that suggest useful and socially appropriate purposeful intent. If basic parental guidance does not alleviate the problems, evaluation by a child psychiatrist or other mental health professional with specific experience with infant's and toddler's emotional and behavioral development is warranted. Ongoing parent and/or child psychiatric treatment in collaboration with the multidisciplinary treatment team is the most effective treatment.

7. Psychotropic Medication

This form of treatment is generally not needed or advisable for infants and toddlers. Behavioral management, environmental adjustments, and consistency in parenting are more effective therapeutic interventions given the long-term nature of the problems. Disorders with neurologic impairments that include high levels of irritability or self-injurious behavior and that are unresponsive to behavioral management may warrant the use of small doses of phenothiazines.

BEHAVIORAL PROBLEMS

Presenting symptoms are generally in the realm of daily behaviors that are not acceptable. Difficulties in sleeping, feeding, stubbornness or oppositionality, irritability, thumb sucking, hair pulling, crying, clinging, temper tantrums, breathholding, head banging, and toileting problems are noted by parents.

It is essential that the diagnostician determine if multiple etiologies contribute to the disorder to ensure adequate psychological as well as pediatric medical attention. On some occasions, the etiology may be unrealistic expectations by the parents given the child's age.

1. Consultation with Parents

After determination of the etiology of the behavior, the pediatrician should review the comprehensive assessment, addressing the physical and psychological components of the problem as well as the strengths and capabilities of the child. For example, the infant presenting with difficulties in feeding may have gastroesophageal reflux and pain but be developing well mentally while having distorted behaviors whenever the parent tries to feed him. Additionally, irritability, sleep problems, and oppositional parent-child interactions may be occurring. The parents need to understand the primary problem and the secondary behavioral reaction so as not to believe that their child is pervasively disordered or is trying to sabotage their every effort at parenting. A further example would involve a child with a sleep disorder who cannot calm himself. Discussion with the parent about the areas of satisfactory development while addressing the child's neurologic make-up can prevent dysfunctional parent-child relationships. Consultation should take into account the parents' own feelings about the area of the child's difficulty and the possibility that they themselves or their families may have had difficulties in this area, thus limiting their capacity to implement a treatment plan.

2. Therapeutic Interventions

Treatment must be tailored to the individual infant-caretaker dyad, including the environmental, financial, and family situations. The parents should help establish the array of interventions feasible for treatment. These can range from hospitalization with a behavioral refeeding program for a child who has been traumatized and refuses to eat, to the temporary use of a sedative to assist a child in initiating sleep while giving the parents some rest so that they may start a more positive cycle of a structured repetitive bedtime schedule. Clarity in the parents' minds about the specific approach to the behavioral problem and physician support to continue the plan for even as little as a 3- to 4-day period may be sufficient to help a young child master a problem and progress positively again. Additionally, increased attention to the area of difficulty in and of itself may be therapeutic. If developmentally consistent suggestions do not result in symptom relief, referral to a child psychiatry service for in-depth evaluation and determination of more complex treatments such as parent-child psychotherapy, behavioral treatment, parent group treatment, or a therapeutic nursery is warranted. Often the recalcitrant behavior problem has its roots not in the child but in psychopathology of the parent or family or a combination of these and environmental circumstances. Suggestions for consistent limit setting, adequate affection, acceptance of respite care, and treatment of parental psychiatric disorders—including anxiety and depression—may require extended pediatric work for parents to accept the recommended referral.

3. Environmental Manipulation

If the child's behavior is thought to be the result of external stresses, such things as an inappropriate match between a child's temperament, developmental needs, and the day-care program, suggests that a change in the day-care may be needed. Many changes in primary caretakers, hospitalizations, household moves, and other family stressors may need to be addressed with psychotherapy. This will assist the young child and the parents in regaining a sense of mastery while helping the child develop some areas of control appropriate for his developmental phase. The particular treatment plan can be as complex as the life circumstances that the child and his family bring to the situation. An expert grasp of normal child development, a capacity to observe a child and his caretaker's interactions, and skill in eliciting a history combine to establish an accurate diagnosis and etiology. With this, the formulation of the treatment plan often becomes readily apparent to both parents and physician.

PARENT-CHILD PROBLEMS

Given the integral relationship between the caretaker and the child during infancy and toddlerhood, disorders may originate there. Such symptoms as nonorganic failure to thrive, breath-holding, Munchausen's syndrome, emotional, physical, and sexual abuse, and some head-banging are examples of this. In general, the treatment is highly complex, necessitating multidisciplinary professional collaboration, as disorders and distress occur in the parent as well as the child.

1. Emergency Intervention

Determination and implementation of emergency procedures to prevent further damage or death are critical. Consultation with child psychiatry services and/or protective service agencies will specify available re-

sources. Hospitalization to rule out life-threatening physical injuries, toxic exposure, and nutritional intake are more effective than prematurely confronting parents about suspected inadequate parenting. The physician should be knowledgeable regarding circumstances for mandatory reporting of abuse and neglect.

2. Consultation with Parents

Discussion with parents should cover the comprehensive scope of the child's health and development, with an empathetic explanation of the parent-child disorder being formulated using the wording provided by the parents. This is especially difficult if the parent places all responsibility for the problem on difficulties within the child. This circumstance requires ongoing sensitive pediatric work with a parent and referral to a mental health service that will slowly move from the parent's view of a problematic child to an understanding of the more realistic socially reciprocal caretaking of early childhood. At that juncture (unless protective interventions were instituted without the parents' consent), a fuller array of psychotherapeutic services is available for treatment. Given the high failure rates of treatment in these circumstances, it is essential that the pediatric-psychiatric team anticipate the need for a plan that allows the parent to move back and forth between the two services. Parents who are more receptive to some responsibility in the disorder may still have difficulty following through on management suggestions and may need child psychiatric consultation or treatment to facilitate successful treatment.

3. Multidisciplinary Interventions

Involvement of social services, legal systems, early intervention programs, nursery schools, and child psychiatric services are needed given the complex circumstances that maintain parent-child disorders. In the less serious disorders, the strengths and weaknesses of the child can be used as a guide in redesigning the caretaking needs to ensure that a gratifying, mutually reciprocal parent-child relationship is established. To prevent the return of the adverse parent-child circumstances, one must teach the parents about normal development while simultaneously helping them manage their own disappointments and frustrations. Parents with these difficulties often need referral for psychiatric evaluation and treatment for their own psychological disorders. The use of stable day-care may help break a negative cycle in parenting while more intense parental therapy is undertaken.

EMOTIONAL DISORDERS

Parents reporting emotional difficulties note that their child tends to have more of one particular mood, often an unpleasant mood, or to have great intensity of emotions. They describe the child as "too much on the go," "not able to calm down," extraordinarily stubborn, always crying, sad, or depressed. They may report such behaviors as clinginess, whininess, and an inability to "leave the parent alone." All of these symptoms may arise from the entire range of organic to purely psychosocial etiologies of disorders, and thorough review of all areas of the infant's or toddler's development is essential to ascertain the etiology.

1. Consultation with Parents

Explanation of the findings from the evaluation with a description of vulnerabilities, strengths, temperament, and developmental and physiologic contributants to the disorder is needed. The parents' desire for a simple explanation should be resisted unless that is clearly the case. This wish may reflect their worry that some features of their parenting may be contributing to the disorder.

2. Therapeutic Interventions

If clear environmental or parenting style circumstances are the etiology of the disorder and can be easily modified, appropriate suggestions should be made. If inadequate resolution results after a brief period, referral to infant/toddler psychiatric services for psychotherapy, behavioral therapy, and evaluation for psychopharmacologic treatment is warranted. This is especially true if there is family history of such things as manic-depressive illness, depression, autism, and psychosis. At times, hospitalization may be necessary if the parents cannot ensure safety and protect the self-injurious child. Children with certain temperaments may need adjustments in their schedules, anticipation of transition periods, and respite care.

3. Parental Guidance

Whether a child responds to brief pediatric treatment or is referred to a mental health service, inclusion of the parent in the care is essential. Parents should be told how young children learn to identify internal emotional states and discharge these feelings in a manner that increasingly approximates verbal rather than physical discharge. Children must be helped to identify their emotional states by simple parental description. A parent could comment that a child "seems upset" or is "angry" or "sad."

Channeling a child's emotional energy, making suggestions, and providing activities to help direct feelings in a constructive fashion are essential. For example, aggressive feelings can be directed toward hammering pegs or vigorous coloring. The child who gets easily overexcited can be helped by a parent's anticipating these periods and providing activities of lower energy levels. Physically holding or hugging a small child until he or she can calm down ensures that the message of containment is implemented. Parents who are aware of what brings on the various emotional states and who institute the appropriate adjustments have a much greater likelihood of weathering the developmental phases as well as teaching their child how to manage his or her feelings.

TOURETTE SYNDROME
(Tourette's Disorder; Gilles de la Tourette's Disease)
STEVEN DEMETER, M.D.,
and RUTH D. BRUUN, M.D.

Tourette syndrome is a neurologic disorder manifested primarily by multiple motor and phonic tics. It occurs worldwide and in all races. It is usually inherited in an autosomal dominant fashion, with males, however, being affected at least three times as frequently as females. Sporadic cases also occur.

In affected families, a wide array of symptoms of various degrees of severity can be observed, suggesting that the different manifestations are genetically linked, although with variable penetrance. Those most severely affected have tics involving nearly all skeletal muscle groups, resulting in striking muscular jerks and vocalizations that may occur almost continuously. Those with milder cases may have multiple motor or phonic tics but not both (chronic motor or phonic tics). The mildest cases may be manifested by only a single kind of movement (simple tic) that occurs infrequently and can be so subtle as to be hardly noticeable. Although simple tics, characterized by seemingly meaningless muscular contractions and vocalizations, occur most commonly, complex tics, consisting of apparently intentional motor activity such as clapping, fist clenching, hopping, and kicking also can occur. Other complex symptoms include palilalia (spontaneous repetition of one's own words or sounds), echolalia (repetition of words or sounds heard), and echopraxia (imitation of behaviors seen). Coprolalia (involuntary cursing), once considered a characteristic symptom of Tourette syndrome, is frequently not present. Complex symptoms are usually accompanied by simple tics. Tics can be suppressed to some extent by conscious effort, especially in milder cases, and usually abate during sleep, intense concentration, and physical exertion. Emotional stress accentuates the symptoms.

Tics are usually first noted between 2 and 15 years of age, but may begin earlier or later. The muscles of the face and neck are most commonly involved. Symptoms are usually most intense in the years around puberty and tend to subside to a variable degree by adulthood. They may abate completely, but, more commonly, persist throughout life. Exacerbations can occur after years of total or partial remission. Overall, progressive neurologic deterioration does not occur. Stuttering, enuresis, minor EEG abnormalities, and soft neurologic signs can occur in some affected individuals. In addition, some people with Tourette syndrome have been known to exhibit attention deficit disorder with and without hyperactivity, aggression, specific learning disabilities, and depression.

Obsessive-compulsive symptoms, which may take the form of ritualistic behavior, also may be present and can occur in individuals free of tics. These traits tend to have a later onset and are likely to persist. However, not all individuals who have tics or obsessive-compulsive disorder necessarily have Tourette syndrome; presumably, the majority do not. It has not been resolved whether the association of some of the aforementioned conditions with Tourette syndrome is coincidental or integral.

The pathophysiology of Tourette syndrome is not understood. The similarities it has to other hyperkinetic states and its response to dopamine-blocking drugs suggest that it is characterized by a hyperdopaminergic state. However, dopamine metabolites are actually reduced in the cerebrospinal fluid of affected individuals. That paradox can be resolved by postulating dopamine receptor supersensitivity rather than increased dopamine production as the basis for the hyperdopaminergic state. Other neurotransmitters may also be affected.

Autopsy studies of Tourette syndrome are scarce. In one case report, underdeveloped neurons were reported in the basal ganglia. In a more recent case study, the neuropeptide dynorphin was reported to be markedly reduced in the basal ganglia. However, those observations require confirmation by additional independent studies.

The diagnosis of Tourette syndrome is strictly clinical at present. However, it is usually straightforward when multiple motor and phonic tics are present, particularly if other members of the family also are affected.

Most cases of tics and Tourette syndrome are mild, and in those situations the first approach is the education of the child and the family, with general reassurance about prognosis. When the symptoms are more severe, families and children are best engaged in the process of long-term monitoring, establishing the waxing and waning course, and assessing whether the symptoms are interfering with development and adaptation in an important way. With the establishment of a clinical relationship and education, familial tensions may be reduced and harmony re-established; behavior may also improve. For those children whose symptoms interfere with functioning and normal development, more intensive treatment may be required.

Pharmacologic intervention is a very successful treatment in many patients. The most effective medications are neuroleptics, which primarily inhibit the dopamine system. Unfortunately, side effects involving motor and cognitive functioning sometimes preclude or limit their use. Some patients do not respond to medication or do not require it. Mental blunting and parkinsonism, although reversible, are commonly reported. A more ominous complication is tardive dyskinesia, postulated to be a drug-related dopamine receptor supersensitive state, which most often involves the facial muscles and tongue. That complication, although infrequent, can be permanent and refractory to treatment.

Haloperidol, a potent dopamine blocker, has been the traditional agent used in the treatment of Tourette syndrome and is often effective in unusually low doses. However, pimozide may have fewer side effects on cognition and mood. Fluphenazine may also have fewer side effects than haloperidol. All of the dopamine-blocking agents are given in a single daily dose.

Clonidine, an alpha$_2$-adrenergic agent, also has been reported to be effective and does not produce unacceptable side effects or tardive dyskinesia in most individuals. The only double-blind study to investigate the effect of clonidine did not find it to be useful for tics, although replication of that finding will be necessary, since it contradicts clinical experience. However, it may be the preferred drug for people with attention deficit disorder and for those whose tics are exacerbated by marked anxiety.

Stimulants such as methylphenidate and dextroamphetamine can precipitate or aggravate tics. Therefore,

while they can be helpful for symptoms of attention deficit disorder, stimulants should be used with caution with a child who has Tourette syndrome, who has a first-degree relative with Tourette syndrome, or who has a close relative with tics. Tricyclic antidepressants have also been reported to be of value for the treatment of attention deficit disorder. There are individual reports that preservatives or other food additives can worsen Tourette syndrome, but they have not been investigated in rigorous scientific studies.

The Tourette Syndrome Association is a voluntary health organization dedicated to fostering research and education on Tourette syndrome and providing service to patients and their families. The Association offers research grants, endorses postmortem studies in an effort to discover the pathologic basis of Tourette syndrome, and can be of assistance to potential donors and recipients of tissue as well as others who need information or help.

For further information contact:

Tourette Syndrome Association
42-40 Bell Boulevard
Bayside, New York 11361
(718) 224-2999

AUTISM*

D. A. ALLEN, Ed.D.
and I. RAPIN, M.D.

Autism is a pervasive developmental disorder that involves serious deficits in socialization and interpersonal communication accompanied by a variety of perseverative and/or stereotypic behaviors and abnormal preoccupations. Autism is not a disease. Rather, it is a behavioral syndrome that reflects the dysfunction of as-yet-undetermined brain system(s). Autism is a spectrum disorder inasmuch as children with the diagnosis may exhibit a wide range of abnormal behaviors. The severity of the disorder varies as a function of both the number and kinds of autistic features exhibited and the level of cognitive competence in a given child.

The pediatrician has an important role in the diagnosis and management of the autistic child, since he is almost always the first professional to see the child. Many autistic features are observable in infancy, and parents are quite likely to detect and report to the physician that they are concerned about abnormal behaviors or developmental delays within the first year of life. Other parents report developmental arrest between the ages of 12 and 36 months after apparently normal early development. This arrest is followed by regression in the areas of language, socialization, and play without discernible cause and without loss of motor skills. The first obligation of the physician is to pay careful atten-

*Supported in part by Program Project Grant NS 20489 from the National Institute of Neurologic Diseases, Communication Disorders and Stroke, US Public Health Service. The assistance of Carl Feinstein, M.D., who reviewed the manuscript, is gratefully acknowledged.

tion to such parental concerns. A detailed developmental history is a must.

The second obligation is to confirm as early as possible any suspicions of autistic behaviors by referring the family to a diagnostic center for a full multidisciplinary evaluation to determine more precisely the exact nature and extent of the child's deficits. The work-up must include a full speech/language assessment, neuropsychological testing, and a thorough behavioral observation, including, whenever possible, a psychiatric evaluation. The physician must ensure that specific genetic abnormalities such as fragile X syndrome, tuberous sclerosis, phenylketonuria, and Rett syndrome have been considered, since they mandate genetic counseling. Conditions that require specific therapies must be ruled out, notably absence seizures and hearing loss, since these conditions can co-occur with autism and they also affect language development. Any autistic child who does not speak well must have his hearing tested definitively, because missing even a partial hearing loss would jeopardize any therapeutic effort directed at the child's inadequate communication skills. It is an error to ascribe autistic symptomatology to lack of hearing and its consequent communication disorder; even severely hearing-impaired children in whom the diagnosis is missed do not demonstrate autistic symptoms. Hearing-impaired children with autistic symptomatology are multihandicapped, with dysfunction of both the brain and the ear (as, for example, in rubella embryopathy). The same is true of blind children; those with autistic symptomatology suffer from both blindness and autism, rather than autistic symptoms due to visual deprivation, although it is true that some nonautistic blind children make repetitive movements and may not look toward the person speaking to them unless specifically taught to do so.

Once the diagnosis of autism has been confirmed, the pediatrician should be prepared to assume the responsibility of assisting the parents by co-ordinating the many services that will be needed throughout childhood. In order to assume the pediatric management of the autistic child, it is crucial that the physician be informed of the availability of services in his community. The Education For All Handicapped Children Act of 1975 and the resulting Public Law 94-142 mandate that any child determined to be handicapped is entitled to "specially designed instruction, at no cost to parents or guardians, to meet the unique needs of a handicapped child, including classroom instruction, instruction in physical education, home instruction, and instruction in hospitals and institutions." In addition, related services, including transportation for such services, are to be provided free of charge. These services include speech/language therapy, audiology, physical, occupational, and recreational therapies, and psychological and counseling services. Medical services necessary for diagnosis and evaluation are also provided for under this law. Most parents are not aware that they are entitled to these educational and therapeutic services. Since the accessibility and means for obtaining these services vary by state and community, it is incumbent upon the pediatrician to inform the parents how to proceed.

Also, since the law provides for only those services required by each individual child, the physician in conjunction with the educational professionals and psychologists in the child's school district must document the need for such services.

The kinds of programs needed for an autistic child are determined by such factors as the age of the child, cognitive status, and physical condition. The severity and type of impairment in language as well as the extent of social/emotional/behavioral abnormalities must also be considered. Optimally, a child's needs should be met by educators and therapists who are specialists in autism. However, such optimal conditions may not exist within the home community. In such cases, the parents may need the assistance of the physician to lobby for or help to establish appropriate programs or to facilitate admission to an available program in a community nearby.

No child is too young to enter a remediation program. Taking a "wait and see" position is not a useful one for the family pediatrician. Autism is a chronic, life-long condition that children do not grow out of. On the other hand, with early intervention, many children can be helped to attain their highest possible level of functioning. Many communities provide infant stimulation programs that work with parents and children together, either at home or in a center. For toddlers and preschool children, a therapeutic nursery program that serves the needs of the autistic child and provides intensive parental counseling is the treatment of choice. Therapeutic nurseries regularly address, through a combination of individual and group work, the deficits in language, socialization, and play. Behavioral management and/or behavior modification techniques are used to assist the child to establish mutual focus and self-control. The young autistic child, perhaps more than any other type of handicapped child, places extraordinary demands on his family. A well-informed, supportive pediatrician can be of great help to the parents in the early years.

By the time an autistic child reaches school age, the parents of children who have received treatment and remediation in the early years often become experts in the care and management of their child. This expertise is frequently accompanied by frustration that the school personnel seem to know less about their child than they do. In addition, as the child becomes physically more mature, the kinds of demands made on the family may be quite different. Some autistic children become quite aggressive with parents and siblings. Here again, parental counseling, in some cases together with adjuvant medication of the child (see below), is often critical to maintaining the child in the home setting. Some communities offer sibling support groups as well as parent groups. The physician should become familiar with the Autism Society of America (ASA). This national group provides useful information to parents and professional persons through its state and local chapters.

It is important that the pediatrician monitor the family situation. Although some families are able to function well with their autistic children, in far too many cases parents continue to attempt to care for severely afflicted children until the marriage dissolves and siblings are severely affected. In such cases, the pediatrician should be knowledgeable about alternative living arrangements, such as residential schools, and be prepared to support the parents in placing the child.

By adolescence it will be clear whether or not the child will be able to function independently. Some high-functioning autistic individuals can be gainfully employed and manage their own affairs. More commonly, they continue to need some adult supervision. Many communities in metropolitan areas are currently establishing group homes for autistic adolescents and adults. Again, parents should be informed about their alternatives.

It is common for autistic children to have symptoms reflecting the malfunction of other brain systems besides those that make us characterize them as autistic. Those that are treatable may have to be addressed before the child is amenable to remedial educational and behavioral interventions. Unfortunately, many of the stigmatizing or troublesome symptoms of autism, such as stereotypy, perseveration, humming, smelling, staring at lights, and, and of course, aberrant social behaviors, are not amenable to pharmacologic intervention today. The associated symptoms for which pharmacology has something to offer are seizures, tics, attention deficit disorder with hyperactivity (ADHD), explosive behavior, mood disorders, anxiety, and, perhaps, self-mutilation.

A major problem when considering pharmacologic intervention in autistic children is that the disorder almost always reflects a static encephalopathy. Symptoms persist, unlike those of the adult psychoses that tend to wax and wane with exacerbations and remissions. Before committing a child to medical intervention, one needs to be sure that one is not buying relief of symptoms for the present at the expense of long-term permanent side effects. Since some symptoms—for example, aggressive behaviors—are often situationally determined and are more likely to occur in the less stringently structured milieu of the family than at school, one must always consider behavioral approaches to management as an alternative to pharmacology.

Some 10 per cent of autistic children have clinical seizures, and they must be treated as one would in a nonautistic child, including obtaining an EEG. Autistic children without clinical seizures whose language is very impaired or who are mute, especially those whose parents report deterioration of language in the toddler or early preschool years, must undergo EEG while sleeping; some of them may be suffering from the syndrome of acquired aphasia with epileptiform EEG discharges, a syndrome particularly often associated with profound lack of comprehension of acoustic language (verbal auditory agnosia, or word deafness). These paroxysmal EEG abnormalitites are usually bilateral and are especially likely to be present during sleep, when they may dominate the tracing. Nonparoxysmal EEG abnormalities do not warrant anticonvulsant therapy. A trial of adequate doses of anticonvulsants such as carbamazepine, valproate, or phenytoin, documented by blood levels in the therapeutic range, may be justified in children without seizures whose EEG tracing is frankly epileptiform. The physician must explain to the parents that prescribing anticonvulsants is controversial in this situation and that the treatment may be ineffective. There is no clear end-point in children who do not have clinical seizures, since there is likely to be a poor correlation between the appearance of the EEG and the child's language. The recommendation to give anticonvulsants a trial is motivated by the report of an occasional child whose language does improve with this approach. Although anticonvulsants do not affect the child's autistic symptoms directly, effective communication is essential to educational intervention, and any treatment that might improve it is warranted in such severely handicapped children.

Occasional autistic children have tics; either isolated tics or the full-blown Tourette syndrome is encountered in some children with learning disabilities. Medications are used only when tics and vocalizations are severe enough to cause social problems in school or at home. Tics may respond to haloperidol (Haldol) used together with benztropin (Cogentin) or clonidine (Catapres) in children who do not tolerate haloperidol without parkinsonian side effects. The dose is increased until the desired effect is achieved; then, after several weeks, it is decreased slowly to the smallest effective dose. Tics tend to wax and wane, so that long-term medication is indicated only in severely affected children. There is no indication that medication alters the natural history of Tourette syndrome.

Many autistic children suffer from attention deficit disorder with hyperactivity (ADHD), which is often associated with sleep disturbance. The use of stimulant drugs, the most widely used pharmacologic approach to the treatment of ADHD in nonautistic children, is controversial in autistic patients. As in nonautistic children, methylphenidate (Ritalin), dextroamphetamine (Dexedrin), and pemoline (Cylert) have unpredictable effects. Stimulants may render some children even more hyperactive than before, whereas others may be overly sedated and depressed. Large doses of these drugs may exacerbate autistic behaviors and stereotypies or even precipitate a paranoid state with hallucinations. However, when stimulants are used cautiously, starting with a small dose that is increased slowly, some autistic children benefit just as much as nonautistic children, so that a trial is clearly justified.

There is a larger experience with methylphenidate and dextroamphetamine than pemoline, but long-term stimulant medication appears to be safe, with the notable caveat that it must be discontinued slowly (over several weeks), since children may become depressed if it is withdrawn too fast. The rule is that the smallest dose that produces the desired behavioral effect is the one used. The starting dose of methylphenidate is 5 mg bid (morning and midday), increasing at the rate of 5 mg/dose no sooner than once a week so as to have a representative sample of behavior to evaluate effectiveness. Doses larger than 20 mg bid are rarely used. Dextroamphetamine is used exactly like methylphenidate, but the effective dose is half that of methylphenidate. Both these drugs are available in a sustained-release form that has the advantage of smoother release in some children. In others the greater timing flexibility of the short-acting form is preferable. Pemoline is a longer-acting drug than methylphenidate and dextro-amphetamine. The starting dose of pemoline is 18.75 mg in the morning; the maximum dose rarely exceeds 75 mg/day. The sleep disturbances of autistic children do not respond well to chronic administration of chloral hydrate or barbiturates, drugs that often increase agitation in hyperkinetic children. Some hyperkinetic children actually sleep better with stimulants.

Aggressive, impulsive behavior is often a major problem in autistic children. Aggression is frequently motivated by frustration but may also occur spontaneously with no obvious precipitant. Parents may lack knowledge of how to manage this kind of undesirable behavior. Autistic children who have not learned that aggression and tantrums will not be tolerated while they are small present severe problems once they are too big to be physically restrained. Physicians are then frequently pressed to prescribe neuroleptics or anticonvulsants to those children whose temper outbursts are mistaken for seizures. Physicians need to be aware that large doses of phenothiazines or butyrophenones are required to decrease severe behavior disturbances, doses large enough to have sedative effects and doses that are likely to produce tardive dyskinesia if taken over many years. These large doses may also lower seizure threshold in the sizeable minority of autistic children who have a tendency to seizures. Physicians also need to know that these medications must be withdrawn very slowly, over many weeks, if they have been taken chronically in high dose, in order to avoid severe emergent movement disorders and agitation. Small doses of haloperidol (Haldol), of the order of 1 to 4 mg/day, are effective in some cases and have less sedative effect than thioridazine. Small doses of thioridazine, such as 10 mg tid, are marginally effective, so that improvement is as likely due to a placebo as to a pharmacologic effect. (The same is true of very small doses of stimulant drugs.)

Thioridazine in higher doses, e.g., 50 mg tid or more, is frequently prescribed to autistic children with severe behavior disorders and to hyperactive patients who do not respond to stimulants. Thioridazine is less likely than haloperidol to produce acute dystonic side effects, but it has very significant and undesirable sedative effects. Some child psychiatrists recommend haloperidol in relatively high dose (5 to 8 mg/day) for relatively short courses in autistic children whose behavior is so out of control as to jeopardize school attendance, in the hope of making the child amenable to behavioral intervention. A number of severely affected older autistic children are chronically medicated with thioridazine, chlorpromazine, and/or haloperidol. Most of these adolescents or young adults are in custodial situations at home, in group homes, or in other institutions. This approach must be considered a solution of last resort.

There was a great deal of hope that fenfluramine (Pondimin) would improve the behavior of autistic children because of its antiserotonergic activity. Although a few children respond to the drug, overall its effect has been disappointing. Because of the small number of effective drugs to modify behavior in autistic children, other drugs such as thiothixene (Navane) are being tried. Thiothixene has the advantage of being less sedative than thioridazine, and it does not carry as much risk of dystonic reactions as haloperidol; its disadvantage is that it may decrease seizure threshold. Clinical experience with it is still limited.

Unprovoked explosive behavior and major temper tantrums may respond to propranolol (Inderal) and other beta-blockers in children in whom these drugs are not contraindicated by a history of asthma. This is a novel indication for propranolol. One may start at a dose of 20 mg bid and work up to the maximum dose that does not produce bradycardia or arterial hypotension. A combination of propranolol and desipramine (Norpramin) may be more effective in some aggressive autistic children than propranolol alone. Beta-blockers are indicated in children in whom panic or extreme anxiety plays a role in precipitating behavioral explosions.

Some autistic children and adolescents are depressed. They may respond favorably to the use of such antidepressants as imipramine (Tofranil), nortriptyline (Pamelor), desipramine, or amitriptyline (Elavil). Some agitated autistic children, especially if there is a family history of manic-depressive illness, may respond favorably to lithium.

Many autistic children are anxious. Anxiety may contribute to explosive and hyperkinetic behaviors. In addition to the beta-blockers, drugs such as lorazepam (Ativan) and aprazolam (Xanax) are sometimes prescribed by child psychiatrists and physicians familiar with psychopharmacology. As is true of psychotropic drugs in general, anxiolytic drugs produce physiologic dependence, and therefore they must be tapered slowly after prolonged administration so as not to precipitate significant worsening of the symptoms for which they were prescribed in the first place.

One of the most distressing symptoms in severely affected autistic children is self-mutilation. Self-mutilation may take the form of head banging, self-biting, or hitting the head with the hands or fists to the point that the child has lumps over both temples. Self-mutilation may increase when the child is frustrated or anxious. It does not respond well to tranquilizers unless they are prescribed in sedative doses. Propranolol, the antidepressants, and antipsychotic drugs may help some children. Because of the hypothesis that self-mutilation may be due to excessive levels of endogenous endorphins, a trial of the oral opiate antagonist naltrexone (Trexan) has been suggested. Such a use must be considered experimental.

Clearly, the average pediatrician will not be familiar with many of these psychotropic agents and will need to seek a consultation with a child psychiatrist with experience in psychopharmacology. A major pitfall, and one to be strenuously avoided, is to try one drug, then add another and another in an attempt to address each of the child's symptoms. Polypharmacy results in dull, overdrugged children and occasionally in life-threatening toxicity. As is true in the case of anticonvulsants, one needs to try one drug at a time and push it to either clear improvement or undesirable side effects, then withdraw it slowly before trying another drug, unless symptoms are so severe as to mandate transient drug overlap.

Child psychiatrists, psychologists, and special educators with special training in behavioral management techniques are often helpful in assisting the parents with the management of children. Some high-functioning autistic children and adolescents can benefit greatly from adjunctive supportive psychotherapy. These intelligent autistic children, after appropriate early intervention, may be educated later on with normal or learning disabled children. Because this is a spectrum disorder, it is important to prescribe for each individual child, not for diagnosis. On the other hand, as more severely affected autistic children grow older, some of them become violent or overtly psychotic and therefore require psychiatric hospitalization for optimal management of psychotropic medication in a controlled environment. The most severely impaired cannot be managed in the community and require long-term residential placement.

Autism is the most complex of the developmental disorders of brain function. It mandates behavioral, educational, and medical interventions. It is the result of a multidetermined encephalopathy that is not well understood and is not curable with today's knowledge. This is not to say that it is hopeless, however, since many of its symptoms may be ameliorated. Prognosis is a function of both the severity of the disorder in the individual child and the effectiveness and timeliness of the interventions provided.

PICA

RICHARD B. GOLDBLOOM, M.D., F.R.C.P.(C)

The term *pica* is actually the Latin name for the magpie (*Pica pica*), a bird that is notorious for its habit of collecting all variety of foreign materials. As applied to humans, pica refers to the idiosyncratic craving for and compulsive ingestion of foreign material of any kind, most often material of no food value. An array of "phagia" terms commonly denotes the particular materials craved and ingested, e.g., geophagia (eating earth or clay), amylophagia (starch), pagophagia (ice), geomelophagia (raw potatoes), coprophagia (feces), and trichophagia (hair). Other foreign substances that have been the objects of pica include plaster, paint, paper, crayons, matches, grass, and specific foods.

Treatment must be directed at both the causes and the effects of pica and at commonly associated problems. In children, pica occurs most commonly in association with iron deficiency, and there is considerable (although not conclusive) evidence to suggest that in such children pica may be the result rather than the cause of iron deficiency. Interestingly, the foreign material craved by the individual with pica is rarely a good source of the deficient nutrient, e.g., iron. It has been

observed repeatedly that pica ceases rapidly when the iron deficiency is treated, and iron treatment for pica was recommended as early as A.D. 1000. Zinc deficiency had also been found in association with pica. It has been suggested that pica may be due to depletion of cytochromes or other essential iron-containing enzymes in the brain. However, pica occurs most commonly in lower socioeconomic groups and in families under psychosocial stress.

Depending on the substance ingested, problems resulting from pica may include lead poisoning from ingestion of lead-containing plaster or paint; mercury poisoning from paper pica; trichobezoars or phytobezoars with gastrointestinal obstruction, or perforation and peritonitis due to the foreign material; parasitic infestations, especially ascariasis and toxocariasis from geophagia; and hypokalemia from clay ingestion. The treatment of each of these conditions is described elsewhere in this book.

To evaluate the overall treatment needs of a child with pica, particular attention should be paid to the following: (1) socioeconomic status and psychosocial problems; (2) adequacy of physical growth (growth delay may reflect inadequate caloric intake and/or zinc deficiency); (3) repeated examination of fresh stool specimens for ova and parasites and examination for eosinophilia if geophagia is present; (4) determination of iron and zinc status, the latter especially if hypogeusia (decreased taste acuity) is present.

Comprehensive treatment can then be tailored to the problem complex of the particular child. If iron deficiency is present, it may be treated by giving oral iron as ferrous sulfate, 25 mg/kg/day (providing 5 mg elemental iron/kg/day) for 2 months. If oral iron therapy is not well tolerated or if there are problems of compliance, intramuscular iron may be considered, as described in the article on iron deficiency. Milk intake should be severely curtailed or even eliminated for a time. Depending on social conditions, which should be evaluated in detail, a brief hospital admission may be necessary to ensure adequate diagnosis and treatment of all problems that may have caused or resulted from pica.

The treatment of pica in children with significant developmental retardation may present special problems requiring a custom-tailored approach to management. Treatments reported to have been successful include removing the object of pica, brief (e.g., 30 sec) periods of physical restraint, praise when the child exhibits more acceptable behaviors, and other forms of reinforcement. Where necessary, consultation with a behavioral psychologist may offer valuable assistance in developing individualized treatment "packages" for such patients.

PSYCHOSOMATIC ILLNESS

JUDITH ROBINSON, M.D.

Psychosomatic disorders are defined as those disorders in which emotional factors lead to changes in somatic functioning. These disorders may be divided into two general types: somatoform disorders and psychophysiologic disorders. In somatoform disorders, physical symptoms suggest a physical disorder for which there are not demonstratable organic findings or physiologic mechanisms and for which there is positive evidence or strong suspicion of contributory psychological factors. Unlike factitious illness or malingering, the symptom production is not thought to be intentional or under conscious control. In psychophysiologic disorders, there is confirmed evidence of a physical disorder with a physiologic mechanism thought to be triggered, sustained, or exacerbated by stress.

Somatoform disorders are divided into five categories. There is no correlation between the type of stress and the type of disorder. These categories include conversion disorder, psychogenic pain disorder (a conversion disorder in which the symptom is pain), body dysmorphic disorder (preoccupation with some imagined defect in appearance in a normal-appearing person), hypochondriasis (preoccupation with the fear of having a serious illness), and somatization disorder (recurrent and multiple somatic complaints of several years duration for which medical attention is ardently sought but for which there is no underlying physical disorder). Although more prevalent in adults, all of these disorders may be seen in children.

Conversion disorder represents the classic form of somatoform disorder and is the one most commonly seen in children. It involves a loss of physical functioning suggestive of a physical disorder but is in actuality the expression of an emotional need or conflict. Usually the symptoms affect the sensory organs or voluntary muscles and are suggestive of neurologic disease; however, they may also involve the autonomic or endocrine system. Most often the patient is monosymptomatic and the symptom has appeared abruptly. When the patient presents, both the child and family tend to put much pressure upon the physician for a biomedical explanation, even though initial evaluation may indicate no evidence for this. There is usually a lack of psychological-mindedness and an active avoidance of talking about emotional issues. Even when psychological stressors have been identified, these patients and their families tend to minimize their impact and to deny any relationship between them and the development of symptoms.

The conversion symptom benefits the patient psychologically in many ways. It may serve to keep conflict or need out of awareness and consequently bind anxiety (i.e., if one is preoccupied with one's somatic needs, one can avoid dealing with one's psychological needs). More directly, it may provide an escape from something noxious or a path to something gratifying (e.g., if one cannot use one's leg which is "paralyzed," one can hardly be expected to stay at overnight camp, and one's parents may even have to cut short their own vacation to attend to the medical problems). Furthermore, it may, under any circumstances, gain the patient attention, support, and comfort. Usually there is a temporal relationship between the stress and the development of symptom formation. In some instances, the symptom is symbolic of the problem and is a partial solution to it (e.g., a person who has viewed a traumatic event may develop "blindness"). In other instances, the symptom may be modeled from a previous illness of the patient himself or someone close to him. In the latter, the symptom may have developed in an attempt to avoid something unpleasant or to gain solicitous attention given in the past under similar circumstances.

In the past, it was believed that an attitude of "la belle indifference" was almost pathognomonic of this disorder. Current thinking is that this feature, although frequently present, is of little diagnostic value, since it is often found in patients with biomedical illness who have difficulty dealing with their feelings about their illness. The epidemiology of conversion reactions in a childhood population differs from that in an adult population. There seems not to be a uniformly high female to male ratio, but rather there is an equal sex distribution among the prepubertal population, with the higher incidence in females increasing with adolescence. Additionally, most authors do not describe a pattern of histrionic personality in children with this diagnosis.

Children with anxiety, affective illness, and psychotic processes may all present with psychosomatic symptoms ranging from headaches and stomachaches to conversion reactions. Psychological testing may be very helpful both in eliciting or confirming stressors and in establishing a questionable psychiatric diagnosis.

PROGNOSIS AND TREATMENT

Each manner of presentation of symptoms has a different implication for prognosis and treatment. Most children show rapid remission. It is estimated that up to 90 per cent show recovery within 1 year. A good prognosis is associated with acute symptoms of recent onset precipitated by a stressful event that can be elicited. Patients with good premorbid psychological and physical health do best. The longer the symptoms persist and the stronger the patient's and family's investment in discovering a physiologic basis for the symptoms, the more complex the treatment and more guarded the prognosis. In some instances, the development of psychosomatic symptoms is part of a larger psychiatric problem such as schizophrenia, and treatment should address the major mental illness.

Optimally, involvement of the psychiatrist as part of the treatment team should begin as early as possible. Since many patients initially diagnosed as having somatoform disorders are later found to have an organic illness, the diagnosis should be based not solely upon negative physical findings but also upon positive psychological findings consistent with the diagnosis of somatoform disorder. Once the diagnosis has been definitively established, the patient and family should meet with the combined medical-psychiatric team to discuss both the diagnosis and the treatment plan. Patients and family must be gently helped to understand the illness. Confrontation is not helpful and often invites antagonism. Caregivers and patients and their family must keep in mind that psychosomatic symptoms are "real," are not signs of malingering, and are not under the patient's conscious control.

It is important that the pediatrician and psychiatrist work jointly to treat the patient. Turning over the patient to the psychiatrist implies that the symptoms are not "real" and that the patient is not valued by the pediatrician. Often such an act engenders feelings of rejection and resentment in the patient. Such feelings may be acted out by seeking a second opinion.

Continued medical and psychiatric collaboration allows a two-pronged approached to treatment. Psychiatric intervention focuses upon understanding the patient's life situation and listening for the possible symbolic meaning of the symptom as well as the unbearable affect against which the symptom defends. Psychiatric intervention helps the patient raise to consciousness and put into words what had previously been expressed through the body alone and to tolerate feelings that had previously been intolerable. Medical intervention provides a more direct approach to symptom relief. The pediatrician assumes the role of reassuring the patient that he will be well by "prescribing" a regimen of physical therapy with specific suggestions of how symptoms will resolve (e.g., first you will be able to bear a little weight on your foot and then soon be able to walk a few steps). The pediatrician provides a program for the patient to gradually surrender his symptoms without the loss of self-esteem. A combined psychiatric-medical approach seems to be a particularly effective treatment modality. In some cases, psychopharmacologic intervention may be useful. This is especially true when there is evidence of anxiety, depression, or major psychiatric illness.

Treatment should begin as soon as the diagnosis is certain; delay fosters secondary gain. The treatment must always involve both the child and the parents, particularly since the development of conversion symptoms is often in response to stress within the family. Although acute individual and family intervention is always indicated, ongoing psychiatric treatment must not be recommended solely because of a conversion disorder. After the symptoms resolve, an assessment must be made regarding the degree of psychopathology and the current needs.

As the development of physical symptoms fills the psychological need for the child, it may also fill a need for the parent. The Munchausen's by proxy syndrome is a variant of somatoform illness in which the parent has a psychological need to have a sick child. In this syndrome the parent makes the child appear ill and then presents the child for evaluation and treatment. There is a striking symbiotic tie between parent and child in these cases; the children are at serious risk both physically and psychologically. Management of this problem is a medical emergency that involves a multidisciplinary treatment team. A full discussion of this syndrome is beyond the scope of this section.

Unlike the somatoform disorders, psychophysiologic disorders present with confirmed evidence of physical dysfunction. According to the DSM III-R, this diagnosis can be made when psychologically meaningful stimuli are seen as temporally related to the initiation or exacerbation of a physical condition; the physical condition is either demonstrable organic pathology (e.g., diabetes

mellitus) or through a known pathophysiologic process (e.g., headaches). Common examples of psychophysiologic conditions include asthma, tension and migraine headaches, and ulcer pain.

There is no evidence that a particular stress causes a particular physiologic manifestation; however, certain people seem more prone to physiologic manifestations of stress than others. Often there is a familial history of psychophysiologic disorders with the same target organ.

Psychophysiologic conditions are complicated and often chronic. In many cases, the illness and its treatment create additional stresses that further exacerbate the physical problem. A combined medical-psychiatric care team from the onset provides the best approach to these patients, who must be told, when the diagnosis is made, that the problem is "real" and that stress affects it. Ideally, the consulting psychiatrist should evaluate the patient and family as soon as the diagnosis is made in order to better understand the psychological factors contributing to the medical condition. The extent of further psychiatric intervention must be determined on an individual basis. Such intervention ranges from periodic appointments with the psychiatrist or clinic social worker during routine clinic visits to recommendations for individual or family psychotherapy. Groups for children with similar disorders (e.g., diabetes, Crohn's disease) are often useful. As in somatoform disorders, the child should be encouraged to return to a full range of social and academic activities as soon as possible.

CHILDHOOD SLEEP DISTURBANCES AND DISORDERS OF AROUSAL

GABOR BARABAS, M.D.

Abnormalities in sleep behavior and sleep pattern represent a relatively frequent chief complaint in a general pediatric practice. Parents most frequently complain that their children are having difficulty in falling asleep or that they are restless during sleep, with frequent or early awakening. Nightmares also are relatively common. Such sleep disturbances are generally transient and are related to stages in development and certain environmental and psychological factors. For instance, it is not unusual for a young child to develop sleep disturbances upon moving to a new home, starting school, or after the loss of a family member or a close pet. On occasion, sleep disturbances may be symptomatic of more serious psychological conflicts or problems within the family unit.

These "behavioral" phenomena are categorized as sleep disturbances or abnormal sleep behavior patterns. Another group of sleep abnormalities are generally considered to be independent of environmental and psychological factors and are categorized as disorders of arousal. These symptoms tend to occur during specific stages in sleep and are more often thought of as being "organic" and associated with intrinsic biochemical disturbances. This distinction between sleep disturbances and disorders of arousal, however, is in many ways fictitious, for fever, fatigue, emotional tension, depression, and sleep deprivation can affect biochemical changes in the brain and therefore can influence the intrinsic organic nature of sleep.

Somnambulism. The management of sleepwalking can pose problems to the physician and family. On rare occasions it can present a physical threat to a child, so that all windows and doors have to be secured. A child may climb out of a window or wander into the street and may risk serious physical harm. In such situations, relocating the child's bedroom to the ground floor when possible is advisable. In children with frequent somnambulism, diazepam, 2.5 to 5.0 mg before sleep, can dramatically suppress symptoms. While this has been my clinical experience, and while other clinicians also attest to the efficacy of benzodiazepines in individual cases, the few systematic studies that exist on this subject fail to demonstrate a consistent beneficial effect. Benzodiazepines suppress Stage 4 sleep, thereby decreasing the time spent in the sleep state during which sleepwalking characteristically occurs.

Pavor Nocturnus. Night terrors, like sleepwalking, may respond dramatically to diazepam by suppression of Stage 4 sleep. Families need to be reassured of the benign nature of this symptom, for to be witness to it can be a frightening experience for a parent. They need to be further reassured that night terrors are usually not associated with psychological problems and that, with rare exceptions, children invariably outgrow the tendency. In contradistinction, persistent nightmares in a child warrant further investigation into family dynamics and potential psychopathology.

In general, pharmacotherapy for sleepwalking or night terrors should be reserved only for severe cases in which the potential for bodily harm exists or when emotional pressures are significant enough to warrant such intervention.

Jactatio Capitis Nocturnus and Sleep-Rocking. Like night terrors, nocturnal head-banging and rocking in sleep tend to affect younger children than sleepwalking does. Therapy does not appear to be necessary. Parents need to be reassured regarding the head-banging. It must be kept in mind that some retarded children engage in stereotypic rocking and head-banging. On rare occasions infants and toddlers suffering from headaches may bang their heads. However, this tends not to be limited to sleep alone, and it is obvious that such a diagnosis is an extremely difficult one to entertain and almost impossible to substantiate. Of assistance is the fact that head-banging from pain is associated with overt evidence of pain while nocturnal head-banging is not accompanied by any apparent discomfort.

Enuresis. The management of enuresis is discussed elsewhere in this book. It suffices to mention that in recent years imipramine has gained the most popularity in the pharmacologic approach to therapy. Its actions are related to parasympathetic effects on the bladder with an increase in bladder capacity. Some effects may also be related to an influence on sleep stages.

Sleeptalking. This appears to be the most frequently encountered "disorder of arousal." Because of its be-

nign nature, it does not pose a management problem and is viewed by most families with amusement.

Bruxism. Nocturnal teeth-grinding can be a bothersome symptom. It has occasionally been linked to temporomandibular joint disease and resultant facial pain. This association, however, has hardly been established. In some children, a dental appliance may be necessary to prevent the teeth-grinding.

Nocturnal Seizures. Some children suffering from epileptic seizures also experience nocturnal seizures. When these are witnessed, the nature of the symptoms is generally apparent. Generalized convulsions associated with urinary incontinence may be seen, as well as various rudimentary motor seizures with tonic spasm, myoclonus, or focal symptomatology. Rolandic seizures begin between 6 and 10 years of age. They frequently present as focal twitching of the face, during which consciousness is often retained, followed by slurred speech. The electroencephalogram is often diagnostic.

Some children have only nocturnal seizures. When not witnessed, they may masquerade as enuresis. The presence of tongue biting and postictal somnolence with muscle aches upon awakening may suggest this condition. Sleep lowers seizure threshold, accounting for nocturnal seizures in susceptible individuals. *Sleep myoclonus* is a benign jerking of the trunk and extremities that occurs commonly upon falling asleep and needs to be differentiated from nocturnal myoclonic seizures. Once again, the electroencephalogram is often helpful in making this distinction.

VOICE, SPEECH, AND LANGUAGE DISORDERS

SYLVIA ONESTI RICHARDSON, M.D.

Therapy for voice, speech, and language disorders should be administered by qualified speech clinicians (also called speech-language pathologists). The physician's primary responsibilities are in the prevention and early diagnosis of speech, language, and voice problems; in parent counseling; and in the appropriate, timely referral of patients to qualified speech therapists and clinics.

VOICE DYSFUNCTIONS

Hypernasality of voice quality usually is associated with the velopharyngeal incompetence of a child with a cleft palate, even a submucous cleft. Such a child should be followed by a speech therapist who can supervise the home program from the age of 3 months to 2 years, regardless of the type of operative or nonoperative treatment. The parents must be taught how to help the child develop non-nasal speech.

If the hypernasality is not due to anatomic defect (functional) and is serious enough to create a problem for the child, a speech clinician can teach the patient to use the soft palate by doing blowing exercises. Parents also can help at home. To learn to direct the breath stream through the mouth and to help strengthen the palatal muscles, the child should spend several periods a day in blowing activities such as blowing soap bubbles, keeping a feather aloft, blowing boats in the bath-tub, and blowing a Ping-Pong ball across a table.

Hyponasality, or "adenoidal speech," in which "n" sounds like "d," "m" sounds like "b," and "ng" sounds like "g," can be caused by excessively enlarged adenoids or any nasal or nasopharyngeal obstruction. This usually disappears if the adenoidal mass becomes smaller or if adenoidectomy is performed. If excessive nasality occurs postadenoidectomy and persists for more than 8 weeks, speech therapy should be considered to help the child relearn to use the soft palate correctly.

Hoarseness may appear in children 8 to 10 years of age, especially boys, because of development of tiny nodules between the anterior and middle thirds of the vocal cords. These may be due to prepubescent endocrine changes, allergy, or too much yelling in the Little League outfield. Treating any allergy or requiring the child to stop yelling or singing loudly is usually successful, although difficult to enforce in the latter case. If such hoarseness persists and the nodule shows a slow reduction in size, a speech clinician can teach the child to alter voice pitch until healing is effected. This disturbance usually disappears spontaneously when change of voice occurs around the age of 12 or 13 years.

DISORDERS OF ARTICULATION

Dysarthria is due to neuromotor involvement of the muscles used for articulation, phonation, or respiration. Dysarthria in children is usually due to cerebral palsy. In such a case the child will benefit from an interdisciplinary approach, including the pediatrician, child neurologist, physical and occupational therapists, speech/language pathologist, and infant teacher. The child with *articulatory dyspraxia* is able to carry out the movements necessary for articulation spontaneously but has difficulty in directing them for voluntary imitation of movements (motor planning) or for reproduction of the correct articulatory sounds when hearing is normal. *Dyslalia* includes those defects of articulation which appear to be functional in origin rather than attributable to damage to the brain or failure of neurologic maturation for speech. In this article we are concerned with the latter.

Indications for the physician's referral to a speech and hearing clinic for further evaluation and possible therapy are as follows: (1) Articulation is mostly unintelligible after age 3 years. If the causes appear to be chiefly environmental or functional, a good nursery school can be therapeutic if recommended by a speech clinician. (2) There are many substitutions of easy sounds for difficult ones after age 5 years. In such cases, psychological evaluation may be sought to determine mental age or reasons for retention of infantile speech patterns. Speech therapy is influenced by the cause of the disorder, as is parent counseling. (3) The child is omitting, distorting, or substituting any sound past age 7 years. Speech therapy consists largely of ear training and teaching the child to produce the sounds correctly in isolation and then in combination with other sounds.

Audiologic evaluation is important in *every* case and

is particularly indicated when the speech is characterized by omission of sounds or word endings or if there has been a history of chronic otitis media. Assuming that hearing is normal and the problem is one of dyslalia, the majority of articulatory defects in children under 7 years of age can be handled at home by the mother, in nursery school, or in the classroom. However, such management should be recommended and supervised by a qualified speech clinician.

Home management must be handled skillfully without pressure, or not at all. All members of the family are instructed to use clear, precise speech to provide suitable models. At first, two or three 15-minute periods can be set aside daily when one member of the family reads aloud, leafs through picture books naming the pictures, plays games involving imitation of different animal sounds, and engages in similar activities. As the child begins to identify pictures correctly, these may be cut out and placed in a scrapbook for review. As stated above, the parents should confer with a speech therapist for guidance.

Most children with dyslalia show marked improvement in articulation between the first and second grades and some between the second and third grades. Thus the child's maturation *within a good speech environment* is often the best course of therapy for simple articulatory defects.

A note on "tonguetie": Parents and others still seem to think a child is "tonguetied" if there is any kind of speech problem. If a child can articulate t, d, n, or l; can say "no," "ta-ta," and "da-da"; or can lick a lollipop, the speech problem is not due to tonguetie alone, if at all. If there is a true tonguetie and the lingual frenulum is bound down to the lower central incisors, the treatment is surgical—not a scar tissue–producing snip with a pair of scissors.

STUTTERING

The physician's ability to determine the child's position in the continuum from developmental nonfluency to established stuttering is important in planning treatment.

Effective parent counseling by the physician is the first step in treatment of the problem of nonfluency. He can explain to the parents the developmental nature of early nonfluency and provide instructive reading for them.

Treatment of nonfluency in preschool children is indirect, aimed at the child's environment rather than the child. The parents must help to change the conditions that precipitate or perseverate stuttering episodes, including problems in the home that tend to produce anxiety in the child. The parents are advised to encourage the child to speak during fluent periods, to allow ample time for him or her to speak, to maintain eye contact when the child speaks, and to be responsive listeners. Comments like "Slow down, Johnny," or "For heaven's sake, stop and think before you try to talk" are to be discouraged—as is any suggestion that the child modify his speaking.

The effectiveness of the treatment is directly proportionate to the consistency the parents are able to maintain. For this reason, counseling with a speech therapist must be regular and must continue until the problem is resolved.

When nonfluency has progressed to the point at which children think of themselves as stutterers and develop struggle reactions to speech, such as circumlocutions to avoid a sound on which they usually block, facial tics, and grimaces or other evidence of avoidance or anxiety reactions, the treatment is direct and may involve combined speech therapy and psychotherapy.

SPEECH AND LANGUAGE DELAY

Treatment of speech and language delay depends upon definitive diagnosis, and this may be considered one of the most difficult diagnostic problems in pediatrics.

Treatment for delayed speech development may vary from counseling parents to sending the child to a good preschool or to play therapy in a speech clinic. Psychiatric treatment may be indicated before speech therapy is attempted. Direct speech therapy is usually not recommended before a child has reached a general developmental level of about 4 years.

Deafness and mental retardation must be ruled out. Intervention programs for the child with hearing impairment must be instituted as soon as diagnosis is made. Such programs include amplification, total communication, oral speech/language therapy, and infant stimulation. Mentally retarded children usually present a picture of retardation in all areas of development, especially when the IQ level is below 70. Improvement in speech and language may occur with development and maturation, but training in prelinguistic sensory-motor skills is most helpful. The parents of these children often need to understand that speech therapy per se is of no value to the child until he or she has had adequate prelinguistic experience and has developed the necessary motor coordination of the articulatory muscles to produce speech.

The term *language disorder* is used to include dysphasia, dyslexia, and dysgraphia. Dysphasia is the inability or limited ability of a child to use spoken symbols for communication. To plan treatment for the young dysphasic child, one must determine whether the primary problem is receptive (understanding speech), expressive (self-expression with speech), some combination of these two, or global (lacking "inner language"). The last condition represents a severe disorder in which the child cannot use symbols internally for thinking, and prognosis is poor regardless of therapy.

The dyslexic child has a problem in the reception of written symbols, and the dysgraphic child has a problem with expression of written symbols. Developmental dysphasia, dyslexia, and dysgraphia are closely related conditions and may be found together in the same patient or in members of the same family. Some children learn to speak adequately and are not recognized to be dyslexic until they fail to learn to read in school.

Therapy for any language disorder requires a total program in which the environment can be suitably structured and the therapy can be tailored to suit the child's individual needs. Speech therapy alone, or any

other single kind of therapy, is inadequate and unsuitable for such a child. An experienced team of specialists is usually required for reaching a diagnosis and for recommending appropriate language therapy.

Treatment plans for very young children with language disorders usually include sensory-motor activities: training in the motor bases of behavior, such as posture, the development of laterality and directionality, and the development of body image; training in perceptual skills, such as form perception, space discrimination, stereognosis, and recognition of texture, size, and structure; and training in auditory perception (listening), visual perception (looking), and kinesthetic perception (muscular memory of movements, positions, and posture). The child with a language disorder usually requires assistance in learning these skills, which are developmentally antecedent to language production per se.

Speech and hearing clinicians are now involved in the development and application of new assessment and intervention techniques for high-risk and developmentally delayed infants. They are valuable members of the interdisciplinary teams involved with parent-infant programming.

For those with severe communicative disorders, a number of augmentative systems are available. Manual communication using signs has been employed with mentally retarded, cerebral palsied, and autistic children. Communication boards may be used to facilitate communication for those with extensive motor problems. When such systems are used, the speech and language clinician's task is essentially the same as when oral language is taught—to train comprehension and production of language using the augmentative system.

The American Speech-Language-Hearing Association (ASHA) can provide information concerning speech correction facilities throughout the United States. Speech, language, and hearing specialists who are certified by ASHA are listed geographically and alphabetically in its annual directory, which is available at The American Speech-Language-Hearing Association, 10801 Rockville Pike, Rockville, Maryland 20852.

DISORDERS OF LEARNING
RUSSELL D. SNYDER, M.D.

Disorders of learning or learning disabilities occur in a heterogeneous group of school children and adults. Thus, it is unlikely that there will ever be one all-encompassing therapeutic modality. Considerable controversy exists regarding the etiology of the problem and the efficacy of the various therapies.

Disorders of learning are usually not circumscribed problems. Affected individuals manifest significant difficulties in one or several areas of performance. Problems may be found in the acquisition of skill in reading, listening, speaking, writing, mathematics, or reasoning. The disorder is not the direct result of mental retardation, sensory impairment, emotional disturbance, socioenvironmental influence, or attention deficit disorder. The development of subgroups, although potentially useful in therapy, has proven elusive.

The problem results in part from the emphasis of educational institutions on the necessity for success in the use of the written symbols of language. The problem is a behavioral and educational problem, and its biological basis remains controversial. It is a problem identified by educators, educational diagnosticians, and psychologists. Only secondarily does the physician become involved. However, because of the presumption of a biological basis and because of the significant family and social impact, physicians should become extensively involved. The student needs an advocate, counselor, and co-ordinator. The physician can fill these roles and assure access to rational and appropriate services at school or outside of school. Disorders of learning may lead to the development of secondary conditions in need of medical attention such as low self-esteem, depression, and acting-out behavior.

The major disorder of learning which is of concern to parents, educators, and physicians is reading disability, also known as developmental dyslexia. Developmental dyslexia and learning disability are sometimes considered synonymous terms, although purists would disagree. Disorders of learning exist in other areas such as music, athletics, and mathematics. However, difficulties in these other areas seldom become clinical problems.

Contrary to general perceptions, students disabled in reading are seldom nonreaders; rather, they are inefficient, slow, and poor readers. They are usually not students who seek reading activities. They may never become proficient in using the visual symbols of language. However, they usually attain levels of skill which enable them to handle commonly encountered reading materials with an acceptable degree of comprehension.

GENERALLY APPROVED THERAPIES

Special Education

Experts generally agree that the most effective interventions for disorders of learning are educational. This may include a diagnostic educational evaluation by a multidisciplinary team. The evaluation is performed to determine level of academic achievement and to direct the interventions. This is followed by the design of an individualized educational program (IEP). An attempt is made to build on strengths while remediating weaknesses and to teach strategies for learning. Tutoring, special classes, resource rooms, and full-time classes for the learning disabled may be appropriate. Other professionals besides educators may become involved. A speech therapist may be required to intervene in language disability and auditory processing disability. An occupational therapist may attempt to improve motor disability. A program should be long enough in duration to achieve meaningful results. This means that the program should continue for 1 or more years.

Private tutoring may be the most successful form of intervention, probably related in part to its anonymity. Support and encouragement are very important aspects

of management. Help may be needed in dealing with academic pressures and related social problems. Attention must be paid to the attainment of social success as well as academic success. Encouragement of nonacademic skills and out-of-school activities is appropriate. Family expectations for academic performance need to be realistic. Vocational and career counseling may be important interventions for the adolescent or adult. Educational intervention should be a pleasant and rewarding experience for the student.

The language arts consist of reading, writing, speaking, and listening. Speaking and listening hold equal importance with reading and writing for success outside the educational system. It is disappointing that educators pay so little attention to ability in speaking and listening and place overwhelming emphasis on reading and writing. Many affected individuals do well in oral-aural communication, and they should be encouraged in this modality.

Most of the learning-disabled population respond to some extent to a carefully structured, relatively traditional approach to their language problems. Caution must be exercised when a program claims results that are "too good to be true." Any program should reflect sensitivity to the needs of the individual.

Gains that occur with time and development are mistakenly attributed to therapy. In addition, there are nonspecific gains from the increased attention that the student receives. There is little realization among therapists of normal variation and of the need for use of control populations.

Psychopharmacology

Available pharmaceuticals include methylphenidate, dextroamphetamine, and pemoline. These stimulants do not directly treat the learning disability. They can lessen hyperactivity and distractibility in a student with an attention deficit disorder and make the student more amenable to classroom learning (see chapter on Attention Deficit Disorder for a more detailed discussion). However, not all children with a disorder of learning have attention deficit disorder. Tranquilizers and antidepressants do not appear to be effective unless major psychological problems coexist.

Psychological Therapies

Social, emotional, and family problems may accompany learning disability. If the problems are secondary to frustration and failure, intervention will not be useful unless the underlying cause is addressed. Psychological therapy, when appropriate, must be undertaken as part of an educational program. Individual psychotherapy may be indicated, or group and family therapy may be more appropriate. Such therapy must be constantly reevaluated to assure that the therapy is appropriate and not becoming another experience in frustration and failure.

Bypass Technique

Until more effective therapies appear, it is necessary to teach these children how to live with their problem and how to bypass it. If learning-disabled students are not taught bypass techniques, they will often learn such techniques themselves. A course with lectures may be more beneficial than a course with a heavy reading requirement. A multiple-choice test may be easier than an essay response. Oral examinations may be more appropriate than written examinations. Acceptable performance may be achieved if additional time is allowed. A typewriter may be easier than writing. Asking may be easier than looking up. Audiovisuals may be more useful than books.

Different students are probably receptive to different modalities of learning. Different modalities of learning during normal childhood development are just beginning to be recognized and certainly occur in those with learning disabilities. Excessive reliance on the printed word may be excluding some children from the educational system. Students should be allowed to show what they know rather than give evidence of their disability.

Students can be challenged to learn by doing rather than by just reading or listening. Activities could include drama, music, art, media/video, athletics, and field trips. This type of teaching would probably be beneficial to students of all reading abilities. The great tragedy of many programs is the absence of emphasis on a student's strengths.

Traditional Medical Therapies

Correction of any complicating medical problem is a necessity. Such complications include any chronic or acute disease, recurrent ear infections, defects in vision or learning, seizures, tics, sleep difficulties, depression, enuresis, encopresis, and allergies.

CONTROVERSIAL THERAPIES

The incomplete success of the generally approved therapies leads parents and teachers to search for alternate therapies. A great temptation exists, often born of desperation, to utilize any available therapy.

Neurophysiologic Retraining

Neurophysiologic retraining rests on the assumption that by stimulation of specific sensory inputs or by exercising specific motor patterns, improved function of the nervous system can be attained. The improvement is presumably acquired by retraining of the nervous system, with development of new circuits. Although widely practiced, the benefit from neurophysiologic retraining is uncertain and may be an additional burden for an already overburdened student.

Patterning

Patterning assumes that failure to pass through certain sequences of development in an orderly fashion reflects poor neurologic organization and may indicate brain damage. Remediation occurs through imposition of patterns of passive movement, rebreathing of expired air through a face mask, and restriction of fluid, salt, and sugar intake (Doman-Delacato). Patterning requires a large investment of time and personpower and is without experimental verification.

Optometric Visual Training

Visual training assumes that reading difficulty is a problem in peripheral visual perception and co-ordination. The presence of a visual defect should be excluded by a medical eye examination. Reading appears to be a peripheral visual process, although it is actually a cortical process. There is no known scientific evidence to support claims for improvement in reading based on eye muscle exercises, laterality training, balance board, or perceptual motor training. Eye problems such as jerky eye movements, strabismus, or poor eye-hand co-ordination do not cause reading disabilities. These therapies may only delay more appropriate remediation. Deficiencies in visual perception or in visual-motor functioning are as common in the general population as they are in learning-disabled children. Uneven visual pursuit movements may be compensatory for difficulty appreciating all the letters in a word at once; training to track symbols more evenly could interfere with this spontaneous compensation.

Vestibular Stimulation

Vestibular dysfunction is difficult to define. No relation has been demonstrated between an abnormality in the vestibular system and learning disabilities. Vestibular training consists of spinning or rocking. There is no evidence that vestibular responsivity correlates with academic performance or that vestibular function can be modified in a significant fashion by vestibular training.

Orthomolecular Medicine

Megavitamins. The use of megavitamins is based on the theory that some children have a genetic abnormality that produces a requirement for a specific nutrient that is greater than that of the general population. Benefit has not been established by experimentation. Megavitamins are ineffective in the management of learning disabilities, do not improve intellectual function, and have potential toxicity, especially when taken for a prolonged period of time.

Trace Elements. There is no support for the claim that deficiencies in trace elements cause learning disabilities or that learning disabilities improve with the addition of trace elements to the diet. Hair analysis is an inaccurate method for determination of mineral-deficient states.

Hypoglycemia

No data are available to support the view that treatment for hypoglycemia improves a disorder of learning.

Food Additives and Preservatives

Although elimination of food additives and preservatives may have a small success with attention deficit disorder, it has little place in the management of learning disabilities (see chapter on Attention Deficit Disorder).

Refined Sugars

Intake of refined sugars does not appear to be associated with classroom behavior or learning disabilities.

There is no basis for recommending a diet low in sugar for learning disabilities.

OTHER THERAPIES

Dyslexic subjects can identify letters in a wider peripheral visual field than controls, but the dyslexic subjects have a masking of letters between the foveal field and the near periphery. Dyslexics seem to learn to read outside of the foveal field used by normal subjects. This suggests the possibility of developing an alternative reading strategy for dyslexic children, teaching them to read using the part of the retina where letter identification is more accurate.

Interactive computer video displays enjoy some popularity. An attempt is made to teach words from context. This technique is in exploratory stages.

The theories regarding immune or endocrine abnormalities as an etiology of disorders of learning are as yet only theories. Any intervention in these areas solely to improve learning is unwarranted.

PROGNOSIS

A disorder of learning is a chronic problem, often persisting into adult life and requiring long-term attention and follow-up. The effects of the disorder are seen in adulthood as lower levels of school attainment, academic success, and social success.

SUMMARY

Remedial instruction in reading remains the keystone of therapy. However, such therapy must not be approached in a punitive fashion, must be a rewarding experience for the child, and must seek and emphasize strengths. Unsubstantiated treatments should be avoided. The primary goal is to develop the student's abilities, instill confidence, and restore self-esteem.

ATTENTION DEFICIT DISORDER

RUSSELL D. SNYDER, M.D.

Attention deficit disorder may occur with or without hyperactive behavior. The hyperactivity is often the feature that directs attention to the child. Attention deficit disorder seldom occurs in isolation but is part of a collection of problems in higher cortical function, which may include difficulty with cognition, communication, and social competence. In contrast to disorders of learning, in which therapy is educational and psychological in nature, attention deficit disorder has in addition pharmacologic intervention.

Pharmacologic approaches are sometimes appropriate for hyperactivity, impulsiveness, easy distractibility, and short attention span. While medication helps some of these children complete school-related tasks and makes them more receptive to the classroom setting, medication does not improve their basic intellectual capacity.

STIMULANT MEDICATION

Stimulant medication decreases aggressiveness, improves goal-directed activity, improves sustained attention, decreases impulsivity, improves learning of rote material, and improves performance on fine motor tasks in some children. Medication may be used in children showing attention deficit disorder without hyperactivity. The response to medication is not specific for attention deficit disorder; normal children show some of the same responses.

Merely writing a prescription for stimulant medication is not adequate management. Medication is not the panacea sought by educators and parents. Medication is indicated only when the problem is of sufficient magnitude that functional impairment is occurring and the problem is chronic. Impairment may be at school, at home, or in relationships with peers. Pharmacologic agents should not be used as the sole therapeutic modality but as part of a total program to modify behavior both at school and at home. Counseling, psychological help, behavior modification, family therapy, classroom placement, physical education, and activities outside of school are all important.

Pressure is great to modify the behavior of children who are disruptive in the classroom or at home. The physician must guard against indiscriminate prescribing at the request of school personnel and other professionals.

Methylphenidate

Methylphenidate is a mild central nervous system stimulant that is structurally similar to amphetamine. The initial dose is approximately 0.3 mg/kg/day, which can be gradually increased to 0.6 mg/kg/day. The medication should be administered once or twice a day, usually morning and midday. The maximum dose is about 0.8 mg/kg/day. Doses above 1 mg/kg/day appear to produce deterioration in performance and attention. Clinical response occurs about 2 hours after a dose. Tolerance may develop. Always titrate the dose to the child.

Methylphenidate is not recommended for children under 6 years of age, although it is commonly prescribed in this younger group. When used in younger children, it should probably be given only in the most severe cases which have not responded to a structured preschool setting. Some mentally retarded individuals with hyperactivity respond to the medication.

Seventy-five per cent of children with attention deficit disorder and hyperactivity benefit from use of a central nervous system stimulant, compared with 40 per cent on placebo. Withholding of medication on weekends and holidays may prevent some of the negative results of the medication. Parents can be permitted some discretion regarding a third daily dose. The use of a long-acting preparation does not seem to produce any added benefit.

Dextroamphetamine

Dextroamphetamine has a clinical response similar to that of methylphenidate. The peak effect occurs 3 to 4 hours after a dose. The recommended dose is one-half the dose of methylphenidate. Use of this long-acting preparation for hyperactivity has been disappointing. Dextroamphetamine is not recommended for children under 3 years of age. Tolerance may develop.

Pemoline

Pemoline, a mild central nervous system stimulant, is structurally unrelated to methylphenidate and relatively free of sympathomimetic activity. The dose is approximately 2 to 3 mg/kg/day. Once-a-day dosing is satisfactory. A single morning dose is usually all that is required. Clinical effect is not apparent for 3 to 4 weeks after the start of medication. Pemoline appears as useful as methylphenidate or dextroamphetamine and may have fewer undesirable side effects. It may be the most appropriate medication for adolescents, in whom the possibility of drug abuse is higher.

Caffeine

Caffeine is a mild central nervous system stimulant and readily available in beverages. It does not appear to be of benefit in children with attention deficit disorder.

ADVERSE RESPONSES TO STIMULANT MEDICATION

Weight loss may be noted at the beginning of therapy, which is probably secondary to reduction in appetite. Transient nocturnal wakefulness has occurred. Some children develop abdominal pain, irritability, nervousness, and increased sensitivity to criticism. There may be regression to a more infantile form of behavior. Hallucinations and depression have been noted. A small elevation in heart rate and blood pressure may occur, but this is inconsistent. An insignificant reduction in height has resulted but only when medication is given in very high doses. These medications may produce involuntary movements. Methylphenidate has been implicated in the precipitation of Tourette's syndrome and should probably not be used in a child with tics or with a family history of tics. Exacerbation of symptoms of schizophrenia, depression, and autism has occurred with these medications and upon withdrawal of the medications. Stimulant medications do not appear to precipitate seizures in children with seizure disorders.

Dependence is rare. Children who have taken these medications do not have a higher incidence of drug abuse in later life. Methylphenidate and dextroamphetamine have been abused as "street drugs." A vocal lobby has been insisting that physicians and pharmaceutical companies are working together to drug children into submission.

ANTIDEPRESSANTS

The tricyclic antidepressants improve the symptoms of attention deficit disorder in some patients. Imipramine and desipramine have been used. Response to these medications has not been as consistent as the response to central nervous system stimulants. Their greatest usefulness may be in the older child with attention deficit disorder, school failure, social adjustment difficulty, and depression.

DIET

Food additives and preservatives have been implicated in the etiology of hyperactivity. Elimination of foods containing artificial colors and flavors, salicylates, and certain other additives has been proposed as treatment for hyperactivity (Feingold diet). The diet seems to hold no physical danger. Dietary management may be helpful to a small subset of hyperactive children (1 to 2 per cent).

ENVIRONMENTAL MANIPULATION

Environmental manipulation is appropriate before the use of medication. The management of environmental aspects is probably more important than any pharmacologic management. The classroom setting must be able to cope with the special requirements of these children. The teacher must be tolerant of a child who does not respond to the usual classroom controls. This may require a special classroom and a special curriculum. These children usually respond to a more structured classroom. Individual tutoring may be helpful. The institution of behavior modification techniques is of some benefit. Counseling may be necessary for the student and the student's family.

Teachers should be discouraged from attributing classroom success of a medicated child to the medication. A child with attention deficit disorder is just as worthy of praise for individual accomplishments as any other child. Whether classmates should know that the child is on medication constitutes an important issue. This is a reason for an attempt to avoid the midday dose given in school.

Attention deficit disorder is associated with disorders of learning, and any program for management should not neglect this aspect. Greatest success occurs when a plan combines medication with environmental manipulation in a program specifically designed for children with attention deficit disorder.

OTHER THERAPIES

Orthomolecular therapy is discussed in the chapter on learning disabilities. This therapy is not useful for attention deficit disorder.

Lead intoxication is not the cause of the symptoms in most children with attention deficit disorder. However, lead intoxication should be considered in children with a history of pica or significant environmental exposure. Treatment consists of removal from the toxic environment.

PROGNOSIS

Consideration in management should be given to the possibility of an unfavorable long-term outcome. Low self-esteem, persistent impulsivity, alcohol abuse, poor academic achievement, and frequent court appearances have been noted in follow-up of some cases. In treatment, it is necessary for the physician to realize that this is a chronic condition with implications for adult life.

3

Nervous System

HEAD INJURY

RICHARD H. STRAUSS, M.D.

Five million children suffer head injury in the United States each year, 250,000 of whom are hospitalized; 4000 die and 15,000 have prolonged hospitalization and rehabilitation. Approximately 5 per cent of all hospitalized children are admitted because of head injury. Most of those patients are hospitalized for assessment of neurologic status and for monitoring the development of intracranial complications; less commonly they are hospitalized for immediate treatment of their injuries. Despite these figures, over 99 per cent of children with head injury have normal outcomes, and of children in coma secondary to head injury, at least 60 per cent of the survivors return to their preinjury condition. Most minor head injuries are treated by pediatricians (or parents, babysitters, or school nurses, who may contact a pediatrician) in emergency rooms or in offices.

EXTRACRANIAL INJURY

Scalp lacerations should be inspected for foreign material, cleaned, and repaired with suture material or sterile tapes, making certain the apposed wound is free of hair. If lacerations extend to the skull or beyond, further investigation may be warranted to check the integrity of the dura and the brain. Tetanus immunization status should be reviewed and appropriate treatment provided.

Hematomas of the scalp usually resolve within several weeks after the injury (although some go on to calcify). Aspiration of subgaleal hematomas or cephalohematomas is not recommended and may in fact be a cause of further hemorrhage or infection. Some scalp hematomas have sharply edged borders so similar to the edges of a depressed skull fracture that a tangential skull x-ray view may be necessary to differentiate the two.

SKULL FRACTURE

Many patients who have suffered minor head injury have skull x-rays taken, even though the patients appear normal on examination. Those x-rays sometimes demonstrate linear skull fractures. Unless the history of the accident is unusual or unknown, or the child has abnormal findings on physical and neurologic examinations, hospitalization is not required. (Temporal swelling/fracture and swelling/fracture across the sagittal suture, pathways that cross important blood supplies, are indications for hospitalization in the view of some experts.) Guidelines for parents ("head injury sheets"), to be used while observing their child at home, and availability of the pediatrician to answer parents' questions are reasonable alternatives to hospitalization. Observation over a period of several hours in an office or emergency room with repeated neurologic examinations before discharge home with a "head injury sheet" is another acceptable alternative to hospitalization. Skull x-ray examinations are not necessary or diagnostically helpful for patients with minor head injury. Similarly, lumbar puncture is not a useful procedure for diagnosis or treatment of the child with a head injury.

Depressed skull fracture should be considered when a palpable depression or a large swelling is felt on the skull. Tangential skull x-ray is usually adequate for diagnosis unless there are other abnormalities on examination suggesting intracranial injury, which would make emergency unenhanced computed tomography a more desirable examination. Surgical elevation of a depressed skull fracture depends on the depth of the depression (greater than 5 to 10 mm), the presence of a dural tear or compound fracture, and the presence of neurologic abnormalities. Whether elevation of a depressed skull fracture stems the occurrence of post–head injury epilepsy is not known.

Diastatic fractures occur along the lambdoid and sagittal sutures in young children, and in the absence of other neurologic findings rarely lead to problems; therefore, they require no specific treatment other than the guidelines already mentioned.

Basilar skull fracture involves the basal sections of the frontal, ethmoid, sphenoid, parietal, or occipital bones. Basilar fractures are more often diagnosed from physical findings (mastoid or periorbital ecchymosis, CSF otorrhea, CSF rhinorrhea, hemotympanum) than from radiographic studies. Basilar skull fracture is associated with dural tear and communication with the paranasal sinuses or the middle ear, so that patients are at risk for the development of meningitis. Studies have not shown that antibiotic prophylaxis (against the most common infecting organism, *Pneumococcus*) decreases the incidence of meningitis following basilar skull fracture. Cerebrospinal fluid rhinorrhea and otorrhea usually cease spontaneously by 1 week after the injury. Should a CSF leak persist longer than 2 weeks, radionuclide examination of the CSF can help localize the leak. Patients with hemotympanum should have tympanographic and audiologic follow-up after discharge from the hospital or office. Hospitalization is not necessary when basilar skull fracture is unaccompanied by more serious injuries (or CSF leak).

Children with linear, diastatic, and basilar skull fracture associated with dural tear are at risk for the development of "growing fractures" several months after the accident, and they should be followed clinically and radiographically.

INTRACRANIAL INJURY

The child who has sustained a mild closed head injury with a period of unconsciousness not longer than 5 minutes can usually be observed at home if the results of physical and neurologic examinations are normal and reliable observation at home can be guaranteed over the next day (with "head injury sheets" that tell parents how to monitor changes in level of consciousness, motor activity, pupillary activity, behavior, sleep habits, and breathing patterns). In addition, parents should be told to observe carefully for neurologic and behavior changes and fever over the next few weeks. If reliable observation in the home cannot be guaranteed, hospitalization is necessary. In either situation, hourly observation over a period of 6 to 24 hours should be instituted, and if the child remains stable, observation may become less frequent. Should a change in the level of consciousness occur, neurologic examination must be repeated, and CT scanning to check for the presence of an intracranial hemorrhage or cerebral edema should be done. The decision to admit a comatose child is not a difficult choice. It is much more difficult to determine the risk that a healthy-looking child has of developing an intracranial complication following minor head injury. The child with minor closed head injury who has abnormal findings on neurologic examination even in the absence of obvious head injury should not be sent home. Any child who has altered consciousness, focal central nervous system abnormalities, or signs of worsening illness should be hospitalized and should undergo CT scanning.

Severe closed head injury has many anatomic forms, several of which are discussed in other sections of this text. It is frequently (but not always) associated with prolonged (longer than 5 to 10 minutes) loss of consciousness, altered state of consciousness (disorientation, unarousability, delirium), seizures, focal neurologic signs, abnormal vital signs, persistent headache, and other physical signs of major trauma. In addition to localizing and describing the intracranial injury by CT scanning, and determining whether it is a surgically remediable lesion, intensive care to the injured brain must be provided to optimize blood flow to the brain and to minimize the possibility of herniation and ischemia. At the same time, support of other body systems must be maintained and neck stabilization must be secured. Endotracheal intubation provides airway protection and a route for pulmonary toilet and mechanical ventilation as well as a means for hyperventilation (Pco_2 approximately 25 to 30 mm Hg) to decrease arterial Pco_2, thereby avoiding cerebral vasodilatation and increased intracranial pressure (normal ICP is less than 15 mm Hg, or 200 mm H_2O). Intubation itself is a noxious stimulus, and it should be done by the most experienced person present in order to avoid acute severe rises in ICP. Intubation should be preceded by hyperventilation with 100 per cent O_2. Arterial Po_2 should be maintained at a level greater than 100 mm Hg.

Fluid and electrolyte therapy must be titrated to the patient's skin perfusion, heart rate, urine production, insensible water loss, weight change, and degree of cerebral edema/increased ICP, but as a rule, two-thirds fluid maintenance is a reasonable starting point. Hypovolemic shock does not usually result from head injury unless there is major scalp bleeding. Shock is treated with volume infusion even in the presence of increased ICP. Serum electrolytes and osmolarity should be monitored frequently in order to avoid (or treat) hyponatremia (caused by inappropriate ADH secretion) or severe hyperosmolarity. There is no evidence that corticosteroids help reduce cerebral edema/increased ICP secondary to severe head injury. Antacids (0.5 ml/kg via nasogastric tube every 2 hours if gastric pH is less than 4) should be given to patients with severe head injury irrespective of steroid administration.

Increased ICP can be avoided in some patients and treated in other patients by simple maneuvers designed to maintain cerebral perfusion pressure (CPP) over 50 mm Hg. From the equation, CPP = mean arterial pressure − ICP, it is apparent that if ICP rises or mean arterial pressure falls, cerebral perfusion pressure and cerebral blood flow may become inadequate. (Invasive monitoring of ICP and arterial pressure is necessary if cranial nerve dysfunction, apnea, posturing, and/or Glasgow Coma score less than 8 are present.) Methods to decrease ICP are elevation of the head to 30 degrees, midline positioning of the head so that venous return is not impeded, avoidance of noxious stimuli, a trial of intravenous lidocaine (1.5 mg/kg/dose) before endotracheal suctioning, chest percussion and endotracheal suctioning that follow hyperventilation, maintenance of normal temperature to avoid shivering, paralysis with pancuronium (0.1 mg/kg intravenously, given every 1 to 3 hours as needed), and sedation with diazepam (0.1 to 0.25 mg/kg/dose IV every 1 to 2 hours) or morphine (0.05 to 0.1 mg/kg/dose IV every 2 to 4 hours) or midazolam (0.1 to 0.2 mg/kg/dose IV every 1 to 2 hours) unless sedation is believed to interfere with accuracy of the neurologic examination.

Acute ICP elevation over 20 mm Hg can be treated with hyperventilation, hypertonic osmotic agents (mannitol 0.25 to 2.0 gm/kg/dose IV over 20 minutes every

1 to 4 hours; glycerol 10 per cent in a maintenance dextrose-electrolyte solution, 0.25 to 0.50 gm/kg/dose intravenously over 30 minutes every 2 hours, or by continuous infusion: 0.5 gm/kg over 30 minutes, then 0.5 gm/kg glycerol over 90 minutes, every 2 hours), and drainage of small aliquots (0.5 to 1.0 ml) of CSF. Osmotic agents may be given along with furosemide or ethacrynic acid (1 mg/kg/dose intravenously). Craniectomy, hypothermia, and pentobarbital infusion may be considered if other treatments fail. If inadequate mean arterial pressure is the cause of low cerebral perfusion pressure, intravenous fluid administration and pressor agents may be necessary as well as measurement of central venous pressure.

Phenytoin (15 to 18 mg/kg intravenously as a loading dose, no faster than 0.75 mg/kg/min, then 5 to 7 mg/kg/day orally or intravenously over 30 minutes, divided in two daily doses) is recommended as an anticonvulsant when seizures occur in children with head injury because it does not usually have an effect on the level of consciousness. It is unclear how long anticonvulsant therapy should continue, so patients treated with phenytoin should be followed for subsequent seizures even beyond the 6- to 12-month seizure-free period of suggested anticonvulsant treatment. Patients with early seizures, those occurring in the first week after head injury, are less likely to develop subsequent epilepsy than those patients with seizures developing after the first week.

Nutritional status should be discussed early in the patient's hospitalization, and consideration should be given to hyperalimentation or nasogastric feeding when it becomes clear that the patient will not be able to take food by mouth.

Approximately 10 per cent of survivors of prolonged coma following severe head injury have persistent, severe intellectual and motor deficits. Early diagnosis of intracranial injury, cerebral edema, and increased ICP helps lead to definitive care of those problems, thereby improving the outcome of patients with severe closed head injury. Some patients with mild or moderate head injury may develop subtle learning disorders and behavioral problems despite seemingly excellent recovery; such patients may benefit from psychometric evaluation and appropriate treatment.

CEREBRAL EDEMA

EMILY D. FRIEDMAN, M.D.,
and DARRYL C. DE VIVO, M.D.

Cerebral edema is most commonly seen in the pediatric population in the setting of trauma, but it may also complicate encephalitis, Reye syndrome, hypoxic injury, poisoning, and stroke. If early vigorous treatment is instituted, the vicious circle, whereby brain swelling aggravates ischemia of adjacent, marginally perfused brain, can be interrupted. Children, unlike adults, can recover to nearly normal and sometimes *entirely* normal levels of functioning if cerebral edema is recognized early and treated aggressively.

Steps in the management of cerebral edema fall under the following headings: positioning, hyperventilation, fluid management and osmotic agents, blood pressure control, thermoregulation, and CSF drainage. High-dose barbiturate therapy to control intracranial pressure is a last, but sometimes effective, measure.

Positioning

On first presentation to the ER or ICU, the patient should be positioned head up at 30 degrees from the horizontal and in neutral, eyes-forward position. Exceptions to this rule occur when spinal cord injury is suspected or the patient is in shock. Then, the supine position is preferred. Head elevation is the single most rapid and efficient maneuver to lower raised intracranial pressure (ICP). Eyes-forward positioning of the head ensures that jugular venous drainage can be maximal, whereas turning the head 60 degrees can compress the ipsilateral jugular vein.

During the early phases of injury, increases in cerebral blood volume are a major cause of increased brain volume and elevated ICP. Therefore, treatment is directed toward (1) reducing cerebral blood volume to the minimum needed to ensure adequate perfusion and (2) reducing the swings in blood volume that occur secondary to impaired autoregulation seen in injured brain. With head elevation, gravity helps lower cerebral blood volume.

Hyperventilation

In the setting of acute cerebral edema with a child who has CT scan evidence of increased ICP (and no surgically treatable lesion), it may be wise to intubate the child in order to obtain hyperventilation. Second to positioning, the most effective treatment for cerebral edema is controlled hyperventilation to reduce the P_{CO_2} initially to 28 to 30 torr, and if necessary to 25 torr. Here again, intracranial volume is reduced by vasoconstriction causing decreased blood volume. The P_{O_2} should be maintained at or above 100 torr if possible. A comatose child should be paralyzed (with a nondepolarizing muscle relaxant such as vecuronium, 0.1 mg/kg), and the lethargic child warrants an anesthetic such as thiopental, 5 mg/kg, prior to endotracheal tube placement. Sedation should be continued as long as hyperventilation is required, since suctioning and pulmonary toilet are noxious stimuli that raise systolic arterial pressure (SAP) and may thereby elevate ICP when cerebral autoregulation is impaired. Coughing elevates ICP, and therefore suctioning should be gentle. Small doses of morphine sulfate (0.1 to 0.15 mg/kg) are ideal prior to suctioning or other stimuli. P_{CO_2} should not be reduced below 22 torr because cerebral vasoconstriction to this degree may worsen brain ischemia.

Fluid Management and Osmotic Agents

The rationale for using osmotic agents is to create a hyperosmolar gradient between the blood and brain so that water is removed from the brain tissue compartment. This gradient will reduce brain volume. Mannitol is used at doses of 0.25 to 0.5 gm/kg and administered intravenously at 4- to 6-hour intervals. Increasing the dose usually is not more effective but may prolong the dosing time interval. During osmotic diuresis, serum osmolarity and electrolytes should be checked every 4 hours. Most patients tolerate a serum osmolarity between 290 and 320 mOsm/L. The serum sodium should not exceed 150 mEq/L. Total 24-hour fluid intake and output should be carefully monitored.

Occasionally SIADH (syndrome of inappropriate antidiuretic hormone secretion) occurs in the setting of cerebral edema, and the safest treatment for this "water intoxication" is to restrict intravenous fluids (one-half to two-thirds of daily maintenance). The intravenous composition should be 5 per cent glucose in half-normal sodium chloride. Diabetes insipidus following trauma, often an end-stage phenomenon, carries a grim prognosis. Aqueous Pitressin, 0.1 to 0.25 ml (1 to 5 units), is given subcutaneously two to three times daily to control free water loss.

Placement of an intracranial pressure monitoring device (Richmond screw, Ladd epidural catheter, or Camino ventricular monitor) aids in the management of the patient by providing minute-to-minute ICP measurements. Mannitol dosing can then be determined by using ICP criteria: ICP greater than 20 (for longer than 5 to 10 minutes) warrants a mannitol dose. However, these monitors do require surgery and pose an infection risk, so experienced personnel should insert them.

Blood Pressure Control

The systolic arterial pressure should be maintained between 100 and 160 mm Hg. Since autoregulation may be impaired in the injured brain, changes in systemic blood pressure will be immediately transmitted to the brain. Systolic blood pressure above 160 mm Hg may (1) elevate ICP and (2) threaten hemorrhage into contused brain. Therefore, hypertension should be treated with morphine sulfate (0.1 to 0.15 mg/kg) or hydralazine (1.7 to 3.5 mg/kg IM/IV). Nitroprusside should be avoided, since it causes cerebral vasodilation.

Hypotension should be avoided, of course, since it worsens intracranial ischemia by lowering cerebral perfusion.

Thermoregulation

Hyperthermia (body temperature greater than 38°C) should be treated with a cooling blanket and Tylenol suppositories, since brain metabolic demand and blood flow increase with higher temperatures. Body temperature should not be lowered below normal, and extreme hypothermia warrants a heating blanket.

Cerebrospinal Fluid Drainage

As discussed above, the objective in treating cerebral edema is the reduction of intracranial volume. The removal of CSF after placement of a ventricular drain may make a significant difference in reducing ICP. The drain may be placed in the ventricular cavity by an experienced surgeon while the patient remains in the ICU, and CSF drainage can be regulated by (1) adjusting the height of the drainage chamber relative to the patient's head or (2) placing a one-way valve in the tubing between the ventricular drain and the drainage bag. Antibiotics (oxacillin 50 mg/kg/day or vancomycin 40 mg/kg/day) directed against common skin pathogens such as *Staphylococcus epidermidis* should be given intravenously if ventricular drainage is initiated. In general, the drain should be removed after 7 to 8 days because of the risk of CSF infection.

High-dose barbiturate therapy for uncontrollable ICP is a last resort when all other measures have been fully exhausted or patients have become refractory to treatment. This requires a highly experienced ICU team. A loading dose of pentobarbital (3 to 5 mg/kg) is given intravenously slowly, and a serum level of 3 to 7 mg/dl is maintained. Complications include hypothermia and hypotension. Barbiturates cannot be abruptly discontinued but must be withdrawn slowly over days.

In summary, cerebral edema should be treated expeditiously and aggressively. The patient should have head elevation and should be intubated for hyperventilation. Mannitol, and if necessary, CSF drainage can both lower persistently elevated ICP. Noxious stimuli should be minimized, and seizures, if they occur, should be controlled promptly with intravenous anticonvulsants (phenytoin sodium 15 to 20 mg/kg or phenobarbital 10 to 15 mg/kg, loading dosages given intravenously slowly). Steroids are used, since they may have a "protective" effect on brain tissue, but the mechanism is unknown. Dexamethasone is the preferred steroid, given intravenously in large doses of 0.2 to 0.4 mg/kg every 4 to 6 hours.

EXTRADURAL AND SUBDURAL HEMATOMA

JAMES M. DRAKE

EXTRADURAL HEMATOMA

Extradural hemorrhage occurs between the skull and dura as a result of tearing of an artery or vein. The artery is usually the middle meningeal or one of its branches. Venous sources include the dural venous sinuses, meningeal veins, emissary veins, or the diploë of the bone itself.

Extradural hematomas are rare, occurring in approximately 2 per cent of children hospitalized for head injury. Their importance is twofold: (1) the rapidity with which these patients may deteriorate, and (2) the good outcome that may be expected should the hematoma be evacuated in time. All efforts should therefore be made to identify these patients early and direct them to prompt neurosurgical care.

Extradural hematomas occur most commonly in children over the age of 10 years. This may be related to the difficulty with which the dura is stripped in younger children. Vehicular injuries are the most common traumatic event in this age group, whereas falls are more commonly responsible in infants and younger children. Unfortunately, there is often nothing that distinguishes children harboring one of these hematomas from the full spectrum of mild to severe head-injured patients.

The classic loss of consciousness, followed by a lucid period, followed by progressive signs of transtentorial herniation, occurs in less than one third of patients.

Skull fractures are seen on plain radiographs in only half of patients. CT scanning reveals the "lentiform" high-density lesion most commonly in the temporoparietal area. The CT scan also reveals the shift of the midline structures, the size of the basal cisterns, and the presence of other lesions such as parenchymal hemorrhages and edema. In acute hematomas, a low-density swirl within the clot indicates ongoing arterial hemorrhage.

Extradural hematomas may be "delayed" and not seen on an initial CT scan. Persistent symptoms in a head-injured child should prompt reinvestigation. Asymptomatic or "chronic" extradural hemorrhages are occasionally detected days following injury. Neurosurgical advice regarding their management should be sought.

The occurrence of drowsiness, hemiparesis, and pupillary dilatation are ominous signs of transtentorial herniation. These children require immediate intravenous access, intubation and hyperventilation, and the administration of mannitol 1 gm/kg concurrently with urinary catheterization. In this setting, evacuation of the hematoma is urgent. In centers remote from neurosurgical care, immediate burr hole exploration must be considered prior to transport.

The outcome following evacuation of these lesions is generally excellent. Major morbidity or death still occurs in about 10 per cent of patients either from delay in treatment or from concurrent injury to the brain or other organ system.

SUBDURAL HEMATOMA

Subdural hemorrhage occurs in the potential space between the arachnoid and dura. This space is freely distensible, and these clots tend to spread over the convexity of the hemisphere. They result either from the tearing of a draining cortical vein which traverses this space or from laceration of a cortical artery or vein following direct injury to the brain.

In the acute form, a large clot compressing the underlying hemisphere and producing shift of the midline structures is in fact unusual. More commonly there is a small "slick" of subdural blood. In this case, the depression of consciousness is a result of coexisting parenchymal injury, which may be any combination of diffuse shear injury, cortical contusions and hemorrhage, and edema. These hematomas occur after the usual forms of accidental trauma in children. They can also occur following birth trauma, in which case they are commonly in the posterior fossa.

Subdural hemorrhage is an important marker of nonaccidental trauma in infants. The hemorrhages are thought to occur with the violent shaking of the head. Retinal hemorrhages are commonly associated. Direct cranial trauma including skull fracture or parenchymal injury from blows to the head may coexist.

Management includes the same resuscitation measures as for any head-injured child, including the search for other organ system injuries. Seizures are a frequent accompaniment, and prolonged or repeated seizures should be treated with anticonvulsants. For children under 2 years of age, intravenous phenobarbital is given as a 10 to 20 mg/kg loading dose, followed by a 5 to 10 mg/kg/day maintenance dose. Children over 2 can be treated with phenytoin, 15 mg/kg loading dose followed by a 5 to 10 mg/kg/day maintenance dose.

CT scanning is crucial in assessing the extent of injury and planning treatment. Large subdural hematomas require evacuation. Otherwise children with a Glasgow Coma Scale score of less than 8 require admission to a neurosurgical intensive care unit and intracranial pressure monitoring. Elevated intracranial pressure is treated by elevation of the head, maintenance of normothermia, hyperventilation to a P_{CO_2} of 25 to 30, and muscle paralysis. If these measures fail to control the intracranial pressure, then mannitol 1 gm/kg by intravenous bolus up to 4 gm/kg in 24 hours is given. This can be followed by furosemide, 1 mg/kg/dose up to four doses per 24 hours. These patients require close monitoring of fluid and electrolyte balance. Steroids have not been proven to be of any benefit, nor has "barbiturate coma," although the latter is still employed when all other efforts to control intracranial hypertension have failed.

The outcome in children with acute subdural hematomas is largely determined by the other coexisting brain injuries. Over half the patients presenting with a Glasgow Coma Scale score of less than 7 die or are left severely disabled.

Chronic subdural hematomas have undergone some degree of clot dissolution through degradation. Long-standing subdural hematomas have an external vascularized membrane that is prone to rebleeding. Young infants may present with only an enlarging head. Older children may present with signs of raised intracranial pressure and contralateral weakness. Children with coagulopathies are at increased risk following minor trauma. These collections need to be distinguished from benign enlargements of the subarachnoid space, postmeningitic effusions, and subdural empyema. Treatment consists of drainage, either via a burr hole or by a subdural peritoneal shunt. Recurrence of subdural hematoma is rare, and a good outcome is to be expected.

INTRACRANIAL HEMORRHAGE

MICHAEL J. NOETZEL, M.D.

Intracranial hemorrhage encompasses all forms of bleeding within the head, including bleeding into the parenchyma of the brain as well as subarachnoid, subdural, and epidural hemorrhages. The diverse nature of intracranial hemorrhage is reflected in its multiple etiologies and modes of presentation, although certain specific age-dependent factors and clinical syndromes can be identified.

NEONATAL PERIOD

Intracranial hemorrhage represents a significant problem in neonatal medicine owing to its high frequency and resultant serious neurologic sequelae. Periventricular-intraventricular hemorrhage is the most common and serious hemorrhage in the premature infant, occurring in 40 to 50 per cent of newborns less than 35 weeks' gestation.

Ideally, management of periventricular-intraventricular hemorrhage consists of preventative measures, either to eliminate premature birth or to minimize prophylactically those factors responsible for the hemorrhage. At present, however, treatment is for the most part supportive. Every effort should be made to maintain normal cerebral perfusion and thus decrease the possibility that the hemorrhage will be extended. A prerequisite of successful management is the normalization of arterial blood pressure through careful fluid balance. Acidosis, hypoxia, and hypercapnea, all of which may cause cerebral hyperperfusion, must be minimized by controlled respiration. For similar reasons, seizures and apnea must also be recognized early and effectively managed. Elevated intracranial pressure, if documented at the time of CSF exam, may be treated by serial lumbar punctures. This latter form of therapy may also be of benefit in slowly evolving posthemorrhagic ventricular dilatation, as are medications that decrease CSF production, such as acetazolamide* (100 mg/kg/day), furosemide (1 mg/kg/day), and glycerol (1 to 2 gm/kg q6h).

Newborns with rapidly progressive ventriculomegaly usually require an external ventriculostomy. Since the incidence of infectious complications increases significantly after 5 to 7 days, the ventriculostomy must be removed at that time. Such a temporizing measure may allow resolution of other critical problems that render the child a poor risk for surgical placement of an internal shunt. On occasion the ventriculostomy may actually prevent the development of hydrocephalus. More commonly, however, the progressive nature of the condition necessitates utilization of a ventriculoperitoneal shunt.

Other forms of neonatal intracranial hemorrhage, while not as common as periventricular-intraventricular hemorrhage, have similar pathogenic and clinical features. In incipient herniation, rapid surgical evacuation of a subdural or intraparenchymal hemorrhage may prove life-saving. Cerebral convexity hematomas can often be treated with only subdural taps, in which a blunt 22-gauge 1/2-inch needle is carefully placed through the lateral edge of the anterior fontanel into the subdural collection of blood. Indications for repeated taps include recurrence of neurologic symptoms or disproportionate head growth. Primary subarachnoid hemorrhage usually requires only the supportive measures previously described, unless the rare complication of hydrocephalus supervenes.

INFANTS AND CHILDREN

Trauma is the major cause of intracranial hemorrhage in infants and children. Unfortunately, many of the traumatic injuries are nonaccidental, resulting from child abuse.

Initially management should be directed toward ensuring adequate ventilation and circulation. Once the patient's condition has been stabilized, a computed tomographic (CT) scan should be obtained. In cases of clear-cut trauma with incipient brain stem herniation, subdural taps prior to CT evaluation may be both diagnostic and life-saving. Conversely, lumbar punctures have little role in the management of traumatic intracranial hemorrhage unless infection is a consideration. In any event, they should be avoided, at least until a mass lesion has been excluded by CT examination. Epidural and, less frequently, subdural hematomas may require surgical evacuation of the blood clot, especially when there is progressive deterioration. Intracerebral hemorrhage can usually be managed conservatively with strict limitation of activity and close observation in an intensive care unit. The fluid status should be monitored carefully, as diabetes insipidus or inappropriate antidiuretic hormone secretion can follow from trauma. A clinically significant increase in intracranial pressure requires placement of a monitoring device. The elevated pressure is then managed initially by controlled ventilation to lower P_{CO_2} to 22 to 25 mm Hg and by fluid restriction. High doses of barbiturates can also be employed to reduce cerebral edema, as can hypothermia. In patients with diffuse hemorrhage, osmotic agents such as mannitol (1 to 2 gm/kg of a 20 per cent solution administered intravenously over 15 to 20 minutes) and furosemide (1 mg/kg intravenously) may also be helpful in decreasing cerebral edema. Such agents are contraindicated in focal hematomas unless used as a temporizing measure prior to surgery, since they may cause rebleeding.

In all types of intracranial hemorrhage, the immediate goal of therapy is to stabilize the child. Surgical evacuation of accessible aneurysms is at present the most prudent course producing the lowest subsequent morbidity and mortality. In addition, an infectious source of the aneurysm such as subacute bacterial endocarditis should be sought and treated appropriately. In arteriovenous malformations, the indications for surgery are less clear, reflecting to a large degree the often inaccessible location of the malformation.

Another common cause of intracranial hemorrhage in children is bleeding into an area of infarction, usually the result of arterial or venous thrombosis. Such a pattern may be seen in children with sickle cell anemia, congenital cyanotic heart disease, and abnormal lipoprotein metabolism. Treatment consists of supportive measures as previously defined. Careful management of fluid status is especially critical in sickle cell disease, congenital cyanotic heart disease, and other high-viscosity states, since excessive restriction of fluids may produce extension of the hemorrhagic infarction while liberalization may potentiate cerebral edema. In hemorrhage secondary to emboli or a hypercoagulable condition, anticoagulation in the form of heparin (100 units/kg IV q4h) may be of value. Maintenance therapy would then consist of dipyridamole (Persantine), aspirin, or warfarin sodium (Coumadin).

---

*This use of acetazolamide is not listed by the manufacturer; in addition, this dosage is higher than manufacturer recommends for other uses.

Systemic diseases may produce intracranial hemorrhage, usually as a result of a hypocoagulable state. Approximately 25 per cent of children with hemophilia sustain central nervous system hemorrhage, often following incidental head trauma. Persistent complaints, usually headaches, should be evaluated with a CT scan. Treatment consists of previously described support and the administration of appropriate clotting factors to achieve a level of 50 per cent of normal. Intracranial hemorrhage is also common in leukemia, although the bleeding may reflect either hyperviscosity (acute leukemia with increased numbers of circulating white cells) or hypocoagulability (advanced stage of the disease with resultant thrombocytopenia). In both situations, fresh frozen plasma should be administered to increase the level of circulating platelets, in addition to treatment with standard chemotherapeutic measures.

HYDROCEPHALUS

MICHAEL J. NOETZEL, M.D.

Hydrocephalus is characterized by an increased amount of cerebrospinal fluid (CSF) within the ventricular system, often under elevated pressure. The causes of hydrocephalus are varied, but all result in either an impairment of CSF absorption within the subarachnoid space (communicating hydrocephalus) or an obstruction of CSF flow within the ventricles (noncommunicating hydrocephalus). Regardless of the cause, early diagnosis and appropriate long-term management of hydrocephalus are imperative given the progressive cerebral damage that can result from this condition.

The management of hydrocephalus centers on three major areas: initial relief of the hydrocephalus, treatment of complications arising from shunting of CSF, and management of problems related to the effects of hydrocephalus on normal psychomotor development. A mass lesion such as a tumor or cyst not uncommonly may cause obstruction to the flow of CSF. In these instances, the hydrocephalus may be corrected by surgical removal of the mass.

Shunt Procedures. Most children with hydrocephalus, however, require primary drainage of the CSF from the ventricles to an extracranial compartment, usually the peritoneum or vascular system. The majority of shunt systems today consist of a ventricular catheter, a flush pump, a unidirectional flow valve, and a distal catheter. A reservoir is often added to allow direct access to the ventricular system for instillation of chemotherapy agents or antibiotics and removal of fluid. The valves open at predetermined CSF pressure levels and are selected to fit an individual patient's need. High-pressure valves (60 to 120 mm H_2O) are utilized to prevent complications from rapid decompression of the ventricles, most commonly subdural hematomas. Long-standing hydrocephalus in most children can be treated with medium-pressure valves (40 to 60 mm H_2O). Low-pressure valves (0 to 40 mm H_2O) are often used in small infants.

A single shunt procedure is rarely curative; revisions are usually required, since fixed catheter lengths can accommodate only limited growth. The ventriculoperitoneal (VP) shunt is the preferred form of initial management, especially in neonates and young infants, since there is a greater allowance for excess tubing, thus minimizing the number of revisions. The ventriculoatrial (VA) shunt is usually reserved for those older children whose somatic growth is nearly complete. The VA shunt is contraindicated in patients with cardiopulmonary disease or elevated CSF protein (over 250 mg/dl) and should be avoided when the CSF has been recently infected.

Elective lengthening of a shunt should be a routine procedure in the management of all children with extracranial shunts. If the initial shunt is placed within the first 3 to 4 months of age, revisions at 18 to 24 months, at 4 to 6 years, and at an age when approximately 80 per cent of adult height is reached (usually 10 to 12 years) are recommended. Compared with emergency shunt revisions, elective procedures are performed with fewer complications and, as part of a management program predicated on frequent clinical and radiologic evaluations, have been shown to control hydrocephalus and preserve brain function better.

SHUNT MALFUNCTION. The most commonly observed shunt complication is mechanical obstruction, which occurs in 20 to 40 per cent of children with shunts. The obstruction may occur at either end of the catheter but usually is the result of obstruction within the ventricles. Distally the malfunction is often secondary to thrombosis (VA shunts) or linear growth, which displaces the catheter from the peritoneum (VP shunts). Shunt obstruction may present as an emergency; the clinical manifestations are those of acutely raised intracranial pressure, often with a worsening of a previously noted neurologic deficit. In the more indolent cases, alterations in behavior such as lethargy, irritability, a sudden drop in grades, and episodic emesis are common. In some children, progressive cranial enlargement is the only evidence of obstruction. Once the obstruction is confirmed, surgery should follow promptly even if the site of the obstruction is not perfectly clear. Temporizing measures such as frequent reservoir pumping or irrigation are of little benefit and may in fact accelerate decompensation and adversely affect outcome.

SHUNT INFECTIONS. Infectious complications of extracranial shunts occur with a frequency of 5 to 15 per cent. Septicemia, bacterial endocarditis, wound infection, shunt nephritis, meningitis, and ventriculitis usually result from concurrent infection at the time of shunt placement or introduction of the organism during surgery. Meningitis and ventriculitis are of greatest concern, since central nervous system infection complicating shunted hydrocephalus is a significant predictor of poor intellectual outcome. The period of greatest risk for infection is 1 to 2 months after shunt placement, but an infection can occur at any time. The most common pathogens isolated are *Staphylococcus epidermidis* and *S. aureus* acting alone or in concert with other gram-positive organisms.

Appropriate antibiotics, as determined by organism

sensitivity, are mandatory and should be administered systemically or intraventricularly. Many clinicians agree with the dictum that any infection requires expedient removal of the entire shunt device and, if necessary, institution of an external drainage system through which to instill antibiotics or remove fluid and control intracranial pressure. Recent studies, however, have shown that almost 50 per cent of infected VA shunts can be treated successfully with high-dose combined systemic and intraventricular antibiotics without resorting to shunt removal. Such a regimen requires a reservior through which antibiotics can be instilled and, in most instances, the capability of measuring an antibiotic's minimum inhibitory concentration in both the CSF and blood.

Medical Therapy. Attempts at nonsurgical management of hydrocephalus have been disappointing except in newborns with progressive ventricular enlargement secondary to intracranial hemorrhage. As many as 50 per cent of these infants spontaneously exhibit stabilization or resolution. Therapeutic measures such as serial lumbar punctures or medications that decrease CSF production may improve this figure. In any event, the decision to proceed with a shunt in this clinical setting must be weighed carefully. In older children, acetazolamide and isosorbide have been of some benefit, both in the treatment of very slowly progressive hydrocephalus and as temporizing measures in acute hydrocephalus when prompt surgery is contraindicated.

Other Problems in Management. On the average, the overall IQ in children with hydrocephalus is slightly lower than normal, in the range of 90 to 95, although a wide spectrum is seen. Deficits are usually more pronounced in nonverbal intellectual skills. The degree of overall impairment appears to relate to the rate at which hydrocephalus develops, the duration of raised intracranial pressure, the frequency of complications (especially shunt infection), and in all probability the etiology of the hydrocephalus. All children with hydrocephalus should therefore have a psychometric evaluation performed at some time prior to the start of their education, with the aim of establishing both realistic goals and an appropriate educational program through which the child's potential might be realized.

A child with hydrocephalus is also at greater risk for developing an emotional problem such as an anxiety neurosis or antisocial-conduct disorder. These difficulties are amenable to treatment through early intervention, especially family counseling.

The management of hydrocephalus in children is a demanding task often requiring a multidisciplinary effort. The aim of the management program should be to maximize the potential of each child. In this regard, an awareness of complications common to hydrocephalus and its treatment by extracranial shunts are essential. Prompt initial treatment, routine shunt revisions, prevention and early treatment of shunt infection, and maximization of intellectual development should be cornerstones of a management program which, if properly enacted, will enable a child with hydrocephalus to experience a normal or nearly normal life.

MYELODYSPLASIA
GARY J. MYERS, M.D.

Abnormal development of the neural tube affecting the spinal cord can occur as an isolated event or can be associated with vertebral abnormalities. Its most severe forms compatible with survival are spina bifida (myelomeningocele) and the caudal regression syndrome. In extreme cases of open spine (rachischisis), those affected do not survive.

Approximately 1 infant in every 1000 live births in the United States has open spina bifida. The recurrence risk in subsequent pregnancies is markedly increased (5 per cent) and rises even higher if one parent has spina bifida. Prenatal counseling of parents at risk should always be offered. Evidence is accumulating that pre- and postconceptual consumption of vitamins may reduce the incidence of spina bifida. However, experimentally hypervitaminosis can also cause spina bifida. Currently this is the only truly preventive measure known.

INITIAL MANAGEMENT BY THE PRACTITIONER

Survival of infants born with spina bifida has increased dramatically and now exceeds 90 per cent. In addition, technological advances have improved their functional abilities and long-term outcome. The early care and attitudes of health professionals may have a profound and lasting effect. Early optimism tempered with realism is a wise course. The outcome for a given child is difficult to predict, and a negative or discouraging attitude is not helpful to a family destined to care for a handicapped child for many years.

Most infants with open spina bifida are born in community hospitals. However, the specialized knowledge and consultants needed to properly care for such children are generally located in regional centers. The diagnosis is usually obvious and transfer to a specialized center is indicated. However, urgent transfer is needed only if the back lesion is actively leaking cerebrospinal fluid or an associated life-threatening anomaly is present (cardiac or gastrointestinal malformation). Surgical closure of the back lessens the risk of meningitis, but there is no evidence it improves the outcome in other ways. Initially attention should focus on decreasing the infant's risk of infection and helping the family understand, adjust, and knowledgeably participate in the decisions that need to be made. Infants with spina bifida generally appear normal except for the back lesion and perhaps lower extremity deformities. Both parents need an opportunity to see, hold, and become attached to their infant. They should also be counseled about the problems associated with myelomeningocele and given the opportunity to jointly participate in decisions concerning treatment. The Baby Jane Doe case confirmed the family's right to participate in decisions and stimulated many hospitals to establish a bioethical review committee. Any final decision about how aggressive care and treatment should be, especially if limited intervention seems indicated, requires the opinions of specialists with experience in treating this disorder.

The initial medical assessment should focus on the following: (1) the open spina bifida and its associated problems (hydrocephalus, spinal lesion, paraplegia, orthopedic deformities, genitourinary abnormalities); (2) acquired problems, whether associated (meningitis) or not (hypoxia, hemorrhage); and (3) other malformations (cardiac, gastrointestinal).

The spinal lesion should be inspected first. If leakage of cerebrospinal fluid (CSF) is present, early surgical closure should be considered to lessen the risk of meningitis. The sac itself should be kept sterile prior to surgery. It can be covered with gauze and kept moist with sterile saline. A ring placed around the defect made of cotton wadding and gauze will allow the infant to be held and even lie on the back without further damage to the sac. Montgomery straps are used to hold the ring in place. If meningeal infection is suspected, CSF should be aspirated and examined. Aspiration is done by starting the needle lateral to the lesion in normal skin and running it parallel to the back through subcutaneous tissue into the sac. Associated vertebral anomalies above or below the defect are common and scoliosis can be present at birth.

The head is next examined for separation of sutures. The occipitofrontal head circumference should be recorded daily. A cranial ultrasound or CT scan will document any ventricular enlargement. Ultrasonography is an excellent method of following ventriculomegaly serially. Placement of a shunt is not an emergency in the newborn, but shunting should be considered when there is clear evidence that the hydrocephalus is progressive. A cranial CT scan may document the presence of an Arnold-Chiari malformation. Clinically the presence of cranial nerve abnormalities (abnormal eye movements, laryngeal dysfunction, hyperactive gag) will support this diagnosis.

The level and extent of spinal dysfunction deserve careful evaluation. Most lesions involve the midlumbar region, but high lumbar or sacral involvement is also common. There is marked individual variation. Consequently, specific muscle testing is required. Voluntary muscle movement must be distinguished from reflex activity resulting from an isolated functioning spinal cord segment that is not under voluntary control. The level of sensory loss may differ from that of motor loss. Incontinence of urine and stool is nearly universal except in cases of hemimyelocele. However, the type of bladder or rectal involvement varies widely. Imbalances of muscle innervation can lead to dislocation of the hips, club foot, or other orthopedic abnormalities of the spine, hips, or lower extremities.

In addition, a careful evaluation for other abnormalities should be performed. The presence of dysgenetic features or cardiac malformations might suggest a chromosomal problem. If inoperable or lethal defects are found, supportive care performed locally may be best for all concerned. The information gained by this initial assessment will help the practitioner in early management, facilitate consultation, and determine the need for and timing of referral.

INITIAL MANAGEMENT BY THE SPECIALIST

Transfer to a specialized center should occur in the first few days of life, generally when the family has had an opportunity to understand the situation, at least partially. Referral should be to the spina bifida team, usually the pediatrician, so that the overall picture will not be lost by a narrow focus of attention. Other team members such as the nurse, social worker, physical therapist, neurosurgeon, urologist, and orthopedist are then called upon to evaluate the infant and make recommendations. After the evaluations, a consensus opinion should be reached. A comprehensive plan is then formulated and presented to the family along with the evaluation results.

First priority should be given to helping the family understand the defect and reach a decision about closure of the back lesion. Inclusion of the mother in this process, even if via telephone, is important, since she will likely be the primary caretaker for many years. Until a decision is reached and surgery performed, the sac should be kept sterile and moist. Occasionally multiple major defects or an extensive back lesion leads the family and spina bifida team to feel that aggressive treatment is not indicated. Such a decision should be made only after the hospital's bioethical review committee evaluates the situation and concurs. This decision can be reversed later if the infant stabilizes or other considerations become more important. Most infants have the back surgically repaired.

A shunting procedure for hydrocephalus should be performed if serial cranial ultrasonography or a rapidly increasing head circumference documents progressive hydrocephalus. Occipitofrontal head circumference should be measured daily and plotted. Should elevated CSF pressure lead to CSF leakage through the back repair, an early shunt may be necessary. Shunts successfully reduce intracranial pressure but can lead to shunt dependence and serve as loci of infection, and their malfunction can result in acute life-threatening increases of intracranial pressure. Avoidance of a shunt, if feasible, is in the long-term interests of the child.

The genitourinary tract deserves early and regular evaluation. Preservation of renal function is essential to long-term survival. Infections of the bladder or kidneys and retrograde pressure leading to hydronephrosis need early recognition and aggressive treatment. A urine culture, serum BUN and creatinine, and radiologic studies (IVP, VCUG, renal sonogram) should be done.

Early orthopedic care is indicated, since scoliosis and joint deformities, especially in the lower extremities, may be present at birth. In infancy the deformities may not be so fixed. Consequently, serial casting of such defects as club feet may be more effective and reduce the need for later surgery. Similarly, early treatment may help the hip joint to form properly, and the progressive dislocation that sometimes occurs may be avoided. The longer orthopedic treatment is delayed, the less likely it is that surgical treatment of musculoskeletal abnormalities can be avoided.

MANAGEMENT AFTER INFANCY

Responsibility for Care. Ongoing care by an interdisciplinary team with experience treating children with spina bifida and their families provides optimal medical expertise. However, such a team of experts should not displace or intimidate the primary care physician. Specialized expertise should be neither under- nor overvalued. These experts are often located at some distance and oriented to a single organ system, periodically change responsibilities, and are often very busy. They may not understand the child in the context of his family or local environment. It is in the areas of psychosocial care, a comprehensive overview, and time for counseling and discussion that the primary care physician can and should make a major contribution. The fundamentals of primary care for the chronically ill include the following six basic canons:

Care: genuine, personal, and professional
Communicate: establish mutual trust
Customize: each child is unique
Counsel: help the family understand their choices
Coordinate: guide and assist
Continue: provide longitudinal stability

The primary care physician is in an optimal position to provide these essentials while simultaneously utilizing the expertise of the spina bifida team and its specialists for assistance.

The Head. The majority (approximately 66 per cent) of individuals with spina bifida have intelligence within the normal range. This is a valuable asset for a child handicapped in other ways and one that should be recognized, reinforced, and built upon. Although CNS infections often lower intellectual capability, it appears that shunt revisions and the rate of early head growth do not. The expectations of parents and others need to be tailored to this ability. Some children with a normal intellect, however, do have learning disabilities. Visuomotor perception problems are prominent. Attention to learning ability and appropriate school arrangements can greatly improve the child's chances for both learning and socialization with peers. Public Law 94-142, which mandated that public schools provide education to all handicapped children, facilitated the correct school placement.

Progressive hydrocephalus generally occurs early and requires shunting in roughly 75 per cent of children with spina bifida. Cranial ultrasonography through the anterior fontanelle provides a safe, easy, reliable way to serially document changes in ventricular size and the need for a shunt procedure. Ventriculoperitoneal shunts have reduced complications and the need for frequent revisions. However, blocked shunts do occur and, if not promptly recognized and corrected, can lead to death. The main signs of shunt blockage are drowsiness, headache, vomiting, irritability, and changes in neurologic condition. Neurosurgical consultation or evaluation should be promptly obtained if any of these signs are present and especially if they are persistent.

Musculoskeletal System. Skilled orthopedic care is a cornerstone for helping the child with spina bifida. It should begin early and be longitudinal, since deformities may be present at birth or result from growth or prolonged muscle imbalance. Involvement of muscles can result in flaccidity or spasticity. There is great diversity in individual patterns of involvement. In addition, the pattern may change over time. Deterioration of neurologic function may indicate tethering, a lipoma, or other complications. Imbalance of muscles about a joint, such as the hip, can result in dislocation. The dislocation may be present at birth or occur gradually as normal hip flexors and adductors (L1-L3) act unopposed by hip extensors and abductors (L5-S1). Unequal forces acting on knees, feet, or spine can also result in progressive deformities.

Sitting, standing, and mobility all require certain joints to be stable and body parts to be properly aligned. For example, plantigrade feet improve standing balance and more evenly distribute the weight over the soles to lessen the risk of pressure sores. Similarly, if hips or knees are not fully extended, the trunk cannot be balanced, while if the hips cannot be flexed, sitting is difficult. Viewing the world from an upright position such as sitting or standing is important in development. In addition, truncal stability is essential for full use of the upper extremities. Recent developments in bracing using lightweight materials have made standing and independent mobility feasible for most of these children. These are important experiences for them, especially during the developmental years, even though many choose a wheelchair as a more practical solution when they reach their teens.

Many orthopedic procedures such as casting and surgery are prolonged and disruptive of school, family, or social life. Coordination of care and selection of priorities are especially important in this area, since the problems being addressed are seldom urgent.

Genitourinary System. Social acceptability, the concept of self, and long-term survival are all affected by how well the genitourinary system is managed. An experienced urologist is needed on the spina bifida team, and regular evaluations, including radiography, throughout life are indicated.

Continence is needed for socialization and acceptability, as well as prevention of skin damage in the perineal area. Abdominal pressure to empty the bladder (Credé's method) has been replaced by clean intermittent catheterization (CIC), a simple and reliable method that ensures total emptying of the bladder. If performed regularly, it prevents overflow incontinence and ureteral reflux secondary to retrograde high pressure. CIC can be performed by parents or learned by young children. Ensuring full bladder evacuation decreases the risk of infection. Medications can be used with CIC to improve bladder storage and continence. The use of CIC has nearly eliminated the need for surgical urinary diversion. However, CIC has limitations (it must be performed regularly in a clean manner). Implanted artificial sphincters have been designed and used, but they need careful regulation to avoid serious problems.

Infections are a significant problem in these children and require prompt, vigorous therapy. Because of the spinal cord dysfunction, signs such as local pain may be absent. A urinary tract infection should be considered anytime a child with spina bifida is ill. A urinalysis and urine culture are needed to rule out this possibility.

Sexual function is possible in many individuals with spina bifida. Most females are fertile, able to have normal sexual activity, and capable of bearing children. Sexual function in males depends on their individual pattern of denervation. Some have erections and ejaculations and can have fairly normal sexual activity. Many are sterile as a result of either chronic prostatitis or retrograde ejaculation. Urologic care may improve male sexual functioning.

Bowel Control. Rectal continence is important for social acceptability and the concept of the self. With time and consistent effort it can be achieved in most children with spina bifida. Regular bowel evacuation with no stool leakage between bowel movements is the goal. It requires good dietary and toileting habits. Constipating or laxative foods must be avoided and systematic toileting procedures developed. Medications may be needed. Achievement of bowel control is often a lengthly procedure but one that is rewarding to all concerned.

Summary. The outlook for children with spina bifida has steadily improved in recent years. Although they have multiple problems, much can be done to help them and their families. Proper treatment requires the expertise of specialists, preferably in coordination with a spina bifida team. The pediatrician or general practitioner, however, can play a significant role.

BRAIN TUMORS

A. LOREN AMACHER, M.D.

New Techniques. Some recent technologic refinements hold great promise for allowing neurosurgeons to safely biopsy deeply placed mass lesions in the brain. Established concern for the long-term effects of radiotherapy and chemotherapy upon the immature brain makes it essential to obtain diagnosis of cerebral masses before recommending therapies that may be detrimental to the intellectual development of children who survive treatment of brain tumors. Reliable diagnosis of medulloblastoma may be possible from cerebrospinal fluid cellular sediment obtained from the ventricles of a child with a posterior fossa mass. Chemical-hormonal markers such as AFP and hCG-beta in raised concentration in the CSF from patients with pineal region or suprasellar masses may indicate a tumor of germinal cell origin. As many such tumors are exquisitely sensitive to radiotherapy or chemotherapy, open biopsy may be obviated.

CT-guided stereotactic biopsy of deeply placed or otherwise poorly accessible lesions is proving to be a safe and reliable technique for determining histology. Examples of tumors that are prime candidates for this procedure are pineal region masses, tumors of the thalamus and hypothalamus, and tumors abutting the brain stem. CT-guided stereotactic surgery is applicable for drainage of cysts and for the placement of interstitial radiation carriers for brachytherapy.

Vastly improved resolution of ultrasonic images of discrete cerebral structures, including mass lesions, makes it practicable to consider *ultrasound-guided biopsy* for any lesion that has sufficiently contrasting density from surrounding brain to create a visible image on the viewing screen. The probes containing the image-creating crystals are small enough to allow the surgeon to visualize and biopsy a tumor through a small craniotomy. A substantial advantage of the technique is that the surgeon can view a real-time image while advancing an instrument to the lesion within the plane of the ultrasonic slice. Image resolution is good enough now that it is possible to watch the jaws of a microsurgical biopsy forceps opening and closing within the desired target. Pulsations of nearby larger arteries often are discernible.

Magnetic resonance imaging (MRI) of the brain has a decided advantage over CT scanning for lesions within the posterior fossa or spinal canal. Since bone produces only a faint image with MRI, bone artifact is reduced substantially, making visualization of brain stem and spinal cord tumors in particular more dramatic and convincing. Nontoxic agents of high magnetic moment such as gadolinium have enhanced the diagnostic precision of MRI; new programs such as serial inversion null synthesis (SINS) hold great promise for giving MRI a diagnostic specificity unobtainable with other imaging techniques.

Stereotactic technique combined with finely collimated and focused beams of ionizing radiation delivered through several small ports is the basis for *stereotactic radiosurgery* of brain tumors and other lesions, notably arteriovenous malformations. The advantage of this technique is that high tissue doses of radiation can be delivered in a very steep isodense spectrum to small volumes of tissue, thereby minimizing serious radiation damage to surrounding normal tissue. The radiation-induced obliteration of vascular lumina takes many weeks to months; during this interval, AVMs remain at risk for rebleeding.

The substantial pool of experience in craniofacial surgery for traumatic and congenital craniofacial disorders has led to innovative approaches to tumors at the base of the brain and in front of the brain stem. For example, temporary removal of the zygomatic arch permits the surgeon to approach the interpeduncular fossa from a more anterior and inferior aspect. Tumors that may be more accessible as a result include craniopharyngioma and chordoma.

Certain tumors of the central nervous system may be approached more safely and completely through smaller exposures or be resected more completely when ancillary equipment such as carbon dioxide laser or an ultrasonic aspirator is used. Intrinsic spinal cord tumors, for instance, may be exposed with less damage to normal tissue by carrying out the myelotomy by laser radiation. Tumor removal is enhanced by laser evaporation or ultrasonic aspiration.

Brain Tumors in the Very Young. The incidence of cerebral neoplasms in infants has been reported variously as a distinct rarity or as approximately the same as at other times during childhood. At least one observer has expressed concern that tumors in babies may occur more frequently in communities in which certain chemicals are manufactured. No data clearly support this hypothesis.

To qualify as a truly congenital lesion, a tumor must be present at birth or produce symptoms within a few weeks of birth. Many such neoplasms are of primitive ectodermal origin and were usually classified as medulloblastoma in older taxonomic nomenclatures. These small-celled, extremely cellular tumors may arise at any site where primitive undifferentiated cells occur, including the surface of the cerebellum, the posterior medullary velum, the pineal area, and in or around the third ventricle. They are usually aggressive and difficult to control.

Ependymomas appear to occur with uncommon frequency in infants, and they may be spread diffusely throughout the subarachnoid space at diagnosis. Hydrocephalus and cranial nerve palsies are the common presenting signs for ependymomas and primitive ectodermal tumors.

Malignant gliomas of poorly differentiated origin have a propensity for deep midline structures. The clinical description of an irritable infant with loss of subcutaneous fat, motor delay with or without spasticity, voracious appetite, and large head with a bright-eyed appearance frequently suggests a tumor of the hypothalamus, which gives rise to the diencephalic syndrome.

Treatment of malignant CNS tumors in babies is likely to be frustrating and unrewarding. Seldom are the lesions resectable in their entirety, and vigorous radiotherapy and chemotherapy carry substantial risks of damage to normal tissue. Experience suggests that children who survive the tumor and its treatment pay a price in terms of physical and intellectual development. Nevertheless, long-term survivors are recorded, 10 to 30 or more years from treatment, and some have done very well.

Benign tumors of the CNS presenting in infancy include papillomas of the choroid plexus, neuroglial cysts, dermoids, and benign teratomas. Aggressive surgical therapy for such lesions is usually very efficacious, unless the anatomy at the base of the brain is distorted grossly by such lesions as infiltrative teratomas or dermoids. Antecedent hydrocephalus may require a preresection shunt procedure, and the hydrocephalus may remain shunt-dependent after the tumor is removed.

Intracranial dermoids may be connected to the skin surface by a dermal track, particularly when the tumor is located in the posterior fossa or at the midline base of the frontal fossa. These tracks may allow entry of skin organisms with abscess formation within the tumor and a great risk of contamination of the subarachnoid space. Meninigitis arising from this mechanism is likely to be polybacterial and recurrent. The external os of the track is in or close to the midline and is discernible as a small pit that usually has short, thick protruding hairs. A diligent search over the midline skin of the posterior fossa may necessitate shaving the hair. Tracks presenting on the nose may have their external os between the glabella and the junction of the middle and lower thirds. There may be a visible bulge above

the external os, often with a history of recurrent inflammation. Intermittent extrusion of a creamy, thick exudate from the os is not uncommon. Such tumors obviously are congenital, although their clinical presentation may be delayed for years.

Tumors Associated with the Neurocutaneous Syndromes. The genetically related neurocutaneous syndromes of neurofibromatosis and tuberous sclerosis are commonly associated with neoplasms of the CNS. In areas where there is a genetic pool with several family pedigrees having manifestations of these disorders such tumors are frequent. Because the spontaneous mutation rate in the gene responsible for neurofibromatosis is high, sporadic cases are almost as common as familial ones. Tumors of Schwann-cell origin involving lower cranial nerves (especially the eighth), optic nerve gliomas, and meningiomas are the hallmarks of CNS neurofibromatosis. The classic tumor seen with tuberous sclerosis is the giant-cell astrocytoma arising from the environs of the foramen of Monro and obstructing it. Hamartomas of deep grey matter and cortex are extremely common in tuberous sclerosis, perhaps acting as seizure foci. In neurofibromatosis, CNS tumors may be multiple and of varying histology. Bilateral acoustic nerve tumors are of particular note, as removal of both usually results in permanent deafness. Sarcomatous change in the Schwann-cell derivative tumors may arise in as many as 10 per cent of such lesions.

Intracranial neoplasms in the form of hemangioblastomas are a common finding in patients with the von Hippel-Lindau syndrome. The tumors may be cystic, commonly occur in the cerebellum and upper spinal cord, are slow growing but frequently multiple, and may be curable.

Hydrocephalus occurring in children with neurocutaneous syndromes is not necessarily due to tumor. Aqueduct stenosis occurs with an increased frequency in these conditions. And it is well to recall that extracranial tissue of neurectodermal origin exhibits a greater than usual incidence of neoplasms such as chemodectomas, pheochromocytomas, and secreting neuroblastomas. Initial symptoms in such cases may mimic intracranial pathology.

The tumors associated with the neurocutaneous syndromes are congenital in the sense that they are preprogrammed by genetic anomalies. The symptoms and signs that declare their existence do not frequently arise before later childhood or adolescence.

Suprasellar Tumors. The histologic diversity of these tumors in children is remarkable. Personal experience with these lesions in a 30-month interval has included ependymoma (2 yrs), gangliocytic hamartoma (3 mos), Rathke-pouch cyst (5 yrs), juvenile astrocytoma (8 yrs), germinoma (11 yrs), and prolactinoma (13 yrs). Ectopic primitive ectodermal tumor, chiasmic glioma, craniopharyngioma, malignant teratoma, dermoid tumor, and lymphomatous deposits are other possible inhabitants of this region. For spherical masses in the suprasellar area, MRI provides rapid differentiation from giant aneurysms.

The visual loss associated with suprasellar, perichiasmatic tumors usually is insidious and often profound before being noted by a parent or teacher. The child may be very reticent to complain of visual loss and often is adept at dealing with the problem by using islands of good vision to the fullest. Three of the children alluded to above presented with profound visual loss in the form of a chiasmal junctional syndrome. Therein, one eye is blind to all but light perception and, perhaps, gross movement while the other eye has a dense temporal field defect and, often, severely reduced visual acuity. The blind eye usually shows optic atrophy, whereas the other eye may demonstrate the virtually pathognomonic "double-peak" papilledema—a medial wedge of atrophy separating upper and lower swollen disc. This particular visual syndrome occurs when pressure on one optic nerve and ipsilateral anterior chiasm includes the contralateral nasal retinal fibers that loop into the base of the optic nerve under pressure. Unfortunately, optic apparatus decompression may accomplish very little in relieving this cause of severe visual disability in children.

BRAIN ABSCESS

MARVIN L. WEIL, M.D.

Pyogenic organisms gain access to the brain substance by one of three routes: (1) the blood stream, in association with bacteremia or septic emboli, especially with a cardiopulmonary malfunction, most commonly cyanotic congenital heart disease with a right-to-left shunt; (2) extension of contiguous infections, such as leptomeningitis or infections of the middle ear or the paranasal sinuses, either directly from osteomyelitis or as a result of septic thrombophlebitis of bridging veins; or (3) as a complication of a penetrating wound. Children with chronic pulmonary infections are more prone to develop brain abscesses. Treatment of any brain abscess should include a diligent search for the source of the infection. Multiple brain abscesses should also raise the question of immunodeficiency. Multiple blood cultures should be taken in order to identify the causative agent.

The most common causative organisms are *Staphylococcus aureus* and *S. epidermidis*, anaerobic and microaerophilic streptococci, beta-hemolytic streptococci, alpha-hemolytic streptococci, pneumococci, *Bacteroides*, and other gram-negative rods—particularly *Haemophilus* species. Infections caused by *Aspergillus, Nocardia, Actinomyces, Leptothrix,* and *Cryptococcus* occur less often. Abscesses caused by *Corynebacterium, Mycobacterium,* and protozoans such as *Entamoeba histolytica* and *Toxoplasma* are even rarer except in the immunocompromised host. Approximately 6 to 20 per cent of abscesses are caused by mixed flora. Anaerobic as well as aerobic organisms may cause brain abscesses derived from otitis media or from infections in the petrous or mastoid regions.

Abscesses resulting from hematogenous spread may be localized within any part of the brain, but most commonly at the junction of gray and white matter of the cerebral hemispheres. By contrast, abscesses derived from contiguous sources tend to be superficial and close to the infected bone or dura. Multiple abscesses occur in 6 per cent of patients, usually when sepsis or congenital heart disease is the predisposing cause.

TREATMENT

Medical therapy without surgery has been successful during the stage of cellulitis or early abscess formation. Initial antibiotic therapy should include coverage of anaerobic as well as aerobic organisms. Penicillin G (400,000 units/kg/24 hours) and metronidazole (loading dose 15 mg/kg, maintenance 7.5 mg/kg q6h) or chloramphenicol (100 mg/kg/day) should be started as soon as possible. Oxacillin (150 to 200 mg/kg/day) or methicillin (150 to 200 mg/kg/day) should also be started until it is established that a beta-lactamase–producing *Staphylococcus* is not involved. Failure of prompt improvement beginning within 24 hours or deterioration of clinical status is an indication for surgical intervention. When an abscess is fully established, surgical treatment is usually required. Focal lesions for surgical intervention may be established either by the presence of advancing neurologic signs, percussion tenderness on tapping the skull, a slow wave focus on EEG, focal radionuclide brain scan, or radiographic image or contrast studies. Magnetic resonance imaging is particularly useful. The area in question is surgically tapped and any abscess is aspirated. The aspirate should be examined for aerobic and anaerobic bacteria, mycobacteria, fungi, and parasites. Subsequent antibiotic therapy is guided by laboratory determination as to etiology and antibody sensitivity. Needle aspiration and antibiotic therapy can be adequate therapy for some cases. Effective antibiotics with good brain tissue penetration, such as some of the third-generation cephalosporins, may be preferred. Treatment is usually continued for a minimum of 3 weeks but often is continued for 4 to 6 weeks. Intravenous fluid is usually limited to 1500 ml/m² in order to minimize cerebral edema. Increased intracranial pressure or brain herniation may require hyperventilation, mannitol or furosemide, muscle paralysis, or intracranial pressure monitoring. A short course of steroids to reduce life-threatening edema may safely be administered.

Open surgical drainage may be required, or excision may be necessary. Total excision of brain abscesses has been beneficial and may be associated with decreased mortality when compared to drainage or medical treatment. Care must be exercised to avoid rupture of an abscess in the ventricular system with resultant ventriculitis.

Patients with an increase in intracranial pressure and danger of brain stem herniation should have a careful selection of anesthetic agents because halothane, trichlorethylene, and methoxyflurane may cause a considerable rise in intracranial pressure in patients with space-occupying lesions. Signs of brain herniation which require urgent intervention may develop at any time.

Because of the cortical injury due to the brain abscess or its therapy, patients are at risk of seizures during treatment. Seizure prophylaxis with phenytoin (loading dose 18 mg/kg, maintenance dose 5 to 9 mg/kg/day in two divided doses) should be instituted for the period of acute therapy. Residual defects such as seizure activity, localized neurologic abnormalities, mental retardation, and hydrocephalus may require specific therapy. No relationship exists between the development of seizures and the age of the patient or the mode of surgical therapy.

SPINAL EPIDURAL ABSCESSES

MARVIN L. WEIL, M.D.

Epidural abscesses may develop from contiguous infection of structures that surround the brain and spinal cord. They may arise from local infection or secondary to congenital anomalies such as dermal sinuses. Bacteremia and trauma have also been implicated. About one third of cases involve staphylococcal organisms.

Infection of the spinal epidural space is extremely rare in childhood. Infection is usually limited to the dorsal surface of the cord except in its lower sacral portion, where the space completely surrounds the cord. The anatomy of the space limits extension to vertical spread and produces extradural compression. This may result in a clinical course that may be acute and rapidly progressive or chronic. The former, more common in children, requires urgent intervention and is usually the result of a metastatic infection, whereas chronic lesions are most commonly caused by a direct extension of a spinal osteomyelitis. Paraplegia may be complete within a few hours or days.

The history of neurologic signs may be difficult to differentiate from that of acute transverse myelitis. A similar clinical picture may be produced by intradural extramedullary tumors. Careful, rapid evaluation is essential prior to institution of therapy. A history compatible with infection in association with focal pain in the region of the spine, especially if associated with neurologic symptoms of spinal cord or root involvement, should suggest this diagnosis. Blood cultures during the period of diagnosis may reveal the causative organism.

Lumbar puncture should not be performed. Aspiration may be done carefully with a large-gauge needle and frequent aspiration of the spinal needle so as not to miss any pus in the extradural space that might be carried subdurally. The risk of spread of the infection to the subdural or subarachnoid space contraindicates this procedure except under radiographic guidance. A myelogram confirms the presence of an extradural mass.

A spinal epidural abscess that has produced neurologic deficit should be regarded as a surgical emergency in view of the possible rapid progression of potentially irreversible consequences. It is treated by immediate laminectomy with decompression and drainage.

Antibiotic therapy is an adjunct to relief of pressure upon the spinal cord and nerve roots. Therapy is similar to that for brain abscesses except that staphylococcal infections are more frequently encountered. If tuberculosis of the spine is suspected, antituberculous therapy

should be instituted pending identification of the causative organism.

CEREBROVASCULAR DISEASE IN INFANCY AND CHILDHOOD

GAIL E. SOLOMON, M.D.

The sudden onset of hemiplegia in a previously well child, often under the age of 2 years, is the hallmark of strokes in children. These strokes are frequently idiopathic but sometimes have distinct predisposing factors. They present not only with the sudden onset of hemiplegia but also with fever, headache, seizures, and even coma, depending upon the type of pathology—whether arterial thrombosis, embolus, venous thrombosis, or hemorrhage, the location of the pathology, and the degree of maturation of the developing nervous system. The predisposing factors include congenital heart disease, systemic and local infections, hematologic disease, neurocutaneous syndromes, drug abuse, trauma to the head and neck, aneurysms, and arteriovenous malformations.

Cyanotic congenital heart disease, especially tetralogy of Fallot and transposition of the great vessels, is the most frequent predisposing condition to cerebral vascular occlusion. Rheumatic heart disease, subacute bacterial endocarditis, atrial myxoma, rhabdomyosarcoma, mitral valve prolapse, and patent foramen ovale all are associated with cerebral emboli.

Upper respiratory illness, throat infections, mycoplasma pneumonia, viral encephalitis with coxsackie A-9, herpes simplex, and rubella may produce inflammatory arteritis of the carotid artery and its intracerebral branches. Pyogenic infections of the ears and mastoids sometimes lead to lateral sinus thrombosis, whereas infections of the face, nose, and eye may produce cavernous sinus thrombosis. Meningitis as well as diarrhea and dehydration predisposes to cerebral vein and sagittal sinus thrombosis.

Hematologic diseases including sickle cell, polycythemia, thrombocytopenia, leukemia, and coagulopathies may produce either occlusive or hemorrhagic strokes. Collagen vascular diseases such as lupus erythematosus and Takayasu's disease also predispose to stroke. Even metabolic disease such as homocystinuria may induce endothelial injury and platelet adhesiveness, leading to stroke. Diabetes mellitus, rare cases of progeria, and mitochondrial myopathy with lactic acidosis have been associated with childhood stroke. Ulcerative colitis, nephrosis, and steroid therapy itself may predispose to a cerebrovascular accident. Neurocutaneous syndromes including neurofibromatosis, tuberous sclerosis, and Sturge-Weber syndrome have all been associated with childhood cerebrovascular disease. Hypertension in children can also cause stroke.

Drug abuse and drug toxicity, especially cocaine-crack, phenylpropanolamine ("black beauties"), phencyclidine (PCP, "angel dust"), lysergic acid, mescaline, heroin, amphetamine, and even alcohol can lead to ischemic or hemorrhagic stroke.

Trauma to the head and neck, for example when a child falls with an ice cream stick in the mouth, can cause carotid occlusion in the tonsillar fossa. Vertebrobasilar occlusion may result from trauma or chiropractic manipulation of C1-C2. Vertigo, ataxia, cranial nerve palsies, and hemiplegia or a "locked in" syndrome may ensue. Children with ligamentous laxity, Down's syndrome, or achondroplasia are more prone to vertebrobasilar occlusions.

Hemorrhagic stroke occurs after head trauma or secondary to arteriovenous malformations (AVMs) and rarely aneurysms. Posterior fossa AVMs are unusual. Rarely, pontine telangiectasia or a spinal AVM may present as a stroke.

Strokes must be differentiated from brain tumor, abscess, subdural hematoma, encephalitis, complicated migraine, and Todd's paralysis after partial seizures. Rarely, migraine itself may lead to stroke.

Diagnostic evaluation must include a detailed history and comprehensive physical examination searching for underlying predisposing conditions. Laboratory investigations should include complete blood count, sickle prep, platelet count, coagulation studies, ESR, ANA, fasting blood sugar, and a biochemical profile. Urinalysis and urine cyanide nitroprusside for homocystinuria are helpful.

In patients with emboli a search for underlying cardiac disease by means of chest radiograph, ECG, echocardiogram, and Holter monitor may be needed.

Computed transaxial tomography (CT) scan defines an infarcted area of the brain as a region of decreased density, usually not apparent until 12 hours after the onset. CT scan shows whether the infarct is ischemic or hemorrhagic and if there is subarachnoid, subdural, or parenchymal blood. Contrast-enhanced scans after hemorrhage has resorbed may delineate aneurysms larger than 1.5 cm in diameter. AVMs may be calcified and enhanced after contrast. Magnetic resonance imaging (MRI) is more sensitive than CT in early detection of infarcts and in the diagnosis of venous sinus and cerebral vein thrombosis. MRI shows vascular malformations in the brain without injections of contrast.

Cerebral angiography is definitive in visualizing occlusions, small vessel disease, telangiectatic patterns of moya-moya, AVMs, and aneurysms. The supraclinoid portion of the carotid artery is often the site of occlusion. There may be associated collateral circulation in the basal ganglia called moya-moya (a puff of smoke), which indicates progressive disease and identifies possible candidates for external carotid–internal carotid artery (EC-IC) anastomosis. Branch occlusion suggests a good prognosis. If angiography is needed in a patient with sickle cell disease, sickled hemoglobin must be reduced to 20 per cent by transfusion before angiography is done.

Spinal tap is usually negative in thrombosis and embolus but does document hemorrhage by showing red cells and xanthochromia. If a child has focal neurologic deficit with increased intracranial pressure, first do a CT scan to exclude a mass effect, thus avoiding cerebral herniation after spinal tap.

Supportive care is the key factor in treatment. One must provide adequate airway, avoid aspiration, ensure adequate oxygenation, and provide and monitor hydration and electrolytes. Reduce fever with antipyretics and treat the underlying systemic disorder. Maintenance fluids should be restricted to 1200 ml/m^2/24 hr for the first 2 to 3 days in order to prevent an increase in cerebral edema. Solutions may vary from 0.2 to 0.4 per cent saline with 5 per cent glucose. Potassium (20 mEq/L) is added to the maintenance solution if the patient shows adequate renal function. If the child is febrile, he or she should be cultured and treated with widespectrum antibiotics until a specific infectious etiology is found.

In neonates with a large AVM or vein of Galen malformation, treat congestive heart failure with digitoxin and furosemide. Cardiac arrhythmias must also be treated. If there is a coagulopathy, specific factors or transfusions are required. In sickle cell disease, transfusion must be given to lower the percentage of sickled hemoglobin.

Children with acute stroke may show signs of increased intracranial pressure when the brain swells from the effects of acute infarction or hemorrhage. If there is cerebral edema leading to progressive clinical deterioration, treat the patient with intravenous mannitol 20 per cent in a dose of 1.5 gm/kg over 20 minutes. The dose can be repeated in 4 to 6 hours. This is a temporary measure, since there is often a rebound effect; corticosteroids therefore should be started as well. Intravenous dexamethasone (Decadron) 0.5 mg/kg should be given right after the initial dose of mannitol; then give 0.25 mg/kg q8h for 72 hours and taper over 3 to 4 days. If there is impending herniation, use hyperventilation with intubation, decreasing the PaCO$_2$ to 25 mm Hg.

Status epilepticus is a medical emergency. Specific antiepileptic medication should be given intravenously to stop seizures because hypoxia, acidosis, and increased metabolic needs lead to brain damage. Give oxygen by mask or nasal catheter and insert an airway if possible.

Phenobarbital 15 mg/kg should be given slowly intravenously over 5 min. If the seizures continue after 15 min, an additional 5 mg/kg can be slowly administered. If seizures persist, after another 15 min give IV phenytoin (Dilantin), 15 mg/kg slowly at a rate less than 50 mg/min. In young infants, give at a rate no more than 1 mg/kg/min. Heart rate, blood pressure, and respiration must be closely monitored. The patient should then be placed on maintenance phenobarbital, with the level maintained at 20 to 40 µg/ml. If phenytoin maintenance is needed, the level should be held between 10 and 20 µg/ml.

An alternate treatment for status epilepticus, particularly in older children, adolescents, and patients in whom monitoring of mental status is essential in the management, is to start with diazepam (Valium) 0.3 mg/kg, not to exceed 10 mg. If seizures persist or recur, give an additional dose of diazepam after 15 min. Since diazepam is short-acting and is not a maintenance drug, immediately after the initial injection of diazepam give phenytoin, 15 mg/kg at a rate not to exceed 50 mg/min through a different intravenous site. If there is no response to phenytoin, phenobarbital can be added. The use of diazepam and phenobarbital together is reported to produce significant respiratory depression. Patients must be closely monitored and intubated and given respiratory support if necessary.

Embolic phenomena can be treated with anticoagulants. If there is hypertension, bleeding diathesis, or hemorrhagic infarction, anticoagulants should be avoided. A suggested regimen for anticoagulation in the appropriate patient is continuous infusion of heparin at 10 to 15 units/kg/hr. Partial thromboplastin time (PTT) should be kept about two to three times normal and checked daily. After 5 days of heparin, Coumadin (sodium warfarin) is given in a 5- to 10-mg loading dose followed by 2 to 3 mg/day. When prothrombin time (PT) is between 20 and 30 sec or twice normal, usually in about 4 days, the heparin is discontinued.

Anecdotal reports in two patients with moya-moya suggest that a calcium-channel blocker, verapamil, might be useful in treating strokes. Another report suggests that verapamil may also reverse diffuse vasoconstriction that occurs as a result of ingestion of LSD, mescaline, or phencyclidine (angel dust). Further study is necessary.

Surgery is the treatment of choice for aneurysms, accessible vascular malformations, and large vessel disease of the cervical carotid artery. Large AVMs may have to be embolized by the neuroradiologist as a palliative measure or prior to surgery in order to decrease their size and make surgery feasible. In moya-moya patients, external carotid–to–internal carotid artery (ECA-ICA) anastomosis may improve prognosis.

After the initial emergency treatment, long-term therapy should include physical and occupational therapy. Rehabilitation should be started early, with splints and passive range-of-motion exercise to prevent contractures even in the first week in hospital. Mobilization should begin as soon as possible.

Platelet hyperaggregability has been associated with strokes, which suggests a potential role for antiplatelet medication such as acetylsalicylic acid (aspirin), especially if the patient has transient ischemic attacks (TIAs). Further study is essential to assess this therapy.

Children with sickle cell disease and strokes are benefited by transfusions to maintain the sickle hemoglobin at less than 20 per cent to prevent further strokes. With hypertransfusion, the iron and iron-binding capacity level must be monitored. Deferoxamine may be required for iron chelation from the heart and liver.

Prognosis in stroke depends upon the etiology of the stroke and the location and size of the infarct or hemorrhage. Most patients have residual deficits. Management involves a multidisciplinary approach with antiepileptic drugs, special education, and psychological and speech therapy.

BENIGN INTRACRANIAL HYPERTENSION

MELVIN GREER, M.D.

Impairment of vision is the major concern underlying the need for treatment of the child with benign intracranial hypertension (pseudotumor cerebri). About 10 per cent of all patients with this syndrome have suffered from irreversible partial or complete loss of vision.

Diagnostic studies including neuroimaging procedures (computed tomography, magnetic resonance imaging), electroencephalography, and spinal fluid examination with pressure measurements are among the tests done. They will exclude other known causes of intracranial hypertension: intracranial mass, hydrocephalus, meningoencephalitis, demyelinating diseases, and encephalopathies of toxic or metabolic origin. Visual evoked response testing provides an important initial assessment of optic nerve involvement as well as a valuable guide to the course and effects of treatment.

Specific diagnostic studies are helpful in identifying a specific cause for benign intracranial hypertension. Table 1 lists known conditions that have been associated with the syndrome. Selective radiographs and blood tests may provide the answer and lead to specific treatment. Visualization of the intracranial venous pathways (arteriography or venography) is important in children with benign intracranial hypertension. In contrast to adults, occlusion of the sigmoid or lateral sinus in association with chronic mastoiditis is a common cause for the condition. Antibiotic treatment alone is not sufficient to eliminate the mastoid infection and restore the patency of the draining intracranial sinus. Mastoidectomy is necessary to remove the chronic inflammatory tissue overlying the occluded sinus. Any thrombus suspected at the time of surgery should be left alone. Recanalization will take place. Ligation of the distal portion of the sinus or jugular vein, thrombectomy, or the use of anticoagulation designed to prevent embolization or clot propagation is of no value and is risk-laden.

Hormone replacement therapy in those unusual conditions in which benign intracranial hypertension is associated with endocrine disturbances will effect a resolution of the neurologic problem. Reinstitution followed by very gradual reduction of adrenocortical steroid treatment is the therapy advocated for the child whose steroid treatment given for another illness had been terminated, giving rise to the signs and symptoms of benign intracranial hypertension.

Other specific treatment approaches need to be instituted in those circumstances in which an association between a known physical condition and benign intracranial hypertension exists. The obese adolescent is to be put on a weight-reduction diet, the child with a hematologic problem requires directed therapy, and in those in whom an exogenous factor (e.g., drugs) is believed to be the contributory cause simple discontinuation is sufficient.

Lumbar puncture is indicated for diagnostic as well as therapeutic purposes. Normal results with respect to cells and chemical constituents are reassuring. Spinal

TABLE 1. Conditions Associated with Benign Intracranial Hypertension

Intracranial venous drainage obstruction
    Mastoiditis and lateral (sigmoid) sinus obstruction
    Extracerebral mass lesions
    Congenital atresia or stenosis of venous sinuses
    Head trauma
    Cryofibrinogenemia
    Polycythemia vera
    Paranasal sinus and pharyngeal infections
Cervical or thoracic venous drainage obstruction
    Intrathoracic mass lesions and postoperative obstruction of
      venous return
Endocrine dysfunction
    Pregnancy
    Menarche
    Marked menstrual irregularities
    Oral contraceptives
    Obesity
    Withdrawal of corticosteroid therapy
    Addison's disease
    Hypoparathyroidism
    "Catch-up" growth after deprivation, treatment of cystic fibrosis,
      correction of heart anomaly
    Initiation of thyroxine treatment for hypothyroidism
    Adrenal hyperplasia
    Adrenal adenoma
Hematologic disorders
    Acute iron-deficiency anemia
    Pernicious anemia
    Thrombocytopenia
    Wiskott-Aldrich syndrome
Vitamin metabolism
    Chronic hypervitaminosis A
    Acute hypervitaminosis A
    Hypovitaminosis A
    Cystic fibrosis and hypovitaminosis A
    Vitamin D–deficiency rickets
Drug reaction
    Tetracycline
    Perhexiline maleate
    Nalidixic acid
    Sulfamethoxazole
    Indomethacin
    Penicillin
Prophylactic antisera
Miscellaneous
    Galactosemia
    Galactokinase deficiency
    Sydenham's chorea
    Sarcoidosis
    Roseola infantum
    Hypophosphatasia
    Paget's disease
    Maple syrup urine disease
    Turner's syndrome

fluid measurement provides only an initial gauge of the intracranial pressure and should not deter the treating physician from initiating therapy by withdrawing sufficient fluid to allow the pressure to drop to a normal level. Once reassured by neuroimaging studies that a mass or hydrocephalus does not exist, the volume of fluid removed is of no consequence regarding herniation of intracranial contents. Moreover, the restoration of normal intracranial pressure, albeit perhaps temporarily, is accompanied by an improvement in the subjective complaints of headache, dizziness, and blurred vision.

Subsequent lumbar punctures are performed on the basis of these subjective complaints plus the assessment of visual function, including the results of visual evoked responses. A single lumbar puncture may be sufficient in the treatment of the patient; the hole in the lumbar dural membrane may allow continuous drainage to the adjacent tissue to maintain a lesser pressure and subsequent resolution of the complaints. On the other hand, two to five lumbar punctures during the course of a 2-week period may be necessary.

The appearance of papilledema is not a useful guide to the need for repeated lumbar punctures. It is the persistence of the patient's symptoms and the evaluation of visual function which indicate the need for other therapeutic approaches if it is believed that lumbar puncture treatment alone has not been successful. In those patients in whom complaints persist, a re-evaluation of the initial diagnostic investigation needs to be undertaken. By and large, benign intracranial hypertension is a self-limiting condition once the cause has been recognized and its treatment initiated. The lumbar puncture is a nonspecific means of lowering the intracranial pressure until the inducing mechanism has been resolved. In those patients in whom no known cause has been determined and the symptoms persist for a longer period of time than anticipated, other measures need to be considered to preserve vision.

The reduction of intracranial pressure by diverting spinal fluid via a lumbar-peritoneal shunt has been successful in some patients who are refractory to lumbar puncture treatment. Subtemporal or suboccipital cranial decompression, designed to allow expansion of intracranial contents under pressure in a fixed cranial vault, is no longer done because of the risks of surgery and the postsurgical sequelae.

Another surgical approach, designed to reduce pressure on the optic nerves, is to decompress the nerves within their orbital canals. Effective in some patients in whom lumbar punctures or shunting has proven to be inadequate, the optic nerve decompression procedure does not resolve the intracranial hypertension. It may, however, prevent nerve damage until the underlying problem spontaneously resolves.

There is little rationale to the use of drugs designed to reduce intracranial hypertension. After all, hyperosmolar agents such as mannitol, urea, or glycerol are effective in reducing cerebral edema in certain instances in which a remedy to an acute cerebral process exists, such as in the preparative state to the removal of a brain tumor. In subacute conditions such as benign intracranial hypertension, intravenous hyperosmolar agents would need to be given over an extended number of days. This would create risks for other organ systems such as the kidney and heart in addition to potentially aggravating intracranial hypertension because of the rebound effect to be noted 6 to 8 hours after such an infusion.

Moreover, the nature of brain swelling in benign intracranial hypertension is not vasogenic or cytologic. It is believed to be interstitial. It is perhaps for this reason that other drugs such as adrenocortical steroids have proven ineffective. In like manner, carbonic anhydrase inhibitors or diuretics such as furosemide have not been of value despite animal research, which has shown them to reduce spinal fluid production in the early phase of treatment. Certainly, such drugs would have an adverse effect when given over an extended number of days.

NEUROCUTANEOUS SYNDROMES
MANUEL R. GOMEZ, M.D.

To date more than 50 neurocutaneous syndromes (NCS) have been described. Some of them are listed under such headings as inherited metabolic diseases, DNA repair disorders, or hereditary neuropathies, among other categories, and will not be described in this section.

Tuberous Sclerosis

Tuberous sclerosis (TS) is a hamartiosis and hamartomatosis of autosomal dominant inheritance, variable expressivity, and high penetrance. Approximately half of newly recognized cases are due to new mutation. Through genetic linkage studies the TS gene has been mapped to 9q34 (long arm of chromosome 9 near the gene locus for ABO blood types) in certain families and to 11q22-q23 (long arm of chromosome 11 near the NCAM gene) in other families. There are still families informative for markers in these two chromosomes, but no linkage has been found.

The symptoms and signs in TS are due to the hamartias and hamartomas located in different organs and depend on the number and size of these lesions. The phenotype of patients with cerebral involvement also depends on the location of the lesions within the brain. These cerebral lesions are associated with seizures and mental retardation or with intracranial hypertension if they obstruct the CSF circulation. When this occurs, it is usually at the foramina of Monro. Cardiac hamartomas or rhabdomyomas may obstruct blood flow. Renal hamartomas may cause chronic renal failure by replacing parenchyma, and the tumor may bleed spontaneously.

There is no specific treatment for TS. Symptomatic treatment listed according to the affected organs is outlined in Table 1.

The treatment of infantile spasms and myoclonic seizures should be started as soon as possible after the diagnosis of these symptoms is made and confirmed by electroencephalography. A trial of valproate of no more than 1 week's duration is in order, but if this fails, adrenocorticotropic hormone should be given intramuscularly in dosage of 150 U/m²/day in two divided doses for 7 days, followed by 75 U/m²/day in a single intramuscular dose for another week and then 75 U/m²/every other day for 2 more weeks. After this, the dose should be continued on alternate days, slowly decreasing it over a 6- to 8-week period. If there is a seizure relapse as the ACTH is being tapered, the dose should be increased to an amount equal to or greater than the dosage that maintained the seizures under good control. After there is again a seizure remission, the dose reduction should continue, but by smaller steps

than before. During the period of ACTH reduction and after its discontinuation, the patient should be treated with an anticonvulsant medication and preferably with valproate or nitrazepam. Relapses following successful completion of the ACTH course require a second course of ACTH with a longer and more gradual period of withdrawal. Side effects and complications of the ACTH therapy are common but rarely require stopping it. They are hypertension, glycosuria, hypokalemia, irritability with persistent crying, cushingoid features, acne, cataracts, peptic ulcers, osteoporosis, and obesity.

Tonic, atonic, generalized tonic-clonic, partial motor, or complex partial seizures should be treated with anticonvulsant medication: Valproate, clonazepam, or carbamazepine and, rarely, acetazolamide may be found useful. Less often phenobarbital and phenytoin may be effective, although the former may be accompanied by hyperactivity severe enough to require discontinuation.

There is a correlation between early onset and severity of seizures and mental subnormality in patients with TS. This is frequently demonstrable as and recognized by delay in motor and language acquisition. Early intervention infant stimulation and special education programs should be made available both for the benefit of the patients and for the tranquility of the parents, who may find it difficult to cope with the retardation and abnormal behavior.

Finally, genetic counseling should be provided to the parents. It is necessary to ascertain if any parent has TS by completely examining the skin and fundi and imaging the brain with CT or MR and the kidneys with ultrasound or CT.

Neurofibromatosis 1

Neurofibromatosis is the most common of the neurocutaneous syndromes and is reported to have a prevalence of 1 in 3000, or three times greater than TS. It is of autosomal dominant inheritance with high penetrance and variable expressivity. Here we will refer only to neurofibromatosis 1, or so-called von Recklinghausen neurofibromatosis, since neurofibromatosis 2, or bilateral acoustic neurofibromatosis, is a separate entity that rarely causes symptoms during childhood.

Neurofibromatosis 1 (NF1) can be diagnosed when a patient has at least two of the following clinical features:

—Six or more café-au-lait spots over 5 mm in greatest diameter in subjects who have not yet reached puberty, and over 1.5 mm in greatest diameter in postpubertal individuals.

—Multiple axillary or inguinal freckles.

—At least one plexiform neurofibroma or two neurofibromas of any type.

—Optic nerve and/or chiasmatic glioma.

—Two or more iris pigmented nodules demonstrable with slit lamp.

—Thinning of long bone cortex with or without pseudarthrosis.

—Dysplasia of the sphenoid.

—A first-degree relative with NF1 by the above criteria.

Treatment is always symptomatic and may be medical

TABLE 1. Treatment for Tuberous Sclerosis

Symptoms	Treatment
Seizures	
Infantile spasms	Valproate (VA), adrenocorticotropic hormone (ACTH); see text
Myoclonic	Clonazepam, ACTH, VA
Atonic, tonic	Ethosuximide, acetazolamide, VA
Tonic-clonic	Phenobarbital, phenytoin, VA
Partial seizures	Carbamazepine; surgical treatment is seldom indicated
Intracranial tumors	
Nonobstructing giant-cell tumors	Surgical removal may be necessary for seizure control
Cortical tubers	
Obstruction of CSF pathways	Shunting and/or tumor removal
Cardiac rhabdomyoma	
Asymptomatic	No treatment needed
With obstruction	Surgical removal
With arrhythmia	Antiarrhythmic drugs
Renal angiomyolipomas	
Asymptomatic	No treatment needed
Persistent hematuria	Embolization, partial or total nephrectomy
Retroperitoneal bleed	Nephrectomy
With uremia	Dialysis
Large obstructive renal cysts	Surgical removal
Hypertension	Antihypertensive drugs
Pulmonary lesions	
Spontaneous pneumothorax	Pleurocentesis
Recurrent pulmonary hyperinflation	Respiratory therapy, O_2
Retinal hamartoma	None
Skin lesions	
Facial angiofibromas	Removal with laser beam or abrasion
Shagreen plaques	Cosmetic surgery
Forehead plaques	Cosmetic surgery

or surgical. An experimental medical treatment is now under way to control the pruritus with the drug ketotifen. There is no other medical treatment. Anticonvulsant medication may be required in the exceptional patient with NF1 who has seizures. The surgical treatment may be for cosmetic reasons or to eradicate tumors within the cranium, face, orbits, neck, spinal canal, thorax, or abdomen. Radiation treatment is contraindicated in the majority of lesions, although it has often been used for treating optic gliomas, astrocytomas, and extracranial lesions. It should be remembered that a large amount of radiation produces permanent damage to the cerebrum of young children and that postradiation encephalopathy may have worse consequences than the optic glioma itself. A shunting procedure may be needed when there is aqueductal stenosis or obstruction of the third ventricle by a chiasmatic glioma. Hormonal replacement is necessary when there is pituitary-hypothalamic axis insufficiency. Malignancy is a complication of NF1. The frequency of malignant transformation of neurofibroma to neurofibrosarcoma has been estimated at about 5 per cent. Other malignant tumors may be angiosarcoma, malignant fibrous histiocytoma, and liposarcoma. Wilms' tumor, rhabdomyosarcoma, juvenile chronic myelogenous leukemia, and perhaps neuroblastoma have been reported with more frequency among NF1 patients than in the general population. The appropriate treatment for these lesions with radiotherapy or chemotherapy is necessary.

Patients with NF1 often suffer recurrent headaches in the absence of increased intracranial pressure. In these patients it is necessary to obtain a head CT or an MRI. Some of the headaches have a vascular characteristic and may resemble migraine. Intracranial vascular anomalies and vascular occlusions have been reported with more frequency in NF1 than in the general population. They may present with hemiplegia or other neurologic deficit of sudden onset. Patients with NF1 who have received radiation therapy for intracranial tumors are particularly prone to develop vascular occlusions.

Special methods of education or behavior modification techniques should be offered to the patient with learning or behavior disorders. Psychometrics and evaluation by an educational psychologist are often necessary in children with NF1.

Genetic counseling to the patient and his family is mandatory. Through linkage studies the NF1 gene has been mapped to the long arm of chromosome 17, a useful finding that may be applied to prenatal diagnosis in those families informative for markers located near the gene locus.

Von Hippel–Lindau Disease

Von Hippel–Lindau disease (VHD) is also a hamartiosis and is usually included with the neurocutaneous diseases, although it rarely affects the skin. Like other hamartioses, it is of autosomal dominant inheritance.

Characteristically, the patients with VHD develop retinal and cerebellar hemangioblastomas; renal, pancreatic, and epididymal cysts; and renal carcinoma. The diagnosis can be made when a patient has a hemangioblastoma of the central nervous system or retina and one of the other aforementioned lesions or has a direct relative with this disease.

Treatment of the intracranial hemangioblastoma and

other tumors is surgical. Radiotherapy is of little benefit, but it is recommended for patients who are inoperable, such as those with a hemangioblastoma in the medulla. Since the disease is autosomal dominant and has a high penetrance, individuals at risk should be examined at least once a year for the hemangioblastomas, and, if present, they should be eradicated surgically. The use of MRI of the head contrasted with gadolinium is the preferred neuroimaging method.

Nevoid Basal Cell Carcinoma Syndrome

This is another autosomal dominant disease also known as the Gorlin-Goltz or just the Gorlin syndrome. It is characterized by a skin lesion on the basocellular nevus of the face, neck, and upper trunk, which makes its appearance between puberty and the fourth decade of life. The lesions rarely regress, and some may undergo malignant transformation. The patient often develops the very characteristic odontogenic keratocysts by the first decade of life and generally after the age of 7 years. Their development continues during the second and third decades. The cysts are symptomless unless they become infected. They may be associated with pathologic fractures of the mandible or the maxilla. In addition, some patients have one or more of the following tumors: ovarian fibroma or fibrosarcoma, cardiac fibroma, meningioma, ameloblastoma, leiomyoma, craniopharyngioma, adrenal cortical adenoma, lymphangiomyoma, rhabdomyosarcoma, fetal rhabdomyoma, seminoma, melanoma, neurofibroma, and maxillary fibrosarcoma. These require surgical treatment. Some patients may develop lymphatic cysts of the mesentery, gastric polyps, spindle cell epithelioma, or hamartomatous cysts of the lung, and other patients have congenital blindness due to corneal opacities, congenital cataracts, or glaucoma, and still others may have coloboma of the iris, choroid, or optic nerve, harelip, or cleft palate.

The course of the disease is variable. Only when a medulloblastoma develops is the disease fatal. Its treatment is surgical. Here the prognosis of medulloblastoma is better than in patients with medulloblastoma who do not have the nevoid basal cell carcinoma syndrome. Even when patients do not develop a fatal neoplasia, they may become depressed owing to the continuous development of malignant tumors of the face, requiring frequent intervention which leaves them with many facial scars. Psychiatric treatment may be necessary. Otherwise, the prognosis is not serious, and the patient may live many years. Radiation therapy is contraindicated because it may stimulate development of new skin lesions.

Xeroderma Pigmentosum

This autosomal recessive inherited disorder is caused by a defect in the repair of damaged DNA. The defect causes acceleration of aging of tissues exposed to solar light and premature degeneration of neurons.

The clinical findings are hyperpigmented spots of the skin or freckles, hypopigmentation, telangiectasia, xerosis, desquamation, atrophy, and, following exposure to sunlight, erythema bullae. Among the various types

of neoplasias and preneoplastic lesions are actinic keratosis, basal and spindle cell carcinomas, malignant melanomas, keratoacanthomas, angiomas, fibromas, and sarcomas. In the eyes there may be blepharitis, erythema, eyelid pigmentation and keratosis, a loss of eyelashes, atrophy of the lids leading to entropium or ectropium, papillomas or epitheliomas of the lid borders, basal or spindle cell carcinoma, conjunctivitis, epiphora, edema, pigmentation, telangiectasias, dryness of the conjunctiva, keratitis, synechiae, and iris atrophy. All these lesions appear after exposure of the skin and eyes to the sunlight, usually in the first months of life. By the age of 4 years most of the patients have clinical signs of the disease. A short exposure to sunlight during infancy causes an acute reaction with erythema and vesiculation of the skin. Although this reaction may be transient, subsequently the pigmented lesions appear, increase in number, and become confluent. The skin becomes dry and desquamates and at the end the neoplasias appear.

Neurologic signs develop in some of the patients. In the most severe form there is microcephaly, mental deterioration, ataxia, spasticity, choreoathetosis, and hyporeflexia progressing to areflexia due to a peripheral neuropathy. There may also be delay in growth and sexual development.

Treatment consists of protecting the patients from solar radiation. The diagnosis must be made very early and should be suspected when an infant or small child has suffered an intense erythematous skin reaction after a short exposure to sunlight. Once the diagnosis is confirmed, either because there is a positive family history or through diagnostic laboratory testing that shows a deficient DNA repairing fibroblasts, the patient should be well-protected from ultraviolet radiation, solar light, and fluorescent light of approximately 313 nm wavelength. The most damaging radiation is that of 340 nm wavelength, which does not go through ordinary glass but does penetrate through clouds. The patient should not be exposed to smoke from cigarettes because it has been demonstrated that cultured fibroblasts of these patients, when exposed to the carcinogen present in tobacco smoke, do not repair the damage produced to the DNA. The neoplastic lesions of the skin should be treated with cryotherapy, liquid nitrogen, cryosurgery, electrocoagulation, curetting, or surgical removal. Radiation therapy should not be used to treat the neoplasias.

Incontinentia Pigmenti

Incontinentia pigmenti is a disease that affects almost exclusively females and is inherited from the mother. This type of inheritance may be explained by an X-linked dominant gene that is lethal to homozygotes. Incontinentia pigmenti is manifested by skin lesions that appear in the first days of life as an erythematous macular or papular skin eruption. The lesions become vesicular and later bullous and sometimes pustular. Several crops of lesions appear within the first 2 weeks of life. Later, between the third and sixth weeks of life, the lesions become keratotic or verrucous. Finally, between the twelfth and thirty-sixth weeks of life the skin takes on a dark gray or chocolate color, and this pigmentation has the appearance of designs made on the skin with a brush in curious shapes such as streaks, whirls, and flecks, among others. They are more prominent over the lateral surface of the trunk and limbs and more on the lower than the upper limbs. The pigmentation may persist for several years and usually disappears by the second decade of life.

In 50 to 80 per cent of patients there are lesions in the central nervous system, eyes, teeth, or bony skeleton. The CNS is affected in 30 to 50 per cent of patients. The most common clinical finding is psychomotor retardation. The degree of retardation is variable. Other patients develop symptoms early in life of generalized or focal type. Other findings are spastic diplegia and microcephaly.

The treatment of patients with incontinentia pigmenti is symptomatic. The skin lesions need no treatment other than prophylaxis of infections. Seizures during the acute stage of the disease need anticonvulsant therapy. At a later stage when the child has developmental retardation, spastic paralysis, or mental subnormality, the appropriate services of education and physical therapy can be offered. Similarly, if there are skeletal problems such as scoliosis, hip dislocation, contractures of tendons, and limb deformities, orthopedic treatment may be required. Ophthalmologic service may be necessary when there are refractive errors, strabismus, or cataracts. Finally, genetic counseling should be offered to the parents, as well as the children who may become future parents, before they approach the childbearing age.

Sturge-Weber Syndrome

Sturge-Weber syndrome (SWS) is a nonhereditary congenital malformation of the cephalic venous microvasculature. The complete syndrome consists of facial, cerebral, and ocular signs, which result from telangiectatic venous angiomas on the face, leptomeninges of the cerebrum, and choroid, usually all on the same side. In its incomplete form it may affect one or two of the three tissues.

In the first weeks or months of life the first cerebral symptoms to appear are partial motor seizures. The seizures may or may not become generalized. As patients get older, the seizures may become more frequent and severe. Postictal transient hemiparesis lasting minutes or hours is common, and it may later be replaced by permanent hemiparesis or hemiplegia.

Buphthalmos or glaucoma associated with choroidal angioma is present in 30 per cent of patients with SWS, and more than 50 per cent of these have buphthalmos. The glaucoma may be bilateral even when the facial nevus is unilateral.

The prognosis depends on the severity and extension of the cerebral and ocular lesions. The cutaneous nevus may need cosmetic treatment with the laser beam. The cerebral lesions, when unilateral and associated with intractable seizures that do not respond to anticonvulsant medications, are surgically treatable with lobectomy or hemispherectomy, preferably when the patient is still young and there has been no neurologic deterioration. Glaucoma is medically or surgically treated.

ACUTE ATAXIA
JAMES F. SCHWARTZ

Acute ataxia may occur with primary cerebellar disease or may be a result of disease of other parts of the nervous system. Ataxia should be distinguished from vertigo or dizziness, the subjective feeling of unsteadiness, which is rarely associated with either objective evidence of ataxia or other signs of brain stem or cerebellar disease.

Accurate diagnosis of the disorder producing ataxia is necessary in order to determine specific therapy. Prior or concurrent febrile illness, rash, recurring headaches and early morning vomiting, and a history of drug ingestion or exposure are all historical clues that may indicate the likely diagnosis. Careful neurologic examination is mandatory, with particular attention to the level of consciousness and the presence or absence of signs of increased intracranial pressure, including papilledema, pupil abnormalities, and sixth nerve palsy in addition to ataxia. Other cranial nerve deficits, meningeal signs, and muscle strength, tone, and reflexes are all important in the evaluation of an ataxic child. General physical findings that may be helpful in determining the cause of the ataxia include characteristic rashes such as varicella or vesicular eruptions, which may occur with some enteroviral infections, and lymphadenopathy and splenomegaly as seen with infectious mononucleosis.

Selective tests including urine drug screens, determination of anticonvulsant blood levels, spinal fluid examination, viral serologies and cultures, CT scans, and MRI may be necessary to pinpoint a diagnosis.

Increased Intracranial Pressure/Hydrocephalus and Brain Tumors. Hydrocephalus related to congenital malformation or other non-neoplastic causes of obstruction of CSF circulation may have ataxia as a major finding. Emergency ventriculoperitoneal shunting may cure the ataxia as well as relieve the hydrocephalus. Tumors arising within the cerebellum and the fourth ventricle, such as medulloblastoma, ependymoma, and cystic astrocytoma, commonly have gait ataxia as a major manifestation. Headache and early morning vomiting may be associated symptoms indicative of increased intracranial pressure caused by ventricular obstruction. CT scans or MRI may show ventricular enlargement as well as reveal the presence and size of a cerebellar or fourth ventricle tumor. Administration of dexamethasone, 0.5 mg/kg/day given in four divided doses intravenously, may be helpful in reducing brain swelling associated with increased intracranial pressure followed by ventriculoperitoneal shunting, prior to direct surgical approach to the tumor. The steroids and shunt may not only relieve signs and symptoms of increased pressure but may also result in diminution in the ataxia. Following shunting, direct surgery on the tumors is necessary for biopsy or removal. If removal is not possible, radiation and/or chemotherapy is indicated. The latter may produce significant improvement, especially in patients with medulloblastoma and, to a lesser degree, ependymoma. Primary tumors arising within the brain stem, most commonly in the pons, usually present with ataxia as well as single or multiple cranial nerve palsies and lateralized long track findings, usually without signs of increased pressure. MRI is the diagnostic imaging procedure of choice to determine the site and extent of the tumor. The primary treatment of these tumors is radiation, currently given as hyperfractionated therapy, which may produce significant improvement in the ataxia and other neurologic signs, but it only very rarely results in cure. If radiation is ineffective, chemotherapy is often administered, although this treatment is rarely effective in producing significant clinical improvement or cure.

Acute Cerebellar Ataxia. Acute cerebellar ataxia may be a sequela of various viral infections, including, in particular, varicella or various enteroviruses and exanthems. It has an acute onset, most commonly affecting children under the age of 6 years, and is usually not associated with any neurologic findings other than irritability. Fortunately this disease is most commonly self-limited, requiring no treatment, with spontaneous improvement in the ataxia occurring within a period of 7 to 10 days. In rare instances, ataxia may be severe and persistent and the child may also develop myoclonic jerks. This latter, more serious, persisting form of acute cerebellar ataxia is also associated with rapid jerky eye movements (opsoclonus), and this disorder is then referred to as myoclonic encephalopathy. The severe ataxia, myoclonus, and opsoclonus may respond to daily injections of ACTH gel, 20 to 40 U/day; long-term ACTH therapy may be necessary. Myoclonic encephalopathy may also be associated with occult neuroblastoma, which tends to be in a paraspinal location. Treatment of the neuroblastoma with chemotherapy and surgery may result in alleviation or cure of the tumor as well as the ataxia.

Meningitis. Ataxia occurs as a complication of meningitis, particularly *Haemophilus influenzae* meningitis, in about 10 per cent of cases. It is a self-limited disorder, usually clearing spontaneously within 1 to 2 months after recovery from meningitis, and no specific medical or surgical treatment is required.

Drug Intoxications. Drug ingestion or intoxication is a not uncommon cause of ataxia. Various sedative-hypnotic agents when ingested accidentally or in attempted suicides may cause ataxia along with lethargy and impaired level of consciousness. Usually no treatment is necessary other than the usual supportive measures, including intravenous fluids and ventilatory support. Administration of sufficient sodium bicarbonate intravenously to produce an alkaline urine may enhance the urinary elimination of barbiturates. Acute ethanol intoxication requires no treatment. Overdose of the anticonvulsant drugs phenytoin and carbamazepine, either as a result of an acute ingestion or because of chronic overdose by patients on these drugs for treatment of seizure disorders, may result in ataxia, with phenytoin drug levels usually greater than 25 μg/ml and carbamazepine drug levels greater than 14 μg/ml. This latter form of drug intoxication with carbamazepine usually occurs with patients who, in addition to this drug, are given erythromycin for treatment of infection; the interaction between these two drugs invariably results in intoxicating levels of carbamazepine. The treatment requires immediate discontinuation of erythromycin and withholding the carbamazepine for 24 hours. Subsequently, the carbamazepine may be started once again at the previous dosage and the ataxia should promptly subside. In the case of phenytoin- and carbamazepine-induced ataxia not associated with erythromycin, treatment requires omission of at least one dose of the offending drug and reduction of the maintenance dosage of medication to achieve a more therapeutic level.

Metabolic Diseases. The rare inborn errors of metabolism—maple syrup urine disease (MSUD), disorders of the urea cycle, and multiple carboxylase deficiency (biotinidase deficiency)—may present with ataxia as well as somnolence. In the case of MSUD, recurring ataxia with somnolence usually reflects dietary lapse with accumulation of ketoacids as a result of increased ingestion of the branched-chain amino acids. It usually responds to administration of intravenous fluids and withholding of all protein intake for a period of 24 to 48 hours. Biotin administration to patients with multiple carboxylase deficiencies who present with ataxia and rash may alleviate the ataxia.

Weakness. Children with weakness of acute onset may present with ataxia as their major complaint. Ascending weakness of the legs and trunk along with loss of reflexes and elevated spinal fluid protein is characteristic of the Guillain-Barré syndrome. A variant of this disorder, the Miller-Fisher syndrome, may be associated with ataxia, areflexia, and loss of ocular movements. Steroids have no place in the treatment of the Guillain-Barré syndrome. Careful attention to respiratory function may be necessary with ascending paralysis, and assisted ventilation may be required if the weakness involves intercostal muscles as well. Plasmapheresis may be indicated with progressive severe Guillain-Barré syndrome. Other acute causes of weakness include tick paralysis, for which the treatment is removal of the tick; transverse myelitis, for which steroids may be of some benefit; and spinal cord compression manifested initially by ataxia as well as obvious weakness, reflex changes, sensory loss, and loss of bladder/bowel function. MRI of the spine is indicated in this clinical setting, and surgery is performed if an intrinsic or extrinsic spinal mass lesion is detected.

DEGENERATIVE DISEASES OF THE CENTRAL NERVOUS SYSTEM
PHILIP J. BRUNQUELL, M.D.

Although degenerative diseases of the central nervous system are a heterogeneous group, they share two common features: pathologically there is a progressive, more or less symmetric breakdown of cells in the nervous system, and clinically there is progressive loss of motor and/or intellectual function. Neurons, glia, or myelin sheaths may be primarily affected, but the majority of these conditions represent neuronal degenerations. The ages of onset, rates of progression, and initial clinical manifestations vary. In the later stages of these diseases, however, patients may appear remarkably similar, and therapeutic measures tend to address common clinical problems.

The diseases can be classified into two broad groups: those that are associated with an underlying biochemical defect and those that are not. As research methods become more precise and more biochemical mechanisms are identified, many diseases are being reclassified from the latter category into the former. It is important to distinguish between the two groups because specific therapies are available for some of the disorders in which a biochemical basis is known.

SPECIFIC THERAPY

The goal of specific therapy is to reverse, ameliorate, or circumvent the underlying metabolic defect. Although this approach is currently possible for only some of the diseases, as more biochemical bases are identified, the prospect of having more successful, specific therapies increases correspondingly.

For most of the biochemically based degenerative disorders, an abnormal gene serves as the template for a defective protein, usually an enzyme. The enzyme deficiency may cause accumulation of its substrate, deficiency of the end product, accumulation of substances via alternate metabolic pathways, or a combination of these factors. Specific therapies have attempted to address each of these biochemical processes.

Gene Manipulation

Currently the most effective way to address biochemically based CNS degenerative disease is to prohibit gene expression through either retrospective or, preferably, prospective genetic counseling. Since many of the biochemical disorders follow mendelian (usually autosomal recessive) modes of inheritance, the risks of recurrence can usually be accurately predicted. Furthermore, for many of these conditions, prenatal detection by transabdominal amniocentesis is possible, and the option of therapeutic abortion can be considered. Prospective counseling depends on screening large populations to detect individuals in the preclinical stages of their diseases (e.g., neonatal metabolic screening programs) or screening segments of the population at risk for transmitting specific disorders (e.g., heterozygous carriers of Tay-Sachs disease).

Beyond genetic counseling, direct gene manipulation holds distinct promise. As gene mapping techniques reveal the chromosomal loci of biochemically based degenerative diseases, and as cloning of "corrected" genes becomes possible, the ultimate goal of gene replacement may not be as unrealistic as once was perceived.

Enzyme Manipulation

Both direct and indirect approaches to this form of therapy have been attempted, with varying measures of success. Indirect approaches include cofactor administration and organ allotransplantation. The direct approach of enzyme replacement remains highly experimental at the current time.

Many enzymes require vitamin or metal cofactors to achieve biological activity. Cofactor administration may increase a deficient enzyme's catalytic activity and produce clinical improvement, as in the administration of vitamin B_{12} in methylmalonic acidemia and biotin in propionic acidemia. Allotransplantation of an organ that manufactures the deficient enzyme may be limited by the organ's capability for enzyme synthesis: Sufficient enzyme may be produced for its own use but not for other organs of the body, including the brain. Recently, however, encouraging results have been noted in patients undergoing bone marrow transplantation for a number of conditions, including Gaucher's disease and some of the mucopolysaccharidoses.

Attempts at direct enzyme replacement have been limited by problems with enzyme purification, peripheral inactivation, and tissue targeting. At present, research is aimed at overcoming these obstacles, as in the delivery of enzymes in lipid envelopes (liposomes), the entry of enzymes into the CNS via transient osmotic opening of the blood-brain barrier, and the linkage of enzymes to cell receptor–specific ligands, thus permitting receptor-mediated endocytosis.

Substrate Removal

In many cases, a patient's condition may improve when the accumulating substrate is eliminated or restricted from the diet. Dietary restrictions may be general, such as the reduction of protein in patients who have disorders of the urea cycle, or more specifically, such as the elimination of galactose in galactosemia or the reduction of phenylalanine in phenylketonuria. The amount of substrate to eliminate from the diet and the length of time to continue the restriction vary with the underlying metabolic defect; for some disorders there is a lack of consensus on these issues.

Occasionally biochemically based degenerative disease may present as an acute, overwhelming encephalopathic illness. This is especially true of conditions presenting in the neonatal period. Emergency removal of excess substrate may in some cases prove life-saving. Peritoneal dialysis, hemodialysis, or exchange transfusion has been useful in a number of disorders of amino acid metabolism, particularly those that are resistant to pharmacologic intervention.

Elimination of Accumulating Substances by Creating Alternate Metabolic Pathways

Administration of certain compounds may permit the disposal of accumulating substances via pathways other than the one catalyzed by the deficient enzyme. In urea cycle disorders, for example, lowering of serum ammonia has been achieved by administering sodium benzoate. Nitrogen-containing compounds that, by virtue of the metabolic defect, cannot be excreted as urea and would ordinarily accumulate as ammonia are conjugated to benzoate to form hippurate, which is then easily excreted in the urine. Another example is the lowering of copper accumulation in Wilson's disease by the administration of the heavy-metal antagonist penicillamine. Penicillamine is a chelating agent that forms a complex with copper, thus competing with body ligands for binding of the cation and permitting enhanced urinary copper excretion.

End-Product Replacement

The clinical symptoms of enzyme deficiency may result not only from substrate accumulation but also from deficiency of the end-product produced by the reaction catalyzed by the deficient enzyme. Replacement of the end-product may, in turn, ameliorate the symptoms or, if administered in the preclinical stage, prohibit the clinical appearance of the disease. Early thyroid hormone replacement in patients with congenital hypothyroidism may, for example, avert clinical catastrophe.

In most cases of biochemically based degenerative disease, the mother's metabolism protects the fetus in utero. Postnatally, when the infant relies on its own metabolism for survival, neural tissue is placed in jeopardy. The effectiveness of the strategies described above depends therefore upon early, accurate diagnosis. Whether the physician is amplifying enzyme activity by cofactor administration, restricting dietary substrate, eliminating accumulating substances by creating alternate metabolic pathways, or supplying missing end-products, intervention must be instituted before irreversible brain damage has occurred.

SYMPTOMATIC THERAPY

The goals of therapy aimed at treating the symptoms of degenerative disease are to maximize remaining function, promote patient comfort, minimize the risk of secondary illnesses, and facilitate nursing care. The implementation of these goals needs to be continually redefined as the patient's disease progresses. The views of the parents or guardians are crucial to this process of redefinition, and therefore it is incumbent upon the physician to discuss with them the clinical manifestations, the therapeutic ramifications, and the natural history of the disease so that they will be equipped to make informed decisions. Plans for emergency management need to be considered prior to any abrupt, life-threatening decline. Some hospitals have guidelines for the selective emergency management of terminally ill children. Such guidelines seek to ally the recommendations of the physician with the desires of the family while providing opportunity for the ongoing reassessment of the management plan as the child's disease progresses.

The remaining sections describe issues pertinent to the care of these patients.

Dysphagia

Much of the failure to thrive seen in children with degenerative disease of the nervous system is due to insufficient caloric intake caused by the inability to suck and swallow in a co-ordinated fashion. Nasogastric feedings are a useful temporary measure, but for chronic use a gastrostomy is usually required. Caloric needs may vary widely. Immobile patients may require substantially less than those who, although bedridden,

manifest nearly continual adventitious movements such as chorea or athetosis.

Respiratory Function

With progression of the underlying disease, the child typically becomes prone to episodes of atelectasis and aspiration. Chest physical therapy and postural drainage amplified by the use of mucolytic agents and expectorants are frequently required. Tracheostomy may be necessary to promote respiratory toilet. Mechanical ventilatory support is most appropriate during the initial phases of the patient's illness when pneumonia and other pulmonary problems tend to represent transient setbacks.

Seizure Control

Although patients with degenerative disorders of the central nervous system (and gray matter diseases in particular) are prone to seizures on the basis of their underlying condition, seizures secondary to reversible causes such as hypoglycemia, electrolyte disturbance, or infection need to be considered because they are unlikely to respond to conventional anticonvulsant therapy unless the precipitating cause is addressed. For seizures that arise from the primary degenerative process, the choice of a particular anticonvulsant will depend on the clinical and EEG manifestations of the patient's seizures. As many patients with degenerative disorders exhibit myoclonic seizures, valproic acid may be of particular benefit. However, some children with inborn metabolic errors may be at particular risk for valproate-induced hepatic failure, and therefore alternative anticonvulsants should be considered in this group.

During the evolution of the child's illness a variety of unusual postures and movements may emerge, not all of which represent seizure activity. Referral of the patient to an EEG-videotelemetry laboratory may be helpful in distinguishing epileptic from nonepileptic behavior. The results of such studies may lead not only to more accurate therapy for seizures but also to the avoidance of unnecessary medication for those events that are not seizure-related.

Behavior

Agitation, irritability, and aggression may become severe enough to require medical management. Before considering whether to administer minor or major tranquilizing agents, the physician needs to rule out the possibility that the patient may be reacting to discomfort from a reversible cause, such as dental abscess, other occult infections, obstipation, or bony dislocation. When tranquilizing agents are indicated, doses need to be carefully titrated to the patient's condition. For example, some patients with degenerative disease may spontaneously and unpredictably alternate between hyperkinetic and hypersomnolent states. The toxic effects of tranquilizing medications may be exacerbated when superimposed on the latter condition.

Neuromuscular Care

Muscle spasticity and contractures are hallmarks of many degenerative diseases of the central nervous system. While the maintenance of ambulation may be a viable goal early in the course of the patient's illness, as the disease progresses this expectation becomes increasingly unrealistic. Nonetheless, neuromuscular therapy may still be useful to address separate issues. For example, spasticity with contractures and bony dislocation may cause pain and thus merit treatment, and relief of adductor spasm of the lower extremities may be necessary to permit perineal hygiene.

Overall, management can be viewed in a hierarchical order of invasiveness beginning with physical therapy, advancing to bracing with or without the addition of spasmolytic therapy, and culminating in surgical intervention such as tendon lengthening. Spasmolytic therapy is rarely useful alone and is limited by the occurrence of drug-induced side effects such as sedation from diazepam and baclofen and hepatic dysfunction from dantrolene sodium. Of the surgical procedures, selective spinal dorsal root rhizotomy is currently being evaluated as a promising means of alleviating spasticity. Regardless of which approach is used, care must be taken in those circumstances in which spasticity is necessary to sustain an upright posture or maintain balance in ambulation, as excessive reduction in tone in these instances may further compromise motor function.

Skin Care

Decubitus ulcers should be prevented by proper positioning, frequent turning, protection of bony prominences, treatment of dependent edema, and maintenance of good nutrition. The skin should be kept dry and a protective ointment, such as petroleum jelly, should be applied to the areas exposed to moisture. If ulcers develop, mechanical and/or lytic enzyme débridement is necessary if necrotic tissue is present. Application of radiant heat and massage around the area of ulcer may improve circulation and facilitate healing. Protective dressings are applied, and use of water- and oxygen-permeable synthetic materials may be helpful (e.g., Op-site).

Bladder Management

Intermittent catheterization is the most common method for managing the neurogenic bladder. Chronic drug therapy is often limited by toxicity. Of the relatively safer medications, imipramine hydrochloride may be useful to reduce detrusor muscle hypertonicity, and oxybutynin chloride* may increase vesical capacity, decrease the frequency of uninhibited detrusor muscle contractions, and delay the initial desire to void in patients with uninhibited neurogenic and reflex neurogenic bladder. Occasionally, a surgical measure such as transurethral resection of the bladder neck is indicated. Since prolonged immobilization may lead to hypercalcinuria, maintenance of a high fluid volume is important to prevent kidney stone formation. Acidification of the urine may not only help to prevent infection but may also keep mineral salts in solution.

---

*Manufacturer's precaution: The safety and efficacy of oxybutynin chloride (Ditropan) have been demonstrated for children 5 years of age and older; there are insufficient clinical data for children under age 5, and Ditropan is not recommended for this age group.

Bowel Management

Fecal impaction is very common in patients with CNS degenerative diseases. Adequate hydration, natural dietary laxatives, glycerine or bisacodyl suppositories, and stool softeners such as dioctyl sulfosuccinate are useful measures. Digital removal of stool and enemas may be required.

Infectious Diseases Surveillance

The child's resistance to infection is typically lowered by immobility, poor nutrition, and compromise of protective physiologic functions such as coughing, gagging, and complete bladder emptying. Acute infections, even those outside the nervous system, can produce an abrupt decline from the patient's current level of neurologic functioning, which may often be reversed upon adequate treatment of the infection. The role of occult infections in causing chronic agitation and irritability has already been mentioned.

Psychosocial Support

The presence of CNS degenerative disease in a child places an enormous emotional and financial burden on the family. For the child who is cared for at home, respite care for the parents can be of immense benefit in allowing them to renew their physical and emotional resources. Parent support groups can ameliorate the isolation that families experience in caring for their afflicted child. For some conditions, such as Tay-Sachs disease, national foundations exist which can provide further support services. Financial assistance for such items as adaptive equipment, medications, and nursing care should be explored.

One of the most important therapeutic measures that the physician can employ is to avoid retreating from the patient and the patient's family when the terminal stages of the illness arrive. The presence and concern of the physician are never more fully appreciated than when the technologic methods of treatment are no longer relevant to the destiny of the child.

CEREBRAL PALSY

LAWRENCE T. TAFT, M.D.

Although cerebral palsy per se is a motor disorder, associated nonmotor handicaps, such as mental retardation, often prove more disabling. The specific strategies necessary for the child to develop to his full potential are only partly determined by the type and extent of the cerebral dysfunction. At least as important in the selection of optimal strategies are the child's family and social milieu.

The first goal in pediatric management should be to maximize the coping abilities of the child and family. Several general principles are particularly important in achieving this goal: (1) Past success is a powerful motivator for future effort. Thus, whenever possible, the child should be placed in situations that optimize his chances for success. Failure depresses and tends to lessen motivation; failure must be avoided. (2) The importance of achieving functional motor improvements, such as independent ambulation, should not be unduly stressed. (3) Co-ordination of the diagnostic and treatment modalities involved is essential. (4) Achievement of the rights of the child and his family vis-à-vis governmental and other institutional support may require active advocacy on the part of the health care provider.

INITIAL DIAGNOSIS

The parents must be told of the problem in a compassionate and empathetic manner as soon as the diagnosis is suspected or confirmed. They should be given as much information about the cause, treatment, and prognosis as is available. When, as frequently occurs, the prognosis for independent ambulation and/or functioning cannot be accurately stated, the parents should be told of the limitations of early prognosis. Upon hearing the words "Your child has cerebral palsy," the initial reaction of the parents is commonly extreme grief. Listening may continue, but comprehension often suffers. Thus, it is often necessary to repeat the explanations and to answer the same questions over several subsequent sessions to ensure that the parents understand the situation and have no misconceptions.

At the time of the informing interview, let the parents know that you will be referring the child to a nearby "early intervention center." Many of these programs are home-based. If center-based, they require the parent to bring the child to only one session per week. Explain that the center will educate the parents further about cerebral palsy, will explore the problems the infant and the family usually have in coping, and will offer intervention strategies that will optimize the child's intellectual and motor functioning. The parents will act as therapists, under the tutelage of the intervention center staff. The advantage of immediate referral is that it does not leave the parents with a sense of complete hopelessness after they are informed of the diagnosis. It offers immediate and essential family support.

The Committee on Children with Handicaps of the American Academy of Pediatrics has concluded that early intervention programs mitigate the denial that families experience after learning of the diagnosis and, consequently, allow for an earlier adaptation.

SPECIFIC INTERVENTION STRATEGIES

Motor Performance

Many techniques are used to improve motor function or prevent complications. The purpose may be to modify the dyskinetic movements, to decrease the hypertonus, or to develop specific skills. Treatment includes physical, occupational, and speech therapies, adaptive devices such as braces, medications, chemical neurolysis to decrease tone, and orthopedic intervention to correct the musculoskeletal abnormalities that develop in the growing child with cerebral palsy.

Physical Therapy

Physical therapy for cerebral palsy can be broadly categorized into two major types: The first is to maintain the range of motion of the joints and to increase muscle strength; the second is to favorably modify the abnormal tone and movements.

The first, most traditional, type includes passive and active stretching of joints to maintain a full range of motion and prevent musculoskeletal deformities; strengthening exercises by active movements against increasingly greater resistance to counteract the weakness of specific muscle groups; and the teaching and encouragement of the voluntary performance of specific tasks, especially those related to daily living. Parents can be taught to be "therapists." As the child gets older, he himself can assume responsibility for many of these therapies.

Techniques that attempt to favorably influence tone and posture are more controversial. They are best known by the names of the individuals who have described them, e.g., Bobath, Rood, Kabat, Bronstrum, Fay. Bobath neurodevelopment physical therapy (NDPT) appears to be the most commonly used by physiatrists and physical therapists. It attempts to inhibit persistent primitive reflexes and to modify tone by the use of applied sensory stimuli—tactile, vestibular, and proprioceptive. An example of the inhibition of a primitive reflex is modification of the dysfunctional posture caused by a persistent obligatory symmetric tonic neck reflex. When this reflex is present, the trunk extension that often occurs in these children activates extension of the upper extremities. This latter posture does not allow the child to engage in hand-to-mouth activities or to learn eye-hand co-ordination. With the Bobath technique, the child is placed in a position that encourages trunk flexion. This activates the symmetric tonic neck reflex in a manner to cause flexion of the upper extremities, thereby facilitating the child's use of his hands and, it is hoped, making him more functional. With active use of his hands, he can improve eye-hand co-ordination and also increase his sensory experiences.

A recent clinical trial concluded that short-term motor outcome in infants with spastic diplegia given 12 months of NDPT was not improved over a control group given 6 months of infant stimulation plus 6 months of NDPT. Chronic stimulation of spastic muscles before abnormal intrinsic muscle development occurs has been reported to improve motor performance and gait.

Occupational Therapy

Occupational therapy is often prescribed to improve a youngster's ability in self-help activities. Adaptive equipment may be recommended to facilitate functional use of the hands. Adaptive seating is utilized to maintain trunk stabilization, allowing better use of the upper extremities.

Speech and Language Therapy

Many infants with cerebral palsy have difficulty sucking, chewing, and/or swallowing. This may result in markedly slow feeding, aspiration, and poor weight gain. Speech therapists with training and experience with infants utilize proper positioning and sensory stimulation of the oropharyngeal areas to help ameliorate the problem. Empirically, there appear to be successes that cannot be explained by maturation. Also, coping by infant and mother is made easier when feeding becomes a pleasurable activity.

Early identification of a delay in expressive language is important, and these infants should receive the benefit of referral to a speech therapist. The mother is taught how to stimulate language development as part of the daily routine care of the infant. A hearing loss must be ruled out.

If articulation is abnormal, a speech therapist should be consulted.

Drug Modification of Tone

Successful use of medication to decrease tone (to improve voluntary control of movement) has been limited by drug side effects. Diazepam (Valium) usually has a marked sedative effect before it favorably ameliorates hypertonus. However, when anxiety increases involuntary movements, especially athetoid, Valium may be beneficial. Dantrolene, which acts directly on the muscle to limit its contractility, also may cause sedation. However, the major concern with Dantrolene is that the desired decrease in muscle tone is often associated with marked muscle weakness. In addition, Dantrolene is hepatotoxic, and liver function must be carefully monitored while the child is on this drug. Baclofen, a gamma-aminobutyric acid derivative, is believed to inhibit neurotransmitter impulses. It has mild sedative effects with no significant toxic effects. Studies in children are limited and have not proved its effectiveness in improving motor function. A trial of therapy may be indicated, especially in children with severe hypertonus. Use of a muscle relaxant may also benefit the caretaker of the cerebral palsied child. For instance, a child with severe adductor spasticity is difficult to diaper. The spasticity may be minimized with the use of the appropriate drug.

Local therapy to improve tone has included the use of phenol. Because of phenol's neurolytic properties, injection of the drug around the motor nerve results in partial denervation. This effect may last from a few weeks to a few months. It may especially help to alleviate a spastic equinus foot or severe hip adductor spasm. However, repeated injection of the solution is contraindicated. Use of the phenol solution may allow a more accurate prediction of the functional result achievable through surgery.

Orthotic and Adaptive Equipment

Bracing is used for two purposes: to prevent contractures and to maintain joint stability as an aid in achieving an erect posture. Although lightweight braces are now available, bracing is becoming a less popular mode of therapy.

There are numerous adaptive devices to aid in independent functioning. Occupational and physical therapists can evaluate the patient to determine the need for these devices and the type that would provide more independent self-care abilities.

In the past decade, computers have made it possible to develop electronic aids that may permit the most severely motor handicapped individual to gain some control of his environment. A movement of the head or an eye blink can permit a severely quadriplegic individual to turn a page or open a door. Rehabilitation engineers are being utilized on rehabilitation teams to assess each individual as to whether a specifically designed environmental control apparatus will aid the individual to function more independently.

Wheelchairs may be self-driven or propelled by caretakers. The latter are called travel-chairs and usually are most appropriate for the severely handicapped child. The chair can be aligned to permit maximal stability of the trunk and to minimize reflexive spastic responses such as hyperextension. The traditional, independently propelled wheelchair has segments to support the leg, seat, and back. These can be adjusted to minimize abnormal postures. The specific type of wheelchair and adaptive equipment should be prescribed by an experienced professional.

Biofeedback

Biofeedback involves the patient's active participation in an attempt to control motor activity through sensory feedback mechanisms. There are very few controlled or long-term studies of the duration of the effects achieved. However, there have been some suggestions that biofeedback has helped hemiplegic cerebral palsied children of normal intelligence to attain a more symmetric, more cosmetic gait.

Electromyographic auditory feedback training of the orbicularis oris and an auditory signal to cue swallowing have been shown to be effective in decreasing drooling. Further experience with this technique is necessary before being able to endorse its therapeutic value. However, a trial of therapy is indicated as a first endeavor to correct drooling, since there are no complications. Drugs and surgical interventions have many associated risks.

Inhibitory Casting

Attempts have been made to realign partially deformed ankles by use of a walking cast applied for a period of 4 to 6 weeks. The foot is maintained in a more normal anatomic position, which, in spastic cerebral palsy, necessitates sustained stretching.

There is clinical evidence to indicate that inhibitive casting does result in an increase in ankle dorsiflexion and range of motion. However, this gain is usually lost after 4 to 5 months in spite of the use of rigid ankle orthoses worn during waking hours.

Orthopedic Surgery

Orthopedic surgery is often recommended to correct deformities due to the neuromuscular imbalance of cerebral palsy. Heel-cord lengthening, adductor tenotomies, and hip flexor and hamstring releases are done to improve posture and function. There is still controversy regarding the optimal timing of these procedures as well as which procedures are most effective.

Many cerebral palsy centers have a gait analysis laboratory and utilize this type of evaluation to assist in the decision-making as to the type of orthopedic surgery that might offer the best result. The gait analysis is also used to monitor the results of the intervention.

Neurosurgery

Chronic cerebellar stimulation to modify hypertonus has been attempted. Results have been disappointing. Selective posterior rhizotomy to reduce hypertonus and therefore to facilitate movement is now being done at many neurosurgical centers. The posterior roots of the lumbar plexus are exposed and stimulated. The observed electromyographic response aids in identifying those fibers that appear to be facilitating muscle responses. These fibers are resected. Results of this type of surgery appear encouraging in that muscle tone is reduced with improved motor ability. More must be learned as to the short- and long-term effects and the selective indicators to achieve the best results.

Health Maintenance

Cerebral palsied children should benefit from the health maintenance routines offered to children without handicaps. For example, they should be immunized according to the standard recommended schedule. In addition, there are a number of screening tests and areas of anticipatory guidance that are particularly relevant to the care of disabled children.

Routine screening for auditory abilities is essential. Over 70 per cent of athetoid cerebral palsied youngsters, secondary to bilirubin encephalopathy, have high-frequency hearing loss. Thirty per cent of all other cerebral palsied children have sensorineural hearing impairment. Early recognition of and appropriate intervention for these problems are important for the prevention of additional difficulties.

Vision screening should be stressed during routine examinations. Strabismus is present in over 75 per cent of cerebral palsied individuals. Early recognition and referral to an ophthalmologist will help prevent amblyopia ex anopsia. Ophthalmoscopic examination should be done to evaluate for cataracts and to judge whether a refractive error exists. Nearsightedness is commonly found. When the child is cognitively ready, visual acuity should be tested with the use of "E" or Snellen charts.

There should be routine assessments of the range of motion of spastic joints. Tightness or limitation in the full range of joint motion requires a referral to a physical therapist. The parents can be taught to passively stretch the child's joints to prevent irreversible contractures.

The presence of scoliosis must be monitored. A high prevalence is noted, especially in quadriplegic patients.

Leg length discrepancies should be assessed in hemiplegic infants and children. Over 50 per cent of patients with hemiparesis due to congenital insult have a leg length discrepancy. In an ambulatory child, early recognition and correction of an inequality of leg length by the use of a sole lift helps prevent the development of scoliosis.

Advice must be given to parents regarding the importance of preventing obesity in the child. The limitation of physical activity that results from a neuromotor handicap often results in excessive weight gain.

During each health maintenance visit, the parents should be asked if there are any recurrent episodes in which the child appears to be unaware of his surroundings. These may be seizure manifestations. Over one half of children with cerebral palsy develop epilepsy. Some types of psychomotor seizures may not be recognized as such, being attributed to aberrant behavior.

Assisting Psychosocial Adjustment

Anticipatory guidance of the parents may help minimize adverse psychosocial adjustment of the child and family members. Parents should be advised not to act solicitously toward the child. Doing so can cause the child to develop a self-concept of dependency and helplessness. Parents should be encouraged to discipline the child as they would a healthy youngster.

Preschool children frequently believe their handicap is punishment for some wrongdoing. The pediatrician should explore this issue with the child and, if there is evidence that this is the case, the youngster should be informed that his problem is not related to a punishment or previous bad behavior. As the child grows older, his inability to compete physically and socially may lead to isolation from his peers. Attempts should be made to find recreational or social activities in which the youngster may successfully interact with peers and, it is hoped, develop more positive social relationships.

Education

Early intervention centers for infants are quite abundant. In almost all states mandatory education for handicapped youngsters must be offered from 3 years of age. Parents of young cerebral palsied children should be encouraged to have their child enrolled in these preschool programs. However, if the disability is minimal, as is often found in hemiplegic patients, and if the youngster does not have a significant cognitive deficit, a normal nursery school placement is preferable.

Mainstreaming children who are capable of competing with their normal peers is preferable to special class placement. However, if there is any suggestion that the child is finding it difficult to maintain his self-esteem because of an inability to compete academically with his peers, he should be placed where he can experience success and better maintain his self-esteem. Children in wheelchairs can be successfully mainstreamed if they have the necessary cognitive abilities.

Nonverbal Communication

Many children with cerebral palsy have difficulties with expressive language, owing to severe dysarthria, verbal dyspraxia, or expressive aphasia. The inability to control one's environment through the use of language can be very depressing. With the use of communication devices as substitutes for spoken or written language, significantly language-impaired children can make themselves understood. There are many devices that resemble calculators which the child can use to make selected inquiries or responses. The use of nonverbal communication has had amazing success. Many children who are thought to be retarded or withdrawn have demonstrated unexpectedly high cognitive abilities. Successful nonverbal communication has also resulted in positive personality changes. The children become more interested in relating to their peers and caretakers. An infant who has evidence of a severe motor dysfunction of the oropharyngeal muscles should be offered nonverbal communication aids. This will not inhibit later development of the ability to communicate verbally.

Recreation

Recreational and social programs geared to the handicapped are necessary so that the child does not become homebound. Parents should be referred to the regional voluntary health agency, such as the United Cerebral Palsy Association or the state Developmental Disability Council, to learn where and what programs exist.

Day care and sleep-away camps are also available and should be utilized.

Vocational Training

Adolescents should receive vocational training. Parents should be advised to urge their child's educators to find a suitable vocational training program. This should not be delayed until graduation. If the handicap is so great as to preclude functioning in competitive employment, sheltered workshops should be considered.

SPINAL DISEASES

FRANCIS S. WRIGHT, M.D.

The spinal cord may be affected by several pathologic conditions, all resulting in varying degrees of weakness, sensory loss, bowel and bladder dysfunction, and other autonomic symptoms. The major objectives in the treatment of spinal cord diseases are to prevent further neurologic impairment, avoid non-neurologic complications that interfere with recovery, maximize neurologic functional recovery, and provide early rehabilitative procedures.

In patients presenting with signs and symptoms of spinal cord dysfunction, it is essential that spinal cord tumor, epidural abscess, and arteriovenous malformation be excluded. These entities are best diagnosed by MRI techniques but also may be detected by myelography and metrizamide CT scanning.

If the patient presents with symptoms of rapidly progressing spinal cord dysfunction, an emergency neurosurgical consultation is indicated.

SPINAL CORD TRAUMA

Any patient who is unconscious or has multiple injuries should be suspected or assumed to have a spinal cord injury until proven otherwise. Consequently, the initial treatment should be to provide spinal column immobilization with a soft cervical collar and sandbags placed on either side of the neck for possible cervical spine injury, and the patient should be supported on a rigid frame with shoulder and pelvic girdle support for possible thoracic and lumbar injury. The cervical spine

must be protected during airway stabilization. If respiratory function is deteriorating as a result of intercostal and/or diaphragmatic dysfunction, intubation should be performed by the nasotracheal route if possible, with the head supported in a neutral position to avoid any manipulation of the head. If the nasotracheal route is inadequate, a tracheostomy may be necessary. Cardiovascular status needs to be monitored continuously. Careful attention should be given to blood pressure, oxygen and carbon dioxide concentration, and possible anemia. Acute spinal cord injury often results in a loss of autonomic nervous system function with an impairment in vasomotor and sympathetic tone. Consequently, bradycardia, functional hypovolemia, and hypotension frequently develop. These effects may be initially treated with intravenous atropine followed by dopamine or dobutamine. The hypovolemia is treated with volume expansion.

Once the patient's condition is stabilized, radiographic examination of the spine should be performed in areas of suspected injury. Cervical spinal radiography should be performed in all patients with multiple trauma or major head injury. The cervical spine should be immobilized and a lateral cervical spinal radiograph obtained. A CT scan may provide additional information. In severely injured patients, neurosurgical, orthopedic, and general surgical management is essential.

The initial neurologic examination should assess the extent of spinal cord injury. Special attention should be given to respiratory movements to detect the typical "see-saw" respirations characteristic of intercostal muscle paralysis. This pattern may be recognized by the failure of the rib cage to expand in conjunction with the abdominal expansion during the inspiration phase so that the chest appears to sink while the abdominal wall is rising, resulting in a "see-saw" movement. The neurologic examination should include assessment of the level of consciousness. Cranial nerve function should be evaluated. The extent of motor weakness should be documented. Spontaneous movements may indicate the level of dysfunction. If the spinal cord injury is at the thoracic level, the patient moves only the upper extremities and demonstrates a paraplegia. In addition, the patient does not experience pain or discomfort to painful procedures such as bladder catheterization or movement of an obviously fractured leg. Sensory testing should be carried out with response to touch and pin prick to establish a sensory level. Position and vibration senses should be evaluated for posterior column function. To test the integrity of the sacral cord, perianal sensation and rectal tone should be evaluated. Generally in acute spinal shock the tendon reflexes are depressed or absent.

In addition, a sweat level may be detected by stroking the skin upward over the trunk with the dorsum of the hand until an increase in resistance is perceived, which indicates the autonomic sweat level. Hypothermia is common in children with spinal cord injury. This may be managed with a hyperthermia blanket.

The bladder size should be evaluated, since acute urinary retention is very common. A greatly dilated bladder may interfere with respiration in a patient who is dependent solely on diaphragmatic movement. An indwelling catheter should be placed.

Axial skeletal traction is needed if there is any bony vertebral malalignment. General care for the spinal cord injured patient is similar to that described for the patient with acute myelitis.

SPINAL CORD TUMOR

Extramedullary tumors affecting the spinal cord usually can be completely removed surgically. Intramedullary tumors of the spinal cord may benefit from neurosurgical decompression, especially with the improved surgical capability of the operating microscope and with ultrasonic aspirator removal of tumor, leading to subsequent improvement in spinal cord function. Additional chemotherapy or radiation treatment may be indicated. Prior to surgery, spinal cord edema resulting from the mass lesion may be treated with dexamethasone, 0.5 to 1.5 mg/kg/day in four divided doses.

TRANSVERSE MYELITIS (MYELOPATHY)

This syndrome is characterized by sudden, progressive weakness and impaired sensation of the legs which evolve over hours to days and are associated with bowel and bladder dysfunction. It is essential that spinal cord compression resulting from a tumor, epidural abscess, or arteriovenous malformation be excluded.

The acute management of this condition involves continued assessment of vital signs and evaluation for neurologic progression. In addition, early rehabilitative procedures should be carried out that will diminish long-term disability. The vital signs should be monitored every 2 hours, or more frequently if they are changing rapidly. Since myelitis often involves the thoracic cord, there may be impairment of respiratory function. The patient should be placed on a cardiac monitor, and in addition the vital capacity should be measured at frequent intervals. Blood gas determinations may be useful in assessing respiratory function. Neurologic function should be assessed at frequent intervals with regard to progressive weakness and ascending sensory level. Maintenance intravenous fluids should be administered. Since the patient has urinary incontinence, an indwelling catheter should be inserted. Urinary tract infections should be treated with appropriate antibiotics. Because of the sensory loss over the trunk and pelvis, pressure sores may develop. Consequently, the patient should be placed on an air mattress and turned frequently. Heel pads may be used to prevent further skin injury.

Physical therapy should be initiated as soon as the patient's condition is stabilized. The goals of physical therapy are to maintain flexibility in the extremities, increase strength in all extremities with resistive exercises, and develop independent ambulation with minimal assistive devices. The patient's nutritional status should be monitored with regard to caloric intake during the period of inactivity to provide sufficient nutrition while preventing excessive weight gain. If the patient is experiencing pain, analgesics should be prescribed.

Patients often experience a reactive depression, and psychological intervention is appropriate.

CONGENITAL DEFECTS

Atlantoaxial instability, syringomyelia, diastematomyelia, narrowed lumbar spinal canal, and tethered cord syndrome all may produce static or progressive spinal cord symptoms and signs. These are diagnosed by MRI techniques. Altantoaxial instability may be diagnosed by upper cervical spine radiographs demonstrating an increased (5 mm or more) atlantodens interval. Neurosurgical treatment is indicated if there is evidence of spinal cord compression or progressive symptoms.

SEIZURE DISORDERS
GREGORY L. HOLMES, M.D.

A seizure can be defined as a sudden, involuntary alteration in neurologic function secondary to an abnormal discharge of neurons in the central nervous system. Epilepsy refers to a chronic condition in which a patient experiences recurrent unprovoked seizures. Epilepsy is not a single disease but rather a sign of underlying brain dysfunction. Seizures secondary to a provoked brain insult, i.e., febrile seizures and those associated with hypoglycemia or other temporary disorders, do not fall under the definition of epilepsy but are considered provoked seizures.

Epilepsy is a common disorder. The incidence of epilepsy is highest in the first two decades of life. Approximately 75 per cent of patients with epilepsy have the onset of seizures before age 20 years.

Although the ketogenic diet and epilepsy surgery both have a role in the management of epilepsy in a minority of children, the principal mode of medical therapy of childhood seizures is drug management. This discussion will be confined to the pharmacologic management of children with seizures.

STATUS EPILEPTICUS

Status epilepticus is defined as continuous, repeated, or recurring generalized (or lateralized) convulsive seizures without recovery of consciousness, lasting at least 30 minutes. The salient points contained within the above definition are the following: (1) The seizure type is usually major motor: tonic, clonic, or tonic-clonic. (2) Consciousness is not recovered between serial convulsions. (3) The convulsion lasts at least one-half hour. The definition of status epilepticus implies that it is a self-sustaining process that will not spontaneously cease unless "neuronal exhaustion" supervenes.

Tonic-clonic status epilepticus is a neurologic emergency. Clinical and experimental studies dictate that an attack of tonic-clonic status epilepticus be stopped as soon as possible. It should not be allowed to last longer than 60 minutes if severe, permanent brain damage or death is to be prevented. Significant mortality rates after tonic-clonic status epilepticus have been reported in both children and adults. The longer tonic-clonic status continues, the more difficult it is to control and the higher the incidence of neurologic sequelae or morbidity.

Convulsive status must not be allowed to progress beyond 20 minutes—the so-called transitional period. If convulsive status epilepticus continues beyond 60 minutes despite antiepileptic drug (AED) treatment, the patient should be placed under general anesthesia. Adequate cardiorespiratory function and brain oxygenation must be provided to prevent selective cell damage in the cerebellum and amygdala; when present, secondary metabolic complications such as hypoglycemia, electrolyte imbalance, lactic acidosis, dehydration, and hyperpyrexia must be corrected.

In addition, the causes and immediate trigger of status epilepticus must be appropriately treated and corrected at the same time the patient is undergoing treatment of the tonic-clonic status. For example, a child with status epilepticus secondary to meningitis needs immediate treatment of the meningitis as well as the status epilepticus.

A patient in status epilepticus should be treated in an intensive care unit where adequate nursing and physician aid are readily available and emergency facilities for resuscitation are present. The first step is to protect the child from injury by placing him or her on a well-padded bed. The child should be placed on his side and an oral airway inserted. Other foreign objects such as spoons are to be avoided. This helps avoid aspiration of gastric contents and facilitates oropharyngeal suctioning, if required. In status epilepticus, respiratory effort frequently becomes ineffective and progressive cyanosis ensues. Mechanical ventilatory support may then be required. Cardiac function and blood pressure should also be closely monitored.

A secure intravenous line, preferably an indwelling catheter, should be placed. Before beginning the infusion, blood should be obtained for the following: glucose, urea nitrogen, sodium, potassium, chloride, carbon dioxide, magnesium, and calcium. If appropriate, AEDs, toxicology screen, and pH and osmolality determinations may be valuable.

Therapy may be either *specific*—directed at the cause of the convulsions—or *symptomatic*—directed at the seizures themselves. Most often, one begins with symptomatic treatment and, as the cause is uncovered, institutes specific therapy.

Drug Therapy

The selection of AEDs in treating status epilepticus varies from center to center. Although the most efficacious sequence of AEDs in status epilepticus has not yet been established, it is imperative for the physician to have a plan and to be familiar with the doses and side effects associated with the drug. All AEDs must be given by the intravenous route, as intramuscular absorption is slow and less predictable, especially if the patient is hypotensive.

I would recommend that the physician start with a benzodiazepine, either diazepam or lorazepam. If diazepam or lorazepam stops the seizures, it is necessary to administer an AED that has a longer half-life and can also be used as a maintenance AED. In the event that lorazepam or diazepam is not effective, I would then administer phenytoin. If the seizures continue, I would administer phenobarbital until a level of 40 µg/ml is achieved. If status epilepticus continues, I would then give the child rectal paraldehyde. Recommended dosages are given in Table 1. General anesthesia is recommended if these drugs are not effective.

Although diazepam has been the standard benzodiazepine used in status epilepticus for a number of years, lorazepam is being increasingly used. The effect of diazepam is rapid, achieving high brain concentrations within 5 minutes. However, the serum half-life is brief, about 15 minutes. Apnea is a potential side effect, and it is more likely to occur if the patient has previously received barbiturates. The dose may be repeated twice at 10-minute intervals.

Lorazepam is a new benzodiazepine that appears to have a great deal of promise for treatment of status epilepticus in both children and adults. The drug has a longer-acting antiepileptic effect than diazepam. In addition, the respiratory depression may be less common than with diazepam. Further clinical trials are necessary to determine whether lorazepam is superior to diazepam in the treatment of status epilepticus. Lorazepam may be repeated twice at 10-minute intervals.

Phenytoin is a very effective first-line drug used for status epilepticus. Maximal brain concentrations are reached in 10 to 30 minutes. One major advantage of phenytoin is that it causes minimal hypnotic effect and therefore has minimal effects on consciousness. The drug should not be administered at a rate greater than 50 mg/min. Serious side effects occurring with rapid infusion of phenytoin include hypotension, bradycardia, and cardiac arrhythmias that may lead to cardiac arrest. If an arrhythmia or bradycardia occurs during infusion of phenytoin, the drug should be stopped briefly and then continued at a slower rate when the heart rate returns to baseline. Potential cardiac toxicity may be aggravated by systemic acidosis and hyperkalemia. Since toxic phenytoin levels may actually exacerbate seizures, further phenytoin should not be given after the loading dose unless serum levels are less than 20 µg/ml.

Phenobarbital has also been extensively used in status epilepticus and is considered the drug of choice by many physicians. Maximum brain concentration is reached in about 1 hour. Side effects include depression of consciousness, respiratory depression, and occasionally hypotension. Phenobarbital doses may be repeated, although once levels exceed 40 µg/ml there is a greater risk that respiratory depression will occur.

TABLE 1. Doses of Medication Used to Treat Status Epilepticus in Children

Drug	Initial Dose	Subsequent Doses
Lorazepam	0.05–0.1 mg/kg	Repeat 2 ×
Diazepam	0.3 mg/kg	Repeat 2 ×
Phenobarbital	20 mg/kg	Give 5 mg/kg increments
Phenytoin	20 mg/kg	Give 5 mg/kg increments up to level of 20 µg/ml
Paraldehyde	0.3 mg/kg (per rectum)	Repeat 2 ×

Paraldehyde continues to be used in status epilepticus unresponsive to the benzodiazepines, phenytoin, and phenobarbital. The drug is available only for rectal administration, since the intravenous/intramuscular preparation is no longer available. The drug is administered at 0.3 ml/kg mixed in mineral, olive, or peanut oil. The drug must be kept in the rectal cavity for at least 20 minutes. Unused paraldehyde should be discarded, since in the presence of air the drug is oxidized to acetic acid.

Following adequate control of seizures, the patient should be placed on maintenance doses of appropriate AEDs.

NEONATAL SEIZURES

Although the proper treatment of neonatal seizures is important, it is equally important, if not more important, that the etiology of the seizures be determined as soon as possible. After ventilation and adequate glucose levels are assured, initial goals are to establish the underlying cause and institute appropriate therapy. The availability of accurate and timely chemistry screening panels has largely obviated empirical infusions of glucose and calcium as the first steps in treatment. Chemical abnormalities should be corrected when documented and AEDs given to the infant with recurrent seizures. Treatment recommendations are given in Table 2.

Phenobarbital is the most widely used drug in the treatment of neonatal seizures. The half-life of phenobarbital varies widely, ranging from 45 to 173 hours in newborns. With maturation, the infant's ability to metabolize phenobarbital improves dramatically. The initial loading dose should be 15 to 20 mg/kg intravenously. Neither the loading dose nor the maintenance dose of phenobarbital appears influenced by gestational age or birth weight. Because of the long half-life, phenobarbital can be given once or twice daily. Although therapeutic levels have not yet been firmly established, most infants require serum levels between 10 and 40 μg/ml to suppress seizures. When seizures continue despite levels of greater than 40 μg/ml, it is unlikely that further administration of phenobarbital will be helpful, and an additional AED should be administered. The maintenance dosage of phenobarbital is 3 to 4 mg/kg daily (given either orally or intravenously).

The second drug of choice in neonatal seizures is phenytoin. Like phenobarbital, the range of half-life for phenytoin is extremely large in newborns. The greatest variability and widest range of phenytoin half-life are encountered in the first week of life, varying in

one study from 6 to 140 hours. The apparent half-life decreases with postnatal age from an average of 58 hours in the first week to 20 hours in the fourth week. As in older children, phenytoin follows nonlinear kinetics in the newborn period. Loading doses of 15 to 20 mg/kg intravenously are required to achieve serum levels of 15 μg/ml. Unfortunately, phenytoin is not well absorbed in the gastrointestinal tract in newborns, and it is often difficult to obtain therapeutic levels using the oral route. Intramuscular administration of phenytoin is irritating and results in unpredictable plasma levels. Therefore, in the neonatal period the only reliable method of administering the drug is through the intravenous route. When phenytoin is administered intravenously, a recommended maintenance dose is 3 to 4 mg/kg/day. Although data are not available concerning the clinical efficacy of phenytoin as the initial drug in the treatment of neonatal seizures, most neurologists and neonatologists agree that it is an effective medication in infants whose seizures are not controlled by phenobarbital.

Lorazepam has recently been used in some centers to treat neonatal seizures. Lorazepam may be preferable to diazepam, since it has a longer half-life and may cause less respiratory depression than diazepam. Although a definite dosage has not been established, most authors have recommended a dosage of 0.05 to 0.10 mg/kg for the acute management of neonatal seizures. Lorazepam has not been widely used as a maintenance AED.

Although primidone has not been evaluated as the initial AED in the treatment of neonatal seizures, it has been reported to be effective in neonates who have not responded to phenobarbital and phenytoin. Primidone is unique in infants, since there is limited metabolism of primidone to phenobarbital. An oral loading dose of 20 mg/kg is recommended.

There is not a strong consensus as to when AEDs should be discontinued after neonatal seizures are controlled. Since there is some concern, based on laboratory experiments, that AEDs may be injurious to the developing brain, prolonged use of AEDs after neonatal seizures is no longer recommended. In addition, many seizures in neonates are short-lived and do not require long-term AED administration. I would recommend the following approach to withdrawing AEDs following control of seizures in neonates: (1) Discontinue phenytoin prior to removing intravenous lines. (2) Discontinue phenobarbital prior to discharge from nursery if neurologic examination and electroencephalogram (EEG) are normal. (3) If the child is discharged on phenobarbital, reassess at 3 months; discontinue phenobarbital if the EEG does not demonstrate paroxysmal abnormalities. (4) If the child continues on phenobarbital, discontinue at age 6 to 12 months if seizure-free.

CHRONIC ANTIEPILEPTIC DRUG THERAPY

The first step in the treatment of seizures is to firmly establish the diagnosis of epileptic seizures. There are many nonepileptic conditions that resemble seizures. If the physician is not certain of the diagnosis, it is better to refrain from labeling the child as having epilepsy

TABLE 2. Treatment Recommendation For Neonatal Seizures

With hypoglycemia:
　Glucose, 10% solution: 2 ml/kg IV
Without Hypoglycemia:
　Phenobarbital: 20 mg/kg IV
　　If necessary, additional phenobarbital: 5–10 mg/kg IV to achieve level of 40 μg/ml
　Phenytoin: 20 mg/kg IV
　Lorazepam: 0.05–0.1 mg/kg IV

and starting potentially toxic medications. The second goal of the physician in evaluating children with recurrent seizures is to determine the type of seizure the patient is having. This is very important, since the type of seizure the patient has determines the type of workup, prognosis, and AED of choice. For example, children with partial complex seizures need CT or MRI scans as part of their evaluation, have a generally poor prognosis with regard to remission of their seizures, and are treated initially with carbamazepine, phenytoin, or phenobarbital. Conversely, children with absence seizures rarely have structural lesions associated with their seizures and do not require CT or MRI scans, often outgrow their seizures, and respond to ethosuximide or valproic acid.

Following the determination of seizure type, the physician should determine whether he wishes to initiate chronic AED therapy. Since many children do not have a recurrence after their first seizure, it is not necessary to empirically begin chronic therapy. In patients with idiopathic partial, tonic, or generalized tonic-clonic seizures who are neurologically normal and have a normal EEG, I recommend that treatment not be started unless the child has a second seizure. Since patients with absence, tonic, atonic, and myoclonic seizures rarely have only one isolated seizure, I recommend that treatment begin following the diagnosis in these children.

The physician who cares for children with epilepsy must understand the basic principles of antiepileptic therapy. Although the use of AEDs is more difficult in the pediatric population than in adults, application of a few key principles enables the physician to markedly improve the effectiveness of pharmacologic therapy.

General Principles of Drug Therapy

Following the administration of a single dose of an AED, a peak plasma concentration is reached when the absorption phase is almost complete. The time to peak plasma concentration is dependent on the absorption fraction. While the drug is being absorbed, it is undergoing biotransformation by the liver. However, since the rate of absorption is much higher than the elimination rate, there is accumulation of the drug in the body. With time the amount of drug in the gastrointestinal tract decreases, and therefore the absorption rate decreases. Simultaneously, the biotransformation and excretion of the drug increase and the serum concentration falls.

In first-order enzyme kinetics, the rate of biotransformation increases linearly with concentration of the drug. Most AEDs, in conventional doses, follow first-order kinetics. Enzymatic processes proceed in this fashion as long as there is adequate enzyme present. However, with a sufficiently large amount of substrate, all of the enzyme that is present is saturated, and the process follows a different mathematical formula. In this situation the rate of the biotransformation is constant regardless of the drug concentration. This process is termed zero-order or nonlinear kinetics and is a practical problem only with phenytoin.

When elevated levels of phenytoin are reached, saturation of enzyme systems occurs and zero-order kinet-

ics dictate that a given maximum quantity of drug can be handled per unit time until the drug concentration falls below this saturation level. In the saturated state, the half-life is strikingly prolonged in comparison with the half-life of the same drug at a lower serum concentration. With low doses of phenytoin there is a linear increase in concentration with increasing doses (first-order kinetics). However, with saturation of the hepatic enzymes, the kinetics change to zero-order, and a small increase in dosage results in a large increase in plasma concentration. This is an important clinical point, since phenytoin can rapidly become toxic if large increments are given once serum levels are above 10 to 15 µg/ml. Once the drug concentration becomes toxic, the elimination of the drug is constant and unrelated to serum concentration until the hepatic enzymes are no longer saturated.

In the chronic treatment of epilepsy, AEDs are administered orally on a long-term basis. Following initiation of therapy, the drug accumulates in the body until the rate of elimination equals the rate of administration. Over this period of time, body and plasma concentrations increase until they reach a steady state or plateau. The steady state is a balance between accumulation and elimination of the drug and results in a stable level below which the concentration in the serum does not fall. Serum therapeutic levels of AEDs are based on steady-state levels (Table 4).

During repeated administration of a drug, the two primary variables that determine the steady state are dosage and the interval between doses. With repeated administration of an AED at an interval equal to its half-life, the concentration increases to a constant level or steady state. The approximate time to reach a steady state is five times the drug's half-life. Conversely, once an antiepileptic drug is stopped, it takes five half-lives to remove 95 per cent of the drug from the body. This principle should be kept in mind when ordering serum AED levels (Table 3). For example, there is little reason to order a phenobarbital level 7 days after starting or changing the dosage, since the steady state is not reached for 14 to 21 days.

Although the optimal dosage schedule for an AED involves many factors, the most important one is the drug's half-life. AEDs with short half-lives should be administered more frequently than those with longer half-lives. For example, carbamazepine has a short half-life and should be administered on a two- or three-times-a-day schedule, whereas phenobarbital, with a longer half-life, need be given only once a day. However, some drugs that theoretically could be given on a once-daily basis are sometimes administered more frequently because of local gastrointestinal effects. Ethosuximide, for example, is given two or three times a day, since administering the full dose at one time causes gastrointestinal distress in many patients.

For many AEDs a slow decline in steady-state levels occurs over a period of weeks or months following the initial establishment of a steady state. Initially, enzyme activity remains constant but eventually may expand its capacity to metabolize drugs as either a steady or an increasing substrate load is presented. With increasing

TABLE 3. Summary of Pharmacokinetic Data of Frequently Used Antiepileptic Drugs

Drug	Peak Time of Effect (hr)	Plasma Protein Binding (%)	Half-Life (hr)	Dosage in Children (mg/kg)	Dosage Interval	Time to Steady State (days)	Therapeutic Plasma Levels (μg/ml)
Carbamazepine	3–6	70–80	8–25	10–30	tid-qid	3–4	8–12
Clonazepam	1–4	47–80	20–40	0.1–0.2	tid	4–8	20–80 ng/ml
Ethosuximide	1–7	0	24–36	15–40	tid-qid	7–10	40–100
Phenobarbital	5–15	40–60	37–73 45–173 (neonates)	2–4	qd	14–21	15–40
Phenytoin	4–8	69–96	5–18 10–60 (neonates)	4–8	bid (children) qd (adults)	7–10	10–20
Primidone	1–3	15–20	5–18	10–25	tid-qid	7–10	4–12
Valproic acid	1–4	80–95	4–14	30–60	qid bid (enteric-coated)	1–2	40–150

availability of enzyme (termed induction of hepatic metabolism), there is an increased rate of biotransformation with a subsequent decrease in half-life and serum concentration. Induction of metabolism may account for the erroneous comment that an AED has "lost its effectiveness" after several months of use when, in fact, an increase in dose is all that is needed. It is important to obtain "routine" AED levels every 6 months to 1 year, even if the patient is seizure-free and not having side effects.

Rational Use of Antiepileptic Drugs

Treatment should always be initiated with a single AED. The drug dosage should then be increased to the therapeutic level or until clinical toxicity is reported. The goal of therapy is to suppress seizures without inducing intolerable side effects. If the first AED does not work or results in bothersome side effects, slowly taper the first drug while simultaneously introducing a second AED. Although sometimes it is difficult to avoid polytherapy, the aim should be to have the patient on a single AED. Monotherapy in epilepsy is likely to result in higher blood levels, fewer side effects, and better control than polytherapy.

One of the most important developments in the treatment of epilepsy was the introduction of serum drug levels. These levels are very useful in determining when and how much the dosage should be changed and evaluating possible drug-induced side effects.

Laboratories report the total amount of AEDs in the plasma. This includes both the protein-bound and free levels. The free fraction (non–protein-bound) is the portion that is available for entry into the brain. With AEDs that have a high percentage of protein binding, the "free" level may correlate better with efficacy and side effects than the total drug concentration.

Serum drug levels are especially valuable when patients are on phenytoin, phenobarbital, carbamazepine, and primidone. With these drugs there is a close relationship between efficacy and toxicity with therapeutic levels. Serum AEDs are also very helpful when the patient is taking other drugs in addition to the AED or is on more than one AED, since there are innumerable drug interactions that occur. Table 4 lists indications for obtaining drug levels.

Frequently Used Antiepileptic Drugs

The vast majority of children can be managed medically with one of the following seven AEDs: phenobarbital, phenytoin, primidone, carbamazepine, ethosuximide, valproic acid, and clonazepam. Table 5 lists the efficacy of the AEDs in the various seizure types.

Phenobarbital and Primidone

Phenobarbital and primidone are the two barbiturates most commonly used as AEDs. Phenobarbital has been used in most seizure disorders, whereas primidone has been used primarily in partial complex seizures. There is a debate whether primidone offers any advantage over phenobarbital. Phenobarbital is also effective as prophylaxis against febrile seizures. Although recently physicians have been avoiding phenobarbital in favor of other AEDs, it remains an inexpensive, safe medication.

Phenobarbital comes in tablet form of varying doses as well as a suspension (20 mg/5 ml), whereas primidone is available in 50- and 250-mg tablets and oral suspension (250 mg/5 ml). Phenobarbital serum concentrations of 15 to 40 μg/ml are necessary for a reasonable therapeutic effect. Serious toxic side effects are usually produced by concentrations of phenobarbital exceeding 60 μg/ml. Primidone's therapeutic plasma concentration is 5 to 12 μg/ml. Primidone is metabolized by the liver to two metabolites, phenylethylmalonamide (PEMA) and phenobarbital, both of which have antiepileptic properties. For that reason, a phenobarbital level is usually obtained when checking the serum level of primidone.

TABLE 4. Indications for Antiepileptic Drug Blood Level Determinations

1. To determine serum level at steady state following initiation of therapy
2. Following addition of another AED
3. When interaction with non-antiepileptic drugs is suspected
4. When drug biotransformation or elimination is altered as a consequence of a secondary disease
5. When the therapeutic effect is not achieved or symptoms of toxicity are observed
6. When noncompliance is suspected
7. When suspected maturational changes in absorption, biotransformation, or elimination occur
8. When significant weight gain or loss occurs

TABLE 5. Efficacy of Antiepileptic Drugs Used in Various Seizure Types

Drug	Simple Partial	Complex Partial	Generalized Tonic-Clonic	Absence	Myoclonic	Tonic
Carbamazepine	+	+	+	0	0	+
Clonazepam	±	±	±	+	±	±
Ethosuximide	0	0	0	+	0	0
Phenobarbital	+	+	+	0	0	+
Phenytoin	+	+	+	0	0	+
Primidone	+	+	+	0	0	+
Valproic acid	±	±	+	+	+	+

+ = Effective; ± = Somewhat effective; 0 = Not effective.

The oral maintenance dosage of phenobarbital in children is 2 to 6 mg/kg/day. The adult dosage is 90 to 220 mg/day. The initial dose in children should not exceed 90 mg regardless of weight. The administration of a loading dose is an effective maneuver for reaching therapeutic plasma concentrations more rapidly. Oral loading can be achieved by administering twice the maintenance dose for 4 consecutive days. The usual dose of primidone in children is 10 to 25 mg/kg/day. Loading with primidone is not recommended.

Phenobarbital's half-life in adults is 46 to 136 hours and in children 37 to 73 hours. Because of the long half-life it takes 2 to 3 weeks for phenobarbital to reach a steady-state therapeutic level. Once-a-day dosing, usually at bedtime, is quite adequate except in infants. PEMA has a plasma half-life of 10 to 36 hours, and primidone is usually given in two to four divided doses.

By far the most common side effect of these agents is sedation; however, with continued therapy, tolerance to this effect usually develops. The most common side effects of the barbiturates include irritability, hyperactivity, sleep disorders, and cognitive abnormalities. With close questioning we have found that over 50 per cent of parents or patients report these side effects. Other side effects such as rashes or allergic manifestations occur in less than 1 to 2 per cent of patients. Side effects of primidone are believed to be dose-related and occur with serum levels exceeding 15 μg/ml. Effects frequently seen include sedation, nausea, emesis, diplopia, dizziness, and ataxia. These effects can be minimized by initiating therapy at a low dose and increasing the dosage to a therapeutic level.

Routine laboratory monitoring is not necessary with the use of phenobarbital. Since a megaloblastic anemia has been associated with primidone therapy, CBCs are recommended every year while on this drug (Table 6).

Phenytoin

Phenytoin, like the barbiturates, has been used as a first-line AED for many years. It remains a relatively safe, inexpensive, well-established AED. The drug is used primarily in generalized tonic-clonic and partial seizures (both simple and complex) as well as in some of the other, rarer seizure types. Indications for the use of phenytoin parallel those for carbamazepine and phenobarbital.

The drug comes in 30- and 100-mg capsules and 50-mg chewable tablets. Although an oral suspension is available, it is not recommended for use since the bioavailability of the suspension differs from that of the tablets and capsules. Furthermore, the concentrations of the suspension may vary unless the bottle is shaken very well. The plasma half-life of phenytoin is 10 to 34 hours in adults and 5 to 18 hours in children. Steady-state therapeutic levels are achieved 7 to 10 days after initiation of therapy. Optimum control without clinical signs of toxicity occurs with serum levels between 10 and 20 μg/ml. Because of the long half-life of phenytoin, the drug needs to be given only once or twice a day. The usual initial daily dose in the pediatric age group is 5 mg/kg/day, with a maximum of 300 mg daily. Rapid attainment of therapeutic serum levels can be achieved by giving four doses of 5 to 6 mg/kg every 8 hours.

Major side effects include gingival hypertrophy, hirsutism, and, in some children, behavioral changes and cognitive dysfunction. In toxic doses nausea, emesis, nystagmus, ataxia, and lethargy may be present. Phenytoin may cause a mild elevation of liver enzymes (SGOT/SGPT), which does not necessarily require discontinuation of the drug if there is no other evidence of liver or systemic disease. Rashes associated with phenytoin are not infrequent and should lead to prompt discontinuation of the drug, since the child may go on to develop serious problems, including the Stevens-Johnson syndrome. Other serious side effects include rare hematologic abnormalities including thrombocytopenia, anemia, leukopenia, and lymphadenopathy. Since lymphadenopathy may lead to a malignancy, the drug should be withdrawn if this complication arises.

Recommended routine blood studies are given in Table 6.

Carbamazepine

Carbamazepine recently has emerged as one of the most frequently prescribed AEDs. The efficacy of this drug in the treatment of partial seizures (both simple and complex) and generalized tonic-clonic seizures as well as the lack of significant side effects has resulted in the popularity of this drug.

Carbamazepine comes in both 100- (chewable) and 200-mg tablets and a suspension of 100 mg/5 ml. A

TABLE 6. Recommended Laboratory Monitoring for Patients on Chronic Antiepileptic Drugs

Drug	Tests
Carbamazepine	**CBC** before and 2 weeks, 1 month, 2 months, 3 months after start of therapy; then every 6 months
	SGPT before and 1 month after start of therapy; then every 6 months
Clonazepam	**CBC** before and then every 6 months after start of therapy
Ethosuximide	**CBC** before and 1 month, 2 months after start of therapy; then every 6 months
Phenobarbital	None recommended
Phenytoin	**CBC** before and yearly after start of therapy
	SGPT before and yearly after start of therapy
Primidone	**CBC** before and yearly after start of therapy
Valproic acid	**CBC** before and 1 month, 2 months after start of therapy; then every 6 months
	SGPT before and 2 weeks, 1 month, 2 months, 3 months after start of therapy; then every 4–6 months

dosage of 10 to 30 mg/kg is required in most children. Peak serum levels are reached within 4 to 5 hours. Carbamazepine has a half-life of 14 to 27 hours in adults and 8 to 25 hours in children. Although a twice-daily dosage schedule can be used, the rapid achievement of peak concentrations often leads to acute, unpleasant side effects. Three and sometimes four doses per day are better tolerated. Initiating treatment with small, multiple doses followed by incremental adjustments over 1 to 2 weeks reduces the risk of toxicity and encourages patient compliance. As with all AEDs, maximum dosage is titrated by evaluating seizure control versus side effects.

Many controlled and uncontrolled studies confirm the beneficial effects of carbamazepine. Primary efficacy has been demonstrated in the treatment of generalized tonic-clonic as well as partial seizures with elementary and complex symptoms. Comparative double-blind studies with phenytoin and phenobarbital have shown them to have similar efficacy, although one may be effective when the other has failed. Combination phenytoin and/or phenobarbital with carbamazepine may be more effective than the single agent in some patients, but combination therapy should not automatically be used unless the single-drug regimen has proven ineffective.

The pediatric dosage is in the range of 10 to 30 mg/kg/day. Therapeutic serum levels of 8 to 12 µg/ml are usually well tolerated; however, patients may complain of side effects with levels as low as 4 µg/ml. Conversely, other patients require and tolerate levels greater than 12 µg/ml.

Bothersome side effects are common until a stable dose and dosing schedule are achieved. Visual disturbances such as diplopia or blurred vision may be the most troublesome clinically and can usually be correlated with the peak serum concentrations. Reduction of the dosage or adjustment of dosage intervals may be necessary. Although aplastic anemia and serious liver toxicity are rare and overemphasized adverse reactions, hematologic and hepatic parameters should be monitored closely during the first 6 months of use (Table 6). Rashes may also occasionally occur. Carbamazepine has been reported to exacerbate seizures in some children.

There is disagreement regarding whether carbamazepine has a positive psychotropic effect. It is now clear that carbamazepine has fewer adverse side effects on behavior, alertness, and cognition than phenytoin, phenobarbital, and the benzodiazepines. It is possible that the mood elevation and increased alertness seen when switching patients from other AEDs may reflect better seizure control and withdrawal from sedating and cognitive impairing compounds.

Ethosuximide

Ethosuximide has proved over the past two decades to be a safe and effective AED used for absence seizure. Ethosuximide is generally ineffective in other seizure types.

Ethosuximide, which comes in both a liquid (250 mg/5 ml) and capsule (250 mg) preparation, is well absorbed and reaches a peak level 1 to 4 hours after oral administration. The rate of metabolism and half-life are age-dependent and are 14 to 27 hours in adults and 24 to 36 hours in children. Based on the half-life, the drug can be given once a day to achieve a steady-state plasma level but is often given more frequently to reduce local irritative effects on the stomach (including gastric discomfort, nausea, vomiting, and anorexia). The drug can be started at a low dose and increased slowly until seizure control or toxicity ensues. Plasma levels of 40 to 80 µg/ml appear to offer optimal protection for typical absence seizures.

Dose-related effects of ethosuximide include fatigue, dizziness, and headaches. Rare idiosyncratic side effects include rashes, hiccoughs, leukopenia, and pancytopenia. It is recommended that CBCs be followed while the child is on ethosuximide (Table 6).

Clonazepam

Clonazepam is the most frequently prescribed benzodiazepine used in the chronic therapy of epilepsy. Although it is a relatively broad-spectrum AED, significant behavioral side effects limit its usefulness. Because of these side effects, clonazepam is rarely used as the initial AED in the treatment of epilepsy.

Clonazepam is rapidly absorbed from the gastrointestinal tract and reaches peak concentrations in approximately 1 to 4 hours. While available, clonazepam serum levels are of limited usefulness, since there is not a close relationship between serum level and seizure control or toxicity.

Side effects associated with clonazepam include drowsiness, ataxia, and behavioral and personality changes. The behavioral disturbances in children can be quite marked and include hyperactivity, irritability, moodiness, and aggressive behavior. Although lowering the dose may reduce some of these side effects, in many children the adverse effects still persist. Clonazepam may bring about increased salivation and bronchial secretions, leading to respiratory distress and pneumonia in some pediatric patients.

Table 6 lists the recommended laboratory studies for patients taking clonazepam.

Valproic acid

Valproic acid is a broad-spectrum AED and an excellent first-line drug in generalized tonic-clonic, absence, myoclonic, and infantile spasms and serves as a second-line drug in partial seizures.

Valproic acid is rapidly absorbed from the gastrointestinal tract with peak plasma concentrations reached within several hours after administration. Because of the short half-life, serum levels fluctuate widely, making interpretation of valproic acid levels difficult. For that reason drug levels should be drawn at a consistent time. Trough levels, i.e., levels drawn shortly before a dose is to be given, are preferred by many neurologists. Although some studies have demonstrated efficacy with single dosing, less fluctuation in blood levels is achieved by two- or three-times-a-day schedules. Less frequent dosing is satisfactory if the patient has no side effects and is seizure-free.

Valproic acid comes in both a liquid (250 mg/5 ml)

and capsule (250 mg). Enteric-coated tablets (125 mg, 250 mg, and 500 mg) are also available and are generally preferable to the capsule if the child is able to swallow the tablets, since this form allows slower absorption and less fluctuation of the serum levels. The enteric-coated form may be administered on a twice-a-day schedule. Valproic acid has recently been released as sprinkles (125 mg) which can be mixed with food. This preparation is helpful for children who cannot tolerate the liquid form or swallow tablets.

Treatment should be started with a divided dose of 15 to 20 mg/kg, which is slowly increased by 5 to 10 mg/kg/day weekly until seizures are controlled, toxicity occurs, or the child is on a daily dose of 60 mg/kg/day. Levels between 100 and 150 μg/ml may be required for seizure control. When valproic acid is used as the sole AED, these levels are usually well tolerated. The drug should always be given with food.

Side effects of valproic acid include mild sedation, nausea, vomiting, and anorexia. These side effects may occur at the beginning of therapy but are usually transient or may respond to a slight decrease in dosage. Hair loss, weight gain or loss, and menstrual irregularities have been reported with the drug.

Cases of stupor and coma associated with therapeutic valproic acid levels have been reported. These symptoms may occur when valproic acid is used alone or in combination with other drugs and in most cases appear to be secondary to hyperammonemia. If children become lethargic on valproic acid, an ammonia level should be obtained. Reductions in dosage may then result in clinical improvement.

The major serious adverse reactions are hepatic failure and pancreatitis. Many children on valproic acid develop mild elevations of liver enzymes. This side effect is usually dose-dependent, and the transaminases usually return to normal with reductions in the dosage. Unfortunately, some children have an idiosyncratic reaction and develop severe liver failure and death. The majority of deaths were in infants or children who had a wide variety of seizure disorders and were on AEDs in addition to valproic acid. If there is an idiosyncratic reaction, it usually occurs within the first 6 months of therapy.

It is essential that a serum transaminase (SGOT, SGPT) be obtained prior to initiation of treatment and at regular intervals while the child is on the medication (Table 6). If liver function tests are normal after 6 months, they can be checked every 4 months thereafter. Children with elevations of a transaminase two or more times the upper limit of normal for that test, or with clinical symptoms of hepatic dysfunction, should have the medication discontinued. Pancreatitis has been associated with valproate therapy, and serum amylase levels should be checked when patients develop abdominal pain while on the medication. Finally, rare cases of leukopenia and thrombocytopenia have been reported; thus, routine monitoring of CBCs and platelets is recommended.

Choosing the Appropriate AEDs

Although there are no strict guidelines about which particular AED should be used for each of the various seizure types, there is a consensus as to the group of AEDs that is indicated for each of the seizure types. Table 7 lists the AEDs used for each of the seizure types in the order I prefer. Regardless of the drug chosen, the physician must be aware of all the side effects that may be encountered.

Stopping AEDs

There has recently been a tendency for physicians to withdraw AEDs following seizure control sooner than in the past. Factors reported to be associated with a high risk of relapse by some but not all authors have included a long duration of epilepsy before control, mental retardation, abnormal neurologic examinations, the onset of seizures before the age of 2 years, and an abnormal EEG prior to discontinuation of the AEDs.

The decision of when to taper AEDs should be individualized for each child. For example, children with typical absence seizures and benign rolandic epilepsy have a very high remission rate, and tapering after several years of seizure control appears reasonable. Even if the child has a seizure during tapering or following discontinuation of the AED, the consequences are minor. In children who have had frequent, prolonged, generalized tonic-clonic seizures prior to seizure control, the physician may wish to treat for a longer seizure-free period before tapering the medications. As a general rule I try to withdraw AEDs after the child has been seizure-free for 2 years. While the speed of withdrawing AEDs has not yet been established, a reasonable approach is to taper over a 3- to 6-month period of time.

HABILITATION OF THE CHILD WITH EPILEPSY

Since epilepsy is a disorder of the brain, it is not unexpected that brain dysfunction will be manifested in ways other than seizures. Children with epilepsy are at risk for learning disabilities and behavioral problems. The underlying cause of the seizures, the seizures themselves, or the AEDs employed may contribute to these problems. In addition, children with epilepsy have an increased incidence of low self-esteem, depression, anxiety, and high absenteeism from school. Unfortunately, children with epilepsy are often subjected to ridicule and rejection by classmates and teachers. Recognition and management of these problems, in many instances, are as important as, if not more important than, the control of the seizures.

The physician caring for the child with epilepsy must be aware of potential problems and be willing to spend a considerable amount of time with parents and other family members in addition to becoming involved with the child's educational program.

Once the diagnosis is established the physician should carefully explain the terms *epilepsy*, *convulsion*, and *seizure*, since many parents and children have gross misconceptions of what these terms imply. In addition, parents may be totally mistaken regarding the etiology or outcome of the seizures. It is not uncommon for parents to believe their child will die during a seizure or that the seizures will result in mental retardation. Since parents often fear that their child has a brain

TABLE 7. Drugs of Choice in the Various Seizures Types

Simple Partial	Complex Partial	Generalized Tonic-Clonic	Typical Absence	Atypical Absence	Myoclonic	Tonic
Carbamazepine	Carbamazepine	Carbamazepine	Ethosuximide	Valproic acid	Valproic acid	Phenytoin
Phenytoin	Phenytoin	Valproic acid	Valproic acid	Clonazepam	Clonazepam	Valproic acid
Valproic acid	Valproic acid	Phenytoin	Clonazepam			Carbamazepine

tumor, this should be openly discussed. A description of typical events during a seizure is helpful, and guidelines should be given as to when emergency care is necessary. Although epilepsy, by its very nature, is unpredictable, thorough education does allow some feeling of control.

Early identification of academic difficulties is important, and it is recommended that school personnel be notified about the child's seizures. Although some parents do not wish the school to be notified, the parents should be told that this is usually in the best interest of the child. It is important for a medical professional to speak with the child's teacher in order to give guidance regarding the clinical manifestations of the seizures and potential side effects of the AEDs the child is taking. School personnel can play a very important role in the child's management, and having the teacher as a partner is helpful. At the first sign of academic difficulties, the child should be evaluated with psychological tests. If the child has a learning disability, special education may be required.

Unnecessary dependency can become an additional burden for the child with epilepsy and for the parents. Physicians have an important role in minimizing restrictions on the child's activities and in encouraging the parents to allow appropriate independence to develop. For example, most children with epilepsy can ride bicycles and participate in physical education classes. However, the children should take showers as opposed to tub baths. Decisions to restrict activities should be made according to each individual's needs, with consideration of seizure frequency, type, timing, and the patient's age.

FEBRILE CONVULSIONS

N. PAUL ROSMAN, M.D.

FEBRILE SEIZURES, RECURRENCES, AND LATER EPILEPSY

Febrile seizures (FS), seizures triggered by fever in the absence of intracranial infection, occur in at least 2 to 4 per cent of children between 3 months and 5 years of age. Most of these seizures are generalized and most are brief. The causative fever is usually greater than 38.9°C, and in most children the seizure occurs within the first 12 hours of fever. One child in three with an FS has at least one recurrence. When the first FS occurs before 1 year of age, 50 per cent recur; also, younger children are more likely to have frequent recurrences. Recurrences are also more frequent when there is a family history of FS. Half of the recurrences happen

within 6 months, 75 per cent within 1 year, and 90 per cent within 2 years.

Children with FS are at increased risk for later epilepsy, with the risk continuing to increase as children grow older; thus, by age 5 years, 2 per cent have afebrile seizures, and by age 25 years, 7 per cent. Major risk factors for later afebrile seizures include FS that are complex (focal *or* longer than 15 minutes *or* recurrent within 24 hours), an abnormal neurologic examination, and epilepsy in parents or siblings. It is appropriate to try to prevent FS, for they are upsetting to children and parents, they may cause brain injury, and with frequent FS the risk for later epilepsy increases (although it is unknown whether frequent FS cause later epilepsy or whether the child destined to be epileptic is more likely to have frequent FS).

MANAGEMENT OF A CHILD WITH A CONTINUING FEBRILE SEIZURE

Although the large majority of FS have ended by the time the child is seen by a physician, on occasion seizure activity is continuing and sometimes has persisted for more than 30 minutes (status epilepticus). (Although children with FS only infrequently develop status epilepticus, among all cases of status epilepticus in children, FS are a common cause.) If FS are continuing, they must be treated aggressively, since febrile status epilepticus carries with it substantial neurologic morbidity as well as the risk of death. As in other cases of ongoing seizure activity, supportive measures must be provided in order to minimize neurologic morbidity. The child should be placed in a semiprone position and an adequate airway ensured. A plastic or rubber airway should be inserted in the oropharynx and the airway cleared of secretions by gentle suction. Oxygen should be given. If there is any question about the adequacy of respiratory function, endotracheal intubation and assisted ventilation are indicated. An intravenous line should be inserted to obtain blood specimens, maintain hydration, and facilitate administration of medications. A solution containing 5 per cent dextrose in 0.25 per cent normal saline is usually used, with an infusion rate of 1000 ml/m²/day. A nasogastric tube is inserted to empty the gastric contents. The child must be protected against injury from hard objects and from compromising his respirations by pillows and blankets. Clothing should be loosened and excess clothing removed. The fever is treated with sponging with tepid water, cooling blankets, and antipyretics such as acetaminophen. A urinary catheter should be placed if seizure activity persists. Vital signs should be monitored frequently. The most useful anticonvulsants to give to a febrile child who is still seizing are diazepam (Valium), lorazepam (Ativan), and phenobarbital.

Diazepam has a wide range of safety if given carefully and in the absence of other hypnotic drugs. It can control seizures very quickly because it enters the brain in seconds, and peak brain levels are reached in 10 to 15 minutes. Its anticonvulsant effect is rather poorly sustained, however, because of its short half-life (30 minutes); thus, patients not uncommonly need additional doses, and a second, longer-acting anticonvulsant (such as lorazepam or phenobarbital) is often needed to establish a sustained anticonvulsant effect. Further, diazepam may produce unacceptable sedation, hypotension, respiratory depression, laryngospasm, and cardiac arrest, although these complications are more likely if the patient also receives phenobarbital. Diazepam should be given by slow intravenous injection, in a dose of 0.2 to 0.5 mg/kg (maximum dose of 2 to 4 mg in infants and 5 to 10 mg in older children). It is given at a rate of 1.0 to 2.0 mg/min; the initial dose can be repeated every 15 to 30 minutes, if necessary, to a total of three doses.

Lorazepam is a benzodiazepine structurally similar to diazepam but with a much longer duration of action; thus, frequent doses are not needed. It should be given by a single intravenous injection, in a dose of 0.05 to 0.20 mg/kg, at a rate of 1.0 to 2.0 mg/min.

Phenobarbital, although slower-acting than diazepam, has a much more sustained anticonvulsant effect because of its long half-life (50 to 120 hours) and its relatively slow clearance from the brain. Given intravenously, it enters the brain in minutes, with peak brain concentrations reached in 30 to 60 minutes. It usually produces sedation and may cause respiratory and cardiovascular depression, especially if given with diazepam or lorazepam. In addition to its anticonvulsant effect, phenobarbital also has an antipyretic action. Since some children with FS will be placed on continuous phenobarbital prophylaxis, in these children a loading dose of phenobarbital is advantageous. Phenobarbital is given intravenously in a dose of 10 to 20 mg/kg at a rate of 30 to 50 mg/min. If additional doses are needed, one-half the original dose can be given in 1 hour and every 4 to 6 hours thereafter.

If a fourth anticonvulsant is needed as an adjunct to diazepam, lorazepam, and phenobarbital (although this is rarely necessary), *paraldehyde* is particularly useful, for it can be given rectally, by nasogastric tube, intramuscularly, or intravenously (in a 4 per cent solution in water or saline). Given rectally, it is diluted in a 2:1 ratio with cottonseed, peanut, olive, or mineral oil and given in a dose of 0.15 to 0.3 ml/kg. The dose can be repeated in 1 hour and every 2 to 4 hours thereafter.

Once the seizure activity has been controlled acutely, additional *history* should be obtained in an effort to determine the nature of the underlying disorder that caused the fever. Appropriate treatment for the causative illness should then be initiated without delay. If that illness is bacterial meningitis, such treatment may be life-saving. Seizures have been found to occur in 18 to 80 per cent of cases of acute bacterial meningitis; they usually begin within 2 days of the first sign of the meningitis; and such seizures, like FS unaccompanied by bacterial meningitis, are usually generalized, tonic-clonic, and short-lived. It is important to remember that a febrile child who has seized may have done so because of something other than (or in addition to) his fever. One should try to determine if the child has ingested any drugs or toxic substances or if he has a history of previous seizures treated with anticonvulsants that may have been reduced or discontinued. Head trauma, sometimes unnoted, may have been causative. Also, the child may have a neurocutaneous syndrome (such as neurofibromatosis or Sturge-Weber disease) with accompanying skin lesions, signaling a lowered seizure threshold.

The most crucial part of the *examination* is to look for signs of meningitis. As noted earlier, even in older children with meningitis, meningeal signs may be absent. Bacterial meningitis in children is almost always accompanied by signs of acutely increased intracranial pressure. These include an altered mental state, vomiting, strabismus, a "setting sun" sign of the eyes, change in vital signs (increased blood pressure, increased or decreased pulse rate, decreased respirations), and, in the infant, a full and nonpulsatile fontanelle. Signs of accompanying illnesses, such as otitis media, should be sought along with evidences of trauma and skin lesions (brown, white, and red) indicating a phakomatosis. An identification bracelet may indicate the presence of an established seizure disorder. The classic neurologic examination in the child with a FS often discloses transient abnormalities that in this circumstance lack localizing value.

Many *laboratory studies* have been shown to be *un*helpful in the management of the child with FS; these include a complete blood count, blood sugar, serum electrolytes, serum calcium, blood urea nitrogen, urinalysis, and skull radiographs. Unless the examination points to a possible structural brain lesion, a cranial CT scan is usually not useful. Studies that may be helpful include anticonvulsant blood levels (if the child is on treatment for a seizure disorder), various cultures (blood, cerebrospinal fluid [CSF], and other), CSF examination, and a blood sugar (if the CSF is examined). Since no studies have produced unfailing criteria by which meningitis can be excluded on clinical grounds in a child with a FS, there are a number of circumstances in which a *lumbar puncture* (LP) should be done. These include (1) all children with FS with a suspected CNS infection; (2) all children with FS less than 2 years of age (when signs of meningitis not uncommonly are absent); (3) all children older than 3 years of age with a first FS (since it is unusual for an initial FS to present so late); (4) children with complex FS (since complex FS have been found to be much more frequent than simple FS when there is an underlying CNS infection); (5) a child with FS who does not look quite right. In general, if in doubt, do the LP! Further, with suspected meningitis it is sometimes necessary to do a second LP because the CSF may be normal early in the course of a meningitis.

The *electroencephalogram* (EEG) is of limited value in the management of a child with a FS. In those minority of cases in which it is uncertain if a FS has occurred, the EEG can be helpful, because an EEG obtained within a day of an initial FS has been found to be normal in only 12 per cent of patients. Thus, the presence of an EEG abnormality that later disappears serves to confirm the clinical impression of seizure.

PREVENTION OF FEBRILE SEIZURE RECURRENCES

Approaches to Preventing Recurrences

Treatment options in FS prophylaxis include (1) *continuous* treatment, with daily administration of medication, and (2) *intermittent* therapy, with medication given to the child *only* at the times of recurrent fevers. If both approaches are of comparable efficacy, intermittent therapy is preferable, since it is better if medication is administered only a few days a year than on a daily basis.

Candidates for Continuous Prophylaxis

Children to be considered for continuous FS prophylaxis include those in whom intermittent therapy is not feasible because of (1) lack of parent compliance, (2) sudden, rapid elevations in body temperature, and (3) unacceptable side effects from medications that are taken intermittently. Other children who might be considered for continuous prophylaxis are those with a substantially increased risk for later epilepsy. These are (1) children with complex FS, including those with a history of febrile status epilepticus, (2) children with abnormal neurologic examinations, (3) children with a family history of epilepsy in first-degree relatives, (4) children with FS beginning before 1 year of age, (5) children with frequent FS recurrences, and (6) children with highly anxious parents.

Treatment Options in Daily Prophylaxis

Daily administration of oral *phenytoin* and *carbamazepine* has been found to be ineffective in preventing FS recurrences. By contrast, three drugs taken orally have been shown to prevent approximately 80 per cent of FS recurrences: (1) *phenobarbital,* (2) *primidone,* and (3) *valproic acid.* Comparison of these three medications has shown them to be of comparable efficacy.

PHENOBARBITAL. Experience with oral phenobarbital in FS prevention has been greater than with any other anticonvulsant. In doses of 3 to 5 mg/kg/day, phenobarbital has been shown to be effective in preventing FS recurrences. The phenobarbital dose must be sufficient to produce a blood level of at least 15 to 20 μg/ml. The daily dose is usually divided into a morning and evening one, although a once-daily dose at bedtime is usually equally satisfactory. Many studies, however, have demonstrated an unacceptably high frequency of associated side effects in children taking daily phenobarbital (up to 60 per cent of patients). These include irritability, inattention, overactivity, aggression, drowsiness, and sleep disturbances. In some cases, side effects subside with continuance of the phenobarbital; in others, they appear to be dose-related and ameliorated by a lowering of dose; in still other instances, adverse effects appear not to be influenced by the phenobarbital dose. A rash develops in 1 to 3 per cent of patients taking phenobarbital; if it persists beyond a few days or

is associated with fever and/or lymphadenopathy, the drug should be discontinued. Whether or not phenobarbital can produce cognitive alterations and whether any such changes may be irreversible are matters of continuing debate. Additionally, in children in whom continuous phenobarbital prophylaxis is advised, compliance is frequently a problem; even with careful instructions to and encouragement of parents, the compliance rate is only about 65 per cent.

PRIMIDONE. Primidone, at 10 to 25 mg/kg/day, is as effective as phenobarbital in preventing FS recurrences. Primidone is partially metabolized to phenobarbital, however, and as with phenobarbital, side effects frequently limit its use. The daily dose should be divided equally into three or four doses, with enough primidone given to achieve a blood level of 4 to 12 μg/ml or a phenobarbital (primidone-derived) blood level of 15 to 40 μg/ml.

SODIUM VALPROATE. Sodium valproate, at 30 to 60 mg/kg/day, given in three or four equally divided doses to achieve a blood level of 40 to 150 μg/ml, is as effective as phenobarbital and primidone in preventing FS recurrences. The enteric-coated tablet need be given only twice daily because of its slower absorption. Sodium valproate is much less likely to cause behavioral side effects than phenobarbital or primidone, but complications do occur, including gastrointestinal upset, tremor, weight loss or gain, hair loss, pancreatitis, and acute liver failure that may be fatal. Although it is effective in preventing FS recurrences, the rare but very serious side effect of hepatic failure makes it difficult to recommend sodium valproate for FS prevention.

ADVANTAGES OF INTERMITTENT PROPHYLAXIS. Although in some cases daily anticonvulsant therapy may be appropriate for children with FS, there are reasons not to select continuous prophylaxis for FS: (1) Daily anticonvulsant therapy involves expense (purchase of medicines; blood tests; physician visits). (2) Anticonvulsants have side effects; some are frequent and of variable severity (such as behavioral changes with phenobarbital), whereas others are infrequent but very serious (such as hepatic failure with sodium valproate). (3) The long-term developmental consequences of continuing anticonvulsant prophylaxis are uncertain.

Treatment Options in Intermittent Prophylaxis

Fevers are frequent early in life. A Chapel Hill, North Carolina, epidemiologic study of fevers accompanying respiratory infections found the average number of fevers in the first year to be four; in the second year, three; and in the third, fourth, and fifth years, two. Parents, particularly mothers, are skillful in anticipating the onset of a febrile illness, especially in infants. Thus, it seems entirely feasible that at the onset of a febrile illness, a parent could give to a child with previous FS a drug that is rapidly absorbed by mouth and known to prevent FS recurrences. This would obviate the use of continuous medication and its attendant disadvantages.

Unfortunately, children with FS who are given *antipyretics* alone at times of fever appear not to be protected against recurrences, for these seizures recur with equal frequency whether or not antipyretics are given. Intermittent prophylaxis with *oral phenobarbital,* given at times of fevers, has been shown to be ineffective in preventing FS recurrences, in contrast to oral phenobarbital taken daily.

RECTAL DIAZEPAM. Rectal diazepam, given only at times of fever, is effective in preventing FS and as effective as phenobarbital taken daily by mouth; side effects are infrequent with diazepam (about 10 per cent of cases) and rarely are serious, with mild sedation and dizziness most commonly noted. Less often, salivation, drooling, and tracheobronchial hypersecretion are seen. Serious toxic effects (hematopoietic, hepatic, renal) are rare and have followed chronic oral use. Rectal diazepam can be given in either liquid or suppository form. As a liquid, it is rather cumbersome to administer, and rectal administration of liquid diazepam is not an approved method of FS prophylaxis in the United States. Diazepam suppositories, although easier to manage, are not available in the United States.

ORAL DIAZEPAM. Taken by mouth, peak serum diazepam levels in children are achieved rapidly, usually in 30 minutes, which is more rapid than that following administration of diazepam by rectal suppository. In addition, diazepam blood levels are well sustained, with a half-life of 15 to 25 hours in children 2 to 15 years of age.

We are currently engaged in a 4-year, double-blind, randomized clinical trial of oral diazepam, taken only at times of fever, to see if this intermittent therapy will prove to be effective in preventing FS recurrences.

Since 75 per cent of FS recur within 1 year and 90 per cent within 2 years, the *duration of therapy* should be for at least 2 years, or for 1 year after the last FS, whichever is longer.

INFANTILE SPASMS

DANIEL J. LACEY, M.D., Ph.D.

Infantile spasms consist of progressive myoclonic seizures that typically begin in mid-infancy, occur in 1 in 5000 live births, and form one of the most refractory of all pediatric epilepsy syndromes. These seizures are notoriously difficult to treat and are associated with a high (80 to 90 per cent) likelihood of developmental retardation. Initially, isolated flexion or extension spasms can appear as normal startle responses, usually symmetric but occasionally focal. They rapidly increase in number, occur without sensory provocation, and begin to cluster, especially when falling asleep or upon awakening. In the earliest stages the EEG can be normal but rapidly evolves into the classic hypsarrhythmic pattern.

The etiology of the spasms is usually divided into idiopathic (cryptogenic) and symptomatic causes. Examples of the latter include tuberous sclerosis, inherited metabolic disorders, congenital infections, perinatal asphyxia, and developmental CNS malformations. Of these, the only specifically treatable conditions are the metabolic disorders (e.g., PKU).

Management of infantile spasms has been refractory to standard oral anticonvulsants. Valproic acid and nitrazepam have occasionally been successful in small series, but the most effective agents have been ACTH and prednisone. Most child neurologists have preferred intramuscular ACTH gel to oral prednisone, but recent data suggest equipotentiality for seizure control. Doses of ACTH ranging from 20 to 160 u/day have been used, but there is no evidence that higher doses are more effective. Side effects such as hypertension, electrolyte imbalances, and infections are clearly less likely and less severe with lower doses. We typically begin treatment with intramuscular ACTH gel, 20 u twice a day for 2 weeks. If the spasms stop or are markedly reduced, we eliminate the second daily dose and continue with 20 u every morning for another 2 weeks. If after the initial 2 weeks of treatment the spasms are not affected, 40 u/day is given for another 2 weeks. At the end of 4 weeks, if the spasms have stopped, the ACTH is discontinued. If the seizures have not responded, the ACTH is stopped and oral prednisone is begun at 2 mg/kg/day. Similarly, the prednisone is tapered after 4 weeks of treatment. If the spasms are still not controlled after ACTH and prednisone, oral agents such as valproate, nitrazepam, or clonazepam or the ketogenic diet is considered. For a child who has a recurrence of seizures after ACTH or prednisone, the successful regimen is repeated. It must be remembered that many infants with myoclonic spasms have other types of seizures that begin either before or after the onset of their spasms. These seizures may require continuing anticonvulsant treatment in addition to ACTH or prednisone.

Unfortunately, the rapidity of seizure control does not appear to influence the ultimate developmental prognosis. Rather, the presence or absence of underlying anatomic or metabolic pathology of the brain is the most important determinant of outcome. Recent studies report normal development in only 5 per cent of children with abnormal brains (symptomatic spasms) and in only 10 to 20 per cent of those with cryptogenic infantile spasms.

SPASMUS NUTANS

WILLIAM D. SINGER, M.D.

This unusual benign condition begins between 3 and 12 months of age and is characterized by head nodding, nystagmus, and head tilt. For reasons unknown, it begins most frequently during winter months. It is a self-limited disorder with spontaneous remission occurring 4 to 36 months after onset. There is no sex preference. The reported incidence is declining, making this a rare disorder.

Head nodding, often the first symptom noted, may be intermittent or constant and may be either from side to side or forward to back. The nodding is not compensatory for nystagmus. It is accentuated when the child is upright and during ocular fixation, decreasing when supine, and disappearing during sleep. Nystagmus, when present, may be unilateral or bilateral but is more marked in one eye. The movements are rapid and of small amplitude, horizontal, vertical, rotatory, or pendular in character. Combinations of these movements may be seen. The abnormal eye movements disappear when the eyes are covered and during sleep. Head tilt is the least constant finding, occurring in approximately one third of cases.

The diagnosis of spasmus nutans should be reserved for children who are neurologically normal and have no structural or functional abnormality of the eyes. It may be differentiated from the bilateral searching nystagmus associated with marked visual impairment and congenital nystagmus. The latter two are bilateral and do not disappear with advancing age. Congenital nystagmus may be accompanied by head nodding compensating for the abnormal eye movements. The head tilt must be distinguished from that associated with structural abnormalities of the neck, cerebellar hemisphere tumors, and abnormalities of extraocular muscles with malalignment of the eyes.

Computed tomography or magnetic resonance imaging of the head should be performed because of the occurrence of symptoms resembling spasmus nutans associated with optic gliomas and frontal lobe tumors.

HEADACHE

N. PAUL ROSMAN, M.D.

Headache, one of the most frequent human discomforts, is common in children. By age 7 years, more than one child in three will have experienced headaches, and by 15 years they will have occurred in three fourths.

PAIN-SENSITIVE STRUCTURES

There are pain-sensitive structures both outside and inside the cranium. Those that are *extracranial* include the orbits and eyes; ears and mastoid sinuses; nose and paranasal sinuses; pharynx, teeth, and jaw; scalp, including scalp arteries; muscles attached to the skull; cervical nerve roots; and other structures in the neck. *Intracranial* structures sensitive to pain include proximal cerebral and proximal dural arteries; venous sinuses and large veins; dura at the base of the brain; cranial nerves V, IX, and X; and the upper three cervical nerves.

MECHANISMS OF HEADACHE

One or more of the following mechanisms are involved in the production of head pain: (1) *inflammation* (extracranial, as with sinusitis, or intracranial, as with meningitis); (2) *traction/displacement* (intracranial, as with brain tumor); (3) *muscle contraction* (extracranial, as with tension headache); (4) *vasodilation* (extracranial, as with migraine); (5) *neuronal inhibition* (intracranial, as with migraine).

Of the many causes of childhood headache, among the most common are migraine, muscle contraction,

and postconcussive headaches. Less common is headache from sinusitis. Most concerning is the headache of increased intracranial pressure, a diagnosis to be considered in every child who presents with persisting headache.

Migraine

Migraine headaches affect at least 10 per cent of the population. Since most migraine begins in the first decade of life, it is particularly frequent in childhood. The pathogenesis of migraine continues to be elusive. All would agree that there is some interaction between a variety of triggering events and a combination of biochemical, vascular, and neural changes. Of the different factors thought possibly to contribute to migrainous head pain, many believe that accompanying dilation of scalp arteries, resulting in stimulation of pain-sensitive nerve endings, is of major importance. Others have suggested that depression of neuronal activity in the brain may cause loss of endogenous opioid peptides and that this depletion gives rise to the headache of migraine.

The therapies for migraine are many. A number of these influence serotonin (a constrictor of scalp arteries), blood levels of which are known to fall during a migraine attack. In some patients, drugs that potentiate serotonin appear to work, whereas in others serotonin antagonists are helpful. At times, vasoconstrictors are useful, while at other times and/or in other patients, vasodilators seem to be more effective. These apparent paradoxes may be explained by a lack of agreement in results of studies of cranial blood flow measured during migraine attacks (both increased and decreased flows have been reported). Also, efficacy of drugs might be expected to vary with the phase of the migraine attack (aura or headache) when they are administered.

Therapy of Migraine

Many parents come to the physician concerned that their child with recurrent headaches has a brain tumor. When the diagnosis of migraine rather than a structural lesion of brain is made, the "good news" always is therapeutic. Families should be told that the child's headaches are real and, although they are likely to recur, there are many effective therapies. They should also be told that headache frequency usually declines as the child gets older and that the headaches may stop altogether. Occasionally, parental anxiety may be such that the physician feels "pushed" to order diagnostic tests, such as an EEG or a cranial CT scan. Unless the clinical circumstances justify such studies, such pressure should be resisted, for it is not uncommon in such situations to find test abnormalities that bear no obvious relationship to the child's symptoms, thereby compounding the family's anxiety.

There are five approaches to the management of childhood migraine: (1) avoiding triggering events; (2) symptomatic treatment of acute attacks; (3) abortive therapy for acute attacks; (4) prophylactic drug therapy; (5) nonpharmacologic prophylaxis.

AVOIDING TRIGGERING EVENTS. Literally dozens of triggers for migraine attacks have been recorded, yet in most children a specific trigger cannot be found. Categories of precipitants that have been identified include external events, physiologic factors, psychologic factors, dietary substances, and drugs. Included among *external* triggers are stuffy environments, sunlight, heat, noise, smoke, and fluorescent lights. *Physiologic* triggers include fatigue, excess sleep, physical exertion, head trauma, missing meals, intercurrent illness, and menstruation. *Psychological* factors include stress (often school-related) and sometimes removal from stress ("let-down" headache), continuing anxiety, excess excitement, and depression. *Dietary* triggers are most commonly chocolate, milk, eggs, cheese, nuts, citrus fruits, fried foods, pork, grains, seafood, and alcohol. Hot dogs, containing vasoactive nitrates as a preservative, also can trigger a migraine attack ("hot-dog headache"). Of the *drugs* that can trigger migraine in adolescents, oral contraceptives are probably the most common offender. Clearly, while it is not possible to avoid many triggers of migraine, one should make every effort to do so.

SYMPTOMATIC TREATMENT OF ACUTE ATTACKS. Many children have infrequent migraine headaches of only mild to moderate severity, and these are best managed by treating each occurrence symptomatically. Since such children are usually sensitive to light and sound, they should be placed in a darkened, quiet room and encouraged to sleep. Sleep can be facilitated by hypnotics such as chloral hydrate (25 to 50 mg/kg) or flurazepam (Dalmane) (15 to 30 mg/dose). Sedatives such as phenobarbital or pentobarbital (3 to 5 mg/kg) are also helpful in the older child.

The child should be given analgesics for his headache. Aspirin and acetaminophen are particularly useful, with codeine an alternative for more severe headaches. The dose of aspirin in children less than 5 years is 60 mg per year of age; between 5 and 10 years, 325 mg (one adult-size aspirin); after 10 years, 650 mg; these doses can be repeated every 3 to 4 hours. Acetaminophen (Tylenol) is given in a dose of 160 mg in children less than 5 years; between 5 and 10 years, the dose is 325 mg; after 10 years, 650 mg; again, these doses can be repeated every 3 to 4 hours. Codeine is given in a dose of 0.5 mg/kg every 3 to 4 hours as necessary. Children with migraine frequently vomit, which obviously diminishes the absorption of medications given by mouth. In that circumstance, medicines such as aspirin or antiemetics (see below) are better taken in suppository form. Absorption of oral medications in migraine is also lessened by accompanying reduction in gastric motility.

For nausea or vomiting associated with migraine, antiemetics afford relief; of these, chlorpromazine (Thorazine) is particularly effective. Children less than 5 years old can be given 10 mg; those 5 to 10 years, 10 to 25 mg; and those more than 10 years, 25 to 50 mg. The dose can be repeated every 4 to 6 hours. Alternatively, trimethobenzamide hydrochloride (Tigan) can be given in a dosage of 100 to 200 mg tid. Both medicines are available in suppository form. Other antiemetics, sometimes useful, are prochlorperazine (Compazine) and promethazine (Phenergan).

In the child with occasional migraine in whom the pain is quite severe, two proprietary combinations of medication are helpful. One of these is Fiorinal, which contains butalbital (50 mg), aspirin (325 mg), and caffeine (40 mg). This can be given to children older than 10 years with one to two tablets or capsules at once and every 4 hours to a maximum of four (or six with adolescents). This preparation is also available with codeine (in various amounts). The other proprietary medicine is Midrin, which contains isometheptene mucate (65 mg), dichloralphenazone (100 mg), and acetaminophen (325 mg). It too can be given to children older than 10 years, with one to two capsules immediately and then one every hour to a maximum of four. Both of these medicines work by virtue of combined sedative, analgesic, and vasoconstrictor effects.

ABORTIVE THERAPY FOR ACUTE ATTACKS. In children in whom there is a warning (aura) of an impending migraine attack (seen particularly in classic migraine in older children) and in those in whom a migraine headache has already begun (and when previously such headaches have been severe), ergot-containing preparations can be helpful in aborting the acute attacks. These should be used in postpubertal children with attacks generally not responding satisfactorily to symptomatic treatment. Ergot is most effective when taken early in an attack. There are a number of ergot-containing preparations available, many in combination with other drugs, for use by a variety of routes. The key ingredient, ergotamine, is usually present in 1 mg amount, except in sublingual preparations, which usually contain 2 mg. Ergotamine is thought to abort migraine headaches by virtue of its vasoconstrictor action, which combats vasodilation of scalp arteries accompanying the head pain. Ergot-containing preparations are many and varied. Examples include ones that contain ergotamine alone (as with Ergostat, sublingual); ergotamine with caffeine—a cranial vasoconstrictor (as with Cafergot); and ergotamine with caffeine, belladonna—a parasympatholytic antiemetic, and pentobarbital—a sedative (as with Wigraine-PB). One (sublingual or oral) or two (oral) tablets or capsules are taken at the onset of the headache, followed by a half dose every half hour until (1) the headache ceases, or (2) nausea or vomiting develops, or (3) a maximum of four tablets or capsules is used, or (4) a maximum of two tablets in 24 hours, taken 1 to 1½ hours apart, is used (if the sublingual preparation is taken). Ergot-containing preparations rarely abort an attack that has been in progress for several hours with the pain severe. If nausea or vomiting is prominent, sublingual preparations or suppositories should be taken. Ergotamine also can be inhaled or taken by injection. It should probably not be given in cases of complicated migraine, since prolongation of cerebral vasoconstriction may result in brain infarction and permanent neurologic deficit.

PROPHYLACTIC DRUG THERAPY. Daily prophylaxis should be considered in (1) the child with more than one migraine a week that interrupts his regular activities; (2) the child who has one or two headaches a month that force him to bed for a day or more; and (3) children with sufficiently severe migraine to require use of narcotics during most attacks. With all of the drugs listed below, it is best to increase the dosage gradually, over several weeks, before the recommended daily dose is reached.

A variety of medicines is available for migraine prophylaxis, but relatively few have been consistently helpful in children. In the young child with migraine, anticonvulsants are often useful; of these, phenobarbital and phenytoin (Dilantin) have helped most. The dose of either is usually 3 to 5 mg/kg/day, to achieve a phenobarbital blood level of 15 to 40 mg/dl or a phenytoin blood level of 10 to 20 mg/dl. Although electroencephalograms are frequently abnormal in children with migraine, the presence of EEG abnormalities seems not to be correlated with increased likelihood of successful anticonvulsant prophylaxis.

The vasocontrictor propranolol (Inderal), a beta-adrenergic blocker, may be the most effective drug in preventing migraine, particularly in the older child. The usual dosage is 2 mg/kg/day, given in three divided doses. It should not be given to children with asthma or heart disease. Also useful in migraine prophylaxis is cyproheptadine hydrochloride (Periactin), a serotonin antagonist and antihistaminic that also has anticholinergic, calcium-channel blocking, and sedative effects. It should not be given to children with asthma. The usual dose is 0.2 to 0.4 mg/kg/day, taken in three divided doses.

Tricyclic antidepressants, particularly amitriptyline hydrochloride (Elavil), may prevent migraine headaches in children by blocking re-uptake of blood serotonin. The drug seems to be most successful if the child with migraine is also depressed, but that is by no means necessary to ensure efficacy. The usual dose is 2 mg/kg/day, with one third taken in the morning and two thirds at bedtime. It may be several weeks before a clinical effect is seen. Antidepressants that are monoamine oxidase inhibitors, such as phenelzine (Nardil), have been used less often in childhood migraine; they too protect against a fall in blood serotonin levels, in this instance by preventing its degradation. Blood serotonin can also be maintained by daily administration of aspirin, which prevents platelet aggregation, for such aggregation is followed by release of serotonin and its clearance from blood. Dipyridamole (Persantine) can also be used to that purpose. Both of these drugs have been used for migraine prophylaxis much more extensively in adults than in children.

Occasionally, clonidine (Catapres), which unlike propranolol is a vasodilator and an alpha-adrenergic blocker, has been useful in preventing migraine attacks, but here too experience in children is limited.

In adolescents with migraine refractory to other drugs, methysergide maleate (Sansert) is often useful. The drug is a synthetic ergot-like preparation that is a serotonin antagonist and a vasocontrictor. The usual dose is 1 to 2 mg bid to tid. Because of the possibility of complicating fibrosis of retroperitoneal, pulmonary, or cardiac tissues, methysergide should be discontinued for 1 month no less often than every 6 months, before considering its resumption.

To date, experience with calcium-channel blockers, such as nifedipine (Procardia) and verapamil (Isoptin),

has been primarily in adults. These agents, apparently because of their vasodilator properties, can be helpful in migraine prophylaxis. Their efficacy in children has yet to be determined.

All of the medicines noted above are sometimes effective in the treatment of cluster headache, the vascular headache most refractory to therapy. Additional drugs that may be useful in cluster headache include lithium carbonate (Eskalith), indomethacin (Indocin), prednisone, and 100 per cent oxygen inhalation.

NONPHARMACOLOGIC PROPHYLAXIS. These therapies are primarily behavioral and should be considered in older children and adolescents when there is a reluctance to use drugs or when drugs have failed. Further, once learned, these therapies have the advantage of lasting a lifetime. They are of two main types: relaxation training and biofeedback. In all of these behavioral therapies, the child assumes primary responsibility for his own care. During relaxation training, the child learns to relax his skeletal muscles. This is aided initially by cassette tapes, later by visual imagery. Self-relaxation is particularly effective in migraine when stress is a usual trigger. The efficacy of relaxation training can sometimes be enhanced if the child is also provided supportive psychotherapy. This is especially useful in children who are chronically anxious.

In migraine prophylaxis utilizing biofeedback, the child learns to bring under conscious voluntary control those pathophysiologic processes that are normally unconscious and involuntary (and usually subserved by the autonomic nervous system). Operant conditioning is the cornerstone of such therapy. In migraine, skin temperature is characteristically lowered because of accompanying vasocontriction; such changes are also observed in stress from a variety of causes. Thus, one biofeedback approach particularly geared to migraine is thermal in nature. A finger thermistor that senses heat is employed, and the child learns to elevate his skin temperature. During the earlier phases of training, the child is provided visual (and auditory) feedback, monitoring his success in elevating his skin temperature. Later, he learns to effect such elevation without reinforcement. Biofeedback to promote relaxation of skeletal musculature may also be useful in migraine. This is especially helpful if stress is a frequent trigger or accompaniment or if muscle contraction headaches coexist (see below).

Consideration should be given to withdrawal of prophylactic therapy, whether pharmacologic or behavioral, in children whose migraine has been in remission for some months. This is most likely to be effective during the summer. Not infrequently, however, symptoms recur when the child returns to school, necessitating reinstitution of migraine prophylaxis.

Muscle Contraction Headache

Included in this category are psychogenic headaches, tension headaches associated with anxiety, and headaches accompanying depression. Such headaches may be acute and quite responsive to therapy, but often they are chronic and more difficult to treat. Muscle contraction headaches are increasingly frequent from adolescence onward, when they are often the child's only headache type. Not uncommonly, however, they coexist with headaches of migrainous or other causation.

Symptomatic Treatment of Acute Headaches

These can be treated with aspirin, acetaminophen, or, if severe, codeine. Local heat and/or cold often provides relief. Massage is frequently useful, and sometimes a cervical collar helps.

Symptomatic Treatment of Chronic Headaches

Muscle relaxants are often useful. Of these, diazepam (Valium) is especially helpful; in children weighing less than 30 kg, the dose is 1 to 2 mg tid. In heavier children, the dose is 2 to 5 mg tid. Other benzodiazepines such as chlordiazepoxide (Librium) and oxazepam (Serax) are sometimes useful, as is the centrally acting muscle relaxant cyclobenzaprine (Flexeril). Sometimes a cervical collar, with or without cervical traction, may provide relief.

In the child who is chronically anxious, treatment with benzodiazepines such as diazepam (Valium) and psychotherapy are useful. With associated depression, tricyclics such as amitriptyline (Elavil) or imipramine (Tofranil) often help.

Nonpharmacologic Treatment

As with migraine, both relaxation training and biofeedback can be used. With biofeedback, the child learns to lessen contraction of his frontalis, temporalis, and cervical muscles. This learning is initially assisted by reinforcing electromyography, with visual and auditory traces displayed as a challenge to relax. Eventually, the child learns to relax his muscles without such visual and auditory aids.

Postconcussive Headache

In all children who complain of persistent or recurring headache following a cerebral concussion, it is particularly important to exclude underlying intracranial pathologies that could be causative; examples include epidural and subdural hematomas, hydrocephalus, pseudotumor cerebri, and cerebral contusion with accompanying seizures. Another cause of headaches that may follow cerebral concussion is post-traumatic migraine. Other possible contributors to post-traumatic headache include muscle contraction, anxiety, depression, and effects of impending or ongoing litigation.

Clearly the treatment of postconcussive headache is determined by the presence or absence of complicating factors such as those noted above. Treatment should first be focused on the physician's reassuring the parents and the child about the absence of any structural disease of brain (after appropriate testing has been done and determined to be negative). Additionally, it is important to reinforce the need for the child to keep active, continue to attend school, and participate in physical activities within the limits of his capacity. The headaches should be treated symptomatically with aspirin or acetaminophen and occasionally with proprietary medications such as Fiorinal. If there is a continuing source of associated stress, medication such as diazepam (Valium)

TABLE 1. Clinical Symptoms and Signs of Acutely Increased Intracranial Pressure

I N F A	Altered mental state		C H
N T S	Vomiting		I
	Strabismus (CN VI, (III) palsies; "sun setting")		L D
	Altered vital signs (↑ BP, ↓ P, ↓ R) (signs of herniation)		R
	Full fontanelle	Headache	E
	Separated sutures (macrocrania) (papilledema)	Papilledema	N

and psychotherapy often are helpful. Amitriptyline (Elavil) can be used if there is substantial accompanying depression. Impending litigation should be settled as quickly as possible.

Sinus Headache

Sinusitis is an overdiagnosed cause of childhood headache, for it occurs relatively infrequently, particularly in the young child, in whom cranial sinuses are underdeveloped. Treatment is symptomatic and includes nosedrops such as phenylephrine (Neo-Synephrine), nasal sprays such as oxymetazoline (Afrin), oral decongestants such as pseudoephedrine hydrochloride (Sudafed), and histamine-containing proprietary medications, of which Actifed (triprolidine; pseudoephedrine) is particularly helpful. If there is active sinus infection, antibiotics should be given.

Headache of Increased Intracranial Pressure

Such headaches are caused by direct pressure on or dislocation of pain-sensitive structures (arteries, veins, venous sinuses, dura). A mass (as with tumor) may be present, but need not be (as with pseudotumor or hydrocephalus). Symptoms differ depending on whether the increase in intracranial pressure is acute or chronic and whether the patient is an infant or an older child (Tables 1 and 2).

There are several therapies to be considered when managing intracranial hypertension: supportive, specific, medical, and surgical. Of the different supportive therapies with acutely increased intracranial pressure, most important is maintenance of the airway. If possible, the cause should be specifically treated, either medically (as with antibiotics for bacterial meningitis) or surgically (as with brain tumor). Medical therapies for an acute increase in intracranial pressure include passive hyperventilation, mannitol, glycerol, pentobarbital, hypothermia, and steroids. Medical therapies for chronic increase in intracranial pressure include glycerol, steroids, acetazolamide, furosemide, ethacrynic

TABLE 2. Clinical Symptoms and Signs of Chronically Increased Intracranial Pressure

I N	Altered mental state		C H
F A	Vomiting		I
N T S	Strabismus (CN VI, (III) palsies; "sun setting")		L D
	Macrocrania	Headache	R
	Delayed fontanelle closure	Papilledema	E
		Macrocrania	N
	Separated sutures (failure to thrive)	Unfused sutures (open fontanelle(s))	

acid, and isosorbide. Possible surgical treatments include lumbar punctures, subdural aspirations, CSF shunting procedures, ventricular drainage, and decompressive craniotomy.

Clearly, childhood headache is a symptom with many causes and many treatments. The outlook is determined by the physician's ability to make a correct and prompt diagnosis and initiate effective therapy. Most children do well.

GUILLAIN-BARRÉ SYNDROME

FRANCIS S. WRIGHT, M.D.

Guillain-Barré syndrome (GBS) is an acute demyelinating neuropathy resulting in muscular paralysis of variable degree ranging from mild to severe. It is a syndrome of unknown etiology but most often follows a nonspecific viral illness. The onset of the disease is sudden, characterized by pain in the extremities and weakness that may progress to involve all extremities and the muscles of swallowing and respiration.

GBS is a self-limiting process. The outlook for recovery is favorable. However, the mortality rate may be as high as 20 per cent. Death in GBS results from respiratory failure or cardiovascular collapse. Consequently, the major focus of treatment must be on optimal supportive therapy.

RESPIRATORY INSUFFICIENCY

The most important aspect of the treatment of GBS is early treatment of airway obstruction and respiratory insufficiency. Although muscle paralysis may progress rapidly, early indications of respiratory insufficiency are readily apparent. These signs include restlessness, anxiety or apprehension, and lethargy. These clinical features are often present before there is a detectable change in respiratory rate or depth. Optimally, the patient should be treated before the onset of cyanosis, a late sign of respiratory failure.

The progression of weakness to involve all four extremities, resulting in a quadriplegia, is frequently associated with respiratory failure, since the muscles of respiration (intercostal, diaphragm) are often affected as well. Consequently, as the patient manifests shoulder and arm weakness, respiratory insufficiency should be expected. Respiratory function is evaluated by examination of the patient's respiratory rate, pattern, and depth. The patient may be asked to count on a single deep breath or cough as an indication of ventilatory capacity. However, serial vital capacity measurements provide the most accurate assessment of the development and severity of respiratory insufficiency. If the patient's vital capacity decreases below 50 per cent of the expected normal value, respiratory support may be necessary to prevent excessive fatigue. However, if the patient's vital capacity falls below 30 per cent of the expected normal value, prolonged respiratory assistance will be required. Respiratory homeostasis may be monitored by arterial blood gas determinations of serum bicarbonate and oxygen concentrations.

Pharyngeal paralysis is manifested initially by subjective difficulty in swallowing. During the course of the illness, the patient should be asked about any swallowing difficulties and should be observed during the act of swallowing to ensure that function is adequate. If pharyngeal paralysis becomes more severe, the patient will have difficulty swallowing saliva and begin to pool secretions. Isolated pharyngeal paralysis without impaired respiration may be managed by suctioning and body positioning to promote drainage. An oral airway may be helpful. However, if the patient has both pharyngeal paralysis and respiratory insufficiency, a tracheostomy will be required. Optimally, this procedure should be performed on an elective basis when adequate personnel are available to avoid hypoxia. Atropine may be necessary preoperatively to prevent vagally induced cardiac arrhythmia and cardiac arrest from tracheal manipulation.

CARDIOVASCULAR AND AUTONOMIC DYSFUNCTION

Cardiovascular collapse (shock) is a potential cause of fatality in GBS. It is characterized by restlessness, sweating, cyanosis, hypotension, peripheral coolness, and mottled skin. It is important to be aware of this potential complication. Abrupt postural changes and overly vigorous tracheal aspiration should be avoided. Pulse, respiration, and blood pressure should be monitored closely. In the patient with progressing weakness, a cardiac monitor is indicated. Intravenous epinephrine may be required to treat the hypotension.

A wide variety of cardiovascular disturbances have been encountered in GBS including hypertension, hypotension, cardiac arrhythmias, pulmonary edema, and focal myocarditis. Some of these cardiovascular disturbances have been attributed to autonomic dysfunction, either excessive or inadequate activity of the sympathetic or parasympathetic system.

Hypertension resulting from excessive sympathetic activity is the most common cardiovascular disturbance. In addition, sympathetic hyperactivity may also be manifest by agitation, delirium, tachycardia, pupillary dilation, profuse diaphoresis, and peripheral vasoconstriction. If signs of autonomic dysfunction occur in a patient maintained on respiratory assistance, the adequacy of respiratory ventilation should be evaluated to exclude hypoxia or respiratory obstruction as causes for the autonomic dysfunction. Vasodilators or adrenergic blocking agents may be required to treat the hypertension. In rare instances, hypertension may result from increased renin-angiotensin activity. Consequently, evaluation of the renin-angiotensin system as well as catecholamine secretion is indicated in GBS. If excessive catecholamine excretion is present, alpha-adrenergic blocking agents are indicated. Propranolol is indicated if the hypertension results from increased renin-angiotensin activity.

Postural hypotension may reflect inadequate sympathetic activity. The patient experiences vertigo and syncope upon assuming an upright posture, during coughing or straining at defecation, or when emotionally upset. Measurement of changes in blood pressure and pulse during a postural change is a useful means of detecting insufficient sympathetic activity. Gradual postural changes and elastic stockings may counteract the postural hypotension.

Various cardiac arrhythmias occur in GBS, including bradyarrhythmias (sinus arrest, atrioventricular block) and tachyarrhythmias (supraventricular and ventricular). Although these arrhythmias may result from the primary disease, other causes should be excluded, especially inadequate ventilation, electrolyte and acid-base disturbances, pneumonia, thromboembolism, and pneumothorax. In the face of recurrent asystole, a cardiac pacemaker may be required. Digoxin with or without propranolol may be needed to treat the tachyarrhythmias and cardiac failure. Atropine is effective in treating bradycardia.

METABOLIC ABNORMALITY

In addition to the acid-base disturbances resulting from respiratory insufficiency, hyponatremia may occur secondary to inappropriate antidiuretic hormone secretion. Hyponatremia is clinically characterized by delirium, tremors, or generalized seizures. In order to detect this condition, the urinary output should be compared with the water intake on a daily basis, and the serum electrolyte concentrations should be determined repeatedly during the acute phase of the illness. Hypercalcemia may occur in the totally paralyzed patient as a result of the immobilization. Although rare in GBS, impaired level of consciousness or seizures may occur with marked hypercalcemia. Treatment is directed toward reducing calcium intake or increasing urinary calcium excretion.

OTHER NEUROLOGIC AND MEDICAL COMPLICATIONS

Bladder dysfunction rarely occurs. However, during the initial stages of progression of the illness, urinary retention may occur. Intermittent bladder catheterization may be needed.

Papilledema occurs rarely in GBS. This complication results from a communicating hydrocephalus or cerebral edema. The prognosis for recovery from papilledema is favorable. However, an intracranial shunt procedure may be required for the treatment of severe increased intracranial pressure. Frequent serial funduscopic examinations are indicated in patients with GBS. The appearance of papilledema indicates a need for other studies, including a CT scan, lumbar puncture with pressure measurements, and CSF flow dynamics.

Myokymia may occur bilaterally in the face or extremities. This condition is characterized by spontaneous, undulating muscle contractions. Although these are self-limited and do not require treatment, calcium metabolism should be assessed.

Acute glomerulonephritis may develop in GBS. Serial serum BUN and creatinine concentrations and urinary microscopic examinations are indicated.

PLASMAPHERESIS

The removal of circulating substances by plasmapheresis has been demonstrated to shorten the recovery time and may prevent progression of weakness. Artificial replacement fluids or albumin should be used for plasmapheresis, and fresh frozen plasma should be avoided because of the high risk of hepatitis and other infections. At the present time, those patients who are unable to walk unaided or demonstrate significant decrease in vital capacity or pharyngeal muscle weakness should be treated with plasmapheresis. This procedure should be performed only in centers experienced with the technique and possible complications of plasmapheresis.

NURSING CARE

Optimal nursing care is essential for maximal recovery. Adequate tracheal care, suctioning, and normal ventilator function are critical factors for life support. Frequent turning is necessary to prevent the development of atelectasis and pneumonia. An air mattress and skin care obviate the occurrence of decubitus ulcers. Contractures may be prevented by the use of leg splints, trochanteric rolls, and frequent passive range-of-motion exercises. Adequate nutrition should be provided, often requiring nasogastric tube feeding. Thrombophlebitis prophylaxis may require the use of thigh-high elastic stockings. Constipation should be prevented by an adequate water intake and stool softeners. The nursing procedures should be arranged to provide an adequate amount of rest.

PSYCHOLOGICAL ASPECTS

The occurrence of paralysis in a previously well individual represents a threat to his or her body image and may well be perceived as a life-threatening event. The loss of normal health often triggers a series of emotional reactions, including disbelief, denial, anger, anxiety, and depression. The patient needs a great deal of help and support during the initial phase of shock and disbelief. Patients with GBS frequently manifest emotional lability that may have an impact on their emotional adjustment and social relationships with their families and peers. If the maladaptive reactions persist or intensify, psychological consultation is indicated. Offering basic information to the patient and family can facilitate coping with the illness by developing awareness and cognitive mastery. An adaptive adjustment to the illness is enhanced by a full explanation to the patient and family of the progress of the disease, the necessity of certain medical procedures, and the favorable outcome expected. The adolescent's need for privacy should be respected during the nursing care procedures. The patient's feelings of inadequacy and insecurity can be relieved, in part, by allowing them to assume a role in their daily care. Encouragement of independent care of functions such as feeding and partial bathing should be given as soon as feasible.

Communication with a tracheotomized, respirator-dependent patient may be enhanced by means of a Bliss board containing symbols for common functions.

REHABILITATION

The treatment of residual paralysis and contractures requires muscle strengthening, muscle re-education, and stretching exercises. Orthopedic bracing and intensive physiotherapy may modify the late sequelae of joint deformities and contractures. Frequent follow-up examinations with assessment of muscle and joint function are essential in the growing child after an episode of GBS.

OTHER THERAPIES

Corticosteroid therapy does not appear to alter the outcome of GBS, although some authors claim that it may shorten the course of the disease. Further research is needed to determine the benefit of this therapy.

CHRONIC INFLAMMATORY DEMYELINATING POLYRADICULONEUROPATHY

NANCY L. KUNTZ, M.D.

This disorder is characterized pathologically by segmental demyelination, clinically by weakness, sensory loss, and a potentially relapsing, remitting course. The diagnosis is usually made at the time of a "relapse" of what had been considered Guillain-Barré syndrome (acute inflammatory demyelinating polyradiculoneuropathy [AIDP]) or when a single phase of this type of disease process demonstrates clinical worsening for longer than 2 weeks. Weakness can be profound, and, when it involves respiratory or bulbar musculature, can lead to serious complications or death. The weakness caused by this pathologic process can remit spontaneously, as demonstrated by the clinical course in some adults in the placebo/nontreatment groups in clinical treatment trials. This disorder clearly occurs in children and adolescents; however, the literature contains no large series of pediatric cases, and the clinical treatment trials have been limited to adults.

When this disorder begins to progress clinically, it is wise to observe the patient carefully (possibly as an inpatient) until the degree of respiratory weakness and the need for assisted ventilation or airway protection are more clearly established. Inability to handle secretions, declining vital capacity (less than 15 cc/kg in a child or less than 1 liter in an adult-sized patient), or declining peak inspiratory pressure (less than 25 to 30 mm H_2O) suggests the need to consider elective intubation.

Whether any treatment specifically directed toward the inflammatory process should be instituted depends on the degree of weakness encountered. Since the disease process is occasionally mild and occasionally demonstrates spontaneous improvement, one should be certain that serious weakness is developing before instituting plasma exchange or therapy with immunosuppressive drugs and accepting the associated potential risks. Controlled clinical trials have not been performed

to provide us with well-substantiated guidelines; however, weakness marked enough to threaten independent ambulation has worked well as a personal guideline for instituting specific treatment.

Plasma exchange is a theoretically appealing treatment because of the analogy between CIDP and experimental allergic neuritis. For individuals with marked weakness, a series of six total volume plasma exchanges over a 2- to 3-week period is a reasonable first form of treatment. In older children and adolescents, the technique is similar to that in adults. In infants and younger children, technical problems are greater but surmountable. In one large series of plasma exchanges in pediatric patients, the complication rate was 17 per cent and included inappropriate clotting, hemolysis, hypotension, delayed transfusion reactions, infection, and pain at the catheter site. The smaller size and blood volume in infants and young children make vascular access more difficult, sometimes necessitate priming with red cells or albumin, and make blood warming more important. Overall, the technical considerations are great enough to warrant having the procedure performed by an experienced pheresis team in a special unit or the pediatric intensive care unit. The literature contains case reports of dramatic clinical improvement in response to plasma exchange. A large double-blind study of plasma exchange versus sham exchange in adults with CIDP demonstrated modest improvement in some patients and no improvement in others. New separating columns (which can specifically remove selected components of plasma) are undergoing clinical trial and may increase the specificity of the treatment while decreasing the risk by leaving more endogenous plasma proteins untouched.

For cases in which plasma exchange is unavailable or seems inappropriate, serious weakness should lead to treatment with prednisone or other immunosuppressive drugs. A brief burst of high-dose steroid therapy is frequently used (e.g., prednisone 2 mg/kg/day divided into four daily doses for 10 to 14 days). This can be followed by alternate-day therapy for a period of weeks to months depending on clinical response. Variations in the form of steroid therapy and/or use of other immunosuppressive drugs may be appropriate. It should be recognized that all these modes of therapy are empiric, since no controlled trials have been performed in children.

Painful dysesthesia can occur with CIDP, although it is frequently less of a problem than in AIDP or other acute neuropathies. When present, it may respond to usual doses of acetaminophen or it may require carbamazepine or phenytoin in accepted pediatric doses. Supportive nutrition and medical care to minimize the potential complications of prolonged bedrest should be employed. Informal and/or formal psychological support should be provided, as weakness and immobility are very stressful to children and adolescents. Supportive physical and occupational therapy are important during both the acute and recuperative phases of this illness. It is important to help the child and family set realistic goals for improvement and to discourage excessive weight-lifting, which can overuse the weak muscles.

FAMILIAL DYSAUTONOMIA

FELICIA B. AXELROD, M.D.

Many of the clinical manifestations of familial dysautonomia are caused by a deficit in autonomic homeostatic function and sensory appreciation of peripheral pain and temperature. Both deficiencies can be accounted for by the decreased number of unmyelinated neurons noted in sural nerve biopsies and autopsies. Prominent early manifestations include feeding difficulties, hypotonia, delayed developmental milestones, labile body temperature and blood pressure, absence of overflowing tears and corneal anesthesia, marked diaphoresis with excitement, recurrent aspiration pneumonia, breath-holding episodes, ataxia, spinal curvature, and intractable vomiting.

Treatment is directed to specific symptoms and complications.

FEEDING

Breast-feeding is usually impossible owing to the infant's poor suck, uncoordinated swallow, and misdirection of liquids. Experimentation with different nipples and thickened feedings should be tried before deciding to eliminate oral liquids completely from the infant's diet. For infants completely unable to suck and thus unable to maintain hydration, gavage feedings are used as a temporary measure. If the infant accepts spoon feedings well, the gavage feedings can be discontinued. However, if the problem persists, a gastrostomy is indicated to maintain nutrition and avoid dehydration and prevent aspiration.

FEVERS

Labile body temperatures result in brief episodic fevers in response to dehydration, mucous plugs in the bronchi, excessive external temperature, and even stress. Fever often is accompanied by shaking chills, cold extremities, and lack of sweating. Antipyretics may not suffice. Cool extremities should be massaged while cooling the trunk by sponging or even with a hypothermic mattress.

A muscle relaxant often is helpful in reducing anxiety and muscular spasms during hyperpyrexia. Diazepam (0.1 mg/kg/dose) has been found effective.

A persistent fever lasting more than 24 hours requires a search for a source of infection.

VOMITING

Dysautonomic patients have abnormal gastrointestinal motility patterns, making them prone to vomiting. Vomiting occurs intermittently in some patients as part of a systemic reaction to infection or stress. In another group of patients (40 per cent), vomiting assumes a cyclic pattern. These vomiting crises often are associated with hypertension, tachycardia, diffuse sweating, personality changes, and, occasionally, hyperpyrexia. The cyclic pattern can be quite marked and is usually characteristic for that patient. The vomiting may occur once a month or even once a week. The crises can last from

3 to 72 hours and can lead to severe dehydration. Aspiration is an ever-present risk.

Management has five goals: (1) maintenance of adequate hydration, (2) relief of gastric distention, (3) cessation of clinical vomiting with antiemetics, (4) relief of hypertension, and (5) induction of sleep, which seems to be necessary for resolution of the crisis. Despite the loss of copious amounts of gastric fluid, the dehydration is characteristically isotonic. A volume expander, such as normal saline, should be given rapidly upon hospital admission at 10 ml/kg for mild dehydration and 20 ml/kg for severe dehydration. Maintenance and calculated rehydration are given with a solution of one-third normal saline in 5 per cent glucose. Dehydration is best estimated on the basis of weight change. A nasogastric tube should be placed and set on low intermittent suction and continued until the vital signs are stable and nausea has abated.

Diazepam is now considered to be an effective antiemetic for the dysautonomic vomiting crisis. The initial dose is 0.1 to 0.2 mg/kg/dose intravenously. The dose should be effective in normalizing the blood pressure and producing sleep. If the patient does not sleep, then chloral hydrate, 30 mg/kg, can be given as a rectal suppository. Subsequent doses of diazepam are repeated at 3-hour intervals until the crisis resolves. Chloral hydrate can be repeated at 6-hour intervals. Frequent monitoring of blood pressure is indicated, because the choice of subsequent antiemetics will be influenced by the absence or presence of hypertension. Intravenous cimetidine (20 mg/kg/24 hr) is a useful adjunct in reducing emesis volume. The crisis usually resolves abruptly and is marked by normalization of personality and return of appetite. At this point the patient may be allowed to resume a normal diet.

PNEUMONIA

Recurrent pneumonias are frequent. Repeated aspiration is probably the major factor in causing pulmonary disease, with most of the damage to the lung occurring during infancy and early childhood. Gastroesophageal reflux also may be a contributing factor. The signs of pneumonia may be subtle. Cough is not consistently present and is rarely productive. The child is more likely to vomit increased pulmonary secretions. Tachypnea is generally not evident, and auscultation may be unrevealing because of decreased chest excursion. Radiographic examination is often necessary for diagnosis. Pathogens cultured from tracheal aspirations are often uncommon agents, such as *Escherichia coli, S. proteus,* or *Serratia.* Broad-spectrum antibiotics should be used until bacteriologic study permits more specific therapy. In the seriously ill child, blood gases must be monitored to detect CO_2 accumulation, which may be severe enough to cause coma and require assisted ventilation.

Bronchiectasis is a common sequela of repeated pneumonias. Pulmonary hygiene, consisting of postural drainage and inhalation of bronchodilators, is helpful not only in the acute situation but also as a daily routine for children with chronic lung disease. Suctioning is often required because of ineffective cough. Chest therapy should be administered at home by the parents on a regular basis. Chest surgery is rarely indicated, as the disease usually is diffuse. In patients with gastroesophageal reflux, xanthine derivatives are avoided. Fundoplications have been performed if medical management has been unsuccessful.

SPINAL CURVATURE

Spinal curvature (kyphosis or scoliosis or both) develops in 95 per cent of dysautonomic patients by adolescence. Spinal curvature may start as early as 3.5 years or as late as 14 years. There may be rapid progression at any time. The completion of puberty generally halts the progression of scoliosis, as it does in the idiopathic adolescent form, but puberty is commonly delayed in dysautonomia. Spinal curvature further compromises respiratory function, adding the component of restrictive lung disease to bronchiectatic disease.

Annual radiographic examination of the spine is recommended after the child starts to walk. Splinting with a brace is the only effective conservative treatment. The brace must be carefully fitted and the skin inspected daily at pressure points because of the risk of ulceration as a result of decreased sensitivity to pain. The brace may also impair pulmonary ventilation. Most patients rely primarily on the use of their abdominal muscles for adequate pulmonary excursion. A high anterior projection on a brace, compressing the epigastric area, may restrict breathing and even contribute to esophageal reflux. The orthopedist should be alerted to the possibility of these problems. If the brace is not successful in halting progression, or if the patient has a severe curve, spinal fusion is recommended.

CORNEAL ABRASIONS

Corneal complications have been decreasing with the regular use of artificial tears solutions containing methylcellulose. Artificial tears are instilled three to six times daily, depending on the child's own baseline eye moisture, environmental conditions, and whether or not the child is febrile or dehydrated. Moisture chamber spectacle attachments help to maintain eye moisture and protect the eye from wind and foreign bodies. If an ulcer occurs, the eye should be patched. Tarsorrhaphy of the medial or lateral part of the palpebral fissure has been reserved for unresponsive and chronic situations. Soft contact lenses have been found recently to be very effective in promoting corneal healing.

BREATH-HOLDING (SEIZURES)

The phenomenon of prolonged breath-holding with crying in the early years can result in actual cyanosis, syncope, and seizure activity. This is due to lack of awareness that it is necessary for the next inspiration to be initiated; i.e., the patients are manifesting insensitivity to hypoxia and hypercapnia. This may become a manipulative maneuver with some children. Such an episode is frightening but self-limited and, in our experience, has never been fatal. The cyanosis of breath-holding must be differentiated from that which occurs with mucous plugs. Both types of cyanotic spells can produce seizure-like movements and decerebrate pos-

turing. Electroencephalograms usually are normal or nonspecific, and the frequency of either type of spell is unaffected by anticonvulsant therapy.

Owing to the lack of appropriate response to hypoxia and hypercapnia, diving, underwater swimming, and air travel at high altitudes are potential hazards. If the plane's altitude exceeds 39,000 feet, the cabin pressure will be equivalent to more than 6000 feet, and supplemental oxygen probably will be necessary.

AZOTEMIA

A large proportion of patients have a moderate degree of azotemia (20 to 30 mg/dl) and variable values for creatinine clearance. Although these patients do not exhibit clinical signs of dehydration, the urea nitrogen often may be reduced by simple hydration. In four patients whose urea nitrogen was consistently greater than 40 mg/dl and unalterable by intravenous hydration, renal biopsies were performed. These showed significant ischemic-type glomerulosclerosis. The high prevalence of the renal lesion has been confirmed by retrospective analysis of autopsy material. It has been suggested that these slowly progressive lesions are associated with labile blood pressure. Patients are being encouraged to maintain adequate hydration, especially during warm weather. Treatment of postural hypotension is becoming more aggressive (see below).

POSTURAL HYPOTENSION

Episodes of postural hypotension may be associated with actual syncope, complaints of "dizziness," brief loss of vision, or leg cramps. These episodes may also occur with micturition or with sudden change in position, such as after sitting or extended periods in a car or theater.

In addition to increasing dietary salt and fluids, treatment may include use of caffeinated beverages, elasticized waist-high stockings and Florinef, a mineralocorticoid.

ANESTHESIA

Anesthesia for surgical procedures is associated with an increased risk because of extreme lability of blood pressure and diminished responsiveness to hypoxia and hypercapnia. Local anesthesia with diazepam as preoperative sedation is preferred whenever possible. Large amounts of epinephrine should not be infiltrated because of the exaggerated response to sympathomimetic drugs. If general anesthesia is indicated, the gas anesthetics are preferred because of the rapid reversibility of their effects. An intravenous drip is started the night before surgery to ensure adequate circulating volume prior to the administration of anesthesia. An arterial line is inserted for frequent monitoring of blood gases and blood pressure. Profound hypotension should be corrected by decreasing the percentage of gas anesthetic and giving of volume expanders. Rarely has a pressor, such as Neo-Synephrine, been required. Postoperative management can be extremely challenging. To avoid postoperative aspirations, cimetidine (5 mg/kg/dose) can be given and the stomach should be kept decompressed. Patients will require vigorous chest physiotherapy as there is a tendency toward development of mucous plugs and exacerbation of preexisting lung disease. Intubation may need to be extended until the respiratory status stabilizes or there is less reliance on pain medication. Visceral pain is appreciated so that narcotic pain medication may be required for intraabdominal or intrathoracic procedures.

Because dysautonomia is a multisystem disorder, the physician can render the family a great deal of support and comfort by becoming thoroughly familiar with its varied manifestations. Living with the dysautonomic child imposes a great burden upon the parents, who are aware of the serious prognosis and are faced with the care of a chronically handicapped child with repeated life-threatening crises. A sympathetic, artful physician can provide needed reassurance.

INJURIES TO THE BRACHIAL PLEXUS

MURRAY BRAUN, M.D.

NEWBORNS

Brachial plexus injuries occur with difficult extractions of infants after vertex or breech presentation and less often after cesarean section. Fetal hypotonia and macrosomia play a role as well. Anatomic peculiarities of spinal nerves predispose the infant to stretch injuries of the plexus rather than avulsion of roots.

Erb's palsy is the most common type. The upper brachial plexus (C5, C6, C7 nerve root components) is affected. Adduction and internal rotation at the shoulder, pronation of the forearm, and flexed wrist with either slight flexion (paralysis of C5, C6, C7) or complete extension (paralysis of C5, C6) of the elbow is noted. The "waiter's tip" posture is accompanied by diminished or absent deep tendon reflexes. Initial pain in the affected limb(s) and sensory deficit are suspected. Hand grasp may be present, but the traction component is lost. The Moro reflex is absent or asymmetric.

Klumpke's palsy is rarely seen in isolation. The lower brachial plexus (C8, T1 nerve roots) is affected. This involves finger flexors and ulnar intrinsics.

Complete plexus involvement manifests as a motionless, pale or marbled, limp limb. Horner's syndrome (miosis, ptosis, and warm hemiface) denotes either severe lower plexus stretch injury or avulsion. Diaphragmatic paralysis (phrenic nerve involvement) sometimes accompanies upper plexus injury. Various sequelae such as iris dyspigmentation, clawlike hand deformity, limb atrophy, and winging of the scapula are not seen in the neonatal period. Differential diagnosis includes cervical spine injury, cerebral palsy, and arthrogryposis.

Initial investigation includes radiographs to rule out clavicular, humeral epiphysis, and cervical spine fracture and subluxation of the humeral head and fluoroscopy to demonstrate diaphragmatic mobility. Arthrography may further delineate fractures or subluxation of the humerus. Electromyography (EMG) has been recommended from 2 to 3 weeks and at 6-week intervals, since EMG recovery precedes the clinical functional return by several weeks. Two to 3 weeks after injury, intradermal 1 per cent histamine may elicit a flare response (axon reflex), indicating a preganglionic lesion (avulsion). Myelography (spine CT or MRI) may demonstrate meningocele at the intervertebral foramen and a defect of the nerve sleeve.

Therapy is delayed to spare the infant any further stretch to the plexus and includes range-of-motion exercises beginning at approximately 1 week. Electrostimulation has been recommended but is of unproven benefit. Although controversial and even considered experimental, surgical reconstruction by graft or repair has been attempted after 3 months if there is absence of biceps muscle recovery. Results are encouraging in some series. Axonal regrowth continues after 3 months and perhaps explains the satisfactory recovery of some patients beginning only after 6 months or more. Tertiary centers provide intraoperative nerve action and somatosensory potential recording. Plexus repair (sometimes limited to neurolysis) is combined with subsequent joint release and muscle tendon transfers.

CHILDREN AND ADOLESCENTS

Injury of the plexus after the neonatal period is best managed by neurosurgical and orthopedic specialists.

HYPOXIC ENCEPHALOPATHY

BENNETT A. SHAYWITZ, M.D.

In pediatric practice hypoxic-ischemic encephalopathy is seen at all ages. In the newborn period its pathogenesis is usually intrauterine asphyxia, although this may be complicated by postnatal difficulties including recurrent apnea, congenital heart disease, sepsis, and, in premature infants, hyaline membrane disease. Intrauterine asphyxia is typically diagnosed by low Apgar scores at birth, depressed level of consciousness, seizures beginning 6 to 12 hours after birth, and, often, frequent apneic spells. Other clinical features are weakness in the hip-shoulder distribution in full-term newborns and lower limb weakness in premature newborns, and disturbances in feeding and persistent hypotonia. Neuronal necrosis is evident in the cerebral and cerebellar cortices, thalamus, brain stem, basal ganglia, and perhaps in the parasagittal and periventricular areas.

Although postnatal events may exacerbate pre-existing problems, in most cases hypoxic-ischemic encephalopathy is a consequence of intrauterine factors. Thus, effective treatment depends upon the identification of the woman who is at high risk for the development of hypoxic-ischemic encephalopathy and the subsequent careful intrauterine monitoring of the fetus. If signs of intrauterine asphyxia become evident, measures must be taken to deliver the infant by cesarean section as quickly as possible. After birth, the primary focus is prevention of an exacerbation of the hypoxic-ischemic events. Good supportive care must include maintenance of adequate ventilation; this may necessitate intubation and controlled positive-pressure ventilatory support.

Measures must be taken to treat such common sequelae of hypoxia-ischemia as seizures, myocardial failure, and acute tubular necrosis. Seizures should be treated with phenobarbital given as an intravenous loading dose (10 to 20 mg/kg) and then at 5 mg/kg/day to maintain phenobarbital blood levels at 20 to 30 μg/ml. If seizures continue, phenytoin should be added at an intravenous loading dose of 15 mg/kg and a daily maintenance dose of 5 to 7 mg/kg, designed to maintain blood levels between 10 and 20 μg/ml. Myocardial failure is treated with agents to improve cardiac contractility and prevent arrhythmias. Acute tubular necrosis is managed by appropriate fluid therapy, and, at times, dialysis. Sepsis, too, may complicate the immediate postnatal course, and appropriate antibiotics are frequently employed. More specific measures in the treatment of the hypoxic-ischemic insult itself, such as the prevention and treatment of associated brain edema, the use of barbiturates, and the role of glucose therapy, remain controversial in the newborn period. Their role in hypoxic-ischemic encephalopathy in older individuals is discussed below. A significant and often the most difficult part of the management of hypoxic-ischemic encephalopathy in the newborn period is determination of severity of the insult. Such an estimate is critical in providing the physician with a rationale for counseling the parents of the affected infant about the prognosis and potential complications. Thus, the mortality rate ranges between 10 and 20 per cent and the incidence of neurologic sequelae in survivors is estimated at 25 to 45 per cent. These include a variety of spastic motor deficits (cerebral palsy), psychomotor retardation, bulbar difficulties, and seizure disorders. The treatment of each of these complications is formidable and includes, in addition to anticonvulsant agents to treat seizures, physical and occupational therapy, speech therapy, and supportive counseling to the parents. Details of each of these are discussed elsewhere in this volume.

In contrast to hypoxic-ischemic encephalopathy in the newborn period, which nearly always results from intrauterine asphyxia, the disorder in older children may occur after a variety of insults. Thus hypoxic-ischemic encephalopathy is seen in disorders resulting in airway obstruction, such as suffocation and drowning; as a consequence of obstruction of blood flow in the cerebral vessels in strangulation, severe brain edema from a closed head injury, or disseminated intravascular coagulation from sepsis or leukemia; and in sudden decreases in cardiac output, as in myocarditis or hemorrhagic shock. Such an insult immediately deprives the brain of substrate and oxygen for the formation of high-energy phosphate, which is necessary for maintenance of the integrity of the brain. The clinical consequences are immediate and are characterized by sudden loss of consciousness, pupillary dilatation, and, often, generalized convulsions. Although survival with good neurologic functioning has been reported in rare instances (associated with drowning in ice-cold water) of prolonged asphyxia (10 to 20 minutes), several minutes (2 to 4) of anoxia usually result in significant neurologic sequelae, with damage first to mitochondria and neuronal cell body. The neuronal injury is compounded by the development of brain edema and local circulatory disturbances, which further exacerbate the hypoxic-ischemic insult.

As was the case in the infant with a hypoxic-ischemic insult, prevention of further hypoxia by attention to ventilatory support and maintenance of circulatory parameters is critical in these older children. Management of brain edema often plays a critical role in reducing mortality and minimizing neurologic sequelae. Cerebral edema is often difficult to recognize. Papilledema may be observed, but it is far more common after an hypoxic-ischemic insult for brain edema to be suspected and then confirmed after intracranial pressure monitoring. We accomplish this by insertion of a ventricular catheter lead to a transducer. Intracranial pressures are maintained below 20 mm Hg, a pressure chosen to maintain cerebral perfusion pressure (calculated as the difference between mean arterial blood pressure, usually approximately 100 mm Hg, and intracranial pressure) above 60 to 70 mm Hg. Measures taken to reduce intracranial pressure include careful monitoring of fluid intake; administration of Decadron at a loading dose of 1 mg/kg and then a daily maintenance dose of 0.25 to 0.5 mg/kg; and periodic intravenous infusion of mannitol at doses ranging between 0.25 and 1 gm/kg. Mannitol infusion usually results in reductions in intracranial pressure within 5 to 10 minutes and a duration of effect between 30 minutes and 4 hours. We have also employed another diuretic, furosemide, at doses of 1 mg/kg every 3 to 6 hours as an alternative if mannitol does not produce the desired effect.

In addition to the treatment of the complications of hypoxic-ischemic encephalopathy described, investigators have attempted to mitigate the effects of the insult by measures designed to increase the tolerance of the brain to hypoxia. The first such attempt was the use of hypothermia to reduce the energy requirements of the brain. For example, with body temperatures as low as 16°C, cardiac arrest can be tolerated for as long as 30 minutes; this technique has been employed for many years in patients undergoing open heart surgery. However, such extreme hypothermia is accompanied by major systemic complications, and this is not practical, even in intensive care situations. A less severe degree of hypothermia, although effective in experimental paradigms of hypoxia, has proved to be disappointing in the usual clinical situation.

Prognosticating the effects of hypoxic-ischemic encephalopathy remains a difficult problem and, to date, such laboratory procedures as computed tomography, EEG, and brain stem evoked responses have provided little help. In general, rapid initial improvement remains the most reasonable gauge of further recovery; children who remain unresponsive to painful stimuli for 2 weeks after the insult have a bleak outcome.

REYE SYNDROME
JEROME S. HALLER, M.D.

Despite the considerable fall-off of reported cases of Reye syndrome (RS) over the last few years, it is essential that physicians caring for children remember how to identify victims of it both clinically and with laboratory support. It is equally important to be prepared to treat the CNS complications of RS, namely cerebral edema and increased intracranial pressure, and to recognize or at least consider other disorders that may mimic RS. The failure to intervene or to delay therapy can make a difference in the neurologic outcome for these children.

Repeated vomiting with no or minimal temperature elevation; change in mentation with lethargy, restlessness, or combativeness; and confusion progressing to unresponsiveness are the key clinical elements of RS, especially when preceded by a febrile illness or chickenpox. Infants with RS under 1 year of age commonly present with seizures, tachypnea and alteration of consciousness. Vomiting is an unusual event in this age group.

Laboratory confirmation of the diagnosis includes highly elevated serum AST and ALT, blood NH_3 (preferably arterial), and prolonged PT and PTT. Additional tests that can be abnormal are serum CK, glucose, and amylase.

A CNS infection must be ruled out. If there is concern about increased intracranial pressure (ICP) or a space-occupying mass, a CT should be done before a lumbar puncture. The CSF in RS is normal. Protein level is appropriate to the age of the child. Glucose should correspond to peripheral values. Up to 10 WBC may be found without implying infection.

Liver biopsy is not absolutely needed but should be done if the history suggests repeated bouts of RS, and in infants under 1 year in whom urea cycle disturbances or disorders of carnitine metabolism are possible. If a biopsy is undertaken, a piece should be deep frozen for biochemical investigation of the latter disease states. In this regard, it is helpful to obtain a urine specimen for amino and organic acid analysis.

TREATMENT

To date there is no specific treatment for RS. Two components of therapy must be carried out carefully and simultaneously: fluid and electrolyte balance, and monitoring and management of ICP. Children with RS are best cared for in a pediatric intensive care unit (PICU). On admission, serum electrolytes, osmolality, BUN, and creatinine should be determined in addition to the laboratory studies noted above. Fluid loss as a result of vomiting should be corrected if more than 10 per cent dehydration is present. While there are a number of ways to calculate fluid requirements, caution must be exercised; fluid overload is to be absolutely avoided. I am not a believer in "keeping the patient on the dry side." Normal maintenance fluid should be given using 10 to 15 per cent glucose and one-half normal saline with added K as KPO_4, 2 to 3 mEq/kg for 24 hours if PO_4 is less than 5.5 mg/dl, otherwise as KCl when urine is flowing (condom or catheter drainage) at 1.5 to 2 ml/kg/hr. Blood sugar should be maintained at 150 to 200 mg/dl to compensate for the transient errors in gluconeogenesis associated with RS.

The second component in the treatment of RS is the management of increased ICP and cerebral edema. Again, clinical clues in the progression of this problem must be watched for. The appearance of papilledema may lag well behind clinical deterioration. Coma staging is useful if everyone agrees with the numerical staging. I find it preferable to describe the patient's verbal and motor responses, rather than using stages. If, on admission, the child is lethargic, that is, arousable with appropriate directed activity in response to painful or noxious stimulation, watchful waiting is appropriate. If the child becomes unresponsive to verbal stimulation and has nondirected motor responses or posturing to noxious stimulation or arrives in the ICU in this state, ICP monitoring and management are obligatory. In preparation for this, fresh frozen plasma must be administered, 10 ml/kg. The child should be paralyzed with Pavulon, 0.05 to 0.1 mg/kg/q2h. Intubation for respiratory control is essential. PCO_2 should be maintained between 20 and 25 torr. Arterial and central venous pressure lines, nasogastric tube, and bladder catheter should be in place. In the interim, hyperventilation can be used to reduce total intracranial volume. The child should be placed with the head elevated 30 degrees. An intracranial pressure monitoring device must be inserted to monitor ICP and its response to treatment. Although an epidural catheter system is preferable, a subarachnoid bolt or intraventricular catheter transducer system is equally effective. Ideally ICP should be maintained below 15 torr, with a cerebral perfusion pressure (CCP) of 40 torr or better to adequately perfuse the brain. Pressure waves to 20 torr which rise and fall rapidly to 15 torr or less seem to be innocuous. Hyperventilation for 2 minutes is effective intervention if there are pressure waves of the same value but with slow return to normal. Mannitol is the drug of choice when this fails or when there are pressure waves over 20 torr. A dose of 250 mg/kg should be given initially, administered over a 10-minute period, increasing doses of 500 mg/kg to as much as 1.5 gm/kg if pressure does not respond to lesser doses. With subsequent rises, the last lowest effective dose should be used. Serum osmolality must be determined before the next infusion of mannitol or 2 hours after the last dose. A value of over 320 mOsm precludes further use of this agent. The patient must be carefully monitored for dehydration or renal failure. Should mannitol be ineffective, pentobarbital infusion has been used in some centers. A loading dose is 20 mg/kg infused at a rate of 10 mg/kg/hr over a 2-hour period. Maintenance dose is 2 mg/kg/hr to keep the serum level to 25 to 35 μg/ml. A level should be obtained at the end of the loading infusion and then periodically every 8 to 12 hours. An additional loading dose of 10 mg/kg over a 2-hour period may be given if a maintenance level has not been achieved. Bradycardia and hypotension are complicating side effects of this agent. The latter responds to infusions of crystalloid solutions.

When the ICP has been stable at less than 15 torr for 24 hours, the patient can be weaned from the support system. If pentobarbital was used, the infusion can be stopped without tapering dosages. The respirator is next adjusted to permit PCO_2 to return toward normal.

If there is no increase in intracranial pressure, Pavulon can then be discontinued. If over the subsequent 24 hours intracranial pressure remains normal, the monitoring system can be removed and the patient extubated.

Steroids have not been of any use in this disorder, nor, in my opinion, is it necessary to reduce intestinal flora with antibiotics. The contribution of NH_3 from this source is minimal.

These children must have careful outpatient follow-ups. They may recover fully neurologically but have both behavioral and educational sequelae.

4

Respiratory Tract

MALFORMATIONS OF THE NOSE

· MAHA K. BASSILA, M.D.

MALFORMATIONS OF THE EXTERNAL NOSE

Congenital anomalies vary in incidence from the very rare, like arrhinia (nasal aplasia), polyrrhinia (double nose), and nasal clefting—median or lateral, to the more common, such as cleft lip and palate, posterior choanal atresia, dermoid cysts, gliomas, and encephaloceles.

Malformations of the nose can be primary embryologic defects, defects secondary to other facial structures, and interactions that continue to occur between the nose and the other facial components.

Diagnosis of nasal aplasia and the other rare anomalies is easy; however, the other anomalies like choanal atresia or stenosis, hypertelorism, and facial clefts must be looked for. Management consists primarily of providing the infant with an adequate airway, similar to the management of choanal atresia. Reconstructive surgery can be deferred until later.

CHOANAL ATRESIA AND STENOSIS

The incidence of choanal atresia ranges between 1 in 5000 and 1 in 8000 births, with a greater incidence in females (2:1), unilateral more common than bilateral (2:1), and more common on the right side (2:1). The incidence of associated anomalies can be as high as 50 per cent, mainly craniofacial and cardiovascular malformations.

The site of the atretic plate is consistent at the tangential plane in the choana; however, it may be entirely osseous, membrano-osseous (90 per cent), or membranous (10 per cent), with varying thickness between 1 and 12 mm. The characteristics of high arched palate, the lateral nasal walls crowded medially, and shortened anteroposterior nasopharyngeal vault further substantiate the theory of mesodermal cell migration and overgrowth of the palatine bones, in addition to the persistence of the bucconasal membrane. Computed tomography is essential for diagnosis and treatment.

Airway management consists of establishing an oral airway by using a feeding nipple or pacifier with a large hole made at the top with or without a feeding tube as tolerated. The nipple is secured to the head or around the ears with ribbons and elastic bands. The infant can be sent home with this. Mouth breathing is usually acquired at 4 to 6 weeks of age, which will be a good time for definite surgical treatment. In unilateral atresia surgical correction can be deferred until later, provided that the infant or child has no significant respiratory difficulty or cyclic cyanosis.

The preferred approach for surgical correction is the transpalatal route, irrespective of the age. The transnasal approach with the use of microsurgical techniques can be used as well. Preservation of mucosal flaps and stenting of the newly created openings are essential for a successful result. After removal of the stent at 4 to 6 weeks, dilation of the choanae may be necessary, more often with the transnasal approach and more often unilaterally on the more stenotic side.

Dermoid cysts most commonly present as a mass or single pil (sinus) with extruding hair on the nasal dorsum. They constitute 10 per cent of all head and neck dermoids. Treatment of dermoid cysts is simple excision, using a suitable incision overlying the mass. An alternative, more cosmetic approach is through an intraoral gingivobuccal incision and facial degloving.

The dermoid sinuses extend into nasal cartilage and bone and may go into the septum, to the basisphenoid and beyond the cribriform plate to the dura. Diagnosis is made on CT scan with contrast and/or MRI.

Treatment is by complete surgical excision. If dural connection is present, then a subfrontal combined neurosurgical and otolaryngologic approach is utilized.

Dermoid cysts must be differentiated from extranasal gliomas and encephaloceles. Intranasal gliomas and encephaloceles are confused, since both can appear as polypoid masses; however, since encephaloceles maintain a connection to the CNS, softness, compressibility, and enlargement with crying distinguish them from gliomas. Diagnosis is best made on CT scan, looking for a bony defect and widening, and MRI for better delineation of the mass.

Treatment is by combined neurosurgical and otolaryngologic excision. A staged procedure may be required. The otolaryngologic approach depends on the nature and site of the glioma or encephalocele; a lateral rhinotomy may be needed. The use of the microscope may aid in better visualization of the lesion and its intracranial connection.

TUMORS AND POLYPS OF THE NOSE
MAHA K. BASSILA, M.D.

NASAL POLYPS

Benign nasal polyps are infrequently seen in children and should alert the physician to the possible presence of an underlying disorder, mainly cystic fibrosis, rather than the common allergic polyps seen mostly in adults.

After adequate medical treatment and allergy control, intranasal surgical excision with intranasal exenteration of the ethmoid sinuses and creation of nasoantral windows is performed. In older children Caldwell-Luc and transantral ethmoidectomy may be necessary. The intranasal polypectomy and nasoantral windows may need to be repeated for recurrence. Functional endoscopic sinus surgery can be useful in some children. CT scan is necessary prior to the application of the latter modality of treatment.

Antrochoanal polyps are more common than the multiple nasal polyps. They have a characteristic presentation of a progressive unilateral nasal obstruction; depending on the size, they may present as a bilateral obstruction and a hot potato voice because of the extension into the nasopharynx and possibly the oropharynx. Since the antral choanal polyp originates from the maxillary sinus mucosa, it is not seen prior to the age of 4 or 5 years. Surgical excision is indicated and includes a Caldwell-Luc exposure of the maxillary antrum for removal of the antral attachment of the polyp. The nasopharyngeal part can then be removed via the mouth. A nasoantral window is also made.

BENIGN TUMORS OF THE NOSE

Intranasal hemangiomas are the second most common group of intranasal tumors after antrochoanal polyps. Transnasal local excision is necessary to prevent recurrent epistaxis. These are different from the cutaneous hemangiomas in that they are usually not present at birth and do not regress with time. They should be differentiated from angiofibromas and sarcomas.

Angiofibromas are rarely confined to the nose and are better classified as nasopharyngeal tumors. They occur almost exclusively in adolescent males. Diagnosis is made clinically and on CT scan, and, depending on the extension of the disease, complete surgical excision with or without radiation therapy is done. Preoperative vascular embolization is very helpful.

Inverted papillomas are uncommon in children. Treatment is by wide local excision utilizing the lateral rhinotomy approach. Squamous cell papillomas presenting as wartlike masses in the nasal vestibule, local cellulitis, and nasal bleeding may occur. Treatment is by local excision.

Other tumors like glandular mixed tumors may arise from the nasal septum or lateral nasal wall. Biopsy followed by wide local excision is the treatment of choice. Chordomas, neurofibromas, and fibroepithelial polyps are other benign tumors that occur in children.

Rhabdomyosarcoma is the most common intranasal malignancy of childhood. Biopsy followed by surgical excision and chemo- and radiotherapy is the treatment of choice, as with any other head and neck rhabdomyosarcomas. Esthesioneuroblastoma is a rare neuroepithelial malignancy with specific histologic features. Treatment is by surgical excision and radiation.

NASAL INJURIES
MAHA K. BASSILA, M.D.

Nasal trauma in childhood is less apparent than in adults. The difference is that there is a proportionally smaller part of the child's nose contributed by the bony nasal pyramid and relatively greater elasticity of the bones and immaturity of the suture lines. Because of these factors, injuries to the child's nose may go unnoticed or may be considered minor. This may eventually result in arrested growth or gross deformity secondary to malaligned structures.

The treatment of soft tissue injuries is by careful approximation of lacerated and avulsed tissues. Septal hematomas should be carefully looked for and treated with incision and drainage; careful follow-up for possible reaccumulation and infection is important. Radiographs are of no help in diagnosing nasal fractures; the clinical examination is usually enough, looking for epistaxis, ecchymosis, and displacement of cartilage and bone.

The septal dislocation of the newborn can be easily realigned using the surgical blade handle. Septal deviation of childhood, if asymptomatic, is not corrected until adulthood. When symptomatic, conservative septoplasty with incision and displacement of the deviated part suffices. Excision of cartilage is avoided, in order to avoid the possibility of arrested growth and saddling.

Nasal bone fractures can be safely managed by closed reduction. Revision in adulthood may be necessary for both functional and cosmetic results.

EPISTAXIS
STEVEN D. HANDLER, M.D.

While epistaxis is a relatively common occurrence in childhood, it often causes significant anxiety in both the child and his parent. Although bleeding occasionally occurs secondary to the mucosal maceration associated with an upper respiratory infection, nose picking or direct trauma to the nose accounts for most cases of recurrent epistaxis. The most common site of bleeding is the anterior nasal septum, known as Kiesselbach's or

Little's area. Epistaxis originating from the posterior nose or nasopharynx is very rare in children.

Uncomplicated anterior epistaxis most often stops spontaneously or with direct pressure exerted by squeezing the nostrils together. Topical vasoconstrictors such as phenylephrine can be useful in slowing down or stopping epistaxis. A child should be sitting in a chair or slightly propped up on a bed with the head elevated to decrease the blood pressure and venous congestion at the level of the nose. If the child is bleeding profusely, he will probably be more comfortable leaning forward so that the blood runs out his nose and not down his pharynx.

If these simple measures are not successful in stopping the nosebleed, or if the episodes of epistaxis are recurrent, further evaluation and treatment may be indicated. A complete history is one of the most important steps in the proper management of severe and/or recurrent epistaxis. The site of nasal bleeding (one or both sides of the nose), frequency, presence of bleeding from other sites, history of trauma, use of anticoagulants, and family history of bleeding should be ascertained. A careful examination of the nose should be performed to identify the site and cause of bleeding. Good lighting is absolutely mandatory in the examination of the nasal cavity. A headlight is most useful in this examination; however, a halogen-illuminated otoscope with a large speculum can be used to examine the nasal cavity if a headlight is unavailable. Frazier suction tips and material for cauterization and packing should be readily available. Topical vasoconstrictors, such as phenylephrine, can be used to shrink the nasal mucosa to permit better visualization of the nasal cavity, and this may possibly slow or even stop the bleeding. The physician should once again attempt to stop the bleeding with simple pressure exerted by squeezing the nostrils together. Occasionally, a roll of cotton placed beneath the upper lip will stop bleeding by compressing the labial artery. If topical pressure proves unsuccessful, cauterization with a silver nitrate stick or packing of the nose is performed. It is very important to apply the silver nitrate stick directly to the bleeding site and not to adjacent tissue. It is necessary to suction as much blood and secretions out of the way as possible so that the stick is not immersed in a pool of blood. Excess silver nitrate is then gently removed with a cotton-tipped applicator. Absorbable packing such as oxidized cellulose (Gelfoam) is usually adequate to stop most epistaxis. It also has the advantage of not having to be removed, since it will liquefy over time.

Proper management of severe or acute episodes of epistaxis that do not respond to the above maneuvers requires the assistance of an otolaryngologist. Epistaxis that fails to stop with simple pressure or absorbable packing may require deeper cauterization or a more substantial anterior nasal pack of vaseline-impregnated gauze or one of the new nasal tampons. Systemic antibiotics are routinely prescribed to patients with nasal packing in place in order to avoid sinusitis and the rare case of toxic shock syndrome.

If an anterior pack is not sufficient to control epistaxis, and bleeding continues down the pharynx, a posterior nasal pack using gauze or a Foley catheter may be necessary to stop the epistaxis. Any child who requires packing of this nature must be hospitalized for observation of any further bleeding and of any airway obstruction secondary to the nasal packing. Care must be taken not to sedate children with nasal packing because this may decrease muscular tone and precipitate airway obstruction. During the hospitalization, further evaluation of the etiology of the epistaxis is indicated. The nasal packing is removed in 3 to 5 days in a treatment room under controlled circumstances so that the specific site of bleeding may be identified, cautery applied, or the packing replaced if necessary. Recurrent or severe bleeding may rarely require ligation of the internal maxillary or anterior ethmoid artery. Treatment of the child with recurrent epistaxis should include measures to prevent further trauma to the nose which might continue to cause bleeding. A vaporizer placed in the child's room at night will increase the humidity and thereby soften the nasal mucosa. Application of petroleum jelly or antibiotic ointment to the anterior septal areas twice daily can aid in healing irritated nasal mucosa and prevent recurrent epistaxis.

Chronic allergic rhinitis can precipitate epistaxis by the continued inflammation of the nasal mucosa and subsequent bleeding from the fragile underlying vessels. While it is important to control allergic symptoms, avoidance and desensitization therapy are probably the most successful in reducing epistaxis secondary to allergy. Use of topical vasoconstricting drugs, nasal corticosteroid sprays, or systemic antihistamine/decongestant medications leads to drying of the nasal mucosa, which can precipitate or worsen epistaxis.

In children with severe or recurrent epistaxis, causes other than simple nose picking must be ruled out. Nasal septal deviation or perforation, sinusitis, tumor (nasal, nasopharyngeal, sinus), and nasal foreign body can all present with epistaxis. The use of coagulation-inhibiting drugs such as aspirin or ibuprofen may cause epistaxis. Blood dyscrasias such as hemophilia, idiopathic thrombocytopenic purpura, von Willebrand's disease, and hematologic conditions associated with leukemia or the administration of chemotherapeutic agents may lead to severe epistaxis. Treatment must include the correction of any underlying hematologic problem in addition to the utilization of the previously described local measures.

Nasal bleeding is frequently severe in Osler-Weber-Rendu disease (hereditary hemorrhagic telangiectasia), a condition associated with multiple telangiectasias throughout the aerodigestive tract. Treatment of epistaxis associated with this syndrome involves extensive resection of the fragile nasal mucosa and resurfacing the nasal cavity with skin or dermal grafts.

FOREIGN BODIES IN THE NOSE AND PHARYNX

STEVEN D. HANDLER, M.D.

Foreign bodies in the nose and pharynx are a common problem in children. Successful management requires a high index of suspicion in evaluating children with unexplained pain or nasal discharge. While most cases present to the primary physician with a history of the child having been observed placing a foreign object in the nose or mouth, in many instances the presence of a foreign body is unsuspected and may not be detected until the physician begins an orderly evaluation of the child. The dictum that "a unilateral foul-smelling nasal discharge is a foreign body until proven otherwise" is still very pertinent today. The diagnosis of nasal foreign body is made upon anterior rhinoscopy. Radiopaque foreign bodies, such as toys and beads, may be seen on routine sinus radiographs, but most are radiolucent, such as paper, cloth, and pieces of food.

If the parent is aware of the foreign body and can see it in the anterior nose, he may attempt careful removal with a small tweezers. One trick to employ in attempting to remove nasal foreign bodies is to compress the contralateral nasal aperture and to have the child attempt to blow his nose. In this way, many nasal foreign bodies can be blown out safely and comfortably by the child, and instrumentation of the nasal airway is avoided.

If the foreign body is not expelled spontaneously or removed by the parents, treatment by the physician is required. A topical analgesic/vasoconstricting solution such as 4 per cent cocaine or 2 per cent lidocaine with epinephrine should be placed in the nasal cavity on a piece of cotton to provide comfort to the child and to shrink the nasal tissues to improve visibility to the physician. A high-intensity directed light source such as a head light or spotlight focused into the nose is necessary to provide adequate illumination to remove the foreign body. If these are not available, an otoscope with a large speculum may be used in the evaluation of the nasal cavity. If the object is located in the nasal vestibule, next to the inferior turbinate, the primary physician may attempt to remove it. The foreign body can usually be removed with a small blunt hook, ear forceps, or a suction tip. Hygroscopic foreign bodies such as beans, however, may swell with nasal secretions and become very difficult to remove. The foreign body should never be pushed or irrigated into the nasopharynx, where it could be aspirated by a struggling child.

If the foreign body cannot be removed easily or is pushed posteriorly to the posterior nose or nasopharynx, no further attempt should be made to remove it. The patient should be referred to an otolaryngologist for removal of the foreign body under general anesthesia.

The use of a balloon catheter to remove the foreign body is strongly discouraged. The catheter can force the foreign body into the nasopharynx, where it can be aspirated or swallowed by the struggling child.

Special mention should be made of the problems associated with disc batteries (used in calculators, hearing aids, etc.). These batteries leak corrosive material on contact with mucosal surfaces and have been associated with septal ulcerations and perforations. They should be removed immediately.

After removal of the foreign body, a careful repeat examination of the nasal cavity is necessary because there may be a second, unsuspected foreign body deep in the nasal cavity. Once the absence of any other foreign body has been determined, the child is placed on antibiotics to treat the rhinosinusitis that usually accompanies the nasal foreign body.

Foreign bodies of the pharynx are relatively uncommon because either the child swallows the object, or it is expelled by a cough or gag. However, sharp foreign bodies may become stuck in the oral mucosa of the tonsil or pharynx. There is usually a good history of a foreign body so that the physician can search appropriately. Fishbones, pins, or sharp toys are the most common foreign bodies presenting in the pharynx. If the object can be seen and grasped easily with a forceps, it should be removed by the primary practitioner. If this cannot be done easily or bleeding is associated with the injury, an otolaryngologist should be consulted for removal of the foreign body under a general anesthetic.

Occasionally, large boluses of food or large foreign bodies may lodge in the hypopharynx. If the child can phonate and is having no respiratory distress, he should be taken to the operating room for prompt removal under a general anesthetic. No attempt should be made to remove the foreign body in the physician's office. The physician should not stick his fingers into the child's pharynx to attempt removal of a large object, as this may push the object down further and block the airway completely.

If the child with a pharyngeal foreign body is unable to breathe or phonate, a true emergency exists and immediate intervention is required to save the child's life. The Heimlich maneuver or back slaps should be instituted in this instance to attempt to dislodge the material from the hypopharynx and laryngeal inlet.

If there is a convincing history of pharyngeal foreign body such as a fish bone, and no bone is visualized on physical examination or by radiography, management depends upon the severity of the child's symptoms. If the child is having significant distress from a possible foreign body, he should be taken to the operating room for endoscopic examination under general anesthesia. If the discomfort is mild or moderate, the child is kept NPO and re-evaluated again in the morning. If the foreign body sensation has passed, this would indicate that the original injury was a scratch and that the foreign body is no longer present in the pharynx. If the pharyngeal pain is still present, the child should be taken to the operating room for endoscopic examination and removal of the probable foreign body.

The use of balloon catheters to extract pharyngeal foreign bodies is strongly discouraged. The foreign body may scratch or tear the mucosa as it is dragged out. In addition, the object may be pushed farther down and impacted in the pharynx or it can be aspirated by the struggling child.

Disc batteries pose special problems when they become lodged in the pharynx. Corrosive material leaking from the batteries can cause mucosal ulcerations, perforations, and even death. These must be removed on an urgent basis.

Once again, the area from which a pharyngeal foreign body has been removed should be examined thoroughly for a possible second foreign body.

NASOPHARYNGITIS

RICHARD H. SCHWARTZ, M.D.

Upper respiratory infections of the posterior nasal passages (nasopharynx) and the adenoids announce themselves with mucus or purulent rhinorrhea or a mixture of the two. When the nasal discharge is watery and clear or opaque and cloudy in appearance, the etiologic agent is likely to be one of the many viruses—notably rhinovirus, respiratory syncytial virus, adenoviruses, or influenza viruses—that can cause anterior rhinitis. Neonates with profuse and protracted blood-tinged serous or mucopurulent rhinorrhea may be congenitally infected by *Treponema pallidum*. Children less than 4 years old may, on occasion, present with a watery nasal discharge, erythema around the nasal vestibule, and scattered impetiginous papules below the nose and on the upper lip. This constellation of signs is likely to be caused by *Streptococcus pyogenes* (group A *Streptococcus*), which, when accompanied by a smoldering low-grade fever, is called streptococcosis. Nasopharyngitis caused by the group A *Streptococcus* is more common in young children who attend a day-care center or who have school-age older siblings living at home than among those who do not have daily contact with other children. Unimmunized immigrant children from impoverished families who appear very toxic and have a blood-tinged watery or thin purulent nasal discharge should alert the physician to the possibility of nasopharyngeal diphtheria. Fortunately, nasopharyngitis caused by the syphilitic spirochete or *C. diphtheria* is quite rare. Much more commonly, pediatricians encounter children with profuse purulent nasal discharge containing many polymorpholeukocytes and pathogenic bacteria such as the pneumococcus or *Haemophilus influenzae*, 90 per cent of which are nonencapsulated, noninvasive, and nontypable strains.

If the child has purulent nasal secretions accompanied by nasal crusting, a bacterial etiology is quite likely. Increasingly, *Moraxella (Branhamella) catarrhalis* is the causative bacterial agent of purulent nasopharyngitis. *H. influenzae* and *M. catarrhalis* may be resistant to amoxicillin because a significant percentage of these bacteria produce penicillinase enzymes, which inactivate aminopenicillin antibiotics. The role of *Staphylococcus aureus* as an etiologic agent in acute nasopharyngitis is unclear, and most specialists in infectious disease believe that a culture containing *S. aureus*, even in large numbers, does not mandate antistaphylococcal therapy. Although the meningococcus, the gonococcus, *Bordetella*

pertussis, and the measles virus, in the catarrhal stage, can cause nasopharyngitis, even an astute clinician is unlikely to consider these bacterial organisms before laboratory results of the nasopharyngeal culture are known, except in epidemic conditions.

A diagnosis of nasopharyngitis should be considered when there has been purulent nasal drainage for several days, often following 8 or more days of anterior rhinitis. The physician can often express a nickel-sized glob of purulent material merely by squeezing the alae nasi together. Scant purulent nasal secretions that have lasted only a day or two and that disappear soon after the child arises in the morning should not be considered diagnostic of nasopharyngitis. When a child with unexplained fever or an upper respiratory infection is seen, a careful examination of the middle meatus of the nose (a neglected part of the physical examination) may uncover a pool of mucopurulent secretions. On occasion elevation of the soft palate by a tongue depressor may dislodge a rivulet of purulent material that cascades down the posterior pharyngeal wall.

Nasopharyngitis is not synonymous with acute sinusitis; however, nasopharyngitis is often associated with acute ethmoid or maxillary sinusitis, acute otitis media, and acute purulent conjunctivitis. If a young child presents with purulent rhinorrhea, even in the absence of otalgia, it is advisable to examine both tympanic membranes carefully, after removing any accumulated cerumen. When areas contiguous to the nasopharynx are infected, the most common organisms are still the *Pneumococcus, H. influenzae, M. catarrhalis,* and *S. pyogenes,* in that order. Accompanying symptoms of nasopharyngitis/adenoiditis include fretfulness or querulousness, fever, nocturnal cough, offensive breath, and reduced appetite. Babies may have problems with nighttime awakening or develop aerophagia with intestinal colic because of obstruction of the nasal passages. Purulent nasal secretions draining into the stomach may cause mild nausea or abdominal pains. The differential diagnosis of *persistent* nasopharyngitis includes an inappropriate choice of antibiotic, poor pharmacologic compliance, viral etiology, or obstruction of the nasal passages or paranasal sinus ostia. Nasal obstruction may be caused by congenital choanal atresia of one or both nasal passages, the presence of a foreign body in a nasal passage, a nasal polyp, a mucus retention cyst, or a nasopharyngeal tumor. Clues to the presence of a foreign body in the nose are a fetid odor to the nasal secretions and blood-tinged drainage. Careful rhinoscopy after nasal suction and instillation of 0.25 per cent phenylephrine nose drops (0.125 per cent for babies under age 2 years) may permit visualization of the obstructing mass. Children with small nasopharynges such as some with Down syndrome seem to be predisposed to frequent bouts of purulent nasopharyngitis, and these patients may benefit from administration of an antimicrobial at bedtime at the onset of an upper respiratory infection.

Nasopharyngeal cultures may be rewarding on occasion, particularly when they uncover unsuspected group A *Streptococcus* or *B. pertussis.* Nasopharyngeal cultures may have poor specificity with any pathogenic organisms in the middle ear and paranasal sinus bacterial etiology.

Purulent nasopharyngitis remains an arena of either the academician or the experientialist ("In my clinical experience . . ."). Not only are the criteria for its diagnosis imprecise, but there is also great controversy regarding the need for specific antimicrobial therapy. And, if such therapy is indicated, when in the course of the disease does one introduce it? Do antibiotics really prevent the development of acute otitis media (AOM)? If so, is AOM prevented only in those who had been otitis-prone recently? Are antibiotics most helpful when the purulent drainage first appears, or should one wait until several days have elapsed or until there are symptoms or fever or irritability? Does it make a difference if both the child's parents are employed and the child attends a day-care center that will not allow him or her to attend with a "snotty nose"? Few of the answers to these questions have been confirmed by scientific studies. The only published study that attempted to address the question of treatment efficacy found no advantage to cephalexin treatment for purulent nasopharyngitis. However, the antibiotic chosen was not particularly effective against *H. influenzae.*

I generally prescribe an antibiotic for patients who have had profuse purulent nasal drainage for 2 or more days. I give antibiotics when children with nasopharyngitis are otitis-prone or have signs suggestive of paranasal sinusitis, when they attend day-care centers where rules preclude the child's return until the nasal drainage is clear, when I find laboratory confirmation of group A *Streptococcus,* when they are scheduled to travel by aircraft, and when they are about to go on vacation. Amoxicillin in a dose of 40 mg/kg/day may be prescribed; however, as increasing numbers of studies report amoxicillin-resistant bacterial strains, other antibiotics may be needed for treatment of nasopharyngitis, sinusitis, and AOM, at least for infants and preschoolers. Additional antibiotic choices include trimethoprim-sulfamethoxazole, 5 ml/10 kg body weight (do not prescribe if group A *Streptococcus* is the pathogen), amoxicillin-clavulanate combination (same dose as the amoxicillin component), cefaclor (same dose as amoxicillin), erythromycin-sulfisoxazole (same dose as amoxicillin for the erythromycin component), or, if the organism is known to be a pneumococcus or group A *Streptococcus,* penicillin V K.

Symptomatic management may include administration of antipyretics at established dose for age, aspiration of profuse nasal secretions with a bulb syringe, maintaining proper humidification in the child's bedroom, increasing the intake of fluids, and instilling normal saline drops into the nasal passages several times daily. With cooperative children, one or two phenylephrine drops (or sprays) per side (0.125 per cent strength for infants or 0.25 per cent for older children) may provide relief for 3 or 4 hours, but these topical vasoconstricting nose drops/sprays should not be given more than four times daily and they are limited to 5 or 6 consecutive days. A sympathomimetic drug (decongestant syrup or tablet), such as pseudoephedrine or phenylpropanolamine, given orally may help to shrink swollen nasal turbinates. I do not recommend antihistamine drugs for nasopharyngitis, since their value for this condition, in the absence of allergic rhinitis, has not been proven.

RHINITIS AND SINUSITIS

DACHLING PANG, M.D., F.R.C.S. (C), F.A.C.S., *and* ELLEN R. WALD, M.D.

Infections of the upper respiratory tract are the most common reason for seeking medical care. Most of these infections are caused by viruses and require no specific therapy; symptomatic treatment may increase patient comfort. However, other respiratory infections such as otitis media and sinusitis may be primarily bacterial or may be complicated by impaired local drainage resulting in bacterial superinfection.

RHINITIS

Rhinitis, when acute, is caused almost exclusively by respiratory viruses and as such requires no antimicrobial treatment. However, in the newborn period rhinitis may be due to congenital syphilis.

Persistent rhinitis in infants or young children (less than 3 years old) suggests the possibility of group A beta-hemolytic streptococcal infection, or "streptococcosis." Streptococcal infection in this age group often fails to localize in the throat and instead causes a clinical picture of a protracted cold. Occasionally an older child (over 5 years of age) with streptococcal infection presents with persistent nasal discharge and cough.

If streptococcal infection is documented by culture of the nasopharynx or throat, treatment with penicillin for 10 days is appropriate. Dosages of phenoxymethyl penicillin of 125 mg three or four times daily for those under 60 pounds and 250 mg three or four times daily for those over 60 pounds are recommended. In penicillin-allergic patients erythromycin at 40 mg/kg/day in four divided doses is a suitable substitute.

In both infants and older children the likelihood of paranasal sinusitis should be considered as a cause of persistent nasal discharge (see next section on sinusitis). Purulent rhinorrhea may also be indicative of an intranasal foreign body, especially if fetor oris is prominent or if the discharge is unilateral or bloody or both.

Whether bacteria other than group A streptococci may cause purulent rhinitis has not been adequately evaluated. The use of antimicrobial preparations cannot therefore be recommended in the management of the routine upper respiratory infection. However, there are data suggesting that antibiotic prophylaxis (daily or during the course of a cold) may be effective in preventing symptomatic episodes of acute otitis media in otitis-prone children.

Children with persistent rhinitis may be demonstrating symptoms of allergic inflammation or vasomotor rhinitis. Children with the former problem may have a positive family history of allergies or the physical stigmata of allergic problems. Symptomatic treatment with oral antihistamines or decongestants or combination agents may result in prompt improvement. Cromolyn sodium and aerosol steroid preparations may be helpful in older patients with chronic allergic nasal symptoms. Reduction of environmental allergens should always be undertaken. If simple measures of avoidance and symptomatic therapy fail, desensitization may be necessary.

SINUSITIS

There is a paucity of literature on the efficacy of antimicrobial therapy for sinusitis in children. However, in adults, although there are conflicting reports regarding the benefit of antimicrobials, several points emerge. (1) Appropriate antimicrobials eradicate susceptible microorganisms in sinus secretions; inappropriate agents fail to do so. (2) In order to accomplish sterilization of the sinus secretions, a level of antimicrobial agent exceeding the minimum inhibitory concentration of the infecting microorganism must be present in the sinus secretions. (3) In some instances in which adequate antimicrobial levels within sinus secretions are documented, sterilization of secretions is still not accomplished. This observation points to the importance of local defense mechanisms (such as ciliary activity and phagocytosis), which may be impaired in the altered environment within the purulent sinus secretions (decreased partial pressure of oxygen, increased carbon dioxide pressure, and decreased pH.) Therefore, irrigation and drainage of sinus secretions may be required in some patients. (4) There does appear to be a decrease in the serious suppurative orbital and intracranial complications of paranasal sinus disease consequent to the systemic use of antimicrobials, and currently medical therapy with an appropriate antimicrobial agent is recommended in children with acute sinusitis. The recommended treatment is amoxicillin (40 mg/kg/day in three divided doses) or ampicillin (100 mg/kg/day in four divided doses). Both these drugs are relatively safe, inexpensive, and active against the common bacterial pathogens as well as most anaerobic organisms found in the sinuses.

Alternative antimicrobials, which may be useful if the patient is allergic to penicillin or if there is a high local prevalence of beta-lactamase–producing *Haemophilus influenzae* or *Branhamella catarrhalis*, are trimethoprim-sulfamethoxazole* (8 and 40 mg/kg/day, respectively, in two divided doses) or erythromycin-sulfisoxazole* (50 and 150 mg/kg/day in four divided doses) or cefaclor (40 mg/kg/day in three divided doses). Trimethoprim-sulfamethoxazole is not optimal therapy for *Streptococcus pyogenes* and is therefore not the best choice as an amoxicillin alternative in the 5 to 15 year age group, an age group in which *S. pyogenes* is most likely to be encountered. Cefaclor, while a reasonable substitute for amoxicillin in selected patients, has been noted to be ineffective in vitro against approximately 40 per cent of the beta-lactamase–producing *B. catarrhalis*. A new drug combination consisting of amoxicillin and potassium clavulanate (Augmentin) is also suitable for use in

*Manufacturer's warning: Contraindicated in children less than 2 months of age.

patients who have sustained a clinical failure with amoxicillin or reside in geographic areas where there is a high prevalence of beta-lactamase–producing bacterial species. Potassium clavulanate is an irreversible beta-lactamase inhibitor. If this drug combination is used in treating an infection with a beta-lactamase–producing bacterial species, the beta-lactamase will be bound by the inhibitor and the amoxicillin restored to its original spectrum of activity.

In pediatric patients who require parenteral therapy for acute sinusitis but who do not have intracranial or intraorbital complications, cefuroxime at 150 mg/kg/day in three divided doses given intravenously is ideal. This agent is suitable for *S. pneumoniae* and both beta-lactamase–positive and negative *B. catarrhalis* and *H. influenzae*. Cefuroxime is also adequate, although perhaps not ideal for *Staphylococcus aureus* and anaerobes of the upper respiratory tract.

The use of antihistamines and decongestants in the treatment of sinusitis is controversial. There has been no evaluation of the efficacy of these preparations in acute or chronic sinusitis. Although the topical decongestants phenylephrine and oxymetazoline produce potentially undesirable local effects such as ciliostasis, they may provide dramatic relief from symptoms. The effectiveness of these agents with respect to shortening the clinical course of illness in acute sinusitis or preventing suppurative complications is unknown.

Sinus puncture with irrigation and drainage (usually best accomplished by a transnasal approach) often results in dramatic relief from pain and provides material for definitive culture and sensitivity (cultures of the nose and throat correlate poorly with sinus aspirate cultures). In experienced hands and with proper sedation, the procedure is safe and can be accomplished with minimal discomfort. Although a sinus aspiration is not necessary for the management of an uncomplicated case of acute sinusitis, indications for sinus aspiration include clinical unresponsiveness to conventional therapy, sinus disease in an immunosuppressed patient, severe symptoms such as headache or facial pain, and life-threatening disease at the time of clinical presentation.

Orbital Complications

Orbital cellulitis is the most frequent serious complication of acute sinusitis. Despite antimicrobial therapy, it is a potentially life-threatening infection.

Children with stage I disease (see Table 1) can be managed as outpatients by the usual regimen for acute sinusitis, provided that the parents are cooperative and cognizant of the serious implication if prompt alleviation of symptoms does not occur. If the infection has progressed beyond stage I, hospitalization and intravenous antibiotics are mandatory. The choice of antibiotics is guided by knowledge of the usual bacteriology of acute sinusitis. Blood cultures and sinus aspirate should be obtained aerobically and anaerobically, and appropriate antimicrobials should be added if unsuspected organisms are isolated. Surgical drainage is required if there is a subperiosteal or orbital abscess, but orbital cellulitis may respond to antimicrobials without surgical

TABLE 1. Clinical Staging of Orbital Cellulitis*

Stage		Signs
I	Inflammatory edema	Inflammatory edema beginning in medial or lateral eyelid; usually nontender with only minimal skin changes. No induration, visual impairment, or limitation of extraocular movements.
II	Orbital cellulitis	Edema of orbital contents with varying degrees of proptosis, chemosis, limitation of extraocular movement and/or visual loss.
III	Subperiosteal abscess	Proptosis down and out with signs of orbital cellulitis (usually severe). Abscess beneath the periosteum of the ethmoid, frontal, or maxillary bone (in that order of frequency).
IV	Orbital abscess	Abscess within the fat or muscle cone in the posterior orbit. Severe chemosis and proptosis; complete ophthalmoplegia and moderate to severe visual loss present (globe displaced forward or down and out).
V	Cavernous sinus thrombophlebitis	Proptosis, globe fixation, severe loss of visual acuity, prostration, signs of meningitis; progresses to proptosis, chemosis, and visual loss in contralateral eye.

*Modified from Chandler JR, Langenbrunner DJ, Stevens, EF: The pathogenesis of orbital complications in acute sinusitis. Laryngoscope 80:1414–1428, 1970.

intervention. The prognosis for stages I and II is usually good if diagnosis and appropriate therapy are carried out promptly, but residual visual loss due to infarction of the optic nerve may complicate frank abscesses. Severe neurologic sequelae or death may follow cavernous sinus thrombophlebitis.

Intracranial Complications

Intracranial extension of infection is the second most common complication of acute sinusitis. Although the incidence of suppurative intracranial disease in patients with sinusitis is unknown, paranasal sinusitis is the source of 35 to 65 per cent of subdural empyemas. Intracranial infection should be suspected if signs of systemic toxicity and headache do not improve after an adequate course of oral antibiotics and decongestant has been given for the original sinusitis.

Treatment of sinusitis-related intracranial suppuration requires antimicrobials, drainage, and excellent supportive care. There is evidence that preoperative meningitic doses of antibiotics may improve the chances for survival. Since the predominant organisms isolated from sinusitis-related subdural empyema include anaerobic and microaerophilic streptococci, non–group A streptococci, *Staphylococcus aureus*, and a mixture of *Proteus* and other gram-negative rods, the initial antibiotic regimen prior to culture and sensitivity results should be a combination of a penicillinase-resistant penicillin and chloramphenicol. The recently available third-generation cephalosporin cefotaxime (Claforan) may be used in place of chloramphenicol to avoid hemopoietic complications in young infants, although experience with this drug is limited.

Hyperosmolar agents should be given if high intracranial pressure threatens brain herniation. Systemic doses of steroid are prescribed with caution because of the theoretical suppressive effect on granulocytic and immune functions. Anticonvulsants should be given prophylactically to protect against a 79 per cent incidence of associated seizures.

Extradural and subdural empyemas should be drained through a generous craniotomy. The entire collection of pus can be evacuated and the infected bed profusely irrigated with bacitracin solution under direct vision, and, with a judiciously fashioned flap, the opposite parafalcine space can be explored. Extradural and subdural drains are left in place for 3 to 5 days for continuous drainage and intermittent antibiotic lavage. An underlying brain abscess is best handled by intracapsular evacuation and catheter drainage to avoid unnecessary brain damage associated with radical excision of deep-seated lesions within eloquent areas of the brain. In some cases of subdural empyema, the underlying brain is so swollen that the bone flap must be left out for external decompression. Following radical débridement of all osteomyelitic sequestra, the frontal sinus is opened widely, its content exenterated, and its cavity drained.

Postoperatively, intravenous administration of antibiotics should be maintained for a minimum of 2 to 3 weeks. Intermittent antibiotic irrigation of the infected cavities can be done through the catheters until their removal in 3 to 5 days. The shrinking of the abscess or empyema can be followed accurately by serial CT scans.

Despite modern diagnostic and surgical capabilities, the mortality associated with subdural empyema and brain abscess remains over 20 per cent. Causes of death and permanent morbidity are related to delayed diagnosis, recurrent suppuration, missed concomitant lesions, extensive cortical and dural sinus thrombophlebitis, and fulminant bacterial meningitis in infants. Early diagnosis remains the most effective way for improving survival.

RETROPHARYNGEAL AND PERITONSILLAR ABSCESSES

FRED S. HERZON, M.D.

Retropharyngeal abscess is not an uncommon admission diagnosis in major pediatric centers throughout the country. It is, however, an extremely rare discharge diagnosis today.

This is not to say that a child entering with a high fever, stiff neck, drooling, and radiographic evidence of widened retropharyngeal space could not have a retropharyngeal abscess. If an abscess is present, general anesthesia, intraoral incision, and drainage are indicated, with strict attention to protection of the airway. Parenteral antibiotics would be dependent upon culture results, with broad coverage given until bacterial identification is obtained.

Peritonsillar abscess, on the other hand, is the most common intraoral abscess in children today. The abscess occurs in association with tonsillitis and pus formation in the peritonsillar space between the capsule of the tonsil and the superior constrictor muscle. Diagnosis is made by observing unilateral bulging of the tonsil, deviation of the uvula, and trismus. It is confirmed by needle aspiration of the abscess at a point midway between the base of the uvula and the posterior molar. As much pus as possible is removed by aspiration. In over 90 per cent of the cases this results in resolution of the abscess within 24 to 48 hours, without further drainage. Penicillin, parenterally or orally, is the drug of choice, and hospitalization is unnecessary for resolution of this disease. In 59 peritonsillar abscesses treated in a 10-year period at the author's institution, at no time did culture results influence the outcome of the disease. Therefore, I do not advise sending the pus for culture and sensitivity. The recommendation for tonsillectomy after resolution of the peritonsillar abscess is still subject to some controversy.

THE TONSIL AND ADENOID PROBLEM

RICHARD B. GOLDBLOOM, M.D., F.R.C.P.(C.)

The decision to perform or not to perform tonsillectomy and/or adenoidectomy (T&A) remains one of the most subjective in the pediatric family practice and otolaryngologic repertoires, and the tenacity with which individual opinions are held often seems inversely proportional to the volume of supporting scientific evidence. Over the past decade the trend has been toward conservatism in recommending either procedure. This is reflected by a steady decrease in the number of T&A's performed annually. Parenthetically, the declining number of these operations has been paralleled by a progressive increase in the rate of myringotomy and tube insertions. Thus, the total number of pediatric otolaryngologic procedures performed annually under general anesthesia has not changed substantially.

A decision to perform these operations on a child should never be taken lightly. A small but significant number of fatalities associated with T&A continue to occur every year. Postoperative hemorrhage is not uncommon, and other serious unanticipated complications, such as malignant hyperthermia, can turn an ostensibly simple intervention into a major catastrophe. Therefore, such surgery should never be looked upon as "minor" and should be carried out in hospitals that offer skilled pediatric anesthesia and postoperative care. In most instances, an elective T&A is a decision in favor of a procedure that carries a small but definite mortality in order to benefit a condition that carries none. Probably the only absolute indication for surgery is the occurrence of obstructive sleep apnea associated with CO_2 retention, hypoxia, pulmonary hypertension, and cor pulmonale—an uncommon syndrome. Antecedent

peritonsillar abscess (quinsy) has been considered a strong indication for tonsillectomy in the past, but this assumption has not been adequately tested.

Among children with *severe* recurrent throat infections (representing less than 10 per cent of patients referred for tonsillectomy), a recently reported large-scale controlled study suggests that surgery is followed by significantly fewer throat infections during the first 2 postoperative years as compared with unoperated controls, with the difference tending to disappear in the third year. However, in this study many of the subjects who did not undergo operations also had markedly fewer throat infections during follow-up, and most that did occur were minor. Differences in the number of sore throat days or in the number of days of school absence were modest or insignificant between operated and unoperated children. Thus, even for children with severe recurrent throat infections, the evidence of benefit from tonsillectomy is modest and transient and must be weighed against the risks of the procedure. It has been estimated that at most only one or two children with the frequency and severity of throat infection required for inclusion in this study would be seen annually in a pediatric or family practice.

Despite continuing debate, there is no convincing evidence of benefit from adenoidectomy in the treatment or prevention of recurrent otitis media. On the other hand, there is good evidence to support the efficacy of daily sulfonamide prophylaxis for this purpose. One absolute contraindication to adenoidectomy is the presence of a cleft palate (typically associated with recurrent otitis media), since removal of the adenoid further exaggerates the defect in palatopharyngeal closure, thereby increasing the nasal escape of air, which creates serious speech problems for these children. The presence of a bifid or notched uvula should also be regarded as a likely contraindication to adenoidectomy, since it is often accompanied by a submucous cleft or related anomalies.

Physicians sometimes feel pressured by the parents' insistence that something be done for their child who has recurrent throat or ear infections, snores at night, or has other symptoms attributed to enlarged or infected tonsils or adenoids. It has now been well-documented that parental perceptions of the frequency of antecedent sore throats in their child are unreliable guides to the subsequent frequency of sore throats under close observation. From the physician's viewpoint, it is always easier and quicker to recommend surgery than to discuss the pros and cons of surgery with patients (or guardians), defer a decision, or attempt less dramatic alternatives. The temptation to take the expeditious route should be resisted.

Parental tolerance for recurrent respiratory infections in their children varies greatly. The parents' diminished tolerance or exasperation may be conditioned by familial factors unrelated to the child or by anecdotal reports of dramatic improvements following surgery. A thorough understanding of the family is essential to making a decision that is in the child's best long-term interest. If the basis for conservatism is fully explained to parents, they will usually accept and respect such caution.

The natural process of involution of tonsillar and adenoidal lymphoid tissue in the prepubertal years is usually associated with decreasing frequency of throat and ear infections. In this age group, a decision to defer surgery is often rewarded by progressive and spontaneous clinical improvement.

Aside from any beneficial impact that tonsillectomy and adenoidectomy might have on the frequency of throat and ear infections, our knowledge about possible deleterious effects of such surgery on the immune system is fragmentary. Prior to the advent of the polio vaccine, it had been well established that previously tonsillectomized children who contracted poliomyelitis were at increased risk for bulbar involvement. Children who underwent tonsillectomy have been shown to be at increased risk for colonization by *Neisseria meningitidis*, but it is not yet known whether children thus colonized (or their associates) are at increased risk for invasive meningococcal disease. The presence of virus-specific cellular reactivity in tonsillar lymphocytes is associated with significant clinical protection during close household contact with varicella-zoster virus. These observations are mentioned here simply to underline the possibility that the long-term effects of tonsillectomy and adenoidectomy may extend well beyond the pharynx and are still poorly understood. Taken together, the foregoing considerations favor increasing caution and conservatism in recommending tonsillectomy or adenoidectomy in the majority of children.

DISORDERS OF THE LARYNX

GEORGE H. ZALZAL, M.D.,
and KENNETH M. GRUNDFAST, M.D.

GENERAL CONSIDERATIONS

Improved instruments for endoscopy, new techniques in laryngeal surgery, and changing concepts in medical management have engendered advances in the current therapy of laryngeal disorders. Since the larynx of a normal child is the region of the upper airway with the smallest lumen, any abnormality or condition causing additional narrowing can lead to dangerous airway obstruction. When stridor, retraction, labored respiration, and nasal flaring indicate the presence of a compromised upper airway, therapy for laryngeal disorders primarily involves a series of critical decisions regarding the timing and relative necessity for intubation or tracheostomy. It is better to recognize impending severe airway obstruction early than to rely on emergency measures for regaining an adequate airway when severe obstruction occurs. Speculations regarding adequacy of the airway and inferences from radiographs do not constitute sufficient information for decision-making. Similarly, arterial blood gas determination usually is not a critical factor in deciding whether endoscopy and alternate airway are required. If one waits to see evidence of significant hypoxemia or hypercarbia in order to conclude that there is marked upper airway obstruction, a precarious situation may rapidly become an acute, life-threatening emergency. The best way to determine the relative adequacy of an airway is to view the lumen directly and to determine the precise nature and location of the obstruction. Needless delay before proceeding to endoscopy can be counterproductive. Endoscopy carries minimal complications when performed adequately. Flexible endoscopy of the larynx is important to visualize vocal cord mobility and laryngeal dynamics, especially in laryngomalacia. Rigid endoscopy is superior to flexible endoscopy for examination of the subglottis, trachea, and bronchi. Although medical management can be important, establishing or maintaining an adequate airway precedes and supersedes decisions regarding choice of medication. The total approach to management of laryngeal disorders depends on the etiology and severity of the disorder and the age of the child. The younger the child (and the smaller the diameter of the airway), the more life-threatening are disorders that involve impingement of the glottic and subglottic space.

CONGENITAL

When a neonate has stridor, a hoarse cry, cough, aspiration, dysphagia, or signs of a compromised airway, a congenital laryngeal disorder should be considered, and consultation with an otolaryngologist is warranted. In considering congenital laryngeal disorders, it must be clearly understood that use of the term "congenital laryngeal stridor" merely connotes that a newborn child has a harsh, high-pitched respiratory sound; it does not indicate that a discrete diagnosis has been made or that an etiology has been determined. The first step, then, in management of the neonate with stridor is one of determining etiology. One of the most common congenital laryngeal disorders is laryngomalacia. In this condition, an abnormally compliant epiglottis along with portions of the aryepiglottic folds tend to get drawn into the larynx during inspiration. The findings at endoscopy are diagnostic, and treatment is usually expectant. Keeping the infant in a prone position may be helpful. Usually children outgrow the problem between the first and second year of life. In children with severe laryngomalacia with associated cyanosis, apnea, feeding difficulties, and failure to thrive, surgical intervention is needed. Epiglottoplasty is a procedure to be considered instead of tracheotomy. The procedure entails trimming of the redundant mucosa over the arytenoids, aryepiglottic folds, and epiglottis. Tracheostomy for laryngomalacia is rarely necessary.

Unilateral or bilateral vocal cord paresis or paralysis can be present at birth. Bilateral vocal cord paralysis is usually secondary to central nervous disorders, whereas unilateral vocal cord paralysis is usually traumatic or iatrogenic (cardiac surgery). The impairment of vocal cord mobility may be part of a general neurologic disorder or the result of compression of the vagus nerve rootlets within the foramen magnum, as in the Arnold-Chiari malformation. Trauma to the neck during birth can damage the vagus or recurrent laryngeal nerve, in turn causing impaired vocal cord movement. The underlying cause of impaired vocal cord mobility should be sought. Neonates with unilateral vocal cord paralysis have a hoarse cry and moderate impingement of the airway but usually do not require tracheostomy. Neonates with bilateral vocal cord paralysis can have a hoarse or nearly normal cry with high-pitched stridor; usually tracheostomy is needed to maintain an adequate airway.

Congenital subglottic stenosis can be secondary to a small cricoid ring or thick submucosal layer. If the subglottic lumen is extremely small, tracheostomy may be necessary early in life, with surgical reconstruction of the subglottic region during the first few months of life. The subglottic lumen may be expected to enlarge as the child grows, but the presence of a tracheotomy for a long time can lead to tracheal stenosis and collapse and even death secondary to obstruction. Acquired subglottic stenosis is usually more severe than congenital subglottic stenosis and is best treated surgically. Other congenital disorders of the larynx include cysts, webs, clefts, and hemangiomas. Cryosurgery and more often carbon dioxide laser are being utilized in the treatment of localized subglottic hemangiomas. Also, a trial of prednisone 2 mg/kg/day, or 60 mg/m²/day in three divided doses, can be given to promote regression of subglottic hemangioma, provided that the stridor is not severe. If the stridor decreases in response to prednisone, then the dose is gradually changed to a maintenance dose of 1 to 2 mg/kg of prednisone in a single dose given every other day. Although it is reported that these doses of prednisone can be given safely for up to 6 months, possible adverse effects such as adrenal suppression, Cushing's syndrome, increased susceptibility to infection, and growth disturbances must be considered. No single method is universally effective. Radiotherapy should not be used in treatment of subglottic hemangiomas.

To determine the etiology of a congenital laryngeal disorder, it is often necessary to view the endolarynx. Although it has been common practice to attempt diagnostic laryngoscopy in the neonatal nursery with an anesthesiologist's folding laryngoscope, better and safer methods are now available. Rod-lens telescopic fiberoptic illuminated ventilating pediatric bronchoscopes have greatly facilitated laryngotracheobronchoscopy in the newborn. Despite a traditional reluctance to allow a neonate to undergo endoscopy, the new and improved optical systems give the modern endoscopist an accurate magnified view of laryngeal and tracheal abnormalities with minimal risk. Sometimes tracheostomy can be avoided with propitious use of newly devised microinstruments and microcautery for excision of webs and removal of cysts.

TRAUMATIC

The incidence of laryngeal injuries in childhood has increased. Intrinsic injuries secondary to aspiration, burning fumes, and lye ingestion are life-threatening if not attended to quickly. A child riding a minibike or trailbike can be hit in the anterior neck by a branch or clothesline, sustaining laryngeal fracture or laryngotracheal separation. Such injuries are acute emergencies and, depending on the type of injury, immediate tracheostomy rather than endotracheal intubation may be necessary.

IATROGENIC

The left recurrent laryngeal nerve is in jeopardy of being injured whenever a child undergoes cardiac surgery. If the child develops hoarseness, stridor, or both postoperatively, indirect laryngoscopy is warranted to assess mobility of the vocal cords. If hoarseness or aspiration caused by vocal cord paralysis presents significant problems, polytef paste (Teflon) can be injected to change the position of a lateral-lying vocal cord.

When endotracheal intubation is required for a prolonged period, there is risk of developing subglottic stenosis. Although the pathogenesis of this acquired form is not entirely clear, it is likely that trauma to the mucosal surface is a factor. Neonates can remain intubated for several weeks without developing subglottic stenosis; older children cannot. It appears that children with Down's syndrome do not tolerate intubation well. Systemic and intralesional steroids, as well as a variety of surgical procedures, are being utilized in the treatment of acquired subglottic stenosis. Most forms of therapy for subglottic stenosis are complicated, and many ultimately provide less than optimal results. It is important to take preventive measures. Endotracheal tubes should be of proper size, preferably with no cuff or a low-pressure cuff. Intubated children should be well sedated in order to reduce the chance that head movements will cause the tube to traumatize the laryngeal and tracheal mucosa. When it is determined that children older than 2 months will require prolonged intubation, tracheostomy should be considered. A rational decision must be based upon the patient's general condition and the projected duration of need for assisted ventilation; it is preferable to wait until extubation can be attempted rather than immediately converting to a tracheostomy.

INFECTIOUS

The most common infectious disorders that compromise airflow through the larynx are epiglottitis and laryngotracheobronchitis (croup). Therapy for croup and epiglottitis is discussed in the next article. When the airway obstruction from croup is more severe and the child is taken to a hospital emergency room, a mixture of 2.5 per cent racemic epinephrine diluted 1:8 with water can be administered nebulized through an open plastic hose held near the face or through a face mask.

Recently there have been reports of pulmonary edema associated with croup and epiglottitis. The pulmonary edema may develop at the time that the severe upper airway obstruction is relieved, either by intubation or tracheostomy. The etiology is being investigated, and it appears to involve hemodynamic and pulmonary interrelationships that are complex. Prevention of the pulmonary edema must begin as soon as the artificial airway is inserted. Continuous positive airway pressure (CPAP) should be applied to the airway immediately after the obstruction is relieved and gradually diminished during the following 24 to 36 hours. Sometimes fluid restriction and diuresis are necessary.

NEOPLASM

Benign squamous papilloma (also known as juvenile laryngeal papilloma or recurrent respiratory papillomatosis) is the most common laryngeal neoplasm in children. There is evidence that a virus may be involved in pathogenesis. Although immunotherapy has been attempted, surgical excision remains the most reliable method of treatment. Interferon has been found to cause only temporary relief from this disease. The carbon dioxide laser is now being utilized to ablate the papillomatous lesions. The laser, however, has no inherent curative power. Rather, it is a very precise surgical tool that enables removal of minute areas in a relatively blood-free field. The laser's ability to avoid damaging adjacent normal tissue and to remove all lesions present at a given time makes it valuable in preserving laryngeal structure and function in those children who often must undergo numerous endolaryngeal surgical procedures because of relentlessly recurrent papillomas.

ALLERGIC

Allergic edema can involve the supraglottic or subglottic larynx. Supraglottic allergic edema with marked swelling of the mucosa covering the arytenoids can present a clinical picture similar to that of epiglottitis. Supraglottic angioedema can develop rapidly when an atopic child ingests a drug or food known to be allergenic or when the child is exposed to an offending inhalant or when horse serum is administered. Allergic supraglottic edema usually responds quickly to subcutaneous administration of 0.01 ml/kg of 1:1000 epinephrine to a maximum dose of 0.3 ml epinephrine along with a single intramuscular or intravenous dose of 100 mg hydrocortisone sodium succinate.

Subglottic allergic edema is also known as "nocturnal spasmodic croup." It is distinguished from other forms of croup by its sudden onset, absence of fever, and complete or almost complete remission of symptoms during the day. Relief of symptoms often can be achieved with use of diphenhydramine hydrochloride as elixir of Benadryl, 5 mg/kg/day or 150 mg/m²/day given in three to four divided doses. Sometimes it may be necessary to give 0.2 ml of 1:1000 epinephrine subcutaneously as a single dose. If the symptoms do not subside within 12 hours following treatment, the child probably has infectious laryngotracheobronchitis, which requires different treatment.

VOICE DISORDERS

Improper use of the vocal cords can cause voice abnormalities. Any child who has hoarseness persistent for more than 8 weeks or a quality of breathiness with speech should undergo indirect and possibly direct laryngoscopy. Persistent yelling and shouting may lead to the formation of vocal cord nodules. In children, it is preferable to treat vocal abuse and vocal cord nodules initially with speech therapy rather than with surgical excision of the lesions. Often the child has acquired poor speech habits that can be corrected. If speech therapy is unsuccessful after a trial period of 6 to 12 months, surgical removal of vocal cord nodules is a reasonable treatment, combined with postoperative speech therapy. The vocal cord nodules may recur if the faulty speech is not corrected; thus surgery should not be considered frequently. Children with cleft palate have a specific problem—they may strain to produce voice volume within the larynx in order to overcome volume lost through air escape at the nose. Thus, children with persistent abnormal nasal emission following cleft palate repair may be prone to vocal cord nodules. In some children, vocal abuse can be a manifestation of underlying psychological problems that need investigation. Inappropriately loud or soft voices may be associated with hearing loss or noise-polluted environments.

THE CROUP SYNDROME
(Supraglottitis, Viral Laryngotracheobronchitis, Spasmodic Croup, Bacterial Tracheitis, Laryngeal Injuries)

DENNIS C. STOKES, M.D.

The term *croup syndrome* denotes a group of conditions of viral, bacterial, or traumatic origin. The characteristic features of croup are acute upper airway obstruction at the level of the larynx, which leads to stridor (usually inspiratory), cough, and changes in the voice or cry. Fever and associated signs of systemic illness may be present when croup is of infectious origin. Obstruction in the croup syndrome may involve the supraglottic structures (the epiglottis, arytenoids, and the aryepiglottic folds, or false cords), the subglottic area, or (rarely) the true vocal cords.

ACUTE VIRAL CROUP (LARYNGOTRACHEOBRONCHITIS)

Most cases of croup are viral in origin; parainfluenza viruses types 1 to 3 are the most common isolates. The typical patient with viral croup is a male infant younger than 3 years who develops low-grade fever, stridorous breathing, and a barking cough following an upper respiratory infection. The symptoms are often mild during the day but worsen at night, with varying degrees of airway obstruction and distress (primarily due to subglottic edema).

The first step in treating any infant or child with airway obstruction is to assess the adequacy of the airway by examining color, respiratory and pulse rates, and severity of retractions. Patients who require an emergency airway must be transported rapidly to a setting where a skilled team (which may include an anesthesiologist, otolaryngologist, pediatric surgeon, or intensivist) is available to place an emergency airway (by endotracheal intubation, tracheostomy, or cricothyroidotomy).

The vast majority of children have only mild obstruction with viral croup and can be managed successfully at home. Supportive therapy is the mainstay of therapy for viral croup. Humidification of inspired air to relieve the symptoms of croup is a common practice, although controlled studies of this mode of therapy are lacking. Humidification should be provided by a cool mist vaporizer or croupette. Temporary relief can often be provided by taking the child into a closed bathroom filled with steam from a hot running shower. Adequate oral fluid intake is also essential; failure to maintain adequate fluid intake can be an indication of severe obstruction and respiratory fatigue and indicates need for hospitalization.

In addition to humidification, hospitalized patients may require supplemental oxygen because of the frequency of hypoxemia (presumably due to diffuse airway involvement) in more severe cases. A quiet environment should be provided (but not at the expense of careful observation), and mild sedation may be necessary if the child is agitated.

Racemic epinephrine delivered by air- or oxygen-powered nebulizer (0.25 to 0.5 ml of 2.25 per cent racemic epinephrine diluted in 3.0 to 4.0 ml normal saline) provides immediate relief of symptoms of airway obstruction in patients with moderate distress. However, the effect is generally short-lived (<2 hours), and rebound worsening of obstruction can occur. Therefore, use of racemic epinephrine should be reserved for hospitalized patients. The use of intermittent positive-pressure breathing (IPPB) provides no advantages over nebulization in the delivery of racemic epinephrine and increases the theoretical risk of barotrauma.

Corticosteroids are not generally recommended for viral croup, although their efficacy is debated. Dexamethasone, 0.5 to 1.0 mg/kg for two or three doses, has been recommended for patients with severe obstructive symptoms, and studies have shown neither clear benefits nor adverse effects in viral croup. Antibiotics are not indicated in uncomplicated viral croup, as opposed to their use in the severe form of obstruction secondary to bacterial tracheitis. Ribavirin has in vitro activity against parainfluenzae, but there is no evidence that it is effective in viral croup.

Endotracheal intubation until the obstruction subsides is necessary for patients with severe obstruction. Generally, the smallest polyvinylchloride endotracheal tube that will allow adequate gas exchange while permitting a small leak around the tube should be used. The endotracheal tube is typically removed after 48 to 72 hours (the subglottic area cannot be examined directly with the tube in place) to judge adequacy of the airway. Preparations must be made to reintubate in case of recurrent obstruction, which can develop for as long as 12 to 48 hours after extubation. In rare cases of prolonged obstruction, a tracheostomy may be necessary to maintain an airway until the obstruction resolves.

SUPRAGLOTTITIS (EPIGLOTTITIS)

Supraglottitis (or epiglottitis) is an acute infectious disorder of the upper airway, generally caused by *Haemophilus influenzae* type b, that primarily involves the epiglottis and adjacent areas. The typical patient with supraglottitis is 3 to 6 years old and presents with an acute febrile illness, with pharyngitis and dysphagia.

Drooling and anxiety are often prominent. Signs of airway obstruction may be surprisingly mild initially but can rapidly progress to complete airway obstruction. Supraglottitis can also occur in both young infants and adolescents, although the clinical history may be very atypical (more prolonged course, predominance of pharyngitis symptoms).

Supraglottitis is a true medical emergency because of the suddenness with which complete obstruction can develop. Every practitioner and emergency room should have a protocol in place for managing patients with suspected supraglottitis. A patient seen in the physician's office should be transported by the physician to the nearest emergency facility equipped to handle placement of an emergency airway. The team of anesthesiologists, otolaryngologists, and operating room personnel should be assembled as soon as possible.

The child with suspected supraglottitis must be kept in a comfortable environment, such as the parent's arms, for all examinations and procedures. Blood drawing and intravenous catheter placement should be deferred until an airway is secured in patients with severe obstruction. Arterial blood gases are not indicated in the child with suspected supraglottitis, although pulse oximetry may be an atraumatic method to follow trends in oxygenation. Some children may be cooperative and permit a quick visualization of the epiglottis, but no attempt should be made to force a view of the epiglottis because of the risk of precipitating complete obstruction. The failure to visualize the classic "cherry red" swollen epiglottis does not rule out supraglottitis because other structures may be more severely involved with edema and inflammation.

If the patient's condition is stable, a lateral soft tissue radiograph of the neck should be obtained if the diagnosis is uncertain, with a physician in constant attendance. An anteroposterior view may be useful to demonstrate the subglottic narrowing that is more typical of viral croup. If the diagnosis of supraglottitis is confirmed or strongly suspected on the basis of the radiograph, the patient should be transported immediately to the operating room for placement of an airway. However, negative or equivocal radiographic studies should never rule out the diagnosis when clinical suspicion of supraglottitis is strong.

In the operating room, every attempt must be made to keep the child comfortable and to reduce anxiety. A parent should be allowed to stay with the child, and the staff can dispense with masks, which may further frighten the child. Anesthesia is induced with halothane-oxygen by face mask, administered with the child sitting in the parent's lap. If the child is frightened by the anesthesia mask, initial sedation with intravenous or intramuscular ketamine or intravenous midazolam may be more effective and permit rapid orotracheal intubation and initiation of anesthesia. When swelling of supraglottic structures is severe, application of pressure on the chest may force bubbles of secretions out the glottis opening to help guide intubation of the trachea. Preparations in the operating room for possible emergency tracheostomy must always be made in case of complete airway obstruction. After examination and confirmatory cultures (bacterial, viral) of the epiglottis and supraglottic structures, the orotracheal tube should be changed to a cuffless polyvinylchloride nasotracheal tube (one size smaller than that ordinarily used) to reduce the risk of accidental extubation and minimize airway trauma.

Management of the patient after an airway is secured mandates having a skilled ICU team trained to manage the patient with a nasotracheal tube in place, prevent accidental extubations, and reintubate the patient if necessary. If such an ICU team is not available on a 24-hour basis, the patient must be transported to a tertiary center with this capability. Sedation and restraints may be desirable to prevent accidental extubation, but paralysis and mechanical ventilation are generally not required. In a few centers, intubation followed by tracheostomy is still used for airway management. This is an acceptable, although less desirable, alternative to maintaining nasotracheal intubation.

As soon as the diagnosis of supraglottitis is made, the patient should receive antibiotic therapy with ampicillin (200 to 300 mg/kg/day IV in four divided doses; daily adult dose 6 to 12 gm) and chloramphenicol (50 to 100 mg/kg/day in four divided doses; daily adult dose 2 to 4 gm). Chloramphenicol is continued only if subsequent antibiotic sensitivity testing of blood or epiglottis cultures confirms *Haemophilus influenzae* that is a beta-lactamase producer. Chloramphenicol levels should be monitored if it is continued. Second- and third-generation cephalosporins, including cefotaxime, cefuroxime, moxalactam, and ceftriaxone, are also effective therapies for invasive *Haemophilus* infections. Intravenous antibiotic therapy should be continued for 5 to 7 days, followed by 5 to 7 days of oral antibiotic therapy. These antibiotic choices should provide coverage for the other possible causes of bacterial supraglottitis (*Streptococcus pneumoniae*, group A beta-hemolytic streptococci). Corticosteroids are not indicated in the treatment of supraglottitis.

After 1 to 3 days of antibiotic therapy, extubation is generally possible. This determination can usually be made by the presence of a sizable leak around the endotracheal tube and by direct examination of the epiglottis by flexible fiberoptic nasopharyngoscopy.

Supraglottitis secondary to *H. influenzae* type b may be accompanied by invasive disease elsewhere, including pneumonia, meningitis, and septic arthritis. Rifampin prophylaxis should be given in households that include an unimmunized child younger than 5 years. Because most young children now receive immunization for *H. influenzae* type b, the development of supraglottitis should prompt further investigation of the child's immune status to assess the possibility of an immunodeficiency.

BACTERIAL TRACHEITIS (NECROTIZING TRACHEITIS, PSEUDOMEMBRANOUS CROUP)

Bacterial tracheitis (necrotizing tracheitis, pseudomembranous croup) is a severe inflammatory disease of the trachea and main bronchi. It is generally due to bacterial pathogens, principally *Staphylococcus aureus*, as well as group A beta-hemolytic streptococci, *S. pneumo-* niae, *H. influenzae*, and some viruses. The cause of the acute airway obstruction is necrosis and sloughing of airway mucosa and an inflammatory exudate ("pseudomembrane"). Although it is most common in infants and toddlers, the disorder may occur in any age group. The copious thick secretions cause severe airway obstruction that constitutes a medical emergency. The diagnosis is generally made by culture and examination of the trachea by bronchoscopy or at emergency tracheostomy. Radiographs may show airway narrowing or abnormal shadows within the tracheal air column. Treatment includes aggressive airway management to remove secretions and broad-spectrum antibiotic coverage for possible bacterial pathogens, including *S. aureus*, *S. pneumoniae*, and beta-hemolytic streptococci.

SPASMODIC AND ALLERGIC CROUP

Spasmodic croup is recurrent croup that occurs with no apparent infectious etiology. The onset is generally sudden, occurring at night, and there is no viral prodrome. Some patients may have an allergic basis for their croup. This condition is generally benign; therapy is merely supportive and includes humidification and oral hydration. Corticosteroids and racemic epinephrine are effective in spasmodic croup but should be reserved for the rare patient with severe obstruction who requires hospitalization.

Some forms of hyper-reactive airway disease (asthma) often include a large component of upper airway obstruction. Such patients are recognizable by the presence of signs of both upper and lower (intrathoracic) airway obstruction and by improvement in their stridor and wheezing with inhalation of beta-2 agonists, such as metaproterenol.

ACUTE LARYNGEAL INJURIES

Foreign Bodies. Airway foreign bodies often lodge at the laryngeal level or, occasionally, in the trachea and give rise to acute inspiratory stridor. The diagnosis depends on a high index of suspicion in patients with a possible history of foreign body aspiration, on recognition of the atypical croup history, and on careful radiologic examinations. The foreign body must be removed in the operating room by an experienced otolaryngologist to prevent possible dislodgement and complete obstruction of the trachea or larynx.

Burns. Ingestion of hot liquids may burn the epiglottis and produce acute upper airway obstruction similar to that seen with bacterial supraglottitis. As in the case of supraglottitis, securing an adequate airway by nasotracheal intubation or tracheostomy is the major and immediate concern.

Postintubation Croup. Prolonged endotracheal intubation can cause subglottic edema. Various therapies have been recommended to reduce or prevent this sequela, including corticosteroids, racemic epinephrine, furosemide, and vasoconstrictors. Although none is associated with major side effects, their effectiveness over humidification has not been proven in carefully controlled studies.

RECURRENT CROUP

Patients may develop recurrent croup due to separate episodes of viral croup or, more commonly, due to spasmodic croup. Patients with recurrent croup frequently also show evidence of airway hyper-reactivity to other stimuli. Congenital malformations, such as hemangiomas and mucoceles, often present with recurrent or unusually severe episodes of croup. Recurrent stridor, usually with infection, is common among graduates of neonatal nurseries with mild acquired subglottic stenosis. Management of these forms of recurrent croup depends on recognition of these lesions by careful history, physical examination, and use of diagnostic procedures such as radiography, followed by referral to an experienced otolaryngologist.

CROUP IN THE IMMUNOCOMPROMISED HOST

Croup in the immunocompromised host, such as patients with cancer or AIDS or those who have undergone bone marrow transplantation, is more likely to be due to unusual opportunistic pathogens such as *Candida albicans*. An aggressive approach to diagnosis, including the use of flexible fiberoptic endoscopy (with cultures and biopsies), is necessary to guide appropriate therapy.

PNEUMOTHORAX AND PNEUMOMEDIASTINUM

WILLIAM E. TRUOG, M.D.

PATHOPHYSIOLOGY

Neonatal pneumothorax and pneumomediastinum develop when pulmonary alveolar or acinar walls rupture and gas migrates into the pulmonary interstitium. Gas then moves along perivascular lymphatic and bronchiolar sheaths until reaching the mediastinal or pleural spaces. Partial or complete collapse of the lung follows when air enters the pleural space, accumulating between the lung and the inner chest wall. Air reaching the mediastinal space may remain contained there or dissect into subcutaneous tissue, pleural space, retroperitoneum, pericardium, or intravascular spaces, producing additional morbidity or death.

A baby's first postnatal breathing efforts must generate high transpulmonary pressure in order to move air into the previously gasless lungs. Airway fluid, surface tension, and the elastic recoil of the lung all may limit air entry. Uneven distribution of ventilation, as may occur in the lung undergoing transition to postnatal life, produces overinflation of localized areas, predisposing to airway rupture. Neonatal pneumothorax and pneumomediastinum are the two most common forms of air leak complications that may result either spontaneously, from neonatal pulmonary diseases, or from the use of positive-pressure ventilation.

Pneumothorax may be either unilateral or bilateral. Either can produce a life-threatening emergency because of compression of pulmonary veins at the hilum of the lung, resulting in diminished cardiac output with diminished systemic perfusion, hypotension, systemic arterial desaturation, and death if the air collection and vascular compression remain untreated.

DIAGNOSIS

Pneumothorax can produce a variable effect on vital signs, ranging from no overt changes to an immediately life-threatening condition. Usually there is evidence of respiratory embarrassment with dyspnea or tachypnea. Some signs of pneumothorax in an adult (shifted mediastinum, or tracheal shift away from the midline) are often not present in a neonate, especially a premature or mechanically ventilated neonate. Diminished breath sounds on the ipsilateral side can sometimes not be easily appreciated in neonates. Unilateral pneumothorax also can sometimes be identified by transillumination of the involved hemithorax if the procedure is carried out in a darkened room. A "normal" transillumination study does not exclude a pneumothorax, however. Diagnosis is made definitively by evacuation of air under pressure from the pleural space or by chest radiography. The latter can often be accomplished by a single anteroposterior (AP) radiograph of the chest, but for the most accurate evaluation of the location and extent of the pneumothorax, both lateral and AP views of the chest are helpful. Occasionally a cross-table lateral radiograph helps detect a small pneumothorax. Skin folds appearing on radiographs may be confused with a partially collapsed lung. Identifying extension of the skinfold line beyond the thorax and confirming the appearance of lung markings peripheral to the skinfold line help eliminate confusion. The extent of lung collapse associated with unilateral pneumothorax need not correlate with presence or degree of clinical signs.

Isolated pneumomediastinum rarely causes clinical signs in neonates. Pneumomediastinum is distinguished radiographically from pneumothorax in neonates because the large thymus is lifted off the anterior mediastinum by the collection of mediastinal air, which additionally creates an unusually sharp or clear cardiac silhouette on the affected side. Either or both lobes of the thymus may be elevated, producing a characteristic radiographic appearance, known as the "spinnaker" or "sail" sign. Pneumomediastinum can be differentiated from pneumopericardium, which causes complete encirclement of the heart by air inside the pericardial sac. Air in the mediastinum does not encircle the heart. Both AP and lateral chest radiographs help differentiate these conditions.

THERAPY

Symptomatic pneumothorax, or pneumothorax occurring with extensive parenchymal disease, requires evacuation of air and re-expansion of the lung. Usually this is accomplished by placement of a flexible thoracostomy tube of appropriate size (10 Fr in a full-term infant) in the anterior axillary line, away from the nipple, and with the tip of the tube placed in the anterosuperior location. The baby is rolled slightly with the affected side up to help in placing the tube in the desired location. Following infiltration of local anesthetic into the skin and subcutaneous tissue, a 0.5-cm skin incision is made. Then the tube with a rigid trocar inside is inserted just over the top of a rib into the pleural space. Insertion over the top of the rib helps avoid puncture of a vessel in the vascular bundle which runs beneath each rib. If the pleura is first punctured with a hemostat, that instrument can be used to guide the thoracostomy tube tip inward through the pleural rent. If this technique is used, the tube usually can be inserted without the trocar in place. The thoracostomy tube is sutured in place with a purse-string suture, with the operator exercising care that the tube not be dislodged because of inadvertent traction placed on the tube during the suturing procedure. Prophylactic antibiotics are not administered unless sterile technique has been compromised during the procedure. The distal end of the thoracostomy tube should be connected to underwater drainage providing 10 to 15 cm H_2O negative pressure to help evacuate air. Bubbling of withdrawn air through the water trap should be noted. Repeat chest radiographs are mandatory to confirm correct tube placement.

If pneumothorax produces acute deterioration, then air under pressure can be removed by needle aspiration before placing the thoracostomy tube. This procedure can be performed using a butterfly needle (No. 21 gauge) attached to flexible tubing, with a clamp placed behind the needle tip to prevent inappropriately deep needle insertion. The end of the flexible tubing is connected to a three-way stopcock and syringe, and the air can then be manually evacuated. The end of the flexible tubing of the metal needle can be placed under sterile water to observe the exit of air under pressure and prevent drawing more air into the pleural space during spontaneous ventilation while tube thoracostomy is accomplished. Very large or rapidly accumulating pneumothorax may not be evacuated satisfactorily by this method and may require emergency decompression with scalpel and clamp as described above. Acute deterioration in a neonate often includes development of apnea. Therefore, intubation and assisted ventilation may be necessary before reducing the pneumothorax.

The duration of thoracostomy drainage must be individualized for each baby and will depend on severity of the underlying pulmonary disease. Following radiographic resolution of free pleural air and a period of hours without any bubbling of air through the water trap, the tube can be clamped or placed to water seal drainage without negative pressure. If there is no recurrence of symptoms and no radiographic evidence of reaccumulation of free air, the tube can be withdrawn, with care taken to pull the tube at end inspiration. At this point in the respiratory cycle there is less risk of the infant's creating additional negative pressure as the tube is removed. The dressing applied over the site should include occlusive gauze to help prevent an air leak.

Recurrent ipsilateral pneumothorax following tube placement is an especially difficult problem. Air pockets may become loculated and cannot be drained by the indwelling tube. A second tube can be placed if repositioning the baby (rolling side to side, or head up or down) or gentle manipulation of the already inserted tube fails to relieve the problem. Not every milliliter of trapped air must be removed, and judgment must be used regarding the risks of additional tube insertions

versus risk of deterioration from partially treated pneumothorax.

Some advocate use of 100 per cent inspired oxygen for a period of hours to accelerate the absorption of the nitrogen-containing pleural gas if the pneumothorax occurred during spontaneous breathing of room air and the patient has few or no symptoms. Since 100 per cent O_2 may induce lung injury via the production of toxic oxygen metabolites, this form of treatment is limited to a few hours' duration. The baby is either insufficiently compromised to require any specific treatment or is sufficiently ill to require definitive therapy by tube thoracostomy.

Pneumomediastinum rarely requires evacuation, even when air dissects into the neck. Nonetheless, if an infant with respiratory distress is deteriorating and serial chest radiographs reveal enlarging pneumomediastinum without pneumothorax, then evacuation of the air can be attempted. One approach is by the subxiphoid route, inserting a plastic catheter (No. 20 or 22 gauge) attached in series to a short length of tubing, a three-way stopcock, and a 20- or 30-ml syringe. The mediastinal space is entered following insertion of the needle tip through the skin, advancing the needle at a shallow angle from the mid-subxiphoid location with the tip of the needle aimed toward the middle of the right clavicle. Gentle pressure is applied to the barrel of the syringe until the mediastinal airspace is encountered, at which point air should be readily evacuated.

OTHER CONSIDERATIONS

Most neonates who develop a symptomatic pneumothorax have a readily discernible underlying explanation, usually a history of aspiration of meconium-stained amniotic fluid or maternal blood, presence of hyaline membrane disease, or need for positive-pressure assisted ventilation (either bag and mask or bag and endotracheal tube) following perinatal asphyxia. In the absence of a perinatal history consistent with problems leading to the development of a pneumothorax, and especially if the pneumothorax is recurrent or bilateral, consideration should be given to the possibility of pulmonary hypoplasia, sometimes associated with renal disorders. Renal ultrasonography should be considered in such infants to identify associated renal anatomic anomalies. The most severe and readily recognized form, renal aplasia–pulmonary hypoplasia syndrome, is rapidly fatal.

Potential complications of a pneumothorax and its treatments are listed in Table 1.

CONCLUDING COMMENTS

Pulmonary air leaks are common problems in the sick newborn. Pneumothorax is not limited to the intensive care setting. Any infant with a mild degree of respira-

TABLE 1. Possible Complications of Tube Thoracostomy

Perforation of liver, spleen, pericardial sac, heart, or lung parenchyma
Hemothorax or hemoperitoneum from vascular perforation
Infection, including entry site cellulitis or abscess
Creation of bronchopulmonary fistula

tory distress may develop pneumothorax, which may progress to produce significant pulmonary compromise or more rarely cardiovascular collapse. Therefore, all institutions caring for neonates must have medical personnel immediately available to correct this potentially life-threatening complication.

PLEURAL EFFUSION

JOHN G. BROOKS, M.D.

Pleural effusions are usually first detected by physical examination or chest radiography. Key aspects of optimal management are (1) determining the disorder leading to the pleural effusion, (2) deciding whether a thoracentesis should be performed for either diagnostic or therapeutic purposes, (3) beginning appropriate antibiotic or other treatment of the causative disease process, and (4) deciding whether to initiate continuous, closed-system chest tube drainage.

THORACENTESIS

A diagnostic thoracentesis is usually indicated if infection is the most likely cause of the effusion, particularly if ultrasonography or radiography indicates that a significant amount of nonloculated (i.e., freely movable) fluid is present, if *Staphylococcus aureus* or group A streptococci are suspected, or if the patient has failed to show clinical response to 2 to 3 days of appropriate antibiotic therapy. Since long-term complications with parapneumonic effusions due to *Streptococcus pneumoniae* are rare, a diagnostic thoracentesis may sometimes be omitted if this diagnosis is firm. Diagnostic thoracentesis may not be necessary if the effusion is probably due to congestive heart failure or nephrotic syndrome unless infection of the pleural fluid is suspected. Immunocompromised hosts are more likely to warrant a diagnostic thoracentesis. Any patient with pleural fluid of unknown etiology should receive a diagnostic thoracentesis if he is failing to improve after 2 to 5 days.

After localization of the pleural fluid by physical examination, ultrasonography, and/or radiography, the thoracentesis should be performed using careful sterile technique, local anesthesia, and an 18- to 20-gauge needle and external catheter (e.g. Intracath) with a short bevel and a sharp point. The patient should sit forward or, less commonly, lie in the lateral decubitus position. The needle should be attached to a 10-ml syringe via a three-way stopcock to minimize the risk of air entering the pleural space. If the patient is sitting, the needle should be introduced in the posterior axillary line at a level at or above the eighth intercostal space, depending on the size and location of the fluid. When the patient is in the decubitus position with the lateral chest protruding slightly beyond the edge of the bed or table, the needle should be introduced in the dependent lateral chest wall well above the level of the diaphragm. In either case the needle should enter the skin near the middle of a rib and then be introduced over the top of the rib into the pleural space not more than about 5

mm to avoid lacerating the lung. Fluid should be collected anaerobically in a heparinized syringe for measurement of pH (and stored on ice until time of measurement), and other samples should be analyzed for protein, LDH, glucose, cultures, cell count and differential, stains, CIE, and in some cases, amylase. If tuberculosis is likely, a pleural biopsy should be considered.

A therapeutic thoracentesis, performed in the same manner, is indicated if the patient has a significant amount of fluid that is likely to be causing respiratory distress. Depending on the patient's size, not more than 100 to 1000 ml should be removed at a time to avoid major abrupt fluid shifts and shock. The major complications of thoracentesis are pneumothorax, infection, and laceration of the lung, liver, or spleen. If the patient starts to cough, the needle should be removed but a catheter can remain in place.

ANTIBIOTIC THERAPY

Antibiotic therapy, often initiated prior to the diagnosis of pleural effusion or empyema, should usually be adjusted to cover the three major pathogens—*Haemophilus influenzae, S. aureus,* and *S. pneumoniae*—until specific bacteriologic, fungal, viral, or mycobacterial sensitivities are established or until a specific organism can be identified as the most likely cause of infection. Cefuroxime provides adequate initial coverage in most normal hosts. Parenteral administration provides sufficient antibiotic concentrations in the pleural space, so intrapleural administration of antibiotics is not indicated. The duration of antibiotic therapy depends on the causative pathogen and the patient's clinical response to therapy. Courses of at least 7 to 14 days are recommended for *H. influenzae* infection, and at least 3 to 4 weeks for *S. aureus* and mixed bacterial empyemas. In patients with group A streptococcal empyema, other parameters of clinical response which should be monitored include hematocrit, reticulocyte count, and erythrocyte sedimentation rate.

CHEST TUBE DRAINAGE

Continuous closed chest tube drainage is indicated in any of the following situations: (1) empyema due to *S. aureus* or group A *Streptococcus pyogenes;* (2) patient requiring repeated therapeutic thoracentesis for rapid pleural fluid reaccumulation causing respiratory compromise which cannot be managed by less invasive, more specific measures; (3) pleural fluid pH less than 7.0. Most patients with empyema (pus and/or organisms in the pleural space) are treated with continuous closed chest tube drainage. The chest tube should be positioned to allow dependent drainage and should usually remain in place until ongoing fluid drainage is less than 10 to 20 ml/day.

More aggressive interventions such as decortication and chemical pleurodesis are only very rarely indicated. Spontaneous resorption of the inflammatory pleural peel usually occurs, although the process may take at least 6 to 12 months.

CHYLOTHORAX

H. GORDON GREEN, M.D.,
and DALE COLN, M.D.

External trauma (including birth trauma), cardiac or other intrathoracic surgery, or pressure from enlarged lymph nodes or tumors may lead to disruption of the thoracic duct or its tributaries. Chylous fluid from the thoracic duct escapes from the mediastinum into the pleural space. The interval between injury and onset of symptoms may be days or even weeks. The abundant loss of fluid, characteristically containing sudanophilic lipids except in newborn infants, is accompanied by considerable protein loss as well. Large volume losses can cause fluid volume deficits and severe nutritional compromise, particularly in the younger patient.

A thoracic tap may be both diagnostic and therapeutic. The site of thoracentesis depends upon physical and radiographic findings. After proper skin preparation and local anesthetic infiltration, the needle is inserted through the chest wall near the superior margin of the appropriate rib, avoiding the intercostal nerve and vessels lying at the inferior margin. Penetration of the pleura may be perceived as a slight "pop" or giving-way of resistance. Drainage of the chylous fluid should be as complete as possible, as documented by post-tap radiograph.

Medical management can bring about decreased drainage through the duct, allowing it to seal. Continued conservative treatment is appropriate if lung compression or mediastinal shift does not compromise cardiac or respiratory function.

Repeated evacuation may be required to relieve the respiratory distress associated with reaccumulation of fluid and compression of one or both lungs and/or mediastinal shift.

If tube thoracostomy drainage is required, attention must be paid to nutritional status and may become even more important as proteins, lipids, lymphocytes, and immunoglobulins are drained away. Losses must be overcome through vigorous dietary management, including emphasis on protein, carbohydrate, and medium-chain triglycerides substituting for long-chain fats. Medium-chain triglycerides are absorbed not through the lymphatics but directly into the portal venous stream from the gastrointestinal tract. While long-chain fats contain 9 calories per gram, medium-chain triglyceride oil supplies only 8.3 calories per gram due to fewer available units of acetyl CoA. Particular attention must be directed to restoration of electrolyte balance and to repletion of protein stores and of the fat-soluble vitamins.

In some cases, healing of the injured thoracic duct requires bypassing the lymphatic system with total parenteral nutrition. Calories and nitrogen can be supplied through an intravenous combination of dextrose solution, amino acids, and lipid emulsion. Oral feedings may then be resumed slowly, using medium-chain triglyceride oil. (A hybrid mixture of long-chain and medium-chain fatty acids is under investigation and may prove useful in this transition.)

Dyspnea, a friction rub, or pallor may be noted. The severity of respiratory embarrassment corresponds roughly with the rate of accumulation and the volume of chylous effusion. Repeated thoracentesis may be successful, but the risk of infection or pneumothorax increases with repetition. If there is a large volume or rapid recurrence, placement of a pliable catheter through the anterior intercostal space under local anesthesia allows for drainage and approximation of the parietal and visceral pleura to seal the leak from the duct. Radiography is often helpful in determining optimal placement of the thoracostomy tube. Ultrasonography may help in determining completeness of drainage. If the volume of drainage exceeds 40 ml/kg/day, thoracotomy with suturing of the duct is indicated. Lesser rates of drainage which do not decrease within 5 days require surgical ligation of the duct.

If the injury is to the pericardial lymphatic system, especially after cardiac surgery, then chylopericardium can occur. Pericardial aspiration or pericardiotomy may be required to relieve cardiac tamponade.

INTRATHORACIC CYSTS

ROBERT M. FILLER, M.D.

Intrathoracic cysts may be acquired or congenital in origin. They cause symptoms because they occupy space and press on normal structures or because they become infected. However, many cystic lesions produce no symptoms at all and are discovered incidentally.

ACQUIRED CYSTS (PNEUMATOCELES)

These lesions usually result from pulmonary infection, most commonly staphylococcal pneumonia. Occasionally they are seen following pulmonary contusion. Although most acquired cysts are small, cysts of 5 to 10 cm in diameter are not unusual. In most cases they are self-limited, and spontaneous resolution within a few weeks of origin is the rule. In the very rare case in which the cyst expands rapidly and causes respiratory distress (or pneumothorax), chest tube insertion can relieve symptoms. In others no treatment is necessary. Pulmonary resection is almost never indicated.

CONGENITAL CYSTS

Mediastinal Cysts

The most common mediastinal cysts, bronchogenic and enteric cysts, are of foregut origin.

Bronchogenic cysts, which are so named because they are lined by ciliated columnar epithelium and have cartilage in their wall, occur in the mediastinum, esophagus, and lung. Bronchogenic cysts that present in the mediastinum usually occur adjacent to the trachea or major bronchi. They do not ordinarily connect with the airway lumen, but the mucus-filled cyst may compress the airway and produce symptoms of stridor, air trapping, and pneumonia. Complete excision is indicated for the symptomatic lesions. The cyst is often in the middle mediastinum near the midline and may be difficult to find on exploration of the mediastinum. Resection of the major airways is almost never necessary. Bronchogenic cysts that occur in the esophagus can be found in the wall of the esophagus between the muscularis and mucosa. They rarely cause symptoms, but the mere presence of a mass usually provides sufficient indication for excision. At surgery the cyst can be shelled out of the wall of the esophagus after its muscular coat is opened longitudinally. Since the lesion does not involve the mucosa, the lumen of the esophagus need not be entered. Bronchogenic cysts that originate in pulmonary parenchyma are discussed below.

Cysts of enteric origin occur in the posterior mediastinum and may communicate with the intestinal tract below the diaphragm or with remnants of the embryonic neurenteric canal, which arises in the upper thoracic vertebrae. Even in cases in which the enteric cyst does not communicate with the spinal canal, a vertebral malformation is usually evident by radiography. This radiographic finding is diagnostic of the anomaly. Because enteric cysts can present as lesions with an air-fluid level, these cysts may be confused with lung abscess or empyema. As a result, they have been treated mistakenly by chest tube drainage. Complete excision is necessary for cure. At the time of surgery, extensions to the intestinal tract below the diaphragm and to the spinal canal in the chest must be located and removed appropriately.

Lymphangioma, thymic cyst, cystic teratoma, and pericardial cyst are some of the other less frequently occurring cystic lesions in the mediastinum. Excision is required in most cases, both for diagnosis and to prevent or relieve compression of normal structures in the thorax.

Lung Cysts

Congenital cysts of the lung are usually of lung bud origin, and most are thought to originate by entrapment of a portion of the developing lung bud. Most unilocular and multilocular cysts have the same histologic pattern as the bronchogenic cysts of the mediastinum and esophagus already described. These cysts communicate with the airway so that they contain air and often become infected. Surgical excision is necessary for cure. Chest tube drainage is to be avoided, since it may complicate definitive treatment. Usually lobectomy is necessary, although partial lobectomy may be possible in those cases in which only a small segment of normal lung tissue is involved.

Congenital adenomatoid malformation (CAM) of the lung is the other common cystic lesion in the lung. CAM is characterized as a lesion of various-sized cysts arising in terminal respiratory structures. These cysts, which communicate with the airway, often involve more than one lobe of the lung and tend to occupy more space in the chest than bronchogenic cysts. In the most severe cases, the cysts are so large that uninvolved lung segments are compressed and hypoplastic. As in children with diaphragmatic hernia, the degree of pulmonary hypoplasia may be incompatible with life. In those cases in which only one lobe is involved, lobectomy is

the most appropriate approach. However, when multiple lobes are affected multiple lobectomies would permanently compromise pulmonary function. In these cases, a staged approach has been successful in some cases. The largest cysts are unroofed at the initial operation, relieving the compression of the residual normal lung. If and when the cyst recurs (usually several months later), complete cystectomy can be accomplished without sacrificing as much normal lung tissue as would have been sacrificed originally.

TUMORS OF THE CHEST
ROBERT M. FILLER, M.D.

Neoplasms of the chest that develop in childhood involve the mediastinum and the pulmonary parenchyma.

MEDIASTINAL TUMORS

Neurogenic tumors are the most common mediastinal tumor and present in the posterior mediastinum. Most often they are found incidentally when the infant or child with respiratory symptoms is being evaluated by chest radiography. Except for massive tumors and those dumbbell-type tumors that involve the spinal canal and cause cord compression, mediastinal neurogenic tumors rarely cause symptoms.

Neuroblastoma. In the younger child, neuroblastoma is the predominant histologic type. The primary treatment is surgical excision. If the tumor is completely excised, no chemotherapy or radiation therapy is given, and cures approaching 100 per cent are reported for children under 18 months of age. For the child with a dumbbell neuroblastoma, treatment varies, depending on the presence of signs and symptoms of spinal cord compression. In those with cord compression, emergency laminectomy is necessary as a first step. At thoracotomy, usually 7 to 10 days later, the intrathoracic portion of the mass is removed. This order of surgery is reversed when the intraspinal component of the tumor is small and there are no signs of cord compression.

Radiation therapy and chemotherapy are employed for those children in whom the entire tumor cannot be excised. Repeated courses of cyclophosphamide and vincristine are used in those with localized residual disease. More complex chemotherapy protocols are being tried in institutional and multicenter group trials for disseminated disease. Radiation doses to areas of residual tumor range from 1000 to 2400 rads, depending on the patient's age.

Ganglioneuroma is the benign variant of neuroblastoma and is usually found in the older child. It may represent maturation of a neuroblastoma. Surgical excision is curative.

Lymphoma. Lymphoma is the most common tumor in the middle and anterior mediastinum in children. Primary treatment of these tumors is described elsewhere in this book. Surgery is generally not indicated for the treatment of either Hodgkin's or non-Hodgkin's lymphoma, although the surgeon is often called upon to obtain tissue specimens for a histologic diagnosis.

Occasionally a patient with mediastinal lymphoma presents with the "superior mediastinal syndrome" and severe respiratory obstruction. In these high-risk patients intravenous high-dose steroid therapy is instituted at once, and biopsy is delayed. When a therapeutic effect from steroids is obtained (usually in 1 to 2 days), one can proceed with biopsy. In the child with an extremely large mediastinal mass, steroid therapy alone may not relieve the respiratory problems, and emergency radiation therapy may be necessary. Since the rapid resolution of lymphoma may result in hyperuricemia, allopurinol, intravenous hydration, and alkalinization of the urine are advised for these patients.

LUNG TUMORS

Primary Tumors. Primary tumors of the lung are rare in childhood, but *bronchial adenoma* is the most common type. These tumors are recognized as low-grade adenocarcinomas. The carcinoid-type tumor accounts for 80 to 85 per cent of all adenomas seen in childhood. Children with these tumors present with infection or atelectasis in the lung supplied by the affected bronchus. These lesions can be seen by bronchoscopy and biopsied, but attempts at complete excision via the bronchoscope are not recommended for definitive treatment because most tumors grow through the bronchial wall. Most adenomas require pulmonary resection for cure. Lobectomy is used for lesions localized to a lobar bronchus or peripheral lung. Bilobectomy and pneumonectomy may be necessary when an adenoma in a main bronchus extends into a lobar bronchus or extraluminally to adjacent structures. Sleeve resection of the bronchus without pulmonary resection should be considered for the small adenoma confined to a central bronchial segment, provided that infection has not destroyed the distal lung.

Secondary Tumors. Secondary tumors of the lung are relatively common in children, especially those originating from Wilms' tumor and osteogenic sarcoma.

Initial therapy for pulmonary metastases from *Wilms' tumor* includes radiation therapy (1500 rads to both lungs) and chemotherapy (usually actinomycin D and vincristine). More complex chemotherapy is used for those patients whose tumor is of "bad histology." Additional radiation is given to sites of persistent tumor. Resection is undertaken when tumor persists or recurs after medical treatment, provided that complete removal is technically possible.

Recent experience for patients with pulmonary metastases from *osteogenic sarcoma* has shown that by combining an aggressive surgical approach with the standard chemotherapy program approximately 40 per cent of patients can be salvaged. Surgical resection of lung metastases is most effective in those patients with the fewest number of lesions, and in those in whom metastases develop many months after initial diagnosis of osteogenic sarcoma. However, the presence of a large number of metastatic deposits is not a contraindication to surgery per se, since many cures have been reported even after the resection of more than 10 lesions from each lung. The indications and timing for surgery have varied in individual cases and among different institutions. Our feeling is that metastatic lung lesions should be excised prior to the institution of other therapy in the following circumstances: (1) when lesions persist despite adequate standard chemotherapy; (2) when metastases are isolated (less than five) and appear late (greater than 6 months from diagnosis); and (3) when the metastatic tumor mass is large and unlikely to respond to chemotherapy. Surgery is delayed in favor of chemotherapy for those who have received inadequate or no prior chemotherapy and for those in whom pulmonary metastases are detected within 3 months of the original diagnosis. In the latter situation, lung metastases are excised as soon as rapidly growing lesions are stabilized by chemotherapy. Our experience has shown that there is little hope for the patient who develops multiple metastases soon after diagnosis and in whom chemotherapy fails to halt their growth.

One of the important principles of surgery when dealing with metastatic lung lesions is to preserve as much lung tissue as possible, since most patients usually have more than one metastatic lesion, and others are likely to develop in the future. Wedge resection of the involved lung is usually adequate, but lobectomy and even pneumonectomy are sometimes required. Cure is unlikely unless all gross tumor is excised. When bilateral lesions are present, they can be excised at one operation by exposure through a median sternotomy. Alternatively, bilateral tumor nodules can be resected through two separate lateral thoracotomies spaced 1 week apart. In patients in whom pulmonary metastases recur after successful surgical excision, repeat resection is indicated as long as the volume of residual lung is sufficient to support life.

PULMONARY SEQUESTRATION

ROBERT C. STERN, M.D.

Although an occasional asymptomatic patient can be treated conservatively, the usual treatment for sequestration is surgical excision. Intralobar sequestrations (equal incidence in each lung; more frequent in lower lobes) often present as pneumonia. Chest films may show an air-fluid level. The boundary with the surrounding lung tissue may be obscured by inflammation. Antibiotics are needed to control the infection prior to definitive diagnostic procedures and surgery. Extralobar sequestration (90 per cent of cases involve the left lung; usually retrocardiac location) may present as an incidental finding on chest roentgenogram. Work-up should include angiography to confirm the diagnosis and minimize the risk of inadvertent severing of a major feeding artery during surgery. The possibility of associated congenital malformations (e.g., diaphragmatic hernia) should be considered. Intralobar sequestrations usually require lobectomy; however, if there is no infection, a localized resection is occasionally possible. In extralobar sequestration, simple surgical resection of the sequestered tissue is often possible.

RIGHT MIDDLE LOBE SYNDROME

NANCY C. LEWIS, M.D.

The right middle lobe syndrome (RMLS) characterizes patients with persistent or recurrent RML collapse and is the best-known form of persistent atelectasis in childhood. The spectrum of diseases causing RMLS is the same as for children with persistent collapse of other lobes. Several anatomic features combine to make the RML bronchus vulnerable to collapse. It is of relatively narrow caliber and has an acute take-off angle from the bronchus intermedius, as well as being surrounded by a cuff of lymph nodes. These nodes drain the entire right lung and can compress the RML bronchus as they enlarge in response to infection. In addition, the RML is relatively isolated and may be separated from other lung tissue by complete fissures. This impairs collateral ventilation, which in turn interferes with what would otherwise be normal resolution of an inflammatory process. Inflammation and secretions in peripheral airways of the RML may predispose to atelectasis that cannot be offset by ventilation through collateral airways.

Appropriate treatment should be based upon an understanding of the etiology of the atelectasis. Atelectasis may result from (1) obstruction of the airway lumen directly (from aspiration, foreign body, mucous plug); (2) airway wall edema and inflammation (infections, asthma); (3) narrowed airway secondary to scarring (bronchopulmonary dysplasia, bronchiolitis obliterans); or (4) extrinsic compression (enlarged nodes, commonly secondary to infection). Atelectasis associated with acute lower respiratory infections is usually short-lived, clears before the infection, and requires no specific therapy.

Chronic or recurrent atelectasis requires careful investigation for an underlying cause. A history of pneumonia, asthma, or recurrent respiratory infections may be obtained. Atopic or asthmatic children constitute the largest group of patients with RMLS, with edema of bronchial mucosa, hypertrophy of bronchial glands and excessive secretions, or bronchospasm causing bronchial obstruction. Evaluation should include total IgE measurement and spirometry. Maximal expiratory flows are often decreased and may improve after bronchodilator therapy. A CBC with differential count and sputum cultures may be helpful in determining the presence of infection. Additional testing for persistent RML collapse should include quantitative immunoglobulins to rule out immune deficiency, sweat chloride to detect cystic fibrosis, sinus films to look for chronic sinus disease, and possibly an esophagram to look for evidence of a vascular ring or gastroesophageal reflux. A Mantoux skin test should be included in the evaluation.

Appropriate therapy must be directed at any underlying lung disease, including bronchodilators for children with asthma, antibiotics for bacterial infection, or gamma globulin for known hypogammaglobulinemia. Aggressive treatment with oral or inhaled bronchodilators followed by chest physiotherapy and postural drainage is usually indicated. There is no evidence to support the use of IPPB treatments. Most cases are likely to resolve spontaneously within 2 to 3 months. Protracted collapse predisposes to infection and increases the likelihood of structural changes in the airways, which may result in fibrosis or bronchiectasis. If atelectasis persists after several months despite optimal medical management, bronchoscopy is indicated for diagnosis and treatment. Fiberoptic bronchoscopy is of value to differentiate between central obstruction (e.g., mucous plug, foreign body), bronchial stenosis or bronchomalacia, and external compression. Findings often include mucosal edema and inflammation with narrowing of the airway lumen. The RML bronchus is often patent, suggesting obstruction of multiple peripheral airways from mucus plugging as a cause of the atelectasis. Secretions should be obtained for culture and measurement of lipid-laden macrophages (increased with chronic aspiration) and a brush biopsy done for ciliary motility studies. In rare instances, when medical treatment and bronchoscopy are ineffective and the atelectasis has persisted for longer than 6 months, lobectomy may be justified. Bronchography should be performed only if surgery is seriously being considered.

Aggressive therapy should decrease the frequency of RML collapse. Chronic bronchodilators should be considered for asthmatic children who have a propensity for RML atelectasis.

BRONCHITIS AND BRONCHIOLITIS

DAVID B. NELSON, M.D., M.SC.

Acute bronchitis, inflammation of the bronchial mucosa, is a mild self-limited disease that has cough as its primary symptom. Viral infections are the primary cause of bronchitis; therefore, specific therapy is limited and treatment is aimed at symptomatic relief. Therapy, when necessary, should be directed at cough control. In most children, fluids alone may be sufficient; however, if the child's cough either keeps him awake at night or results in vomiting, the use of a cough suppressant is indicated. Preparations containing either codeine sulfate or dextromethorphan are the most helpful. Decongestants and antihistamines are of no value.

Bronchiolitis, an inflammation of the bronchioles, results in small airway obstruction. The illness is characterized by tachypnea, wheezing, hyperinflated lungs, and often hypoxia. Like bronchitis, bronchiolitis is usually caused by a viral infection, with the respiratory syncytial virus (RSV) accounting for 50 to 75 per cent of diagnosed cases. Except for *Mycoplasma* pneumonia, a relatively rare cause of bronchiolitis, there is no specific antimicrobial therapy. If *Mycoplasma* pneumonia is suspected, then erythromycin, 30 to 50 mg/kg/day in four divided doses, will help shorten the clinical course.

Other antibiotics are useless in the treatment of bronchiolitis and should not be used. The interstitial pneumonia seen in children with bronchiolitis is caused by the infecting virus. Secondary bacterial pneumonia is extremely rare.

The majority of children with bronchiolitis can be managed as outpatients. Parents should be advised to give their child fluids and be instructed to look for signs of respiratory distress. Decongestants and antihistamines should not be prescribed.

If the child has significant respiratory distress or is hypoxic, he should be hospitalized. The mainstay of hospital treatment is good supportive care: hydration and oxygen. All hospitalized children should receive sufficient humidified oxygen to maintain their arterial Po_2 at 80 to 100 mm Hg. This usually requires an FiO_2 of between 30 and 40 per cent. Mist alone is of no value and may actually increase airway resistance.

An antiviral drug, ribavirin, is now available for treatment of severe RSV infections. The drug, which is teratogenic in animals, is delivered by way of aerosol; therefore care must be taken to avoid exposing pregnant caretakers to the drug.

Intravenous hydration should be given, since the infants have significant respiratory distress and are usually too ill to maintain adequate oral hydration. The child should receive maintenance fluids with correction of any fluid deficit. Overhydration may be harmful and should be avoided.

Although hypercarbia and respiratory failure are rare in bronchiolitis, 1 to 2 per cent of hospitalized children require mechanical ventilation. Assisted ventilation should be considered in a child with clinical deterioration as evidenced by increased work of breathing or by increasing Pco_2. Any child requiring mechanical ventilation for bronchiolitis should be cared for in a pediatric intensive care unit experienced in managing severely ill children.

Studies evaluating the efficacy of bronchodilators such as aminophylline for bronchiolitis have been inconclusive. However, at least one study has shown a definite clinical improvement with epinephrine. This suggests that sympathomimetic agents may be of some benefit. Bronchial smooth muscle is sparse in children younger than 1 year, the age when children are at greatest risk of having severe bronchiolitis. Because of the relative lack of smooth muscle in young children, bronchospasm is not a major component of this disease. Edema, inflammation, mucus, and sloughing of epithelial cells rather than bronchospasm lead to the classic obstructive signs seen in bronchiolitis. With this underlying pathophysiology aminophylline should theoretically have little effect. However, in selected cases of severe illness aminophylline* may be useful. If used, aminophylline should be administered at a rate of 0.4 to 0.5 mg/kg/hr following an infusion of 5 mg/kg administered over 30 minutes. Because of aminophylline's relatively low therapeutic index in infants and its variable and to a degree unpredictable metabolism in young

children, it should be used only when blood levels can be monitored closely. The level should be maintained in the 10 to 20 μg/ml range. Aminophylline should never be used for the outpatient management of bronchiolitis, since the risk of complications far outweighs any possible therapeutic benefit. Steroid therapy has been studied and is of no value in treating bronchiolitis.

Since RSV is contagious, children hospitalized for bronchiolitis should be isolated from other patients. Children hospitalized with certain chronic illnesses, particularly those with lung and cardiac problems, are at particular risk of developing severe disease with this infection.

ASPIRATION PNEUMONIA

JOHN T. McBRIDE, M.D.

Pneumonia related to aspiration or inhalation of material into the lungs commonly occurs in three clinical pediatric settings. Children of any age may acutely aspirate a large quantity of material from the pharynx. This is most often seen in the intensive care unit in children whose level of consciousness is depressed, and the material aspirated is usually regurgitated gastric contents. Toddlers who accidentally ingest any of a variety of hydrocarbons are often unable to prevent the material from entering the lungs because of its low surface tension and subsequently develop pneumonitis. In addition to these two acute aspiration syndromes, chronic aspiration bronchitis/pneumonitis occurs in various high-risk children and a few otherwise apparently normal children who habitually allow small amounts of food to enter the airway.

ACUTE ASPIRATION PNEUMONITIS

As soon as a child has been observed or is suspected to have aspirated regurgitated gastric contents or other material, the nasopharynx should be suctioned and a nasogastric tube placed to empty the stomach and prevent recurrent aspiration. If a large amount of material or material which includes large particles has been aspirated, laryngoscopy or bronchoscopy and direct suctioning of the trachea with a large-bore catheter should be considered. If the child is unconscious or obtunded, an endotracheal tube should be inserted to allow regular suctioning and to protect the airway. In any case, a regular program of chest percussion and postural drainage with or without suctioning should be instituted.

Once the airway is clear and further aspiration prevented, therapy is primarily supportive. Oxygen should be administered to maintain arterial oxygen saturation greater than 90 per cent. If this requires more than 80 per cent oxygen or if carbon dioxide retention and acidosis develop, mechanical ventilation should be begun with positive end-expiratory pressure. Inhaled beta-adrenergic bronchodilators may be used for bronchospasm in standard doses up to every 4 hours (or more frequently with cardiac monitoring) if a clinical

---

*Manufacturer's warning: Safety and efficacy for use in children less than 6 months of age have not been established.

response is apparent. Intravenous aminophylline (0.9 to 1.1 mg/kg/hr after a loading dose of 5 to 7 mg/kg) or oral theophylline (15 mg/kg/day in three or more divided doses) may also be helpful but may encourage gastroesophageal reflux and should be used cautiously for children in whom recurrent aspiration is possible. Corticosteroids are not indicated.

Although many clinical features of acute aspiration pneumonia suggest infection (pulmonary infiltrates, fever, leukocytosis), bacterial pneumonia is uncommon in the first 36 to 48 hours following aspiration. Therefore, antibiotics need not be given unless the material aspirated is known to be grossly contaminated, such as pus from a ruptured peritonsillar abscess. It is important, however, to monitor patients closely in the days following aspiration for signs of bacterial superinfection, such as changing pulmonary infiltrates, recurrent fever or leukocytosis, or general clinical deterioration. If superinfection is suspected, a Gram's stain of sputum or tracheal secretions should be examined. Mouth flora is the most frequent cause of bacterial pneumonia following aspiration. Unless other organisms are likely, penicillin alone in moderate doses is adequate as initial therapy if the child has not been previously hospitalized and is not in some other way a compromised host. If so, penicillin (or clindamycin if *Staphylococcus* is suspected) and an aminoglycoside such as tobramycin should be given. If experienced personnel are available, bronchoalveolar lavage, transtracheal aspiration, or direct lung puncture for Gram's stain and culture should be considered when a clinical response is not apparent within 24 to 48 hours of initiating empiric therapy.

HYDROCARBON ASPIRATION

The initial decision in the management of children with acute hydrocarbon ingestion is whether or not to remove the ingested material from the stomach. The risk of further pulmonary aspiration during vomiting or gastric lavage usually represents a greater danger than systemic toxicity from gastrointestinal absorption. Therefore gastric emptying is indicated only when the material ingested includes other toxic substances (such as heavy metals) or when there is a definite history of an unusually large volume of ingested material (more than 1 ml/kg body weight). If so, induced vomiting is acceptable if the child is fully conscious; otherwise, gastric lavage is indicated, preferably after tracheal intubation to minimize the risk of further aspiration.

Children with hypoxemia and respiratory distress after acute hydrocarbon ingestion should be hospitalized for observation and treatment. Those with mild or no respiratory symptoms may be safely observed in the office or emergency department without laboratory or radiologic studies. Those who are asymptomatic after 4 to 6 hours may be discharged without further evaluation and the parents instructed to bring the child back if respiratory symptoms recur. Children who remain symptomatic or are progressively symptomatic 6 hours after ingestion should admitted for observation, and a chest radiograph should be obtained.

The treatment of children with hydrocarbon aspiration pneumonia is otherwise the same as that for acute

gastric aspiration: oxygen to correct hypoxemia, tracheal intubation and mechanical ventilation with positive end-expiratory pressure for respiratory failure, aerosolized beta-adrenergic bronchodilators and/or theophylline for bronchospasm, and general intensive care measures. Corticosteroids and prophylactic antibiotics have no role in the acute management of this syndrome. Bacterial superinfection occasionally develops after 24 to 48 hours and is treated in the same way as superinfection after gastric aspiration.

CHRONIC ASPIRATION

Repetitive aspiration of small quantities of food or oropharyngeal secretions may cause pneumonia or bronchitis and eventually bronchiectasis. Chronic aspiration may occur in apparently normal children but is most common in those with neurologic handicaps or structural abnormalities of the airway or oropharynx. In either case, acute symptoms related to chronic aspiration usually present against a background of chronic bronchitis and recurrent lower respiratory tract symptoms.

Acute pneumonia with or without fever in children with chronic aspiration syndrome may be viral, bacterial, or noninfectious, and differentiation among these etiologies is often difficult if not impossible. Initial empiric treatment with a broad-spectrum antibiotic such as amoxicillin or trimethoprim-sulfamethoxazole is usually justified. Aggressive chest physical therapy and aerosolized bronchodilators are often helpful. Theophylline may also be useful but should be avoided in children in whom gastroesophageal reflux is suspected. Progression of symptoms despite empiric therapy should lead to more aggressive diagnostic measures.

The most important aspect of the management of children with this problem is the elimination of further aspiration following appropriate diagnostic studies to identify the specific cause. Surgical correction of structural abnormalities or gastroesophageal reflux, medical management of reflux with metoclopramide or bethanechol, gastric tube feedings, improved oral feeding strategies, and other specific measures may each be helpful in individual children.

BRONCHIECTASIS
ROBERT C. STERN, M.D.

Bronchiectasis (permanent dilatation of the subsegmental airways, usually with associated noneradicable infection) is a "final common pathway" of many lung diseases and virtually always represents a medical (or psychosocioeconomic) failure. For example, the patient may have a disease for which available treatment is inadequate (e.g., cystic fibrosis), may have a long-neglected problem (e.g., an untreated foreign body), or may not have complied with medical advice (e.g., failure to obtain adequate protection from pertussis and/or rubeola). Thus, in all patients with bronchiectasis, there are two general goals: (1) optimal treatment of the underlying disease (e.g., removal of foreign body, comprehensive treatment of cystic fibrosis, correction of hypogammaglobulinemia, etc.); and (2) treatment directed at the bronchiectasis itself. The first goal will not be discussed here; the reader is directed to other sections of this book for discussion of individual disease entities. With regard to the second goal (direct treatment of the bronchiectasis itself), the vicious circle that tends to perpetuate and aggravate the lesion should be attacked in every possible way. The individual components of such a therapeutic regimen are outlined below.

Infection should be aggressively treated, since it leads to additional direct injury to the airway wall, results in further accumulation of retained secretions (hypersecretory state), causes local and occasionally systemic hypoxia, and is associated with various systemic manifestations, such as fever, anorexia, and fatigue. Furthermore, spread of infection to adjacent airways is an ever-present threat. Sputum cultures, Gram stains, and cytologic examination should be undertaken, at least as part of the initial work-up. In some diseases, such as cystic fibrosis, sputum cultures at regular intervals may be helpful. Since the infection in bronchiectasis is largely within the airway (and not in a tissue that has a true blood supply), large doses of appropriate antibiotics may be needed to achieve sufficient antibiotic penetration into the respiratory secretions. In many patients, chronic (even continuous) antibiotic use may be necessary, since the infection can never be totally eradicated. Trimethoprim-sulfamethoxazole, tetracycline (for older patients), antistaphylococcal penicillins, and the like may be indicated. Concern about emergence of future resistant organisms is usually subordinate to the need to control the infection that is already there.

Measures to facilitate expectoration of secretions benefit the majority of these patients. Postural drainage with vibration and clapping should be taught to the family/patient. Some authorities are satisfied with relatively short treatment sessions that involve treating entire lobes, but segmental positioning seems to be more effective, either because the positions themselves are more accurate or because the entire treatment period is longer. Obviously, for localized disease, chest physiotherapy may be needed only for one or two lobes. In the case of young children in particular, initiation of this treatment often requires hospitalization so that a respiratory or physical therapist can do the treatment first (on the unenthusiastic young patient) and then allow the parents to gradually take over. Patients with severe disease may need one or more daily treatments for long periods of time, perhaps for life. Others improve to the point at which they need this treatment only during exacerbations of infection or when they have acute upper respiratory infections. Patients, particularly toddlers, who have problems with gastroesophageal reflux may have a difficult time with postural drainage, particularly with the head-down positions, and the therapy may have to be modified to accommodate the fine line between achieving optimal clearance of secretions and avoiding the risks of aspiration of gastric contents and the nutritional stress of vomiting meals. Efficacy of repeated bronchoscopic "wash-outs"

has not been definitively documented. Similarly, although maintenance of normal hydration is important, no substance (including iodides and glyceryl guaiacolate) has yet been shown to be a clinically effective expectorant in patients who are not dehydrated. Furthermore, the possibility of inducing thyroid disease with chronic iodide therapy is an additional reason not to use them.

Aerosols may be useful, particularly in patients with hyper-reactive airways. These may be most effective if done just prior to postural drainage/clapping treatments; however, in patients with gastroesophageal reflux, care must be taken to minimize the problems caused by the tendency of most bronchodilators to aggravate reflux. The clinician must also remember that, in some patients, a paradoxical worsening of pulmonary status may occur with aerosolized bronchodilator use if reduction in bronchomotor tone is associated with impairment of the cough reflex. Antibiotic aerosols have limited usefulness except in cystic fibrosis, in which they appear quite effective in some patients. Mucolytic drugs (e.g., N-acetylcysteine) are usually unnecessary; they may cause bronchospasm and, in any case, adequate drainage can usually be achieved without them.

Surgical resection may be indicated, especially for localized saccular bronchiectasis (which is usually even less likely to show anatomic reversal than the cylindrical type). Surgery is ideal for the patient who does not have a progressive underlying disease (e.g., a patient with a foreign body that has been removed), has excellent overall pulmonary function, and who has very severe but localized disease that is responding poorly to medical management. Poor candidates are those who have severe underlying disease (e.g., cystic fibrosis), diffuse bilateral involvement, and marginal pulmonary function. The decision in most cases, of course, is less clear-cut, but the overall approach to the issue of possible surgery should be as described above.

General measures include the following: Routine immunizations should be kept current, particularly for those diseases (e.g., rubeola) that are known to cause or aggravate chronic pulmonary disease. Most patients with bronchiectasis should receive influenza vaccine every year. Active sinus disease should be considered; if present, aggressive local treatment (e.g., decongestants, surgical drainage) may be useful. Finally, patients in whom cystic fibrosis has been excluded, but in whom Young's syndrome (early-onset chronic pulmonary disease with bronchiectasis, associated with progressive obstructive aspermia) is still being considered, should be offered the opportunity to "bank" their sperm for future use (if semen analysis shows that spermatozoa are still present).

ATELECTASIS

DENISE J. STRIEDER, M.D.

The word *atelectasis* means imperfect lung expansion and is synonymous with collapse. Partial atelectasis should be managed as promptly and as vigorously as complete atelectasis. The responsible mechanism is either bronchial obstruction with subsequent absorption of alveolar air distal to the obstruction or lack of distending transpulmonary pressure. Involvement of the right middle lobe is caused by the same mechanisms and responds to the same management as that of any other lobe. I will review the treatment of atelectasis according to mechanism and then separately consider the role of oxygen therapy and that of surgery.

BRONCHIAL OBSTRUCTION

Foreign body aspiration calls for rigid tube bronchoscopy performed under general anesthesia by an experienced thoracic or otolaryngologic surgeon, in possession of special kinds of forceps needed to grasp and remove foreign bodies. Even in the absence of suggestive history, the finding of lobar or pulmonary atelectasis in a previously well child suggests the possibility of a foreign body and indicates bronchoscopy as the only means to rule out foreign body aspiration. Similarly, bronchoscopy deserves consideration in the event that lobar atelectasis persists during recovery from aspiration pneumonia or near-drowning, to look for and remove a possible foreign body.

Mucoid impaction as a complication of prolonged mechanical ventilation has become rare since the advent of effective humidifiers. This obstruction also is best removed at bronchoscopy. Mucoid impaction as a result of chronic airway disease, such as asthma or cystic fibrosis, usually is a manifestation of allergic bronchopulmonary aspergillosis and responds to medical treatment of the underlying disease; the mucous plug becomes fragmented and is coughed up.

Bronchial stenosis, whether congenital or acquired (e.g., sequela of endobronchial tuberculosis), often leads to atelectasis. Bronchodilators are useless. Antibiotics are helpful when there is evidence of infection. However, medical treatment is usually disappointing: The atelectasis tends to be recurrent or persistent.

In the absence of any stenosis or discrete plug obstructing a lobar or segmental bronchus, retained secretions suffice to cause atelectasis, particularly in young children. Treatment is that of the underlying disease. For asthma, bronchodilators and corticosteroids are given by the systemic route, as nebulized adrenergic and steroid drugs help the functioning lung but do not reach the atelectatic region. For cystic fibrosis, hypogammaglobulinemia, and the dysmotile cilia syndrome, the main component of treatment is antibiotics effective against the organism(s) isolated from sputum, which in the case of *Pseudomonas aeruginosa* should be given intravenously (ciprofloxacin is effective by the oral route, but its use is limited to exceptional circumstances); chest physiotherapy and bronchodilators are often helpful; parenteral gammaglobulins are helpful only in patients with hypogammaglobulinemia, including those with IgG_2 deficiency, who are not well controlled with antibiotics alone.

Extrinsic compression of a bronchus can also cause atelectasis. In children, the usual culprit is lymphadenopathy, secondary to recurrent or persistent lung infections. Treatment is that of the underlying infection, but time must be allowed for regression of the lymphadenopathy. When the responsible agent is *Mycobacterium tuberculosis*, a 1-month course of prednisone, 0.5 mg/kg/day in a single morning dose, is given in addition to isoniazid and rifampin, to hasten the shrinkage of involved lymph nodes and the restoration of bronchial patency. When the responsible agent is an atypical mycobacterium, management depends on the drug susceptibility of the organism and the extent of the disease process; atelectasis is rare and the risks and benefits of prednisone in its treatment are not known.

Various tumors can cause atelectasis by filling the bronchial lumen or compressing the bronchial wall. The presence of an unsuspected tumor will be recognized when bronchoscopy is done to rule out foreign body aspiration. Initial treatment is surgical.

INSUFFICIENT TRANSPULMONARY PRESSURE

Breathing with consistently normal or small tidal volumes leads to diffuse, spotty, but progressive atelectasis. To re-expand collapsed alveoli, we need from time to time to take large breaths, as we do with physical activity while awake and with sighs while asleep. During mechanical ventilation in children, one needs to apply a positive end-expiratory pressure (PEEP) of 3 to 5 cm H_2O and to superimpose intermittent mechanical sighs. Higher levels of PEEP, used in the management of the respiratory distress syndromes, are contraindicated when lung mechanics is normal or nearly normal (e.g., neurologic indications for mechanical ventilation). No PEEP should be applied when the need for mechanical ventilation results from airway obstruction (e.g., bronchiolitis, asthma). Once lobar atelectasis has occurred, the respirator settings should not be changed for that reason; particularly, PEEP should not be increased, as this would increase the right-to-left shunt through the atelectasis. All elements of management should be reviewed and optimized and chest physiotherapy intensified. Intermittent insufflations, given with a self-inflating bag, make it possible to apply a large positive pressure (15 to 30 cm H_2O) for a longer period of time than that allowed by the respirator's intermittent sighs; sudden release of the pressure coupled with chest vibrations can be used to mimic cough. As a rule, however, the atelectasis resolves when the illness necessitating the mechanical ventilation resolves.

Following thoracic or abdominal surgery, patients are reluctant to take large breaths, which favors the onset of atelectasis. Splinting, bronchial hypersecretion, and reluctance to cough make things worse. Reluctance to expectorate complicates neck and throat surgery, including tonsillectomy and adenoidectomy. Treatment and prevention include the same measures: (1) positioning to minimize dorsal kyphosis and abdominal pressure; (2) voluntary cough, deep inspirations, chest physiotherapy, blow bottles, incentive spirometry, and early ambulation, and (3) pain management. Pain is responsible for the child's reluctance to move, breathe deeply, cough, and raise secretions. Postoperative pain does not respond to acetaminophen, which helps mostly by controlling fever. Codeine, which is a weak analgesic and a strong cough suppressant, is to be used only when cough suppression is desirable, which is rarely. Effective analgesia requires oral meperidine, subcutaneous morphine sulfate, or intercostal nerve block. Antibiotics are indicated when sputum is purulent and in the presence of fever and leukocytosis. Results of sputum smear and culture should guide the choice of antibiotic.

Left lower lobe atelectasis after cardiac surgery is predominantly the result of insufficient transpulmonary pressure and may occur even in the absence of bronchial hypersecretion. It resolves spontaneously as the child resumes physical activity.

Postpneumonic atelectasis is seen occasionally in young children. The alveolar exudate drains out of the affected lobe or segment, which is left airless. Re-expansion requires strong inspiratory efforts that the child is not likely to volunteer while in the hospital. This too resolves with the resumption of physical activity, although at times resolution may be delayed for months.

A similar mechanism accounts for the atelectasis often associated with pulmonary infarction. Hemorrhage causes airlessness, and large inspiratory efforts are prevented by pain. The atelectasis resolves with treatment and lysis of the thromboembolus and healing of the infarct.

All processes capable of reducing overall lung volume may be complicated by lobar atelectasis. Examples are pneumothorax, large pleural effusions, thoracic tumors, circumferential burns, kyphoscoliosis, and neuromuscular disease involving the respiratory muscles. The loss of one lobe causes the transpulmonary pressure across the rest of the lung to rise, so that, as a rule, there is no domino effect. Treatment, both medical and surgical, is addressed to the primary disease process.

Atelectasis of a whole lung rapidly follows unilateral intubation. Once the tracheal tube is properly repositioned, a few deep insufflations usually suffice to re-expand the affected side.

OXYGEN THERAPY

Regardless of its mechanism and its cause, acute atelectasis is associated with right-to-left shunting through the atelectatic lobe. The magnitude of the shunt is limited: both the loss of volume and the local hypoxic vasoconstriction raise the local vascular resistance and, therefore, reduce blood flow through the affected lobe. This phenomenon calls for redistribution of pulmonary blood flow to unaffected lobes, which, if they are free of disease, can increase their perfusion without any appreciable rise in pulmonary artery pressure. If the lobes free of atelectasis are diseased, as in cystic fibrosis, supplemental oxygen with an FIO_2 of 0.25 to 0.30 relieves the hypoxic vasoconstriction of the ventilating lobes and allows flow redistribution to take place. The residual hypoxemia is due to shunting through the atelectasis and responds poorly to higher inspired oxygen concentrations, which should not be used.

SURGICAL EXCISION

When bronchial obstruction is due to a tumor, lobectomy may be unavoidable, but not always. If the in-

volved bronchus is rather long (e.g., left main stem bronchus) and the tumor rather small, it may be possible to save the lobe or lung with a sleeve resection.

Bronchial stenosis often causes considerable morbidity. In that case, once the diagnosis is solidly established, surgical resection of the involved lobe or segment should be carried out without much delay. Because of subsequent compensatory growth, the long-term functional outcome of lobectomy is better when the operation is performed in children than in adults.

In cystic fibrosis, hypogammaglobulinemia, or immotile cilia syndrome, bronchiectasis may be complicated by recurrent or persistent lobar atelectasis and again cause considerable morbidity. Lobectomy should be considered in those children who are in a well-preserved state of nutrition, who have sufficiently good lung function to undergo surgery without the need for postoperative mechanical ventilation, and in whom CT imaging of the lung shows the remaining lobes to be less severely affected than the atelectatic lobe.

In children who otherwise have normal or nearly normal lungs, incidental atelectasis (e.g., postpneumonic or postoperative) may persist for months, even for several years, and eventually resolve spontaneously. As long as the child is asymptomatic or has only rare bouts of lower respiratory tract infection which are easily managed, surgery is not indicated.

EMPHYSEMA
MICHAEL A. WALL, M.D.

Emphysema can be defined in an operational sense as any condition that leads to dilatation of distal air spaces. Such dilatation may be accompanied by destruction of alveolar walls, as occurs in adults secondary to cigarette smoking. In this condition smoking leads to lung inflammation, attraction of neutrophils, and release of neutrophil elastase, which breaks down alveolar walls. An analogous situation occurs in individuals with alpha$_1$-antitrypsin deficiency. Alpha$_1$-antitrypsin is an abundant and important protease inhibitor in normal human serum. The major function of this protein is to inhibit the action of neutrophil elastases and prevent autodestruction of tissue. Many genetic variants or Pi types of alpha$_1$-antitrypsin have been described. The most common normal Pi type is MM. Pi types S and Z, the most common abnormal variants leading to clinical manifestations, result from point mutations in the structure of the molecule. Individuals who are homozygous for these abnormal Pi types secrete very little alpha$_1$-antitrypsin from the liver and thus have low levels of circulating protease inhibitor activity. This allows neutrophil elastases to work unopposed on lung elastin, leading to emphysema. Commonly Pi ZZ individuals present in the third to fifth decades of life with dyspnea, airways obstruction, and radiologic evidence of hyperlucency. Very rare cases of symptomatic alpha$_1$-antitrypsin deficiency have been reported in children. Alpha$_1$-antitrypsin replacement therapy is now available for symptomatic patients. Smoking definitely hastens the progression of lung disease in deficient individuals, and perhaps the major therapeutic modality available to child health care providers is strong, personalized non-smoking counseling.

Far more common than alpha$_1$-antitrypsin deficiency as a cause of emphysema in children are congenital and acquired forms of distal air space dilatation. Of the congenital forms, congenital lobar emphysema (CLE) and cystic adenomatous malformation (CAM) are the most common. Both can present in the newborn period as respiratory distress caused by massive unilobar hyperexpansion. The hyperexpansion causes mediastinal shift and contralateral atelectasis. In CLE there is usually a single cyst caused by aplasia or dysplasia of bronchial cartilage leading to expiratory bronchial collapse and a ball-valve phenomenon. In CAM multiple cysts are present, but again the condition is unilobar in nature with respiratory distress caused by hyperexpansion and atelectasis. In both conditions lobectomy is the definitive therapy and should be considered in the setting of respiratory distress or other physiologic compromise. Some patients with small lesions do not become symptomatic in the newborn period and may not need surgery.

In premature infants requiring ventilatory support, pulmonary interstitial emphysema (PIE) is fairly common. This condition is caused by rupture of alveolar air into the interstitium and lymphatics. Reduction of airway pressure, if consistent with maintaining adequate gas exchange, should be attempted. On occasion the condition is localized enough that selective intubation of the contralateral lung can be performed, allowing the hyperinflated area to slowly deflate. In life-threatening situations in which the lesion is sufficiently localized, lobectomy may be indicated.

In older children distal air space dilatation is usually caused by generalized or localized airways obstruction. Asthma, cystic fibrosis, and bronchiolitis are the most common childhood examples of conditions leading to generalized air trapping and alveolar hyperexpansion. Bronchoscopy is usually not helpful in the diagnosis of conditions leading to generalized air trapping, and therapy is directed toward relief of bronchospasm and mucous plugging. Localized hyperlucency seen on a chest radiograph suggests a congenital lesion such as CLE; an intrabronchial lesion such as foreign body, granulation tissue, mucous plug, or tumor; or extrinsic bronchial compression caused by a lymph node, tumor, or large vessel. A foreign body or mucous plug may cause complete bronchial obstruction with lobar atelectasis. In this instance, an adjacent lobe often hyperexpands to partially compensate for volume loss (compensatory emphysema). In the setting of localized air space dilatation whose cause is not obvious on a chest radiograph, bronchoscopy should be performed for diagnostic and sometimes therapeutic purposes. Flexible bronchoscopy can be performed on virtually any child, and therapeutic maneuvers such as suction of a mucous plug or laser resection of granulation tissue can be performed through such an instrument. If a foreign body is highly suspected, rigid bronchoscopy should be performed, as grasping forceps cannot be advanced through the small-diameter flexible pediatric bronchoscopes.

PULMONARY EDEMA

GERALD M. LOUGHLIN, M.D.

Pulmonary edema describes the accumulation of excess fluid in the extravascular spaces of the lung. In normal circumstances, the balance of physical factors controlling the movement of fluid from the pulmonary capillaries is such that only a small amount of fluid filters out of the vascular compartment. This fluid is generally removed quite efficiently by the pulmonary lymphatics. The causes of pulmonary edema can be separated on the basis of derangements in this balance of forces. Knowledge of the underlying pathophysiology can be quite helpful in developing a rational approach to therapy. The usual causes can be categorized into six major groups: (1) increase in pulmonary capillary pressure—this generally occurs secondary to cardiac dysfunction such as myocardial infarction, severe mitral stenosis, fluid overload, or pulmonary veno-occlusive disease; (2) altered permeability of the pulmonary capillary endothelium, usually secondary to infection, circulating toxins, or oxygen toxicity; (3) decreased plasma oncotic pressure—dilution or protein wasting are usual contributing factors; (4) inadequate lymphatic drainage; (5) increased negative interstitial pressure in response to marked airway obstruction or following re-expansion of a collapsed lung—excess intravascular volume may also be a contributing factor; and (6) finally, a group of causes in which the underlying mechanism responsible for the accumulation of edematous fluid is not known, as is seen in pulmonary edema secondary to high-altitude exposure, heroin use, or CNS injury.

Initial therapy of the patient with pulmonary edema regardless of the etiology must focus on increasing oxygen delivery. Pulmonary edema results in hypoxemia secondary to altered matching of ventilation and perfusion. All patients should receive supplemental oxygen delivered by either nasal cannula, oxygen hood/tent, or face mask with an oxygen reservoir. Patient preference and oxygen requirement may influence decisions regarding choice of delivery system. Monitoring oxygen delivery is essential. Oxygen saturation monitors are useful for the patient with mild to moderate hypoxemia. Critically ill children may require use of indwelling arterial lines and pulmonary artery catheters to monitor cardiac output and oxygen delivery to tissues.

Delivery of positive pressure to the airways has been shown to be effective in improving oxygenation secondary to pulmonary edema from a variety of causes, particularly that due to leaky pulmonary capillaries. In some older children and adolescents, this pressure can be delivered via a tight-fitting face mask. Patient tolerance and pressure requirements limit usefulness of this technique. For patients with more profound hypoxemia, endotracheal intubation with administration of continuous positive airway pressure is indicated. The addition of positive-pressure ventilation may be required if there is also evidence of inability to maintain adequate ventilation. Careful monitoring of oxygen delivery is essential so that the optimal range of positive pressure delivered can be determined. Controlled administration of positive pressure is important to reduce effects on cardiac output and minimize barotrauma. Use of high levels of positive pressure demands monitoring of cardiac output.

Morphine, 0.1 to 0.2 mg/kg/dose IV or IM, may also be useful in reducing anxiety associated with pulmonary edema and may lead to improved ventilatory patterns. Peripheral vasodilation, which also occurs, reduces venous return and left ventricular end-diastolic pressure.

Diuretic therapy in the form of furosemide (1 to 2 mg/kg IV or IM q12h) is the most effective means of reducing intravascular volume. It is quite useful in situations of actual or relative volume overload. It may be less effective in situations of pulmonary capillary injury but is useful with edema due to increased negative interstitial pressure complicated by volume overload. This situation is encountered commonly in management of infants with bronchopulmonary dysplasia or children with croup or epiglottitis.

Beyond general supportive therapy, one should attempt to attack the underlying cause. Specifically, pulmonary edema secondary to increased negative interstitial pressures from overcoming the increased resistance seen in croup, epiglottitis, or asthma is best treated by avoiding fluid overload and by aggressive therapy to reduce airway obstruction. Diuretics may be helpful if the patient has received excess fluids. Pulmonary edema secondary to myocardial dysfunction may respond to a combination of therapies. Diuretics, inotropic agents such as dopamine or dobutamine in the acute setting, or digitalis for chronic therapy may improve left ventricular function, thus increasing renal blood flow and diuresis. In low doses (1 to 5 µg/kg/min), dopamine increases renal blood flow. At higher doses (5 to 15 µg/kg/min), peripheral vasoconstriction occurs as well as increased inotropic effects and increased renal blood flow. At higher doses (>20 µg/kg/min), alpha-adrenergic effects dominate and renal blood flow is reduced. Dobutamine (2.5 to 15 µg/kg/min, maximum recommended dose 40 µg/kg/min), on the other hand, can result in a greater increase in inotropic effects without comparable increases in peripheral resistance. To prepare the infusion of both medications, a convenient approach is to use the formula

$$\frac{6 \times \text{wt (kg)} \times \text{desired dose (µg/kg/min)}}{\text{IV infusion rate (ml/hr)}} = \begin{array}{l} \text{mg of drug} \\ \text{to be added} \\ \text{to 100 ml of} \\ \text{IV fluid} \end{array}$$

In a situation in which maximum inotropic stimulation of myocardial function is not sufficient, some patients may respond to afterload reduction with either nitroprusside (0.5 to 10 µg/kg/min titrated to blood pressure) or hydralazine (0.1 to 0.5 mg/kg/dose q4–6h).

Reduction in afterload increases cardiac output and diuresis, thus reducing pulmonary vascular congestion.

Sepsis, which causes pulmonary edema secondary to the adult respiratory distress syndrome, also requires combination therapy. Antibiotics to treat the infection supplemented by diuretics, oxygen, and positive airway pressure as described above are required. However, it should be kept in mind that, since the pathogenesis of the pulmonary edema is related to significant increases in capillary leak, diuretic therapy may be of limited value. Positive pressure can be helpful and, as mentioned, should be titrated to improve pulmonary function and gas exchange without impairing cardiac function or causing barotrauma. Administration of colloid solution to hypotensive patients with pulmonary edema secondary to capillary leak should be approached cautiously, since this colloid may simply leak into the interstitium and thus contribute to more edema formation.

In summary, the primary focus of the therapy of pulmonary edema is to improve oxygenation. Supplemental oxygen, diuretics, and positive airway pressure are the mainstays of therapy. Management is facilitated by knowledge of the underlying pathophysiology.

PULMONARY THROMBOEMBOLISM

ROBERT C. STERN, M.D.

Pulmonary embolism is not a primary lung disease; the embolus, usually clotted blood, orginates elsewhere and reaches the lung via the venous system and the pulmonary artery. Although the treatment of the thromboembolic state and the resultant pulmonary problem are discussed here, any underlying extrapulmonary disease obviously must be correctly diagnosed and appropriately treated as well. Thus, for example, if pulmonary embolus is diagnosed in a neonate, the possibility of its having arisen from an intravenous catheter, or as a complication of an arteriovenous fistula secondary to a surgically implanted device (such as a shunt), congenital heart lesion, or maternal diabetes should be considered. In an adolescent, on the other hand, recent abortion, trauma, drug abuse, and use of oral contraceptives, among other predisposing problems, should come to mind. Treatment directed at the pulmonary embolus itself or the resultant pulmonary infarction or pulmonary hypertension is more likely to be successful if the primary problem is well treated. Although the treatment of nonthrombotic emboli (e.g., marrow, air, catheter fragments) is not specifically discussed in this article, for the most part, the general principles are still valid.

GENERAL SUPPORTIVE TREATMENT

Supplemental oxygen should be given in sufficient concentration to maintain arterial hemoglobin saturation above 90 per cent. Patients who have systemic hypotension should be given inotropic agents such as dopamine. Chest pain can be severe, and analgesics may be indicated. Sedation may be justified in some patients.

MASSIVE EMBOLUS IN A CRITICALLY ILL UNSTABLE PATIENT

If the embolus is massive, the patient is acutely decompensating (totally inadequate pulmonary perfusion and systemic hypotension that cannot be corrected by inotropic agents), and anticoagulation has failed or is contraindicated, emergency surgery (pulmonary artery embolectomy and interruption of the inferior vena cava) may be attempted as a desperation measure but is unlikely to be successful. However, surgical interruption of the distal inferior vena cava can be useful in some patients with lower extremity thrombosis and recurrent showers of emboli. These gravely ill patients may also benefit from thrombolytic therapy (e.g., urokinase or streptokinase); however, this treatment does not appear to be useful in patients whose embolus occurred longer than 72 hours before. Furthermore, because there has not been sufficient experience with these agents in children to allow definitive discussion of dosage, safety, or efficacy, their use in children is not recommended by the manufacturers. Despite the logic of many of these treatment measures, the prognosis for these patients remains very poor.

SMALL EMBOLUS IN A STABLE PATIENT

In patients who are stable and not critically ill, the immediate goals of treatment are to prevent additional thrombus formation with anticoagulants and to minimize the risk of additional embolism while the existing thrombus is given a chance to attach to the peripheral vessel wall. The former necessitates treatment with anticoagulants; the latter is addressed largely by physical measures, including bed rest. Most patients who survive and stabilize long enough to begin "routine" heparin treatment do well.

Once the diagnosis of pulmonary thromboembolism is established, heparin should be given by continuous intravenous infusion (loading dose: 50 to 75 units/kg; continuing dose: 25 units/kg/hr). Dosage adjustments may be needed frequently, based on the results of the activated whole blood clotting time (therapeutic goal: approximately twice control value) or the activated partial thromboplastin time (APTT; therapeutic goal: 1.5 times control value). This initial anticoagulant treatment should be continued for 7 to 10 days. Another decision, whether to continue (low-dose) heparin or other prophylactic anticoagulation, must then be based on the status of the disease or condition that was ultimately responsible for the patient's pre-embolus thrombotic state. The presence of additional risk factors for recurrent thromboembolism, such as obesity, positive family history of pulmonary thromboembolism or thrombotic state, recent surgery, and trauma, should be considered in this decision to use low-dose heparin. In general, it is safer to proceed with low-dose heparin or warfarin (Coumadin; therapeutic goal: prothrombin time 1.5 times control) for a reasonably long course (e.g., 3 to 6 months). Future development of risk factors, particularly if several such factors are simultaneously present, should prompt consideration of reinstitution of low-dose heparin even if there has not (yet) been a recent recurrence of pulmonary embolus.

PRIMARY PULMONARY HEMOSIDEROSIS
ROBERT C. BECKERMAN, M.D.

Primary pulmonary hemosiderosis, commonly called idiopathic pulmonary hemosiderosis, or IPH, is a rare lung disorder in children characterized by recurrent bouts of spontaneous alveolar hemorrhage. These episodes may be triggered by respiratory infections or by hypersensitivity reaction to cow's milk protein. In general, however, there are no consistent triggers, underlying mechanisms, or definite predisposing diseases that appear to cause the pulmonary hemorrhage. Although IPH may sometimes occur in families, there is no defined pattern of inheritance. All other causes of pulmonary hemorrhage must be ruled out before the diagnosis of IPH is made. These causes include pulmonary vasculitis (e.g., systemic lupus erythematosus), heart failure with pulmonary venous hypertension, systemic coagulopathy, and pulmonary renal syndromes (e.g., Goodpasture's syndrome). With each episode of pulmonary hemorrhage, the child (usually between 1 and 7 years of age) first experiences coughing followed by either hemoptysis or hematemesis, and dyspnea at rest and on exertion; he/she is usually observed to be pale and tachypneic. Fine end-inspiratory crackles and occasionally focal bronchial breath sounds are heard on auscultation of the chest. Splenomegaly and digital clubbing may be present, especially if the disease has been longstanding and if the patient has developed pulmonary fibrosis.

While the chest roentgenogram usually demonstrates transient or migratory fluffy infiltrates during the acute phase of bleeding, an underlying interstitial pattern of lung disease predominates as the acute bleeding resolves. During episodes of hemoptysis, pulmonary function often demonstrates airflow obstruction and a baseline restrictive ventilatory pattern typlified by a low forced vital capacity. Between episodes of hemorrhage, pulmonary function tests either are normal or demonstrate a restrictive pattern of lung disease (low forced vital capacity with elevated FEV_1/FVC). The index of lung function that most sensitively indicates the ongoing interstitial process and correlates with dyspnea on exertion is a decreasing arterial oxygen saturation during exercise stress. Moderate to severe anemia of the microcytic hypochromic type is usually associated with a modest reticulocytosis. If the pulmonary hemorrhage is triggered by milk protein hypersensitivity, immunologic laboratory abnormalities may include high levels of precipitating antibodies to cow's milk proteins, high IgE, a positive RAST for cow's milk protein, and, very rarely, selective IgA deficiency. The syndrome of hemosiderosis associated with cow's milk protein has been called Heiner's syndrome and almost always presents in infancy. The diagnosis of IPH must be supported by the demonstration of hemosiderin-laden macrophages either in bronchial or gastric washings or in an open lung biopsy specimen. The lung tissue should be evaluated by routine hematoxylin and eosin, collagen, and iron stains, fungal and AFB smears, immunofluorescent studies to look for antigen-antibody complexes or for linear deposits of antibody along the alveolar capillary membrane, and electron microscopic examination to look for breaks in the capillary endothelial lining.

Primary cardiac disease as the cause of hemosiderosis must be ruled out by echocardiography, and systemic lupus erythematosus, by the absence of antinuclear antibody. Goodpasture's syndrome may also be excluded by lack of antibasement membrane antibodies and/or immune complexes in the serum. The episodes of pulmonary hemorrhage may be life-threatening and may cause profound anemia, hemorrhagic shock, and respiratory failure. They may also recur or be chronic in nature. An open lung biopsy should be done before therapy is instituted in order to establish the diagnosis of IPH and to rule out other underlying diseases as mentioned above.

In cases of acute pulmonary hemorrhage in which respiratory distress is associated with hypoxemia, supplemental oxygen should be administered to the child. Mechanical ventilation may be necessary when there is severe pulmonary hemorrhage leading to refractory hypoxemia and respiratory failure. Positive end-expiratory pressure may have specific benefit by reducing alveolar bleeding in patients who have severe pulmonary hemorrhage. Transfusion of packed red blood cells may be necessary when there is acute anemia secondary to pulmonary bleeding, since hemoglobin in the sequestered alveolar cells may not be readily available for oxygen transport purposes. A milk elimination diet should be tried even if the diagnosis of cow's milk–induced pulmonary hemosiderosis is not proven.

If the first episode of pulmonary hemorrhage is severe, then corticosteroid therapy should be initiated as soon as possible after the diagnosis of IPH has been established. Although no control trials have proven the benefits of corticosteroids in children with IPH, most children improve dramatically after corticosteroids are initiated. Whether corticosteroids have any beneficial effect on the long-term prognosis of the disease remains uncertain. I recommend using 2 mg/kg/day of prednisone by mouth or methylprednisolone intravenously in four divided doses. If the child's disease responds to steroids, a dosage of 2 mg/kg/day given once daily in the morning should be continued for 2 weeks and then tapered to the smallest daily or alternate-day dose that will suppress the signs and symptoms of the disease.

Cytotoxic immunosuppressive therapy using both azathioprine and cytoxan has been tried in several cases with variable success. If bleeding continues after several days of adequate corticosteroid therapy, either oral azathioprine, 2 to 3 mg/kg/day, or cyclophosphamide, 2 mg/kg/day, should be added to the steroids. Repeated transfusion of packed red blood cells may be necessary for supportive therapy during recurrent pulmonary hemorrhage. Oral iron replacement should be given until an adequate hemoglobin level is restored. The

hemoglobin in the lung tissue and air spaces that is engulfed by macrophages is poorly utilized in making new erythrocytes.

Prospective laboratory follow-up should include CBC, reticulocyte count, spirometry, and arterial oxygen saturation by pulse oximetry at rest and during and after exercise as indicators of response to initial therapy and to withdrawal of therapy, and of disease stability. Sleeping respiratory rate logs that the parents keep at home may provide useful data about changing pulmonary status. Administration of low-flow humidified oxygen at night may be necessary if the interstitial pulmonary component is chronic and if the child develops pulmonary hypertension and cor pulmonale.

Inhalation of sodium cromolyn, plasmapheresis, and iron chelation therapy have been suggested as potentially useful modalities of therapy for selected patients with IPH but have not been proven to be effective in changing the course of the disease or its complications. IPH is characterized by exacerbations and remissions of pulmonary hemorrhage but usually becomes a chronic pulmonary disorder. Repeated episodes of alveolar and interstitial hemorrhage may result in progressive interstitial pulmonary fibrosis and its associated exertional dyspnea. The prognosis for IPH in childhood, however, seems better than in adults if aggressive therapy is initiated early in the course of the illness.

CONGENITAL DIAPHRAGMATIC HERNIA
ELI R. WAYNE, M.D.

The most common thoracic surgical emergency seen in the neonatal intensive care unit is congenital diaphragmatic hernia. Congenital diaphragmatic hernia occurs in about 1 in 2500 live births. The hernia occurs on the left side in 90 per cent of cases in most series. The defect in the diaphragm is variable in size but is most commonly located in the posterolateral portion of the left hemidiaphragm. In the majority of patients there is a fairly well-developed anterior portion of the diaphragm with aplasia or absence of the posterior one-half of the diaphragm. With left-sided diaphragmatic hernias, the spleen, stomach, transverse colon, small intestine, and left lobe of the liver are located within the chest. Hernias on the right side usually contain primarily liver, with variable amounts of small and large intestine. The lung on the side of the hernia is hypoplastic and usually does not expand immediately upon evacuation of the viscera from the chest. The branches of the bronchial tree are decreased in number, thereby resulting in fewer alveoli than normal. The weight of the lung on the side of the diaphragm at autopsy is markedly decreased, but the weight of the contralateral lung is also markedly decreased, indicating that there is bilateral pulmonary hypoplasia.

CLINICAL PRESENTATION AND DIAGNOSIS

Maternal ultrasonography may lead to the discovery of diaphragmatic hernia in the fetus. However, in most cases the affected infant is born without suspicion of the diagnosis prenatally. Most infants with congenital diaphragmatic hernia develop respiratory distress within the first 5 minutes of birth. On physical examination the abdomen is noted to be scaphoid, and the anteroposterior diameter of the chest is increased on the side of the hernia. Also, breath sounds are most likely absent on the ipsilateral side and bowel sounds can be heard in the chest. The point of maximal impulse of the cardiac beat is displaced to the side opposite the hernia. The infant then becomes increasingly tachypneic, cyanotic, and then hypotensive.

Chest radiographs establish the diagnosis in almost all infants with congenital diaphragmatic hernia. Typically only a small portion of lung is visible in the chest, with multiple gas-filled intestinal loops filling the thoracic cavity. The heart silhouette is also displaced to the contralateral side. The mortality in patients with congenital diaphragmatic hernia presenting in the first 6 hours of life is approximately 50 per cent in most large series.

PREOPERATIVE TREATMENT

Although the degree of preoperative respiratory difficulty may vary, certain actions are recommended for monitoring and preparation of the infant with congenital diaphragmatic hernia. A nasogastric tube is placed into the stomach to minimize distention of the bowel. Additionally, an umbilical artery catheter for monitoring postductal blood gases is placed and, if feasible, an arterial cannula in the right radial artery is used to measure preductal gases. In most cases endotracheal intubation is indicated, and gentle, rapid hand ventilation must be utilized to prevent the development of a pneumothorax in both the ipsilateral and contralateral hemithoraces. Supplemental oxygen up to 100 per cent may be necessary to maintain adequate arterial blood gas saturations. After a brief period of stabilization, the patient should be operated upon for repair of the diaphragmatic defect.

OPERATIVE TREATMENT

Once the patient has been moved to the operating theater, the entire abdomen and chest are draped. A left subcostal incision is then constructed and carried down into the peritoneal cavity. The viscera then are usually easily reduced out of the chest. Great care should be taken not to damage solid structures such as the spleen. Once the viscera have been reduced out of the chest, the anesthesiologist is instructed to gently bag the endotracheal tube, thereby gradually increasing the pressure so as to aid in expansion of the left lung. Following this a search is made for the rim of the posterior portion of the left diaphragm. The diaphragm is then closed with silk sutures in an interrupted fashion. A chest tube is then placed into the intrathoracic space and placed on underwater seal. In some cases, because of the severe respiratory distress, we believe that it is unwise to close the muscles of the anterior abdominal wall, and a ventral hernia is created to allow the abdominal viscera to expand into the hernia defect rather than pressing on the newly repaired diaphragm. For patients

with right-sided congenital diaphragmatic hernias, either a transthoracic or a transabdominal approach may be utilized. It is our preference in most cases to use a transabdominal approach even for the right-sided hernias, although some investigators have used a transthoracic approach.

POSTOPERATIVE CARE

The postoperative management of a newly repaired diaphragmatic hernia represents perhaps a greater challenge than the intraoperative repair itself. Because of the altered anatomy and physiology of the neonatal lung, constant attendance by a neonatologist is necessary to react to the changes in the blood gases. The development of pulmonary hypertension with right-to-left shunting across the patent ductus arteriosus and the foramen ovale occurs frequently in patients with congenital diaphragmatic hernia. This can be managed with the use of Priscoline, a pulmonary bed vasodilator. Unfortunately, with prolonged use of Priscoline the patient becomes resistant to its effects, and it is usually of little value after the first 24 hours of its administration. Because of this, great attention must be paid to maintaining the patient's arterial oxygen tension at least at 100 mm Hg. This is thought to minimize the development of pulmonary hypertension and right-to-left shunting across the ductus and foramen ovale. The onset of the shunting can be documented by comparing blood gases from the right radial and umbilical artery cannulas. Once the shunting does develop, all efforts must be made to reverse it immediately. In addition to the use of Priscoline, which commonly drops the blood pressure, we use dopamine to maintain blood pressure and peripheral perfusion. Large amounts of fluid are also necessary because of the peripheral vasodilation caused by the Priscoline. The chest tube is used only to keep the mediastinum in the midline, and it is seldom necessary to place it on suction. Another effective tool to maintain adequate levels of oxygen tension is hyperventilation, with rates frequently over 200 per minute. In addition to the use of dopamine to support systemic blood pressure, the use of dobutamine has now been recommended because of the fact that dopamine seems to potentiate the pulmonary hypertension. Patients who ultimately survive have been weaned from most pharmacologic agents by 4 to 5 days of life, although ventilatory assistance and high FIO_2 may be needed for several more weeks.

RESULTS OF SURGICAL AND NEONATAL MEDICAL THERAPY

As previously mentioned, most centers report a mortality of approximately 50 per cent in babies who present with respiratory distress secondary to a diaphragmatic hernia within the first 6 hours of life. Despite the newest modalities in therapy, we have been unable to decrease this mortality figure. The recent use of extracorporeal membrane oxygenation (ECMO) has given much hope for a new generation of patients with severe diaphragmatic hernias. We have had limited experience with it at our institution but will continue to use this modality in the hope of improving the mortality figures in this disease.

5

Cardiovascular System

CONGESTIVE HEART FAILURE

DAVID R. FULTON, M.D.

When ventricular dysfunction causes symptoms of exercise intolerance, pulmonary congestion, or growth failure, congestive heart failure is present. The therapeutic approach is dependent on identification of the underlying cause of the myocardial dysfunction. Structural heart disease is the most common etiology for congestive failure and in the case of congenital disease generally presents within the first several months of life. Viral myocarditis, pericarditis, Kawasaki disease, acute rheumatic fever, acute bacterial endocarditis, toxic shock syndrome, sepsis, and anthracycline toxicity are common causes of acquired congestive failure. When possible, treatment of the underlying abnormality may hasten resolution of the cardiac symptoms and should be used in conjunction with other pharmacologic support. Rhythm disturbances may lead to acute congestive heart failure, and their therapy is discussed elsewhere.

ACUTE CONGESTIVE FAILURE

Viewed most simply, congestive failure is either acute or chronic. In acute disease, the cause may be volume overload, pressure overload, or primary myocardial or pericardial disease.

Inotropic Therapy

The rapid onset of congestive heart failure is frequently accompanied by altered myocardial contractility with diminished myocardial performance. Improvement is most rapidly accomplished by intravenous inotropic agents. Dopamine and dobutamine are preferred because of their rapid onset of activity, minimal proarrhythmogenic effect, potential for titration, and often predictable alpha-adrenegic effect on peripheral vasculature. Dopamine at low doses of 3 to 5 μg/kg/min potentiates renal vasodilatation, which can improve renal blood flow and subsequent diuresis. In mid-range doses (5 to 15 μg/kg/min), dopamine has positive inotropic effect on the myocardium, with positive chronotropy as well. At doses beyond 15 μg/kg/min, dopamine

may exert alpha-adrenergic activity, raising systemic or pulmonary vascular resistance. To minimize this effect, dobutamine 5 to 10 μg/kg/min can be added to the lower doses of dopamine (2 to 7.5 μg/kg/min). Isoproterenol, a potent beta-agonist, may be utilized for acute failure at 0.1 to 2.0 μg/kg/min, but its chronotropic and arrhythmogenic effect may exacerbate symptoms, so doses must be titrated carefully. Amrinone, a nonglycosidic, phosphodiesterase inhibitor, appears to exhibit potent inotropic and vasodilatory effects. Since safety and efficacy in pediatrics have not yet been determined, its use should be reserved for cases of failure of the above agents. In postoperative cardiac patients we have used an intravenous loading dose of 0.75 mg/kg/bolus over 5 minutes followed by continuous infusion at 5 to 10 mg/kg/min. Platelet counts should be monitored for thromboctyopenia, which is reversible after discontinuation of the drug. Digoxin is usually not favored for acute congestive heart failure, particularly in the presence of metabolic derangements or acute myocarditis, which increase myocardial sensitivity to the drug.

Diuretics

The use of diuretic therapy in acute congestive heart failure should be prudent and based upon the underlying diagnosis. In the case of volume-overload lesions such as left-to-right shunts at the ventricular or ductal level, furosemide, 1 mg/kg/dose, may improve cardiac function and congestive symptoms of pulmonary edema by decreasing preload. The same may be true in acute pressure-overload lesions such as left ventricular outflow tract disease, i.e., critical aortic stenosis or coarctation of the aorta; however, volume preservation may be advantageous in these settings, and furosemide should be used cautiously. In the case of impaired primary myocardial dysfunction in acute myocarditis with cardiac decompensation, the use of diuretics should not be considered initially, since maintenance of ventricular preload may be essential for preservation of adequate cardiac output.

Afterload Reduction

In the presence of impaired myocardial function with low cardiac output and elevated systemic vascular resistance, various arteriolar vasodilators have been of great benefit. In the acute setting, intravenous nitroprusside 0.25 to 5.0 µg/kg/min is used while monitoring heart rate, blood pressure, atrial filling pressures (CVP or pulmonary capillary wedge tracings), and urine output. The blood pressure and filling pressures may fall after starting therapy owing to arteriolar vasodilatation and venous pooling. Volume challenges should be used to raise filling pressures in order to sustain cardiac preload. Use of a thermodilution pulmonary artery catheter to measure cardiac output during nitroprusside infusion should be mandatory. Measurements of cardiac output and systemic vascular resistance permit judicious titration of inotropic agents, vasodilators, and fluid replacement. When nitroprusside is used beyond 24 hours, serum thiocyanate and cyanide levels must be monitored for proper dose adjustment.

Transfusion

Increasing the hematocrit for patients with congestive heart failure improves the oxygen-carrying capacity to tissues whose perfusion may be inadequate. In addition, raising the hematocrit increases blood viscosity and has been shown to result in an increase in pulmonary vascular resistance, which in turn decreases the magnitude of left-to-right intracardiac shunting.

Prostaglandin E

In the newborn period left ventricular outflow tract obstruction is a frequent cause of myocardial decompensation. In particular, aortic arch lesions—severe coarctation and interrupted aortic arch—may produce severe left ventricular dysfunction as the ductus arteriosus narrows and cardiac output falls. Ensuing metabolic acidosis from diminished tissue perfusion may aggravate congestive failure. When the diagnosis is established, prostaglandin E (PGE) is started immediately at 0.05 to 0.1 µg/kg/min. Central apnea may occur during the initial 30 minutes of use, so preparation must be made for possible intubation. Prophylactic intubation prior to interhospital transport is well warranted. Peripheral vasodilatation is frequently seen and may result in hypotension. Initial treatment should be fluid bolus rather than discontinuation of the drug. Titration of the dose may be necessary to avoid persistent hypotension. Concomitant administration of sodium bicarbonate, 0.5 to 1.0 mEq/kg/dose, is indicated until improved peripheral perfusion reverses lactic acidemia.

Surgical Therapy

When the primary cause of congestive heart failure is identified, surgical intervention is indicated as soon as practical. When cardiothoracic surgery in infants is not available, arrangement for transport to an identified center is crucial. Balloon dilatation valvuloplasty and surgical valvotomy for critical aortic stenosis, as well as surgical repair of coarctation of the aorta and interrupted aortic arch, are life-saving procedures. Stabilization with inotropic agents and PGE and correction of acid-base balance for a short period of time before proceeding to surgery may improve the outcome.

Pericardiocentesis

Acute hemodynamic decompensation may occur in the presence of acute pericardial fluid collection or progressive constrictive pericarditis. The causes are varied, but in younger children most often the etiology is viral or bacterial. Compression of the cardiac chambers leads to impaired diastolic ventricular filling with resulting diminished cardiac output. When hypotension is present, immediate intervention is indicated. Intravenous access is mandatory and volume infusion should be administered as 10 ml/kg over 15 to 30 minutes. A pericardiocentesis should be performed by a skilled operator. Utilizing a long spinal needle or angiocatheter, the pericardial space is entered from either the subxiphoid position or the fifth left intercostal space in the mid-clavicular line. Ideally an exchange J-wire can be advanced through the needle to the pericardial space and a multiperforated side hole catheter advanced over the wire. This maneuver permits stabilization of access through which large amounts of fluid can be removed. During evacuation of the pericardial space, vital signs must be carefully monitored. Fluid bolus is required if the blood pressure falls further during fluid removal. If the effusion is purulent, antibiotic therapy should be started and consideration given to surgical evacuation of the abscess. If the effusion is serous or serosanguineous, the catheter may be left in place in sterile fashion and used for further fluid removal.

CHRONIC CONGESTIVE HEART FAILURE

Following stabilization of the acutely ill child with congestive heart failure, therapy is directed toward chronic management. As in acute decompensation, selection of therapy depends on the underlying etiology.

Inotropic Support

The standard therapy for inotropic support is digoxin. Although its efficacy for volume overload lesions has been challenged, digoxin is still used almost universally. Loading doses of digoxin are based on body weight, but owing to pharmacokinetic differences for age, various regimens are employed (Table 1). In general, digitalization is scheduled over a 16- to 24-hour period with one half of the total digitalizing dose given initially, followed by one fourth of the dose given 8 to 12 hours later and an equivalent amount 8 to 12 hours after the second dose. Maintenance doses can be started 12 hours after digitalization and are divided into two equal daily doses. In situations in which gastrointestinal absorption is uncertain, the intravenous route is pref-

TABLE 1. Digoxin Doses in Pediatric Practice (IV)

	Loading (µg/kg/day)	Maintenance (µg/kg/day)
Prematures	15–20	5
Neonates* (0–1 month)	20–30	5–10
Infants (1–12 months)	40	10
Children (>12 months)	40	10–15

Data from Nyberg L, Wettrell G: Digoxin dosage schedules for neonates and infants based on pharmacokinetic considerations. Clin Pharmacokinet 3:453–461, 1978, with permission.
*Full-term newborns birth to 1 month of age.

erable, noting that the oral dose is 75 per cent of the parenteral dose. When not needed acutely, oral digitalization can be performed by starting maintenance doses without loading. In cases of renal insufficiency, maintenance doses should be adjusted according to parameters of renal function. Assessment of digoxin effect by electrocardiographic tracings is important, particularly after completion of digitalization. Digoxin effect is often manifested by prolongation of the PR interval with changes in ST segments and T waves and should not necessarily be considered a sign of toxicity. Toxicity in children is not common but includes gastrointestinal symptoms—anorexia, nausea, vomiting. Other symptoms include drowsiness and visual changes. Rhythm disturbance may often be the first and only indication of toxicity and may be either supraventricular, ventricular, or conduction abnormalities. When new rhythm abnormalities occur after starting digoxin, toxicity should be suspected and serum potassium, BUN, and creatinine should be determined and corrected when possible. Discontinuation of digoxin should occur if any rhythm is thought to be toxic in origin.

Diuretic Therapy

Chronic diuretic therapy is a useful adjunct to digoxin in the management of chronic CHF. Use of diuretic enables moderation of fluid restriction, which secondarily permits optimization of caloric intake. Various combinations are possible; however, chronic therapy with either furosemide (1 to 2 mg/kg/day) or chlorthiazide (20 to 30 mg/kg/day) must be accompanied by potassium supplementation (1 to 2 mEq/kg/day); alternatively, a potassium-sparing diuretic (spironolactone, 2 to 3 mg/kg/day) should be used. Serum electrolytes should be monitored after introduction of combined therapy until a stable state is reached. These drugs may need to be discontinued during acute gastrointestinal losses.

Afterload Reduction

Maximization of therapy to reduce preload and enhance inotropy may not improve CHF sufficiently to permit growth or reduce symptoms of exercise intolerance or dyspnea. A rise in afterload results in increased vascular wall stress and in turn myocardial wall stress, further limiting myocardial performance. In the chronic setting of congestive failure from left-to-right intracardiac shunts or dilated congestive cardiomyopathy, hydralazine, a vasodilator that acts to relax smooth muscle and produces selective arteriolar vasodilation, is given orally as 0.25 to 2.0 mg/kg/dose every 6 hours. The most frequently noted side effects include reflex tachycardia, postural hypotension, and gastrointestinal complaints. A lupus-like syndrome may occur in children as in adults and appears to respond to discontinuation of the drug. Captopril, an angiotensin-converting enzyme inhibitor, promotes vasodilation by decreasing angiotensin. The dose for children is 0.1 to 2.0 mg/kg/dose orally given every 8 hours. Side effects include hypotension with dizziness, rash, and neutropenia.

Nutrition

Children with chronic congestive heart failure have increased caloric requirements to achieve adequate growth. Failure to thrive is a common occurrence in infants with large left-to-right intracardiac shunts as well as in those with dilated cardiomyopathy. Often growth is insufficient with caloric intake of less than 150 to 175 kcal/kg. Early supplementation of formula to 28 to 30 cal/kg by addition of polycose, medium-chain triglyceride, or rice cereal is beneficial. If volume increases are not possible because of tachypnea, fatigue, or pulmonary edema, then further slow increase in caloric density to 36 cal/kg is indicated. Diuretic therapy is a valuable adjunct in maximization of calories when volume restriction is not practical. If oral feeding is not well tolerated, other routes of alimentation are used, including bolus nasogastric or continuous nasojejunal feeding. When possible, oral feeding is continued to prevent loss of this skill. Rarely, gastrostomy tube or central intravenous alimentation is necessary.

Transplantation

In cases of refractory congestive heart failure from severe left ventricular dysfunction, cardiac transplantation is becoming an accepted alternative. Challenges remain in improving transplant immunology and increasing public awareness to provide for donor sources. Success in the adult population will continue to stimulate efforts for similar results in children.

CONGENITAL HEART DISEASE
ALEXANDER S. NADAS, M.D.

For the 1990s, the current pediatric therapy of congenital heart disease is cardiac surgery. Most cardiac surgery is corrective—a few operations are still palliative—but there is no *medical* cure for congenital heart disease. Looking into my murky crystal ball, I sometimes see the vague outlines of prevention of congenital malformations of the heart, but this surely will not happen before the millenium.

It may be worth spending a brief paragraph on the significance of the problem. With the virtual disappearance of rheumatic fever from the United States due to a variety of medical and socioeconomic factors, congenital heart disease is the most common type of pediatric heart disease in this country today. The ratio of admissions of congenital to acquired heart disease to the Children's Hospital in Boston is close to 100:1 today. This figure is an approximate one and may not be valid for all institutions, but it is the only one available to me. The overall incidence of congenital heart disease in the United States is generally estimated at 8/1000 live births. Other figures for other parts of the Western world are quite similar. Roughly, one third of these patients become critically ill within the first year of life, another third may get sick later on, and the final third may never experience significant handicaps from their cardiac malformation. It may be said that at present birth

TABLE 1. Diagnostic Frequencies in Infants*

Diagnosis	Infants	
	Number	*Per Cent*
Ventricular septal defect*	374	15.7
D-Transposition of great arteries*	236	9.9
Tetralogy of Fallot*	212	8.9
Coarctation of aorta*	179	7.5
Hypoplastic left heart syndrome*	177	7.4
Patent ductus arteriosus*	146	6.1
Endocardial cushion defect*	119	5.0
Heterotaxis (dextro-, meso-, levo-, asplenia)	95	
Pulmonary stenosis*	79	3.3
Pulmonary atresia with intact ventricular septum*	75	3.1
Atrial septal defect secundum	70	2.9
Total anomalous pulmonary venous return*	63	2.6
Tricuspid atresia*	61	2.6
Single ventricle	58	2.4
Aortic stenosis	45	1.9
Double-outlet right ventricle	35	1.5
Truncus arteriosus	33	1.4
L-Transposition of the great arteries	16	0.7
Other heart disease	117	4.9
No significant heart disease	24	1.0
Primary pulmonary disease	106	4.5
TOTAL	2381	100

* Indicates defects discussed in the text.

rates, close to 40,000 babies are born with congenital heart disease in the United States and one third of these need urgent attention within days, weeks, or months after birth.

In the following paragraphs the conventional, and largely meaningless, classifications of congenital heart disease will be disregarded. Instead, the malformations will be presented according to age of manifestation and incidence. According to long-established principles of this volume, diagnosis will not be discussed in detail, although where important the tools of diagnosis appropriate for the entity will be identified. Emphasis will be on the course of action to be taken, and the risks and benefits of surgery in our institution today will be given. We will restrict the discussion to the most common lesions, both in infancy and in childhood, making up at least 75 per cent of the total.

INFANCY

The following discussion is based on our experience with infants who were so ill that they either died, had to be operated upon, or had to undergo cardiac catheterization within the first year of life in one of the six New England states. Clearly, some babies could be entered by several of these criteria.

Ventricular Septal Defect. This most common cardiac malformation does not need surgical treatment unless the baby is in congestive heart failure manifesting respiratory distress or failure to thrive. Without these signs accurate diagnosis and surgery may be safely postponed beyond the first birthday. If a baby in congestive heart failure is suspected to have a ventricular septal defect on the basis of physical examination, the diagnosis should be confirmed by ECG, radiography, ultrasonography, and catheterization. If through vigorous anticongestive measures, including diuretics (furosemide), digitalis (digoxin), and oxygen, the respiratory distress can be overcome and the baby starts gaining weight, surgery may be postponed, in the hope that the defect will get smaller or even close spontaneously. By watching the baby closely through weekly and later monthly office visits, the pediatrician is in the best position to monitor the infant's progress. If the clinical course is satisfactory and the baby progresses within an acceptable growth channel, there is no reason why surgery could not be postponed beyond the first year of life, assuming that pulmonary vascular obstructive disease can be excluded with reasonable certainty by electrocardiography and echocardiography. A baby with intractable congestive heart failure needs corrective surgery within the first weeks or months of life. Hospital mortality is less than 2 per cent; probability of complete closure among the survivors is 90 per cent.

Transposition of the Great Arteries. The second most common defect among infants is transposition of the great arteries. It always needs surgical correction or palliation. There are many varieties of transposition, but irrespective of anatomic details and in contrast to ventricular defect, *all patients have to be operated upon.* The most common form of the malformation is the patient *without a ventricular septal defect* (± 60 per cent); these are babies who are quite cyanotic within hours

TABLE 2. Incidence of Congenital Heart Disease Among Children Seen at Children's Hospital in Boston

Diagnosis	Number	Age (years)			
		0–5	*5–10*	*10–15*	*15–20*
Ventricular septal defect*	1950	25%	21%	21%	21%
Pulmonary stenosis*	1066	7	14	16	17
Tetralogy of Fallot*	857	10	9	9	8
Aortic stenosis*	774	3	8	12	17
Patent ductus arteriosus*	678	15	7	3	2
Atrial septal defect secundum*	671	6	13	9	7
Coarctation of the aorta*	464	5	7	7	4
Mitral disease	372	2	4	7	7
Transposition of the great arteries	351	8	3	2	2
Endocardial cushion defect*	315	5	3	3	3
Single ventricle	133	2	2	1	1
Malposition	80	1	1	1	1
Other	943	11	8	9	10
TOTAL CASES	8654	3324	1574	1424	1128

*Indicates defects discussed in the text.

after birth, with unimpressive physical findings and normal chest x-ray and ECG. The echocardiogram is diagnostic. In most institutions, as soon as the diagnosis is established, the baby is taken to the cardiac catheterization laboratory for physiologic studies, angiography, and balloon septostomy (rupture of the interatrial septum to promote mixing between systemic and pulmonary blood flow). In our institution, if the diagnosis is transposition of the great arteries with intact ventricular septum, an arterial switch operation is performed within the first week of life. This early correction is proposed to challenge the left ventricle (in transposition, the pulmonary ventricle) before the fetal hypertrophy undergoes involution. If the patient arrives to our institution at some weeks or months of age, having survived through atrial mixing, a two-stage approach is proposed. First, a band is placed on the pulmonary artery to promote hypertrophy of the left (pulmonary) ventricle; 7 to 10 days later the great arteries are switched over to the appropriate ventricles (aorta to left ventricle, pulmonary artery to right ventricle). In patients with transposition and a ventricular septal defect, the baby's arterial oxygen saturation is usually relatively adequate (over 80 per cent) because of mixing through the naturally occurring ventricular defect and the iatrogenically created atrial defect. Consequently, surgical treatment is not as urgent in these as in the ones with an intact ventricular septum; also, the large ventricular defect allows for systemic pressure in the left ventricle (pulmonary ventricle), which maintains hypertrophy of the left ventricle. The condition in these babies is also being corrected in our institution through an arterial switch operation and closure of the ventricular defect. Hospital mortality for both types of transposition is less than 5 per cent, and 5-year follow-up is very encouraging.

In institutions where the surgical preference is an atrial baffle operation (Mustard or Senning), those patients with an intact ventricular septum are being operated on at 2 to 3 months of age while those with a ventricular defect at 3 to 6 months of age. Hospital mortalities are comparable, but sick sinus syndrome some years later is quite common. In addition, there seem to be additional problems relating to the competence of the tricuspid valve as well as the myocardial performance of the systemic ventricle, which makes the arterial switch operation considerably more desirable in those with a ventricular defect.

Tetralogy of Fallot. The third most common lesion manifesting itself in infancy is tetralogy of Fallot. Rarely is cyanosis critical within hours or days of life; in most instances it is noted within weeks or months and may be compatible with reasonable growth and development. The diagnosis may be suspected through physical examination, radiography, and ECG; ultrasound is diagnostic. Corrective surgery is being performed, electively, by 1 year of age in our institution; some centers still prefer to palliate initially with correction at around 2 years. Operative mortality, through one-stage correction or through a combined two-stage approach, should not be higher than 5 per cent. Long-term results, now encompassing three decades, are excellent, with some

concern for late appearance of arrhythmias. Early appearance of hypoxic spells or severe exercise intolerance may force one's hand for early intervention at months, weeks, or even days of life. Preoperative catheterization is usually performed for adequate morphologic and physiologic detail although we do not consider it mandatory, given the high resolution of the two-dimensional echocardiogram.

Coarctation of the Aorta. In the majority of instances, coarctation of the aorta causes congestive heart failure in infancy. In a minority (20 per cent) it remains dormant through childhood and even adolescence. Although aggressive medical management of congestive failure in infancy may be transiently successful, in our institution we believe today that after initial treatment with diuretics, with or without digitalis, corrective surgery is necessary within days or weeks. Diagnosis is strongly suggested by absent, or delayed, femoral pulses in an infant with congestive failure. Relative hypertension in the right arm with severe cardiac enlargement and right ventricular hypertrophy in the electrocardiogram complete the clinical diagnosis; a two-dimensional echocardiogram clearly localizes the aortic obstruction. Preoperative catheterization for anatomic and physiologic detail is recommended but is not mandatory. Operative mortality is less than 5 per cent and long-term outcome is promising. Reoperation should not be necessary in the majority of those operated upon in infancy today. We do not recommend balloon dilation for "virginal" coarctations.

Hypoplastic Left Heart Syndrome. This syndrome is a highly lethal combination of valvular atresias and hypoplasias involving the mitral and aortic valve, resulting in more or less underdevelopment of the left ventricle. Babies with this syndrome become critically ill with congestive heart failure, metabolic acidosis, and hypoxia as soon as the ductus arteriosus closes, surely within the first week of life, sometimes even within hours. The outcome is fatal without operative intervention and somewhat better with surgery. The Norwood operative technique involves two stages. The first stage has to be performed within hours or days after birth and carries an approximately 50 per cent mortality. The second stage, with another 50 per cent mortality, has been proposed for the first or second year of life. Other centers have reported lower mortality rates. Experience is quite limited with this approach but given the uniformly fatal outcome of the malformation and a few survivors of the second-stage surgery with good postoperative hemodynamics, it may be worth consideration in a few selected centers with a large patient population. Another approach being proposed is early heart transplantation; experience with this is even more limited. The wise pediatrician who knows the family well may decide, after discussion with the parents, to choose not to intervene at all; after all, there *are* insolvable problems. The diagnosis is suspected clinically in a baby with symptoms as described, poor peripheral pulses, and a very large heart with pulmonary vascular engorgement. Characteristically, the echocardiogram is diagnostic; cardiac catheterization is mandatory for anatomic and physiologic details only for those who are to undergo surgery.

Patent Ductus Arteriosus. All newborns have an open ductus. In less than 1 per cent of full-term infants the ductus remains open beyond the first week of life. The incidence of a hemodynamically significant patent ductus arteriosus in prematures is 20 per cent overall; the smaller the baby and the more respiratory distress it has, the more likely it is to have an open ductus. On the basis of studies within the past decade, one may state without hesitation that prematures in whom a large ductus arteriosus does not close under usual medical management of congestive failure within approximately 48 hours should be given indomethacin by mouth or, when available, intravenously. If after treatment with indomethacin the ductus remains open, surgery with an operative risk of less than 1 per cent is recommended. The ductus arteriosus in full-term infants usually does not manifest itself within the first month of life. The diagnosis is suspected in a baby with congestive heart failure and bounding pulses, a systolic murmur with or without a diastolic component (rarely is the typical continuous murmur heard), a large heart with pulmonary vascular engorgement, and combined ventricular hypertrophy on the cardiogram. The echocardiogram is diagnostic. Indomethacin is ineffective beyond the first month of life. Surgery with or without preoperative catheterization is safe (hospital mortality less than 1 per cent) and curative.

Atrioventricular Canal. Congestive failure and cyanosis early in infancy are the usual manifestations of atrioventricular canal. The diagnostic feature is the superior axis of the electrocardiogram (between −30 and −90 degrees). There are regurgitant murmurs present and radiographic views show a large heart with pulmonary vascular engorgement. Close to three quarters of the babies with this defect who come to surgery are infants with Down's syndrome. The question of whether infants with Down's syndrome ought to be handled as aggressively as babies without chromosomal abnormalities used to be one of the most difficult dilemmas in pediatric cardiology. In the 1990s the law speaks very clearly. Down's babies with congenital heart disease have to be treated without regard for issues of quality of life. Given the propensity of these babies for cardiac failure as well as pulmonary artery hypertension, elective surgery is recommended beyond 6 months of age and much earlier if congestive heart failure is uncontrollable. Surgical mortality, depending on the age and the complexity of the anatomy, is between 5 and 10 per cent. No good long-term follow-up study of these babies is available.

Valvar Aortic Stenosis. The occurrence of valvar aortic stenosis with critical obstruction in a young infant is a real emergency. Without skillful operative intervention, these babies succumb within weeks or months. The presenting symptoms are congestive heart failure with poor cardiac output, which is not too dissimilar from hypoplastic left heart and even critical coarctation. The principal difference is that in these babies the cardiogram shows severe left ventricular hypertrophy with strain. The echocardiogram is diagnostic. It may be worth noting that the characteristic murmur of aortic stenosis may not be present until the baby's cardiac output has increased through treatment with vigorous anticongestive measures. Our present management consists of catheter-balloon dilation as a palliative and sometimes even curative procedure with negligible mortality and high degree of success. Surgery in those in whom ballooning failed, or was not attempted, is successful almost always but may also not be curative; repeat valvotomy and even aortic valve replacement may not be avoidable within the first one or two decades. Operative risk is less than 10 per cent.

Valvar Pulmonary Stenosis with Intact Ventricular Septum. Valvar pulmonary stenosis with an intact ventricular septum does not cause symptoms in infancy unless the obstruction is severe enough to result in right ventricular pressure of at least systemic level. In this case, the baby is cyanotic (right-to-left atrial shunt) and has the typical murmur of pulmonary stenosis, and the chest film shows a large globular heart with ischemic lung fields. The ECG indicates severe right ventricular hypertrophy, usually with P pulmonale, and the echocardiogram is diagnostic. Cardiac catheterization is recommended, on clinical diagnosis, in order to attempt balloon dilation of the pulmonary valve. This is highly effective and quite safe, with almost no mortality or complications. In our institution surgery is seldom necessary.

Pulmonary Atresia with Intact Ventricular Septum. Pulmonary atresia with intact ventricular septum presents itself with severe, even critical cyanosis as soon as the ductus arteriosus (the only source of pulmonary flow) closes. The clinical picture is quite similar to that of valvar pulmonary stenosis except that the electrocardiogram shows a mean frontal plane axis between +30 and +90 degrees without significant right ventricular hypertrophy. Also, cyanosis is more severe and the murmur is not that of pulmonary stenosis but rather of tricuspid incompetence. Emergency surgery is recommended (a Blalock-Taussig shunt plus opening of the right ventricular outflow tract) as a life-saving measure, but the mortality is relatively high (over 10 per cent) and cure unlikely. At this writing, this is a highly unsatisfactory situation in all but those with only marginally hypoplastic right ventricle.

Total Anomalous Pulmonary Venous Return. This disorder is one of the most difficult diagnostic problems in pediatric cardiology. These babies are very sick very early, within the first few days of life. Their heart size is normal. The lung fields are congested, but it may be difficult to know whether this in fact is pneumonia or pulmonary venous engorgement. Cyanosis may vary from severe to trivial. Murmurs are unimpressive. The ECG shows severe right ventricular hypertrophy. Sophisticated echocardiogram of the two-dimensional variety frequently pinpoints the diagnosis, but it has to be emphasized that this is the lesion most easily missed, not only by clinical examination and echocardiography but even at cardiac catheterization unless one's index of suspicion is very high. Surgery is mandatory following diagnosis. In our department, palliative measures like atrial septostomy are not recommended. Corrective surgery is highly effective, with a mortality of less than 5 per cent and good long-term outlook.

Tricuspid Atresia. There is no good explanation as to why tricuspid atresia, physiologically not very different from pulmonary atresia with intact ventricular septum, has a so much better prognosis. The clinical picture is similar, except for the usually smaller heart and an ECG with a mean frontal plane axis that is designated as a QRS between -30 and -90 degrees. Surgery, consisting of a Blalock-Taussig shunt within the first weeks or months of life, depending on the severity of the cyanosis and the limitation of exercise tolerance, can be carried out with a risk of less than 5 per cent. The "curative" Fontan operation at a risk of less than 5 per cent can be performed anywhere between 2 and 5 years of age, or even earlier, depending on the effectiveness of the previous Blalock-Taussig shunt. Long-term follow-up extending through 10 to 20 years seems to be satisfactory.

CHILDREN

Ventricular Septal Defect. Patients with a ventricular septal defect seldom present as an emergency with congestive heart failure beyond infancy in the United States today. Mostly they are referred on account of a murmur. How far one should investigate these patients if they are asymptomatic is one of the more difficult problems in the field. At the present time, given an asymptomatic child, I would not proceed beyond obtaining an electrocardiogram and probably (not certainly) a chest radiograph. If the results of both are normal, I would forget about it, although the more timid and trusting of our colleagues may recommend dental prophylaxis. If the ECG or chest radiography examinations show some abnormality, echocardiography is highly recommended. If these studies suggest a ventricular septal defect of significant size, cardiac catheterization should be performed. Surgery for those with pulmonary hypertension (pulmonary arterial mean pressure over 20 mm Hg) and a net left-to-right shunt is mandatory; for those without pulmonary artery hypertension but with a pulmonary to systemic flow ratio arbitrarily beyond 1.6 to 1, surgery may be advisable. In those few patients with pulmonary artery hypertension and no left-to-right shunt, those with the so-called Eisenmenger syndrome, surgery is contraindicated. Operative risks in uncomplicated cases should be 1 to 2 per cent, with elimination of the left-to-right shunt a virtual certainty. The course of pulmonary hypertension, if any, depends on many known and unknown factors.

Secundum Atrial Septal Defect. Patients with this relatively simple anomaly seldom present in infancy. It is the most common lesion to be discovered in childhood and adolescence or even in adulthood. Sophisticated pediatricians will suspect the diagnosis from the "fixed" splitting of the second sound, in association with the characteristic ejection murmur, and an early diastolic rumble, modest cardiac enlargement with pulmonary vascular engorgement, and an electrocardiogram showing right intraventricular conduction delay. A two-dimensional echocardiogram will show the size and shape of the opening in the atrial septum, particularly in younger children with thin chest walls. I believe all

atrial defects detectable by clinical means should be closed at some time before the end of the second decade. Surgical mortality is less than 1 per cent; long-term results are excellent. Successfully closed atrial defects do not need dental prophylaxis. In our institution, given a clear-cut clinical profile, preoperative cardiac catheterization is omitted except for therapeutic purposes. Recently a clam-shell device has been used, which is introduced into the left atrium through the inferior vena cava, occluding the defect. We have had good luck with this approach; there is no mortality, few complications, and it is highly effective.

Endocardial Cushion Defect

ATRIAL SEPTAL DEFECT PRIMUM. This disorder is a somewhat more complex and potentially more serious defect than the secundum variety, most likely on account of its frequent association with a cleft mitral valve, resulting in mitral incompetence. The diagnosis is based on auscultatory findings, an electrocardiogram with a mean frontal plane axis between -15 and -60 degrees, and cardiac enlargement. There is some urgency about operating on these patients on account of the potential risk of the development of pulmonary hypertension and the effect of mitral regurgitation. Operative mortality is around 1 to 2 per cent, and long-term outlook is almost as favorable as that of the secundum variety. Antibiotic prophylaxis is recommended even after apparently successful surgery.

COMPLETE ATRIOVENTRICULAR CANAL. The complete atrioventricular canal variety of the endocardial cushion defect is a more serious problem. These patients have already been discussed in the infant's group, since they frequently present as ventricular defects with a superior frontal plane axis in severe heart failure in a young baby. Surgery is mandatory, with an operative mortality beyond infancy of close to 5 per cent. A "cure" cannot always be expected. Mitral valve replacement may be necessary in the second or third decade and late arrhythmias (atrial fibrillation) are not uncommon.

Patent Ductus Arteriosus. Two or three decades ago this was the most common congenital cardiac malformation referred to pediatric cardiac centers. These days, many, even most, of the patients are being treated in infancy. Still, an occasional child with a classic ductus murmur does appear in the office of the pediatrician. If the clinical findings, the ECG, and the x-ray are classic, no catheterization is necessary except, as in secundum atrial defect, for curative purposes. An umbrella device is introduced through a cardiac catheter, which obstructs the ductal orifice. The procedure is safe and effective. The surgical risk is well below 1 per cent, and one can expect to achieve a perfectly normal circulation for the rest of the child's life.

Tetralogy of Fallot. This is by far the most common cyanotic defect to present beyond infancy. The typical clinical picture, the murmur, the radiograph, and the electrocardiogram allowed Dr. Helen Taussig to make this diagnosis with great accuracy through many decades without cardiac catheterization. Many thousands of children all over the world benefited from the shunt operation bearing her and Dr. Blalock's name. Today the Blalock-Taussig shunt is rarely indicated for children with tetralogy of Fallot. Since complete correction is the preferred operation, cardiac catheterization is necessary to furnish appropriate anatomic and physiologic details. The operative risk is around 2 per cent, and long-term results are excellent.

Coarctation of the Aorta. Next to atrial defect of the secundum variety, coarctation of the aorta is the most common congenital cardiac malformation to be discovered in childhood. The reason for this is the reluctance of pediatricians to obtain blood pressure measurements in infants. Also, regrettably, feeling for the femoral pulses, like noting the right radial pulse, is still not an automatic part of pediatric physical examination. Whenever a coarctation of the aorta is discovered, it should be operated upon—the earlier, the better. The long-term results are better the younger the patient is at the time of surgery. At our institution, those with the classic clinical picture do not undergo preoperative catheterization. Operative risks are estimated at 1 to 2 per cent and long-term results are good, although a certain percentage need reoperation.

Valvar Pulmonary Stenosis. Valvar pulmonary stenosis should be treated surgically if the right ventricular pressure is at least 50 per cent of the systemic arterial pressure. The best clinical tool for estimating the severity of pulmonary valvar obstruction is the electrocardiogram; patients beyond infancy presenting with clear-cut right ventricular hypertrophy in the chest leads almost certainly have a significant increase of right ventricular pressure. Given the characteristic auscultatory and radiologic findings, surgery can be, and has been, performed without catheterization. The two-dimensional echocardiogram with Doppler flow measurement further improves the accuracy of the clinical assessment. Still, in most cases, traditional cardiac catheterization is performed preoperatively. The recent introduction of the use of balloon angioplasty makes this approach a more logical one. Within the framework of cardiac catheterization, balloon fracture of the pulmonary valve can be accomplished and thoracotomy can be avoided. There is no mortality so far with this noninvasive management of pulmonary stenosis, and the surgical mortality is also less than 1 per cent. Long-term results are excellent.

Valvar Aortic Stenosis. Valvar aortic stenosis commonly first presents in childhood. The diagnosis is easily made through the typical murmur of aortic stenosis coupled with left ventricular hypertrophy in the cardiogram. The x-ray contributes relatively little to the clinical picture and is of little use in quantitation in this age group. Echo-Doppler cardiogram is very helpful in determining the gradient across the valve. Still, most centers, justifiably, perform cardiac catheterization less for diagnosis than for balloon dilation, as indicated in the section on infants. All patients with a resting gradient of over 50 mm Hg with or without left ventricular strain in the ECG should be ballooned. Gradients of under 25 mm Hg do not need intervention. Those with gradients between 25 and 50 mm Hg with normal ECG should probably be managed conservatively and do not need surgery. To postpone aortic valve replacement, surely necessary for calcific aortic stenosis, as far as possible, we are inclined to propose a valvotomy even for those patients with moderate aortic valve obstruction. Surgery is safe (between 1 and 2 per cent mortality), but need for re-operation is likely in the third or fourth decade. Very careful, at least yearly, follow-up is mandatory, and careful antibiotic prophylaxis is essential.

THE CHILD AT RISK OF CORONARY DISEASE AS AN ADULT

JAMES J. NORA, M.D.

Because of lively debate on the issue of pediatric preventive programs for coronary disease, it must be stated that the following recommendations may be opposed by some. In the absence of 70-year longitudinal studies, one can always assert that the evidence for the efficacy of a specific or even a general preventive program is not available. With this disclaimer, I present the approach we follow on our service.

1. For the majority of children and families, specific preventive programs are not required beyond a general commitment to a life-style that embraces exercise, ideal weight, stress control, a reasonably prudent diet (but not necessarily adhering consistently to the prudent diet shown in Table 1), and abrogation of smoking. However, it should be noted that this prudent diet is the diet recommended by the U.S. Senate committee on nutrition for *all* Americans.
2. For high-risk children from high-risk families, the commitment to prevention cannot be casual. Those at high risk should be deliberately sought out at an early age and should have a preventive program

TABLE 1. A Prudent Diet

1. Avoid overweight, consume only as many calories as you expend: if overweight, decrease calories and increase expenditure.
2. Increase consumption of fruits, vegetables, and whole grains (complex carbohydrates and "naturally occurring" sugars) from the present 28 per cent of calories in the average diet to about half (48 per cent) of your caloric intake.
3. Decrease consumption of refined and other processed sugars and foods high in such sugar by almost half (about 45 per cent) to account for only about 10 per cent of total calories.
4. Decrease consumption of foods high in total fat from 42 per cent of calories to 30 per cent.
5. Specifically reduce saturated fat in the diet (from the present 16 per cent to 10 per cent) and partially replace this with polyunsaturated and monounsaturated fat to account for the remaining 20 per cent of fat intake, by reducing intake of animal fat from meats and high-fat dairy products. Eat more fish and poultry, and select lean meats low in fat (e.g., trimmed ground round in place of hamburger). Low-fat and non-fat milk may be substituted for whole milk except in those infants whose diet is almost entirely milk.
6. Reduce cholesterol to about 300 mg per day. (The major dietary sources of cholesterol are egg yolks, meats, whole milk, and high-fat dairy products.) For children, the major dietary source of cholesterol is whole milk.
7. Decrease consumption of salt and foods high in salt content.

TABLE 2. Diet for Those With High Cholesterol Levels That Do Not Respond Adequately to the Prudent Diet

1. Avoid overweight, as in the prudent diet.
2. Increase consumption of complex carbohydrates (fruits, vegetables, grains) to about half (48 per cent) of total caloric intake, as in the prudent diet.
3. Decrease refined sugar and other processed sugar to about 10 per cent of total calories, as in the prudent diet.
4. Decrease total fat intake to 30 per cent of calories, as in the prudent diet.
5. Reduce saturated fat and take twice as much polyunsaturated fat (P/S = 2/1), as in the prudent diet.
6. Reduce cholesterol to 100 mg; this is lower than in the prudent diet.
7. Reduce salt consumption, as in the prudent diet.

TABLE 3. Diet For Those Who Have Both High Cholesterol and High Triglycerides That Do Not Respond Adequately to the Prudent Diet

1. Reduce weight to the lower limits of the desirable weight range.
2. Maintain complex carbohydrate consumption (fruits, vegetables, grains) at about half (48 per cent) of total calories, as in the prudent diet.
3. Eliminate as much as possible refined sugars and processed foods high in sugar—certainly hold this to less than 5 per cent of calories. This is lower than in the prudent diet.
4. Decrease total fat intake to 30 per cent of calories, as in the prudent diet.
5. Reduce saturated fat, as done in the other diets, to the point that twice as much polyunsaturated fat is consumed as saturated (P/S = 2/1).
6. Reduce cholesterol to 100 mg per day, much lower than in the prudent diet.
7. Reduce salt intake, as in the prudent diet.

designed to attack the specific risk factors. We recommend that at between 1 and 2 years of age (or at later pediatric ages if necessary) the following be done.

a. Obtain a family history of onset of coronary disease or stroke in first- and second-degree relatives before age 65.
b. Obtain family history of hypertension in first- and second-degree relatives and begin annual "tracking" of patient's blood pressure.
c. Obtain serum cholesterol level.
d. For those with a family history of early-onset coronary heart disease or stroke and a cholesterol level about 160 mg/dl, the cholesterol study should be repeated and the prudent diet initiated if the cholesterol level is found to be above 160 mg/dl on the second determination.
e. For those without a family history, the cholesterol level may be "tracked" at annual visits for 2 years. If the elevated level persists over 160 mg/dl, the prudent diet should be instituted and consistently adhered to.
f. Young children *with a positive (or unknown) family history* who do not respond to a prudent diet by lowering cholesterol (being sure that the prudent diet is truly being followed) should receive the following additional evaluation and therapeutic approach.
   (1) A study of total cholesterol, high-density lipoprotein (HDL) cholesterol, low-density lipoprotein (LDL) cholesterol, and triglycerides in the child for phenotyping.
   (2) An initial study of cholesterol levels in first-degree family members (parents, siblings) to help distinguish between the dietary-resistant monogenic and the dietary-responsive polygenic forms. This differential diagnosis will be discussed in the next section.

(3) If the family pattern is compatible with the polygenic forms, diet alone (with the healthful life-style indicated in Item 1) is all that is usually necessary. However, a diet stricter than the prudent diet may be required for some families. These diets are provided in Tables 2 and 3. Diets for elevated triglycerides alone are rarely needed for polygenic forms, and the contribution of high triglycerides to coronary disease is small compared with cholesterol. If a child has elevated triglycerides in spite of being ideal weight but does not simultaneously have high cholesterol, we do not usually suggest a special diet beyond the prudent diet.

3. Distinguishing monogenic from polygenic forms of hyperlipoproteinemia.
   a. Monogenic forms in heterozygotes generally have the following features:
      (1) Higher levels (e.g., cholesterol in childhood of 260 mg/dl rather than 200 mg/dl).
      (2) Do not respond well to diet alone.
      (3) Show bimodality in cholesterol values in family studies. A "classic" monogenic family of six first-degree relatives (adults and children) would have the following cholesterol values: 300, 290, 310, 180, 195, 175—as though the cholesterol levels were coming from two different populations or families.
   b. A "classic" polygenic family of six first-degree relatives (adults and children) would have the following cholesterol levels: 220, 240, 255, 215, 260, 205—as though the cholesterol levels were all from the same bell-shaped distribution curve.
   c. The monogenic forms should fit comfortably into the lipoprotein phenotype classification of Fred-

TABLE 4. Phenotyping Hyperlipoproteinemias

Phenotype	Cholesterol	Triglycerides	Serum	Electrophoresis	Ultracentrifugation
I	↑	↑	creamy	Chylomicrons	Chylomicrons
IIa	↑		clear	Beta ↑	LDL ↑
IIb	↑	↑	± cloudy	Beta ↑, pre-beta ↑	LDL ↑, VLDL ↑
III	↑	↑	± cloudy	Broad beta	Intermediates
IV		↑	± cloudy	Pre-beta ↑	VLDL ↑
V	↑	↑	creamy	Chylo, pre-beta ↑	Chylo, VLDL ↑

rickson and the W.H.O., with the caution that possible underlying diseases such as hypothyroidism and lupus must be eliminated before concluding that the lipoproteinemia is a primary rather than a secondary disorder. See Table 4 for a classification of phenotypes.

4. Treating monogenic hyperlipoproteinemias in heterozygotes.
    a. This is the most difficult and controversial area.
    b. Even strict dietary measures are usually insufficient.
    c. We do not usually consider medication except for patients with cholesterol levels above 240 mg/dl in children and 270 mg/dl in young adults on a 100-mg cholesterol diet.
    d. If medications are then used, we first consider what medications are showing successful results in the parents and older siblings, because there is doubtless considerable heterogeneity among the monogenic disorders. If a regimen works well for one family member, it is more likely to work in first-degree relatives.
    e. A resin (such as cholestyramine or colestipol) in combination with nicotinic acid or either agent alone is used in children (with considerable caution, starting with very low doses, looking for adverse reactions, and being prepared to discontinue if results are unsatisfactory). A dosage schedule is not offered for these drugs because one has not been established for children. If management with drugs is undertaken as the lesser of two unfavorable alternatives, it may be wise for the primary physician to work with a consultant experienced in this area.

5. Treating monogenic hyperlipoproteinemia IIa in homozygotes. These rare conditions require intensive diagnostic evaluation at the hands of experienced consultants. Portacaval shunt has been the most efficacious approach in our experience.

CARDIAC ARRHYTHMIAS

WELTON M. GERSONY, M.D.

Childhood cardiac rhythm disturbances are recognized more often now because diagnostic methods have improved. Furthermore, there are more surgical survivors after repair of congenital heart disease, and some of these patients may be prone to rhythm disturbances.

The major risk of a cardiac rhythm disorder is that a severe tachycardia or bradycardia may lead to decreased cardiac output, a more severe arrhythmia, syncope, or sudden death. When there is apparent ectopic cardiac activity, the major issue is whether there may be deterioration into a life-threatening tachyarrhythmia or bradyarrhythmia. Some rhythm abnormalities, however, such as single premature atrial and ventricular beats are common among children without heart disease and in the great majority of instances do not pose a risk. Thus, accurate differential diagnosis of cardiac arrhythmias is critically important prior to most decisions about further studies, pharmacologic treatment, restriction of physical activities, and prognosis.

An increasing number of pharmacologic agents are available for the treatment of significant rhythm disturbances in children (Table 1). Problems with frequency of administration, compliance, side effects, and variable responses remain, and selection of an antiarrhythmic agent still involves a great deal of empiricism. However, for most rhythm disturbances, treatment regimens with single agents that reliably control the abnormal rhythm pattern are available. Surgical intervention to eliminate bypass tracts associated with pre-excitation syndromes or unusually electrically active areas in the heart is available, but this approach is reserved for situations in which extreme measures are necessary to control a life-threatening rhythm disorder. Finally, implanted pacemakers are currently more reliable and less prone to technical failure than in the past.

BRADYCARDIA

Bradycardia in older children and adolescents is defined as a heart rate of less than 60 beats per minute. Sinus bradycardia may occur because of abnormalities in sinus node automaticity, central nervous system disease, hypoxia, metabolic disease, drug effects, or injury to the sinus node region. However, sinus bradycardia is most often seen as a normal phenomenon, especially in a well-conditioned athlete. The cause of bradycardia that is of the most concern is complete heart block. Atrioventricular (AV) conduction is blocked at the level of the AV node or His-Purkinje system. This results in an intrinsic ventricular rhythm that is independent of atrial activity. The atrial rate is always faster than the ventricular rate, and the electrocardiogram shows no consistent relationship between the P wave and the QRS; the P wave is seen to "march through" the QRS. In most instances of complete heart block, the heart rate is between 30 and 40 beats per minute.

Sinus Bradycardia

When sinus bradycardia is secondary to a noncardiac pathologic process, the underlying disorder requires urgent management and no specific therapy is required for the bradycardia. For example, in the presence of a subdural hematoma resulting in central nervous system–mediated sinus bradycardia, successful evacuation of the hematoma will result in the re-establishment of a normal cardiac rate. Similarly, sinus bradycardia as a result of a high degree of physical conditioning is a normal response and requires no attention.

Sick Sinus Syndrome

The sick sinus syndrome occurs when abnormalities in impulse production in the sinus node and/or atrial conduction pathways result in a slow cardiac rhythm. In many patients, the conduction is variable depending on activity, release of catecholamines, and/or sympathetic or parasympathetic stimulation. A 24-hour electrocardiogram may reveal periods of sinus rhythm, sinus slowing, atrial escape rhythms, and/or supraventricular tachycardia. The latter may be referred to as

TABLE 1. Commonly Used Antiarrhythmic Drug Schedules in Pediatric Patients

Drug	Oral Administration		Intravenous Administration*		Comments and Side Effects	
	Maintenance Dose†	Maximal Maintenance Dose	Loading Dose	Maximal Dose	Comments	Side Effects
Digoxin	0.01–0.02 mg/kg/day DD‡ q12h	0.5 mg	0.025–0.05 mg/kg in 3 DD q4–8h	0.5 mg	Oral loading dose 0.04–0.07 mg/kg/day DD q8h See text for age-related differences	APD's, VPD's, conduction defects, bradycardia, nausea, vomiting, anorexia
Quinidine sulfate	20–60 mg/kg/day DD q6h	2.4 gm	—	—		Nausea, vomiting, diarrhea, cinchonism, QRS and QT prolongation, AV block, asystole, syncope, thrombocytopenia, hemolytic anemia, blurred vision, convulsions, allergic reactions, exacerbation of periodic paralysis, enhancement of digoxin effects
Quinidine gluconate	20–60 mg/kg/day DD q8–12h	2.0 gm	10–15 mg/kg as 250 µg/kg/min	20 mg/min to 1.0 gm	Oral test dose 2 mg/kg	
Procainamide	50–100 mg/kg/day DD q4–6h DD q6h†	6.0 gm	10–20 mg/kg as 300 µg/kg/min	20 mg/min to 1.0 gm	Intravenous maintenance 20–80 µg/kg/min	PR, QRS, QT prolongation, anorexia, nausea, vomiting, rash, fever, agranulocytosis, thrombocytopenia, Coombs-positive hemolytic anemia, lupus erythematosus–like syndrome, hypotension, exacerbation of periodic paralysis
Disopyramide	8–12 mg/kg/day DD q6h DD q12h†	1.2 gm	—	—	—	Anticholinergic effects, urinary retention, blurred vision, dry mouth, QT and QRS prolongation, exacerbation of periodic paralysis, negative inotropic effects
Phenytoin	3–6 mg/kg/day DD q12h	600 mg	10–15 mg/kg as 250 µg/kg/min	20 mg/min to 1.0 gm	—	Rash, gingival hyperplasia, CNS manifestations, ataxia, lethargy, vertigo, tremor, macrocytic anemia
Lidocaine	—	—	1 mg/kg repeat q5 min × 3	50–75 mg	Intravenous maintenance 30–50 µg/kg/min	CNS effects, confusion, convulsions, high-degree AV block, asystole, coma, paresthesias, respiratory failure
Verapamil	4–10 mg/kg/day DD q8h	480 mg	0.075–0.15 mg/kg q20 min × 2	5 mg	—	Bradycardia, asystole, high-degree AV block, hypotension, congestive heart failure, enhancement of digoxin effects
Propranolol§	1–4 mg/kg/day DD q6h	Not established	0.1–0.15 mg/kg	1 mg/min to 10 mg	Long-acting beta-blocking agents (nadolol, atenolol) are preferred for long-term therapy (less frequent administration and CNS side effects)	Bradycardia, loss of concentration or memory, bronchospasm, hypoglycemia, hypotension

From Gersony W, Hordof AJ: Cardiac arrhythmias. *In* Dickerman JD, Lucey JF: Smith's The Critically Ill Child: Diagnosis and Medical Management. 3rd ed. Philadelphia, WB Saunders Co, 1985.

*Intravenous administration of antiarrhythmic drugs should always be given slowly with constant monitoring of blood pressure and electrocardiogram, particularly in patients with compromised cardiac, renal, or hepatic function. Dose must be modified in patients with abnormal renal or hepatic function.

†Sustained-release preparations available for clinical use.

‡Divided doses.

§Manufacturer's warning: Safety and efficacy of propranolol for use in children have not been established.

the bradycardia-tachycardia syndrome. The sick sinus syndrome may occur spontaneously in the absence of associated congenital heart disease and has been reported in siblings. It is most commonly seen after surgical correction of congenital heart defects, especially after the Mustard operation for transposition of the great arteries. This operation involves removal of the atrial septum. Clinical presentation as well as management depends on the heart rate. Many patients remain asymptomatic without treatment. Dizziness and syncope can occur during periods of marked sinus slowing with failure of adequate escape rhythms but also may be observed during supraventricular tachycardia. More often, the heart rate will decrease to the range of 30 per minute during sleep. Treatment varies according to clinical presentation. If drug therapy other than digoxin is deemed necessary to control tachyarrhythmia, most agents that are used (e.g., propranolol, quinidine, procainamide) will suppress sinus and atrial ventricular nodal function to the degree that symptomatic bradycardia may be produced. Thus, a demand ventricular pacemaker to protect against bradycardia may be required if drug therapy is needed for suppression of tachyarrhythmia. However, the majority of patients have only periods of bradycardia and, if no symptoms are associated with this, treatment is unnecessary. However, in the presence of symptoms or unacceptable bradycardia (less than 30 beats per minute) pacemaker insertion may be required.

Complete Heart Block

Congenital heart block is a not infrequent abnormality and may be identified in utero. In most instances, no treatment is required during the neonatal period and beyond. Indeed, individuals may live into old age without symptoms or necessity for treatment of any kind. When complete heart block is associated with congenital heart disease, temporary or even permanent cardiac pacing may be required in the newborn period or later in life. However, in most instances, even in the presence of heart disease, a slow, stable cardiac pacemaker arising from the His-Purkinje system, especially with a narrow QRS, tends to be stable for an indefinite period.

Rarely, a patient with congenital heart block will have a syncopal episode. When this occurs, pacemaker therapy should be instituted.

Acquired Complete Heart Block

When complete heart block occurs secondary to surgical repair of a congenital heart defect, permanent pacemaker therapy is virtually always necessary. When heart block is noted immediately after operation, temporary pacing is instituted and is continued for 2 to 4 weeks. If spontaneous normal AV conduction does not return, permanent pacing is instituted prior to discharge from the hospital.

Drug Therapy. Atropine (0.01 to 0.02 mg/kg intravenously; maximum 1.0 mg) is effective in treating supraventricular bradycardias. The same dose is used to enhance AV conduction in transient heart block. However, in unusual circumstances, the acceleration of sinus rate may exceed the improvement of AV conduction caused by the atropine and may result in a rate-related increase in the degree of block with a reduction in the ventricular rate.

Isoproterenol is used for the treatment of supraventricular bradycardia and atrioventricular block. It is the agent of choice for symptomatic complete heart block until a cardiac pacemaker can be introduced. Isoproterenol is titrated to desired effect or until toxic effects are observed. The usual dosage range is 0.05 to 0.5 μg/kg/min. Beta-adrenergic stimulating agents should be used with caution in patients with hypoxia or acidosis and in those who are taking digitalis preparations.

Cardiac Pacing. Cardiac pacemakers are used for treating patients with bradyarrhythmias, to control the cardiac rate, and recently have also been used to convert cardiac arrhythmias. Most of the modern pacemaker's functions can be controlled by external means after its insertion. In children, the most common indications for cardiac pacing are complete heart block, either postsurgical or congenital, and sick sinus syndrome. The latter is common after open heart surgery for transposition of the great vessels (Mustard procedure). However, most patients do not require a pacemaker.

Pacing is most commonly carried out from the right ventricle; however, recently, atrial pacemakers have been used more frequently, with pacing wires inserted in the right atrium. The pacing wires can be inserted either transvenously or via a thoracotomy on the epicardial surface of the heart. In infants, either epicardial or transverse endocardial wires are employed for long-term pacing. In older children and adults, transvenous pacemaker insertion is the preferred method of electrode placement.

In addition to having the ability to pace the heart, modern pacemakers have a sensing system that allows them to sense the patient's spontaneous rhythms. The most commonly used ventricular pacemakers are the R-wave–inhibited pacemakers. If the pacemaker senses the spontaneous R-wave of the patient's inherent rhythm, the output of the pacing mechanism is inhibited. The rate at which the pacemaker will discharge and be inhibited is preset. The pacing mode of the noncompetitive stimulation pacemaker will be inhibited at all spontaneous rates that are more rapid than the set pacemaker rate. This inhibition theoretically prevents the occurrence of competitive arrhythmias. Noncompetitive atrial P-wave–inhibited pacemakers are also available.

The newest, most sophisticated type of pacemaker produces atrioventricular sequential pacing at all pacing rates. These pacemakers require two leads, one in the atrium and one in the ventricle. The atrial and ventricular leads are both used for pacing and sensing. In a patient with normal sinus rhythm the pacemaker functions by sensing the atrium and stimulating the ventricle. However, should the patient have severe bradycardia or sinus arrest, these pacemakers function as atrioventricular sequential and synchronous pacemakers at a preset low rate. This pacemaker provides for every contingency of cardiac pacing under all physiologic conditions and is replacing all other types of atrioventricular sequential pacemakers.

Automatic antitachycardia pacemakers are used in extreme circumstances for patients with tachyarrhythmias that are refractory to standard medical or surgical intervention. These pacemakers can be activated in response to symptomatic tachycardia. Automatic implantable cardiac defibrillators are available which deliver an electric shock to terminate ventricular tachycardia or fibrillation. Prior to use of these types of pacemakers, detailed intracardiac electrophysiologic testing must be carried out to ascertain whether a particular type of pacing will terminate the tachyarrhythmia.

TACHYARRHYTHMIAS

Supraventricular Tachycardias

In most infants and children who have supraventricular tachycardias without associated cardiac diseases, adequate hemodynamic status is maintained for extended periods. Therefore, in a hemodynamically stable patient a gradual approach for termination of the tachycardias can be carried out. The length of time that these arrhythmias will be tolerated is a function of (1) the underlying state of the myocardium, (2) the rate of the tachycardia, and (3) the duration of the abnormal rhythm. It should be emphasized that electrical cardioversion is the treatment of choice in any patient in whom the cardiac output is significantly compromised.

The first measure is that of vagal stimulation. Initiation of a strong vagal discharge by inducing the diving reflex is the most effective maneuver to enhance vagal tone in children. In a neonate or infant, induction of the diving reflex is carried out by suddenly placing an ice-cold wet towel or washcloth on the patient's face and holding it there for several seconds. In older children, facial immersion in ice-cold water is similarly effective. Other vagal maneuvers, such as carotid sinus massage, stimulating the gag reflex, inducing vomiting, or ocular pressure, have not been as effective in infants as in older children and adults. Often a "vagal maneuver of choice" may exist for each patient, even a bizarre method such as a headstand.

Other measures to induce an increase in vagal tone include the intravenous administration of (1) an adrenergic agent such as phenylephrine in order to increase systolic blood pressure and initiate a responding baroreceptor reflex and (2) an acetylcholinesterase inhibitor, such as edrophonium (Tensilon) that enhances vagal tone by inhibiting the breakdown of acetylcholine by the enzyme acetylcholinesterase. Digitalis is the drug of choice for patients in whom antiarrhythmic drug therapy is to be used to convert supraventricular tachycardias. Once again the mechanism of action is that of vagotonic effect. Digoxin is the most versatile agent and can be administered intravenously, intramuscularly, or orally. The mode of administration is dependent upon how rapid an effect is required. It has a relatively rapid onset of action when used intravenously and has a long enough half-life that it does not have to be given very frequently when administration is long-term. Digoxin is administered intravenously as a total digitalizing dose of 25 to 50 µg/kg in divided doses, with a maximum

total digitalizing dose of 1 mg. The oral dose is 40 to 70 µg/kg in divided doses, with a maximum dose of 1.5 mg. The lower dose is recommended for neonates. Premature infants and patients with renal failure must be evaluated on an individual basis, and even lower doses are required because of decreased rates of excretion.

Digoxin is generally administered in divided doses, with a quarter to a half of the "digitalizing" dose given initially, followed in 2 to 8 hours by subsequent doses. The timing of the doses depends upon how rapidly it is necessary to convert the supraventricular tachycardia to sinus rhythm. The onset of action of intravenous digoxin is approximately 30 minutes, and the peak action occurs within 2 hours. Therefore, if the arrhythmia remains unchanged 2 hours after the initial dose, one can give a second dose of digoxin intravenously at that time.

Once conversion of the tachyarrhythmia occurs, digitalization of the patient can be completed at a more leisurely rate, and even orally rather than intravenously. For an oral dose, a third greater than the intravenous dose should be calculated. Maintenance digoxin dosage is a quarter to a third of the digitalizing dosage and usually is between 10 and 20 µg/kg/day orally, with a maximum maintenance dosage of between 0.25 and 0.5 mg/day. Digoxin has a relatively long half-life of 36 hours, and therefore the maintenance dose is administered either once daily or in divided doses twice daily.

Atrial flutter or fibrillation is also treated with digoxin, which slows the ventricular rate on the basis of the vagotonic effect. Rarely, digoxin converts atrial flutter to sinus rhythm. However, digoxin often converts atrial flutter to atrial fibrillation, resulting in a slower ventricular rate.

Digoxin must be used with care in patients with the pre-excitation syndrome in general, and not at all in those who have short antegrade effective refractory periods of the bypass tract. Digoxin may further shorten the antegrade effective refractory period of the bypass tract, resulting in enhanced conduction to the ventricle, particularly in patients with atrial fibrillation. This effect can result in very rapid ventricular rates that can lead to ventricular tachycardia or fibrillation. This mechanism is very uncommon in infants and children. However, it is a significant potential risk in older children and adults. Another concern about the use of digoxin is the potential for post-digitalis cardioversion-induced ventricular arrhythmias. This possibility is only theoretical and in practice is very uncommon in children. It would be of major concern in patients with severe underlying heart disease and would be unlikely to occur in patients with no structural heart disease unless digoxin had been given in near-toxic doses.

Verapamil is extremely effective in terminating supraventricular tachycardias, particularly those involving the AV node. Verapamil is a blocker of the slow inward current carried primarily by calcium. Since the action potentials of the AV node are "slow response type" calcium-mediated action potentials, verapamil is very effective in treating rhythm disturbances that originate in this region. Its advantage over digoxin is that it has a very rapid onset of action (3 to 5 min) and the effects are seen immediately. However, the immediate effects can also dissipate fairly rapidly, and subsequent doses may be required. The usual dose of verapamil is 0.075 to 0.15 mg/kg intravenously, with a maximum dose of 5 mg. It can be repeated between 10 and 30 minutes following the initial dose. Verapamil is also useful in slowing the ventricular response in patients with atrial flutter and fibrillation, particularly as an adjunct to digitalis therapy. However, verapamil has been shown to shorten the effective refractory period of the bypass tract in patients with pre-excitation syndrome, and therefore the same risks are present for these patients that exist with digitalis. Although verapamil has been proved to be more efficacious than digitalis in the immediate pharmacologic conversions of supraventricular tachycardias, it also has a higher incidence of side effects, particularly in infants, including a high degree of AV block, extreme bradycardia, asystole, hypotension, and congestive heart failure. The adverse cardiovascular effects can generally be overcome by treatment with beta-adrenergic agents such as isoproterenol and parenteral administration of calcium. Verapamil is also available as a long-term oral preparation. The starting oral dosage in children is approximately 4 mg/kg/day in three divided doses. This dosage can be increased until either therapeutic or early "toxic" effects are seen. The upper limits of the dosage for long-term oral preparation is approximately 10 mg/kg/day in infants and young children, but this limit has not been definitely established.

A third antiarrhythmic drug that can be used immediately for the treatment of supraventricular arrhythmias is the beta-adrenergic blocking agent propranolol. As with the other agents, the major effects are on the AV node. The blocking of sympathetic input to the AV node results in an unbalanced parasympathetic (vagal) effect. The intravenous dose of propranolol* is 0.1 to 0.15 mg/kg. The maximum immediate dose should not exceed 5 mg, and the maximum rate of administration should not be greater than 1 mg/minute. This dose can be repeated in approximately 20 to 30 minutes if no effect is seen. As with verapamil, side effects can include a high degree of AV block, extreme bradycardia, asystole, hypotension, and congestive heart failure. The adverse cardiovascular effects can be effectively treated with a beta-adrenergic agent such as isoproterenol.

On occasion, supraventricular tachycardia may be detected in utero. If the arrhythmia persists, the fetus may develop congestive heart failure that is manifested by evidence of hydrops fetalis. The administration of an antiarrhythmic drug such as digoxin to the mother at usual therapeutic doses will often convert the arrhythmia to sinus rhythm in utero. Thus, early delivery by cesarean section is avoided.

Electrical cardioversion using defibrillation and DC cardioversion is the emergency treatment of choice for any patient with a supraventricular tachycardia in an unstable hemodynamic state or severe congestive fail-

ure. This includes most forms of supraventricular tachycardia, atrial fibrillation, and atrial flutter with rapid ventricular response. Cardioversion is also used for elective conversion of these arrhythmias in stable patients who are refractory to routine long-term antiarrhythmic therapy. Such patients should be "anesthetized" by an agent such as diazepam or thiopental prior to the attempted cardioversion. Electrical cardioversion of an awake, fully alert patient is "unkind." The usual dose for cardioversion is 1 to 2 watt-seconds/kg.

Electrical conversion of supraventricular arrhythmias can also be carried out by electrical pacing. Supraventricular tachycardia can be converted either by inducing properly timed premature atrial beats or by rapid atrial pacing. Atrial flutter or fibrillation is best converted to sinus rhythm by means of electrical cardioversion. Atrial flutter also can be converted using rapid atrial pacing of the atrium at rates significantly faster than the flutter rate (entrainment).

Long-Term Management. Long-term therapy of supraventricular tachycardias can be carried out with a variety of antiarrhythmic drugs either alone or in combination. These include digoxin, beta-blocking agents (propranolol, nadolol, atenolol), verapamil, quinidine, procainamide, disopyramide, and other newer agents.

Long-term treatment of atrial flutter or fibrillation is commonly carried out with either digoxin to control the ventricular rate or a combination of digoxin and quinidine to prevent recurrence of the flutter or fibrillation. When treating atrial flutter, one should "protect the AV node" by digitalizing the patient prior to instituting quinidine therapy. This treatment prevents the occurrence of a more rapid ventricular response, which may follow quinidine administration because of the potential anticholinergic effects of quinidine on the AV node and slowing of the flutter rate. In addition, because of the interaction between digoxin and quinidine, the dose of digoxin must be decreased 25 to 33 per cent when quinidine therapy is prescribed for a "digitalized" patient.

A form of therapy that may be useful in selected refractory cases is surgery. Patients with pre-excitation syndrome who display life-threatening or refractory arrhythmias require careful endocardial and epicardial mapping to determine the location of the bypass tract, followed by surgical division. This procedure has been successful in patients with drug-resistant cardiac arrhythmias due to pre-excitation and recently has also been utilized successfully in patients with refractory atrial tachycardias secondary to ectopic atrial foci. The focus is removed surgically after careful mapping, which locates the area of disease from which the arrhythmia originates.

VENTRICULAR ARRHYTHMIAS

The management of the child with a ventricular arrhythmia is dependent upon the severity of arrhythmia, the associated hemodynamic effect of the arrhythmia, and the presence of associated cardiac and extracardiac disease. Premature ventricular depolarizations in a child with a normal heart, whether they are uniform with fixed coupling, uniform without fixed coupling,

---

*Manufacturer's warning: Safety and efficacy of propranolol for use in children have not been established.

multiform, or even couplets, do not require emergency therapy. This applies even if the premature ventricular depolarizations are in a bigeminal pattern unless they are interfering with cardiac hemodynamics or are a precursor to the development of ventricular tachycardia or fibrillation. In patients with abnormal cardiac function or conditions such as the prolonged QT syndrome, suppression of the ventricular ectopy is recommended. Ventricular tachycardia should be treated in most patients regardless of their hemodynamic state. Occasionally, if a child does not have associated heart disease and the tachycardia is "nonsustained" or well tolerated, long-term antiarrhythmic drug therapy may not be required. If the patient with ventricular tachycardia has severely compromised hemodynamics, electrical cardioversion with 1 to 2 watt-seconds/kg is the treatment of choice. For ventricular fibrillation, it is the only treatment available.

If the patient is stable enough that emergency electrical cardioversion is not immediately necessary, an intravenous access route should be established and treatment with intravenous lidocaine is instituted. The initial dose should be 1 mg/kg as a rapid bolus. The maximum amount administered in one dose should never exceed 75 mg. Lidocaine is effective in suppressing ventricular arrhythmias in approximately 85 per cent of pediatric patients. When recommended doses are used, lidocaine has no significant electrophysiologic effects on the AV conduction system, and other than suppression of the ventricular arrhythmia, changes in the PR interval, QRS duration, or QT interval are not seen. If the initial dose does not result in conversion of the arrhythmia, a bolus can be repeated every 5 to 10 minutes to a maximum dose of 3 to 5 mg/kg. Generally, if three doses do not convert the arrhythmia, then lidocaine is not going to be useful. Once lidocaine has been demonstrated to be effective, the intravenous bolus should be followed by an intravenous infusion at a rate of 30 to 50 μg/kg/min. It takes approximately three to five half-lives to reach the steady state of intravenous infusion (lidocaine half-life of approximately 90 min). If ventricular ectopy returns after 1 or 2 hours following the start of the intravenous infusion, rather than increasing the infusion rate, one should give another bolus of lidocaine at half the initial dose, or 0.5 mg/kg. Since the infusion may not have reached steady state at this time, the lidocaine level may have fallen below the therapeutic range. In patients with ventricular tachycardia that does not respond to intravenous lidocaine, the drug of choice is intravenous procainamide, given as a loading dose of 300 μg/kg/min and infused at a maximal rate of 20 mg/min to a maximum dose of 20 mg/kg (mixed as 1 gm of procainamide in 100 ml of normal saline). Once procainamide has been demonstrated to be effective, the loading dose should be followed by an intravenous infusion of 20 to 40 μg/kg/min.

To properly evaluate the efficacy of any of the antiarrhythmic drugs, one should obtain plasma drug levels to ensure that the dose being administered is resulting in therapeutic blood levels for that particular agent. Dosing schedules for children have not been well standardized and in most instances have been adapted from adult dosing schedules. Since there are significant differences in both the pharmacokinetics and responsiveness of the developing heart, one has to be very careful in extrapolating adult dosage to the child's dosage.

The choice of antiarrhythmic agent for the long-term suppression of ventricular arrhythmias in children must often be made on an empiric basis. There are no detailed studies of drug efficacy available to help determine the best choice of antiarrhythmic agents and the proper dosages for pediatric patients of different age groups.

Most patients are treated with quinidine or procainamide. Disopyramide has also been an effective agent. The development of sustained-release preparations has been helpful in encouraging compliance in patients taking antiarrhythmic agents. Newer antiarrhythmic drugs such as amiodarone and mexilitene await further evaluation to determine their place as effective and safe alternative therapy in children.

Surgical treatment of ventricular tachycardia in children is rarely required. However, surgical excision of an arrhythmogenic focus located at the right ventricular outflow tract has been carried out successfully. In addition, surgery has been carried out in children with arrhythmogenic right ventricular dysplasia and cardiac tumors.

MITRAL VALVE PROLAPSE

VICTORIA L. VETTER, M.D.,
and CHERYL C. KÜRER, M.D.

Mitral valve prolapse refers to the abnormal motion of one or both of the mitral valve leaflets into the left atrium during ventricular systole. Pathologically, the mitral valve leaflets are redundant, with myxomatous infiltration and degeneration. The chordae are elongated and thin and the valve annulus is dilated. When associated with chest pain, dyspnea, palpitations, anxiety attacks, skeletal deformities including pectus excavatum and scoliosis, and asthenic body habitus, the entity has been labeled the mitral valve prolapse syndrome. An increase in adrenergic tone, elevated serum catecholamine levels, and autonomic imbalance have been noted in these patients.

Mitral valve prolapse has become the most common cardiac diagnosis made in children, with an incidence of approximately 5 per cent. There appears to be an autosomal dominant pattern of inheritance with age- and sex-dependent (female > male) gene expression. Mitral valve prolapse may be isolated or seen in association with other disorders, including congenital heart defects such as secundum atrial septal defects, acquired heart defects such as rheumatic carditis, or connective tissue disorders such as Marfan's or Ehlers-Danlos syndrome.

Most pediatric patients present with a systolic murmur or mid-systolic click, although some present with chest pain, fatigue, exercise intolerance, anxiety attacks, palpitations, dizziness, or syncope. Prolapse of the mitral valve produces unique auscultatory findings consisting of a midsystolic click and/or late systolic murmur that may have a honking or whooping quality. The murmur and click, which may be intermittent and vary with position, are best appreciated with the patient standing, when the decrease in ventricular volume accentuates the prolapse of the mitral valve. The clinical diagnosis of mitral valve prolapse can be confirmed by echocardiography in 80 to 90 per cent of cases. Electrocardiographic abnormalities including ST-segment and T-wave changes and QTc prolongation are frequent in children with mitral valve prolapse. Supraventricular and ventricular arrhythmias may occur and are best appreciated by using 24-hour ambulatory monitors or exercise stress tests, which should be obtained in patients with symptoms or known or suspected arrhythmias.

Appropriate drug therapy is recommended in patients with symptomatic or life-threatening arrhythmias. Beta-blockers have been effective in treating many of these arrhythmias in children. Sudden death, although rare, has been reported in children and is presumed to be secondary to ventricular arrhythmias. It occurs in less than 1 per cent, most frequently in patients with documented serious ventricular arrhythmias, prolonged QTc interval, history of syncope, or family history of sudden death. In addition to cardiac arrhythmias and sudden death, the other major complication of mitral valve prolapse in childhood is bacterial endocarditis, which may result in severe mitral regurgitation. Antibiotic prophylaxis is indicated in children with a clinical diagnosis of mitral valve prolapse whether regurgitation is present or not, as mitral regurgitation may be an intermittent phenomenon. Neurologic manifestations, including migraines, are seen in childhood, but other more severe complications, such as transient ischemic attacks and cerebral vascular accidents, are rare.

The natural history of mitral valve prolapse during childhood is generally benign. Management of the asymptomatic patient requires reassurance regarding the favorable outcome and proper instruction regarding bacterial endocarditis prophylaxis. No restriction of physical activity is indicated in asymptomatic patients. Infrequent cardiac follow-up is indicated in asymptomatic patients to assess changes or evaluate symptoms if they occur. Symptomatic patients should be followed more frequently based on the nature of their associated complications.

CARDIOMYOPATHIES AND RELATED DISEASES

ROBERT H. FELDT, M.D.

The widespread use of echocardiography has enabled earlier and more accurate diagnosis of myocardial diseases. This technique has also added to the understanding of the extent and variety of these diseases.

Hypertrophic cardiomyopathy can present in infancy and childhood. A family history of cardiomyopathy and/or sudden death may lead to the diagnosis in asymptomatic children by use of echocardiography as a screening technique. Controversy exists as to whether or not asymptomatic children should be treated, but they should be followed for symptoms and/or signs of deteriorating cardiac function. Verapamil has been useful in patients with symptoms and echocardiographic evidence of diastolic ventricular dysfunction. Ultimately, cardiac transplantation will be a consideration for a number of these patients.

Dilated cardiomyopathy in children is diagnosed when lesions such as myocarditis, anomalous origin of a coronary artery, and the dilated type of endocardial fibroelastosis are excluded. Familial clusters of this disease have been reported. The diagnosis can be suspected when cardiomegaly or congestive heart failure occurs and other forms of heart disease are excluded. Typical echocardiographic features are enlargement of cardiac chambers, especially the left ventricle, and reduced estimate of ejection fraction. Anticongestive therapy for those in congestive heart failure has been shown to elicit a favorable response. Such patients may also benefit from reduction of afterload with captopril, hydralazine hydrochloride, or related drugs. Anticoagulation should be considered for those with significant cardiomegaly, as arterial embolic episodes have been reported. Dilated cardiomyopathy is frequently a progressive disease despite all forms of medical therapy. The overall mortality rate is high. These patients are candidates for cardiac transplantation when there is evidence that their ventricular function is deteriorating.

Cardiomyopathy in infants of diabetic mothers can be recognized in early infancy by its echocardiographic features of myocardial hypertrophy and decreased ventricular function. The syndrome represents a wide spectrum of myocardial involvement that is often self-limited, but deaths due to congestive heart failure have been reported. Treatment is largely supportive. Echocardiographic features of myocardial hypertrophy without obstruction may be present for a number of weeks after birth, but usually the echocardiogram becomes normal by 6 months of life.

Cardiomyopathy secondary to carnitine deficiency should be suspected in infants and young children with cardiac enlargement, frequent infection, failure to grow, and hypotonia. Low plasma carnitine levels establish the diagnosis. Successful therapy includes L-carnitine therapy of 50 to 350 mg/kg/day in an oral solution of 100 mg/ml concentration in four or more divided doses. Complete recovery has been reported.

Other forms of cardiomyopathy exist in pediatric patients, but they are not fully understood. Cardiomyopathy secondary to doxorubicin hydrochloride therapy for certain malignancies has been well documented. Unfortunately, there are no reliable methods to monitor potential toxicity during therapy other than serial endomyocardial biopsies. Dose levels and duration of doxorubicin therapy associated with cardiomyopathy have varied from patient to patient. Furthermore, new evidence is accumulating that cardiomyopathy may develop years after cessation of apparently successful doxorubicin treatment.

Tachydysrhythmias are also known to cause cardiomyopathy in children. The frequency of this syndrome is unknown, but careful monitoring of ECGs is indicated for patients presenting with cardiomyopathy of unknown cause. Rapid resting heart rate, abnormal P axis on ECG, or a history of palpitations or tachycardia may be an important clue to detection of such tachydysrhythmias. Successful treatment results from suspecting the diagnosis and submitting these patients to detailed electrophysiologic studies, and then appropriate treatment with antiarrhythmia medication or with surgical ablative techniques.

PERICARDITIS

Pericarditis in infants and children may be due to bacterial infection (purulent pericarditis). Purulent pericarditis most frequently occurs in infants and young children and can cause death if not recognized and treated early. High fever, malaise, and respiratory distress are all frequent presenting symptoms. Often there are other sites of bacterial infection including pulmonary infections, meningitis, osteomyelitis, and localized abscess, in descending order of frequency. Bacteria normally found are *Staphylococcus aureus,* pneumococci, and *Haemophilus,* in descending order of frequency.

Diagnosis is made by positive cultures obtained from pericardial fluid, blood, or other sites of infection. ST-segment and T-wave changes on ECG may be seen. Echocardiography will document the presence of pericardial fluid. Cardiac catheterization is rarely necessary. In addition to appropriate parenteral antibiotic therapy, the pericardial space must be evacuated.

Tuberculous pericarditis occurs in patients at risk and is diagnosed by a high index of suspicion and appropriate skin testing and cultures. Nontuberculous and fungal pericarditis (histoplasmosis) are uncommon.

All forms of infective pericarditis predispose to constrictive pericarditis, which may rapidly develop in infancy or childhood or, rarely, present as constrictive pericarditis without obvious antecedent infections. Significant constrictive pericarditis invariably requires operation to partially remove the pericardium.

Nonbacterial pericarditis is thought to be of viral etiology, although the offending agent is not always identified. Coxsackie B group viruses are most commonly implicated when a virus is found. The clinical picture is similar to that of bacterial pericarditis, although symptoms may develop more slowly and the child may have less severe fever. A pericardial rub or distant heart sounds on auscultation may suggest the diagnosis as well as associated pericardial effusion. Enlargement of the cardiac silhouette on radiography mandates the use of echocardiography to establish the diagnosis as well as to document the volume of pericardial effusion present, which may require pericardiocentesis for evacuation.

Bacterial cultures must be taken from pericardium, blood, and other suspected infected sites to exclude purulent pericarditis. Nonsteroidal anti-inflammatory agents have been proven to be effective. Salicylates are

considered superior to indomethacin. Patients receiving salicylate therapy need to be observed closely for symptoms of Reye syndrome.

Occasionally, the disease recurs and may recur multiple times. Corticosteroids have been effective for patients with multiple recurrences, but such therapy does not necessarily prevent further recurrences. Only rarely is pericardiectomy necessary.

Pericarditis is also seen in patients with uremia, patients who have received thoracic radiation, and patients with connective tissue diseases such as rheumatoid arthritis and systemic lupus erythematosus.

A form of pericarditis is seen frequently following cardiac surgery (postpericardiotomy syndrome). This disease is manifested by fever, pericardial friction rub, and distant heart sounds, although all of those signs may not be present. Echocardiography may detect accumulation of pericardial fluid, although minimal amounts of fluid will not exclude this diagnosis. The diagnosis may be suggested by enlarged cardiac silhouette on radiography. Pleural effusions are common. Cultures of fluid, blood, and other suspected sites are invariably negative. The white blood cell and differential counts are too variable to be specific, although leukocytosis is common.

Treatment consists of salicylates in therapeutic doses with careful monitoring of the patient for signs of Reye syndrome. Postpericardiotomy syndrome is usually self-limited, but chronic and recurrent cases are not uncommon. Corticosteroids have been used for a chronic relapsing course. Rarely, operation with pericardiectomy is necessary. Constrictive pericarditis has been reported as a rare complication in the late postoperative period.

SYSTEMIC HYPERTENSION

DAVID GOLDRING, M.D.,
ALAN M. ROBSON, M.D.,
and JULIO V. SANTIAGO, M.D.

Hypertension is the major health problem in our country, because it has been estimated that approximately 20 to 25 million people have hypertension and that about 250,000 die each year from the complications of this disease. Traditionally, hypertension has been classified as either primary or essential when the cause is unknown and as secondary when it is associated with or a consequence of renal, endocrine, or congenital vascular disease. Even in secondary hypertension, the specific cause is incompletely understood. The above classification profoundly affects the decision and results of therapy. For example, treatment for primary hypertension is usually effective, but it must be emphasized that the therapy is symptomatic. By contrast, for some forms of secondary hypertension the treatment may be curative. One must also keep in mind that the decision to treat a hypertensive patient depends upon the level of blood pressure which justifies a diagnosis of hypertension. This level of blood pressure is arbitrary. For example, the World Health Organization has recommended that 140/90 mm Hg be designated borderline hypertension and 160/95 mm Hg and higher as definite hypertension in adults. These values are inappropriate for infants and children, whose blood pressure is lower than that of the adult and increases progressively with growth. A reasonable working guideline might be as follows: The pediatric patients whose blood pressures are persistently between the 90th and 95th percentile for age and sex be considered suspect and those individuals whose pressures are persistently above the 95th percentile for age and sex be classified as hypertensives. Suggested blood pressure levels that we have used to identify suspect hypertensives are shown in Table 1.

PRIMARY HYPERTENSION

If the above arbitrary definitions of hypertension are used, the most common type in the pediatric population is primary hypertension. During a 5-year period, we measured the blood pressures in approximately 20,000 subjects, 14 to 18 years of age, in the St. Louis metropolitan area; one student was found with coarctation of the aorta and one with hypertension due to hyperthyroidism, but approximately 1000 suspected primary hypertensives were found.

Although the cause is unknown, effective symptomatic therapy is available.

The decision to use pharmacologic therapy in asymptomatic primary hypertensive pediatric patients must be examined from a different perspective than that used for the adult. Therapy may be more effective in the young, early hypertensive, and it may be possible to arrest or even cure the disease in the pediatric patient; this has not been possible in the adult. On the negative side, the undesirable, sometimes serious side effects of all antihypertensive drugs are well known, so that the risk-benefit ratio must be very carefully considered. The drug therapy must be a lifetime commitment, and there is no information about what serious untoward effects these drugs may have upon a young, growing subject. Finally, in a 10-year follow-up of approximately 100 young primary hypertensives we found that in 30 per cent the blood pressure spontaneously returned to normal levels. In the light of the above, we feel that the nonthreatening, safe, therapeutic regimen discussed below is the preferred course to follow in the young primary hypertensive.

Weight Reduction. It has been shown in studies that at least 50 per cent of young primary hypertensives are obese. The pathogenesis of the hypertension with obesity is unknown. In recent studies of adult obese hypertensives, significant reduction in systolic and diastolic pressures was achieved by weight reduction. There are no reported similar studies in pediatric patients, but we would recommend this approach in view of the above experience with hypertensive adults. Patient compliance would be difficult. Expert guidance by the physician is important, and the effectiveness of a weight-reduction program would be enhanced by consultation with a nutritionist, a social worker, and in some instances a psychiatrist.

Exercise. Regimens of dynamic exercise have been shown to normalize blood pressure in some adult primary hypertensives. We have just completed a study on a group of 30 adolescent primary hypertensives who all experienced a drop in systolic and diastolic pressures during and after an exercise regimen of 6 to 8 months. The mechanism for lowering blood pressure with dynamic exercise is incompletely understood. It has been suggested that several months of dynamic exercising produces a relatively hypokinetic circulatory state, which is probably due to the negative inotropic effect of reduction in heart rate and to adaptations in the neuroendocrine system, which results in increased vagal tone and decreased release of norepinephrine and epinephrine.

The regimen we suggest to our young patients is summarized in the following instructions. Supervision and surveillance are provided by weekly visits to the physician. This helps with patient compliance in this dramatic change in their life-style.

ENDURANCE EXERCISE TRAINING

For endurance exercise training to be effective in helping to lower your blood pressure, a few simple guidelines must be followed:

1. The activity should exercise a large amount of your muscle mass. Exercises which meet this requirement are running, cycling, and swimming.

2. The activity must elevate your heart rate to at least approximately 160 beats per minute. This can be measured by taking your pulse for 6 seconds *immediately after exercise* and multiplying it by 10. The pulse can be felt either at the wrist or in the neck below the angle of the jaw. Your doctor can help you locate the pulse if needed.

3. The activity must continue for 30 to 45 minutes at least every other day but preferably five times per week. If you select running, you should build up your endurance so that you run approximately 3 to 5 miles a day five times per week. If you select bicycling, you should build up your endurance so that you ride 10 to 15 miles a day five times a week. If you select swimming, you should build up your endurance so that you swim 1 to 2 miles a day five times per week.

The tendency is to start out much too quickly, which will elevate your heart rate too much and not allow you to continue for 40 minutes. The idea is to start slowly. Find the running, swimming, or cycling pace which results in a heart rate of approximately 160 beats per minute.

TABLE 1. Approximate Guidelines for Suspect Blood Pressure Values

| Supine Position—Lowest of Three Readings | | | |
Boys and Girls			
Age in years	3–5	6–9	10–14
Blood pressure mm Hg	>110/70	>120/75	>130/80

| Seated Position—Average of Second and Third Readings | | | |
	Girls		Boys
Age in years	14–18	14	15	16–18
Blood pressure mm Hg	>125/80	>130/75	>130/80	>135/85

Eventually you will have to increase your pace as your fitness level begins to increase. At this point, it is still essential that you attain a heart rate of approximately 160 beats per minute.

There are no shortcuts to physical fitness. It requires a sincere and serious promise to stick with the program, but it offers a way to lower your blood pressure without taking medicine.

Isometric exercise such as hand-grip and certain forms of weight lifting are not recommended for the adult primary hypertensive who may have in addition either known or silent coronary artery disease. In the young primary hypertensive the incidence of coronary artery disease is very low; therefore, isometric exercise does not pose a risk. However, more studies are needed before these exercises should be recommended for the young primary hypertensive.

Diet Modification (Blood Lipids). Some years ago a number of investigators proposed that elevated blood lipids predisposed an individual to the development of atheromatous coronary artery disease. Elevated blood lipids as well as hypertension were thus considered risk factors. Reducing the intake of foods with a high cholesterol content and drug therapy such as clofibrate, colestipol, and nicotinic acid to lower the blood cholesterol has been recommended for adults with hypertension to protect them against the development of atheromatous coronary artery disease. This subject is still controversial for the adult subjects. Therefore, advising radical changes in the diet for infants and children with primary hypertension to reduce the risk of developing coronary artery disease in adulthood is not justified, because we do not know what serious harm may come to the young individual from this drastic modification of the diet.

Dietary Salt Restriction. There is considerable circumstantial evidence suggesting a link between a high dietary salt intake and hypertension in genetically predisposed individuals. The degree of salt restriction required to produce a significant reduction in blood pressure is unknown. It is believed by some that a diet containing 50 mEq of salt per day may be effective in reducing blood pressure. The degree of salt restriction would be unpalatable, and most children would not comply. We therefore suggest that mothers do not add salt to food in cooking and that they restrict food with high salt content.

Other Forms of Therapy. Smoking should be prohibited, and contraceptive drugs, steroids, amphetamines, and liberal use of nose drops should be discontinued. Behavior modification methods such as biofeedback, relaxation techniques, and psychotherapy are of questionable benefit.

An occasional patient might be considered a candidate for drug therapy as described below under renal hypertension, e.g., a young primary hypertensive who is obese and has a strong family history of hypertension who has not responded to nonpharmacologic therapy and whose pressure is progressively rising.

Unfortunately, the treatment of hypertension in the young will continue to be symptomatic and weakly effective until the pathogenesis of primary hypertension is better understood.

SECONDARY HYPERTENSION

Renal Disorders

Secondary hypertension most often is the consequence of a renal lesion. It may present as an acute event, sometimes requiring treatment as a medical emergency. Alternatively, it may represent a problem of long-term management. Since the approaches to these two situations are different and the drugs used also differ, each will be discussed separately.

Management of Acute Hypertension and Hypertensive Crises. Patients who fit into these categories have no previous history of hypertension or have an acute increase in blood pressure above their previous stable values. Typically, blood pressure levels are elevated well above the 95th percentiles for age. When such an increase is associated with symptoms or signs of an encephalopathy or heart failure, it must be treated as a medical emergency. However, it is important to remember that children are more susceptible to the changes of malignant hypertension at lower blood pressure levels than are adults. Thus, we consider any child who presents with a systolic pressure of 170 mm Hg or greater or a diastolic pressure of 120 mm Hg or greater to be at risk of major complications and to require urgent treatment. Such urgent treatment may be indicated at even lower blood pressure values in the neonate or infant. The only exception to this general rule would be the patient with coarctation presenting in childhood, without heart failure.

Causes of such acute severe elevations in blood pressure include acute poststreptococcal and other acute glomerulonephritides, hemolytic uremic syndrome, collagen vascular diseases, especially when affecting the renal vasculature, chronic pyelonephritis, segmental renal hypoplasia, infantile polycystic kidneys, and renovascular diseases. The initial approach to treatment is the same, regardless of the underlying etiology.

Sodium retention plays an important role in the genesis of the hypertension in many of these patients. Thus, attempting to decrease body sodium content by limiting sodium intake and by increasing urinary sodium losses with diuretics often represents an important adjunct to therapy with antihypertensive drugs. However, it is inappropriate to rely upon this approach alone to treat severe acute hypertension. These measures take too long, frequently days, to become effective. Dietary sodium restriction alone can only prevent sodium retention from becoming worse, and the kidney typically responds poorly to diuretics in many of the renal diseases causing acute severe hypertension. The loop diuretics are the most potent. Our preference is to use furosemide 0.5 to 1.0 mg/kg given either orally or parenterally. On occasion we have used larger doses without problems. The thiazide diuretics are less effective.

The drug that we usually use first is hydralazine. It is a vasodilator that also increases cardiac output and has the advantage of not decreasing renal blood flow even when blood pressure is lowered. Side effects are those seen with vasodilators, namely flushing of the skin, headaches, tachycardia, and palpitations. They occur infrequently in children. The drug is well absorbed when given by mouth, and an effect typically is seen within 1 to 2 hours. The initial oral dose is 0.25 mg/kg and can be repeated every 4 to 6 hours. The total daily dose can be as high as 4.5 mg/kg/day. An effect from a dose of hydralazine of 0.15 mg/kg may be seen within a few minutes when given intravenously and within 15 to 30 minutes when given intramuscularly. Doses may be repeated within 30 to 90 minutes, but oral therapy should be implemented as soon as possible. The intravenous injection of hydralazine often is effective in reducing blood pressure in patients refractory to the drug given orally.

The combination of reserpine, 0.02 mg/kg/day to a maximum dose of 1 mg given intramuscularly every 12 hours, with hydralazine may be effective if hydralazine alone does not lower blood pressure satisfactorily. When reserpine is used, the dose of this drug is kept constant and the frequency of dosage of hydralazine is modified according to the patient's response. Some begin therapy with this combination of drugs. We avoid reserpine when possible because of its side effects, which include symptoms of depression in older children, drowsiness, nasal congestion, and stimulation of gastric secretion, which may result in peptic ulceration and bleeding from the gastrointestinal tract. It should not be used in patients in whom surgery is anticipated.

Patients who do not respond to the regimens outlined above should be treated next with diazoxide. The initial dose is 5 to 10 mg/kg given by rapid intravenous infusion over 1 to 2 minutes. A slower rate of administration usually is ineffective, because the drug is protein-bound. The dose can be repeated 30 minutes later if there is no response. The length of action of the drug typically is from 4 to 24 hours, although an effect for 36 hours or longer may be seen. Side effects are rare, although nausea and hyperglycemia have been reported. Hypotension does not occur unless frequent repeated small doses of the drug are given, usually in combination with other antihypertensive drugs.

Sodium nitroprusside is an effective intravenous antihypertensive agent that we use in patients who do not respond to any of the above drugs. Its onset of effect is immediate, and the response lasts for as long as the drug is infused. To prepare it for use, 50 mg are diluted in 1 liter of 5 per cent dextrose in water (50 μg/ml). The solution is infused at a rate of 0.5 to 8.0 μg/kg/min. The rate of infusion is titrated according to the blood pressure response. The drug is not stable when exposed to sunlight, so the bottle and infusion lines should be wrapped with aluminum foil throughout the infusion. Blood pressure should be monitored constantly throughout the infusion. Whenever possible the drug should not be administered for longer than 48 hours, especially in patients with renal failure, since the drug is metabolized to cyanide, which normally would be excreted by the kidney. If the drug has to be administered for 48 hours or longer, blood thiocyanate levels should be monitored after this period of time, and, if renal failure is present, cyanide may have to be removed by dialysis.

Very few patients do not respond to the preceding approach. Those who do not respond typically have hypertension in association with markedly elevated levels of plasma renin activity (PRA) and do respond to the angiotensin-converting enzyme (ACE) inhibitor captopril. The recommended starting dose is approximately 0.33 mg/kg three times a day. Neonates may require a smaller starting dose of 0.1 mg/kg. The drug is not stable in solution and should be given in tablet, or crushed tablet, form. If response is poor, the dose is increased in stepwise fashion, usually at 24-hour intervals, until a satisfactory response is obtained. The total daily dose should not exceed 6 mg/kg. The effectiveness of the drug often can be potentiated by the use of furosemide (1 mg/kg/day in two divided doses) and propranolol* (1 mg/kg/day in four divided doses, increasing to a maximum of 5 mg/kg/day). We prefer, however, to use a single drug, rather than a combination of drugs, when possible. Few acute side effects have been observed with captopril. Long-term complications include proteinuria and a decrease in the white blood cell count. If either abnormality develops, the drug should be discontinued. An alternate ACE inhibitor, enalaprilat, is given by IV injection and can be used if oral therapy is not appropriate.

The preceding, sequential approach to therapy is designed to control acute hypertension and to reduce the risk of major complications developing from the elevated blood pressure. Once blood pressures have been reduced below the 95th percentile for age, the physician should consider whether there may be a surgically treatable cause for the hypertension and, in those patients in whom hypertension is likely to be chronic, begin to introduce the appropriate drugs for long-term control of blood pressure.

Renovascular lesions are the most likely cause of secondary hypertension that can be controlled by surgery. They should be considered in any patient with very severe hypertension and in those with elevated PRA levels. Nowadays, such lesions can usually be demonstrated most satisfactorily after an intravenous injection of contrast agent and digital vascular imaging in centers where the appropriate equipment is available. This methodology avoids the much more invasive technique of renal arteriography. There has been considerable interest in the use of percutaneous transluminal angioplasty (PTLA) to treat patients with vascular stenoses, including those of the renal artery. This method appears to have limited value in children, since many of the renal artery lesions occur at the origin of the renal vessels and typically involve the abdominal aorta. There have been reports of successful treatment of mid-artery lesions in children using PTLA. It is not clear, however, whether such stenoses will return with time. Treatment of segmental lesions within the renal parenchyma can be particularly difficult. Successful selective embolization of a stenotic intrarenal artery in a child has been reported and would appear preferable to nephrectomy. In all cases, the surgical success de-

---

*Manufacturer's note: Data on the use of propranolol in the pediatric age group are too limited to permit adequate directions for use.

pends on the experience of the surgeon in this kind of work.

Management of Chronic Hypertension. The major difficulty in managing hypertension on a long-term basis is patient compliance. It is self-evident that if a drug is to be effective it must be taken regularly. Compliance is less a problem in the younger child, since most mothers ensure that the physician's advice is followed closely. Most problems are experienced in teenage patients. Compliance can be improved if the drug regimen is simple, is free from side effects, and is relatively inexpensive. A suitable regimen must be supplemented by extensive education of the patient and the family about hypertension, about the prescribed drugs, and about the reasons for prescribing those drugs. It is sometimes very hard to convince asymptomatic patients that they need to take potent drugs, usually for the rest of their lives. Follow-up should be as convenient for the patient as possible.

Antihypertensive drugs can be considered in three basic groups: vasodilators, diuretics that reduce volume, and those that modify release, metabolism, or function of pressor systems such as the renin-angiotensin system. The same principles about determining whether hypertension is volume or pressor-related and treating with a drug that has an appropriate action applies to children as to adults. Again, as in adults, if a drug from one major group is ineffective and a second drug is to be added, it is better to use a drug from a different group than from the same group. Thus, if a patient has a less than satisfactory response to a vasodilator and has a component of volume expansion, it is usually better to add a diuretic to the therapeutic regimen than another vasodilator. If secondary hyperreninism develops, the addition of a drug such as propranolol would be appropriate. However, such an approach often results in a confusing or cumbersome regimen that contributes to poor patient compliance. Thus, we prefer, whenever possible, to use maximum doses of a single drug rather than to use multiple drugs.

It is difficult to recommend specific regimens to treat hypertension. Each patient must have an approach individualized to his or her needs. Below we consider the major groups of drugs and our experience with them.

Vasodilator Drugs. Hydralazine may be used on a chronic as well as an acute basis. Its effectiveness, however, is limited in most patients with secondary hypertension. Its major value in our clinic is to treat night-time hypertension in patients treated primarily with guanethidine. Dosage and side effects have already been outlined. The protracted use of hydralazine in high doses may result in a syndrome resembling systemic lupus erythematosus (SLE). Typically, but not always, this reverses when hydralazine is discontinued. For this reason we do not like to use this drug in patients with SLE even though there is no evidence that hydralazine exacerbates SLE in patients on concomitant immunosuppressive therapy.

Minoxidil is a vasodilator that is a valuable addition to our armamentarium, since patients resistant to other drugs frequently respond to it. The recommended initial dose is 0.2 mg/kg as a single daily dose. This may be increased in increments of 50 to 100 per cent every 2 or 3 days until blood pressure control is achieved. The effective dosage range usually is between 0.25 and 1.0 mg/kg/day, with a recommended maximum daily dose of 50 mg. It is advised that a patient receive a beta-blocker such as propranolol before starting minoxidil. Since minoxidil induces fluid retention, which can be severe and result in pericardial effusions and tamponade, a diuretic such as furosemide should be used concurrently. The side effect that is most distressing to patients and their families is hypertrichosis. Many patients are unwilling to accept the severe overgrowth of hair over their face and forehead, and female patients dislike this growth on other parts of their bodies. Because of its side effects and the inability to use minoxidil as a single drug, we reserve this drug for patients who are resistant to other drugs.

Prazosin* has a direct effect on vascular smooth muscle and also has features of an alpha-adrenergic blocking agent. Therefore, reflex tachycardia typically is not a major complication when prazosin is used to lower blood pressure. The initial dose in older children is 1 mg two or three times a day. This may be increased slowly until an adequate response is obtained. Daily doses above 20 mg rarely increase the efficacy of the drug, although some patients may benefit from doses as high as 40 mg/day. There has been relatively little experience with this drug in younger children, and the size of the smallest capsules (1 mg) makes it difficult to provide a suitable starting dose for very small children. The effects of the drug are enhanced by simultaneous use of diuretics and beta-adrenergic blocking agents. Postural hypotension has been the most important side effect. Blood pressure should be monitored with the patient in the supine and in the upright positions. The patient should be alerted to the possibility of postural symptoms, and if they do occur, the patient should be advised to assume the recumbent position. Such side effects should alert the physician to the need to modify drug dosage. The major advantages of prazosin are the few side effects experienced with its use and the need for only twice-a-day dosage. However, in our experience, it is not as potent as other drugs. When used in large dosage, tachycardia and fluid retention may occur. Drugs that inhibit the transmembrane influx of calcium ions decrease peripheral vascular resistance and may be an effective adjunctive therapy. For example, nifedipine† may be started in an oral dose of approximately 0.5 mg/kg/day given in three individual doses. The dose can be later increased to 1 or 1.5 mg/kg/day.

Drugs Affecting Adrenergic Activity. Propranolol‡ has been found to be an effective antihypertensive agent in children. It is thought to act as a beta-adrenergic blocking agent. Since the renin-angiotensin system is regulated in part by beta-adrenergic activity, it was

*Safety and efficacy of prazosin in children have not been established.

†This use of nifedipine is not listed in the manufacturer's directions.

‡Manufacturer's note: Data on the use of propranolol in the pediatric age group are too limited to permit adequate directions for use.

thought originally that propranolol worked through this mechanism. More recent studies have indicated that other modes of action must be involved too. The drug is readily absorbed from the gastrointestinal tract. The initial dose should be between 0.5 and 1.0 mg/kg/day. Originally it was advised that the total dose should be divided into four doses a day; more recently, twice-daily doses have been found to be effective. Doses can be increased on a daily or every-other-day basis until a suitable response occurs. Daily doses as high as 16 mg/kg/day have been used. The major complication has been the development of heart failure. The drug should not be used, therefore, in any patient with heart disease or pulmonary disease, especially if heart failure is present. We do not use propranolol as a drug of first choice when treating chronic hypertension, because we have been disappointed with it when used alone. However, it is a most useful adjunct to other antihypertensive agents.

Several other beta-adrenergic blocking agents have been developed. The one that offers definite advantages for children is nadolol,* since it is effective when taken once a day.

Guanethidine blocks sympathetic activity and has a prolonged serum half-life, which permits a single daily dose. This is a major advantage when treating hypertension in children. It works only when the patient assumes the upright position and therefore is of very limited value in neonates and infants. In children between the ages of 2 and 10 years we usually use a single daily dose of 5 mg to start. In older children this dose should be 10 mg/day. Effects are rarely seen for 3 or more days. Thereafter, the dose can be increased in increments of 5 or 10 mg/day at weekly intervals. Most patients respond to a dose of 25 mg/day or less; occasional patients require up to 50 mg/day. The major side effect is postural hypotension, typically when the patient arises in the morning or stands up abruptly. Sitting with legs over the edge of the bed for a few seconds before standing up or standing up slowly usually eliminates this side effect. Diarrhea is a side effect in a small minority of children. Fluid retention has been reported with the drug but has not been a problem in our experience. The drug should not be used in any patient receiving a monoamine oxidase (MAO) inhibitor. When monitoring the effectiveness of guanethidine, blood pressure should be taken with the patient in the supine and the upright positions as well as after exercise to determine its postural effect. One major disadvantage of the drug is that it has little effect when the patient is asleep. This can be rectified by having the patient propped up on pillows when asleep. Alternatively, a small dose of hydralazine can be added to the regimen in the evening. Recently we have found that some teenage male patients in whom blood pressure is controlled by guanethidine have discontinued this drug when they became sexually active because of its side effect on inhibiting ejaculation. We now warn teenage males about this problem and convert their control, usually to prazosin, if it appears that this side effect may pose a problem. Extensive personal experience with guanethidine has demonstrated that this drug often is a most effective agent which can be used alone and requires only a single morning dose, helping to ensure compliance.

Methyldopa is a moderately potent antihypertensive agent that probably works by interfering with the production of the neurotransmitter norepinephrine. Its absorption is very variable, and it results in a positive direct Coombs' test in 20 per cent of patients. The first two patients we treated with this drug developed hemolytic anemia. Although this is a rare occurrence, it limited our enthusiasm for the drug. Other patients complain of a sedative effect when starting methyldopa, an effect that may or may not lessen with time. Methyldopa has been reported to be effective in controlling hypertension in children, especially when taken with a diuretic to limit sodium and water retention, which is sometimes seen when the drug is taken alone. The recommended starting dose is 10 mg/kg/day taken in three divided doses. The dose can be increased stepwise every 3 to 5 days up to 40 mg/kg/day. The maximum recommended daily dose is 2 gm.

Other drugs in this group include reserpine and clonidine. Used on a long-term basis, reserpine produces drowsiness, symptoms of depression, and nasal stuffiness. It must be stopped several days in advance of any operation requiring a general anesthetic. Its routine use is not recommended, although it may have a role in some patients resistant to or unable to take other drugs. Clonidine acts on alpha-adrenergic receptors. It too may produce drowsiness. Other side effects include dryness of the mouth and rebound hypertension if the drug is stopped abruptly. We have had limited experience with the drug but have not found any advantage for it in comparison to guanethidine or prazosin.

Drugs Modifying Renin-Angiotensin System. Beta-adrenergic blocking agents such as propranolol interfere with renin release, and at least part of their action is through this mechanism. More recently, drugs have been developed that inhibit the enzyme responsible for the conversion of angiotensin I to angiotensin II, which is the pressor substance. The drug in this category which is absorbed when taken by mouth and which is now available by prescription is captopril. Recent observations suggest that it is effective by acting on both the renin-angiotensin and the kinin systems. Its use in acute hypertension has been detailed already. We have found it to be an extremely valuable agent in the management of chronic hypertension too, especially that which is renin-mediated. The initial dose is 1 mg/kg/day divided into three doses, and this is increased in stepwise manner, at 8-hour intervals if necessary, until effective blood pressure response is observed. The maximum dose should not exceed 6 mg/kg/day. The use of beta-adrenergic blocking agents and diuretics will often potentiate the effect of captopril, and all antihypertensive agents other than those in these two groups should be discontinued before captopril is used. We have been most pleased by the effectiveness of the drug and by

---

*Safety and effectiveness of nadolol in children have not been established.

patient acceptance. To date, we have not seen proteinuria or decreased WBC count, the two complications
that require discontinuing the drug.

Drugs Acting on Volume. Hypervolemia may contribute to chronic hypertension in many patients, or
fluid and sodium retention may occur secondary to the
use of several of the vasodilator drugs. Thus, the use
of diuretics has an important role in the management
of hypertension.

The most frequently prescribed diuretics are the
thiazides. Their effect in hypertension appears to be
through their action to increase urinary losses of sodium
and water. The drugs are well absorbed when taken by
mouth and are relatively free of side effects. Potassium
wasting with or without hypokalemia may occur with
prolonged use. Hyperuricemia, a common complication
of using thiazides in adults, is seen infrequently in
children. Nor have hyperglycemia and hypercalcemia
been reported as a complication of thiazide use in
children. Hydrochlorothiazide will be used as an example of a typical thiazide. The starting dose is 2
mg/kg/day taken in two equally divided doses, the second one of which should be given no later than early
afternoon to avoid nocturia. The dose may be doubled,
but one should wait for at least 7 to 14 days before
increasing the dose, since the maximum therapeutic
response may take this long to develop. Unfortunately
many children with secondary hypertension have a
renal cause for their elevated blood pressure and therefore do not respond optimally to the thiazides.

Chlorthalidone is chemically unrelated to the thiazides but has very similar actions. Its major advantage
is that it has a longer length of action and is effective
when taken only once a day.

Furosemide acts on the ascending limb of the loop of
Henle and thus is referred to as a loop diuretic. It and
ethacrynic acid are the most potent diuretics known.
Although furosemide has a short plasma half-life, it
needs to be given only once a day, in the morning. The
usual starting dose is 0.5 to 1 mg/kg/day. There has
been little published experience to show that larger
doses given for protracted periods of time in children
are safe, but to date we have not experienced any
problems. The major complication is potassium wasting,
necessitating oral potassium supplements. Most effective potassium preparations are extremely unpalatable.
We have found that the use of a salt substitute on foods
is best tolerated by our patients. Caution in administering any potassium supplement must be exercised in any
patient with renal insufficiency in case hyperkalemia
develops. Concern has been expressed that furosemide
may be ototoxic, but there is little evidence to support
this concern when the drug is used as outlined above.

Spironolactone is a competitive inhibitor of aldosterone. When used in conjunction with a thiazide diuretic
or furosemide, it potentiates the diuresis and may have
a slight potassium-sparing effect. We sometimes use it
for this purpose but do not believe that it is an effective
antihypertensive agent when used alone. The starting
dose may be up to 3.3 mg/kg/day in single or divided
doses. Effects from the drug may not be seen for 3 or
more days, and maximum effectiveness may take up to
14 days to develop.

Triamterene is a nonsteroidal potassium-sparing diuretic. We do not use it, since most of our hypertensive
patients have renal disease, and we are concerned about
the potential of this drug to induce significant hyperkalemia.

Any patient in whom a diuretic is indicated should
also receive a salt-restricted diet. It is not practical to
restrict sodium intake to levels as low as 0.5 gm (20
mEq)/day in nonhospitalized patients. We have found
that usually the best one can accomplish is to restrict
intake to around 35 to 50 mEq/day. It is important to
emphasize to parents that the higher the sodium intake,
the greater the dose of diuretics needed. We do not
recommend attempting to control chronic severe or
moderately severe hypertension with dietary sodium
restriction alone. It rarely works; if a benefit is seen,
this usually is short lived, since most patients find that
adhering to a low-salt diet is extremely arduous.

Summary. The therapeutic regimen that is developed
should be as simple and as free from side effects as
possible. Preferably, a single drug should be used.
Guanethidine and prazosin are valuable for this reason.
We are now using captopril more often, especially in
patients with renin-mediated hypertension. Some favor
the use of calcium-channel blockers. Minoxidil may
prove effective in patients resistant to other drugs.
When a second drug is needed, we use a diuretic and
dietary sodium restriction if volume expansion or sodium retention appears to be an etiologic factor in the
hypertension. A thiazide diuretic or chlorthalidone is
used if a moderate diuresis is required; furosemide for
a more vigorous diuresis. If secondary hyperreninemia
appears to be responsible for a reduced effect of the
primary antihypertensive drug, we add propranolol to
the regimen, but we have begun to use nadolol because
it is effective when taken once a day.

Endocrine Disorders

Since some children with hypertension caused by
endocrine disorders can be cured with appropriate
surgical or medical therapy, consideration should be
given early in the course of diagnosis or therapy to the
possibility that hypertension may have an endocrine
cause in all hypertensive children. Some of the more
important causes of endocrine hypertension are briefly
outlined in Table 2.

Pheochromocytoma usually presents as sustained
rather than intermittent hypertension. Pheochromocytomas may present as isolated cases or in association
with Sipple's syndrome (medullary carcinoma of the
thyroid and bilateral pheochromocytomas). High perioperative morbidity requires expert use of alpha- and
beta-adrenergic blocking agents as well as careful monitoring of the hydration status. Surgical removal is the
treatment of choice.

Two syndromes associated with congenital adrenal
hyperplasia can cause hypertension in young children.
They are caused by the accumulation of desoxycorticosterone (11β-OH deficiency) or mineralocorticoids
(17α-OH deficiency) due to an increased secretion of
ACTH secondary to deficient cortisol production.

Approximately 80 per cent of children with Cushing's

TABLE 2. Causes of Endocrine Hypertension

Endocrine Disorder	Clinical Presentation	Therapy
1. Pheochromocytoma	90% sustained hypertension	Alpha-adrenergic blockade (phenoxybenzamine, phentolamine)
	80% headache, 65% sweating	Beta-adrenergic blockade (propranolol)
	35% intermittent abdominal pain	Careful monitoring of hydration status intraoperatively
2. Congenital adrenal hyperplasias	Hypertension	Replacement glucocorticoids
	Rapid growth	
(a) 11β hydroxylase deficiency	Virilization in females	
	Elevated 11-desoxycortisol and DOC	
(b) 17α hydroxylase deficiency	Hypertension	Replacement glucocorticoids
	Hypokalemic alkalosis	
	Ambiguous genitalia in males	
	Delayed puberty in girls	
3. Cushing's syndrome	Growth failure	Surgical removal of adrenal or pituitary tumor
	Signs of glucocorticoid excess	
4. Hyperaldosteronism	Hypokalemia in sodium-repleted state	Surgery (for isolated tumor) or spironolactone
	Low renin, high aldosterone	
5. Hyperthyroidism	Systolic hypertension, emotional lability, goiter, increased sweating, increased height for age, weakness, tremor, tachycardia, elevated T_4, T_3, FT_4, and RT_3U	Surgical excision of thyroid gland or medical treatment with propranolol, propylthiouracil, or methimazole (Tapazole)

syndrome due to bilateral adrenal stimulation by ACTH or to an isolated adrenal tumor will be hypertensive. Treatment consists of surgical removal of the tumor responsible for excess cortisol or ACTH production.

The presence of a low plasma renin in a salt-repleted patient with hypertension should lead to a suspicion that the patient has a form of congenital adrenal hyperplasia or hyperaldosteronism. These disorders are often responsive to appropriate glucocorticoid or spironolactone therapy or to surgical removal of an aldosterone-producing tumor.

Systolic hypertension is sometimes a manifestation of hyperthyroidism, and treatment may either be surgical or medical, as noted in Table 2.

Congenital Vascular Disease

Coarctation of the Aorta. Coarctation of the aorta is a congenital malformation characterized by constriction of the aorta distal to the origin of the left subclavian artery. Characteristically, there is hypertension in the upper limbs and hypotension in the lower extremities. It is generally agreed that surgical correction be carried out in the infant who presents with congestive heart failure due to coarctation of the aorta and a left-to-right shunt such as a patent ductus arteriosus or a ventricular or atrial septal defect. Thus, a volume overload is imposed upon a pressure-overloaded left ventricle. The critically ill infant in congestive heart failure should be started upon treatment for the heart failure. The baby should then be evaluated by cardiac catheterization and angiocardiography. If the diagnosis of coarctation of the aorta is verified, the baby should be operated upon. The time elapsed from admittance to operation should be 24 to 48 hours.

There is also general agreement that surgical correction is imperative in patients with isolated coarctation in the age range of 5 to 8 years when the aortic lumen has achieved approximately 50 per cent of the cross-sectional area of the adult aorta. A second operation will therefore not be needed in adulthood, even if the anastomotic site does not grow with age. Most patients have generalized hypertension postoperatively, which spontaneously returns to normal values in 2 or 3 weeks in approximately 90 per cent of patients. Although some authors have advocated antihypertensive therapy during this period, I have seen no evidence to support such treatment. Nor is there evidence to support the suggestion that antihypertensive drug treatment is of any value in the preoperative state. About 10 per cent of patients have persistent generalized hypertension even if the aortic obstruction is completely relieved. The reason for this is unknown. It may be that these patients are destined to develop primary hypertension.

HYPOTENSION

HERBERT S. HARNED, Jr., M.D.

The pediatric practitioner must be able to assess rapidly the severity of hypotensive states. To recognize hypotension, he must be aware of the normal range of blood pressures in children of differing age groups and be knowledgeable about the proper cuff sizes, manometric techniques, and interpretations of Korotkoff and Doppler sounds and flush methods. Recognition of shock must be made from observing tachycardia, thready pulses, venous collapse, delayed capillary filling, pallor, coldness and moisture of the skin, obtunded consciousness, and oliguria. These findings indicate inadequate oxygenation and perfusion of vital organs and call for immediate action.

Although the various etiologies of severe hypotension with shock require certain specific therapies, especially with septic, anaphylactic, or neurogenic shock, certain general measures must be directed toward the rapid reversal of this life-threatening state.

Recent knowledge of the treatment of shock has been derived from experience in ICU settings. Treatments in this relatively ideal setting will be presented initially. From this perspective, the practitioner can extrapolate appropriate therapeutic measures and monitoring techniques which might apply in his particular circumstances. An organized approach is needed, with one person as the leader. The more assistants he can mobilize, the better the chance of reversal of a case of severe hypotension. At least four active physicians or knowledgeable ancillary intensivists are desirable to handle a severe hypotensive episode.

Shock often is the precursor of cardiopulmonary arrest, and similar therapeutic measures are initiated to those needed for the latter condition. An approach using the initials VIP for "ventilation-infusion-pump" has set proper priorities.

First, immediate attention to ventilation is vital, with realization that the Trendelenburg position (head down) is often detrimental. Improving the state of ventilation, by ensuring a proper airway, administration of oxygen, and hyperventilating the patient to lower alveolar and arterial Pco_2 and combat detrimental acidosis and hypoxemia, offers a direct treatment of the basic problem in shock, i.e., decreased cellular oxidation. In an ICU setting, the person most skilled in endotracheal intubation and ventilatory management should immediately be assigned to the task of evaluating the need for establishing an orotracheal airway.

Suctioning, use of an oral airway, passage of a nasogastric tube for gastric decompression, mouth-to-mouth insufflation, use of self-inflating and reservoir-type resuscitation bags, use of face masks, and use of 100 per cent oxygen need to be implemented as necessary if ventilation is inadequate. The decision concerning endotracheal intubation may be difficult, but this procedure must be done if the severely compromised patient is not improved within minutes. Even though evaluation of ventilation is absolutely essential, severe respiratory depression often develops relatively late during a hypotensive episode and attention needs to be paid to other therapeutic measures.

If the heart rate falls below 40 and severe shock is apparent, external cardiac massage is indicated. Immediate ECG monitoring needs to be instituted and systematic blood pressure recordings taken. An arterial sample for Po_2, Pco_2, and pH determinations may be taken. Additional, more precise monitoring techniques need to be instituted and proper intravascular lines established for administering fluids and drugs. Lack of access for giving drugs limits immediate treatment to such nonsclerosing medications as epinephrine and atropine, which can be administered intramuscularly, lingually, or endotracheally as well as by stat intravenous injection. The stat doses of these medications are as follows: epinephrine (0.1 ml/kg/dose of a 1:10,000 solution or 10 µg/kg) and atropine sulfate (0.01 to 0.03 mg/kg/dose).

The first line to be placed is a venous line preferably, using the most propitious site. Soon after this is in place, a central venous pressure (CVP) line must be established and, concurrently, an arterial catheter for manometric recording of intra-arterial pressures and periodic sampling for blood gases and electrolytes, especially valuable if the course is protracted. A 12-lead ECG and chest radiograph are done as soon as possible.

With the establishment of the peripheral venous line, the therapeutic options are greatly enhanced, for it is now possible to administer emergency medications optimally. Also, isotonic crystalloid solutions such as 0.9 per cent NaCl solution or Ringer's lactate (20 ml/kg) or colloids such as 25 per cent salt-poor albumin (1 gm/kg) diluted to 5 per cent with isotonic saline preferably, plasma, or whole blood (10 ml/kg) infused over 15 minutes can be administered as a CVP line is being placed. These infusions are given to combat the second major feature of shock, poor peripheral perfusion.

While fluids are being administered through the venous line, the CVP and arterial lines should become activated. With the CVP for guidance, one can ascertain rapidly whether there is a cardiogenic element in the shock state of the patient. A bolus of crystalloids or colloids, administered into the peripheral venous line and to be repeated if necessary, can indicate the degree of myocardial failure induced when the CVP has been raised. Also, the bolus increases cardiac filling in all states in which decreased circulating blood volume is the cause of decreased cardiac output. Periodic fluid challenges can be given, using 2 to 4 ml/kg infusions over 10 minutes and attempting to bring the blood pressure back to normal. The rate of change in the CVP as well as its absolute value should be assessed concurrently. If the infusions do not result in any improvement in the hypotension and peripheral perfusion, one must be very concerned about the cardiogenic nature of the shock state. The CVP indicates right ventricular filling pressures, but these may differ widely from those on the left side, which may be estimated better by placement of a pulmonary wedge pressure line. This latter procedure requires special expertise for use in infants especially and may be reserved for special conditions in which complex inotropic and vasoactive drugs are to be used.

In many cases, poor cardiac function may be a temporary condition caused by metabolic acidosis, hypoglycemia, hypocalcemia, or hyperkalemia, and these possible factors should be considered and appropriately treated. If peripheral perfusion has been poor, one can assume the presence of lactic acidosis from anaerobic glycolysis and should give $NaHCO_3$ solution (1 to 2 mEq/kg IV). This $NaHCO_3$ therapy has several immediate favorable effects, including (1) improvement of cardiac contractility, (2) potentiation of the sympathetic-adrenal responses to shock and of the actions of administered sympathomimetic drugs, (3) reversal of local acidosis with improved vasoconstriction of small arterioles, and (4) amelioration of the myocardial effects of potassium toxicity if this exists. Administration of $NaHCO_3$ may need to be repeated if the state of shock remains profound and if blood gas determinations continue to show severe acidosis. Adequate ventilation must be maintained to eliminate excessive CO_2 with this bicarbonate loading. Also, $NaHCO_3$ solutions chemically neutralize sympathomimetic drugs and must never be given in the same line without proper measures to avoid such a deleterious reaction. $NaHCO_3$ solutions are sclerosing and should be given only through adequate intravascular lines, as is also the case with calcium and glucose solutions. Use of glucose to supply needed substrate for myocardial metabolism is often forgotten in the melee of resuscitative efforts. If a blood Dextrostix determination shows less than 45 mg/dl, then 25 per cent glucose (2 ml/kg IV) is given, followed by an infusion of 10 per cent glucose.

All of the measures described above should have been completed within 20 minutes. In addition, after several bolus doses of epinephrine have been given at 5-minute intervals, selection of effective inotropic agents for use during the ensuing hours must be considered if a precarious state continues. Decisions as to the preferred agent can be complex and may require consultations with cardiologists and anesthesiologists.

As a widely used treatment, a continuous epinephrine infusion, administered by an accurate infusion pump, has several advantages, including stimulation of cardiac rate and contractility and increase of peripheral vascular resistance with improved coronary flow. The infusion can be prepared rapidly by adding 5 ml of 1:1000 aqueous epinephrine to a 250-ml bottle of 5 per cent dextrose to make up a solution of 20 μg/ml. The infusion is started at 0.1 μg/kg/min (or 6 μg/kg/hr) and increased to as much as 1.5 μg/kg/min. An infusion chart must be prepared and kept current by one member of the ICU team responsible for recording and calculating the drug dosages. Disadvantages of epinephrine include its tendency to cause tachycardia with increased myocardial O_2 consumption and its arrhythmogenic effects in severe hypoxic states.

Two newer drugs are being used widely for the treatment of hypotension, but the nuances of their complex effects in infants and children are still being evaluated.

Dopamine (Inotropin)* infusions have proved to be useful in cases of hypotension of cardiogenic origin especially. This agent significantly enhances myocardial contractility, heart rate, automaticity, and atrioventricular conduction (beta$_1$-adrenergic effects), but additionally has unique "dopaminergic effects" that can be favorable. Vasodilatation occurs during low doses (2 to 5 μg/kg/min) in the renal, splanchnic, coronary, and cerebral vascular beds, a property especially useful in improving renal perfusion. In higher doses (10 μg/kg/min), needed to augment cardiac output, vasoconstriction occurs and peripheral and pulmonary vascular resistance increase.

Dobutamine (Dobutrex)* also has properties that make it an effective agent in treating cardiogenic shock. This synthetic drug increases myocardial contraction without increasing the heart rate and produces peripheral vasodilatation in doses as high as 10 μg/kg/minute. Careful monitoring and liberal fluid infusions may be needed to maintain the blood pressure as systemic blood flow is improved. In infants below 1 year of age, its inability to increase heart rate may limit dobutamine's effectiveness.

These two agents have superseded other inotropic agents to a degree and appear to be relatively safe with

*Safety and effectiveness for use in children have not been established.

proper monitoring. They are often given concurrently through different venous lines.

On the other hand, isoproterenol (Isuprel) has very strong beta$_1$-adrenergic effects, which may result in tachyarrhythmias, especially in children on digoxin therapy. Its strong systemic vasodilatory effects can also result in increased hypotension in the hypovolemic patient. However, isoproterenol is still the agent of choice in patients with bradyarrhythmias not responding to atropine.

Digoxin is a slower-acting inotropic agent that is not as potent as the sympathomimetic drugs. It is also a dangerous drug in acute hypotensive states and has well-established toxic properties. Its primary effectiveness is in conditions in which prolonged action is desired, as in low cardiac output states from cardiac failure.

When vasoconstrictor effects are desired primarily, norepinephrine (levarterenol, Levophed) infusions, starting at 0.1 μg/kg/min with stepwise increased doses, may be used. Phenylephrine (Neo-Synephrine) infusions of 0.5 to 1.5 μg/kg/min are also gaining acceptance. These drugs constrict the renal and mesenteric vessels so that their prolonged use causes progressive impairment of perfusion of these regions.

When left ventricular pump failure is the major factor in hypotension, outflow resistance can be decreased effectively by primary vasodilator therapy. Special attention must be paid to the intra-arterial pressures, which must be monitored closely to maintain a pressure adequate for coronary perfusion. The systolic pressure should be maintained not lower than three fourths that expected for the child's age as a guideline for dosage of these powerful agents. Sodium nitroprusside (Nipride) infusions, starting at 1 μg/kg/min and increasing to as high as 10 μg/kg/min, are widely used, especially in adults with severe myocardial dysfunction. With prolonged high doses, one must beware of inducing thiocyanate toxicity manifested by vomiting, sweating, and muscle twitching or of cyanide poisoning causing intractable acidosis. It is highly advisable to monitor the use of this agent by insertion of a Swan-Ganz catheter for continuous estimations of left ventricular filling, as delineated by the pulmonary capillary wedge pressures. Passage of this flow-directed catheter is accomplished readily in the older child and adult but is often difficult to achieve in the young child without the assistance of a pediatric cardiologist, anesthesiologist, or intensive care specialist. Fluoroscopic guidance may be needed, but the catheter can be located in the right ventricular outflow tract and pulmonary artery by echocardiography. Combined use of dopamine or dobutamine and sodium nitroprusside has been effective, especially in severe pump failure, but obviously needs particularly careful monitoring. Nitroglycerin solutions appear to be safer substitutes for nitroprusside infusions when preload reduction and venodilation are desired. Initial infusions of 1 μg/kg/min can be increased to as high as 20 μg/kg/min in severe conditions.

If bradycardia develops in association with hypotension, a stat dose of atropine (0.01 to 0.03 mg/kg IV) may be useful, but emergency placement of a transvenous pacemaker by a cardiologist may be necessary. Calcium, most reliably given in the form of $CaCl_2$ (0.2 ml/kg of a 100 mg/ml 10 per cent solution), must be administered intravenously with the aim of strengthening cardiac contraction through another mechanism than that of beta-adrenergic stimulation. One must be aware that this agent should never be given in the same line as $NaHCO_3$ because calcium carbonate will be precipitated. Also, it should be given cautiously to digitalized patients, since these two drugs potentiate each other. It is also an extremely sclerosing material and should only be given through well-established intravenous lines.

Cardiac arrhythmias may cause pump failure and require specific diagnosis and treatment. A variety of causes for these disorders may be identified. Electrolyte imbalance, especially potassium deficiency or excess, acidosis, alkalosis, digitalis toxicity, hypoxia, fever, hypovolemia, presence of pericardial fluid, and irritation from CVP or pulmonary wedge pressure catheters are treatable. Primary arrhythmias, such as paroxysmal tachyarrhythmias, may also require selective therapies, such as the drug regimens and external cardioversion and defibrillation discussed elsewhere. Not to be forgotten is the occasional effectiveness of sharp blows to the chest of the older child in reversing known ventricular tachyarrhythmias, and the vagal stimulating maneuvers (facial immersion, carotid massage, induced gagging, etc.) in reversing supraventricular tachyarrhythmias.

The effects of shock on various organ systems must be weighed in the therapeutic plan, especially if hypotension is persistent. Damage to endothelial cells and alveolar epithelial cells in the lung (shock lung) may result in permeability edema and decreased surfactant production (adult respiratory distress syndrome). Adequate ventilation by endotracheal intubation, use of pancuronium (Pavulon) (0.06 to 0.1 mg/kg/dose IV every 30 to 60 minutes) and sedation (such as morphine 0.1 to 0.2 mg/kg/dose q2–4h), appropriate supplemental O_2, proper airway pressure adjustments, and chest physiotherapy are often indicated. Furosemide (Lasix), 1 mg/kg, increasing to as high as 5 mg/kg/dose, and colloid therapy to raise oncotic pressure may be needed to handle these pulmonary complications of severe hypotension.

The renal blood flow and urinary output must be maintained if possible. Low-dose dopamine* infusions, mannitol (0.5 to 1.0 gm/kg over 30 minutes every 4 to 6 hours), and furosemide are used to combat oliguric renal failure.

If paralytic ileus has occurred, the stomach contents need to be emptied by nasogastric tube. Stress ulcers and erosive gastritis may develop from mucosal ischemia. Antacids such as aluminum hydroxide (Maalox or Amphojel, 5 to 20 ml q4h by mouth) are given to raise the gastric pH to 4.0.

Adequate nutrition must be maintained to provide liver substrates, as well as nutrition, for host defenses against infection. The catabolic effects of shock need special attention if the patient was nutritionally deficient before hypotension developed. Intravenous alimentation may be needed under these circumstances. Glucose therapy may result in increased glycogen synthesis with lipogenesis causing hepatomegaly and abnormal liver function. Infusions of glucose with insulin and potassium have favorably improved cell membrane function and can improve cardiac carbohydrate metabolism.

If treatment is prolonged, concerns will arise about infection from catheters which act as foreign bodies, and difficult decisions must be made concerning antibiotic therapy. Patients with severe hypotension have lowered resistance to infection from a variety of causes. At present, prevention or early treatment with antibiotics aimed at preventing bacteremia is the best therapeutic approach, but treatments to specifically stimulate host defense mechanisms and granulocyte transfusions may find wider use soon.

Special mention must be made of hypotension from sepsis, anaphylaxis, and neurogenic causes. Early in septic shock, increased vascular capacity with peripheral vasodilation produces a picture different from other forms of shock. The skin may be warm and flushed, blood pressure may be normal with wide pulse pressure, and the patient may be febrile, hyperventilating, and having chills. Alpha stimulators, such as epinephrine, norepinephrine, and phenylephrine, are usually ineffective. The preferred treatment as the condition progresses to systemic vasoconstriction appears to be vigorous volume expansion initially and then use of an agent such as isoproterenol or nitroprusside. Concurrent antibiotic therapy, platelet concentrates, fresh plasma or blood, exchange transfusions, and steroids (dexamethasone, 5 mg/kg, or methylprednisolone, 30 mg/kg IV in form of a bolus) must be considered in this shock state especially. The corticosteroid treatment may be repeated every 4 to 6 hours in the severely compromised patient but has not been shown to be effective after 3 days. Another controversial but promising agent is naloxone* (Narcan), an endorphin blocker (given in repeated doses of 0.01 mg/kg IV), which may counteract the deleterious cellular effects of these intrinsic substances. Naloxone is also an effective stimulator of central respiratory drive.

Disseminated intravascular coagulation, present as a major complication of sepsis, may exist to a degree in most severe nonseptic shock states. Treatment is directed against the associated conditions (hypotension, anoxemia, acidosis, and infection), but platelet and fresh frozen plasma transfusions are also indicated. Vitamin K (1 to 5 mg IM or IV) should also be administered. Heparin (100 units/kg/dose q4h or 10 to 25 units/kg/hour as an IV infusion) is advised only when thromboses have been demonstrated.

Occasional episodes of anaphylactic shock are to be expected in the office as well as hospital setting because of the variety of drugs now being administered and other allergens patients may contact. The practitioner must be aware of the variable nature and time of

---

*Safety and effectiveness for use in children have not been established.

*This use of naloxone is not listed by the manufacturer.

occurrence of this condition, the latter varying from minutes to hours after exposure. Usually, symptoms with parenteral drug administration occur within 30 minutes, hopefully while the child is still under observation. The treatment is clear-cut—epinephrine should be given, 0.1 ml/kg IM or IV of a 1:10,000 dilution (or 10 µg/kg), as soon as the diagnosis has been made. Withdrawal of the offending antigen or isolation of its site of injection by a tourniquet should be accomplished. Prophylactic administration of diphenhydramine HCl (Benadryl), 0.5 to 1.5 mg/kg by mouth or intravenously, may be useful. Concern for maintaining an adequate airway, use of aminophylline for persistent bronchospasm, and general circulatory support with fluids and vasopressors have a role in severe cases of anaphylaxis, as they do in other forms of shock.

Many hypotensive episodes detailed above can be reversed readily. Gradual development of hypotension can often be reversed by crystalloid infusions, with the realization that these may leave the vascular compartments significantly within minutes, or with plasma infusions. Attention to maintenance of the hematocrit at 35 to 40 per cent, continuous monitoring of blood pressure, heart rate, ECG, and urinary output (by indwelling catheter), and arterial blood gas determinations are needed. In refractory cases, withdrawal of inotropic agents and decisions as to when respiratory support and monitoring may be discontinued require artful judgments, often involving empirical trials. At least, these decisions can be made deliberately and after discussions with colleagues with special expertise.

Simple syncope can present major problems in differential diagnosis but can usually be identified by its postural nature resulting in inadequate cerebral perfusion and by its rapid recovery when the patient's head is brought to or below heart level. Other neurogenic causes of hypotension, such as head injury and seizures, require special measures detailed elsewhere.

The practitioner must tailor the idealized treatments possible in an ICU setting to his own practice with the realization that patients with severe hypotensive episodes present under suboptimal conditions, often without warning. Since acute shock states require equipment and drugs similar to those needed for other forms of emergency such as primary respiratory arrest states, it would seem wise to establish a "crash cart" in the office with the drugs and equipment detailed in the early part of the above treatment plan for severe shock. The desired equipment, techniques for ventilation, placement of intravascular lines, and emergency drugs are detailed elegantly in the Textbook of Advanced Cardiac Life Support, available through the American and local Heart Associations. This should be required reading by the pediatrician and his support personnel. It would be most desirable for many pediatricians, especially those not familiar with intensive care as it is now practiced in most teaching centers, to participate in the Advanced Cardiac Life Support teaching programs and other similar programs at their hospitals. Organization of the office personnel so that each worker has a defined role in such emergencies is important, as is a thorough knowledge of the effectiveness of the local rescue squad and hospital emergency room. Decisions as to adequacy of equipment and drugs in the office can also be made by studying the equipment on the hospital crash carts, especially that in locations away from the ER and ICU areas.

PERIPHERAL VASCULAR DISEASE

WARREN G. GUNTHEROTH, M.D.,
and D. EUGENE STRANDNESS, Jr., M.D.

The clinical appearance of obstructed blood flow is common to venous disorders as well as peripheral arterial disease. Arterial disease may be simply vasospastic, particularly in children, and a thoughtful approach to diagnosis as well as to selection of treatment is important, since therapy may correctly vary from adjustment of clothing on the one extreme to amputation on the other.

PERIPHERAL ARTERIES

Vasoactive Disorders

Raynaud's Disease. Raynaud's phenomenon with no underlying disease is a vasosplastic disorder of fingers and toes with a characteristic sequence of pallor, cyanosis, and rubor. Criteria for the diagnosis of Raynaud's disease are provocation of the vasospastic disorder by cold or emotion, bilaterality, absence of gangrene, and absence of an underlying primary disease.

Therapy of Raynaud's disease should be conditioned by its generally favorable prognosis. Surgical sympathectomy is rarely, if ever, indicated in the primary disorder. If the symptoms are bothersome, selection of a warm, dry climate may be helpful. Clothing selection should be directed toward conserving body heat rather than just covering the affected extremities; our studies show that cold applied directly to the affected extremity is less likely to produce vasospasm than is general body cooling. The clothing should not be tight-fitting; hard-finish, tightly woven material is essential to block wind, and bulky woolen clothing is necessary for insulation against cold. Stocking caps may be quite helpful in reducing vasoconstriction of the fingers. In adolescent girls, a program of increased physical exercise is probably beneficial. Biofeedback has been successful to some extent in increasing digital temperature and in aborting episodes of Raynaud's, or at least in reducing the severity of the attack.

Medications may be required in more severe cases. The current drug of choice for adults is nifedipine, a calcium channel blocker. (Although this use of nifedipine is not included in the manufacturer's instructions, the use for blocking contractile response of smooth muscle is noted.) In adults, the dose is one 10-mg capsule three times daily; an appropriate basis for children is 0.2 mg/kg three times daily, although there has not been extensive usage in the pediatric age group. The side effects are largely those of vasodilatation, including lightheadedness, flushing, and headache. Improvement is seen in only 50 to 70 per cent of patients, subjectively, but flow in the affected digit does not improve. A 1989 report found equal success with ketanserin, but this serotonin-blocker is not available in the U.S. Its advantage over nifedipine and prazosin is that no generalized vasodilatation is produced.

Studies of the mechanism of cold-induced vasoconstriction implicate alpha$_2$-adrenoreceptors, raising hope for a more specific and effective drug for Raynaud's disease.

When dealing with cold sensitivity, it is important to keep in mind that it may be secondary to some serious underlying problem such as one of the collagen disorders. Exhaustive work-ups, however, are not routinely indicated in a child with good health and mild vasospastic complaints. Although primary Raynaud's disease is a benign disorder, the secondary form may lead to digital artery occlusion, fingertip ulcers, and even gangrene. The occlusion can be recognized by measurement of systolic pressures in the involved finger by either plethysmography or Doppler ultrasound. Finger pressures of less than 70 mm Hg, wrist-to-digit gradients of more than 30 mm Hg, and brachial-to-finger differences of greater than 40 mm Hg are consistent with occlusive disease in the hand or digits.

Chilblains (Pernio). Another disorder of cold sensitivity, chilblains involves itching, localized erythema, and sometimes blisters, occurring over the dorsum of the proximal phalanges of fingers and toes and over the heels and lower legs. It is said that this is a disorder of children in cool, damp climates, but, oddly, we have not seen this problem in Seattle. The disorder is more of a nuisance than a threat to life or limb. Treatment during the acute phase consists of antipruritic medications and a soothing ointment in a lanolin-petrolatum base. Management outlined under Raynaud's disease should be considered for the more persistent cases.

Acrocyanosis. This is probably more common than Raynaud's disease, but the overlap of acrocyanosis with the normal response to cold is greater than in Raynaud's. In acrocyanosis there is a more generalized response of the entire extremity in a glove or stocking pattern, and there is usually only unremitting cyanosis, without the pallor and rubor phases of Raynaud's. Ulcerations are rare, and therapy is rarely required except for cosmetic reasons. When required, therapy is the same as for Raynaud's disease.

Livedo Reticularis. Livedo reticularis and cutis marmorata are even milder peripheral vascular responses to cold, with netlike patterns of cyanosis in arms and legs. Therapy is not usually required, but the general comments pertaining to Raynaud's disease would apply to these conditions.

Erythromelalgia. Although the number of cases of erythromelalgia is smaller than that of Raynaud's disease, the symptoms are so much more debilitating that therapy must be considered briefly. Erythromelalgia presents as a peripheral hyperreaction to heat, the counterpart to reaction to cold in Raynaud's disease. The hot, swollen, and tender hands and feet are extraordinarily unpleasant and led to suicide in a young adult in our hospital. Therapy should be directed toward physical factors as well as medication. Cooling of the body in general, as well as cool soaks to the affected extremities, bring some degree of relief. Ephedrine has been effective in some instances, at 0.5 mg/kg every 4 to 6 hours (average adult dose, 25 mg), preferably with a tranquilizer or a sedative.

Aspirin is definitely worth trying on a regular basis (every 4 hours), not only for its analgesic effects but also because there are indications that endogenous bradykinin may be involved.

Other authorities have suggested that erythromelalgia is a form of "peripheral migraine," and that release of serotonin is responsible. Accordingly, they have suggested antiserotonin medications, such as cyproheptadine. This use of cyproheptadine is not mentioned in the manufacturer's directive, however. For children, an average dose is 0.08 mg/kg (daily dose 0.25 mg/kg). It is available in a syrup containing 2 mg in 5 ml. By the same logic, a trial of propranolol in resistant cases would be justified (adult dose 40 mg q.i.d.).

Causalgia. Although a deep wound with injury to a major nerve trunk leading to "major causalgia" is easily diagnosed, forms of minor causalgia often elude prompt and effective treatment by masquerading as primary vascular disorders. Unilateral vascular disorders, particularly when associated with exquisite tenderness, swelling, and abnormal perspiration, should suggest post-traumatic sympathetic dystrophy, a form of minor causalgia. The vascular disorder is most often vasospastic, but we have successfully treated a boy with a sympathetic dystrophy resembling unilateral erythromelalgia.

Therapy is the same regardless of the vascular disorder: paravertebral sympathetic blockade with injections of 1 per cent lidocaine. If the diagnosis is correct, subjective relief is striking and will last for several hours. Permanent improvement will depend on vigorous physical therapy, beginning at once under the effect of the block, continuing for days or weeks, and usually requiring additional injections at intervals. It is imperative to interrupt the cycle of pain, disuse osteoporosis, and so forth; exercise of the affected limb is the essential therapy. The main function of sympathetic blockade is to permit relatively painless exercise of the limb. Sympathectomy is rarely indicated.

Obstructive Disorders

Trauma. The immediate goal of therapy for traumatic interruption of arterial flow is to prevent loss of tissue and limb. Continuity of the arteries must be restored, spasm relieved, intraluminal clots removed and prevented, and tissue edema managed so that the arterial lumen is not compromised.

Maintenance or restoration of adequate circulating blood volume is of primary importance, not only for the preservation of life but also to permit intelligent assessment of the state of the local circulation. Although actual gangrene is rare in children, a nonoperative approach to vascular injury prolonged beyond 6 to 8 hours may lead to subsequent weakness and atrophy. Thus the ultimate function of the limb should govern the acute management, and early intervention by a skilled surgeon may be truly conservative. Arteriography may be helpful in locating the site and extent of obstruction, but the use of a transcutaneous Doppler flowmeter is less traumatic and may be repeated at will.

Proper surgical technique includes scrupulous débridement; end-to-end anastomosis if adequate vessel length is available to avoid tension, and autogenous vein graft replacement otherwise; complete removal of distal clots; relief of arterial spasm; fasciotomy to control complications of edema and hematoma; and possible anticoagulation with heparin (see under Thrombophlebitis).

An increasingly frequent source of arterial problems is medical cannulation. Poor technique, or overly long cannulation, may lead to embolic problems as well as occlusion. Left heart diagnostic studies via retrograde arterial catheterization have been found to produce leg shortening if the artery clots after the procedure. The instillation of heparin, 100 units/kg in the arterial catheter is helpful, and these patients should be followed closely for arterial pulses and long-term for leg growth.

Congenital Stenosis. Peripheral arterial stenosis rarely produces any definite signs or symptoms when it is congenital, reflecting the remarkable ability of youthful tissues to develop collateral circulation.

Arteritis. Inflammatory disease of arteries may occur locally or as part of a widespread disorder usually called polyarteritis. When smaller arteries are involved, a muscle biopsy is the only means of certain diagnosis. The most effective treatment is identification and removal of sensitizing drugs, infection, or toxin, and in severe generalized arteritis, the use of steroids. Major vessel arteritis that obstructs blood flow may require bypass grafting, depending upon the site and adequacy of collateral circulation.

Fistulas

Trauma. It is quite possible that the most frequent cause of this disorder in the pediatric age group is needle puncture of the femoral vein by physicians. The treatment is obviously surgical, with proper caution that closure of the fistulous connection does not compromise the arterial lumen.

Congenital. Abnormal communications between small arteries and veins, particularly if extensive, pose difficult problems. Because of the extensive and diffuse nature of the fistulas, it is rarely possible to treat by surgical removal. Since these patients often develop edema and incompetence of the superficial veins, it is necessary to treat the patient with gradient support stockings to prevent stasis changes.

PERIPHERAL VEINS

Thrombophlebitis

This is rarely a pediatric problem, but its occurrence is attended by considerable risk to life if treatment is not prompt and effective. The aggressiveness required in the therapeutic approach depends on the extent of the thrombophlebitis, whether it is progressing in spite of medical therapy, and whether pulmonary embolism has occurred.

Massive deep thrombophlebitis (phlegmasia cerulea dolens) involves the entire limb with edema, severe pain, and cyanosis. The presence and quality of the pedal pulses depend on the systemic blood volume and pressure and the degree of edema. In some cases, there may be associated arterial spasm, which can reduce peripheral arterial flow as well. Thrombectomy should not be attempted unless there is a strong question of limb viability. Venous ligation or plication is performed just below the renal vein but is indicated only in those patients with pulmonary embolism that recurs while they are on adequate anticoagulant therapy. The use of fibrinolytic agents, such as streptokinase or urokinase, to promote clot lysis and resorption is useful in adults with massive deep vein thrombophlebitis, but the problems with bleeding are substantial; there is inadequate experience in the pediatric age group to permit a recommendation of fibrinolytic therapy.

Venous thrombosis of the major deep veins is treated with bed rest, elevation, heat, and intravenous heparin. It is now recommended that heparin be given by continuous intravenous infusion to maintain either the whole blood clotting time at 2 to 2.5 times baseline values or the activated partial thromboplastin time at 50 to 80 seconds. An infusion pump is mandatory to avoid fluctuations in the rate of administration.

An oral anticoagulant, such as warfarin, is started when the status of the limb is satisfactory; the prothrombin time should be maintained at 1.2 to 1.5 times the normal control. While the duration of therapy has not been settled, it should be continued for a minimum of 3 months when major venous thrombosis has occurred. With pulmonary embolism, therapy should be continued for 3 to 6 months, or even longer if the patient remains at risk.

If there is any edema in the limb with ambulation, it must be controlled, preferably with tailored, pressure gradient stockings from the level of the foot to the upper thigh.

SMALL VESSEL DISORDERS

Frostbite. Rapid rewarming with moderately warm water (40 to 42°C) should be promptly initiated if the extremity is still frozen or cold. However, for those situations in which the physician may be consulted by radio or telephone, and the patient is still remote from hospitalization, rewarming should not be undertaken unless all danger of refreezing is eliminated. The duration of rewarming required will depend on the depth to which the tissue is frozen; if there is through and through freezing, rewarming of the deeper layers may require over an hour.

The subsequent care requires fastidious hygiene of the injured extremity for a lengthy period; extirpation or amputation should be delayed, since surprising recovery is characteristic of frostbite injuries. Daily care should include gentle cleansing, avoidance of pressure or even light contact, bed rest, and analgesics until the acute inflammation has subsided. After that stage, physical therapy is essential to gradually restore full range of motion; whirlpool baths may aid in this.

DISSEMINATED INTRAVASCULAR COAGULATION AND PURPURA FULMINANS

RICHARD H. SILLS, M.D.

Disseminated intravascular coagulation (DIC) is an acquired failure of hemostasis triggered by an underlying disease process. The excessive intravascular clotting that precipitates DIC can be caused by a wide variety of disorders, including infections, respiratory distress syndrome, and malignant disease. A complex hemorrhagic disorder then develops as a result of depletion of platelets, depletion of Factors II, V, and VIII and fibrinogen, and excessive formation of fibrin split products, which can inhibit fibrin polymerization as well as platelet function. A hemolytic anemia may also develop.

Success in managing DIC is most dependent on the ability to diagnose and treat the underlying disease. If the primary disorder is rapidly and successfully treated, the DIC will resolve without any specific hematologic therapy. Less frequently the primary disorder cannot be quickly managed and specific therapy for the DIC will need to be considered. Examples of this situation include malignant disease and giant hemangiomas. Most commonly, DIC represents a preterminal event, with death due to the primary illness and not the coagulopathy.

It is crucial to realize that no single therapy of DIC has been proven superior to any other. Furthermore, the only controlled study of the treatment of DIC demonstrated no significant improvement in survival or coagulation studies in neonates receiving specific hematologic therapy in comparision with those who received only treatment of their underlying disease. This serves to further emphasize the primary role of treatment of the underlying disorder.

Considering that no therapeutic modality has been proven superior to any other, including no hematologic therapy at all, routine therapy of DIC cannot be recommended except in a few clinical situations. These include potential or actual life-threatening hemorrhage, purpura fulminans or other clinically evident thromboses, and the need for emergency surgery. Laboratory abnormalities in the absence of potentially life-threatening bleeding should not generally be treated.

Platelet and Blood Factor Replacement. Once a decision is made to intervene directly, the initial therapy should consist of replacement of consumed coagulation factors and platelets. Although theoretically this could add "fuel to the fire" and exacerbate the process, practically this has not occurred. The specific replacement therapy should be individualized based on the pattern of relative consumption of platelets, fibrinogen, and Factors II, V, and VIII. The source and dose of these factors, their minimal hemostatic levels, and the expected post-transfusion increments are noted in Table 1. Transfusions should be given to provide at least a minimal hemostatic level. If specific factor assays are not available, the safest approach is to give infusions of platelet concentrates and fresh frozen plasma in the doses indicated. Cryoprecipitate, which specifically concentrates fibrinogen and Factor VII, is given when these factors are more severely depleted. Subsequent transfusions are based on the survival of the infused platelets and factors. This is determined by following the levels of platelets and factors every 3 to 6 hours depending on the severity of the DIC. If specific factor assays are not readily available, the prothrombin time (PT) and the partial thromboplastin time (PTT) are adequate substitutes. The PT should be maintained under 1 to 1.5 times the control value while the PTT should be kept under 1.5 to 2 times the control. Transfusions are often required at least every 12 hours during the active phase of the disease.

Exchange Transfusion. Exchange transfusion is indicated if platelet and factor replacement using simple transfusions fails to control the DIC. Such failure may occur for two reasons. (1) There are limitations on the amount of fresh frozen plasma and/or cryoprecipitate that can be given without causing fluid overload and congestive heart failure. (2) Less frequently, simple transfusions may fail because of high levels of fibrin split products, which contribute to the coagulopathy by inhibiting both fibrin polymerization and platelet function. This situation can be identified by demonstrating evidence of an anticoagulant effect of fibrin split products using a modification of the PTT or PT. Regardless of the reason for failure of simple transfusion, exchange transfusion is more likely to succeed. Much larger amounts of platelets and factors can be provided, and inhibitory fibrin split products will be removed. A single or double volume exchange transfusion with fresh whole citrated blood or packed red cells reconstituted with fresh frozen plasma is generally used. Exchange transfusions are not used as initial therapy of DIC because of the potential risks of the procedure, including catheter-related and metabolic complications, vaso-

TABLE 1. Transfusion Therapy for DIC

Factor	Source	Minimal Hemostatic Level	Usual Dose	Expected Part-Transfusion Increment
Platelets	Platelet concentrates	30,000–50,000/mm³	1 unit/5 kg	50,000–100,000/mm³
Fibrinogen	Cryoprecipitate	100 mg/dl	1 bag/5 kg	150 mg%
Factor VIII	Cryoprecipitate	20–30%	1 bag/5 kg	40%
Factor V	Fresh frozen plasma	10–15%	10–15 cc/kg	15–22%
Factor II	Fresh frozen plasma	15–40%	10–15 cc/kg	10–15%*

*Volume will generally limit reaching a hemostatic level. Fortunately Factor II levels tend to be less severely affected by DIC than levels of Factors V and VIII and fibrinogen.

motor instability, and transfusion related infections due to the greater amount of blood products required.

Heparin. The use of heparin in the treatment of hemorrhagic complications of DIC has fallen into disfavor. Theoretically it arrests the excessive intravascular thrombosis that is causing platelet and factor depletion. Practically there is little evidence that it is beneficial, and it can certainly exacerbate the bleeding diathesis. The use of heparin in hemorrhagic DIC is generally limited to patients with life-threatening bleeding who have failed to respond to both platelet and factor replacement as well as exchange transfusion. Exceptions include DIC secondary to acute promyelocytic or monocytic leukemia, which may respond well to anticoagulation with heparin.

The primary, widely accepted role for heparin in DIC is in treating thrombotic complications, including purpura fulminans and tissue ischemia due to septic shock or major vessel thrombosis. When the use of heparin is indicated, it is given intravenously in an initial bolus of 25 to 50 units/kg followed by a continuous infusion of 10 to 25 units/kg/hr. The higher infusion rates are more likely to be necessary in treating purpura fulminans, but the actual dose of heparin must be individualized. This is best accomplished by measuring heparin levels, but these are often unavailable. The best alternative is to use the PTT to monitor heparin's anticoagulant effect while levels of fibrinogen, Factor VIII, and platelets are used to monitor the severity of the DIC (since these measurements are unaffected by heparin). The PTT should ideally be maintained at 2 to 2.5 times the control, but the initial prolongation of the PTT due to the DIC itself often confuses this regulation of heparin dosage.

If heparin therapy is successful, a response should be measurable in the first 24 hours. The fibrinogen and Factor VIII levels should normalize within 24 to 48 hours, but the platelet count may not reach normal levels for 7 to 14 days. Therapy should be continued until the factor levels normalize, and in the case of purpura fulminans, for at least 2 to 3 weeks. Excessive heparin effect can be neutralized by giving 1 mg of protamine sulfate for each 100 units of heparin estimated to be present in the circulation, but this is rarely necessary. When treating purpura fulminans, replacement therapy with infusions of platelets, cryoprecipitate, and/or fresh frozen plasma may also be required.

Other Therapies. Other therapeutic modalities that have been used in the treatment of DIC include antifibrinolytic agents (aminocaproic acid), antiplatelet agents, dextrans, alpha-adrenergic blocking agents, and antithrombin III concentrates. There is little evidence that they are efficacious, and their use cannot be generally recommended. Antifibrinolytic agents, specifically, are contraindicated in DIC.

Recurrent purpura fulminans in neonates is a rare disorder that is usually due to a homozygous deficiency of protein C. In this situation, acute treatment of the purpura requires infusions of protein C using fresh frozen plasma or Factor IX concentrates known to be rich in protein C. Optimal long-term management of these patients has not yet been determined.

ACUTE RHEUMATIC FEVER

DAVID BAUM, M.D.

When acute rheumatic fever is a serious diagnostic consideration, the patient should be hospitalized. With 2 or 3 days of evaluation, other possibilities usually can be ruled out and the diagnosis made. Carditis, if present, will be recognized and its severity assessed. In the absence of a definitive diagnostic test for acute rheumatic fever, this approach is necessary, since prompt and correct diagnosis is essential for management.

GROUP A STREPTOCOCCAL INFECTION

Since acute rheumatic fever is believed to be a post-streptococcal disorder, eradication of the organism should be accomplished as soon as the diagnosis is made. Treatment is recommended regardless of whether group A streptococci are cultured from the throat. The treatment of choice is intramuscular penicillin G, 1,200,000 units for individuals greater than 60 lb and 600,000 units for smaller children. Oral penicillin V, 800,000 to 1,000,000 units/day in three or four divided doses, administered daily for 10 days, is an acceptable alternative. For those individuals allergic to penicillin, a 10-day course of oral erythromycin, 40 mg/kg/day divided into three or four doses, is recommended.

CARDITIS

Cardiac involvement in acute rheumatic fever is of utmost importance. If sufficiently severe, carditis may result in congestive heart failure and even death. If there is resulting extensive endomyocardial damage with mitral and aortic valvular deformity, the patient usually is disabled and his life expectancy shortened. Because carditis has become a more dominant feature of acute rheumatic fever during the past few years, it is now a matter requiring even greater attention.

Patients with carditis should remain in the hospital where their clinical course can be monitored closely and laboratory support, such as chest radiography, electrocardiography, and echocardiography, is available. Echocardiography is particularly helpful in management, since it allows sequential evaluation of myocardial function, as well as mitral and aortic valve competence. In addition, it is an invaluable technique for the differentiation of pericardial effusion from cardiomegaly, and for monitoring their respective courses.

Management begins with bed rest. Restriction of activity is advised until the diagnosis is ruled out or carditis has subsided. Ambulation should always be gradual after an episode of carditis. The rate at which activity is increased must depend upon the severity of the attack and the response of the patient.

Anti-inflammatory agents are useful in the treatment of carditis during attacks of rheumatic fever. Salicylates and corticosteroids are the drugs in current use. Although both are effective, steroids act more quickly and are more potent. Because steroid side effects can be more troublesome, they are reserved for those patients with more pronounced cardiac involvement.

With myocarditis and little or no cardiomegaly, treatment with salicylates is ordinarily sufficient. Aspirin, not sodium salicylate, should be used. The usual aspirin dose is between 70 and 100 mg/kg/day divided into four doses. Dosage adjustment should be made to maintain blood salicylate levels between 15 and 30 mg/dl. High doses of aspirin are continued until evidence of carditis has subsided and the sedimentation rate has returned to normal. Then medication is withdrawn gradually over a 4- to 6-week period.

Steroid therapy is preferred in patients with carditis who become symptomatic or have moderate to marked cardiomegaly. In such patients, prednisone is administered, 1 to 2 mg/kg/day, divided into two or three doses. Steroids at these high doses are maintained until signs of cardiac inflammation have subsided and the sedimentation rate has returned to normal. Then, steroids should be tapered gradually over a 4- to 6-week period.

Individuals with carditis and congestive heart failure must be treated with steroids. Prednisone is used in the dosage regimen already described. Added measures are required because of the presence of heart failure. Diuretics, oxygen, and sodium restriction often are necessary. If digitalis is used, it should be given with extreme caution, since the inflamed heart seems more sensitive to the drug. As in the case of patients who have other forms of myocarditis, afterload reduction with pharmacologic agents such as captopril seems preferable. The use of afterload reduction should prove particularly helpful when mitral and aortic valvular incompetence are present.

Rebound of the acute disease is not uncommon and frequently is observed a few weeks after drug therapy is stopped. Ordinarily, rebound is self-limited and subsides with a 3- to 4-week course of aspirin, 60 to 75 mg/kg/day. To reduce the possibility of rebound in patients treated with steroids, aspirin in this medium dosage is given as prednisone is tapered. In such cases the aspirin is continued for 2 to 4 weeks after the steroids have been stopped.

ARTHRITIS

Migratory polyarthritis involving the large joints of the body is the most common manifestation of acute rheumatic fever. Rheumatic joint inflammation in patients at bed rest ordinarily is responsive to salicylates in the dosage of 75 to 100 mg/kg/day. Overall improvement and a fall in sedimentation rate usually take place in 1 to 2 weeks of treatment. It is then possible to reduce the salicylate dose and begin ambulation. As soon as symptoms have gone, the patient may be discharged on no medications. If the individual remains asymptomatic over the next 6 weeks, a return to full activity follows. Careful observation for evidence of carditis is advised, since cardiac involvement is frequently associated with rheumatic arthritis.

CHOREA

Chorea is a late manifestation of rheumatic fever, appearing 3 to 6 months after known episodes of group A streptococcal infections. Symptoms may last from 2 to 6 months and frequently become a source of considerable emotional distress for the patient and his family.

Unfortunately, no specific treatment is available. Efforts should be made to reduce physical and mental stress. It is particularly important to provide adequate protective measures to prevent injury when the uncontrolled choreiform movements become violent. One must remember to look for carditis when chorea is present despite the long interval after streptococcal infection.

ERYTHEMA MARGINATUM

This uncommon manifestation of acute rheumatic fever is said to occur only when carditis is present. It is a nonpruritic rash requiring no therapy.

SUBCUTANEOUS NODULES

These small, firm, movable masses are found over extensor surfaces of the elbow, wrist, and knees but also may be suboccipital and along the spine. They are neither tender nor painful and require no treatment.

PROPHYLAXIS

Prevention of streptococcal infections is essential in persons who have had rheumatic fever, because the disease has a tendency to recur. Many patients who have had an episode of rheumatic fever develop a second attack following untreated group A streptococcal pharyngitis. The most effective method of preventing streptococcal infections and subsequent rheumatic fever is by administering intramuscular benzathine penicillin G, 1,200,000 units once per month. Oral penicillin V, 200,000 to 400,000 units twice a day, is a less satisfactory alternative. For those individuals allergic to penicillin, oral sulfadiazine, 1 gm daily for patients more than 60 lbs and 0.5 gm daily for smaller individuals, is recommended. Prophylaxis should be continued until the fifth or sixth decade of life, especially if a patient's acute episode of rheumatic fever was associated with carditis and the individual has residual rheumatic heart disease. Adults with frequent exposure to children of school age or persons known to have frequent streptococcal infections should receive prophylaxis regardless of age.

INFECTIVE ENDOCARDITIS

Individuals with rheumatic heart disease are advised to take antibiotic prophylaxis for dental procedures, surgery of the upper respiratory tract, and gastrointestinal and genitourinary tract surgery and instrumentation. This antibiotic protection should be provided in addition to the prophylactic regimen used to prevent recurrence of streptococcal infections and acute rheumatic fever. Guidelines for antibiotic prophylaxis for infective endocarditis are periodically published by the American Heart Association.

PRIMARY CARDIAC NEOPLASMS

ROBERT M. FREEDOM, M.D., F.R.C.P.(C), F.A.C.C., *and* JEFFREY F. SMALLHORN, M.D., F.R.C.P.(C)

Cardiac neoplasms in infancy, childhood, and adolescence are uncommon, and primary cardiac tumors in childhood account for less than 0.10 per cent of all admissions to the cardiovascular service of the Hospital for Sick Children in Toronto.

As in the adult, the clinical manifestations of primary cardiac neoplasms in childhood are protean. Interest in these uncommon tumors has evolved over the past few decades from histopathologic characterization to clinical recognition, therapy, and in some instances appreciation of natural history. The diagnosis of the cardiac tumor has been facilitated in recent years by the application of cross-sectional echocardiographic techniques and in the older patient by magnetic resonance imaging.

The clinical manifestations of the primary cardiac tumor reflect its location, size, and histologic constitution. Some cardiac tumors are recognized as an incidental autopsy finding, whereas others may lead to fetal hydrops, produce life-threatening cardiac rhythm disturbances, or produce severe mechanical obstruction to the ventricular inlet or outlet. Very small tumors, when located in the region of the atrioventricular node and conduction tissue, may produce atrioventricular conduction disturbances, including complete heart block and very rarely sudden death. Tumors on the left side of the heart may embolize to the cerebral and systemic circulation. Some cardiac tumors can be recognized by fetal echocardiography.

Rhabdomyoma

Although many types of cardiac tumors have been described in the pediatric age range, the most common tumor in the neonate and young infant is the rhabdomyoma. One must remember, however, that the intrapericardial teratoma, the ventricular fibroma, and even the myxoma can occur in the neonate and young infant. Cardiac rhabdomyomas are usually multiple, involve the ventricles or interventricular septum more frequently than the atria, and may obstruct the ventricular inlet and/or outlet. An electron microscopic study of these interesting tumors suggests that rhabdomyomas are derived from cardiac muscle cells and thus may represent hamartomas rather than true tumors. The most common association of the cardiac rhabdomyoma is with tuberous sclerosis, and in 30 to 60 per cent of patients with cardiac rhabdomyoma tuberous sclerosis can be or will be documented. The right-sided cardiac rhabdomyoma may result in tricuspid valve and/or pulmonary outflow tract obstruction. Interference with the tricuspid valve may produce findings of tricuspid regurgitation. Intracavitary left ventricular tumors may cause inflow or outlet obstruction or mitral regurgitation.

Rhabdomyomas tend to be multiple; rarely do they undergo a malignant histologic transformation, but because of their location they may be life-threatening. There is now considerable surgical experience in the resection/removal of cardiac rhabdomyomas, and this is certainly a consideration when dealing with a life-threatening tumor. However, it is evident that some rhabdomyomas, even those that are very large, may undergo spontaneous regression, and because of this a conservative posture may be a sound approach for those patients with extensive biventricular tumors. In older

infants and children identified as having one or more cardiac tumors, the patient should be investigated for tuberous sclerosis.

Intracardiac rhabdomyoma may be an incidental finding in a child with tuberous sclerosis or may result in cardiac symptoms secondary to an arrhythmia or obstruction from the tumor mass. Indeed, in utero diagnosis has been made in fetuses referred for evaluation of an irregular heart rate. The tumor may involve both the atria and ventricles, frequently being multiple. The echocardiographic features are consistent, with the tumor having a broad base and an apparent uniform consistency. A frequent feature is that the tumor appears to involve both sides of the interventricular septum. Inflow or outflow tract obstruction can occur, with Doppler evidence of stenosis, whereas in other cases the superior or inferior vena cava can be compromised. Interestingly, the tumor may regress spontaneously, having reached its maximum size at the time of or even prior to birth. This is substantiated by our own experience in two children, in whom the diagnosis was made in utero. In both cases the tumor appeared to have reached its maximum size in relationship to the remainder of the heart during the third trimester. Echocardiographic evaluation over a 3-year period demonstrated complete regression in one and partial regression in the other.

The rhabdomyosarcoma, a most uncommon malignant cardiac tumor, may have an intramyocardial origin or may present as an intracavitary mass. The clinical findings referable to this tumor reflect the extent of the tumor mass and the involvement of the ventricular inlet or outlet. The outlook for patients with the cardiac rhabdomyosarcoma is poor because these patients tend to present rather late and after the tumor is well established. Similar comments are germane to those few patients with other cardiac sarcomas, including fibrosarcoma, angiosarcoma, and hemangioendotheliosarcoma.

Cardiac Teratoma

Cardiac teratomas contain elements derived from all three germ layers. There is the very real potential for malignant transformation of the teratoma, and those patients whose teratoma contains immature neuroepithelium have a poor prognosis. About two thirds of the cases of an intrapericardial teratoma are identified in infants under 1 year of age. While most cardiac teratomas are intrapericardial, they are still extracardiac, originating in the region of the cardiac pedicle, thus attached to the base of the heart. The tumor, fixed by the aortic pedicle, is usually wedged between the aortic root and the superior caval vein, and both of these vessels can be compressed. In its usual position the intrapericardial teratoma can displace the heart posteriorly and to the left. A pericardial effusion, often massive, is present in the majority of patients. The effusion is generally serous but may be serosanguineous or rarely purulent. Symptoms are usually present, reflecting the very much enlarged, fluid-filled pericardium, with clinical features of both pericardial tamponade and respiratory distress, this latter feature a manifestation of lung compression by the massively enlarged fluid-filled pericardium. The recognition of an intrapericardial teratoma is facilitated by cardiac ultrasonography, and surgical excision is the treatment of choice.

Cardiac Fibroma

The cardiac fibroma is also a tumor of infancy and childhood, although this tumor is somewhat less common in the neonate than the rhabdomyoma. These tumors are usually benign, originate from the ventricular septum or the ventricular free wall, and protrude into the ventricle; the origin is more likely to be in the left ventricle than in the right ventricle. The symptomatology depends on the site of origin and severity of the obstruction. Thus the clinical manifestation is that of left ventricular outflow or inflow tract obstruction more frequently than that of right ventricular outflow tract obstruction. Among some children with a left ventricular fibroma, the presentation may be heralded by paroxysmal ventricular tachycardia. An abnormal cardiac silhouette on chest radiography with a peculiar bulge in this setting should suggest the presence of a left ventricular tumor. These tumors are locally invasive and in some instances may replace a substantial portion of the interventricular septum or free wall. These tumors can be recognized using cardiac ultrasound, selective ventricular angiocardiography, or magnetic resonance imaging. Many of these tumors are resectable, either completely or in large part.

Cardiac Myxoma

Although the cardiac myxoma is the most common cardiac tumor in the adult, this tumor is distinctly uncommon in childhood, and even less common in the neonate and young infant. Myxomas may be familial, and cardiac myxoma has been recognized in a mother and three sons. This tumor can originate on both sides of the heart, but as in the adult, these tumors more frequently originate in the left atrium, on the atrial septal surface in the region of the fossa ovalis. In some patients the presence of an intermittent murmur of mitral stenosis suggests the presence of the pedunculated left atrial myxoma, and this can be rapidly confirmed by echocardiographic examination. Other patients may present with findings of a cerebrovascular accident or event, and a search for the source of systemic emboli will eventually lead to cardiac ultrasound examination and the recognition of a left atrial or ventricular tumor. In an occasional patient, an acute femoral arterial thrombosis with subsequent thrombectomy leads to the diagnosis of cardiac myxoma. The routine application of cardiac ultrasonography greatly facilitates the recognition of the cardiac tumor. Echocardiography reveals a mass with a narrow base, unlike the more frequent rhabdomyoma. The tumors often appear to be very mobile and may be observed occluding the ventricular inlet. Ventricular myxomas are much rarer and may have a broader base, unlike their atrial counterpart. In the older child or adolescent, the presence of a left atrial tumor attached by a stalk or pedicle to the interatrial septum is highly suggestive of myxoma, although we have seen a pedunculated rhabdomyoma originating in this site. Surgical excision is the treatment of choice. Recognition of these tumors is important, as they tend not to regress and may be associated with either systemic or pulmonary emboli. One should remember that a right or left atrial thrombus reflecting a cardiomyopathy should be considered in the differential diagnosis of a cardiac tumor.

THE ECHOCARDIOGRAPHIC APPROACH

Although understanding the morphologic varieties and appearances is important, a systematic echocardiographic approach is essential, as this noninvasive mode of investigation is frequently all that is necessary prior to deciding whether surgical intervention is necessary. Defining the size, number, and location of the tumor(s) is the first step. This requires a detailed assessment, including the inferior vena cava for tumor extension from a Wilms' tumor. Following this, determination of the size of the base provides important clues to the possible type of tumor. The next step is to assess whether or not there is obstruction to either inflow or outflow. This is best evaluated by Doppler technique, as imaging alone may be misleading.

Possibly one of the most important aspects of the study is the evaluation of the extent of involvement of intracardiac structures. This is particularly relevant to ventricular tumors, which may involve the atrioventricular valves such that surgical resection would result in severe regurgitation. If such an approach is followed and combined with clinical features, then an appropriate decision regarding management can be made.

6

Digestive Tract

NURSING CARIES

GEORGE E. WHITE, A.B., D.D.S., Ph.D.,
D.B.A., F.A.G.D., F.I.C.D.

Nursing caries is a disease characterized by rampant caries in the primary dentition, especially extensive destruction of primary maxillary incisors, generally beginning on the facial or lingual smooth surfaces. Carious lesions often occur on the occlusal surfaces of the first primary molars as part of the condition. Eventually the other molars and canines are affected. The disease starts early in life, e.g., 20 to 22 months, and assumes a rapid course.

Nursing caries is thought to be totally preventable by eliminating the source of infection (*Streptococcus mutans*) from the caretaker and eliminating the bottle or breast while the child sleeps. The caretaker can act as a source of infection through contact with the infant. Therefore, the caretaker should be caries-free and be aware of the effects of the baby's sleeping with a bottle in the mouth. The milk or sweetened solution acts as a nutrient for the agent, causing lactic acid to be formed, and frequently carious lesions are the result.

Thus, the chief action for the pediatrician is to inform the parent of the potential destruction of the dentition from the child's sleeping with the bottle. Additionally, the bottle should be discarded at age one.

Information for parents is available through the American Academy of Pediatric Dentistry in the form of posters, slides, cards, video tapes, and films. This information can be given along with other health information, e.g., in prenatal classes.

PREVALENCE

The national prevalence is unknown, since no standard index exists. The current definition, which is derived from clinical description, is early and rampant caries associated with bottle feeding which may be prolonged beyond the usual time a child is weaned from the bottle. In urban populations, estimates of 20 per cent of the children have been reported. Surveys of special groups such as native American or native Alaskan preschool children have shown that more than 50 per cent are affected.

When multiple incisor lesions of the primary dentition are used as the definition of the disease, then the data from Head Start surveys can be used as an epidemiologic index: 15 per cent of children in fluoridated communities and 20 per cent of children in nonfluoridated communities can be affected. It is difficult to know what the correct data are for this disease, but it is safe to assume there are many children who have it. Further, the cost in treatment and danger to the child who has to go to the operating room could be avoided if the parents were properly informed. One source for the information is the pediatrician.

ETIOLOGY

Several predisposing factors are the primary teeth of the infant, night and naptime feeding with a sweetened liquid or milk, and infection with *S. mutans*. For two decades these factors have been known. The bottles have contained juice, soft drinks, Kool-aid, milk, and water with honey.

The association of excessive breast feeding ad libitum with nursing caries has been controversial and is thought to occur at a lower rate than with bottle feeding.

The primary pathogen for nursing caries is *S. mutans*. This pathogen is thought to be transmitted when the caretaker kisses or tastes food for the infant to determine its suitability. When the child sleeps with fermentable carbohydrate on the teeth, *S. mutans* produces lactic acid, resulting in demineralization of the teeth. This is seen clinically as a white spot. Months later the white spot breaks down and a cavity or carious lesion is seen.

INTERVENTION STRATEGIES

1. The parents should be educated about nursing caries. This may occur in a pediatrician's office, pediatric dental office, or elsewhere.

2. The source of the infection should be monitored and removed from the caretaker(s).

3. The infant should not have the bottle when sleeping and not at all past the age of 1 year.

4. Fluoride supplements may help control the disease.

CONGENITAL EPULIS OF THE NEONATE

EDMUND CATALDO, D.D.S., M.S.

The congenital epulis is indeed a very rare oral lesion found only in newborns. It is a benign granular cell lesion that has histologic similarities to the so-called granular cell myoblastoma. However, the congenital epulis is thought to be a distinct entity of undetermined etiology. It arises in the alveolar mucosa of the maxillary and mandibular ridges but is most common in the anterior maxilla. There is an unexplained 9:1 preponderance of females. The lesion presents as a painless, moderately firm, smooth mass varying in size from a few millimeters to several centimeters. The mass is usually pedunculated and may be either nodular or multilobular. There may be multiple separate lesions. Most frequently it is of normal mucosal color but may be erythematous. There are very few lesions that occur on the alveolar mucosa of the newborn, the most common being gingival cysts of the newborn (Bohn's nodules) and eruption cysts from natal and neonatal teeth. These entities, however, can be easily distinguished from the congenital epulis. In addition to causing parental alarm, the larger lesions may inhibit the patient's nutritional intake and respiration. Although there have been reports of spontaneous regression, the recommended treatment is conservative surgical removal. Since the lesion usually has a stalk-like attachment to the alveolus, removal is relatively simple, with no reports of recurrence.

DISEASES AND INJURIES OF THE ORAL REGION

HARVEY A. ZAREM, M.D.

CLEFT LIP

The primary problem with a congenital cleft of the lip is appearance. An infant can function effectively with a cleft lip; it is not a cause of major difficulty in feeding or of a failure to thrive, nor is cleft lip associated with otitis media as is a cleft palate. Although some plastic surgeons repair the cleft lip in the newborn, the majority of craniofacial teams in the United States prefer to close the cleft lip at approximately age 3 months, when an infant better tolerates general anesthesia with less risk than does the newborn. There are no adverse consequences to postponing an operative repair of the lip if there are extenuating circumstances. A bilateral cleft lip presents problems of obtaining a satisfactory aesthetic result years later, and a bilateral cleft involving the alveolus requires extensive orthodontic management. When the bilateral cleft is complete, the mid-portion of the maxilla (premaxilla) is trapped anterior to the collapsed lateral maxillary segments. This produces the typical bilateral cleft deformity, and correction necessitates spreading the maxillary segments and recessing the premaxilla. This process is usually deferred until a mixed or permanent dentition has developed. The columella of the nose is short, the alae of the nose are flared, and the mid-portion of the lip is attenuated. Although techniques have evolved over the last 10 years that permit a greatly improved repair of the bilateral cleft lip, the family must be alerted to the fact that it will take a number of therapeutic efforts over an extended period of time to obtain an optimal result. The teen-age child with unilateral or bilateral cleft lip is usually primarily concerned with the nasal deformity associated with these clefts. It is common for the child to undergo several operative procedures in the preschool years as well as in the teens before achieving a satisfactory aesthetic result.

CLEFT PALATE

A cleft palate presents several problems in addition to that of the cleft lip. Some infants may feed readily despite a cleft of the palate, but many infants do have difficulty with sucking and feeding. A long, soft lamb's nipple is often effective. When the mother has learned to feed the infant patiently, the infant will thrive. If an infant with a cleft palate fails to thrive, it is usually due to frustration on the part of the family over the difficulty of feeding, and it is unwise to attribute a failure to thrive to a cleft of the palate alone. Efforts to educate the family to feed the child and hospitalization with feeding by a trained nursing staff should be tried before assuming that a failure to thrive is due to the cleft palate.

Children with a cleft of the palate have an extremely high incidence of otitis media, even in the neonatal period. Many otologists have recommended that children with clefts of the palate undergo routine myringotomy with insertion of tubes to maintain patency of the drum and to reduce the incidence of otitis media with subsequent hearing loss. The family must be alerted to the incidence of otitis media to facilitate early diagnosis and early treatment with decongestants and antibiotics to minimize the long-term scarring and hearing loss.

The major problem associated with a cleft of the palate is difficulty in speech. Although most craniofacial teams in the United States continue to close the palate at approximately age 18 months, we have frequently chosen to repair the palate at age 1 year in order to accommodate the otologist's need to perform myringotomies. Rather than subject the child to two separate anesthesias, we prefer to combine the two. If the child is thriving, anesthesia and cleft palate repair at age 1 year has been successful, and it is becoming our preference. In addition, speech pathologists believe that early phonation and speech habits can be affected by the cleft palate before the age of 3 years, which was previously doubted. Speech pathologists therefore are enthusiastic about early palatal closure, if it is deemed safe. Effective closure with respect to the anatomy and the use of pharyngeal flaps as well as other adjunctive techniques of palatoplasty and pharyngoplasty have resulted in a significant improvement in the quality of speech of patients with clefts of the palate. Working with the family to encourage them to speak clearly and deliberately with the child to encourage effective speech habits has been a worthwhile effort. If the child does have inadequate closure of the soft palate to the pharynx (velopharyngeal incompetence), several corrective measures are available. A prosthodontist may contribute with the production of a speech bulb that will mechanically aid in the closure of the space between the soft palate and the pharynx, but we prefer to think of this as a temporary measure when other medical problems such as serious cardiac disease preclude operative closure of the palate. When a significant speech defect exists that is not improved with judicious speech therapy following palatal repair, a pharyngeal flap or a pharyngoplasty has been effective in closing the defect and providing adequate speech. Problems with the pharyngeal flap or pharyngoplasty have included inadequate correction with little or no speech improvement, denasal speech, and mild nasal airway obstruction. These problems are usually amenable to additional surgical therapy.

Routine tonsillectomy and adenoidectomy should not be carried out in the child who has undergone cleft palate repair. Frequently the hypertrophic adenoids and tonsils aid in the occlusion of the velopharynx and thereby aid speech by minimizing velopharyngeal incompetence. Concern must also be applied to the child who has a submucous cleft. A submucous cleft (which can be recognized by the bifid uvula, the thin blue midline in the soft palate, and a lack of a nasal spine with notching of the posterior border of the hard palate in the midline) has adequate velopharyngeal closure until a tonsillectomy and adenoidectomy have been carried out. Prior to recommending such an operative procedure, it is necessary to ascertain that the soft palate is normal.

The child born with a unilateral cleft of the lip and palate may expect a normal life pattern in view of the high quality of surgical, orthodontic, otologic, and speech therapy that has evolved today. The child with a bilateral cleft lip and palate, however, presents with a significant number of developmental deformities that produce problems even with excellent dental and surgical care. The midportion of the upper jaw (premaxilla) is prominent in infancy, but hypoplasia of the maxilla and collapse of the maxilla with collapse of the dental arch are frequent accompaniments of the bilateral cleft lip and cleft palate. The adolescent who has had a bilateral cleft of the lip and palate is likely to struggle with deformities of the maxilla and nose and with scars associated with the extreme lip deformity. Although judicious operative repair and sophisticated orthodontia have greatly improved the outcome of these patients in adolescence, the family should be alerted to the significance of the deformity and given encouragement to work with the child in a positive fashion.

Numerous orthodontic, orthognathic, and soft tissue procedures will be needed to accomplish a satisfactory aesthetic and functional result.

MACROGLOSSIA

The term *macroglossia* is applied to an enlarged tongue. Occasionally the diagnosis is made when in fact the problem is a small mandible. The initial and primary concern in macroglossia is the potential for airway obstruction, as in the Pierre Robin syndrome. The major etiologies of macroglossia in children are lymphangioma, hemangioma, and neurofibroma; primary macroglossia may be associated with hyperthyroidism, amyloidosis, and glycogen storage diseases. In a surgical practice lymphangioma seems to be the most common etiology of macroglossia in children presenting at age 4 to 6 years. Small superficial vesicles on the mucosa are characteristic. An open bite and drooling are strong indications for excision of a portion of the tongue.

PIERRE ROBIN SYNDROME

Robin originally described a syndrome that included cleft palate, macroglossia (large tongue), and micrognathia (retruded mandible). The major significance of the Pierre Robin syndrome is the risk of glossoptosis in which the child may asphyxiate by "swallowing his tongue." Approximately 50 per cent of affected children have cleft palate. Respiratory difficulty occurs most commonly at the time of feeding and may be manifested shortly after birth or as late as 1½ to 2 months. The primary anxiety on the part of the treating physician is whether one should be conservative and risk the possibility that one of these respiratory difficulties could be fatal or continue with the conservative approach to tide the child over the first few months of life. The respiratory difficulty usually decreases when the child is on his abdomen and in some instances when an attempt is made to feed the child in the prone position. When this is not feasible, either because of the severity of the deformity or because of the lack of co-operation on the part of the family, an operative procedure to secure the tongue forward has been quite successful in experienced hands. This procedure is temporary and may be reversed after the neonatal period when the danger of respiratory obstruction has passed. Many of the children with Pierre Robin syndrome ultimately have normal mandibular development with correction of the glossoptosis and attain a normal occlusal relationship.

UNUSUAL CLEFTS

Although the most common clefts by far on the face involve the upper lip and palate, numerous other clefts may occur and have been classified from both the therapeutic and the embryologic standpoints. Notching and clefts of the lower lip, alveolus, and tongue; bifid tongue; median cleft of the upper lip; and extensive clefts involving the nose, medial canthus, and orbit are now well recognized.

TONGUE-TIE

A significant number of infants are born with a short frenulum extending from the tongue to the central incisor area of the mandible. The majority of these children are asymptomatic. If the child can protrude the tongue, as in licking a lollipop, the likelihood of tongue-tie affecting speech is minimal. In significant tongue-tie, however, it is appropriate to release the tongue surgically. "Snipping" the tongue-tie is usually inappropriate, since a definitive procedure with Z-plasty and extension of the length of the frenulum is necessary. When the band is extremely thin, simple "snipping" may be effective. In children in whom the indication for surgery is questionable, an experienced speech pathologist may be most helpful.

MACROSTOMIA

The diagnosis of macrostomia is occasionally missed because it is associated with underdevelopment of the mandible. The distance between the midline of the upper or lower lip and the oral commissure is greater on the affected side than on the normal side. It is commonly associated with the first and second branchial arch syndrome (hemifacial microsomia) with hypoplasia of the entire half of the face, including the ear, the temporal muscle, masseter muscle, parotid gland, zygoma, and mandible. The macrostomia can be corrected by Z-plasty. The management of jaw deformity and hemifacial hypoplasia is a complex issue and should be deferred until development of the jaw and eruption of the teeth occur.

JAW DEFORMITIES

Micrognathia

Micrognathia may occur separately or in association with other syndromes such as Pierre Robin syndrome or hemifacial microsomia (first and second branchial arch syndrome). A significant number of micrognathias occur as hereditary features and not necessarily as a feature of a specific syndrome. Unless extreme, jaw development deformities are usually not apparent until the child is 5 to 6 years of age. The child should be evaluated by an experienced orthodontist, who is most capable of assessing dental and jaw development. Treatment of the majority of the children who require operative correction is deferred until full dental eruption, usually at age 18 or older. Severe facial deformities due to extreme jaw abnormality are treated at varying ages, depending on dentition.

Macrognathia

Macrognathia (protruded mandible or prognathism) is also a deformity that is not readily apparent until the child is 5 to 6 years of age. It is characterized by an obtuse angle between the ramus of the mandible and the body of the mandible, and often an open bite. As in micrognathia, the diagnosis, evaluation, and treatment are sophisticated, and the patient should be evaluated by an orthodontist.

Bony Overgrowth of Jaws

A number of disorders with overgrowth of either the maxilla or mandible are not common but present a problem of diagnosis and treatment. Overgrowth of the jaw may be the result of arteriovenous fistula, which is usually apparent by the increased prominence of the vessels, by a bruit in the external carotid and its branches to the involved area, and by the increased warmth of the soft tissues. The management of an arteriovenous fistula involving the mandible or maxilla is difficult. The disease is invariably progressive. Patients may have dramatic episodes of bleeding that require blood transfusions. Frequently it is necessary to ligate the external carotid artery to control the bleeding, but the ultimate treatment is radical excision of the involved parts. This decision is difficult, since the surgery and the deformity are extensive; however, once the diagnosis is established and the course of progression of the arteriovenous fistula and progressive risk of serious hemorrhages have been clarified, definitive treatment should be instituted.

In a number of patients with neurofibromatosis, either local or diffuse (as in von Recklinghausen's syndrome), the face is involved. Overgrowth of the soft tissues and bones on the involved side of the face is the consequence. There is increased bulk of maxilla or mandible with gingival hypertrophy and displacement of the teeth. Management is effected by excising the offending tissues and sculpturing the tissues to correct the deformity. To "cure" the disease would entail an extensive operative procedure with removal of many normal structures and is never advisable. The course of this disease depends on the progression and age of onset of symptoms. The earlier the age of onset and the more rapid the course in youth, the worse the prognosis. Hemifacial hypertrophy, with enlargement of all of the facial structures (including jaw and teeth) unilaterally, presents a similar picture but is without the soft tissue neurofibromas.

Fibrous dysplasia of the jaws is an unusual condition involving the mandible or maxilla, which is enlarged because of the fibrous and noncalcified tissue within the bone. The presence of this entity is often not evident until late childhood, but it is usually self-limited when the child reaches puberty and growth ceases. This disorder must be recognized to avoid a misdiagnosis and radical excision of tissues. Contouring bone to reduce the deformity can be done in order to tide the child over until puberty and skeletal maturation. In some instances the excess bone that had been excised will recur, and this must be appreciated by the family before operative management of children with fibrous dysplasia of the jaws is undertaken.

Orofacial dysostosis is a congenital anomaly expressed in the oral region by alveolar clefts, tongue clefts, cysts of the upper lip, and supernumerary teeth; it is associated with anomalies of the hand and mental retardation.

Infantile cortical hyperostosis (Caffey's disease) is a self-limiting disease of children seen with onset of fever, soft tissue swelling, and periosteal new bone formation of the mandible. It occurs most commonly in the neonatal period (2 to 4 months of age) and could be mistaken for osteomyelitis of the mandible. The clavicles are often involved, and the radiographic picture is one of increased density on the surface of the bone due to new bone formation with overlying brawny induration of the soft tissues. In the mild cases no treatment is necessary except to maintain the comfort of the patient, but in the severe cases treatment with corticosteroids is indicated. It is recommended that the steroid dosage be continued over several months because exacerbations have occurred with early withdrawal of steroids.

TRAUMA

The majority of injuries about the oral region are minor and do not necessitate hospitalization. For the occasional severe injury, the most immediate dangers are exsanguinating hemorrhage and airway obstruction owing to loss of control of the tongue or to the blood. Most bleeding can be stopped by direct pressure.

If a child has eaten solids or liquids within 4 hours prior to the injury, it is generally not wise to consider general anesthesia except in dire circumstances. Emptying time of the stomach is prolonged after injury, so that the time lapse following an injury is often not reliable for judging a safe period. The majority of injuries about the mouth and face can be repaired using local anesthesia if some sedation is given and if the manner of the treating physician and parents is calm. Once the area is anesthetized, the majority of children relax and even doze during the repair.

Anesthesia about the face is often accomplished either by direct infiltration of lidocaine (Xylocaine), 1 per cent with epinephrine 1:100,000, or by regional nerve blocks. The entire upper lip can be anesthetized by injecting the infraorbital nerve bilaterally. These simple nerve blocks are effective, and once the area is anesthetized, the child is usually co-operative.

Prior to the development of antibiotics, surgeons were cautious of closing any wounds that had occurred 4 or more hours prior to treatment. Today it is appropriate to close all facial wounds that are not overly contaminated despite the fact that more than 4 hours may have elapsed from the time of injury to the time of treatment. In animal bites or severe contamination, the use of tetanus toxoid, antibiotics, and judicious closure initially or closure secondarily (within several days of the injury) are appropriate. It is rarely advisable to allow a wound of the face or oral region to heal secondarily because of the resulting scar deformity. If a wound were closed and the degree of contamination underestimated, daily examination would allow the treating surgeon to open the wound at the first sign of infection and prevent a serious consequence.

A major portion of wounds seen in children in the emergency room are puncture wounds of the lower lip from the incisors. This wound lacerates the mucosa, the lower lip musculature, and the skin. This "through-and-through" wound is best cleansed with saline irrigation after local anesthesia and closed primarily. Small wounds may be closed with sutures in the mucosa and in the skin, but large through-and-through wounds should be closed in layers to include fat and muscle. Nonabsorbable soft suture material (preferably silk) should be used in the mouth when it is feasible to remove the sutures postoperatively.

Absorbable sutures cause inflammation in the mouth, and synthetic sutures such as nylon are stiff and extremely uncomfortable to the sensitive mucosa of the mouth. Closure of the muscle may be accomplished by absorbable sutures (Dexon, Vicryl, or catgut), and closure of the skin should be accomplished with nonabsorbable sutures, such as a nonreacting fine (6–0) nylon, which can be removed. In the rare instances in which it is determined that the sutures cannot be removed from the skin, absorbable synthetic sutures such as Dexon or Vicryl are acceptable but only as second choices to the nonreactive synthetic fine nylon. Sutures on the skin of the face should be placed very close to the edge of the wound to avoid suture marks. They should also be removed approximately 4 to 5 days following the injury. The wounds can be supported after suture removal with a porous adhesive tape such as Steri-strips or Clearon. These paper tape closures will remain on the skin for approximately 5 to 7 days.

When the laceration about the lip extends across the mucocutaneous juncture (the white line between the vermilion of the mucosa and the white skin), care must be taken to align the fragments of the juncture. This is best done with the aid of magnifying loupes by aligning the fine white "roll" that is apparent owing to the thick sebaceous glands at the juncture. A small malalignment is conspicuous. When there is a significant loss of mucosa, it is often advisable to excise the wound in a V fashion and close the wound primarily. When there has been a loss of mucosa, such as from a dog bite, it is necessary to consider rotating a mucosal flap from the adjacent lip mucosa, a mucosal graft, or occasionally a tongue flap. Injuries in which there is a significant loss of tissue of the lip are difficult, and the reconstruction to restore mucosa, muscle, and skin is complex. Sometimes it is best to close the wounds in a simple fashion and to defer extensive reconstructive procedures. When the immediate treating physician is not adequately experienced, it is always wisest to do a simple wound closure.

In general, it is preferable for the patient to undergo definitive wound repair at the time of the initial injury. If one allows the wounds to heal initially without definitive repair, scarring must be corrected secondarily. There are often circumstances (such as associated injuries, lack of available facilities and personnel, and the general condition of the patient) that may dictate secondary procedures rather than extensive primary repair. Secondary procedures, which include mucosal flaps, cross-lip flaps, and tongue flaps, should be undertaken only by an experienced surgeon.

Lacerations of the tongue are usually a problem because of extensive bleeding. The bleeding can be controlled by large sutures. The suture material should be silk because it is soft and relatively nonreacting, but this must be done only in the child who will co-operate to allow removal of the sutures.

In all significant injuries of the mucosa of the mouth, including lips, gingiva, tongue, soft palate, and pharynx, several steps have resulted in diminished infection and improved results. The child should be kept on a clear liquid diet for a minimum of 3 days. A clear liquid diet consists of transparent liquids without particles. This prevents food particles from entering the wound as a nidus for infection. It is difficult to convince the family of the child that this diet is compatible with health and well being.

After solid foods have been resumed, it is wise to rinse the mouth after each meal with plain water or a mild salt solution (a quart of warm water in which 1 teaspoon of table salt and 1 teaspoon of baking soda have been dissolved). Frequent washing of the mouth and irrigating of the wounds in this manner have resulted in excellent wound healing. The use of antibiotics in these wounds is variable. Most surgeons agree that the use of an antibiotic for 5 days is safe and has resulted in a diminished incidence of wound infection and inflammation.

In all significant lacerations about the mouth, the treating physician should be aware of possible injury to the parotid duct and facial nerve. Parotid duct injury, if not recognized, can result in parotid secretions into the tissues or in a parotid fistula, which is difficult to manage and often requires secondary procedures. If, on the other hand, the injury to the parotid duct is recognized at the time of the trauma, repair of the duct is simple and effective and is best accomplished under general anesthesia in the young child.

Injuries to the facial musculature or to the facial nerve should be appreciated prior to treatment, especially prior to the administration of local anesthetics. The child should be asked to activate all of the facial muscles of expression, and asymmetry should be carefully noted. If the injury to the facial nerve occurs anterior to a vertical line through the lateral canthus of the eye, the likelihood of recovery of function without surgical repair of the nerve is excellent. However, if the injury occurs proximal to this line, which is proximal to the anterior border of the masseter muscle, it is wise to undertake a search and repair of the nerve. This must be done under general anesthesia with magnification and with microsurgical instruments.

Electrical burns of the mouth are unusual. They usually occur when a toddler places the juncture of an electrical appliance end of an extension cord in the mouth. The saliva acts as a conductor and causes an electrical burn. Severe electrical burns can result in a loss of major portions of the upper and lower lip and gingiva and even injury to the tooth buds and mandible. Fortunately, the majority of these injuries involve only the lips and oral commissure. Electrical injuries to the mid-portion of the upper and lower lip usually heal without severe deformities.

The treatment of the electrical injury to the lip must be definitive. Immediately after the injury, the degree of trauma is usually not evident. The child should be given sedation and antibiotics, and the family must watch the child carefully. Late bleeding from the labial artery can be dramatic and, if it occurs, does so 5 to 7 days following injury. Parents are instructed to watch for bleeding and, if it occurs, to pinch the lip between the fingers and to bring the child to the emergency room immediately.

The majority of surgeons prefer to treat electrical burns with antibiotic therapy and to allow secondary healing. If a deformity occurs at a later date, reconstruction is undertaken electively. The primary reason that this has been a chosen course is that it is often difficult to determine the extent of loss of tissues in the early post-injury phase. About 3 weeks following the injury, the degree of tissue loss is usually evident. If a significant portion of the upper or lower lip at the commissure has been lost, restoration of the bulk of the lip using the tongue as the source of muscle and mucosa can be done as a tongue flap 3 to 4 weeks after injury. This procedure must be carefully executed, but it is effective in extensive electrical burn injuries of the oral commissure.

SALIVARY GLAND TUMORS

DOUGLAS W. BELL, M.D.

Hemangiomas are the most common cause of parotid swelling in the newborn. Eighty per cent are present at birth, with the remainder discovered within the next 6 to 12 months. These benign lesions are diffuse, soft masses in the preauricular area and angle of mandible area. There may be a rapid growth for the first 6 months, but there is also regression because of vessel occlusion. There may be some redness of the overlying skin, but as the tumor regresses, the color subsides. The mass may increase in size with crying or straining. Only in a few cases in which the tumor continues to expand is surgery indicated. This involves a superficial parotidectomy, with identification and preservation of the facial nerve, which courses through the gland.

Lymphangiomas are benign congenital lesions of lymph vessels. Over 90 per cent occur in the cervical region, and many involve the parotid or submaxillary gland. These lesions do not undergo spontaneous regression. Thus, surgical dissection must be utilized to remove all the small cystic lesions. Otherwise, there is a notable recurrence rate, and multifocal lesions develop. Laser therapy may be used at times, and cryotherapy is helpful for intraoral lesions.

If the tumor mass develops later in childhood, the mass is usually firmer, more discrete, nontender, and of variable mobility. The most likely tumor is a benign mixed tumor containing both glandular and ductal elements. If such a mass persists, excisional biopsy with facial nerve protection is necessary.

Only 10 per cent of these masses are malignant. Such tumors expand rapidly and may be fixed to other tissues or may be tender. If there is facial paralysis, the tumor is assumed to be malignant. The most common malignant tumors of the parotid gland are mucoepidermoid carcinomas and sarcomas (rhabdomyosarcomas and undifferentiated tumors). Total parotidectomy with facial nerve preserved may be sufficient. If the nerve must be partially excised, immediate grafting techniques are used. Chemotherapy has made great advances and may be used as primary therapy. Radiation therapy is also part of the "triple attack" on these aggressive tumors. The exact protocol is determined by the cell type, rate of growth, and extent of tumor.

Submaxillary gland tumors are usually the benign

mixed type and occur in older children. More rapid growth would signal a likely malignant potential. In either case, total removal of the submaxillary gland with sparing of the lingual nerve is the best treatment. Any further chemotherapy or irradiation would be decided based on the tumor cell type.

RECURRENT ACUTE PAROTITIS

TONI M. GANZEL, M.D., *and*
FREDERICK M. PARKINS, D.D.S., M.S.D., Ph.D.

Recurrent acute parotitis is an uncommon disorder in children characterized by painful parotid swelling, fever, and purulent discharge from Stenson's duct. The age of onset has been reported to range from 8 months to 16 years, with a mean age at the time of onset of 7 to 9 years. The cause is still unknown, but proposed etiologies include congenital sialectasis, autoimmune disease, ductal trauma, ductal strictures, allergy, and metaplastic transformation of serous secreting cells and intraductal epithelium to mucus-producing cells.

The diagnosis is based on history, physical examination, and sialography, which usually demonstrates sialectasis. Cultures of the mucopurulent material from Stenson's duct frequently grow *Streptococcus viridans*. Based on this finding, antibiotic therapy directed toward this organism is recommended for 7 to 10 days, although the efficacy of this treatment has not been proven. An appropriate antibiotic choice is amoxicillin (40 mg/kg/day in three divided doses). In a penicillin-allergic child, erythromycin (30 to 50 mg/kg every 6 hours) is recommended. Changes to alternative antibiotic coverage may be necessary, depending on culture results. Supportive therapy consisting of acetaminophen for analgesia, warm packs, gland massage, and sialogogues (chewing gum or "sour" candy) should be instituted. Occasionally, Stenson's duct orifice may require probing to facilitate removal of thickened mucous secretions. The duration of the episode is generally 4 to 7 days, and the time interval between episodes varies from weeks to years.

Although there have been sporadic reports of prevention of recurrent episodes by intraductal instillation of antibiotics and by therapeutic use of sialography, no controlled clinical studies have demonstrated that the recurrent episodes can be prevented by these methods. Ligation of Stenson's duct and radiation to the gland have been reported to cause gland atrophy and prevent further infection but have not gained widespread acceptance. Superficial parotidectomy can be performed but should be restricted to the most severe cases owing to the potential risk of surgical injury to the facial nerve. Regardless of therapy, there is a tendency for the disease to undergo spontaneous resolution near the onset of puberty. For this reason, a treatment principle of *primum non nocere* has been advocated.

THYROGLOSSAL DUCT CYSTS

DOUGLAS W. BELL, M.D.

Thyroglossal duct cysts are typically asymptomatic and may pose no problem other than a cosmetic change. The longer the cyst is present, the more likely it is to become infected secondarily from an upper respiratory infection.

In 10 per cent of children in whom the cyst becomes infected, it enlarges, tenderness increases, and it may progress to an abscess. Antibiotics such as amoxicillin or a cephalosporin are usually sufficient with warm compresses. Needle aspiration may be necessary for better culture of the organism if the infection fails to respond to antibiotics. In the extreme case, this abscess ruptures at the skin surface and a draining sinus tract persists. Antibiotics and local dressing care are used to control the infection. Later, the entire sinus tract and the cyst are surgically removed.

Unless the midportion of the hyoid bone is excised, there is a 25 per cent recurrence rate of the cyst. If the cyst is large and little or no thyroid tissue is palpable, it is wise to perform a thyroid scan preoperatively. This is to document the entire thyroid tissue and to avoid possibly removing all the patient's functioning thyroid. The postoperative course is benign, with some dysphagia present only for a few days and no change in speech articulation.

BRANCHIAL ARCH CYSTS AND SINUSES

DOUGLAS W. BELL, M.D.

The typical branchial arch cyst is a smooth, round, nontender cyst along the anterior border of the sternocleidomastoid muscle at any point from the external auditory canal to the clavicle. The cyst may not be noted until it becomes infected—usually in late childhood or adolescence. Then it enlarges and is tender, and the skin become erythematous. Antibiotic therapy usually controls the infection, and the cyst subsides after resolution of the illness. If a sinus tract persists, then it is palpable as a fibrous cord extending along the muscle border. The tract may develop into a fistula, with intermittent drainage onto the neck skin. The treatment of these various cysts and sinuses is surgical excision of the entire tract. It must be traced back to its origin, and the communication with the ear canal or pharynx must be closed.

In evaluating second and third arch fistula tracts, a radiopaque dye is used to identify the entire tract. The internal ostia may be in the tonsil and require a tonsillectomy to solve the problem completely. Knowing the embryology and development, the physician can anticipate any important vessels and nerves that need to be carefully protected during surgery. Antibiotic therapy should precede any surgical treatment so that inflammation is minimized. The excision should be as complete as possible.

DISORDERS OF THE ESOPHAGUS

ARTHUR R. EULER, M.D.

Esophageal disorders may be classified as congenital or acquired lesions. Although this classification is not optimal for some disorders, such as certain types of webs and rings, I will present the general subject of disorders of the esophagus divided into these two large categories.

CONGENITAL DISORDERS OF THE ESOPHAGUS

Congenital esophageal lesions are usually associated with significant morbidity and occasional mortality. These usually become clinically apparent soon after birth when swallowing difficulties develop, although those that present primarily with respiratory tract complications may not present until later. These types of esophageal lesions should be managed in a high-risk neonatal intensive care unit where surgical and medical specialists experienced in the evaluation and treatment of such abnormalities are located.

Esophageal Atresia with Tracheoesophageal Fistula. Approximately 85 per cent of congenital esophageal anomalies are characterized by a blind pouch, usually located in the upper half of the esophagus, plus a communication between a distal esophageal segment and the tracheobronchial tract. The gestational history often has associated polyhydramnios, with the neonatal history being one of drooling, nasal drainage, and slight respiratory distress, followed by significant exacerbations of all these symptoms when the first oral feeding is taken.

Treatment is begun by elevating the head and upper thorax approximately 20 degrees and administering supplemental oxygen as required to maintain oxygenation. The upper esophageal pouch is intubated, evacuated, and subsequently drained continuously with low-pressure suction. Hydration and nutrition are maintained with parenteral fluids until a gastrostomy tube is placed. The latter is usually done under local anesthesia soon after the diagnosis is made. Broad-spectrum antibiotics that cover the types of bacteria usually associated with aspiration pneumonia should be started. These measures lessen further pulmonary complications and provide necessary nutritional support until a definitive surgical repair is performed. This repair should not be undertaken until the neonate's condition is stable, particularly his or her respiratory status.

The surgical approach employed is based on the patient's weight and pulmonary status. Waterston's classification is a useful guide for remembering the appropriate surgical approach. In group A, which contains neonates over 2.5 kg who do not have aspiration pneumonitis or other abnormalities, an immediate single-stage approach via a right thoracotomy incision is appropriate. In group B are two separate clinical groups: those who weigh between 1.8 and 2.5 kg and are well and those who weigh more but have moderate pulmonary disease and/or other moderately severe congenital anomalies. These patients are best managed by an initial period of gastrostomy feedings and medical therapy for their other problems before surgery is undertaken. In group C are those who are smaller (less than 1.8 kg) and/or have severe pulmonary disease or congenital anomalies. These are best managed by a fistula ligation and nutritional support, either parenterally or by gastrostomy, for several weeks before a definite esophageal repair is undertaken.

One difficulty in correcting esophageal atresia lesions is that a primary anastomosis of the proximal and distal segments may be impossible if the intervening gap is very great. Several surgical techniques have now been developed to elongate the two segments, with the goal of avoiding the necessity of a colonic or gastric tube interposition by eventually obtaining a primary anastomosis. End-to-side junctions are preferred because the incidence of side effects is less than with an end-to-end anastomosis.

Postoperatively gastrostomy feedings with glucose water are initiated when evidence of adequate gastric emptying is documented. Salivary secretions are continually and gently suctioned via a nasal catheter, which is usually placed at surgery just above the anastomotic site. Oral feedings are not initiated until 10 to 14 days postoperatively.

Leaks from the anastomotic site are the major and most serious postoperative complication. An initial sign of this is often saliva and/or food in the chest tube drainage. With extrapleural repairs, these leaks usually spontaneously remit so they are only followed expectantly with cessation of oral feedings and institution of parenteral nutrition. With transpleural repairs serious empyema may occur; therefore, in this case, the management consists of a cervical esophagostomy, distal esophageal closure, antibiotics, and chest tube drainage. Although anastomotic leaks occur in the early postoperative period, other problems appear later such as strictures at the anastomotic site. These are treated with repeated bougienage as necessary. A significant factor in the development of these anastomotic strictures is gastroesophageal reflux, which is an almost universal finding. This may be treated with bethanechol (8.7 mg/m² given in three divided doses), but often esophagitis, stricture formation, and pulmonary disease still develop, requiring a Nissen fundoplication. The severity of the complications induced by the gastroesophageal reflux is compounded by the abnormal esophageal peristaltic activity that all such patients have, particularly below the level of the anastomosis. There is no effective treatment for this. A less frequent postoperative complication is a recurrence of the tracheoesophageal fistula. This is treated by a repeat ligation of the fistula.

Esophageal Atresia Without Tracheoesophageal Fistula. This type of atresia is present in less than 10 per cent of patients with these types of congenital esophagotracheobronchial anomalies. The approach is similar to that mentioned previously, with gastrostomy feeding being initiated along with measures to protect against further pulmonary aspiration by applying gentle suction to the proximal pouch. Any pulmonary disease present is treated with appropriate antibiotics and oxygen as required. The definitive surgical approach is as for those with an associated tracheoesophageal fistula.

Tracheoesophageal Fistula Without Esophageal Atresia. This type of anomaly represents a smaller overall number, approximately 4 per cent, of these types of lesions. It is, however, the most difficult to diagnose because there is no abrupt and dramatic onset of symptomatology soon after birth but, rather, usually an insidious course of recurrent pulmonary problems resulting in a delay in proper diagnosis that may range from a few weeks to months. Most of the fistulas can be ligated by a cervical approach because most are located in the proximal esophagus; however, a thoracotomy is required for the remainder.

Laryngotracheoesophageal Cleft. The initial medical therapy for these infants is the same as for those with esophageal atresia and a tracheoesophageal fistula. These infants often have other severe congenital anomalies that require very skillful medical management. The mortality with laryngotracheoesophageal cleft alone is very high, often resulting from a delay in proper diagnosis. Endoscopic evaluation is very important, although the lesion may be confusing at endoscopy. The passage of an endotracheal tube into the larynx may be helpful, since this placement often opens the cleft, confirming the diagnosis. Management can then be either by the endotracheal tube or by tracheostomy. Even with either of these in place, gastroesophageal reflux with aspiration still remains a problem. Maneuvers such as a double gastrostomy have been advocated to prevent this. Definitive early surgical repair should be undertaken as soon as the infant's overall condition permits.

Webs and Stenoses. Esophageal webs are composed of mucosa and submucosa but do not contain muscle. Congenital webs and stenoses are uncommon compared with strictures associated with gastroesophageal reflux. The clinical presentation of both these congenital lesions, however, is very similar to that seen with gastroesophageal reflux–induced strictures. This usually includes vomiting, dysphagia, and/or repeated pulmonary infections. These congenital lesions usually respond to bougienage and rarely require surgical repair. Schatzki rings and other disorders associated with webs, such as the Plummer-Vinson syndrome, are covered in the section dealing with acquired lesions.

Rings. Esophageal and tracheal compression can result from vascular anomalies, including a double aortic arch, an aberrant right subclavian artery, and a right aortic arch with a left ligamentum arteriosum. The resulting constriction may cause partial esophageal obstruction, resulting in dysphagia or vomiting and/or respiratory distress, usually manifested by stridor. Definitive vascular surgery is corrective, but surgery may be delayed until the infant is larger if symptoms are mild.

Duplications. These are usually cystic structures filled with fluid only, but if they are of the neuroenteric type, there are always associated vertebral malformations. With simple duplication cysts, excision via a thoracotomy is all that is required. Careful dissection is mandatory, for cysts may be multiple, may have a separate blood supply from the esophagus, may have a fine connection with the esophagus, and may be associated

with extralobar pulmonary sequestration or diaphragmatic hernia.

Diverticula. Rarely congenital diverticular lesions have been reported to be associated with tracheoesophageal fistula, but most occur alone. They are usually simple protrusions of mucosa and submucosa without any muscular component. Those immediately above the upper esophageal sphincter are called Zenker's diverticula, whereas those in the mid-esophagus or directly orad to the lower esophageal sphincter are called traction and epiphrenic diverticula, respectively. Zenker's diverticula are usually managed with a one-stage diverticulectomy. If the diverticulum is very small, some have advocated a cricomyotomy alone, which is intended to decrease esophageal pressure in the proximal esophagus. In patients with extremely large diverticula, a one-stage diverticulectomy plus a cricopharyngeal myotomy may be considered.

Traction (mid-esophageal) diverticula are most often multiple and are thought to be secondary to an esophageal motor disorder. Unless they are extremely large, therapy is usually not indicated.

Epiphrenic diverticula are also thought to be associated with an esophageal motor disorder. Surgical therapy is directed at removing the diverticulum plus a myotomy aimed at correcting the motor dysfunction such as achalasia or diffuse esophageal spasm.

Sucking and Swallowing Problems. The co-ordination of sucking, swallowing, and breathing requires a high degree of neural sophistication. Many neonates and infants have mild motor dysfunction that requires only a careful history and physical examination to exclude other disorders, plus instructions regarding feeding techniques and reassurance to the parents. In the case of a discrete lesion that is interfering with the patient's ability to co-ordinate these activities, such as a palatal cleft, specific therapy to correct this abnormality should be applied. These patients would also benefit from being fed upright so that gravity can be used to prevent some nasopharyngeal reflux. If specific measures aimed at alleviating such problems are unsuccessful, a feeding gastrostomy should be considered. Unless such disorders are associated with other significant clinical abnormalities, most will improve with age so that most such infants can eventually be returned to oral feedings.

ACQUIRED DISORDERS OF THE ESOPHAGUS

Neuromuscular disorders of the esophagus can be either primary, as in cricopharyngeal dysfunction, or secondary, as in scleroderma.

Cricopharyngeal Dysfunction. This disorder, which involves abnormal upper esophageal sphincter relaxation, is also known as cricopharyngeal achalasia or spasm. Although usually primary in nature, it may be one of the manifestations of a systemic disorder such as familial dysautonomia or generalized neural immaturity, as in a premature infant.

Pharmacologic therapy of this disorder is not usually very helpful, although anticholinergics may decrease salivation somewhat, thereby reducing symptoms. Treatment is directed toward the primary systemic disease. Dilatation has been advocated and may be tried, although a large clinical trial assessing its efficacy has not been reported. Cricopharyngeal myotomy remains the definitive therapy. Before this is undertaken it is vital that the presence of a Zenker's diverticulum and the extremely rare occurrence of an organic lesion be excluded. If the dysfunction is secondary, treatment of the primary systemic disease is extremely important.

Diffuse Esophageal Spasm. This disorder, which has a clinical presentation consisting usually of chest pain and dysphagia plus manometric findings of tertiary contractions, is rare during the pediatric years. Dilatations are not useful, nor does drug therapy give uniform clinical results. Long-acting nitrates in increasing doses have been reported to be helpful in some adult patients. Severe headaches are a serious side effect limiting their use. Calcium-channel blocking agents such as nifedipine may eventually be shown to be the drug class of choice. In severe cases, a long esophageal myotomy may be considered.

Achalasia. Achalasia, or cardiospasm, is a disorder associated with failure of the lower esophageal sphincter to relax properly, with abnormal peristalsis in the smooth muscle portion of the esophagus and eventually often extreme dilatation of the esophageal body (megaesophagus). Pharmacologic treatment with long-acting nitrate compounds such as sublingual isosorbide dinitrate has been reported in adults, but severe headaches have been a significant side effect. Treatment with this type of compound or with a calcium-channel blocker (nifedipine) may be considered in patients who have failed to respond to dilatation and are not surgical candidates, although neither of these drug classes has been extensively used in children with this disorder. The treatment of choice remains pneumatic dilatation or surgical myotomy of the lower esophageal sphincter. Simple bougienage is not effective. Pneumatic dilatation frequently gives sustained periods of relief in some children but requires hospitalization because of the need for sedation and the risk of esophageal perforation. A successful dilatation is usually associated with blood streaking of the pneumatic balloon when it is withdrawn. Dilatation is not appropriate for younger children because of the increased risk of perforation. For older children who do not respond to dilatation or require frequent dilatation, a Heller myotomy is indicated.

If a long myotomy is required, an antireflux procedure such as a Nissen or Thal fundoplication should be considered. However, these antireflux procedures have been associated with severe prolonged postoperative dysphagia, so they should be approached appropriately and performed only by those pediatric surgeons experienced in treating achalasia.

Connective Disease Disorders. Esophageal dysfunction is found in a high percentage of patients with scleroderma and dermatomyositis and in a smaller percentage of those with systemic lupus erythematosus and periarteritis. It is also a significant gastrointestinal manifestation of diabetes mellitus, but since this esophageal complication seems to occur only after the primary disease is present for many years, esophageal dysfunc-

tion is very rare during the pediatric years. All of these diseases, when esophageal complications arise, are associated with abnormal peristaltic activity and low or absent lower esophageal sphincter pressure. This pathophysiology results in gastroesophageal reflux, and subsequent complications, particularly strictures, are common. Therapy is directed at reducing the acid content of the refluxed material by intensive use of antacids or histamine H_2 receptor antagonists. Elevation of the head of the bed and fasting for a few hours before bedtime are also useful.

Metoclopramide (0.5 mg/kg/day) has been used to enhance peristaltic activity and to increase lower esophageal sphincter pressure. Frequent bougienage may be required to treat strictures. Severe cases may require a fundoplication to stop the gastroesophageal reflux and an interposition with colon or jejunum to relieve the stricture.

Patients with chronic idiopathic intestinal pseudo-obstruction syndrome may have a neural, myogenic, or combined etiology for their disease and often have esophageal manometric abnormalities but rarely are symptomatic. Therapy is rarely needed; if it is, it should be directed at whatever esophageal abnormality exists. For example, if gastroesophageal reflux is the reason for the symptoms, the pharmacologic therapy discussed above should be considered.

Patients with cerebral palsy frequently have vomiting and occasionally dysphagia. This usually results from abnormalities in lower esophageal sphincter pressure and peristalsis. Severe gastroesophageal reflux and stricture formation often occur. Therapy should be directed at decreasing the acid content of the refluxed material and increasing peristaltic activity with antacids or histamine H_2 receptor antagonists plus metoclopramide, respectively. Strictures should be treated with bougienage. Fundoplication may be required in cases that do not respond.

Esophageal abnormalities in patients with familial dysautonomia usually are similar to those in achalasia except that peristalsis is preserved. Neostigmine occasionally has been helpful. Measurements to prevent pulmonary aspiration are important, such as elevation of the head of the bed, fasting before bedtime, and sleeping prone. A gastrostomy and fundoplication often are required.

Webs and Rings. Rings differ from webs in that they contain muscle in addition to mucosa and submucosa. The Plummer-Vinson or Paterson-Brown-Kelly syndrome consists of an upper esophageal web and iron-deficiency anemia. Abnormalities in gastric acid secretion and pernicious anemia may also occur. Treatment consists of bougienage and iron replacement. The risk of esophageal carcinoma is high; therefore, the importance of a surveillance program should be explained to the patient.

Schatzki's rings are found in the distal esophagus and have been found at autopsy to mark the junction of esophageal and gastric epithelium, which is abnormally placed above the diaphragm. Often a simple explanation of the abnormal anatomic position of this junction plus instructions regarding the importance of chewing food slowly and the avoidance of swallowing large boluses is all that is required. If this is not sufficient, bougienage is indicated. Rarely pneumatic dilatation is required. Lower esophageal rings, if they can be distinguished from the more common Schatzki ring, should be treated with bougienage. These rings have been reported with the VACTERL syndrome (vertebral, anal, cardiac, tracheal, esophageal, renal, and limb anomalies).

Infectious Diseases. Thrush is the most common childhood candidal infection. With esophageal involvement, nystatin (Mycostatin) 250,000 units suspended in 10 ml of water every 2 hours is indicated. Some have advocated suspending the drug in a viscous solution of 0.5 per cent methyl cellulose and 0.7 per cent carboxymethylcellulose to improve adherence to the esophageal mucosa. With treatment failures, amphotericin, flucytosine, miconazole, or ketoconazole should be considered. Miconazole and ketoconazole are the least toxic of these therapeutic agents. The usual intravenous dosage for miconazole is 20 to 40 mg/kg/day divided into three infusions given over 30 to 60 minutes. Ketoconazole is given as a once-daily oral dose of 3.3 to 6.6 mg/kg. Some studies suggest that a daily dosage of 7 to 10 mg/kg bid or tid may achieve better therapeutic serum concentrations.

Herpetic esophagitis often produces severe odynophagia and, although it is found most often in the debilitated host, it can also be documented in apparently immunologically competent patients. For this latter group, no specific treatment is usually warranted, but symptomatic relief with cool liquid meals and viscous lidocaine is frequently helpful. In severe cases or with debilitated hosts, acyclovir at an intravenous dose of 250 mg/m^2/day may be considered.

Crohn's disease occasionally affects the esophagus. Except for the usual treatment regimen of sulfasalazine and corticosteroids, no specific therapy is available.

The dystrophic form of epidermolysis bullosa can affect the esophagus, causing odynophagia and dysphagia. The latter is usually secondary to upper esophageal webs and strictures. Corticosteroid therapy is often helpful, with tapering of daily therapeutic dosages to maintenance levels being undertaken when relief of symptoms is achieved. Dilatation of strictures is contraindicated. Interposition surgery may be required in severe cases.

Graft-versus-host disease may involve the esophagus and cause severe problems such as chest pain, dysphagia, and reflux symptoms. No specific therapy is available.

Mallory-Weiss Tears. Forceful vomiting or retching, particularly if recurrent and prolonged, can result in mucosal tears associated with hematemesis. Most of these bleeding lesions remit without treatment, but in recalcitrant ones, surgery should be undertaken, although some have advocated that a left gastric artery infusion of vasopressin be attempted first.

Perforation. Esophageal perforations may be spontaneous, as they frequently are during the neonatal period, or induced, as they most often are during childhood. The latter are usually caused by some type of instrumentation, usually of a blind nature, by chest trauma such as occurs in an automobile accident, or by a complication of caustic ingestion. Surgery is the mainstay of therapy except perhaps in the case of a small cervical tear, in which a nonoperative approach consisting of antibiotics, parenteral nutrition, and close observation may be considered. The latter approach would be the exception.

Foreign Bodies. Foreign bodies can be removed from the esophagus in the most controlled and safe manner, with the child under general anesthesia and an endotracheal tube in place. In so doing, the most significant and serious complication occurring during foreign body removal from the esophagus, the aspiration of the foreign body into the tracheobronchial tree, can be avoided. Because of this hazard, the removal of foreign bodies by means of a Foley catheter or while the child is receiving only parenteral sedation without an endotracheal tube in place should be avoided. Most foreign bodies, regardless of shape or size, can be removed endoscopically. A special case, however, is a meat bolus that has become lodged. Meat tenderizer may be considered to help resolve the obstruction. Five ml of papain are given every 30 minutes for 4 to 6 hours. Most often, the obstruction is relieved in 18 to 24 hours. If not, during subsequent endoscopy it can usually be relieved. Meat tenderizer use has been associated with hypernatremia and erosions of the esophageal mucosa, so close observation for the former and endoscopy for the latter should be done.

Chemical Burns. The most commonly ingested chemicals are strong alkalis, usually the sodium or potassium hydroxide contained in drain cleaners. Most other alkalis and acids that children accidentally ingest are not usually associated with a high incidence or severity of esophageal damage. Suicide attempts with strong acids such as concentrated hydrochloric or nitric acid are, however, associated with severe injury. The presence or absence of oral injury is not predictive of the presence or absence of esophageal lesions. Immediate first aid should consist of the ingestion of a liquid such as milk to dilute the ingested substance to reduce further gastric damage and esophageal damage if reflux occurs. Vomiting should not be induced. Parenteral fluids should be started and a chest radiograph taken to exclude mediastinitis. Esophagoscopy should be performed within 24 hours and should be terminated as soon as an area of esophageal burn is encountered. If no lesions are found, the child is discharged without further treatment except for proper poison prevention instruction and psychiatric consultation if this ingestion was a suicide gesture. In those with esophageal lesions, a broad-spectrum antibiotic is started parenterally plus a parenteral corticosteroid such as prednisolone (2 mg/kg/day). As gastrointestinal function returns, both medications are changed to the oral route. The antibiotic is discontinued after 10 days while the corticosteroid is continued for 3 weeks and then gradually tapered. Corticosteroids are not indicated if there is any evidence of mediastinitis or aspiration pneumonitis. A tracheostomy may be required if laryngeal edema is present. A gastrostomy may also be placed at the time of the anesthesia for the endoscopy if severe lesions are seen. In these severe cases, as soon as the patient can swallow, a surgical thread is passed into the stomach. This thread serves as the guide for future bougienage to relieve stricture formation; often, however, severe strictures still develop which require an interposition of colon or jejunum.

Tumors. Most esophageal tumors encountered during childhood are benign, including leiomyomas, lipomas, inflammatory polyps, hemangiomas, hamartomas, and neurofibromas. Rarely leiomyosarcomas, lymphomas, or some other type of gastric cancer may invade the esophagus. All of these tumors are treated by surgical resection. Leukemias are treated by radiation, parenteral chemotherapy, or a combination of both.

Varices. Hepatic disease–induced portal hypertension often results in severe gastrointestinal bleeding episodes. Patients presenting with this type of hemorrhage should be managed in an intensive care unit. Blood for typing and cross-matching of at least two units of blood (depending on the child's size) should be obtained, and both central venous and arterial blood pressure lines should be placed. A pediatric Sengstaken-Blakemore tube should be placed and subsequently monitored by personnel experienced in its use. The usual initial esophageal balloon pressure should range from 30 to 40 mm Hg up to the normal adult pressure of 40 to 60 mm Hg, depending on the child's size. Pulmonary aspiration is a significant complication arising from the use of this tube. Vasopressin should be given via a peripheral vein at a dose of 0.2 to 0.4 unit/1.73m^2/min. Side effects of vasopressin include water retention with subsequent hyponatremia, hypertension, cardiac arrhythmia, and seizure that results from the first two effects. If bleeding continues despite 24 hours of the above treatment or the patient's condition begins to deteriorate, surgery should be undertaken to decompress the portal vascular bed. An alternative that has not been used extensively in pediatric patients is to attempt to obliterate the bleeding varix by injecting a sclerosing agent directly into the vessel. In skilled hands, this technique has achieved a high success rate among adult patients. If a physician skilled in this technique is not available, a variceal-systemic shunt should be placed.

For those patients who do cease bleeding after tube placement and vasopressin administration, elective obliteration of the varices should also be undertaken using a sclerosing solution. This usually requires repeated injections at 2- to 4-week intervals. Side effects of the sclerosing solution include esophageal strictures, ulceration, perforation, and bleeding. Somatostatin, which has shown excellent results in stopping various types of gastrointestinal bleeding in adults, may assume an important role in the treatment of variceal hemorrhage, since it has a low incidence of complications plus a higher efficacy rate than vasopressin.

Esophagitis and Strictures. These lesions are most often caused by prolonged repeated exposures of the esophageal mucosa to acidic gastric contents. If esophagitis is present, a regimen designed to reduce or neutralize the acidic content of the refluxed material

and increase lower esophageal sphincter pressure plus enhance esophageal peristalsis should be undertaken. The former can be accomplished with antacids (30 ml/1.73 m^2/day in six to eight divided doses), cimetidine (1200 mg/1.7 m^2/day in four divided doses), or another histamine H$_2$ receptor antagonist and the latter with bethanechol (8.7 mg/m^2/day in three divided doses) or metoclopramide (0.5 mg/kg/day). Between the latter two drugs, metoclopramide is the drug of choice if delayed gastric emptying is also present, since it increases this function better than bethanechol, which has little effect. Extrapyramidal symptoms occur with metoclopramide hydrochloride use, but these can be stopped with diphenhydramine hydrochloride. Metoclopramide therapy should be terminated if these occur.

In addition to the drug therapy listed above, postural therapy at an angle of 60 degrees should be maintained 24 hours a day in infants. Feedings should be thickened and given more frequently than normal, up to every 3 hours. In older patients elevation of the head of the bed and fasting after the evening meal should be included, along with cessation of smoking. With infants, these regimens should be continued until symptoms have been controlled and esophagitis is healed if it is present. With older children, the therapy should probably be continued indefinitely, although studies supporting this position have not been done in this age group. In patients who do not respond to medical therapy over a period of 3 to 4 months and have severe disease, particularly if associated with any changes compatible with Barrett's epithelium or a stricture, a fundoplication of either the Nissen or Thal type should be considered. If a stricture is present, bougienage is indicated at the initiation of the medical regimen and should be repeated as necessary until the stricture is relieved.

GASTROESOPHAGEAL REFLUX

JOHN J. HERBST, M.D.

Recently gastroesophageal reflux (GER) has become one of the most common gastrointestinal problems recognized in young children. Some amount of GER, especially after a meal, is common and physiologic in both children and adults. The reservoir capacity of the esophagus is only about 6 ml in infants and 180 ml in adults. Since intake in infants is over two times as much on a weight basis as in adults, some vomiting or spitting is common. The challenge to the physician is to identify which children are having significant problems and to treat them appropriately. In the past investigators focused on lower esophageal sphincter pressures as they sought to understand the pathophysiology of GER. It is becoming clear that many factors, including position of the sphincter, angle of entrance of the esophagus into the stomach, gastric emptying, esophageal motility, salivation, swallowing, pharyngeal motor function, presence of a gastrostomy, and central nervous system function, play a role in causing or altering the effects of GER. Excessive spitting and vomiting improve in infants as the size of the esophagus increases and an upright position is maintained at about 1 year of age, whereas spontaneous improvement is less likely in symptomatic children over 2 years of age.

Spontaneous relaxation of sphincter tone is a frequent cause of pathologic reflux. Reflux associated with increased abdominal pressure, as with coughing, or reflux across a lax sphincter pressure, as seen with severe esophagitis, is less common. If esophageal motility is depressed, clearance of acid from the esophagus is delayed, causing increased esophagitis, pain, blood loss, or stricture. Spontaneous salivation and swallowing wash the last traces of acid from the esophagus. Salivation and frequency of swallowing are decreased during sleep, so night-time reflux is often prolonged and associated with severe esophagitis. If there is even minimal inco-ordination of the swallowing mechanism, there may be microaspiration or stimulation of chemoreceptors in the upper esophagus and pharynx, causing gagging, coughing, wheezing, stridor, or other symptoms of respiratory distress. Coughing, choking, hyperextension of the neck, or tongue movements associated with refluxed material in the pharynx may be misinterpreted as signs of primary pulmonary disease, seizures, or other central nervous system disorders rather than as symptoms of GER. Vomiting of large amounts of food may cause loss of weight or failure to thrive.

EVALUATION

Esophageal function and reflux may be evaluated using a variety of methods, including fluoroscopy, upper gastrointestinal scintigraphy, ultrasonography, esophageal motility studies, prolonged esophageal pH monitoring, endoscopy, and biopsy of esophageal mucosa. Not all patients with symptoms of GER need to be studied, and rarely is use of all methods of evaluating patients necessary. A careful history and physical examination can provide much valuable information and for many may be the only evaluation needed, especially if the patient is an infant whose main problem is vomiting or spitting after meals. If it is unclear if the symptoms are caused by GER, if they are persisting despite medical therapy, if they are severe, or if surgery is being considered, evaluation to confirm the presence of abnormal GER or to answer clinically relevant questions is indicated. Since the tests must distinguish between a normal physiologic amount of reflux and an excessive amount, no test is infallible. An upper gastrointestinal series is almost universally available and can give much valuable information. Although results vary, 15 to 20 per cent of patients with GER will not be identified, and at least a 25 per cent rate of false-positive results may be expected. More importantly, other conditions that may cause similar symptoms, such as duodenal bands, stenosis, volvulus, or other causes of partial intestinal obstruction, can be detected. Especially if recorded on videotape, the procedure can evaluate esophageal motility and the swallowing mechanism.

Because some patients have severe vomiting, with weight loss or failure to thrive being the major problem,

and others have major respiratory symptoms and minimal vomiting or spitting, it is obvious that superior esophageal sphincter function and pharyngeal clearance mechanisms are important in determining clinical symptoms. Present methodology has not identified specific motility abnormalities that cause different symptoms. Although tertiary esophageal contractions are increased and lower esophageal sphincter pressure tends to be low in patients with severe esophagitis, motility studies have limited clinical usefulness in evaluating GER.

Gastric scintiscan is simple, relatively noninvasive, and very sensitive in detecting reflux. Because some reflux is physiologic and scanning over the esophagus is relatively brief, it has limitations similar to those of a barium swallow. The test can give evidence regarding gastric emptying, and reflux of the labeled substance into the lung field can document aspiration, but this has not been a very clinically helpful aspect of the test.

Flexible endoscopy can evaluate severe esophagitis. Esophageal biopsy, with or without endoscopy, can document even mild GER. Severe esophagitis with infiltration of eosinophils and polymorphonuclear leukocytes may be noted in biopsies of esophagus without significant endoscopic changes. The milder changes are noted only on biopsies and include increased thickening of the basal layer and increased penetration of the dermal pegs into the stratified squamous epithelium. These changes are noted in only about 15 per cent of patients without symptoms of GER but in approximately 95 per cent of patients with pathologic GER.

Prolonged pH monitoring is considered the gold standard by many but is an expensive, time-consuming test. Since sampling time is long, it is very good at separating pathologic from physiologic reflux. It can document severity and frequency of reflux during asymptomatic reflux, during sleep, and in infants who cannot communicate. A causal relationship can be inferred if pH monitoring demonstrates that symptoms such as cough, apnea, or choking occur at the time of reflux.

TREATMENT

Treatment for patients with reflux may vary from simple postural therapy to major surgery depending on severity of symptoms, and there is no universal agreement on the relative effectiveness of the different modes of therapy.

Diet Therapy. Small, frequent feedings, avoidance of large meals, and careful burping to remove the gastric bubble are important. In extreme cases, short-term use of constant gastric feedings or even transpyloric feeding to decrease the volume of stomach contents available for reflux is helpful. Thickened feedings are recommended on the theory that reflux will be inhibited, but their effectiveness has not been well studied.

Positional Therapy. Placing the patient upright to prevent spillage of stomach contents into the esophagus is intuitive and time-honored in adults and children. Use of an infant seat in the first few months of life may not be effective, since infants have poor truncal tone, slump in the seat, and develop increased abdominal pressure. In infants the prone position is more effective, and raising the head 30 degrees is the best position. A padded post or a harness or a pillow cover with openings for the legs must be used to keep the infant from sliding to the bottom of the mattress. There is no advantage to the head-elevated position if the child is placed on his or her back.

Medical Therapy. If there is esophagitis, neutralizing gastric acid decreases the toxicity of gastric contents to the esophageal mucosa. Studies have shown that when esophagitis is healed, there is increased lower esophageal sphincter pressure and improved clearance of refluxed material. A milk feeding in infants neutralizes gastric contents for approximately 45 minutes. Antacids (15 ml/m^2 of concentrated preparations) administered between feedings are effective but may cause diarrhea. Cimetidine is available as a syrup for infants, the usual dose being 20 to 40 mg/kg/day in four divided doses. Newer H$_2$ blockers such as ranitidine come in tablet form for the older patient. The newer agents do not affect liver metabolism and so are less likely to affect metabolism of other drugs such as theophylline or anticonvulsants that the child may be taking.

Prokinetic agents such as metoclopramide in dosages of 0.10 to 0.15 mg/kg or bethanecol 0.01 mg/kg given four times a day before meals have been shown to be helpful. In some studies it has been difficult to show a decrease in reflux using pH monitoring, but symptoms do improve. Some investigators have noted nervousness, irritability, and tremors as side effects, but these problems are uncommon and respond to decreasing the dose. Cisapride, not yet available in the United States, has been shown to be effective in several studies.

Surgical Therapy. In patients with severe symptoms, meticulous attention should be given to burping, maintaining the head-elevated position for as much of the day as possible, and other aspects of medical therapy. If significant improvement is not noted in 6 weeks, surgical intervention may be considered. Surgery should also be considered if there is a significant esophageal stricture secondary to esophagitis or if there are complications such as apnea or gagging not responding to medical therapy. Inserting a gastrostomy tube increases the risk of abnormal reflux, and most patients being considered for a permanent gastrostomy have swallowing or central nervous system disorders in which GER is common. It is wise to evaluate such patients for GER and consider doing a simultaneous antireflux procedure at the same time if the patient has significant GER.

There are many types of surgical procedures, but a Nissen fundoplication, a Thal procedure, or some variation is the most common. Most modifications deal with how firmly or completely the fundus is wrapped about the esophagus. The goal is to have good control of GER without creating problems with esophageal emptying, such as inability to burp or vomit or the gas bloat syndrome. It is a safe procedure, with several series of over 200 cases reported without an operative mortality. Reflux is usually well controlled, but respiratory symptoms are controlled to the extent that the symptoms were caused or aggravated by GER. As would be ex-

pected, basic motility problems are not cured and about one quarter of patients have some problems swallowing foods such as vegetables, nuts, or chunks of meat. Varying degrees of gas bloat syndrome or inability to belch or vomit occasionally occur but tend to improve with time. A rare but often fatal complication may develop in patients who develop distal obstruction from adhesions or other causes. If they cannot burp or vomit, they may develop severe abdominal distention with obstruction of blood flow and intestinal infarction.

Medical therapy combined with expected improvement as the child develops usually ensures a happy outcome. In a minority of infants with severe problems not responding to medical therapy, surgical intervention cures GER and complications are usually minor or rare.

NAUSEA AND VOMITING
DAVID R. FLEISHER, M.D.

Nausea and vomiting are signals of something gone wrong and should never be treated without considering and reconsidering their causes. Management of most of the disorders consists of removing the causes of vomiting and/or correcting fluid and electrolyte deficits until vomiting subsides. Antiemetics are relatively contraindicated when vomiting is a key indicator of some life-threatening process, e.g., meningitis or adrenal insufficiency, or when they are likely to produce unwanted side effects without significant benefit, e.g., in midgut volvulus. Antiemetics are useful when the causes of vomiting are known and the vomiting is predictable and of limited duration, e.g., in acute gastroenteritis, cancer chemotherapy, or motion sickness.

ANTIEMETIC DRUGS

Antiemetic agents include antihistamines, dopamine antagonists, and a miscellaneous group. Antihistamines—e.g., promethazine, dimenhydrinate, and cyclizine—are effective against motion sickness, probably because of their anticholinergic properties. Dopamine antagonists include phenothiazines and metoclopramide. They suppress the chemoreceptor trigger zone (CTZ) but are generally ineffective against motion sickness. Phenothiazines have both anticholinergic and extrapyramidal side effects. Therefore, Thorazine is preferable to Compazine because it is less likely to cause extrapyramidal reactions. A dysphoric state with feelings of unreality is a side effect of phenothiazines which may be as common as their anticholinergic and sedative side effects and should caution against too liberal a use of these agents as antiemetics or sedatives.

Metoclopramide (Reglan) has a phenothiazine-like action on the CTZ and also affects the motor activity of the upper gastrointestinal tract. It increases the strength of the lower esophageal sphincter mechanism and enhances propulsive motility of the stomach, duodenum, and small bowel without affecting secretion or the motility of the colon. This action is blocked by atropine, and metoclopramide loses its effectiveness when used with anticholinergic antispasmodics. Like phenothiazines, it may cause extrapyramidal reactions and lower the seizure threshold. Metoclopramide blocks the hypotensive effect of dopamine; it should be used cautiously in patients recently treated with adrenergic agents, monoamine oxidase inhibitors, or tricyclic antidepressants.

The pharmacologic properties of trimethobenzamide (Tigan) are similar to those of phenothiazine; it acts on the CTZ, is not useful in labyrinthine disturbances, and may cause drowsiness, extrapyramidal reactions, and lowering of the seizure threshold.

Emetrol, a mixture of glucose, fructose, and orthophosphoric acid, is available without prescription. Its alleged but unproved efficacy is said to result from lessening of stomach motility caused by the presence of a hypertonic sugar solution in the stomach; it should be taken undiluted. A placebo effect may be its most important action. Emetrol's chief virtue is its safety; it has no systemic pharmacologic action, and it does not suppress nausea and vomiting due to serious organic disease. Table 1 summarizes the dosages and side effects of some common antiemetic drugs.

SPECIFIC ENTITIES

Motion Sickness. The combination of scopolamine and amphetamine is most potent for the prophylaxis and treatment of motion sickness but is rarely, if ever, indicated in pediatrics because of its side effects. The antihistamines promethazine (Phenergan, Remsed), di-

menhydrinate (Dramamine), and cyclizine (Marezine), in descending order of potency, suffice. The first dose should be given prophylactically 30 minutes to 1 hour prior to embarkation; further doses should be administered as needed. Side effects are somnolence and atropine-like. These drugs are appropriate for management of vertigo, nausea, and vomiting in other disorders of labyrinthine function. Persistent vomiting may necessitate intravenous fluids and electrolyte replacement.

Acute Vomiting Illness. Suppression of nausea and vomiting may be helpful in the management of acute, self-limited gastroenteritis. Antihistamine drugs are less potent than dopamine antagonists. One dose of chlorpromazine intramuscularly or by rectal suppository may allow the patient to resume oral intake of fluids and antipyretics and get some needed sleep. The risk of Reye's syndrome and meningitis must be considered prior to the use of this potentially hepatotoxic, soporific agent, and the patient's course should be monitored closely with the differential diagnosis of vomiting in mind. Fluids such as ice chips, Pedialyte, and Infalite are preferable to hypertonic fluids or fluids containing fat when oral intake is resumed. Intravenous fluids are necessary for seriously dehydrated children and when attempts at oral rehydration fail.

Functional Vomiting Disorders. Three vomiting syndromes that occur in infancy may mimic organic disease; two of them produce organic complications. They are innocent vomiting, nervous vomiting, and infant rumination syndrome.

Innocent vomiting occurs in 20 per cent of healthy

TABLE 1. Drugs Useful for Control of Nausea and Vomiting

Drug	How Supplied	Principal Side Effects
Antihistamines		
Promethazine (Phenergan, Remsed)	Injection: 25 and 50 mg/ml	Drowsiness, atropine-like
Child: 0.5 mg/kg/dose q12h	Syrup: 6.25 mg/5 cc and 25 mg/5cc	
Adult: 25 mg bid	Tablets: 12.5, 25, and 50 mg	
Dimenhydrinate (Dramamine)	Injection: 50 mg/ml	Drowsiness, atropine-like
Child: 1.25 mg/kg/dose PO or IM, qid	Liquid: 12.5 mg/4 ml	
Adult: 50–100 mg/dose PO or IM qid, 100 mg PR qid	Tablets: 50 mg	
	Suppository: 100 mg	
Cyclizine (Marezine)*	Injection: 50 mg/ml	Drowsiness, atropine-like
Child (6–10 yrs): 1 mg/kg/dose PO or IM tid	Tablets: 50 mg	
Adult: 50 mg q4–6h		
Dopamine Antagonists		
Chlorpromazine (Thorazine)	Injection: 25 mg/ml	Anticholinergic > extrapyramidal, sedation, dysphoria, orthostatic hypotension, lowered seizure threshold
Child: 0.5 mg/kg/dose IM q6h, 1 mg/kg dose PR q6h	Syrup: 10 mg/5 cc	
Adult: 25–50 mg/dose IM or 100 mg PR q6h	Oral concentrate: 30 mg/cc	
	Tablets: 10, 25, 50, and 100 mg	
	Suppository: 25 and 100 mg	
Prochlorperazine (Compazine)	Injection: 5 mg/ml	Extrapyramidal > anticholinergic, sedation, dysphoria, orthostatic hypotension, lowered seizure threshold
Child (> 10 kg): 0.05 mg/kg IM q6h or 0.1 mg/kg PR or PO q6h	Syrup: 5 mg/5 cc	
Adult: 5–10 mg/dose IM or PO q6h or 25 mg PR bid	Oral concentrate: 10 mg/cc	
	Suppository: 2.5, 5, and 25 mg	
Metoclopramide (Reglan)	Injection: 5 mg/ml	Extrapyramidal, restlessness, sedation, lowered seizure threshold
Child: 0.1 mg/kg/dose PO, IM, or IV q6h	Syrup: 5 mg/5 cc	
Adult: 10 mg PO, IM, or IV q6h	Tablets: 10 mg	
Miscellaneous		
Trimethobenzamide (Tigan)	Suppository: 100 and 200 mg	Phenothiazine-like
Child: 100 mg PR, qid		
Adult: 200 mg PR, qid		

*Manufacturer's warning: Safety and efficacy in children have not been established.

infants. They may vomit a small amount or a projectile gush, but the vomitus usually does not contain bile or blood and there is no sign of pain, nausea, or other distress. The vomiting is not lessened when the patient is upright and does not occur more frequently when the patient is supine, in contradistinction to the vomiting of pathologic gastroesophageal reflux. It is not relieved by changing to a protein-hydrolysate formula, as would be expected were the vomiting due to milk or soy sensitivity. There is no weight lag. Vomiting subsides by 12 to 18 months of age. Innocent vomiting may be due to the limited volume the infant's esophagus can accommodate during physiologic gastroesophageal reflux or to retropulsion during antral systole or pylorospasm. Management consists of reassuring the parents and continued vigilance for signs of organic disease.

Nervous vomiting is a form of nonorganic failure to thrive. The vomiting is a visceral reaction to stress or excitement and typically occurs in an infant who is intensely receptive and reactive to environmental stimuli. The mother is typically conscientious and attentive but emotionally and physically exhausted. The reciprocity characteristic of the normal mother-infant relationship breaks down, and a vicious circle occurs in which the mother's anxiety is intensified by the infant's vomiting and weight lag and the failure of conventional antiemetic measures. She becomes less able to soothe her infant, who, in turn, reacts to the increased tension with more vomiting, fussiness, sleeplessness, muscular tension, and episodes of opisthotonos-like arching of his back. He becomes more difficult to hold and to feed. The mother is troubled by ambivalent feelings toward her infant and becomes less tolerant of the irritability and vomiting. The mechanism of nervous vomiting may be an extension of the pylorospasm or antral dysmotility that probably causes innocent vomiting.

The diagnosis of nervous vomiting, like that of most other forms of nonorganic failure to thrive, can be confirmed only by a response to effective management. This may require an unhurried hospitalization that allows time for the weight loss trend to stop. The baby's comfort should be maximized. He should be promptly soothed when fussy and fed an undiluted, nutritious formula on demand, to satiety, even though his vomiting continues. He should be shielded from excessive excitement, especially during feedings and rest periods, which should take place in a quiet, nonalerting atmosphere. Diagnostic procedures should be spaced so as to minimize concentrated stress. Since organic and functional disorders do not preclude each other, an unbiased assessment of each patient is necessary.

Information ruling out diseases of the digestive, urinary, and central nervous systems is needed as a basis for management. Beyond that, the number and intrusiveness of diagnostic studies performed must depend on the evidence of organic disease and, equally important, on the infant's weight, vomiting, and irritability as his comfort improves. Interviews with each parent during the hospitalization permit a deeper appreciation of less apparent sources of distress that impair their ability to sense and satisfy their infant's needs. A conference with both parents at discharge elicits their questions and feelings about what was learned during the hospitalization and enhances collaboration during follow-up until symptoms resolve.

Infant rumination syndrome is a rare but potentially lethal functional vomiting disorder. Rumination is a form of self-stimulation seen in infants over 3 months of age who are unsuccessful at evoking comfort and satisfaction from their mothers. The vomiting does not occur during sleep and is lessened when the infant is engaged in social interaction. It occurs while the baby is awake, quiet, and self-absorbed. There may be other self-stimulating behaviors, such as head rolling, hand sucking, or sound making. Management of infant rumination syndrome requires that the baby receive satisfaction from the mothering environment, thereby allowing the self-stimulation habit to subside. This is best provided by a nurse or nurses maternal enough to enjoy spending time holding, interacting with, and feeding the patient; empathic enough to sense his needs and states; and observant enough to respond early to each episode of rumination by engaging him in reciprocal interaction. A response to such a "therapeutic trial of comfort" consists of reversal of weight loss, improved hydration, and a gradual lessening of vomiting. The patient's mother may react with mixed feelings as her infant improves while cared for by a parent substitute. Good rapport between physician and parent is vital. The parents' permission should be obtained before a special nurse is employed for the purposes of helping with the demanding tasks of infant care and data collection. The nurse's role is that of helper to the physician and the mother, not didactic teacher of superior mothering techniques. The mother's own mothering often improves as her fears for her baby's life subside and she herself feels respected and cared for.

Infant rumination and nervous vomiting differ in that rumination is self-stimulating behavior that occurs in the absence of maternal responsiveness, whereas nervous vomiting is an involuntary, visceral reaction to excessive stress or excitement. Rumination begins beyond 3 months of age, after the infant becomes developmentally capable of self-stimulation, whereas nervous vomiting may begin during the first month of life. The mothers of ruminators tend to be emotionally distant and there is a poverty of interaction with the infant. Mothers of nervous vomitors interact attentively but dyssynchronously with their babies' cues so that their responses heighten rather than lessen tension.

Adult-type rumination is rare in neuropsychiatrically normal children. It typically presents in a child who habitually brings up into his mouth food eaten during a meal 1 to 2 hours before. He chews and reswallows, losing none from his mouth. Adult-type rumination does not seem to cause esophagitis, weight loss, or distress to the child, although it may be very distressing to his parents. It is an otherwise harmless habit. Theoretically, it should be lessened by metoclopramide, but beware of using a potent pharmacologic agent in an escalating power struggle between a parent and a child unwilling to give up this habit.

Oral-defensive vomiting occurs in infants and children

old enough to resist spoon feedings they do not want. Individuals of any age may vomit involuntarily as a reaction to food they "can't stomach" or food they might enjoy but for their feeling that eating it is an obligation they are powerless to resist. Management consists of discovering what motivates the parents to feed coercively, relieving their fears, and having a reflective discussion about how their efforts to get their child to eat might jeopardize rather than protect his nutritional well being.

Contentious vomiting occurs during anger caused by someone the child knows loves and cares for him. The struggles about independence and control characteristic of the "terrible twos" trigger intense emotions. When a child vomits during conflict with his parents, he soon realizes that this accidental occurrence gives them pause. They may view screaming and kicking as "behavior" but vomiting as a symptom of illness. This reflexive vomiting tends to be conditioned and reinforced by the parents' response to it; at first, it is merely part of the autonomic events during the conflict, but soon it acquires purpose. Such vomiting may be a chief complaint of distressed parents concerned that their child may be sick and worried, too, by a feared loss of control in setting limits for their young child. Management aims at reassuring them that the vomiting neither results from nor causes organic disease and discovering and helping to resolve the aspects of the power struggle that are unnecessary or might be better handled with more flexibility. The vomiting begins to disappear when it ceases to frighten or anger the parents.

Two kinds of consciously self-induced vomiting are encountered in older children and adolescents, *vomiting as an act of malingering* and *factitious vomiting*. Malingering is done to deceive parents or other authorities in order to gain something or to be relieved of some obligation. Vomiting as an act of malingering ceases as soon as the manipulative behavior stops working.

Factitious vomiting, exemplified by the bulimic patient, is quite different from malingering. There is a compulsion to vomit and increased anxiety if vomiting is interdicted. The patient may acknowledge the harmfulness of her vomiting, yet she persists because it is too difficult for her to stop. Management ultimately requires psychiatric efforts at uncovering and ameliorating the unconscious motives that fuel the compulsion to vomit. Until this succeeds, surveillance for potassium deficits, Mallory-Weiss tears, gastric perforation, and other injury is necessary.

Children with *the cyclic vomiting syndrome* (CVS) usually experience their first episode between 2 and 9 years of age, although onset during adolescence is not uncommon. Episodes tend to be stereotyped and self-limited, typically begin during the night or on arising, and last 12 to 48 hours, although some have symptoms for as little as a few hours and others for as long as 10 days. Crampy diarrhea and/or mild fever and/or headache may occur during vomiting episodes. Attacks recur fairly regularly in two thirds of the patients and at irregular intervals in one third. Recurrences may be more often than weekly or less than yearly. The majority of patients can identify specific phenomena that trigger attacks, most commonly, noxious emotional experiences, non-noxious excitement such as birthdays and vacations, and colds or flus. The diagnosis is made clinically, since there are no laboratory or radiologic markers of this disorder.

Although family studies and encephalographic data suggest a relationship between CVS, migraine, and epilepsy, therapeutic trials of antimigraine agents and anticonvulsants have generally failed to cure the cyclic vomiting diathesis, prevent attacks, or terminate episodes already in progress. Antiemetic agents may sedate the patient but seldom abolish the nausea or shorten cyclic vomiting episodes. However, recent anecdotal reports suggest that lorazepam may abort or shorten attacks. This benzodiazepine has not been officially approved for use in children and studies of its use in CVS have not been done. Nevertheless, it might be considered for children whose bouts last as long as 10 days, recur more often than once a month, and for whom nothing else is effective. The dose of lorazepam I recommend is 0.05 mg/kg, p.o. or IV, up to a maximum of 2 mg. Attacks may sometimes be aborted by administering a lorazepam tablet p.o. or sublingually before the onset of vomiting, as soon as the characteristic nausea begins. If the patient has already begun vomiting and is hospitalized, an IV infusion is started, and a lorazepam dose is given by IV injection over 5 minutes' time. The desired effect is sedation with cessation of vomiting and then waking up several hours later free of symptoms. Several doses are often required at intervals of 6 to 12 hours before symptoms are relieved.

Water and electrolyte deficits and maintenance needs should be provided for by IV infusion. Patients with prolonged attacks may develop secondary peptic esophagitis and hematemesis because of gastroesophageal reflux due to relaxation of the lower esophageal sphincter mechanism that accompanies persistent nausea and vomiting. Suppression of HCl secretion with IV cimetadine (20 to 40 mg/kg/24 h divided into 4 to 6 doses) is helpful. In addition, the patient with esophagitis may be helped by swallowing a crushed sucralfate tablet (1 gm) suspended in 15 cc of water q. 6 h. Even if the dose is vomited, this agent should adhere to and protect inflamed esophageal mucosa. CVS tends to remit in most patients during adolescence or early adulthood. Establishing the diagnosis is, in itself, therapeutic because it relieves the child and family of the fears caused by such dramatic, incapacitating symptoms. If acute anxiety seems to be a major precipitant, the occasional use of an anxiolytic agent might be beneficial. Psychotherapy for chronically anxious children is helpful if practicable.

Indolent nausea without vomiting, diminished food intake, or weight loss is a chief complaint of some older children and adolescents who are chronically anxious. This symptom is usually functional. Management is directed at the underlying emotional distress.

CONSTIPATION AND ENCOPRESIS

MELVIN D. LEVINE, M.D.

Children are said to be constipated when defecation is inordinately difficult or when the event occurs too infrequently. Commonly their stools are hard and may be difficult to pass. While occasional periods of infrequent or difficult elimination are normal occurrences in childhood, *chronic* constipation can be a source of discomfort, inconvenience, and anguish. Longstanding retention of stool can lead to encopresis, in which a functional megacolon or megarectum develops secondary to obstipation, with resultant loss of control or fecal incontinence, commonly encountered in school children.

Most children with chronic constipation have no other organic pathology. However, in rare instances chronic constipation can be a sign of an anatomic, neurologic, or metabolic disorder. Possible are various forms of imperforate anus in the newborn, sometimes accompanied by vulvar or perineal fistulas. Atopic anus also can impair defecation. Myelomeningocele and other spinal cord defects commonly are associated with this disorder. Although relatively rare, Hirschsprung's disease (aganglionic megacolon) is probably the most widely publicized neurogenic cause of constipation. It is particularly unusual to diagnose Hirschsprung's disease in a school-age child. Metabolic causes include hypocalcemia and hypothyroidism. Certain medications can cause infrequent bowel movements or hard stools. One example is methylphenidate (Ritalin), commonly used to treat attention deficits.

If all of the above organic causes of constipation are ruled out, it is inappropriate to assume that the problem is "psychogenic." Most cases represent neither organic nor psychiatric illness, but rather, a dysfunction, a bad habit, or a constitutional tendency toward sluggish bowel performance. Dietary factors may aggravate the process but are seldom the sole cause.

MANAGEMENT

Newborn and Infancy. It is during the early months of life that the clinician must be most vigilant to possible anatomic causes of constipation that may require surgical intervention. In particular, Hirschsprung's disease may present at this time, often with symptoms of intestinal obstruction or necrotizing enterocolitis. The treatment of choice following appropriate diagnostic work-up generally is a colostomy followed by a pull-through operation late in the first year of life.

The newborn and infancy period also is a common time for symptoms of constitutional constipation to emerge. Treatment should be as noninvasive as possible, in order to prevent the induction of an "anal stamp," a permanent psychological scar associated with the later development of encopresis. The physician should emphasize to parents that the condition is benign, making every effort to minimize their anxiety. Frequent anal manipulations, such as digital disimpaction and the use of suppositories, should be discouraged. In mild cases, parents should be reassured and no therapy instituted.

However, if the infant is uncomfortable and is producing consistently hard stools, one can add dark Karo syrup to feedings. Approximately 1 to 2 teaspoons per feeding generally is adequate. As the baby's diet becomes increasingly diversified, the need for such intervention diminishes. In rare cases, a mild laxative, such as milk of magnesia, may be needed. If so, use as little as possible (starting with ½ tsp a day).

Some infants have considerable discomfort on defecation. A mother may note that her baby constantly strains to have a bowel movement. In some instances, the infant is actually struggling *not to have one!* Such early evidence of voluntary withholding should be noted. Typically, the affected infant hyperextends his legs and clenches his fists while defecating. This may result from discomfort during bowel movements. The physician should ascertain that there are no problems in the perianal area causing painful defecation. The most common offender is chronic diaper dermatitis. Appropriate management of any such condition therefore is important in preventing habitual voluntary withholding.

The Toddler and Preschool Child. Training is the most critical event related to bowel function during this period. Some toddlers develop an aversion to defecation because of coercive or compulsively executed training. Improper training methods can result in constipation. For example, some children have difficulty defecating with their feet suspended in air. They can benefit from the use of telephone books or some other kinds of support while learning to use a toilet. Constipation related to training sometimes must be managed by postponing or modifying the training routine. Some toddlers and preschool children acquire an irrational fear of the toilet. Apprehension may center on the possibility of falling in or encountering "fish monsters" lurking in the bowl.

This can also be a time during which the manifestations of constitutional constipation seem to worsen. Treatment should remain nonaggressive, avoiding especially therapies that entail anal manipulation. Dietary alterations introducing high bulk foods (fruits, vegetables, bran-containing items) may be helpful. If this is ineffective, stool softeners should be given in small doses. Maltsupex is a palatable example. If this fails, small amounts of a mild laxative (such as Senokot granules, ½ tsp a day) can be instituted.

The School Years. There are many reasons why schoolchildren manifest chronic constipation. The phenomenon may be part of a continuing history of stool retention and poor bowel function that began in infancy or the toddler years. Or school itself may be an etiologic or at least aggravating factor. Some youngsters are reluctant to use school bathrooms because they lack privacy. They postpone defecation until safe, in the privacy of home. Some youngsters seem unable to "afford" to do this. That is, although they decline to use the bathrooms at school, they lose the urge when they get home. Over time, these children become constipated, and many develop a functional megacolon. Other schoolchildren acquire constipation because of a frenetic lifestyle. They race to meet the school bus each morning and are tightly scheduled all day. Homework, play, and alluring television shows occupy them until bedtime, leaving little time for something as trivial and uninteresting as defecation. Such children make relatively few trips to the bathroom, and when they do their defecation is partial or incomplete because of their haste. Other youngsters have significant attention deficits. These children are overactive, distractible, impulsive, and impersistent at tasks. They seldom finish anything they start, including defecation. They too ultimately develop chronic constipation.

An understanding of the pathophysiology of the schoolchild's bowel disorder can aid in counseling and management. Alterations in life style, provisions for more privacy of bathroom use in school, and various forms of behavior modification may be critical. In treating schoolchildren with chronic constipation, one should distinguish between those with the complication of incontinence (i.e., encopresis) and those who are fully continent.

SIMPLE CONSTIPATION (WITHOUT INCONTINENCE). Schoolchildren with uncomplicated constipation can be subdivided into those with overt symptoms and those with "occult stool retention." The latter group can be insidious and difficult to diagnose. Occult stool retention is one of the most common causes of recurrent abdominal pain. The diagnosis is often missed, since there may be no history of infrequent or hard stools. A plain supine radiograph of the abdomen in such instances reveals abundant retained feces, the removal of which often is associated with pain relief.

Most cases of uncomplicated chronic constipation can be alleviated by educating the child to use the toilet regularly and to remain in the bathroom long enough to achieve complete emptying. Laxatives such as senna (Senokot, 1 tablet a day) or danthron (Modane, 1 tablet a day) often are helpful. Treatment should be continued for 3 to 4 weeks. If symptoms persist, the child may benefit from the ongoing use of light mineral oil (1 to 2 tablespoons twice a day). In more severe or protracted cases, treatment may need to be more vigorous and long lasting. The regimen suggested for encopresis is recommended under these circumstances.

Encopresis. It is not unusual for schoolchildren with chronic constipation to develop encopresis. Varying degrees of severity are encountered, ranging from multiple large accidents per day to occasional bouts of incontinence or steady but slight leakage. Virtually all children with encopresis have at least intermittent constipation. Although emotional factors may complicate the picture, in most instances encopresis (like enuresis) is not caused by emotional factors. However, children who have suffered from this condition over a long period may become secondarily depressed, anxious, and socially withdrawn. Peer interactions, family harmony, self-esteem, and school performance can deteriorate as a result.

Most cases of encopresis ultimately resolve spontaneously; however, medical treatment can accelerate the cure and thereby diminish the suffering and psychological toll. Management of this condition can be divided into its component steps. The treatment is summarized in Table 1. The following is an elaboration on the steps involved:

1. DEMYSTIFICATION. The first step in treatment is education of the child and parents. The physician should explain normal colonic function, using drawings or diagrams. There can be discussion of the ways in which intestinal musculature propels stool, with consideration of the role of nerves within that musculature in providing signals indicating the need to defecate. It should be explained that some children go through a period when they do not completely empty their bowels. This results in the progressive accumulation of stool with the consequent chronic stretching of intestinal musculature and the loss of tone and strength. It also should be pointed out that the stretching results in diminished feedback from nerves, so that children fail to experience the urge or sensation of needing to move their bowels. A plain film of the child's abdomen can then be reviewed with the patient and parents. The physician can point out the accumulation of "rocks." It then is explained that the good thing about muscles is that they can be restored when they become weak. The treatment strategy is presented. It is pointed out that it is critical to begin treatment by establishing an entirely empty colon. After this, the goal will be to keep it as empty as possible over a period of months so that the stretching can stop and the bowel can gradually return to its normal caliber, with restoration of muscle tone and feeling. It is important to point out that many other youngsters have this problem. A unique aspect of encopresis is that it is rare for any child who has it to have heard of any other who is similarly afflicted. Much anxiety can be relieved through demystification and the revelation that this is not an unusual condition. It also is helpful to emphasize that the problem is nobody's fault and that having it does not mean that a child is crazy, lazy, or immoral.

2. INITIAL CATHARSIS. A complete clean-out is critically important at the beginning of treatment. In most instances this can be performed on an outpatient basis. In severe cases or when there is a very disturbed parent-child relationship, an inpatient program can be instituted. The components of these are summarized in Table 1. Following the initial catharsis the child should have a follow-up plain radiograph of the abdomen to establish that a good clean-out has been achieved. If this shows little or no improvement, the initial catharsis may need to be prolonged. If one begins a maintenance program following an incomplete clean-out, exacerbations are much more likely to occur.

3. MAINTENANCE. After the initial catharsis the youngster should be put on a laxative (Senokot, 1 to 2 tablets per day) or danthrone (Modane, 1 to 2 tablets per day). A stool softener should also be used. Most common and effective is light mineral oil. An average dose is about 2 tablespoons twice a day (for an average 7 or 8 year old). The flavor can be disguised with juice or soft drink. Light mineral oil should never be used when the bowel is impacted, since the lubricant itself is likely to leak around blockages, with the subsequent passage of a gold-colored liquid, which can be disconcerting as it streams down the legs of a schoolchild. In

TABLE 1. Treatment of Encopresis

Treatment Phase		Treatment Program	Comments
Initial Counseling		1. Education and "demystification" 2. Removal of blame 3. Establishment and explanation of treatment plan	Include drawings, review of colonic function, joint observation of radiographs
Initial Catharsis	At Home	1. High normal saline enemas (750 cc bid) 3–7 days 2. Biscodyl (Dulcolax) suppositories bid 3–7 days 3. Use of bathroom for 15 minutes after each meal	Patient admitted when: 1) retention is very severe 2) home compliance likely to be poor 3) parents prefer admission 4) parental administration of enemas is inadvisable psychologically

	Inpatient	1. In moderate to severe retention, 3–4 cycles as follows:
		    a. Day 1—hypophosphate enemas (Fleet's Adult) twice
		    b. Day 2—biscodyl (Dulcolax) suppositories twice
		    c. Day 3—biscodyl (Dulcolax) tablet once
		2. In mild retention, senna or danthron, one tablet daily for 1–2 weeks
			1) Dosages or frequency may need alteration if child experiences excessive discomfort
			2) Admission should be considered if there is inadequate yield

		Follow-up abdominal radiography to confirm adequate catharsis	
Maintenance		1. Child sits on toilet twice a day at same times each day for 10 minutes each time 2. Light mineral oil (at least 2 tablespoons) twice a day for at least 6 months 3. Multiple vitamins, two a day, between mineral oil doses 4. High roughage diet 5. Use of an oral laxative (e.g., Senokot) for 1–2 mo daily in moderate or severe cases	1) A kitchen timer may be helpful 2) A chart with stars for sitting may be good for children under eight 3) Bathroom reading encouraged 4) Mineral oil may be put in juice or Coke or any other medium 5) Vitamins to compensate for alleged problems with absorption secondary to mineral oil 6) Diet should be applied, but not to the point of coercion

Follow-up		1. Visits every 4–10 weeks, depending on severity, need for support, compliance, and associated symptoms
		2. Telephone availability to adjust doses when needed
		3. In case of relapse:
		    a. check compliance
		    b. trial of oral laxative (e.g., Senokot) for 1–2 weeks
		    c. adjust dosage of mineral oil
		4. Conseling and/or referral for associated psychosocial and developmental issues
			1) Duration of treatment program may be as long as 2–3 years or as short as 6 months
			2) Signs of relapse:
			    a) excessive oil leakage
			    b) large caliber stools
			    c) abdominal pain
			    d) decreased frequency of defecation
			    e) soiling
			3) Physician should spend time alone with child
			4) In cases slow to respond, physician should sustain optimism: persistence cures almost all cases eventually

All dosages and frequencies are calculated for an average-sized 7-year-old child. Appropriate adjustments should be made for smaller or larger patients.

fact, if at any point during treatment excessive leakage of mineral oil is reported, one can assume that the youngster is again becoming retentive. In most cases after about a month of maintenance therapy, the laxative can be tapered off or discontinued. The stool softener should be continued for at least 6 months.

4. RETRAINING. A critical part of the treatment is retraining and toilet utilization. The child should be told to visit the bathroom twice a day at the same times each day, preferably after breakfast and supper. A minimum of 10 minutes should be spent therein. The youngster is told that he can read or listen to the radio, but he should try to empty out his bowel completely each time. In children under eight, it sometimes is helpful to set up a system of rewards, using a star chart, suitably embellished for each visit (with extra credit given for success).

It should be emphasized to parents that it is inappropriate to punish a child for having an accident. However, refusal to take medication or resistance to sitting on the toilet should constitute offenses. The child is not to blame for messing but is to blame for not trying to do something about it. Following an accident a child

should be required to clean himself. Underwear should be disposed of properly, although the child should not be expected to wash it, which could be interpreted as punitive.

For the child who soils himself in school, some arrangements may need to be made to provide a change of clothing in the nurse's office. Some youngsters may require a third visit to the bathroom, one that takes place in school. A sufficiently private setting for this should be sought. Most children feel strongly that they do not want school personnel to know about their problem, but most are agreeable to having one schoolperson aware of it. Their greatest fear is that peers will discover this most important secret. Therefore, every effort must be made to sustain their privacy.

5. FOLLOW-UP AND MONITORING. Encopresis is a chronic condition. The pediatrician should establish a strong alliance with the youngster and see him regularly (the frequency depending upon the severity and chronicity of the problem). During return visits, the physician should examine the child's abdomen and talk about management while alone with the youngster. There can be joint discussions with parents. Medication needs to

be "titrated." When exacerbations occur, laxative therapy should be increased or resumed. It is important that parents and the pediatrician be aware that in many cases several years are required for restoration of normal bowel function. Although this can be frustrating, persistence has its rewards. In severe treatment-resistant cases, the physician should periodically review the condition and consider the possibility of complicating psychosocial factors. Referral for a psychological or psychiatric evaluation may help, especially when the child seems to be noncompliant and unable to discuss the problem or when there is evidence that serious family problems are interfering with management. Surgical consultation should be sought in treatment-resistant cases in which aganglionic megacolon is suspected. However, the latter is extremely rare among schoolchildren, whereas slowly responsive encopresis is a common condition.

ACUTE AND CHRONIC NONSPECIFIC DIARRHEA SYNDROMES

DORSEY M. BASS, M.D.,
and W. ALLAN WALKER, M.D.

Diarrhea, defined as excessive loss of fluid and electrolytes in the stools, is one of the most frequent problems confronting the pediatrician in clinical practice. In developing countries diarrhea is the leading cause of death in young children and in the West it remains the second leading reason for "sick" outpatient pediatric visits and nonsurgical pediatric admissions. Although the differential diagnosis of diarrhea is extensive, a brief but complete history and physical examination can usually exclude serious specific causes.

ACUTE GASTROENTERITIS

This usually self-limited illness occurs most commonly during the winter months in children less than 3 years old. The most common cause is rotavirus. The two mainstays of therapy are to treat and prevent dehydration and to avoid excessive nutritional compromise.

In recent years a large number of studies have demonstrated the efficacy of oral electrolyte solutions as therapy for dehydration secondary to diarrhea of any cause. The solutions used in these studies have generally contained higher electrolyte concentrations than the older commercial products. The World Health Organization oral rehydration solution (WHO ORS) contains sodium at 90 mmol/l and glucose at 111 mmol/l, while the older commercial formulations contained less than half the sodium and more than twice the glucose concentration of the WHO ORS. Newer commercial formulations (e.g., Pedialyte, Infalyte) are patterned after the WHO ORS, which is based on better understanding of glucose/sodium—coupled water transport in the small intestine.

These commercial solutions or WHO ORS can be given ad libitum to infants and toddlers with the addition of one bottle of plain or flavored water for every two bottles of solution. Patients with more severe dehydration may benefit from more specific instructions or even supervised administration in the clinic or in hospital. Patients in shock, those with persistent severe vomiting, and those who do not respond to oral therapy need intravenous fluids, but oral therapy should be substituted as soon as possible.

The prevention of excessive nutritional compromise is especially important in the infant with acute diarrhea. Prolonged bowel rest or hypocaloric clear liquid diets can lead to starvation stools, and the malnutrition-dehydration cycle can rapidly accelerate into intractable diarrhea of infancy. Generally, some kind of feeding can be started as soon as rehydration is completed. As lactase deficiency is very common in this setting, small, frequent feedings of soy formula are often successful. In more severe cases or in very young infants, a hydrolyzed formula such as Pregestimil may be indicated. Stool output, pH, and reducing substances can serve as guidelines to advancing the feedings.

Antibiotics have no role in the treatment of acute diarrhea in the absence of documented bacterial infection. Likewise, antiemetics and antiperistaltic medications are more likely to cause toxicity than provide any real benefit. Kaolin compounds merely change the cosmetic appearance of the stools and may camouflage significant fluid losses.

CHRONIC NONSPECIFIC DIARRHEA

Chronic nonspecific diarrhea is a benign symptom complex seen in healthy toddlers with normal growth and development. It is probably the pediatric equivalent of irritable colon syndrome. Many cases remit spontaneously with toilet training, but others continue for years.

The mainstay of treatment is reassurance of the parents. The child's continuing good growth should be stressed by the doctor at every visit. High-residue, high-fiber diets or the use of psyllium compounds can provide some symptomatic relief.

PROTRACTED DIARRHEA OF INFANCY

MARTIN H. ULSHEN, M.D.,
and MITCHELL D. SHUB, M.D.

The vast majority of diarrheal illnesses in infancy are self-limited disorders that respond to simple, supportive care. However, a small group of young infants develop a progressive diarrheal state associated with dehydration, electrolyte imbalance, and protein-calorie malnutrition. This condition, commonly known as intractable diarrhea of infancy, has been defined as an episode of diarrhea lasting more than 2 weeks and occurring during the first 3 months of life. Survival among these infants has improved markedly in recent years as a result of the advent of elemental enteral diets and parenteral nutrition. Therefore, it is now more accurate to refer to this condition as protracted diarrhea of infancy.

Numerous disorders associated with chronic diarrhea can initiate protracted diarrhea of infancy; however, in most instances no etiology is identified. Regardless of the initiating event, prolonged diarrhea in infants rapidly depletes protein and calorie reserves. Malnutrition leads to a loss of intestinal absorptive surface with diminution of brush-border enzymes, a decrease in pancreatic exocrine function, and an altered immune system. Bacterial overgrowth in the small bowel may occur. Nutrient restriction often hastens this sequence of events. Once the intestine is no longer able to efficiently digest food, the diarrhea becomes self-perpetuating.

In planning management of the young infant with protracted diarrhea, the physician must rule out those etiologies that require urgent treatment. Careful evaluation for evidence of enteric or systemic infection should be considered. Hirschsprung's disease with secondary enterocolitis requires early diagnosis and surgical decompression because of the risk of colonic perforation. A small bowel biopsy can be helpful, not only in diagnosis but also in planning therapy. One would be less inclined to vigorously pursue enteral alimentation alone if severe mucosal damage were found. However, overall prognosis appears to correlate poorly with the histologic appearance.

The primary goal of therapy for protracted diarrhea of infancy should be to correct fluid, electrolye, and acid-base imbalances; to treat systemic infection as well as any recognizable etiology of the diarrhea; and to reverse the ongoing catabolic state. No matter what the underlying pathophysiology, there can be no repair or regeneration of damaged intestinal mucosa without proper nutritional support. Much recent evidence suggests that enteral feeding is the preferred source of nutrients. The choice of enteral or parenteral alimentation, used separately or in combination, must be made shortly after admission to the hospital and regularly re-evaluated. Prolonged "bowel rest" is no longer considered the best approach to this disorder. When tolerated, initial treatment with enteral alimentation alone is ideal. This approach has been associated with quicker recovery and shorter hospitalization without the complications of parenteral nutrition. A continuous nasogastric infusion is more likely to be successful than intermittent bolus feedings. Enteral feedings should be introduced as early as possible in those infants requiring initial intravenous treatment. Elemental formulas are available with carbohydrates other than lactose, predigested protein, and medium-chain triglycerides. For an infant with persistent carbohydrate malabsorption, the type and concentration of carbohydrate can be precisely regulated by the use of a modular formula. Both elemental and soy-based modular formulas are available. Use of these formulas allows for slow progression of the quantity of carbohydrate without restriction of other nutrients. The most critical guide to subsequent dietary manipulation is stool output and character; improvement in stool volume and consistency are signs that the diet can be advanced. Typically, formula is given at first at a rate of 25 kcal/kg/day and slowly increased by increments of 25 kcal/kg/day as tolerated. However, some infants may tolerate more rapid advancement of the caloric density of the formula. Daily fluid requirements should be provided (100 to 200 ml/kg/day). Physical signs of hydration, urine volume, and urine specific gravity must be followed closely. However, it should be kept in mind that a malnourished infant may have a decreased ability to concentrate urine and that a dilute urine may not accurately reflect the state of hydration. Continuous enteral feedings may be required for several weeks before cautiously reintroducing bolus feedings.

Those infants who do not tolerate enteral alimentation early in their course require total parenteral nutrition. These very sick infants benefit from the addition of amino acids, multivitamins, and trace metals to their dextrose-electrolyte intravenous solution. Total nutritional support can be provided through a peripheral vein and essential fatty acid deficiency prevented by the use of intravenous fat emulsion. A central venous line is indicated when a course of parenteral nutrition of more than 1 to 2 weeks is anticipated or when access to peripheral veins becomes difficult. In those infants requiring total parenteral alimentation, enteral alimentation should be started as soon as possible to promote small bowel adaptation and repair. Formula can be introduced at full concentration but at a low volume; the rate can then be increased as tolerated. With this approach, optimal nutrient intake can be maintained during the transition from parenteral to enteral nutrition.

Other forms of therapy that have been used in selected cases have included cholestyramine, loperamide (or narcotic antidiarrheal agents such as paregoric), oral nonabsorbable antibiotics, and corticosteroids. None of these therapies has been adequately tested in well-designed, prospective clinical trials; generally, they should not be used except for specific indications. Cholestyramine (1 to 4 gm/day) can be helpful in those cases in which the diarrhea is caused by bacterial overgrowth, toxigenic enteropathogens, or the introduction of excess quantities of bile acids into the colon. The major side effects of cholestyramine include fat malabsorption, metabolic acidosis, and bowel obstruction. Anticholinergics and opiates should be used with caution in conditions associated with rapid motility, as they can precipitate a paralytic ileus with concomitant sequestration of fluid in the intestinal lumen.

Commonly, infants with protracted diarrhea are hospitalized for several weeks or more. Their parents benefit from emotional support, as improvement is often slow. The overall prognosis for protracted diarrhea is quite good; a favorable outcome is related to two factors: early recognition of the condition and effective reversal of the malnourished state. Once children have recovered from protracted diarrhea of infancy, they usually have no long-term effects.

IRRITABLE BOWEL SYNDROME

JOYCE D. GRYBOSKI, M.D.

The irritable bowel syndrome (IBS) is a term used to describe chronic or recurrent abdominal pain associated with constipation and/or diarrhea in children and adolescents who have no demonstrable organic pathology. In younger children the major symptom is chronic, painless diarrhea, often termed "nonspecific" or toddler's diarrhea.

DIARRHEA OF INFANTS AND TODDLERS

Diagnosis of this benign disorder is one made after evaluation for more serious illness, for it is essential to document that there is no evidence of malabsorption, dietary protein or sugar intolerance, or parasitic or bacterial infection. Toddler's diarrhea occurs twice as often in boys as in girls and is characterized by relapses and remissions. Affected children are healthy and growing well but pass two to three (up to 12) mushy or mucoid stools per day. There is often a history of irritable bowel syndrome in one or both parents.

Recent physiologic studies have shown that the normal migrating motor complexes from the duodenum which occur at 1.5-hour intervals and which are inhibited by food or dextrose in the duodenum are not disrupted by these in the child with toddler's diarrhea. Other studies report increased stool bile acids, water, and electrolytes. In some it is postulated that rapid small bowel transit and failure of bile acid reabsorption cause a cholerrheic diarrhea. Plasma prostaglandin $F_2\alpha$ levels are increased in some children, and jejunal biopsies show increased Na^+-K^+ ATPase and adenylate cyclase. Small bowel bacterial overgrowth has been documented in a few children, and scanning electron microscopy has shown increased numbers of bacteria adhering to small intestinal enterocytes.

Although the disorder is considered benign, it causes more problems for mothers than for the children. Reassurance and time are the major therapeutic recommendations. One must be sure that there is adequate although not excessive fat in the diet, since it has been shown that young children develop loose, frequent stools when dietary fat is restricted. Intake of juices containing high concentrations of sucrose or sorbitol (e.g., apple juice) should be restricted. Aspirin and loperamide have been used successfully in European studies. Nonabsorbable, nontoxic clay preparations (e.g., kaolin, atapulgite), through their nonspecific binding properties, may also provide symptomatic relief.

IRRITABLE BOWEL SYNDROME IN OLDER CHILDREN

Although abdominal pain is the major complaint of older children with IBS, there is often accompanying constipation and/or diarrhea. The pain may be generalized, periumbilical, or in the right or left lower quadrants. It is crampy and is not associated with weight loss or wakening of the patient from sleep. It is usually increased by stress, and there is frequently a parental history of irritable bowel syndrome. Often, the children with associated diarrhea pass several losse, mucoid stools in succession shortly after arising.

Originally thought to represent only a hyper-reactive colon, IBS now has been shown to affect the entire gastrointestinal tract. In the esophagus, increased amplitude of peristaltic and nonperistaltic contractions occurs with or just after the onset of esophageal-type chest pain. Anticholinergics and nifedipine, a smooth-muscle relaxant, have provided inconsistent improvement. In adults, low-dosage antidepressants have proved superior to placebo in improving symptoms, and recent success has been reported using biofeedback techniques.

Patients with upper gastrointestinal symptoms of bloating, nausea, and epigastric pain of IBS show either rapid or slow (tachygastria or bradygastria) slow-wave myoelectric frequencies (normal, 3 cycles/min). Metoclopramide and the investigational drug cisapride have restored normal myoelectric activity in a number of patients.

The small intestines of patients with IBS are more sensitive to distention than those of normal controls. Those with diarrhea show rapid small bowel transit and more frequent myoelectric activity, whereas those with constipation have slower than normal transit, abnormal configurations of migrating motor complexes, and failure to convert from a fasting to a fed motor pattern.

The majority of studies have been performed on the colons of patients with IBS which demonstrate excessive nonspecific hyper-reactivity, with a larger proportion of myoelectric slow waves of 2 to 4 cycles/min. (Similar findings are seen in those with lactose malabsorption.) Following a meal, patients have a delayed and prolonged, rather than immediate, increase in colonic motility.

Evaluation must include a careful history and physical examination as well as complete blood count, erythrocyte sedimentation rate, urinalysis, and examination of the stool for pH, occult blood, bacterial pathogens, and parasites. The site of pain is important to define, as well as the frequency and time of occurrence (morning, afternoon, weekday or weekend). In adolescent females a limited pelvic examination should be included and abdominal or pelvic ultrasonography performed depending upon the physical examination. Endoscopic examination is unrevealing unless the pain is localized to the epigastrium or left colon. If there is evidence of weight loss, radiologic examination of the small and large bowel should be performed to rule out inflammatory bowel disease. Lactose intolerance is a relatively frequent cause of abdominal pain and may mimic appendicitis in the adolescent. Fructose and sucrose intolerances are now recognized as factors causing symptoms of IBS. A careful history should be taken for the ingestion of "sugarless" products containing sorbitol or mannitol, since these may cause abdominal pain and diarrhea.

Once the diagnosis of IBS is established, reassurance is essential for the patient. Although emotional factors and stresses are inherent to adolescent life, these are not readily shared with the physician. Detection of early depression should lead to counseling. A high-fiber diet, using true crude fiber of fruits, vegetables, and grains, is superior to the use of medicinal synthetic fiber preparations. Nutritional recommendations lie in the area of 30 gm/day and can best be reached with the aid of a nutritionist. Vegetables contain varying amounts of fiber and the fiber of young vegetables is metabolized differently from that of older ones. Equally important and certainly underemphasized is the importance of water, since its incorporation into the fiber is the ultimate determinant of stool bulk. At least eight 8-ounce glasses of water should be taken daily. For non–water drinkers this can be accomplished using iced tea or fruit drinks. Continuing care is essential for these patients.

RECURRENT ABDOMINAL PAIN

JEFFREY A. BILLER, M.D.

Recurrent abdominal pain is a common complaint in childhood. As defined by Apley, the term refers to three or more discrete episodes of severe abdominal pain over at least a 3-month period. Using this definition, recurrent abdominal pain is reported in as many as 12 to 30 per cent of school-aged girls (peak age, 9 to 10 years) and 9 to 12 per cent of school-aged boys. In only about 5 to 10 per cent of these patients, however, is the pain found to have an underlying organic etiology, divided evenly between urogenital and gastrointestinal disorders.

A thorough history and physical examination are essential in helping to distinguish between organic and nonorganic disease. Details relating to the location (diffuse or localized), severity (incapacitating or mild), radiation of pain, time of occurrence (in school, nocturnal, weekdays versus weekends, during menstrual cycle), and relationship with meals and particular foods may be helpful. In our experience, pain that wakes the patient from sleep is more consistent with an organic etiology. Associated symptoms, including weight loss, constipation, headache, and nausea and vomiting are nonspecific. A detailed review of systems and medical history may suggest a site of organic involvement. A high incidence of abdominal pain is found in parents of patients with pain with a functional etiology. Information regarding the ethnic background and history of migraine or seizures in the family may also provide some assistance in the diagnosis. A detailed social history is vital, with special emphasis on school performance (often requiring direct input of teachers) and parent and sibling interactions. Identification of stresses both at home (parent-parent interaction and parent-child interaction) and at school may point toward an underlying cause. On physical examination, the presence of normal growth and general well-being and absence of signs of systemic or localized disease are consistent with a functional etiology. Most patients will localize their pain to the periumbilical area. The presence of localized right lower quadrant pain (consistent with appendicitis or inflammatory bowel disease) or epigastric tenderness (consistent with peptic related disease) may be more suggestive of an organic etiology.

Laboratory evaluation must be individualized for each patient given the information obtained during the history and physical examination. It is justified, however, to perform a few selected screening laboratory tests in all patients, even in those in whom no clear organic etiology is suspected. These include a complete blood count, an erythrocyte sedimentation rate, urinalysis and culture, and stool guaiac. Further evaluation, including liver function tests, serum amylase, stool for ova and parasites, lactose breath hydrogen test, serum lead level, and radiographic studies should not become part of the routine screening evaluation in these patients. Invasive studies, including endoscopy, laparoscopy, and laparotomy, should be performed only when there is clear direct evidence suggesting their usefulness. Such studies may be detrimental psychologically to many patients with nonorganic causes. Occasionally, observation of the patient in the hospital setting away from the stresses of family and school may be helpful in directing further evaluation.

Once an organic etiology is excluded, therapy must be directed toward understanding the inciting factors, stresses, and motivations for the abdominal pain. This is often not possible until all family members recognize, accept, and understand that the patient is indeed experiencing a real pain that happens not to have any underlying organic cause. Trust and open communication within the family and confidence in the pediatrician may allow the patient to focus away from the abdominal pain and more toward the underlying emotional issue. In some cases, the degree of emotional disturbance in the patient and family is so severe that more formal psychological evaluation and guidance are useful. Medications are rarely helpful in managing nonorganic abdominal pain.

PREOPERATIVE AND POSTOPERATIVE CARE OF PATIENTS UNDERGOING GASTROINTESTINAL SURGERY

LAURIE A. LATCHAW, M.D.

The preoperative and postoperative care of patients undergoing surgery for congenital and acquired gastrointestinal disorders varies with the patient's overall condition, the level of intestine requiring operation, and the urgency of the procedure. Details of the therapy of specific disorders are discussed elsewhere in this text. Certain standard therapeutic maneuvers to ready a patient for the operating room and care for their initial postoperative needs are discussed here.

PREOPERATIVE CARE

Gastric Decompression. The risk of pulmonary aspiration during the induction of anesthesia can be ameliorated by emptying the patient's stomach. In the absence of a bowel obstruction or adynamic ileus, this is accomplished by allowing the patient to have nothing by mouth 8 hours prior to the operation. Infants may be allowed a clear liquid or breast milk feeding up to 4 hours before an operation in some instances.

Emergent operations generally do not permit the required time to empty the stomach and often involve a bowel obstruction or ileus. The stomach of these patients should be suctioned empty with an appropriately sized sump-type nasogastric tube. When barium or food particles fill the stomach, irrigation with normal saline and aspiration through a large-bore tube are indicated.

Prophylactic Antibiotics. Prophylactic perioperative antibiotics are recommended for most operations in which the gastrointestinal tract has a high probability of being opened. Although normal gastric pH is bacteriostatic, patients with a gastric pH greater than 4, such as those receiving H_2 blockers or antacids or those whose acid is neutralized by bile or blood, potentially have viable mouth flora present in their stomachs. One of the cephalosporins may be given intravenously just prior to and for 24 hours after the operation. Similarly obstructed small bowel may have bacterial overgrowth, and prophylactic antibiotics are recommended. Cefotetan should not be given to children, because of reported intraoperative bleeding problems.

The "gold standard" prophylaxis for colonic flora is ampicillin, clindamycin, and an aminoglycoside. In emergency, unprepped colonic surgery, this triple combination should be used unless prohibited by a known allergy or renal dysfunction.

Bowel Preparation. For elective colonic surgery, a mechanical bowel preparation followed by oral nonabsorbable antibiotics is necessary. Mucous fistulas and Hartman pouches should be cleansed with saline enemas and then irrigated with 1 per cent neomycin solution. Mechanical bowel preparation in the Nichol's tradition requires a clear-liquid or low-residue diet for 3 days prior to the operation. Cleansing saline enemas (10 ml/kg) and oral cathartics are given 2 days prior to the operation, and cleansing enemas followed by oral antibiotics (neomycin or kanamycin, 10 mg/kg, q4h × 4 doses, and erythromycin base, 10 mg/kg, q4h × 4 doses) are given 1 day prior to operation. This regimen is time-consuming and uncomfortable and runs the risk of systemic salt disturbances but is effective.

An alternative method is to give 60 ml/kg body weight of GoLYTELY by mouth or nasogastric tube over 3 hours the morning before the operation. This balanced salt solution is not absorbed by the intestines and causes a cleansing diarrhea. Once the effluent is clear of particulate matter, oral antibiotics are given. The patient may have only clear liquids after the bowel preparation is completed and prior to being placed NPO. This method is shorter, more comfortable, and just as efficacious as the traditional bowel preparation. Systemic salt disturbances are uncommon. Infants with shorter transit times require less lengthy mechanical preparation, but either technique may be used judiciously.

Special Consideration in Emergency Gastrointestinal Surgery. True gastrointestinal surgical emergencies involve gram-negative septicemia, massive third space fluid losses, or bleeding. Normalization of fluid and electrolyte disturbances, body temperature, and clotting function must be aggressively achieved prior to the induction of anesthesia. Arterial and central nervous pressure monitoring devices may be needed to aid in the child's expedient resuscitation. Triple systemic antibiotics should be started until operative cultures can dictate more specific antibiotic treatment.

POSTOPERATIVE CARE

Intestinal Decompression and Refeeding. In general, patients undergoing gastrointestinal surgery require intestinal decompression until the return of normal bowel function. Again, a sump-type nasogastric tube on continuous suction is recommended. Nasogastric fluid losses should be measured and replaced intravenously by an appropriate salt solution every 4 hours. One-half normal saline solution of 5 per cent dextrose in water with 1 to 2 mEq potassium chloride per 100 ml is a standard nasogastric fluid replacement. Return of bowel function varies from 8 to 12 hours for the stomach to 3 days for the left colon. Small bowel peristalsis ceases to be effective only if excessive distention or wall edema prevents opposite bowel walls from coapting. This form of "ileus" may last weeks (e.g., following gastroschisis repair).

Re-establishment of bowel function is determined by the passage of flatus and a significant decrease in nasogastric tube drainage. The amounts and frequencies of feedings vary, but clear fluids are used first, followed by full liquids and finally a regular diet for age.

Fluid Management. Management of postoperative fluids can be difficult. Maintenance fluids can be calculated at 1500 ml/m²/day. Replacement fluids for nasogastric tubes and high-output enterostomies should be measured and replaced with appropriate intravenous fluid every 4 hours. Biochemical evaluation of the drainage is helpful in selecting the proper replacement fluid. Unmeasurable "third-space" losses must be estimated. One "best guess" rule to follow is the quadrant method described by Rowe et al. Third-space loss is estimated to be equal to the number of quadrants of the abdomen involved in the operation. For example, appendectomy confined to the right lower quadrant adds a one-fourth maintenance fluid requirement for third-space loss. Free perforation into the peritoneum adds one (4/4) maintenance fluid requirement. A urine output equal to 1 to 2 ml/kg/hour usually indicates adequate postoperative fluid replacement.

Pain Control. Postoperative pain control is just as important for children as for adults. Luckily, many infants and children have excellent pain control with oral acetaminophen, 10 to 20 mg/kg q4h. When oral medication cannot be given, 0.1 mg/kg of morphine sulfate, slowly infused intravenously every 3 hours, affords good pain control. Pain medication should not be ordered PRN in children, since many will not or cannot ask for medication until the pain is severe. Intramuscular injection should be avoided in children whenever possible. Most children are ready to change to oral medication when the nasogastric tube is discontinued.

Fever Management. Except when perianal operations have been performed, rectal temperatures should be taken and recorded every 4 hours postoperatively. Temperatures exceeding 38.5°C should be investigated first by an examining physician. Fevers during the first 24 hours following elective operation are usually secondary to pulmonary atelectasis and are treated by improved pulmonary toilet. Expensive fever work-ups are generally not indicated. Fevers occurring after 24 to 48 hours, however, do require thorough investigation of blood, wound, sputum, and the intra-abdominal cavity. Postoperative urinary tract infection in noninstrumented children is uncommon, as is meningitis.

Activity. The activity level of infants and children postoperatively is generally curtailed only by the need to keep tubes in place and bandages intact. Children should be encouraged to sit up, walk around, and play with adult supervision as much as their operation will allow.

Special Postoperative Considerations. STOMA CARE. A newly created enterostomy is best treated by application of a transparent stoma bag in the operating room. This allows easy observation of the stoma for viability and function as well as preventing it from drying out. Once the stoma begins to function, special protection of the peristomal skin is necessary, especially if a high ileostomy or jejunostomy was created. Cholestyramine may even be needed in some instances to prevent skin breakdown. For low colostomies, "double diapering" may be just as effective and less expensive than using stoma bags.

Tube gastrostomies/jejunostomies should be secured to prevent early dislodgement but require no special care. Gentle cleansing of the exit site once a day and occasional application of silver nitrate may help prevent granulation tissue build-up.

NUTRITION. Parenteral nutrition should be instituted in infants and small children within 2 days of being placed NPO. Older children and teen-agers should not be without nutrition longer than 5 days. The ease of peripheral nutrition using a glucose/amino acid solution along with a fat emulsion renders this policy feasible. For long-term parenteral nutrition, placement of a central venous line, either percutaneously or by cutdown, is preferred.

WOUNDS AND DRAINS. The routine use of peritoneal drains has decreased considerably since computed tomography scanning showed them to be ineffective in preventing fluid collections and abscess formation. Generally drains (a closed suction system) are now placed only into defined abscess cavities. Intraperitoneal drains should be removed when less than 30 ml of fluid drains out over 24 hours.

Postoperative wound care is often the surgeon's personal preference, but most surgeons agree that if closed primarily the skin is sealed within 24 to 48 hours and the dressing can be removed if desired.

Because of the high incidence of infection, grossly contaminated wounds are often left open and loosely packed with saline-moistened gauze. The amount of packing is decreased daily until the wound is closed.

Simple wound infections are heralded by tenderness, followed by erythema, wound separation, and purulent drainage. Opening the wound, irrigating with saline, and packing with saline-moistened gauze once or twice a day eradicates the infection and allows secondary healing. Irrigation and packing the wound with iodine solution or hydrogen peroxide are no more effective than using saline alone and may oxidize healing cells. Iodine solution may also suppress thyroid function in infants and small children.

PYLOROSPASM

GIULIO J. BARBERO, M.D.,
and JOAN DiPALMA, M.D.

Pylorospasm is a descriptive term signifying that the pylorus closes more intensely and suggests an abnormality in gastric motility and emptying. At best, pylorospasm is predominantly a clinical entity, in which no tests or studies can readily confirm a definitive diagnosis. There are two situations in which pylorospasm is suspected. First, pylorospasm is considered partially responsible for the vomiting and abdominal pain seen in peptic ulcer disease and duodenitis. In these cases, the inflammation and ulceration are documented by upper gastrointestinal radiography, endoscopy, and biopsy. Proper treatment of these disorders with a histamine antagonist and an antacid regimen usually manages the accompanying pylorospasm. Another situation is that of the infant less than 3 months of age who presents with recurrent vomiting. Upper gastrointestinal radiography may demonstrate delayed gastric emptying. Investigations for gastroesophageal reflux, infection, and metabolic disease are negative. The impact of pylorospasm in infancy is generally not profound. It is usually more of a nuisance, the vomitus frequently soiling all surrounding clothing and furniture. Fortunately, the degree of vomiting does not produce significant caloric deprivation to impair growth in most cases. Nevertheless, growth of the infant requires careful surveillance. Small frequent feeds may be warranted. Changes of formula composition are of little value. An antispasmodic such as Donnatal Elixir, 0.5 ml four times a day, or an atropine 1:1000 solution, one drop prior to each meal, may be helpful. Metoclopramide hydrochloride, 0.1 mg/kg/dose, has been tried with variable success. Dealing directly with parental fears and concerns is also an important component to management. Environmental factors in the etiology of this uncertain entity are unclear. However, in examining such issues nonjudgmentally and supportively with the parents, a positive therapeutic alliance can frequently occur. Usually, the vomiting symptoms are limited in time and are not protracted. There is little evidence of this entity becoming chronic, but its relationship to other gastrointestinal disorders that may occur later in life is still of some interest.

PYLORIC STENOSIS

GIULIO J. BARBERO, M.D.,
and JOAN DiPALMA, M.D.

Pyloric stenosis is a diagnosis that is reached after careful clinical, laboratory, and, at times, radiologic investigation. Diagnosis is based on the development of forceful vomiting usually 1 to 3 weeks after birth. The vomiting progresses in intensity, often with small and less frequent stools. Gastric waves pass across from left to right of the upper abdomen. The palpation of a pyloric "olive" confirms the diagnosis. Ultrasonography and/or radiography of the upper gastrointestinal area shows a dilated stomach with intensive contractions and a pyloric string sign indenting the antral lesser curvature of the stomach. Once the diagnosis of pyloric stenosis has been made, there are three major components to therapy. First, the infant must be given required restorative care. Second, the hypertrophied pyloric muscle must be corrected surgically. Finally, the patient must be supported while being allowed to reach an adequate oral intake.

Infants with pyloric stenosis can present with clinical and metabolic derangements of varying severity. Some infants show little abnormality, particularly in the early part of the clinical process. These infants require minimal intervention and can proceed to the second phase of therapy. Other infants, because of intense vomiting and a decreased caloric intake, can present with dehydration, hypoglycemia, abdominal distention, or growth failure. The vomiting leads to a hypochloremic, hypokalemic alkalosis. If the vomiting is mild, it may be corrected by oral feedings every 3 hours with a 0.5 normal saline solution with 5 per cent glucose and some added KCl. More severe vomiting and dehydration require intravenous treatment with 0.25 to 0.5 normal saline with 5 per cent glucose at a rate of 125 to 150 ml/kg/24 hours. After urination has been established, KCl can be added at 2 to 3 mEq/kg/24 hours. With severe salt depletion, it may be necessary to increase the amount of sodium chloride by using a 0.75 to 1.0 normal saline solution. Serum electrolytes, as well as the infant's weight and hydration status, should be monitored carefully. Most infants will demonstrate a good response 12 to 48 hours into fluid and electrolyte correction. Occasional patients who show signs of recurrent hypoglycemia and poor nutrition may require parenteral hyperalimentation for several days. Marked abdominal distention can be managed with gastric lavage and gastric decompression via nasogastric suction. Once the infant has achieved an improved physical and metabolic state, the next therapeutic phase can be instituted.

Surgical intervention by Ramstedt pyloromyotomy is the procedure of choice for correction of pyloric stenosis. In this procedure the hypertrophied pyloric and antral muscular layers are incised, leaving the mucosa intact. Two major complications that can arise are the incomplete division of the hypertrophied pyloric muscle and perforation of the duodenal mucosa. The latter is usually detected and repaired by the surgeon during the operative procedure. Both of these complications can become evident in the postoperative period. The procedure's mortality rate is less than 1 per cent. General anesthesia is required in most cases, and the patient should not be fed orally 8 to 12 hours prior to surgery.

Careful observation is imperative in the postoperative period. If the pyloromyotomy has been uncomplicated, nasogastric suction can be discontinued 4 hours after surgery. Two to three ounces of Pedialyte or a 5 per cent glucose solution can then be administered orally every 2 to 3 hours. Feedings can be advanced on the second day to breast milk or full-strength formula 2 to 3 oz every 2 to 3 hours. Infants should be feeding liberally by the third postoperative day. Intermittent vomiting may occur in the first few days post surgery. On rare occasion the emesis may be severe and require continued intravenous replacement therapy and nasogastric suction. If a perforation of the duodenal mucosa is suspected, feedings should be discontinued and nasogastric suction should be reinstituted for a 24-hour period. Oral feeds can then be resumed. If incomplete lysis of the hypertrophied pyloric muscle is suspected, it is best to stop feedings and start nasogastric suction and intravenous hyperalimentation. The infant will be able to feed orally in approximately 1 week. Repeat pyloromyotomy is rarely necessary. An upper GI series is of little value at this point. Radiologic evidence of the pyloric abnormality may persist for months despite adequate surgical intervention.

With careful management during the preoperative and postoperative periods, an excellent outcome can be expected from the surgical approach to pyloric stenosis.

PEPTIC ULCERS

PETER K. KOTTMEIER, M.D.

The present confusion concerning both operative and nonoperative treatment of gastroduodenal ulcers in infants and children is partially related to the assumption that all these ulcers are "peptic ulcers." A correct classification of gastroduodenal ulcers in children is important not only to identify the cause—if possible—but also to select the appropriate therapy. True "peptic ulcers" in childhood are similar to adult peptic ulcers. Another group of children have gastroduodenal ulcers that appear to be neither secondary to stress nor compatible with peptic ulcers. These are loosely grouped together as "acute primary ulcers."

Acute Primary Ulcers. In patients with mild to moderate bleeding, gastric lavage with saline and buffering with antacids or milk will suffice to stop bleeding in most instances. In infants, care should be taken not to induce hypothermia with iced gastric lavage. In acidotic infants, the gastric lavage solution should be either isotonic lactate or isotonic half saline and half bicarbonate to reduce, or at least not to increase, a metabolic acidosis. The administration of isotonic crystalloid solutions, blood, or colloid depends on the amount of blood loss. If the blood loss is significant, either whole blood or packed cells and volume expanders can be used as replacement. In most instances an overreplacement should be avoided, since this may reinitiate gastric bleeding that may have stopped prior to the overadministration of blood.

If the blood loss within 24 hours exceeds the patient's blood volume, or if massive recurrent bleeding occurs, surgery is usually indicated. Since there is no recurrence of the ulcer formation after successful therapy, the most conservative operative procedure necessary to stop the hemorrhage should be used, such as the simple oversewing of isolated ulcers or suture ligation of bleeders. In an occasional infant with diffuse gastric ulcerations, a resection may be necessary, however. The perforation in a patient with a primary acute ulcer is also usually treated successfully by simple closure with or without the use of an omental patch.

A unique type of neonatal ulcer leading to gastric perforations within several days after birth has also been called an acute primary ulcer. Aspiration of the intraperitoneal air will improve diaphragmatic excursion and therefore respiration. The isotonic hypovolemia should be corrected with an initial push of isotonic solutions. The peritonitis, although predominantly chemical at onset, should be covered with broad-spectrum antibiotics. The operative procedure consists of closure of the perforation. If the patient recovers uneventfully, oral feedings can usually be resumed after 5 to 7 days; there is no need for postoperative antacids or other medications.

Chronic Primary or Peptic Ulcers. These usually begin at school age and increase during the teenage years. They represent the childhood equivalent of the adult peptic ulcer. The primary therapy, usually successful, consists of antacids between meals and at bedtime. Either magnesium or aluminum hydroxide can be used. Magnesium hydroxide appears to be a more powerful buffer used to keep gastric pH higher than 4, but serum hypermagnesemia has been reported not only in patients with renal failure but also in neonates, with resulting cardiorespiratory depression. While this is a rare complication, its possibility should be kept in mind with prolonged administration. Sodium bicarbonate, even though a powerful buffer, is contraindicated in view of the resultant alkalosis. Cimetidine appears to be as effective in children (20 to 40 mg/kg in four divided doses) as in adults. There is no proof that special bland diets are of any help; gastric irritants should be avoided, however, including alcohol, aspirin, coffee, tea, and cola-containing drinks. Psychological assistance in children with overlying anxiety problems may be useful. Diazepam (Valium) has been used successfully in children with stress ulcers who have underlying or associated anxiety problems.

As in the adult, there is no unanimity as to the "ideal" operative procedure for peptic ulcers in children. Many investigators emphasize that the natural course of the childhood peptic ulcer is more benign than that of the adult. They report the response to medical therapy to be prompt in most instances. If surgery is necessary, limited operations, such as vagotomy and pyloroplasty, are supposed to suffice. Other series, however, show equally convincingly that childhood peptic ulcers often extend into adulthood and are more difficult to treat in the child than in the adult. Based on increased experience in the adult with selective or highly selective vagotomy, with or without drainage procedure or limited resection, the present trend toward truncal vagotomy plus pyloroplasty in children may change.

The indications for surgery in children with peptic ulcers consist of massive or repeated hemorrhage, perforation, obstruction, and the difficult to define "intractability."

Secondary or Stress Ulcers. In certain groups of patients, such as children with burns or CNS lesions, prophylactic therapy has been shown to decrease significantly the incidence of stress ulcers. The early use of milk feedings, immediately after stabilization of burn patients, can reduce gastric acidity and provide needed calories. The stomach is emptied prior to the nasogastric tube feeding to prevent aspiration. Diazepam (Valium), given orally at 1 to 1.5 mg at 6-hour intervals initially, gradually increased as needed and tolerated, in burn patients, is thought not only to decrease anxiety in burned children, but also to reduce gastric acidity through a direct effect on the hypothalamus. The nonoperative therapy of stress ulcers is otherwise similar to that described in patients with acute erosive gastritis. In contrast to patients with acute erosive gastritis, in patients with bleeding ulcers arterial embolization can serve as either a temporizing or definitive procedure when the general condition prohibits even a limited operative intervention. Stress ulcers can occur in either stomach or duodenum or both areas simultaneously. The majority of bleeding or perforating stress ulcers requiring operative intervention, however, are located in the duodenum. Since there is no recurrence of the ulcer once the underlying stress has ceased, the most conservative operative procedure able to control either hemorrhage or perforation is preferred.

Zollinger-Ellison Syndrome. This syndrome, responsible for multiple duodenal or jejunal ulcers, does occur occasionally in childhood. Non-beta pancreatic islet cells are responsible for the increased gastrin output, leading to a high gastric acidity. The treatment is identical to that in adults: total gastrectomy with esophagojejunostomy.

GASTRITIS

PETER K. KOTTMEIER, M.D.

Infectious gastritis, viral or bacterial, is uncommon even in children with "gastroenteritis." Bacterial gastritis can occur, however, in children with massive sepsis, such as, for instance, in emphysematous gastritis, in which the therapy is directed toward the underlying etiology. Chronic granulomatous disease also occasionally can involve duodenum and stomach. Therapy is supportive, with appropriate antibiotics. Surgery is rarely indicated.

Acute gastritis is most commonly seen after the ingestion of medication or other chemicals. The therapy for acute gastritis after aspirin ingestion consists of the correction of a possible associated coagulopathy, restriction or appropriate selection of oral intake, and the temporary use of gastric antacids. Alcohol-induced gastritis is also self-limiting after the discontinuation of alcoholic intake and symptomatic treatment. Gastritis due to the ingestion of corrosive agents is almost entirely limited to the ingestion of acid solution, such as hydrochloric acid. The attempt to buffer the ingested acid with alkaline solution is useless, since the corrosive effect of the acid is almost instantaneous. The stomach should be put at rest with nasogastric suction after careful insertion of a nasogastric tube to avoid perforation. Diffuse necrosis with perforation is the most likely complication, requiring prompt operative intervention. Gastritis due to lye or alkali ingestion is extremely rare. If it occurs, it is usually associated with esophageal burns and should be treated accordingly: proof of the burn via endoscopy, followed by the administration of steroids and antibiotics for approximately 3 weeks with re-examination.

Chronic gastritis can occur as a protein-losing, benign, hypertrophic gastropathy similar to Ménétrier's syndrome in the adult. It is occasionally associated with cyclic vomiting, viral infections, or eosinophilia, suggestive of a hypersensitivity reaction. Hypoproteinemia and anemia are present in most patients. Therapy consists of the correction of hypoproteinemia, either by infusion of protein or a high protein and low fat oral intake. In contrast to the adult Ménétrier's gastritis, it is usually self-limiting in children, responding promptly to supportive therapy. Bile gastritis, sometimes seen in adults after gastric operations, is rare in children. It can occur after gastrointestinal surgery such as bypass operations or duodenal obstruction. The gastritis due to the exposure of gastric mucosa to bile salts may respond to therapy with cholestyramine, antacids such as aluminum hydroxide, or bethanechol chloride (Urecholine) to stimulate gastric emptying, which is usually delayed. If this fails, a duodenogastric diversional operation is usually indicated to eliminate gastric bile stasis.

Acute Erosive Gastritis (AEG). Although the etiology of AEG is similar to that of stress ulcers, pathologic changes, therapy, and prognosis vary considerably. Stress ulcers are often confined to a single, predominantly duodenal site. Even multiple ulcers are limited to localized areas without the complete and diffuse gastric involvement seen in AEG. Since AEG often occurs in patients undergoing recognizable or anticipated stress, as in postoperative patients or patients with burns or CNS lesions, the therapy should be prophylactic in many instances. Although gastric acidity in children under stress is not necessarily increased, the breakdown of apical mucosal integrity allows back-perfusion of even normal acid, with subsequent gastritis and ulcerations. The breakdown of the mucosal integrity may be related to the diminution of energy source in the stressed patient; part of the therapy consists, therefore, of restoration or maintenance of an anabolic state in the stressed patient, if necessary through parenteral hyperalimentation. To prevent back-perfusion of gastric acid, buffers, such as antacids, or histamine receptor blockers, such as cimetidine, are used individually or together.

In patients in whom AEG has occurred, often leading to life-endangering bleeding, the following therapeutic approach can be used: nasogastric tube suction with intermittent iced saline irrigation until the stomach is cleared of blood clots, followed by the instillation of antacids on an hourly basis. An attempt should be made to keep the gastric pH at or over 4. This can be supported or accomplished by the use of cimetidine, a histamine receptor blocker, which reduces basal and stimulated gastric acid output. It is also assumed to protect mucosal blood flow during hypotension. There is some evidence to suggest that a continuous intravenous infusion of cimetidine is preferable to a bolus infusion or oral administration in patients with AEG. Again, an attempt should be made to keep the gastric pH at or over 4. If the pH cannot be stabilized, uncontrollable sepsis or multiple organ failure is usually present or developing, with an extremely poor prognosis.

Other attempts to control bleeding from AEG consist of the systemic or localized arterial infusion of vasopressors. Arterial embolization, occasionally effective in children with localized duodenal bleeding, is usually not indicated with AEG in view of the diffuse gastric involvement.

Failure of nonoperative therapy requires operative intervention. As in adults, there is no uniformity of opinion as to what operative procedure is the most suitable. In contrast to patients with localized stress ulcers, in whom the most conservative procedure is usually recommended, substantial gastric resection with truncal vagotomy may be necessary for children with massive AEG, not only to control bleeding but also to prevent rebleeding.

Fortunately, the prophylactic use of either antacids or cimetidine to control the gastric pH has reduced markedly the number of patients requiring operative intervention.

MALFORMATIONS OF THE INTESTINE

NANCY E. VINTON, M.D.

Congenital malformations of the intestinal tract can present the pediatrician with emergency situations at birth. Cautionary signs include polyhydramnios in the mother and bilious vomiting, abdominal distention, and failure to pass meconium in the neonate. Gastrointestinal bleeding and obstruction are more often the presenting signs in the older child. Prompt measures must be taken, prior to surgical intervention, to help prevent the high mortality rate still associated with congenital anomalies. Furthermore, the pediatrician may have to deal with sequelae from a surgical correction long after the malformation itself has ceased to be a problem.

MALFORMATIONS PRESENTING AS INTESTINAL OBSTRUCTION

Malformations leading to intestinal obstruction immediately after birth include duodenal web; annular pancreas; stenoses, atresias, or duplications anywhere along the intestinal tract; and malrotation with midgut volvulus. The higher the obstruction, the lesser the degree of abdominal distention but also the more rapid the onset of symptoms and the more urgent the need for intervention. Prompt treatment to relieve the distention from swallowed air and accumulating intestinal secretions avoids possible aspiration and respiratory compromise. Endotracheal intubation may be necessary to protect the infant's airway. Placement of a naso- or orogastric tube (No. 10 French Rapogle tube) effectively evacuates the stomach and prevents further abdominal distention. Only low intermittent suction is used because constant or high-pressure suction frequently results in gastric erosions in neonates. Intravenous ranitidine (1 to 2 mg/kg/day as a continuous or bolus infusion) should be started as additional prophylaxis against upper gastrointestinal hemorrhage and also for prevention of the gastric hypersecretion seen postoperatively if extensive bowel resection has taken place.

Correction of fluid and electrolyte imbalance due to loss of intestinal secretions must be undertaken preoperatively. Gastric outputs are replaced volume for volume with an intravenous solution of one-half normal saline and 30 mEq/L KCl, and maintenance fluids are given on an ongoing basis. If the malformation causing obstruction is malrotation with volvulus, severe acidosis secondary to bowel ischemia may need to be corrected intravenously with a 20 ml/kg bolus of normal saline or even with 1 mEq/kg of sodium bicarbonate. An associated congenital heart defect may be life-threatening and demand priority surgical intervention. In these cases, placement of a central venous catheter for total parenteral nutrition and continued gastric drainage allows deferral of intestinal surgery until it can be safely accomplished.

Surgical techniques to correct malformations causing intestinal obstruction will be mentioned here briefly. The operation is performed under general endotracheal anesthesia. A right upper quadrant transverse incision (with extension to the left of the abdomen in cases of malrotation) is most often chosen because it yields ready access to the entire intestinal tract. Frequently, a gastrostomy tube is placed for chronic decompression of the bowel, protection of the anastomosis, and future enteral feeding attempts.

Duodenal webs are treated with duodenotomy and web excision. In annular pancreas, a bypass operation attaches proximal to distal duodenum so that the sequelae of invading pancreatic tissue are avoided (fistula or pseudocyst formation, peritonitis, and pancreatitis). Areas of stenosis or duplication, if small, are resected and a primary anastomosis is performed. In all of the above cases, a catheter must be passed through the bowel proximal and distal to the anastomosis to ensure that unsuspected webs are not present. Long tubular duplications may be unresectable without impairing the vasculature to the normal intestinal tract. In such cases,

leaving the segment in place after complete mucosal stripping, with or without establishing drainage to the normal bowel, may be adequate therapy to prevent further obstruction or bleeding.

Complete atresia of the intestine (duodenal, jejunal, or ileal) may necessitate significant resection of the dilated proximal segment before primary anastomosis can be attempted. In cases of short bowel syndrome, to salvage as much gut as possible, a tapering procedure along the antimesenteric border approximates the dilated proximal intestinal segment to the more normal caliber distal segment. Dilated, atonic proximal intestine may pose problems as a motility disorder in many children in subsequent years. Discordant motility patterns inherent to small and large bowel may give rise to a functional obstruction at the site of anastomosis between jejunum or ileum and colon. Later management includes use of motility agents such as metaclopramide or cisapride or further surgery to resect amotile segments.

In intestinal malrotation, obstruction occurs from midgut volvulus or from Ladd's bands lying across the duodenum which attach it to the displaced cecum found to the left of midline. With surgery, the bands are lysed and the volvulus is reduced by counterclockwise rotation of the gut around its mesentery. Recurrence of volvulus is rare, and no advantage has been noted with fixation of the mesentery. Intestinal malrotation should be looked for as a frequently associated malformation during surgery for duodenal and jejunoileal atresia. Malrotation presenting with volvulus can happen at any age, even in adulthood, and must always be included in the differential diagnosis of the patient with signs of upper intestinal obstruction, chronic or acute abdominal pain, and/or bilious vomiting.

MALFORMATIONS PRESENTING AS EVISCERATION

Ruptured omphalocele and gastroschisis present an emergency situation in the neonatal period which is unrelated to intestinal obstruction as discussed above. In these infants, initial management is aimed at protecting the eviscerated bowel from heat and fluid loss and from infection. Omphalocele with an intact peritoneal and amniotic sac, however, is not a surgical emergency because there is little risk of contamination, and the surrounding Wharton's jelly acts as insulation to prevent evaporative and heat losses. These infants do not require gastric drainage or intravenous therapy and are usually very stable. Nonoperative management of intact omphalocele is to induce granulation tissue to form over the sac with use of Mercurochrome or silver nitrate. This is a long and tedious process and can be circumvented by initial surgery to free up skin flaps that are then pulled over the omphalocele and sutured closed. In either case, the bowel is left as a ventral hernia until a staged closure of the defect can be arranged.

In gastroschisis and ruptured omphalocele, the exposed bowel must be dealt with immediately. Using sterile gloves, it should be situated centrally on the abdomen to prevent pulling against the vascular pedicle, which causes ischemia. The infant can then be placed up to the axillae inside a Lahey bag, if available. This is a sterile plastic bag with a cinch strap across the top used by abdominal surgeons to hold viscera exposed intraoperatively. The alternative is to cover exposed bowel with sterile saline-soaked gauze to prevent drying and then wrap the bowel with an abundant layer of sterile dry gauze to prevent heat loss. Use of an incubator also helps maintain body temperature and prevent evaporative heat losses. A naso- or orogastric tube is placed to low intermittent suction to prevent abdominal distention with air both pre- and postoperatively. Ventilation by endotracheal tube may be necessary to stabilize the infant, but air leakage around the tube will also increase the probability of abdominal distention. Transcutaneous or peripheral arterial monitoring of oxygenation replaces the usual method of umbilical artery catheterization. Ampicillin and gentamicin are given intravenously to treat possible enteric sepsis. Intravenous access is mandatory prior to transport to another location for surgical intervention.

The aim of operative repair for these malformations presenting as evisceration is to create an internal cavity large enough to hold all of the abdominal viscera. Current techniques utilize Teflon material sutured circumferentially to the abdominal musculature, forming a tubular structure around the exposed bowel. This is then managed either with a drawstring progressively drawn tighter or by sutures repeatedly opened and resutured to take up slack as the abdominal cavity enlarges to hold more intestine. After 7 to 10 days, the Teflon implant is removed because of an increasing risk of infection. Intravenous antibiotic coverage is continued and broadened to include staphylococcal organisms, and topical antibiotics are applied to the operative site throughout this time. The dangers of prematurely forcing the viscera into the small abdominal cavity include respiratory compromise and bowel ischemia.

Gastroschisis is often complicated by the presence of malrotation, intestinal atresia, and enteric fistulas. These complications may not be recognized at the time of initial surgery if the eviscerated bowel is densely adherent and may not become apparent until postoperatively when enteral feedings are attempted. A motility disorder of the remaining intestine also can delay enteral nutrition for months. Hence, all of these infants should have inserted at the time of surgery a central venous catheter for total parenteral nutrition and a gastrostomy tube for later attempts at enteral feeding. Infants with a ruptured omphalocele are not subject to these problems unless the exposed serosal surface of the bowel develops an infection.

OMPHALOMESENTERIC DUCT MALFORMATIONS

Malformations of the umbilicus that remain in continuity with the intestinal tract are the omphalomesenteric duct remnants—granuloma or polyp, sinus or fistula, Meckel's diverticulum or fibrous cord. These anomalies generally are not a problem in the neonatal period but may nonetheless cause life-threatening illness in the pediatric patient. A Meckel's diverticulum can present with massive gastrointestinal hemorrhage from ulceration due to ectopic gastric mucosa; as intes-

tinal obstruction from volvulus, internal herniation, or intussusception; or as diverticulitis with or without perforation. After the child becomes hemodynamically stable, receiving intravenous fluids and antibiotics, abdominal surgery is performed to fully excise the lesion from its origin on the antimesenteric border of the distal ileum. Ileal resection may be necessary if the base of the diverticulum is wide or if there has been some compromise to the adjacent intestine. No sequelae result from this operation unless perforation has led to complications with peritonitis.

Umbilical granulomas may be treated with applications of silver nitrate. Polyps consist of intestinal mucosa and require local resection. Sinus tracts (ending blindly) or fistula tracts (in continuity with bowel and extruding feces) are treated with local antibiotics and débridement to facilitate drainage, but definitive therapy is complete excision through either an intraumbilical or an intraabdominal approach. A fibrous cord remnant from an obliterated omphalomesenteric duct also should be excised, since it can be the lead point around which a volvulus or internal herniation of intestine may occur.

INTESTINAL MALFORMATIONS WITH LATER PRESENTATION

Internal hernias are defects in the mesentery in which small intestine can enter and become incarcerated. They can manifest at any age. During surgery the hernia is first reduced, which may require a further incision of the mesentery to release the incarcerated bowel. The mesenteric defect is then closed with sutures. Intestinal resection is dependent on the degree of damage from prior ischemia.

Umbilical hernia is an abdominal wall defect that occurs due to incomplete development or imperfect closure of the fascia of the umbilical ring. Most close spontaneously by 3 years of age. However, if they are greater than 1.5 cm in diameter at 2 years of age, they should be corrected surgically to prevent the risk of intestinal incarceration. This is accomplished easily by invagination and oversewing of the hernia sac, even as an outpatient procedure.

Mesenteric and omental cysts are usually intestinal lymphangiomas, the majority being mesenteric (70 per cent) and polycystic (85 per cent). They may be asymptomatic at birth but continue to grow in size so that by 5 years of age nearly 60 per cent are detected because of intestinal obstruction or mass effect. Complete resection without removing intestine is recommended but not always feasible if the cyst is too tightly adherent to bowel or too close to the mesenteric blood supply.

FOREIGN BODIES OF THE ALIMENTARY TRACT

E. THOMAS BOLES, Jr., M.D.

In the instance of a history of ingestion of a foreign body, roentgenograms of the chest (posteroanterior and lateral) will locate radiopaque objects in the esophagus, and an abdominal radiograph will identify one that has passed into the stomach or intestinal tract. If a foreign body in the esophagus is suspected but is not radiopaque, a barium swallow study will identify its presence. Foreign bodies in the esophagus should be removed promptly. For rounded objects (e.g., coins, marbles, disc batteries) recently ingested, the Foley bag catheter technique is simple and highly effective. The child is sedated and placed on the fluoroscopic table in the Trendelenburg (head down) position. The catheter is passed into the esophagus beyond the foreign body, the balloon inflated with radiopaque fluid, and the catheter withdrawn under fluoroscopic guidance.

If the foreign body is pointed or sharp or is a disc battery ingested more than 24 hours previously, endoscopic removal under general endotracheal anesthesia should be done. The currently available instruments permit this procedure to be successful in expert hands in almost all instances. Occasionally it may be easier and wiser to manipulate the foreign body into the stomach using the esophagoscope. Either rigid or flexible esophagoscopes may be used depending on individual skill and experience.

A swallowed foreign body that fails to pass uneventfully through the alimentary tract is most likely to become arrested somewhere along the course of the esophagus. If the foreign body reaches the stomach, and that is usually the case, the chances of its becoming arrested in its further passage down the gastrointestinal tract are small. Such an arrest probably occurs in less than 5 per cent of cases. Accordingly, in most instances periodic observation of the patient, who is usually an infant or toddler, is all that is required.

The type and particularly the shape of the ingested object is an important determinant of the possibility of its becoming arrested. Because most of these foreign bodies are visible radiographically, abdominal radiographs are helpful in estimating the possibility of arrest and should be taken routinely. If the object is not radiopaque, it may be outlined by a small barium meal. Rarely a foreign body such as a toothpick may be ingested without symptoms and without knowledge of the parents, only to cause an inflammatory intra-abdominal lesion later as a consequence of ulceration and perforation through the intestinal tract.

If the object is rounded and smooth (e.g., marbles, coins, small plastic toys) the child may be followed on an outpatient basis, since the foreign body will almost certainly pass through safely. Usually this occurs within 2 days, and the parents should be asked to check the stools of the child to assure passage and rejoice in this event. Even open safety pins almost always negotiate the gastrointestinal tract eventually.

Long, thin, pointed foreign bodies are more of a problem. It is possible for these to become impacted at the pylorus, C-loop of the duodenum, duodenojejunal junction, or terminal ileum. Straight pins, bobby pins, and segments of pencils fall into this category. Hat pins are particularly dangerous. Children who have swallowed objects of this type should be observed in the hospital, and the progress of the foreign body documented by abdominal radiographs at 12-hour intervals. If there is failure of progression over a period of 2 to

3 days or if worrisome symptoms develop, the object should be removed. In the stomach and duodenum extraction can often be performed successfully with the use of a flexible fiberoptic gastroduodenoscope. Otherwise, laparotomy with gastrotomy or enterotomy is required to remove the impacted object.

Alkaline disc batteries are a particular concern because the casings are not biologically sealed and corrosive fluid may be released. The larger of these (22 to 23 mm in diameter) may be lodged in the esophagus. The smaller (most less than 12 mm in diameter) usually pass into the stomach. The management of those in the stomach or lower gastrointestinal tract remains somewhat controversial, but generally these pass rapidly through the intestinal tract without causing harm. Therefore, it is reasonable to follow asymptomatic children on an outpatient basis, to have the parents check the stools for the battery, and to repeat the abdominal roentgenograms at 48-hour intervals if the battery has not passed. If still in the stomach at 48 hours, removal with a flexible fiberoptic esophagogastroscope is recommended.

Rarely a foreign body gains access to the intestinal tract through the rectum. In infants most often this is a glass thermometer that escapes upward or is broken off. These require prompt removal, which may be possible by digital manipulation alone. If this is not easily accomplished, proctoscopy under general anesthesia should be performed. In older children a bizarre assortment of foreign objects are at times inserted into the rectum. Often these pass without incident, but if they are large or fragile (e.g., light bulb), their extraction may prove to be a challenging exercise. Proctoscopy under anesthesia is ordinarily required.

Bezoars are masses of hair or vegetable fibers that form a cast in the stomach, sometimes extending down into the duodenum or even upper jejunum. These are usually trichobezoars (hair balls) and occur most commonly in girls. Typically there is no history of eating hair, but clearly this is the mechanism. These patients are often asymptomatic, but symptoms that may develop include loss of appetite, intolerance of solid foods, vomiting, and abdominal pain. The child may show evidence of malnutrition and is often somewhat withdrawn or disturbed. The breath is characteristically fetid. A large, firm, movable mass is palpable in the upper abdomen. A barium swallow with fluoroscopy confirms the diagnosis by outlining the intragastric mass. Treatment is by gastrotomy with removal of the bezoar, which forms a cast in the stomach. The small intestine should be traced down to the cecum to determine whether or not portions of the bezoar have separated from the main mass and lodged downstream.

INTUSSUSCEPTION

J. ALEX HALLER, Jr., M.D., F.A.A.P.,
and CHARLES N. PAIDAS, M.D.

Intussusception is derived from the Latin, meaning "to take up or receive one segment (of intestine) within another." The intussusceptum (inner segment) is that part of the bowel that invaginates. The intussuscipiens is that portion of the bowel that receives the intussusceptum. In children, the most common site of intussusception is the ileocecal area (95 per cent), with ileo-ileal, jejuno-ileal, and colo-colonic sites comprising the remaining 5 per cent. Intussusception in children usually occurs without a demonstrable cause. A typical idiopathic intussusception most commonly occurs between 3 months and 1 year of age. Seventy per cent of the patients are less than 1 year of age; intussusception is the most common cause of bowel obstruction in the 1-month (neonatal) to 5-year (preschool) age group.

Epidemiology

Although a specific etiology is seldom found in the pediatric population (80 to 90 per cent), a lead point for intussusception can be caused by a viral infection (adenovirus) of the Peyer's patches, Henoch-Schönlein purpura, cystic fibrosis, Meckel's diverticulum, polyps (Peutz-Jeghers syndrome), after appendectomy with inverted stump, small intestinal duplication, lymphosarcoma of the ileum or colon, round worms (ascariasis), or after chemotherapy for malignancy. A postoperative, secondary intussusception may be a jejuno-ileal or ileo-ileal invagination and is difficult to diagnose in the postoperative setting. A strong clinical suspicion of this diagnosis, usually within 2 weeks of an operation, is an indication for re-exploration. In contrast to children, adults frequently will have a primary colonic malignancy or benign disease in the small bowel as a specific cause of the intussusception.

Signs and Symptoms

Children usually complain of intermittent abdominal pain which is so severe that they may be aroused from sleep with their legs flexed. This is usually followed by an episode of vomiting, with improvement in the pain symptoms. This sequence, which starts with a gradual increase in pain and frequently ends with a vomiting episode, may recur in 15- to 20-minute intervals. Over time the child becomes exhausted, apathetic, pale, and sweaty, and if severe dehydration occurs secondary to third-space losses, the child may become unresponsive. Infants can develop lethargy, irritability, and pallor along with one or more episodes of vomiting. Early in the natural history of an intussusception the stool may be a milky color secondary to mucus produced by lymphatic congestion. More commonly, arterial inflow with increasing venous outflow obstruction produces engorgement of the invaginated bowel. Persistent arterial inflow leads to edema, breakdown of the mucosa, bleeding, and the characteristic currant jelly stool (mucus and blood). As edema continues, the critical closing pressure of the intestinal arterioles is exceeded and bleeding may cease, giving rise to complete intestinal strangulation, perforation, sepsis, and shock. Vital signs and physical findings depend on the stage of the process. Fever to 39°C is common. In the early stages, the abdomen is soft and nontender. Then, distention occurs over time and always accompanies complete obstruction. A sausage-shaped mass may be felt in the right upper quadrant, with an absence of palpable bowel in the right lower quadrant. Rectal examination may reveal the currant jelly stool and rarely a prolapse of the invaginated intussusceptum.

Laboratory Tests

Laboratory tests are not very helpful in making the diagnosis. Leukocytosis may be present and is generally quite high if the bowel is necrotic. A sweat chloride determination should be performed on all children over 2 years of age who have a repeated history of respiratory tract infections and an intussusception. Plain abdominal radiographs should be obtained to complete the evaluation. A spectrum of radiographic findings can occur, and these include air-fluid levels, dilated small bowel loops, and/or a soft tissue mass in the right upper quadrant. The natural history of an intussusception may be insidious (12 to 24 hours) or abrupt (1 to 2 hours). Thus despite all characteristic signs and symptoms, a careful history and high index of suspicion are necessary.

MANAGEMENT

General Measures of Resuscitation

All patients should be managed with fluid and electrolyte resuscitation. If indicated, the urine output should be monitored using a Foley catheter. A child's stomach should always be decompressed with an indwelling nasogastric tube. We administer intravenous antibiotic therapy (cefoxitin) before hydrostatic reduction is attempted in patients if they have a longstanding bowel obstruction. Surgical indications for immediate exploration include free air in the abdomen, pneumatosis intestinalis, recurring gross blood per rectum, and the presence of symptoms for several days along with septic shock. These children should be taken directly to the operating room following aggressive intravenous fluid therapy, antibiotic administration, and establishment of adequate urine output.

Nonoperative

Children who do not demand immediate exploration (as noted above) should undergo a hydrostatic barium enema under fluoroscopy, preferably with sedation, after the initial fluid resuscitation. A surgeon should be in attendance during the attempt at hydrostatic reduction, and the operating room and anesthesia staff should be alerted. Sedation for children over 12 months of age may include morphine sulfate (0.1 mg/kg) IM, Seconal (1 mg/kg) IM, or a combination of meperidine hydrochloride (1 mg/kg), promethazine hydrochloride (0.5 mg/kg), and chlorpromazine hydrochloride (0.5 mg/kg) IM. A Foley catheter is placed in the rectum, the balloon is inflated with fluid, and the buttocks are taped together. The contrast medium used generally is a suspension of one part barium sulfate in three parts water warmed to body temperature. The height of the barium column should be 36 inches above the abdomen, with hydrostatic pressure of approximately 36 inches for no more than 5 minutes without movement of the intussusceptum. Reduction is defined as complete when there is free flow of contrast material into the ileum. Glucagon (0.02 mg/kg IV) has been evaluated in a double-blind study and was found not to be of significant benefit. Ultrasound-guided hydrostatic reduction and air pressure enema reduction have both been attempted, but present recommendations still favor hydrostatic reduction under fluoroscopic guidance. Success rates of hydrostatic reduction approach 70 per cent. Recurrence rates following radiologic reduction range from 7 to 11 per cent, and the interval to recurrence is highly variable. Any doubts about the completeness of reduction should be resolved by surgical exploration. If a radiographically defined filling defect is discovered as the probable cause of an intussusception, the child should undergo a staged laparotomy. Follow-up for a successful hydrostatic barium reduction consists of adequate return of gastrointestinal patency while in hospital by either the passage of air and stool per rectum or the passage of charcoal followed by discharge at 24 hours. Failed hydrostatic reduction may be attempted again once or twice over a short interval prior to exploration if the child remains stable. A child with recurrent intussusception (two or more episodes) is a candidate for exploratory laparotomy.

Operative

As a general rule, an awake intubation should be performed for a suspected bowel obstruction, and preoperative antibiotics should be administered. Most pediatric surgeons utilize a transverse incision in the right lower quadrant which may be extended across the midline if necessary. The intussusceptum should be milked out carefully from distal to proximal via the intussuscipiens. Extensive serosal splitting, obvious gangrene, or inability to reduce the intussusceptum are indications for resection and usually a primary anastomosis. If manual reduction is accomplished, care is taken to identify any lead points. An appendectomy is usually performed without inverting the stump, since the appendix is frequently involved in the invagination and is edematous. Postoperative care should include continued nasogastric drainage, maintenance of plasma volume, and antibiotics. Since the intestinal wall has been traumatized, an inflammatory response may persist for several days, explaining a persistent low-grade fever. In general, the hospital stay for a laparotomy and manual reduction is approximately 5 to 7 days. If resection is required, the child may be hospitalized for as long as 10 to 12 days.

In summary, the diagnosis and management of intussusception have not changed drastically in 30 years. It is of utmost importance that a surgeon be involved in the care of these cases from the moment of presentation and throughout attempted barium enema reduction because deterioration of the child at any time or failure of hydrostatic reduction is an emergency indication for operative intervention.

HIRSCHSPRUNG'S DISEASE

WILLIAM K. SIEBER, M.D.

Hirschsprung's disease is a congenital anomaly characterized by partial to complete, acute or chronic low intestinal obstruction associated with absence of intramural ganglion cells in the distal alimentary tract.

When Hirschsprung's disease is suspected, prompt surgical consultation for diagnosis and treatment should be obtained. Nonsurgical treatment is ineffective. Cathartics and smooth muscle stimulants such as methacholine (Mecholyl) may be harmful, promoting fatal enterocolitis. Older children with moderate chronic constipation as the only symptom may respond to enemas administered daily or every second or third day. Since the rectum is inactive, impactions occur frequently and may require the use of detergent retention enemas, dioctyl sodium sulfosuccinate (Colace), one part in three parts of saline, followed by a cleansing enema in 12 hours. The dangers of rectal perforation and water intoxication from enemas are well documented. Enemas should be isotonic. Fecal impactions are avoided by preparations that tend to keep the stools soft, such as mineral oil or psyllium hydrophilic mucilloid (Metamucil).

In infancy, acute colonic (90 per cent) or low small bowel obstruction (10 per cent aganglionosis coli) requires emergency relief by enterostomy in the normally innervated intestine just proximal to the aganglionic intestine. Frozen-section control of the placement of the enterostomy requires the aid of a pathologist familiar with the histologic appearance of intramural ganglion cells in infants. The colostomy is done as a loop colostomy or as a divided colostomy with the proximal end brought up to function as a single lumen, the distal end being closed and returned to the peritoneal cavity. When the aganglionic segment is short and involves only the rectum, a right transverse loop colostomy may be done. An emergency colostomy is indicated to prevent the development of enterocolitis, a frequently lethal complication in infancy. A colostomy is done preliminary to definitive surgical treatment in the newborn, in symptomatic infants up to 6 months of age, and in older patients with longstanding symptoms. Definitive surgical treatment is deferred until the infant is over 6 months of age or, in an older child, until general health improves and colonic impactions are completely removed. This usually takes 6 months.

Preparation for definitive surgery includes mechanical emptying of the colon with enemas, a clear liquid diet, bowel preparation with neomycin and erythromycin base, and digital dilatation of the anus.

Definitive surgical treatment involves the resection of the aganglionic intestine and re-establishment of the continuity of the alimentary tract. This is currently done by one of three abdominoperineal procedures—the Swenson, Duhamel, or Soave procedure.

The Swenson procedure is the original and time-tested standard procedure. In this operation, the aganglionic intestine is freed and removed to within 1.5 cm of the pectinate line anteriorly; the procedure includes a sphincterotomy of the internal anal sphincter posteriorly. The normally innervated intestine is then brought down and anastomosed to this remaining rectal stump.

In the Duhamel procedure, the aganglionic intestine is resected down to the rectum. The rectum is sutured closed but left in place. A retrorectal channel is developed, and the normally innervated intestine is pulled through this channel and through an incision in the posterior rectal wall 1 cm above the pectinate line. Half the circumference of the distal rectum is then anastomosed to the posterior half of the pulled-through colonic wall and is opposed to the posterior half of the retained rectum. Clamps are placed intraluminally to remove this common wall, or the wall may be divided by the anastomotic stapler, resulting in an anastomosis of the end of the colon to the posterior wall of the rectum. Variations of the Duhamel procedure involve differences in the type of crushing clamp or suturing method used. In long-segment aganglionosis such as total colonic aganglionosis, the Martin modification of the Duhamel procedure (in which a long side-to-side anastomosis of the pulled-through intestine to the distal aganglionic colon is created) or the right colon patch technique described by Boley may be indicated.

In the Soave procedure (the endorectal pull-through procedure), the mucosa is removed from the rectum down to the skin of the anus. Normally innervated intestine is then pulled through the resultant muscular cuff and anastomosed either directly, as in the Swenson procedure (Boley), or in delay fashion, as a two-stage procedure (Soave), to the anal skin.

The operative mortality associated with these procedures is negligible, and the initial result in all is very good. At present the personal experience of the operating surgeon should determine the best procedure for the individual patient. My preference is the one-stage endorectal (Boley) procedure preceded by an enterostomy in normal intestine just proximal to the aganglionic intestine.

Enterocolitis may occur as a serious complication of Hirschsprung's disease. The sudden abdominal distention, disinterest in nursing, vomiting, and foul diarrhea result in high fever with dehydration and may cause death within 24 to 48 hours. When enterocolitis is suspected, intravenous fluids, gentle copious saline rectal irrigations, antibiotics, and gastric suction followed by decompression by colostomy may be lifesaving. Enterocolitis may first appear after a colostomy has been done for obstruction, or it may appear as long as 6 to 8 years after an uneventful definitive procedure. The Swenson procedure is more likely to be followed by enterocolitis than are the other procedures.

Short-segment Hirschsprung's disease, in which only the lower rectum is aganglionic, sometimes responds to transluminal rectal myectomy (actually an extension of full-thickness rectal biopsy). My experience with this procedure has been disappointing.

INFLAMMATORY BOWEL DISEASE

NANCY E. VINTON, M.D.

Inflammatory bowel disease (IBD) is a term encompassing the entities of Crohn's disease, ulcerative colitis, and indeterminate colitis. Although etiology, presenta-

tion, and pathologic findings may differ, therapy of these types of IBD is quite similar and limited to the same pharmacologic interventions. Steroids, sulfasalazine or its derivatives, and immunosuppressives remain the mainstays of therapy. Initial treatment choices are based on the location, extent, and severity of the intestinal involvement. Recourse to surgery and extraordinary means of nutritional support are usually left for those recalcitrant cases in which there have been multiple drug treatment failures.

Steroids are the drugs of choice for acute-phase management of moderate to severe disease whether involving predominantly the small or large bowel. In the systemically ill child with evidence of an acute abdomen, prompt hospitalization for observation and intravenous fluids and steroids is mandatory. Use of steroids in the acutely ill patient is not associated with any increase in complication rate if immediate surgery becomes indicated. Intravenous hydrocortisone or methylprednisolone may be given as a 24-hour infusion, divided doses, or as a single morning dose. Intravenous ACTH has been found to be effective only in IBD patients who have not been treated previously with steroids. When the patient is stabilized and responding to therapy, the steroids may be given orally in single or divided doses. Less adrenal suppression occurs and no differences in clinical response have been found when a single morning dose of steroid is used. Prednisone and prednisolone have fewer mineralocorticoid effects than hydrocortisone.

A typical course of therapy with prednisone consists of 1 to 2 mg/kg/day (to a maximum of 60 mg/day) for 4 to 6 weeks, followed by tapering of the daily dose by 5 mg every week. A relapse in symptoms during the taper may necessitate a second or even third course of steroid therapy. In these cases it is wiser to taper more slowly—by 2.5 mg every other week. Long-term low-dose steroid therapy during disease quiescence does not improve the relapse rate, extension of the disease, or rate of recurrence after resection. IBD patients do not appear to benefit from alternate-day steroid therapy. Therefore, because of the significant toxic side effects, including growth retardation and osteoporosis, steroids should be tapered completely as soon as possible once active disease is under control. Chronic steroid use may be helpful in those recalcitrant patients whose disease does not ever quite enter remission.

Initial treatment of mild disease and maintenance therapy of IBD consists of sulfasalazine (SAS) at 50 to 75 mg/kg/day qid up to the maximum adult dose of 4 to 6 gm/day. The superiority of a clinical response with 4 gm/day or more is small, especially considering the remarkable increase in toxicity noted at such dosages. Because of the high rate of noxious side effects (nausea, abdominal pain, headache) and drug allergy (rash, bronchospasm, hepatitis, hemolysis, and agranulocytosis), SAS should be started at a low dosage of 10 mg/kg/day and increased slowly over 2 weeks. Of those patients developing a mild hypersensitivity reaction, 85 to 90 per cent can be desensitized by withdrawing the drug and restarting at very low dose and increasing slowly over several weeks. A daily supplement of folic acid, 1 mg/day, should be given because SAS may interfere with absorption of folate in the small intestine.

The active moiety of SAS is probably 5-aminosalicylic acid (5-ASA), produced when colonic bacteria cleave the azo bond of the drug—hence, the rationale for use of SAS in the presence of colonic disease. This includes the vast majority of children with IBD—all patients with ulcerative and indeterminate colitis and about 60 per cent of patients with Crohn's disease. Although there is no evidence of drug efficacy in Crohn's patients with only small intestinal involvement, SAS continues to be used as primary therapy. The second by-product of the azo bond cleavage of SAS is sulfapyridine, which is readily absorbed and accounts for the toxic side effects of the drug. Many alternative preparations now exist which do not contain sulfapyridine in an attempt to alleviate the problems with toxicity. These drugs are pro- drugs, such as diazosalicylate, which is a dimer of 5-ASA, or have pH-dependent enteric coatings that release the active drug in the terminal ileum and colon. Ongoing drug trials may show such drugs to be more effective in Crohn's disease of the small intestine, since they deliver 5-ASA directly to the area involved.

Rectal preparations of steroids and derivatives of SAS are now available for use in those patients with primarily distal intestinal involvement. Rectal suppositories are suitable for patients with ulcerative proctitis. Enema forms of these drugs have been shown to reach the distal left colon, frequently as high as the splenic flexure, and offer an alternative to the 60 per cent of patients with ulcerative colitis confined to the left side. The applicability of rectal preparations for use in younger children is limited by compliance, but they may be appropriate for older adolescents with mild disease. Systemic absorption of rectal steroids depends on the degree of mucosal inflammation and may be as high as 75 per cent, whereas 5-ASA preparations do not seem to be absorbed to any great extent.

Immunosuppressive drug therapy with either azathioprine (AZT) or its metabolite 6-mercaptopurine (6-MP) has a respected place in the treatment of recalcitrant IBD in adults. Although these drugs are not FDA-approved for such use in children, they are now commonly being used at a dosage of 1 to 2 mg/kg/day without significant problems when proper monitoring is undertaken. Their use is still limited to patients who cannot be taken off steroid therapy without relapse or have severe and chronic fistula formation. Temporary continuation of steroids for 2 to 3 months is necessary when starting AZT or 6-MP because of their slow onset of action. About 70 per cent of patients improve clinically and endoscopically, and 50 per cent are able to discontinue steroids during treatment. Beyond the significant steroid-sparing effects of these drugs, their effectiveness in preventing relapse for up to 37 months is dramatic.

Leukopenia is a common dose-related side effect of AZT and 6-MP which can be monitored with a complete blood count every 2 to 4 weeks and that resolves after discontinuation of the drug. Other toxicities include rash, fever, nausea, alopecia, and, in rare case reports, reversible bone marrow depression, pancreatitis, and

hepatitis. There have been no reports of malignant lymphoma or increased predisposition to development of cancer in IBD patients treated with these immunosuppressive drugs.

Intravenous antibiotic therapy has a role in the treatment of children with IBD presenting with systemic illness and abdominal findings suggestive of perforation or abscess. However, it is now clear that oral metronidazole is beneficial in the treatment of Crohn's patients with perineal or perianal disease from fistula formation and in those with bacterial overgrowth syndrome from areas of stenosis. On a dose of 20 mg/kg/day (not to exceed 1 gm/day), about 80 per cent of patients have significant improvement or complete closure of fistulas after 2 to 3 months of treatment. The duration of therapy is not so clear; and fistulas recur in a majority of patients, especially if the drug is not discontinued slowly. Common side effects are metallic taste, nausea, dark urine, urticaria, and furry tongue; an Antabuse-like effect is seen with alcohol ingestion. With long-term use (greater than 6 months), paresthesias may occur but resolve with discontinuation of the drug. Teratogenic and oncogenic effects are common in animal models but have not been reported in humans. Metronidazole is an alternative choice for the patient with allergy to SAS who cannot be desensitized.

Nutritional therapy is an important adjunct to care in children with IBD. Twenty-five to 30 per cent of these children (primarily with small intestinal Crohn's disease) present with linear growth failure. Dietary interventions may be limited by the child's symptoms—anorexia may make compliance with an oral supplementation regimen impossible; age and maturity may make the use of nasogastric feedings unrealistic. In general, dietary restrictions should be recommended based on symptoms—omission of carbonated beverages and gasiferous vegetables in the child with bloating, caffeine and laxative fruits in the child with diarrhea. Low-residue diets should be reserved for those children with known stenotic areas causing partial intestinal obstruction. A lactose-free diet should be advised only on the basis of an abnormal lactose breath hydrogen test, and, if this restriction is necessary, calcium supplementation is mandatory, as milk is the primary source of calcium for most children. Iron, folate, and zinc supplementation may also be required.

Use of total parenteral nutrition (TPN) and bowel rest is an alternate approach for the child who has not responded to the usual medical interventions or has frequent severe relapses. These children are usually at high risk for growth failure and may have accelerated growth with very short-term use of TPN. Although clinical symptoms improve on TPN therapy, disease progression and relapse are usually unchanged on a long-term basis. However, should surgery then be necessary, it is clear that patients treated with prior TPN fare better postoperatively.

Surgery is now considered a last resort by most pediatricians caring for children with IBD, whether Crohn's disease or ulcerative colitis. This cautious attitude is especially appropriate in Crohn's disease with its chronic and relapsing nature. Nonetheless, 90 per cent of Crohn's patients will have undergone at least one resection after 30 years of disease. Surgery has an effective role in the treatment of abscess from a perianal fistula that does not heal with aggressive medical intervention. Strict indications exist for surgery in the child with ulcerative colitis. Toxic megacolon still has a mortality of 30 per cent in those patients who perforate. If this entity is under consideration in the worsening child with unremitting intestinal bleeding with or without signs of an acute abdomen, surgery should be performed within 72 hours, after which time the incidence of perforation increases dramatically. The other strict indication for colectomy in the patient with ulcerative colitis is the presence of dysplasia on biopsy. The incidence of colon carcinoma becomes significant after 10 years of disease and increases by 20 per cent every decade thereafter. Many children fall into this high-risk group while still under the care of a pediatrician, and steps must be taken to ensure that they undergo yearly surveillance colonoscopy.

A high degree of caution must be used when considering antispasmodic and antidiarrheal medications in children with IBD. Commonly used anticholinergics include tincture of belladonna, dicyclomine hydrochloride, propantheline bromide, and clidinium bromide. Narcotic agents frequently used to slow intestinal motility include diphenoxylate, loperamide, codeine, paregoric, and deodorized tincture of opium. These drugs may be used effectively in the child with quiescent disease who still is plagued by frequent loose stools or rectal urgency. The risk arises if the child has a severe exacerbation of disease and continues taking these medications, which may result in ileus with toxic dilatation and possible perforation.

In summary, care of the child with IBD, either Crohn's disease or ulcerative colitis, involves the use of steroids in the acute phase to control active disease and SAS or one of its derivative as maintenance therapy. Refractory disease or complications from fistula formation can be treated effectively with addition of an immunosuppressive drug (AZT or 6-MP) or metronidazole to the treatment regimen. Nutritional support is crucial to recuperate growth failure commonly found in these children. Surgery has a limited but effective role when indicated.

NECROTIZING ENTEROCOLITIS

IVAN D. FRANTZ, III, M.D.

Treatment of necrotizing enterocolitis (NEC) depends upon the severity of the infant's disease. At the most benign end of the spectrum are those infants with "R/O NEC" or "NEC episodes." These infants, in the process of increasing enteric feedings, may demonstrate signs of abdominal distention, gastric residuals, or bowel loops visible through the abdominal wall, sometimes associated with apnea or guaiac-positive stools. This complex may represent the prodrome of NEC or may be only feeding intolerance and usually requires that feedings be discontinued and a nasogastric tube placed. No other therapy may be required, although in some cases further diagnostic investigation is indicated, including abdominal radiographs and evaluation for possible sepsis. If after 48 or 72 hours the findings subside, careful feedings may be reintroduced.

As clinical signs and symptoms become worse or more numerous, more aggressive therapy must be initiated. Any umbilical vessel catheters should be removed to avoid compromise of bowel perfusion. In addition to withholding of feedings and placement of a nasogastric tube, antibiotics must be started in the presence of the usual signs of sepsis, including frequent or severe apnea, hypotension or poor perfusion, lethargy, or abnormal white blood count. Abdominal findings include tenderness, a palpable mass, and abdominal wall erythema. Radiologic confirmation of the diagnosis by the presence of pneumatosis intestinalis or a fixed bowel loop is also an indication for antibiotics. The usual choice of antibiotics is intravenous ampicillin and gentamicin, with some preferring to add clindamycin for coverage of anaerobes. The dosage is as recommended for septicemia. Although oral gentamicin or kanamycin may be given, there is little to recommend this approach.

In the group of infants in whom the diagnosis of NEC is confirmed radiologically or for whom there is a strong suspicion of sepsis, therapy, including withholding of feedings and gastric decompression, must be prolonged. The exact duration of therapy has not been determined and ranges from 7 to 21 days, with 10 to 14 days being usual. Factors influencing duration of therapy include severity of initial presentation, rapidity of response, and personal bias.

Additional supportive therapy may be necessary for those infants with severe hypotension or disseminated intravascular coagulopathy. This includes expansion of the intravascular volume, pressors, and transfusions with platelets or fresh frozen plasma.

There are no absolute indications for surgical intervention, but most would agree that perforation is such an indication. For this reason abdominal radiographs (left lateral decubitus or cross-table lateral) should be obtained every 4 to 6 hours in the acute (first 24 to 48 hours) phase of the disease. Extensive pneumatosis or portal venous gas, although ominous, is not a sufficient indication for surgery. Other relative indicators for operation include a palpable mass, perhaps indicating an abscess, and unremitting metabolic acidosis, hypotension, or disseminated intravascular coagulation.

Most clinicians believe that surgery should be avoided if possible in the acute phase of illness, even if this means that a later operation may be necessary for resection of strictures. The usual operation consists of resection of obviously necrotic bowel and creation of an ostomy. If there are substantial areas of bowel of questionable viability, it may be desirable to do a minimal resection and follow the infant clinically, with the option of a second operation in 24 hours.

During the period that feedings are withheld, whether or not surgery is necessary, adequate fluids and nutrition must be supplied. In many cases peripheral intravenous alimentation with glucose, amino acids, and lipid emulsion suffices to provide 100 kcal/kg/24 hr, but in some cases, particularly in smaller infants, placement of a central catheter may be required.

Upon completion of treatment enteric feedings must be reinstituted with caution. Dilute standard infant formula of appropriate composition for the nourishment of the infant should be given in small quantities and advanced in strength and volume gradually. Infants may have recurrence of NEC as long as 2 or 3 weeks after the initial episode, so they should be carefully observed during refeeding. Some infants may be intolerant of lactose or other components of standard formula and do better when fed a lactose-free or elemental formula. Signs of obstruction on refeeding may be the result of strictures in either medically or surgically treated infants. Strictures demonstrated on contrast study sometimes resolve spontaneously; thus, several attempts at refeeding may be appropriate before surgical relief of the stricture is indicated. A small fraction of infants with NEC treated surgically go on to develop short bowel syndrome. These infants require prolonged parenteral nutrition, and some may never have adequate gastrointestinal function.

PERITONITIS

ANNE KOLBE, M.B., B.S. (HONS.), F.R.A.C.S.,
FADY A. SINNO, M.D.,
and J. ALEX HALLER, Jr., M.D.

Generalized peritonitis in children is a serious condition with an estimated mortality rate of 1 to 2 per cent and substantial morbidity. However, careful initial assessment, appropriate resuscitation, timely surgical intervention, and diligent postoperative care can minimize the complications associated with this condition such that an excellent long-term result can be expected in the vast majority of children.

Peritonitis is inflammation of part or all of the parietal and visceral surfaces of the abdominal cavity. The causes of peritonitis in children are numerous (Table 1), but the presentation, assessment, and management of a child with peritonitis are basically the same regardless of the etiology. To manage a child with peritonitis

TABLE 1. Causes of Peritonitis in Children

Common
Acute appendicitis
Pelvic inflammatory disease
Ischemic intestinal obstruction
Traumatic gastrointestinal perforation

Uncommon
Postanastomotic gastrointestinal leak
Necrotizing enterocolitis
Pancreatitis
Meconium peritonitis
Primary peritonitis
Secondary chronic ambulatory peritoneal dialysis
Secondary urine, bile, or chyle leak
Tubercular peritonitis

it is necessary to understand the basic anatomy and physiology of the peritoneum as well as pathophysiological changes that result from the inflammatory insult.

INITIAL MANAGEMENT

The initial management of a child with peritonitis involves seven basic steps.

1. Fluid Replacement. *All* children with peritonitis are dehydrated. The extracellular fluid volume may be depleted by as much as 10 to 15 per cent of body weight. The aim of fluid resuscitation is to correct this extracellular fluid deficit rapidly, thus minimizing the risks of hypovolemia and allowing early operation on a stable child.

Ringer's lactated solution is an appropriate fluid to use, as it is a buffered solution with electrolyte concentrations that approximate extracellular fluid. Initially 20 cc/kg stat should be given followed by a continuous infusion at two to three times maintenance until homeostasis is restored, as judged by a clear sensorium, good peripheral perfusion, normal blood pressure, fall in pulse rate, an adequate central venous pressure, and a urine output greater than 2 cc/kg/hr. Then the intravenous fluids can be changed to dextrose 5 per cent with 0.5 normal saline with 20 mEq of KCl/liter at 1.5 times maintenance until operation.

2. Antibiotics. Antibiotics must be administered as soon as is practical after the diagnosis of peritonitis is made. The initial choice of antibiotics is empirical but is guided by the knowledge that peritonitis in children is almost always polymicrobial, involving aerobes and anaerobes. The usual organisms isolated from the peritoneal cavity are *Escherichia coli*, enterococcus, Enterobacteriaceae, and *Bacteroides*. On this basis the first-line drugs of choice are the following: (a) gentamicin, 5 to 7.5 mg/kg/day, divided and given IV q8h; ampicillin, 200 mg/kg/day, divided and given IV q4–6h; and clindamycin, 20 to 40 mg/kg/day, divided and given IV q6–8h. All of these drugs achieve the same levels in the peritoneal fluid as they do in the blood. Metronidazole (7.5 mg/kg IV q 6 hours) may be substituted for clindamycin. Recent studies suggest that single-agent therapy with a broad-spectrum cephalosporin or monolactam may be as effective as combination regimens.

3. Nasogastric Decompression. A large-bore sump nasogastric tube must be placed and attached to low-pressure suction. The tube empties the stomach of gastric secretions and swallowed air, which prevents vomiting, reduces the risk of aspiration, and minimizes further respiratory compromise.

4. Sedation. Once the diagnosis is established, all children with peritonitis should be given some form of analgesia and sedation. Either meperidine, 1 to 1.5 mg/kg IV, or morphine, 0.1 to 0.2 mg/kg IV, can be used.

5. Fever Control. Fever results in an increase in insensible fluid loss with ongoing dehydration. High fevers in young children may precipitate febrile seizures. Acetaminophen is usually sufficient to lower the temperature below 38.5°C. In addition, the use of cold sponges, a cooling blanket, or an electric fan may be helpful. Aspirin should not be used, as it alters platelet aggregation and increases the risk of intra- and post-operative bleeding. Aspirin has also been implicated in the pathogenesis of Reye's syndrome.

6. Oxygen. Severely ill children with hypoxemia and acidemia should receive oxygen via a face mask. If ventilation is severely compromised, intubation and mechanical ventilation may be necessary.

7. Emotional Support. In caring for a child with peritonitis, as for any ill child, it is important to remember the emotional impact of the child's illness on both the patient and the parents. A few minutes spent gaining the child's confidence before the initial examination and a brief explanation of proposed management and procedures is invaluable. Also a discussion of the child's illness and management protocol with the parents helps alleviate some of their concerns. This in turn is reflected favorably in their child's behavior.

SURGICAL MANAGEMENT

Operative intervention should be carried out as soon as the initial resuscitative management is completed. The aims of surgery are (1) to confirm the clinical diagnosis, (2) to prevent continued peritoneal contamination by removal of its source, and (3) to remove all foreign material from the abdominal cavity.

At operation, peritoneal fluid is obtained for Gram's stain and culture. The responsible lesion is identified and appropriately managed by closure of the defect, resection, or exteriorization. The peritoneal cavity is carefully and copiously lavaged with warm normal saline to remove all pus, blood, and foreign material and to reduce the bacterial load. No benefit can be demonstrated by the addition of antibiotics to the irrigant in patients already receiving systemic antibiotics. Intra-abdominal drains are used only if a well-formed abscess cavity is encountered. In uncomplicated generalized peritonitis, drains are of no benefit and may, in fact, induce local septic complications. In cases of gross peritoneal contamination, the practice of leaving the skin and subcutaneous layers of the wound open decreases the incidence of postoperative wound infection.

Postoperative Care. The postoperative care of children with peritonitis is aimed at supporting them through the recuperative process and minimizing postoperative complications (Table 2).

In the immediate postoperative period, intra-abdominal sequestration of fluid continues, and temperature and respiratory rate remain elevated, which increases insensible losses. Intravenous fluid is therefore initially administered at 1.5 times maintenance using dextrose 5 per cent with 0.5 normal saline with 20 mEq of KCl/liter. As the child's condition stabilizes, fluids can be changed to dextrose 5 per cent with 0.25 normal saline with 20 mEq of KCl/liter at a normal maintenance rate, which is continued until bowel activity returns and an oral feeding regimen is fully established. In severe, complicated cases of peritonitis it may take many days for the adynamic ileus to resolve. These children are markedly catabolic and will develop severe protein depletion unless intravenous hyperalimentation is initiated.

Nasogastric decompression is maintained until bowel

TABLE 2. Postoperative Complications

Wound
Hematoma
Infection
Dehiscence

Pulmonary
Atelectasis
Pneumonia
Aspiration
Pulmonary embolus

Gastrointestinal
Acute gastric dilatation
Adynamic ileus
Adhesive small bowel obstruction
Intra-abdominal abscess
Anastomotic leak
Stress ulceration of gastroduodenum

Urinary
Retention
Infection

Venous
Phlebitis

activity returns. The volume of aspirate should be measured regularly and replaced intravenously with an equal volume of 0.5 normal saline with 10 mEq of KCl/liter.

As soon as a correctly positioned nasogastric tube that is attached to suction has no significant aspirate the tube should be removed. Leaving a nasogastric tube off suction or clamped for a trial of "gastric emptying" or oral feeding makes no sense. Nasogastric tubes are uncomfortable for a child, they hamper coughing, and they are associated with a significant incidence of otitis media in young children.

Antibiotic coverage may be altered according to the results of the pre- and intraoperative cultures. They should be continued for at least 5 days or until there are no remaining signs of sepsis. These include a normal temperature for 48 hours and a white blood cell count and differential within normal limits. During antibiotic administration appropriate serum levels must be monitored, especially in patients with renal impairment. In immunocompromised patients or those receiving corticosteroids, intra-abdominal and systemic fungal infection should be suspected if there is poor response to antibacterial treatment. A course of intravenous amphotericin B should be initiated early, but only after the diagnosis of intra-abdominal or systemic fungosis is confirmed by appropriate cultures or pathologic examination.

Postoperatively, close attention must be paid to respiratory care. The child should be encouraged to cough and take deep breaths on a regular basis. Young children will usually not do this on demand; however, they can often be coaxed to blow up a balloon or a plastic spirometer, which provides excellent pulmonary physiotherapy.

Adequate analgesia postoperatively is necessary to permit satisfactory pulmonary physiotherapy and to facilitate early mobilization. This is best achieved by using *small, frequent* intravenous doses of a narcotic agent. The dose must be tailored to provide adequate continuous comfort for the patient without excessive sedation.

Intra-abdominal abscesses and wound infection occur frequently after surgery for peritonitis. The wound must be regularly and carefully inspected. Continuing fever, ileus, and a persistently elevated white blood cell count strongly suggest the presence of an intra-abdominal abscess, which must be aggressively searched for by clinical and radiological means and, when found, operatively drained. Occasionally, successful drainage of a localized fluid collection or abscess can be achieved percutaneously by an interventional radiologist under the guidance of ultrasound or computerized tomography. The precise indications for nonoperative drainage have not been determined.

Primary peritonitis is a monomicrobial form of peritonitis that occurs principally in children with nephrotic syndrome or cirrhosis. The infecting organism is usually *Streptococcus pneumoniae, Haemophilus influenzae, Neisseria meningitidis,* or *Escherichia coli.* The treatment consists of antibiotics and supportive measures; and provided objective improvement occurs within 48 hours, operative intervention is unnecessary. Primary peritonitis is an uncommon condition that is clinically difficult to separate from secondary peritonitis due to a surgically correctable lesion. Practically, the diagnosis is most frequently made by laparotomy, but the prognosis is unaltered by this surgical intervention. For these reasons primary peritonitis is a diagnosis of exclusion and should not be made except in a child with a specific predisposing condition. Peritonitis is a common complication of peritoneal dialysis. It usually presents with fever, abdominal pain, and tenderness. The peritoneal effluent is usually cloudy and contains more than 100 white blood cells per cubic millimeter. Gram stain of the effluent will demonstrate organisms in only 25 per cent of cases that eventually show positive cultures. The most frequently cultured organisms are *Staphylococcus epidermidis* and *aureus,* although gram-negative organisms and *Candida* account for 20 to 30 per cent of peritonitis episodes. After evaluating the peritoneal fluid, intraperitoneal antibiotic therapy may be started empirically with a combination of a first-generation cephalosporin and an aminoglycoside (e.g., cephalothin 250 mg/L and tobramycin 4 to 6 mg/L), and continued until bacteriologic identification is available.

NONHEMOLYTIC UNCONJUGATED HYPERBILIRUBINEMIA

WILLIAM SPIVAK, M.D.

Unconjugated bilirubin is a lipophilic molecule that may enter the brain, especially during the neonatal period, and cause either transient or permanent brain dysfunction, especially in low birth weight, hypoxic, acidotic, or septic infants. Older infants with the severe hyperbilirubinemia associated with Crigler-Najjar syndrome are also at high risk. Avoidance of toxic levels of bilirubin is therefore essential in the management of this problem.

PHYSIOLOGIC JAUNDICE

In the adult, the normal serum bilirubin should not exceed 2 mg/dl. By this standard, every newborn has hyperbilirubinemia. In the absence of hemolysis and as long as the serum bilirubin does not exceed 12 mg/dl, indirect hyperbilirubinemia (defined as an indirect bilirubin greater than 85 per cent of total) of the full-term healthy newborn can be characterized as "physiologic" and requires no specific therapy. Since physiologic jaundice usually peaks at day 3 of life, serum bilirubin levels approaching 12 mg/dl during the first 48 hours of life require further monitoring. Phototherapy is indicated for rapidly increasing levels of bilirubin during this period even when levels are less than 12 mg/dl.

BREAST MILK JAUNDICE

Breast milk jaundice, a benign disorder associated with unconjugated hyperbilirubinemia, has been estimated to occur in about 0.5 per cent of otherwise healthy breast-fed babies. However, actual figures for this form of jaundice may be much higher. Typically, serum bilirubin in this disorder rises rapidly after the fourth day of life and peaks at the end of the second week of life. However, recent evidence suggests that breast feeding may be a contributing factor in hyperbilirubinemia during the first 48 to 72 hours of life. Although the serum bilirubin may reach levels requiring phototherapy, kernicterus has not been reported with this entity alone. Even with continued ingestion of the "abnormal milk," serum bilirubin levels decline gradually over a period of 3 to 16 weeks. If phototherapy is necessary for this disorder, it is prudent to discontinue breast feeding; a 24- to 48-hour cessation of breast feeding usually results in a significant reduction in bilirubin levels—a test that is both diagnostic and therapeutic. Resumption of human milk is associated with either a cessation of the previous decline in serum bilirubin or a rise of only 2 to 3 mg/dl.

CRIGLER-NAJJAR SYNDROME

Type I Crigler-Najjar syndrome always presents within the first few days of life with persistent, severe unconjugated bilirubin (usually greater than 20 mg/dl). This form of icterus often leads to kernicterus if not treated with continuous phototherapy and/or hepatic transplantation. There is frequently a family history of severe neonatal jaundice. Type II Crigler-Najjar syndrome is characterized by a less severe form of indirect hyperbilirubinemia (usually 6 to 20 mg/dl) that usually presents during infancy but in some patients is not diagnosed until 2 to 10 years of age. Neurologic complications occur in type II patients but are much less common. The absence of bilirubin diglucuronide from human bile is biochemically pathognomonic of Crigler-Najjar syndrome. The only way to distinguish the two groups (even serum bilirubin levels overlap) is on the basis of the response to administration of phenobarbital (an inducer of microsomal glucuronyl transferase): In type II patients a significant decrease in the serum bilirubin is seen; type I patients have no response.

Patients with Crigler-Najjar syndrome should be treated with aggressive phototherapy during infancy to prevent kernicterus. As the child ages, the weight–to–body surface area ratio decreases and the skin thickens, making phototherapy less effective. Phenobarbital should be used to induce hepatic microsomal glucuronyl transferase in patients with type II disease; however, it is ineffective in type I disease. Exchange transfusion or plasmapheresis may be helpful in the acute case of severe hyperbilirubinemia with neurologic dysfunction. Older patients in this category should be considered for liver transplant. Tin protoporphyrin (a drug that is not yet FDA-approved) is a selective inhibitor of heme oxygenase and in a limited study has been shown to be a safe and effective method of decreasing serum bilirubin levels in neonates with hemolytic anemia. Similarly, since this drug is also effective in Gunn rats (the animal model of type I Crigler-Najjar syndrome), it may offer, in the future, a long-term medical therapy for this disorder. Clinical trials of this drug in children with Crigler-Najjar syndrome should be under way shortly.

PHOTOTHERAPY AND/OR EXCHANGE TRANSFUSION

Appropriate management of the neonate with hyperbilirubinemia is hampered by the fact that the level of toxicity has not been well defined and by the fact that the measurement of serum bilirubin values varies considerably among laboratories. Kernicterus has been reported to occur in sick premature neonates at very low levels of serum bilirubin, even levels lower than the usual recommended values for phototherapy. Therefore, aggressive management of hyperbilirubinemia in the sick neonate often dictates treatment at levels less than recommended by the majority of the literature. Generally, any infant weighing less than 1500 gm should have phototherapy instituted during the first 24 hours of life, regardless of initial serum bilirubin values. Between 1500 and 1999 gm, phototherapy should be started at values of 10 mg/dl. Infants greater than 2000 gm receive phototherapy with serum bilirubin levels above 12 mg/dl. Hemolytic disease or any systemic illness (e.g., sepsis, hypoxia, acidosis) is an indication for phototherapy at lower levels.

Exchange transfusion is indicated when (1) phototherapy is not effective in diminishing serum bilirubin levels, or (2) an infant has early signs of kernicterus, or (3) an infant greater than 2500 gm has a serum bilirubin level greater than 20 mg/dl (neonates with birth weights between 1000 and 2500 gm require exchange transfusion with serum bilirubin levels between 10 and 18 mg/dl).

GILBERT'S SYNDROME

Unconjugated hyperbilirubinemia occurring after the neonatal period is associated with a common disorder (prevalence of 2 to 6 per cent of the population) known as Gilbert's syndrome. Bilirubin levels in this disorder are often elevated to levels of 2 to 8 mg/dl. Serum bilirubin levels may vary in a given individual from normal to 8 mg/dl, although values of 2 to 3 mg/dl are most common. Although this disorder is classically a nonhemolytic form of jaundice, many patients have a subtle form of hemolysis characterized by decreased red cell survival and mild reticulocytosis. Hepatic glucuronyl transferase levels are reduced in this syndrome, and, as a result, an increased proportion of bilirubin monoglucuronide is present in bile. Since older children and adults with this common disorder have a blood-brain barrier that is not permeable to bilirubin, toxic damage to the CNS does not occur. However, because any form of jaundice can be very distressing, reassurance to the patient and parents is necessary after appropriate diagnostic tests have excluded other forms of jaundice. Patients with Gilbert's syndrome should be informed that during times of stress, fasting, or viral illnesses, jaundice may increase to noticeable levels.

CIRRHOSIS

HASSAN HESHAM A-KADER, M.D.,
and WILLIAM F. BALISTRERI, M.D.

Cirrhosis is an irreversible end stage of many forms of liver injury. Having established the diagnosis and confirmed the etiology, it may be possible in some cases to minimize liver damage by treating the cause. Galactosemia, fructosemia, cystic fibrosis, Wilson's disease, obstruction due to choledochal cyst, and total parenteral alimentation–associated hepatobiliary injury are examples of conditions potentially amenable to medical or surgical therapy if detected early. However, in many patients the challenge is to deal with the long-term consequences such as undernutrition and the complications of portal hypertension (ascites, bleeding, and hepatic encephalopathy). The aim of treatment is to reduce discomfort, allow maximum growth, and control complications in anticipation of liver transplantation.

NUTRITION

The nutritional status of the patient with chronic liver disease should be precisely evaluated. In the absence of liver failure, a protein-rich (1.5 to 2 gm/kg/day), low-fat, high-carbohydrate diet is advised. Steatorrhea improves with the use of dietary formula or supplements containing medium-chain triglycerides. Supplementation of fat-soluble vitamins should include vitamin K (2 to 5 mg) every other day, vitamin D_2 (5000 to 8000 IU/day), vitamin E (50 to 400 IU/day as oral alpha-tocopherol), and vitamin A (10,000 to 15,000 IU/day as Aquasol A). Carefully monitoring for sufficiency (or toxicity) allows for adjustment of the dosage. Water-soluble vitamins should be given at twice the daily recommended allowances. Low serum iron levels may be seen and should be treated. Finally, the balance of calcium, phosphorus, potassium, or magnesium may be altered and supplementation may be necessary.

ASCITES

Initially we recommend sodium restriction to 1 to 2 mEq/kg/day. If this maneuver is insufficient, spironolactone (2 to 3 mg/kg/day) is used. Urinary electrolytes are monitored and if the ratio of sodium to potassium does not increase, the dose may be increased up to 10 to 12 mg/kg/day. If the ascites is still uncontrollable, additional diuretics such as thiazide (10 to 30 mg/kg/day) or furosemide (1 to 2 mg/kg every other day to twice daily) may be helpful. Use of diuretics requires repeated measurement of serum and urine electrolytes, serum urea, and creatinine. Large-volume paracentesis followed by albumin infusion may be useful in patients with tense ascites.

GASTROINTESTINAL HEMORRHAGE

Lavage to the stomach should be done when the patient with chronic liver disease and portal hypertension presents with hematemesis or melena. The presence of varices and the site of bleeding should be confirmed. If blood volume is contracted, replacement should be given continuously to avoid overtransfusion. If bleeding continues, vasopressin (0.3 U/kg, maximum 20 U, diluted in 2 ml/kg 5 per cent dextrose) should be administered over 20 minutes followed by 0.3 U/1.73 m^2/min for 12 to 24 hours, then tapered. If the above measures fail, the use of a pediatric Sengstaken-Blakemore tube should be considered. Sclerotherapy seems to be an effective palliative measure that will "buy time" while awaiting definitive therapy. The procedure, which is best done when there is no bleeding, should be repeated at 1- to 4-week intervals. Shunting procedures are difficult and risky and render eventual transplantation more difficult.

ENCEPHALOPATHY

Hepatic encephalopathy is a frequent complication seen in patients with cirrhosis. It may be precipitated by electrolyte imbalance, especially hypokalemia and metabolic alkalosis, gastrointestinal hemorrhage, infection, and the use of drugs such as diuretics or sedatives. Therapy should focus on removal of precipitating factors and reducing ammonia production and absorption. Hypokalemia and metabolic alkalosis should be corrected. Measures to stop bleeding and to remove blood by aspiration and enema will reduce ammonia production. Any infection must be treated, and the drugs mentioned above should be discontinued if possible.

Measures to reduce ammonia production also include protein restriction and oral neomycin in a dosage of 100 mg/kg/day. Lactulose, a nonabsorbable synthetic disaccharide, is our preferred alternative to neomycin. It produces lactic and acetic acids, leading to a drop in pH in the colon and thereby reducing ammonia reabsorption.

Exchange transfusion, hemodialysis, peritoneal dialysis, and plasmapheresis for coagulopathy have been utilized but have not yet been proven to be therapeutically effective. Extracorporeal artificial support may offer hope in the future. Patients failing to respond to the above measures are candidates for liver transplantation.

SPONTANEOUS BACTERIAL PERITONITIS

Spontaneous bacterial peritonitis may occur in patients in whom cirrhosis is complicated by ascites. Symptoms and signs include fever, lethargy, poor feeding, vomiting, diarrhea, diffuse abdominal pain, abdominal distention and rigidity, and diffuse rebound tenderness. However, in up to 15 per cent of patients the condition may be symptomless. Diagnostic paracentesis is indicated in all suspected cases. Antibiotic therapy should be initiated in all patients with polymorphonuclear leukocytes of more than 500 cells/mm^3 of peritoneal fluid and in any patient with signs of peritonitis and polymorphonuclear leukocytes of more than 250 cells/mm^3. Before sensitivity is known, ampicillin and gentamicin should be started. Decreased ascitic fluid pH and increased lactate may help in establishing the diagnosis; however, awareness of the condition remains the key to diagnosis.

LIVER TRANSPLANTATION

Unfortunately in many patients with chronic liver disease and in hepatic failure orthotopic liver transplantation may be the only remaining consideration. Clinical and biochemical indications for liver transplantation include bilirubin greater than 10 to 15 mg/dl, albumin less than 2.5 gm/dl, hepatic encephalopathy, prothrombin time greater than 5 seconds above control, hepatorenal syndrome, recurrent episodes of cholangitis, spontaneous bacterial peritonitis or septicemia, intractable ascites, and the development of focal hepatocellular carcinoma. The requirement for a size-matched donor liver has contributed to the difficulty in obtaining organs for pediatric recipients. However, the use of segmental transplantation has increased the proportion of candidates transplanted and reduced the overall mortality.

TUMORS OF THE LIVER

SHUNZABURO IWATSUKI, M.D.,
and THOMAS E. STARZL, M.D., Ph.D.

Increasing numbers of hepatic mass lesions are found incidentally by advanced imaging technology. Although most of these "incidental" tumors are histologically benign and do not require any therapy, they must be thoroughly investigated. Modern imaging technology is quite efficient in detecting small lesions but is not effective in producing pathognomonic findings of many hepatic lesions other than hemangiomas and cysts. Percutaneous needle biopsy often fails to establish a definitive diagnosis because of its limited sampling, and it can cause serious hemorrhage when unwisely performed for vascular lesions.

Major hepatic resections can now be performed with minimum operative risk (less than 5 per cent), but no surgeon should explore a hepatic mass without having the competence to perform all of the major resections, including a right and left trisegmentectomy.

BENIGN TUMORS

Most of the benign tumors of the liver are asymptomatic and are found incidentally during studies for other disorders or during abdominal operations. The general approach to a small incidental tumor (less than 3 cm in diameter) that is considered benign is close observation after "thorough" investigation. When the tumor changes its imaging characteristics or increases in size during close observation, it must be immediately excised. Larger incidental tumors, other than asymptomatic cavernous hemangiomas, deserve excisional therapy unless unequivocal benignity is confirmed.

Hemangiomas are the most common benign tumors of the liver. Giant cavernous hemangiomas should be treated by surgical excision, particularly when they are symptomatic (e.g., pain, mass-related complaints) or they are found to have a necrotic center inside. The majority of giant cavernous hemangiomas require lobectomies or trisegmentectomies of the liver, but some located on the surface of the liver or pedunculated can be enucleated along pseudocapsular margins without significant loss of normal liver tissue. Ligation or embolization of the feeding hepatic artery and radiation therapy may be hazardous and do not have longstanding effects on the course of giant cavernous hemangiomas.

Infantile hemangioendotheliomas are most often seen in infants during the first 6 months of life and are distinct from cavernous hemangiomas. The lesions should be excised by anatomic hepatic resection whenever possible. Treatment with prednisone, diuretics, and digoxin can be used initially when the patient's condition prohibits surgery or the lesion is too extensive for resection. Response to prednisone may allow surgery to be performed safely in a few weeks. In extensive lesions, radiation to the liver may be used after pathologic diagnosis is confirmed. Favorable responses to steroids, radiation, and hepatic artery ligation or embolization have been reported. The treatment should be vigorous, because complete regression and cure are possible.

Other benign tumors include liver cell adenoma, focal nodular hyperplasia, hematoma, mesenchymoma, teratoma, and fibroma. Radiologic differentiation of these benign tumors from malignant tumors is unreliable. Pathologic confirmation of benign tumors is mandatory for each lesion. Large benign tumors should be treated by surgical excision, particularly when they are symptomatic. Adenoma has a tendency to rupture and cause life-threatening hemorrhage. Some adenomas cannot be easily differentiated from low-grade hepatocellular carcinoma by needle biopsies. If the diagnosis is uncertain, the lesion should be excised with an adequate margin without delay.

Congenital hepatic cysts are usually asymptomatic and do not require any therapy. Although aspiration, internal drainage, marsupialization, fenestration, and sclerotherapy have all been recommended for symptomatic congenital cysts, these approaches are no longer justifiable for the treatment of single or localized multiple cysts because hepatic resections can be performed quite safely now.

MALIGNANT TUMORS

The most common primary malignant tumor of the liver in children is hepatoblastoma. Hepatocellular car-

cinoma is the second most common and usually occurs in older children. Sarcomas of the liver, such as rhabdomyosarcoma and angiosarcoma, are rare. None of these has a favorable outlook, but fibrolamellar hepatocellular carcinoma, which is common in older children and young adults, has a better prognosis than other types of malignancy.

The treatment for all malignant liver tumors is complete surgical excision by anatomic hepatic resection. Hepatic resections of more than the right or left lobe of the liver can be performed quite safely. For example, a large tumor occupying the right lobe of the liver and the medial segment of the left lobe can be resected by right hepatic trisegmentectomy, leaving only the left lateral segment of the left lobe (to the left of the falciform ligament), or a large tumor occupying the left lobe and the anterior segment of the right lobe can be resected by left hepatic trisegmentectomy, leaving only the posterior segment of the right lobe (posterior to the right hepatic vein). These major hepatic resections can now be performed by experienced surgeons with less than a 5 per cent operative mortality.

We have found that computed tomography scan or magnetic resonance imaging is most useful in assessing the extent of the tumor, but it can be misleading, particularly when a large tumor distorts normal anatomic boundaries. If the resectability is uncertain after extensive preoperative investigation, the patient should be referred to a surgeon who is experienced in major hepatic resection rather than undergo exploratory celiotomy by someone who is unprepared to undertake a definitive procedure.

After curative hepatic resection, we usually recommend that patients receive adjuvant chemotherapy for at least 1 year. We have been using combination chemotherapy with doxorubicin, dactinomycin, vincristine, and cyclophosphamide, and often mitomycin or cisplatin. The value of this approach has not been validated in randomized trials, but the patients who have received adjuvant chemotherapy after curative resections of large tumors have seemed to have longer tumor-free survival.

In general, liver transplantation (total hepatectomy and liver replacement) cannot offer good long-term results when applied to large malignant tumors that cannot be removed by subtotal hepatectomy. However, liver transplantation can result in a cure (more than 5-year survival) on more than isolated occasions. The most favorable lesions for transplantation, just as with resection, are the fibrolamellar hepatoma and epithelioid hemangioendothelial sarcoma. On the other hand, most of the patients who have received liver transplantation for other end-stage liver diseases, such as tyrosinemia and alpha$_1$-antitrypsin deficiency disease, and whose malignant tumors were small and incidental, survived tumor-free for several years.

The most common metastatic liver tumors in children are neuroblastoma and Wilms' tumor. Although chemotherapy and radiation therapy may be helpful in treating these metastatic tumors, the lesion should be excised whenever possible, particularly if it is localized to part of the liver. Hepatic resections for metastatic tumors are much safer than those for primary malignancy.

PORTAL HYPERTENSION

SHEILA SHERLOCK, D.B.E., M.D.

Portal hypertension is nearly always due to obstruction to blood flow in the portal venous system. It can be divided into two main categories: presinusoidal, and sinusoidal or postsinusoidal. It is important to make the distinction. In the presinusoidal type of portal hypertension, hepatocellular function is intact, whereas in the second form it is defective, and liver cell failure is liable to be precipitated by hemorrhage. Treatment depends upon accurate localization of the site of obstruction and, if possible, knowledge of the cause.

Management Before and Between Hemorrhages. Apart from any treatment necessary for underlying cirrhosis, the child should be allowed to lead as normal a life as possible and attend ordinary school. Provided the spleen is not too large, games and physical education may be allowed. Particularly vigorous sports, such as football, must be forbidden. The child should not be allowed to become overly tired. The school principal should be informed of the situation, and the parents should not press the child to be too competitive in either work or play.

Note should be taken of fecal color and the parents told to report if it becomes black. Hemoglobin estimations should be done if the child appears anemic or passes black stools. Oral iron treatment is given as required. The cirrhotic child requires occasional estimations of the prothrombin time, and intramuscular vitamin K_1 (5 mg) may be useful from time to time.

Hemorrhage commonly follows an upper respiratory tract infection, and this should be avoided if possible and all necessary inoculations given. If infection develops, it should be taken seriously and broad-spectrum antibiotics given from the start. Drugs containing acetylsalicylic acid must be avoided. Cimetidine is given at the first indication of bleeding.

Undue attention should not be paid to the platelet and leukocyte counts. Although both may be low, the effects on the patient are not definite. Multiple infections are unusual. Low values should not indicate splenectomy.

Management of Hemorrhage. Endoscopy should be done, using a pediatric endoscope. Patency of the portal vein is assessed by ultrasound or CT. Later, selective splanchnic angiography may be necessary.

If the patient is cirrhotic, hepatic precoma and coma may be precipitated by the hemorrhage. This should be anticipated by giving no protein by mouth, keeping the bowels moving freely, giving an enema if necessary, and prescribing oral neomycin, 15 mg/kg four times a day for 3 days. All types of sedation should be avoided. If the child has extrahepatic portal venous obstruction and normal hepatic function, there is virtually no danger of the development of hepatic precoma. The pre-

coma regimen is therefore unnecessary, and sedation can be given as required. It is unusual for these patients to bleed before the age of 4.

Blood transfusion is usually necessary. In patients with extrahepatic portal obstruction, hemorrhages are likely to be multiple over years. The greatest possible care must be taken to preserve peripheral veins for further transfusions and to give absolutely compatible blood.

If liver cell function is adequate, the bleeding usually ceases spontaneously. If liver cell function is deficient and if the bleeding continues, I prefer to use vasopressin* (Pitressin) intravenously, although this route is not recommended by the manufacturer. This drug lowers portal venous pressure by constriction of the splanchnic arterial bed, causing an increase in resistance to the inflow of blood to the gut. It controls hemorrhage from esophageal varices by lowering portal venous pressure. A large dose, 1 unit per 3 kg of body weight, is given well diluted in 5 per cent dextrose intravenously in 10 minutes. Mean arterial pressure increases transiently, and portal pressure decreases for 45 minutes to 1 hour. Control of hemorrhage is shown by the disappearance of blood from gastric aspirates and by serial pulse and blood pressure readings. Abdominal colicky discomfort and evacuation of the bowels, together with facial pallor, are usual during the infusion. If these are absent, it may be questioned whether the vasopressin is pharmacologically active. Inert material is the most common cause of failure. Regular vasopressin injections may be repeated in 4 hours if bleeding recurs, but efficacy decreases with continual use. The ultimate failure of vasopressin to control terminal hemorrhage reflects hepatocellular failure rather than improper method of treatment.

The value of vasopressin is its simplicity of use. In an emergency it can even be used in the home. The short duration is obviously unsatisfactory, and the side effects are unpleasant even if short-lived. However, this dosage is necessary to achieve an adequate reduction in portal pressure.

If vasopressin fails to produce the desired effect, the Sengstaken trilumen esophageal compression tube is used. A special small-sized tube is available for pediatric use. A rubber tube is inflated in the esophagus at a pressure of 20 to 30 mm Hg, slightly greater than that expected in the portal vein. Another balloon is inflated in the fundus of the stomach. The third lumen communicates with the stomach. The tube is passed relatively easily if the pharynx is well anesthetized. When the tube is in position, traction has to be exerted, and this causes difficulty. Too little traction means that the gastric balloon falls back into the stomach. Too much traction causes discomfort, with retching, and potentiates gastroesophageal ulceration.

The compression tubes are very successful in controlling bleeding from esophageal varices. They do, however, have many complications. They should not be left inflated longer than 24 hours. Their use should be

---

*This use of vasopressin is not listed in the manufacturer's directive; 1 unit/3 kg may exceed manufacturer's recommended dosage.

part of a plan of management culminating in either sclerotherapy or surgery. Complications include obstruction of the pharynx with consequent asphyxia, aspiration pneumonia, and ulceration of the pharynx, esophagus, and fundus of the stomach. The tube is not well tolerated by the patient. Skilled nursing is required while the tube is in position.

Emergency endoscopic sclerotherapy may be used after the acute bleeding is controlled. It is usually successful in stopping the hemorrhage but complications are frequent, especially with inexperienced endoscopists. Emergency surgery is rarely necessary. If bleeding does not cease or if it recurs and active intervention becomes essential, the best surgical method is probably esophageal transection. In patients having normal liver function and in whom the splenic venogram or mesenteric angiogram has shown a portal or superior mesenteric vein of adequate caliber, a portacaval or mesocaval shunt may be performed. Emergency shunt surgery has a high mortality rate if the patient has cirrhosis and, if possible, should be avoided in this circumstance. Esophageal transection using the staple gun is occasionally necessary in children with extrahepatic portal vein destruction and exsanguinating bleeding.

Elective Surgery. Prophylactic surgery is not indicated. The patient must have bled from varices before operation can be considered. The choice of procedure depends largely upon the state of the portal venous system as revealed by selective splanchnic angiography. If the portal vein is patent and of adequate caliber, end-to-side portacaval anastomosis is the most satisfactory procedure. In experienced hands this operation carries a low mortality rate (less than 5 per cent). Because of vein size, the operation can rarely be undertaken before the age of 10 years. It carries a small risk of shunt encephalopathy. In children this is particularly small, and in the presence of a normal liver, e.g., obstruction to the portal vein at the hilus of the liver, the risk of encephalopathy is almost nonexistent. In the presence of cirrhosis, the possibility varies with the degree of underlying damage to the liver. The operation should not be performed in the presence of jaundice, ascites, or a past history of hepatic coma. Portacaval shunting renders a subsequent liver transplantation more difficult.

Splenorenal anastomosis may be considered in portal venous occlusion if the splenic vein is of adequate size. It is less efficient than a portacaval anastomosis, because the shunt is small and often occludes. The danger of post-shunt encephalopathy, however, is very small.

Superior mesenteric vein–inferior vena caval shunt is used to treat portal hypertension in patients who have occlusion of the portal and splenic veins, making neither available for anastomosis. The vena cava is transected just proximal to the junction of the two iliac veins, and the distal segment is ligated. The proximal segment is then anastomosed to the side of the intact superior mesenteric vein. Sometimes an intervening graft is used. The selective Warren splenorenal shunt may be particularly useful with predominant gastric varices. Failures may be due to superior mesenteric vein thrombosis, and the mortality rate is about 10 per cent.

Direct attacks on the varices and on various dangerous collaterals are numerous and rarely of lasting benefit. They include splenectomy, transection of the esophagus, partial and total gastrectomy, and partial esophagectomy. In general, they are not recommended. Patients with extrahepatic portal venous obstruction rarely die of exsanguinating hemorrhage. Conservative management usually helps them over the acute episode. Bleeding becomes more infrequent as time allows for the opening of collateral vessels to the renal and lumbar veins. Ultimately, portal pressure may decrease. This possibility may be lessened with repeated operations and removal or transection of such benign collaterals. The operative and postoperative mortality rates of the local operations on varices in a cirrhotic patient with borderline liver function are high, and the ultimate benefit doubtful.

Repeated endoscopic sclerotherapy may be used to obliterate esophageal varices. Three or four sessions at 1- to 3-week intervals are usually necessary. Unfortunately, the esophageal varices recur. Gastric fundal varices are not treated and may increase in size (portal gastropathy).

CHRONIC ACTIVE HEPATITIS
JOSEPH F. FITZGERALD, M.D.

Chronic active hepatitis, also referred to as chronic aggressive hepatitis and active chronic hepatitis, is a continuing inflammatory hepatopathy with the potential to progress to severe irreversible disease (cirrhosis) and death. The goal of therapy is to interrupt the progression to end-stage liver disease.

Initial therapy consists of prednisone alone or prednisone and azathioprine. I prescribe prednisone alone in a dosage of 2 mg/kg/day (up to 60 mg). It is provided as a single morning dose. Remission is defined as a resolution of symptoms with a reduction in the aminotransferase levels (AST/SGOT and ALT/SGPT) to less than 2.5-fold elevation. An alternate-day treatment program (i.e., 2 mg/kg on alternate days) can be instituted when clinical and biochemical remission is attained in order to reduce unwanted steroid side effects. This can often be accomplished after 4 to 6 weeks of therapy. The prednisone can then be reduced in 5-mg decrements every 4 weeks. Clinical and/or biochemical relapse dictates a return to a daily steroid program. An alternate-day program may be reinstituted after tapering of the daily dose has been successful. A typical course of therapy is 15 to 18 months. Hepatic histology is examined early to confirm remission, and 4 to 6 weeks after therapy is discontinued.

Azathioprine is not routinely prescribed but is added when clinical and biochemical remission is not achieved with prednisone alone, or when frequent relapses prevent reduction of the steroid dosage. A single daily dose of 1.0 to 1.5 mg/kg is administered. The CBC and platelet count must be monitored closely in the early therapeutic course. The azathioprine is discontinued when the prednisone is tapered to 5 mg on alternate days.

There is no clear consensus to guide the management of children and adolescents with HBV-associated chronic active hepatitis. Experimental antiviral therapy, aimed at suppression or reduction of hepatitis B virus replication, has severely limited availability. It seems plausible that therapy aimed at suppression of the non–T-lymphocyte response to the virus (as outlined above) may have a place in the management of HBV-associated chronic active liver disease, since this virus is *not* cytopathic. Current opinion, however, embraces the view that immunosuppressive therapy is ineffective in the management of HBV-associated chronic active hepatitis. This matter may not be settled.

DISORDERS OF THE HEPATOBILIARY TREE

ERIC S. MALLER, M.D.,
and W. ALLAN WALKER, M.D.

BILIARY ATRESIA

Extrahepatic biliary atresia is the cause of about one third of all cases of neonatal cholestatic jaundice, having an incidence of approximately 1 in 10,000 to 15,000 live births in the Western world. In 10 per cent of cases, the atresia is of the correctable type, with the patient having either a distal atresia with patent proximal hepatic ducts or cystic dilatation of the ducts at the porta hepatis. In these circumstances, correction is achieved by anastomosis of patent proximal extrahepatic duct remnants or the gallbladder to a Roux-en-Y jejunal loop. In the more common noncorrectable forms of atresia, there are no patent extrahepatic ducts, and the gallbladder is usually absent or only a small remnant. In these lesions, correction is attempted by hepatoportoenterostomy (Kasai procedure), again using a Roux-en-Y jejunal limb brought up and attached to the porta hepatis after dissection and excision of the fibrous extrahepatic biliary tree remnants.

Success rates for this procedure in re-establishing bile flow and clearing jaundice are variable depending upon the series but are reported in Japanese series as high as 70 to 80 per cent. In these patients, a 90 per cent chance of survival with reasonable quality of life to age 10 years is reported if the infant is operated on before 8 weeks of age. Success rates fall to 20 per cent or less if surgery is delayed beyond 3 months of age, probably owing to progression of intrahepatic disease. With the advent of orthotopic liver transplantation as a therapeutic option even in the young infant, some surgeons now advocate forgoing a Kasai procedure altogether in the patient diagnosed late (beyond 3 to 6 months of age) with biliary atresia. This is because the small chance of success at such a late age plus the difficulty and risks of reoperation in the right upper quadrant at a later time for transplantation may make liver transplantation the preferred primary therapy for the patient in these

special circumstances. The untreated infant with atresia, however, faces a dismal mean survival of 11 months without transplantation.

Postoperative cholangitis is a major risk after portoenterostomy and, although often recurrent, even a single episode may contribute to a subsequent poor outcome in a patient who initially appeared to have a good surgical result with clearing of jaundice. The onset of cholangitis may be heralded by fever, leukocytosis with increased band count, and increase in sedimentation rate above the patient's baseline value. The patient may also demonstrate right upper quadrant tenderness, worsening liver function, and decreased bile flow with increasing serum bilirubin and clinical jaundice. However, any or all of these signs, symptoms, and laboratory assessments may be absent, normal, or unchanged from baseline in the post-Kasai infant. Therefore, fever alone, without an obvious source, merits prompt and thorough investigation. Given the significant and sometimes irreversible clinical deterioration experienced by some patients after an episode of cholangitis, some clinicians recommend admission to the hospital for all such post-Kasai patients with fever.

If preliminary investigations fail to reveal a source for the fever, a percutaneous liver biopsy may need to be performed for culture and sensitivity testing and for histologic examination in an attempt to diagnose active, acute cholangitis and isolate a pathogen with specific antibiotic sensitivities to thus guide appropriate therapy. Peripheral blood cultures alone are often inadequate for isolation of a specific pathogen.

In the absence of a specific bacterial isolate from liver or blood culture, broad-spectrum combination treatment with an aminoglycoside and cephalosporin as initial therapy takes advantage of these drugs' relatively good penetration into bile. In our experience, use of gentamicin or tobramycin at 6 to 7.5 mg/kg/day in three divided doses with monitoring of serum levels and cephalothin or cefoxitin when broader coverage of anaerobic pathogens is desired, continued for 10 to 14 days, is adequate therapy in the majority of circumstances.

Fortunately, the incidence of cholangitis appears to decrease markedly by the end of the first year of life. However, until then, many physicians advocate the use of oral suppressive antibiotic therapy as prophylaxis against recurrent cholangitis, using trimethoprim-sulfamethoxazole (10 mg/kg/day of trimethoprim in two divided doses) or another appropriate oral antibiotic such as amoxicillin (40 mg/kg/day in three divided doses) or cefaclor (40 mg/kg/day in three or four divided doses). Cholangitis developing after the first year of life may indicate obstruction of the draining jejunal limb or development of large intrahepatic bile lakes with secondary infection or abscess formation and may require surgical treatment or percutaneous aspiration for drainage of infected intrahepatic fluid collections.

Nutritional therapy in the post-Kasai patient or the patient with chronic cholestasis of any cause is aimed at preventing or ameliorating the sequelae of lipid malabsorption due to decreased intraluminal concentrations of bile salts in the intestine. The use of infant formulas such as Portagen or Pregestemil (the latter having a higher percentage of essential fatty acids) that have a high percentage of their fat content as medium-chain triglycerides, which do not require micellar solubilization by bile salts, aids in providing more usable calories for weight gain and growth while still providing adequate amounts of essential long-chain fats. In the older child a high-protein, low-fat diet is preferred, with medium-chain triglyceride oil supplementation as needed.

Prevention of fat-soluble vitamin deficiencies is achieved by oral supplementation with monitoring of levels to avoid toxicity. Vitamin A as Aquasol A should be given in a dosage of 10,000 to 25,000 IU/day. Vitamin D is administered as ergocalciferol (vitamin D_2) in a dosage of 5000 to 8000 IU/day or 3 to 5 µg/kg/day of 25-hydroxycholecalciferol, especially in the patient with signs of established rickets. Vitamin E is supplemented as oral alpha-tocopherol as either the acetate or succinate ester in dosages of 50 to 400 IU/day to start. In the not uncommon event that adequate levels of vitamin E cannot be achieved by oral supplementation even with high doses of vitamin E (150 IU/kg/day or greater), parenteral supplementation with intramuscular vitamin E may be necessary. A new and still experimental oral preparation of vitamin E, tocopherol polyethylene glycol 1000 succinate (TPGS), has shown great promise in achieving adequate vitamin E levels in patients with chronic cholestasis and reversing some of the sequelae of chronic vitamin E deficiency in a small cohort study group without the pain and inconvenience of intramuscular therapy. Finally, vitamin K is given orally in dosages of 2.5 to 5 mg/day but may need to be given intramuscularly if there is clinical bleeding or the prothrombin time remains significantly elevated, placing the patient at high risk for future bleeding.

Water-soluble vitamin supplementation is also necessary and should be given at twice the recommended daily dosage. Patients are also at risk for mineral deficiencies with chronic cholestasis, particularly calcium deficiency, which is exacerbated by the steatorrhea. While monitoring levels, calcium intake should provide at least 50 to 200 mg/kg/day of elemental calcium as well as 25 to 50 mg/kg/day of elemental phosphorus. Zinc deficiency may be avoided by appropriate supplementation at 10 mg/day if needed. Finally, in the presence of ascites, dietary intake of salt may need to be restricted to prevent excess fluid retention.

Pruritus and xanthomas are particularly troublesome complications of chronic cholestasis. No truly satisfactory therapy exists for the severe, intractable pruritus that may occur in chronic cholestatic liver disease. Simple measures such as skin lubricants, topical corticosteroid or emollient creams, and trimming nails and covering hands are often inadequate. Some of the pharmacologic measures tried include phenobarbital (5 to 10 mg/kg/day), lipid-binding resins such as cholestyramine or cholestipol (0.5 gm/kg/day), and antihistamines such as diphenhydramine (5 mg/kg/day) or hydroxyzine (2 mg/kg/day). Some centers have used carbamazepine (Tegretol) at doses of 20 mg/kg/day as well. Others have resorted to ultraviolet irradiation (UVB) of the skin, plasmapheresis, and even partial biliary diversion by externalized stoma to treat intractable pruritus. Ursodeoxycholic acid, currently approved in the United States only for dissolution of cholesterol gallstones in adults, is a polar bile salt that may have a role in improving bile flow and aiding in the clearance or dilution of toxic bile salts and thus ameliorating pruritus and other complications of chronic cholestatic liver disease.

Portal hypertension and its sequelae, including hypersplenism, ascites, and bleeding from esophageal varices, often accompany chronic, progressive liver disease and cirrhosis. Bleeding varices are treated medically with intravenous vasopressin (Pitressin) in a dosage of 5 to 10 mU/kg/min up to a maximum of 0.4 U/min in 5 per cent dextrose. Complications include systemic hypertension and fluid overload. If this treatment is unsuccessful, the Sengstaken-Blakemore tube may be used with inflation only of the gastric balloon and never for more than 24 hours, with periodic deflation every 6 hours or so to prevent pressure necrosis. Chest radiography should always be done to confirm accurate placement of the tube. Endoscopic variceal sclerosis with various agents now has been used successfully and routinely to control acute variceal bleeding or to prevent recurrent bleeding after the patient has stabilized after an initial bleeding episode. No role currently exists for prophylactic sclerotherapy in children or adults with varices who have not had an initial bleeding episode. Conflicting evidence exists (all in adult studies) regarding the use of beta-adrenergic blocking agents such as propranolol for prevention of a first or subsequent variceal hemorrhage in patients with known varices. When used, a titrated dose is recommended to achieve a 20 to 25 per cent reduction in resting heart rate. Portosystemic shunting procedures in infants and young children are often technically difficult, and long-term results in terms of shunt patency are not promising. The shunts may also interfere with later attempts at liver transplantation and thus should be avoided unless acute intractable bleeding threatens the patient's immediate survival.

As mentioned above, liver transplantation has now become an accepted and widely available treatment of chronic liver failure limited mainly by donor organ availability, especially in the young infant.

DISEASES OF THE GALLBLADDER

Cholecystitis and Cholelithiasis

Cholelithiasis in children is often but not exclusively a complication of chronic hemolytic disease. With the increased use of ultrasonography, there has been an increased incidence reported of gallstones or biliary sludge, often in asymptomatic patients. Many of these patients are young infants who have been receiving total parenteral nutrition and may also have had ileal resection, another predisposing factor to cholelithiasis. Other infants whose neonatal course was complicated by prematurity, sepsis, diuretic use, and/or chronic parenteral nutrition have also been found to have stones, most often pigment stones. There is controversy as to whether asymptomatic large stones found incidentally warrant removal and cholecystectomy, since many stones, especially those found in infants, may subsequently resolve on their own. Since the natural history of these asymptomatic stones in children is not clear, many advocate expectant management in the asymptomatic, healthy patient. Clearly, the child who develops acute cholecystitis should be treated with antibiotics and undergo cholecystectomy. In the patient with cholesterol stones less than 2 cm and with any contraindication to surgery, such as patients with cystic fibrosis, oral medical therapy designed to dissolve gallstones with chenodeoxycholic acid or, more recently, ursodeoxycholic acid may be an option. Data for use in young children are not available, and the recurrence rate may be as high as 50 per cent by 5 years.

Acute cholecystitis in the absence of stones is rare but has been described with typhus, typhoid fever, diphtheria, scarlet fever, shigellosis, viral infection of the gastrointestinal or respiratory tract, and infestation with *Giardia lamblia* or *Ascaris lumbricoides*. Malformations of the biliary tree, sphincter of Oddi spasm, and ectopic gastric mucosa in the gallbladder are also reported associated findings. Antibiotic therapy for 24 to 48 hours followed by elective cholecystectomy is the treatment of choice.

Hydrops of the Gallbladder

Hydrops of the gallbladder may be seen in a variety of infectious conditions, including upper respiratory infections, streptococcal disease, and *Pseudomonas* or *Salmonella* sepsis. It is also a relatively common associated finding in Kawasaki disease and leptospirosis. It may also occur in relatively well infants who are taking nothing by mouth, possibly owing to poor peristalsis and stasis, and often resolves spontaneously after reinstitution of oral feeding. If associated with infection or sepsis, aggressive therapy with antibiotics is essential. If the patient is not toxic and serial ultrasonography shows a decrease or no increase in gallbladder size, the patient can continue to be observed and treated medically. If, however, the size continues to increase, then perforation is a clear risk, and the patient should undergo cholecystectomy.

Choledochal Cysts

This is an uncommon, congenital biliary tract abnormality occurring in approximately 1 in 15,000 births and affecting females three to four times more often than males. The lesion may present in childhood as neonatal cholestasis but more commonly presents in later childhood with pain and variable jaundice. There are several variants ranging from a choledochocele at the ampulla of Vater to diffuse saccular dilatation of the common bile duct to the classic discrete cystic dilatation of a segment of the common bile duct. Complete excision of the cyst followed by choledocho–Roux-en-Y–jejunostomy is the preferred treatment. Simple aspiration of the cyst is unacceptable, as is choledochocystojejunostomy, as both involve an increased risk of cholangiocarcinoma in the retained cyst remnant of approximately 5 per cent. Untreated choledochal cysts

may result in cholangitis, stone formation, or biliary cirrhosis from chronic obstruction and secondary portal hypertension. In spite of adequate excision of the extrahepatic cyst, later complications may ensue from associated intrahepatic ductal abnormalities as well.

Caroli's Disease

Caroli's disease is a disorder characterized by congenital, communicating ectasia and focal cystic dilatation of the intrahepatic biliary tree. It may be seen alone or in association with congenital hepatic fibrosis or choledochal cysts. One-quarter of cases are associated with renal abnormalities, including cortical cysts and medullary sponge kidneys. Cystic disease of the pancreas is also reported. Recurrent episodes of cholangitis and stone formation due to stasis are common and require antibiotic treatment. In the rare instance of cystic abnormalities confined to one lobe or liver segment, hepatic lobectomy may be indicated.

Sclerosing Cholangitis

This disorder is most commonly seen in children in association with ulcerative colitis. However, recent reports describe its association in other disorders, including immunodeficiency syndromes and histiocytosis X. It may involve any or all areas of the intra- or extrahepatic biliary tree, causing strictures, stasis, and subsequent stone formation. The only available treatment is to relieve biliary obstruction by T-tube external drainage, cholecystoduodenostomy or jejunostomy, or strictureplasty of lesions in the extrahepatic biliary tree. Corticosteroids usually offer only temporary relief, if any. Colectomy in patients with ulcerative colitis does not alter this disease course, which progresses from recurring cholangitis and obstruction to biliary cirrhosis, portal hypertension, and an increased risk of hepatic carcinoma. Liver transplantation is now a viable and more frequently used alternative, but recurrent disease in the graft has been reported in some adults.

In children, the most common tumors of the biliary tree are benign papillomas, adenomas, or fibromas and are treated by simple excision. The most common malignant tumor is sarcoma of the botryoid type. Simple rhabdomyosarcoma and cholangiocarcinoma also occur but are rare, and, despite excision and radiotherapy, long-term survival is poor.

Traumatic hemobilia and avulsion of bile ducts with late biliary stricture may be complications of abdominal trauma or child-battering. Avulsion of the bile ducts is treated by surgical drainage and operative repair of the tear. Traumatic hemobilia, resulting from rupture of blood-filled intrahepatic pseudocysts into the biliary tree, is also treated by surgical drainage and pseudocyst excision.

Intrahepatic cholestatic syndromes range from benign recurrent cholestasis to disorders characterized by paucity or hypoplasia of interlobular bile ducts. Those patients with duct paucity in syndromic association with other anomalies such as vertebral arch defects, peripheral pulmonic stenosis, and other findings that characterize the syndrome of arteriohepatic dysplasia seem to have an improved prognosis over those patients with isolated intrahepatic bile duct paucity. Treatment is supportive for the associated cholestasis, as described above for biliary atresia, and liver transplantation is also an option for patients with progressive chronic liver failure.

PANCREATIC DISEASES
KENNETH L. COX, M.D.

ACUTE PANCREATITIS

The general principles of treatment of acute pancreatitis are (1) to treat hypovolemia and electrolyte abnormalities, (2) to relieve pain, (3) to reduce pancreatic secretions, and (4) to remove the precipitating cause.

Correction of hypovolemia should begin immediately, utilizing a large-bore central venous catheter for fluid replacement and to monitor central venous pressure. Hypotension and low central venous pressure should be corrected as rapidly as possible with plasma, dextran, albumin, or whole blood. Shock is the main cause of death in acute pancreatitis. Shock is primarily a result of exudation of plasma into the retroperitoneal space and peripheral vasodilatation caused by increased kinin activity.

After hypovolemia has been corrected, the rate of intravenous infusions should be reduced so as to provide maintenance plus replacement of ongoing losses from nasogastric suctioning and exudation into the peritoneal and retroperitoneal spaces. Monitoring urine output and central venous pressure is a mechanism for assessing the adequacy of the fluid replacement. Major complications of treatment of severe acute pancreatitis are pulmonary edema and congestive heart failure; these usually occur 3 to 7 days after the onset of pancreatitis. Although in many cases the cause is unknown, in some cases fluid overload has occurred because of excessive fluid replacement. Thus, the amount of fluid replacement must be adjusted frequently for changes in intravascular volume.

Serum electrolytes, including calcium and magnesium, serum creatinine, and blood urea nitrogen determinations, will aid in selecting the appropriate electrolyte composition of intravenous solutions. Since between 2 and 17 per cent of patients with acute pancreatitis have renal failure, potassium should not be added to intravenous solutions until stable urine output has been established. In addition to maintenance sodium chloride and potassium chloride of 3 mEq/kg/24 hr and 2 mEq/kg/24 hr, respectively, losses from nasogastric suctioning should be replaced. Although 5 per cent dextrose solutions should be initiated, hyperglycemia and hypoglycemia occasionally seen in severe pancreatitis warrant careful monitoring of urinary reducing substances and blood glucose concentrations and changing the concentration of dextrose in the intravenous solution appropriately. Symptomatic hypocalcemia, i.e., tetany and seizures, should be treated with intravenous calcium gluconate, 0.1 to 0.2 gm/kg/dose (not over 2

gm) as a 10 per cent solution administered slowly and stopped for bradycardia. For asymptomatic hypocalcemia, replacement may be accomplished by adding 10 ml or more of 10 per cent calcium gluconate to each 500 ml of intravenous solution. In severe pancreatitis, serum electrolytes, including calcium, should be measured at least daily so that adjustments in the electrolyte composition of intravenous solutions can be made if necessary.

Pancreatic exocrine secretions are reduced by fasting the patient. Usually feeding should not be reinstituted until abdominal pain and ileus have resolved and serum amylase, urinary diastase, and the amylase-creatinine clearance ratio have returned to normal. If oral alimentation cannot be taken within 5 days, then parenteral nutrition should be given. Since carbohydrate is less of a stimulant to pancreatic exocrine secretion than are protein and fat, the initial diet should consist of carbohydrates only. If the carbohydrate diet is tolerated without worsening or exacerbating symptoms, then a low-fat and protein diet may be given. Again, the diet should be discontinued if symptoms should recur.

Nasogastric suctioning should be used to relieve nausea, vomiting, and abdominal pain. Since there is no evidence that gastric suctioning alters the clinical course of pancreatitis, it is not required in the treatment of mild-to-moderate pancreatitis. However, in severe pancreatitis or marked ileus, nasogastric suctioning should be used.

Relief of the severe abdominal pain associated with pancreatitis not only is important for patient comfort but also may reduce the cephalic phase of pancreatic secretion. Morphine sulfate should be avoided because it may worsen pancreatitis by causing sphincter of Oddi spasm. Meperidine hydrochloride (Demerol) may be administered IV or IM at 1 to 2 mg/kg every 3 to 4 hours for severe abdominal pain. If this does not reduce pain sufficiently, then the effect of Demerol can be potentiated by administering chlorpromazine (Thorazine) at 1 mg/kg IM simultaneously.

Other therapies for acute pancreatitis remain controversial. Prophylactic antibiotics have not been shown to be beneficial. Secondary infection of the pancreas, usually by streptococci, coliforms, or staphylococci, occurs in 2 to 5 per cent of cases of pancreatitis. Identification of the infective organism(s) and the antibiotic sensitivities will allow selection of the appropriate antibiotics. If pancreatic abscess forms, surgical drainage is usually necessary. There is insufficient clinical evidence that suppressors of pancreatic exocrine secretion, such as anticholinergic drugs, glucagon, somatostatin, calcitonin, and tranquilizers, and inhibitors of pancreatic enzymes, such as aprotinin (Trasylol)* and epsilon-amino-caproic acid (EACA), are useful in the management of acute pancreatitis.

Persistence of abdominal pain and of elevation of serum amylase levels for 2 or more weeks after the onset of acute pancreatitis suggests the formation of a pseudocyst. Ultrasonography is an effective method of

---

*Aprotinin is an investigational drug and may not be available in the United States.

identifying pseudocysts, differentiating pseudocysts from inflammatory masses, and monitoring the size of pseudocysts. Many pseudocysts spontaneously resolve in 4 to 12 weeks. If the pseudocyst persists for 6 or more weeks or is enlarging, surgical internal drainage of the cyst into the stomach or upper small intestine has been the treatment of choice. More recently, ultrasonography has been used to guide percutaneous needle aspiration of the cysts and to place catheters for external drainage. This technique may be particularly useful in patients who are poor operative candidates.

Pancreatic fistulas most often occur following pancreatic trauma or drainage of pseudocysts. Most fistulas will spontaneously close. Those that have a high output or interfere with providing adequate oral alimentation often require prolonged periods of fasting and total parenteral nutrition (TPN). Intravenous lipids can be given as a part of TPN therapy since they do not appear to stimulate pancreatic secretion. Rarely, surgical closure of the fistula is necessary.

Chronic and recurrent acute pancreatitis are rarely seen in children. Continued exposure to the precipitating cause, i.e., alcohol, cholelithiasis, child abuse, and so on, or familial pancreatitis must be considered. Hereditary pancreatitis is transmitted autosomal dominantly and is associated with lysinuria and cystinuria in some cases. Most cases of hereditary pancreatitis require total pancreatectomy for control of symptoms. Endoscopic retrograde cholangiopancreatography (ERCP) should be performed if etiology is unknown, since congenital papillary stenosis may be identified and treated by endoscopic papillotomy. ERCP may identify other obstructive abnormalities such as gallstones, choledochal cysts, or duplication cysts that can be surgically corrected. Malabsorption due to pancreatic exocrine insufficiency and, rarely, diabetes mellitus requiring insulin therapy are sequelae of chronic pancreatitis. Malabsorption should be treated with oral pancreatic enzyme replacement therapy. Severe chronic abdominal pain may require prolonged fasting, using home parenteral nutrition or pancreatectomy. Chronic abdominal pain may be reduced by giving before each meal pancreatic enzyme extracts, which inhibit meal-stimulated pancreatic secretion.

PANCREATIC EXOCRINE INSUFFICIENCY

Cystic fibrosis, Shwachman-Diamond syndrome (pancreatic insufficiency and bone marrow hypoplasia), and chronic pancreatitis are main causes of pancreatic exocrine insufficiency in children.

Oral pancreatic enzyme extracts are the primary treatment, independent of the cause. The dose of pancreatic enzyme extract to be administered with meals depends upon the severity of pancreatic exocrine insufficiency, the patient's age, the fat content of the diet, and the type of enzyme preparation. In general, dietary fat restriction is not necessary, and approximately 8000 lipase NF units (one Cotazym capsule or one Viokase tablet) should digest at least 15 gm of dietary fat. Higher doses of enzymes may not improve digestion and may result in hyperuricemia. Ineffectiveness of oral pancreatic enzymes to completely correct malabsorption is

in part due to the suboptimal pH of the stomach for enzyme activity. Reduction of gastric acidity with antacids or cimetidine or protection of preparations with enteric coating (Pancrease or Cotazyms) have been reported to improve enzyme activity.

Deficiency of fat-soluble vitamins D, A, K, and E may occur with severe malabsorption. Clinical manifestations from vitamin deficiencies are rarely seen. Occasionally, bleeding diathesis due to hypoprothrombinemia from vitamin K deficiency and hemolytic anemia from vitamin E deficiency will occur. Prevention of vitamin deficiencies is usually accomplished by reducing malabsorption with oral pancreatic enzymes and by administering a multiple vitamin preparation at twice the minimal daily requirements. Additional supplementation with water-miscible vitamin E, 50 to 100 U daily, and with vitamin K, 0.5 to 5 mg daily, should be given to those who have severe malabsorption or laboratory evidence of deficiency in these vitamins.

Advising patients and families of the appropriate diet for age and dose of oral pancreatic enzymes will usually allow normal growth and development without significant malabsorptive symptoms. Occasionally, additional calories in the form of dietary supplements will be desired, or limited fat restrictions in the diet, i.e., a 15 to 20 per cent fat diet, will be necessary to control steatorrhea. Because elemental dietary supplements like medium-chain triglycerides and predigested protein are unpalatable, children will often refuse to take these preparations, especially for long periods of time. In these cases, nonelemental dietary supplements, such as Ensure, Sustacal, and Meritene, given with enzymes may be more acceptable.

ISOLATED PANCREATIC ENZYME DEFICIENCIES

Isolated pancreatic enzyme deficiencies are extremely rare. Diagnosis is made by pancreatic secretory studies revealing normal concentrations of pancreatic enzymes in duodenal aspirates except for the absence of a single enzyme.

Isolated lipase deficiency is an autosomal recessive disease that presents shortly after birth with oily diarrhea. Standard oral pancreatic enzyme preparations, as are used in cystic fibrosis, will correct the malabsorption.

Isolated amylase deficiency usually presents after 1 year of age. As starch becomes a larger part of the diet, watery diarrhea occurs. Analysis of the stool will reveal reducing substances (Clinitest positive at more than 1/4 per cent) and an acid pH of less than 6.0. The diagnosis can be confirmed with a starch loading test, i.e., failure of blood glucose to rise following ingestion of 50 gm of starch per square meter of body surface area. Treatment consists of starch elimination and supplementation with disaccharides.

Isolated trypsin or trypsinogen deficiency presents shortly after birth with diarrhea, anemia, hypoproteinemia, edema, and severe failure to thrive. Absence of trypsin or trypsinogen results in lack of proteolytic enzyme activity in duodenal secretions. Treatment consists of standard oral pancreatic enzyme preparations.

Isolated enterokinase deficiency is an autosomal recessive disease that also presents in the neonatal period with severe watery diarrhea, failure to thrive, anemia, hypoproteinemia, and edema. Enterokinase is produced in the brush border of the proximal small intestine. Since this enzyme is necessary for the activation of trypsin, duodenal aspirates lack proteolytic enzyme activity, which can be activated by adding enterokinase to the aspirate. Enterokinase can be assayed in the small intestinal biopsies. Standard oral pancreatic enzyme preparations are the required treatment.

CONGENITAL MALFORMATIONS

Annular pancreas is a ring of pancreatic tissue encircling the descending portion of the duodenum. Surgical intervention consists of a duodenoduodenostomy or duodenojejunostomy. The pancreas is left undivided so as to avoid formation of pancreatic fistulas. Pancreatic function is normal in these patients.

Approximately 2 per cent of the population have ectopic pancreatic tissue. Ninety per cent of these occur in the stomach, duodenum, or jejunum. Occasionally, the ectopic pancreas produces abdominal pain, gastrointestinal obstruction, bleeding, or intussusception. When these complications occur, the ectopic pancreatic tissue should be excised.

PANCREATIC TUMORS

Pancreatic tumors in children are very rare. Most are endocrine-secreting tumors, e.g., insulinoma, gastrinoma, VIPoma, and so on.

Ninety per cent of insulinomas are solitary tumors. Severe hypoglycemia often results in irreversible neurologic sequelae. Diazoxide, from 5 to 20 mg/kg/24 hr, will usually prevent hypoglycemia. Most children who have insulinomas during the first year of life will have remission before 5 to 6 years of age. Thus, surgical resection is not usually necessary in these younger children if hypoglycemia is prevented by diazoxide. Earlier surgery is indicated in children with localized tumors seen after 1 year of age or with hypoglycemia that is poorly controlled by diazoxide. Blind resections are often unsuccessful.

Twenty per cent of gastrinomas are solitary and benign. Gastrin secreted by the tumor stimulates gastric acid secretion, resulting in multiple gastric and duodenal ulcers and often diarrhea. Fasting serum gastrin levels may be only marginally elevated but will be markedly elevated (> 400 pg/ml) following intravenous secretin injection or calcium infusion. In adults, cimetidine, an H_2-receptor antagonist, has been shown to be an effective drug for controlling symptoms caused by the gastric hyperacidity. Those whose symptoms are not controlled by cimetidine usually require a total gastrectomy. Since the tumors are usually multiple and difficult to localize, surgical resection is often impossible.

Fortunately, carcinoma of the pancreas rarely occurs in children. However, recent reports from Japan indicate an increasing incidence in pancreatic carcinomas in children. Since clinical manifestations usually do not appear until extensive metastasis has occurred, prognosis of pancreatic carcinoma is poor, with a mean survival of 6 to 9 months after diagnosis in adults. Pancreaticoduodenectomy is recommended for the rare patient who has a small, localized lesion. In those with inoperable disease, supportive therapy consists of providing adequate nutrition and analgesia.

CYSTIC FIBROSIS
LUCILLE A. LESTER, M.D.

Cystic fibrosis is a multisystem disorder associated with generalized exocrine gland dysfunction. Optimum treatment of this disorder at any age can be provided only if its various manifestations and complications are recognized and the wide spectrum of disease severity is appreciated.

Once the diagnosis of cystic fibrosis is confirmed by two positive sweat tests (chloride concentration > 60 mEq/L in at least 100 mg of sweat), coordination of care with a designated cystic fibrosis center often facilitates development of an appropriate regimen. A conference should be held to familiarize the family with the disease process and its treatment, prognosis, and *genetic implications*. Arrangements should be made for instruction in chest physiotherapy, the use of inhalation therapy equipment, the child's special nutritional needs, and the need for vitamin and pancreatic enzyme supplementation.

Following the institution of a care regimen, close follow-up, initially at 2- to 4-week intervals, is required to re-evaluate therapy and answer questions. As the patient's condition stabilizes, less frequent visits are needed. Children who are doing well need to be seen only every 4 to 6 months. At each clinic visit, information should be elicited about frequency and character of cough, sputum production, exercise tolerance, appetite, and recent weight and height changes. Pulmonary function testing should be done when possible, and a minimum yearly chest x-ray examination and liver function tests should be obtained. Exacerbations of the chronic pulmonary disease may thus be detected early and treated in an outpatient setting with oral doses of antibiotics and intensification of the chest physiotherapy regimen. If the patient does not improve, admission to a hospital for parenteral antibiotic therapy, intensive pulmonary toilet, and nutritional support is indicated.

Prevention of complicating diseases is also important. Routine pediatric immunizations should be given to patients who are not acutely ill, even if cough is present. Yearly immunizations against influenza are recommended, but Pneumovax (pneumococcal vaccine, polyvalent, MSD) is not indicated.

PULMONARY THERAPY

For unknown reasons, there is marked heterogeneity in the severity of the pulmonary disease. Since the spectrum of those affected ranges from infants under 6 months of age who present with severely compromised pulmonary status during an episode of bronchiolitis, often caused by respiratory syncytial virus, to adults with nearly normal pulmonary function and lifestyle, specifics of treatment must be individualized. Close supervision and continuity of care permit an anticipatory therapeutic approach. It is generally accepted that a team approach, together with improved antimicrobial agents and more aggressive management of pulmonary complications, has resulted in the recent prolongation of life expectancy.

Chest Physiotherapy. Chest physiotherapy is utilized to facilitate mobilization of the thick mucopurulent secretions from the tracheobronchial tree. In children who produce sputum, it is usually preceded by inhalation therapy. We routinely teach nine-position segmental bronchial drainage techniques at the time of diagnosis, even if there is no evidence of pulmonary disease. The combination of percussion and vibration, together with deep breathing and cough maneuvers in the older child, is performed in each of nine positions, with the average treatment session requiring 20 to 30 minutes. In infants or children with early radiologic signs of bronchial obstruction or chronic cough, we initiate postural drainage once a day. Children 10 to 12 years of age and older should be instructed in how to perform the therapy themselves, and when the patient becomes self-sufficient, it may be helpful to add a mechanical percussor or vibrator to do some of the posterior positions effectively. In school-age children it is difficult to manage more than two sessions per day, but patients with severe bronchiectasis do benefit from three to four treatments per day.

Compliance with daily chest physiotherapy is often poor in the active, seemingly healthy youngster despite repeated attempts to reinforce need and benefits. Recently, along with other centers, we have been substituting or adding a regular program of aerobic exercise such as running, swimming, gymnastics, or tennis for 15 to 30 minutes every other day. Patients with moderate symptomatic involvement should undertake such an exercise program only with medical supervision. The patient's sense of well-being is often enhanced by such activity.

Aerosol Therapy. In patients who cough and produce sputum, whether it is expectorated or swallowed, the addition of aerosol inhalation therapy appears beneficial. This therapy delivers fluid to the lower respiratory tract in an attempt to thin the tenacious mucus and to facilitate its removal, especially during chest physiotherapy. It is also used to administer medications to the lower respiratory tract. Small compressor-driven, hand-held nebulizers can be used, but larger ultrasonic units deliver a greater volume of smaller particle–sized mist to the lower airway. They are more durable and, thus, more practical for long-term daily use.

To enhance the effectiveness of chest physical therapy, a bronchodilator followed by 15 to 20 minutes of a tussive mist is usually employed prior to postural drainage. We routinely add isoproterenol as a 0.05 per cent solution (1 drop/10 kg + 1) to 0.45 per cent saline solution for nebulization treatments. The isoproterenol acts promptly, and its effect dissipates within 30 to 60 minutes. More recently, we have used a 5 per cent solution of metaproterenol or a 0.5 per cent solution of albuterol with good results. Mucolytic agents, such as

N-acetyl-L-cysteine, may be beneficial in some patients. Since it often induces bronchospasm, it is usually given by aerosol with the bronchodilator. One to 4 ml of a 10 to 20 per cent solution of N-acetyl-L-cysteine is administered over 10 to 15 minutes. In the severely ill patient who has been unable to mobilize secretions, the initial N-acetyl-L-cysteine may lead to sudden, rapid mobilization of secretions, which may compromise ventilation. Therefore, the patient should be closely monitored, and nasotracheal suction should be available during and after the administration of the first few doses.

The use of aerosolized antibiotics has been controversial, but a recent enthusiasm has developed for this treatment modality. Prospective, crossover, blinded studies are currently evaluating the effectiveness of different inhaled antibiotic regimens. The most frequently used drugs are the aminoglycosides alone or in combination with a semisynthetic penicillin. We have been administering tobramycin (parenteral solution; 80 mg/ml) by nebulization after chest physical therapy in selected patients. The major benefit of this therapy, observed in our patients with moderate to severe lung disease, is a significant reduction in the necessity for hospitalization. Patients on long-term inhalation therapy with aminoglycosides must be monitored for ototoxicity, nephrotoxicity, and the development of drug-resistant strains of *Pseudomonas*.

Antibiotic Therapy. The progressive, destructive pulmonary disease of cystic fibrosis is initiated by infection in obstructed areas of the lung. Aerosol therapy and bronchial drainage aim to mobilize and remove tenacious secretions. Antibiotics are used to control the chronic infection. We feel strongly that antibiotics should not be used alone or in place of measures to mobilize secretions. Intermittent culturing of expectorated sputum (older children) or nasopharyngeal aspirates at the time of induced coughing (younger children) and determination of antibiotic sensitivity on all isolates of pathogens are the best guides to appropriate antibiotic therapy.

Staphylococcus aureus is usually the first organism to be cultured from the respiratory tract, and many feel that it is the initial and major pathogen in cystic fibrosis lung disease. However, *Pseudomonas aeruginosa*, especially the mucoid strains, almost invariably becomes the predominant organism in sputum. There is evidence that *S. aureus* remains a significant offender, despite the isolation of only *P. aeruginosa* in a given sputum specimen. Intermittently, patients who have harbored only *S. aureus* or *P. aeruginosa* may have *Haemophilus influenzae*, *Escherichia coli*, *Proteus mirabilis*, or *Klebsiella pneumoniae* grow from their sputum. When this occurs, treatment for these organisms should be considered. Patients who have received numerous courses of parenteral anti-*Pseudomonas* antibiotics may develop strains resistant to the aminoglycosides and/or semisynthetic penicillins. Also, multiple drug-resistant *Pseudomonas* strains, such as *Pseudomonas cepacia*, have recently emerged as major problems in some patients with cystic fibrosis.

Significant controversy still prevails over the question of the use of daily prophylactic oral antibiotic therapy. We strongly favor the use of intermittent courses of antibiotics to treat exacerbations of pulmonary symptoms in an effort to delay the early appearance of *P. aeruginosa* and the development of antibiotic-resistant strains. However, patients with severe pulmonary disease and compromised pulmonary function have been found empirically to do better with daily administration of oral antibiotics.

Choice and timing of antibiotic therapy may be difficult, since signs of infection are frequently lacking, making it hard to differentiate between colonization and low-grade infection. Abnormalities on chest auscultation and increasing obstructive disease demonstrated by pulmonary function tests are often the main indications of pulmonary exacerbations. Additionally, findings such as increased cough, significant nighttime cough, increased irritability, decreased activity, poor appetite, and weight loss may also be present. Patients with these findings or with symptoms of an upper respiratory tract infection should be treated with a 10- to 14-day course of an oral antibiotic that has significant anti-*S. aureus* activity. Trimethoprim-sulfamethoxazole is often the first drug we prescribe because it is well tolerated and has to be taken only twice a day. Dicloxacillin, cephalexin, cefaclor, and erythromycin are also frequently prescribed. Tetracycline, particularly doxycycline, is useful alone or in combination with dicloxacillin in patients 9 years of age and older. Chloramphenicol remains a frequently used and particularly efficacious drug because of its high biopenetrability and its action against *S. aureus* and *H. influenzae*. Using short courses limited to 2 to 3 weeks, we have as yet not had hematologic or ocular complications. Ciprofioxacin, a recently released fluorinated quinolone antibiotic, has good activity against *P. aeruginosa* as well as *S. aureus* and has been very efficacious in patients with moderate lung disease. It is recommended for use in children 12 years or older.

Patients with more advanced pulmonary disease who develop acute or chronic symptoms and patients who have failed to improve on an outpatient regimen of oral antibiotics and intensified chest physiotherapy require admission to the hospital for intravenous antibiotics. Patients with only *S. aureus* cultured from their sputum are usually treated with nafcillin alone or nafcillin and gentamicin. In patients with *P. aeruginosa*, we use a combination of a semisynthetic penicillin and an aminoglycoside given intravenously for 10 to 14 days. High doses of aminoglycosides are usually required, and it is often necessary to administer them every 6 hours instead of every 8 hours to achieve levels of 6 to 9 µg/ml 30 minutes after infusion. Trough levels should be less than 2 µg/ml. Some centers favor the addition of nafcillin in patients not improving on the double antibiotic regimen. After hospitalization, we frequently administer another 2 to 4 weeks of oral antibiotics. We have had excellent results with home administration of IV antibiotics to complete a 2-week course or to prolong a course to 3 to 4 weeks. Improved home health care services allows this to work well for highly motivated school-age children or young adults. We have a limited experience with central venous lines or semipermanent peripheral venous access lines for chronic antibiotic administration at home. These catheters for chronic administration of antibiotics are an appropriate treatment approach for a select group of highly motivated patients and families. The intramuscular route is seldom used, since the patient's muscle mass is small and repeated painful injections are poorly tolerated for protracted periods of time.

Treatment of Allergy and Reactive Airway Disease Symptoms. Cystic fibrosis patients have an incidence of allergy equal to that in the general population. The symptoms are often difficult to distinguish from milder pulmonary symptoms of cystic fibrosis. Antihistamines may thicken and dry lower respiratory tract secretions but can be employed for short periods together with decongestants to relieve allergic rhinitis symptoms. Cystic fibrosis patients may develop hyperactive airway disease on an allergic basis. However, those with bronchiectasis may have clinically evident bronchospasm secondary to the chronic inflammation. If pulmonary function testing demonstrates reversibility of obstruction, oral theophylline or beta-adrenergic agents may be helpful. In patients with cold- or exercise-induced bronchospasm, symptoms usually respond to a bronchodilator given 20 to 30 minutes before exposure to cold or exercise. These measures, along with treatment of pulmonary infection, are usually beneficial, but inhaled or systemic steroids or cromolyn may be indicated in selected patients.

Bronchial Lavage. This modality has been recommended as an efficacious way to "clean out" large quantities of mucopurulent material. We feel it has little long-term efficacy, and the severely compromised patient may experience significant hypoxia during the procedure. For these reasons we no longer perform this procedure.

Expectorants. No systemic drug has proved useful in specifically clearing secretions from the lungs. Prolonged use of iodides may be helpful but is limited by the frequent development of goiters. We have not found oral expectorants useful and caution against the use of over-the-counter expectorants or cough preparations. These mixtures often contain antihistamines or cough suppressants, which are potentially detrimental.

PULMONARY COMPLICATIONS

Atelectasis. Lobar or segmental atelectasis is frequently encountered in infants and young children with cystic fibrosis. The right upper and middle lobes and the lingula are most commonly affected. Such atelectasis may be an unexpected finding on a routine chest roentgenogram, but even in asymptomatic patients aggressive treatment with inhaled bronchodilators followed by chest physiotherapy is indicated. Antibiotics are used if atelectasis is noted during the course of an exacerbation and infection. Re-expansion may not occur despite intensive treatment given in the hospital. In such patients we have seen re-expansion after several weeks of continued vigorous bronchial drainage at home. Rigid bronchoscopy with or without lavage is usually without benefit. Removal of the obstruction using a flexible fiberoptic bronchoscope may result in re-expansion and could be attempted.

CYSTIC FIBROSIS   219

Hemoptysis. Blood-streaked sputum is common in cystic fibrosis patients with widespread bronchiectasis. It is usually related to increased bronchial infection, and antibiotics should be prescribed. If mild hemoptysis (less than 30 ml) continues despite antibiotic treatment, hospitalization for parenteral antibiotics is indicated. Postural drainage may be stopped for the first 24 hours and is then gradually resumed. Vitamin K is administered if prothrombin time is prolonged. Massive hemoptysis (500 to 700 ml/24 hr) may occur in older cystic fibrosis patients with more advanced disease. Bed rest, cessation of postural drainage, and blood replacement are urgent steps to be taken. Supportive treatment, including oxygen and parenteral antibiotics, should be instituted. If bleeding persists, an attempt to localize the site of bleeding by bronchoscopy can be tried. This should be followed by percutaneous angiography and embolization of the dilated bronchials on the affected side. Gelfoam and Ivalon (polyvinyl alcohol sponge) have both been used successfully. In patients who continue to have significant hemoptysis, elective embolization of the remaining bronchial arteries is suggested.

Pneumothorax. Spontaneous pneumothorax is a complication most often affecting adolescent and young adult cystic fibrosis patients who have extensive pulmonary involvement. If the pneumothorax is less than 10 per cent of lung volume as determined by chest roentgenogram, and the patient is stable, he can be observed in the hospital. In larger pneumothoraces or in tension pneumothoraces, immediate insertion of a chest tube is mandatory. Owing to the high risk of recurrence, we do chemical pleurodesis after the lung has re-expanded. After appropriate sedation, tetracycline or quinacrine is inserted into the chest tube, and the patient's position is changed frequently to expose as much of the pleura as possible to the irritant medication. If pneumothorax recurs after chemical pleurodesis, open thoracotomy with parietal pleurectomy, oversewing of visible blebs, and visceral pleural abrasion is done. This procedure is tolerated even in severely compromised patients.

Cor Pulmonale. Cor pulmonale, strictly defined as right ventricular hypertrophy, can be detected using echocardiography in patients with mild to moderate pulmonary disease. This hypertrophy progresses slowly with advancing hypoxemia and is probably exacerbated by the increased hypoxemia experienced during exercise and sleep. Nighttime low-flow oxygen at home may delay progression of this cardiac abnormality. Fulminant right heart failure or acute cor pulmonale is a near-terminal event in patients with severe lung disease but often responds to treatment. Humidified oxygen at low flow rates should be administered to maintain the PaO_2 at about 50 torr without depressing the ventilatory drive. Furosemide, 1 mg/kg IV, produces rapid diuresis and can be repeated at 8- to 12-hour intervals. Moderate dietary salt restriction is reasonable in these patients, who may also be receiving intravenous antibiotics with high sodium concentrations. Digitalis is of questionable usefulness, although short-term improvement in ventricular function has been documented. Tolazoline was initially found to be useful for reducing pulmonary

hypertension, but its effectiveness is short-lived and its side effects are undesirable. Newer drugs (hydralazine, nifedipine) with possible pulmonary vasodilating effects may be more promising for use in patients with severe pulmonary hypertension.

Aspergillosis. *Aspergillus* species are most often encountered incidentally in sputum cultures from patients receiving antibiotics for chronic conditions. This finding is thought to represent colonization rather than infection. Invasive aspergillosis requiring antifungal treatment has rarely been documented in patients with cystic fibrosis. In contrast, a hypersensitivity pneumonitis (allergic bronchopulmonary aspergillosis) does occur in cystic fibrosis patients. This complication responds well to steroid therapy, but care should be taken to adjust the basic care regimen to prevent exacerbations of bacterial infection.

Pulmonary Osteoarthropathy. Digital clubbing is commonly observed but is usually only of cosmetic importance. Periostitis of the ends of long bones with new bone formation may be roentgenographically evident in older patients with painful swelling of the larger joints. Aspirin, acetaminophen, and nonsteroidal anti-inflammatory agents such as ibuprofen are effective in relieving the pain and swelling that are exacerbated during active pulmonary infections.

Respiratory Failure. Although usually thought of only as the end result of the chronic progressive bronchiectasis, respiratory failure can be precipitated by acute pulmonary infection in patients with mild to moderate lung disease. Short-term mechanical ventilatory support may be employed for such a patient. In more chronically ill patients developing hypoxia (PaO_2 between 50 and 60 torr on room air), low-flow oxygen by nasal cannula is used. We begin its use during sleep only and extend its use to daytime activities as indicated. Oxygen concentrators or liquid oxygen systems are both convenient for home oxygen administration. This oxygen therapy significantly improves the patients' quality of life by allowing them to be more mobile and less fatigued and dyspneic, and they have decreased headaches and deep bone pain. Mechanical ventilatory assistance appears to be of little benefit for the severely compromised patient with end-stage lung disease. This decision should be completely discussed with family members before the need for ventilatory assistance is clinically obvious. Supportive care, including antibiotics, tranquilizers, chest physiotherapy, and chronic oxygen, is routinely given.

GASTROINTESTINAL THERAPY

Pancreatic Insufficiency. Clinically evident pancreatic insufficiency occurs in most patients with cystic fibrosis, although it may vary in age of presentation and severity. Infants or young children who present with a positive sweat test and frequent, large, foul-smelling stools and failure to thrive do not need a 72-hour fat balance study to document the pancreatic insufficiency. Such infants may be severely malnourished, and we provide them with readily absorbable nutrients by starting them immediately on special infant formulas containing hydrolyzed proteins and medium-chain triglycerides (Pregestimil or Portagen) as well as pancreatic enzyme supplements. These formulas, which can be prepared in concentrations of up to 30 cal/oz, are used to supply the needed extra calories without increased volume. When the special formula is no longer tolerated (around 12 months of age), skim milk fortified with nonfat dry milk powder (20 cal/oz) or 2 per cent whole milk is introduced, and the pancreatic enzyme dose is increased appropriately.

Pancreatic enzymes should be given with meals and snacks. Sufficient enzyme is given to normalize stool number and consistency and to achieve maximal growth. The newer preparations circumvent the problem of gastric acid inactivation by an enteric coating designed to release active enzyme in the duodenum; thus, fewer capsules are required per meal. Young infants, however, are best treated with powdered enzyme mixed with a few teaspoons of formula or strained food (½ to 2 capsules of pancrelipase [Cotazym] per feeding), as the enteric coating of the microspheres may be incompletely removed by the gastric acid in young infants. At age 12 months we change to the enteric-coated microsphere preparations (Pancrease or Cotazym-S, Creon, or Zymase). As the child grows and intake increases, enzyme dosage must be increased, and older infants and children may need from 1 to 5 or 6 capsules/meal. Symptoms of bloating, abdominal distention, crampy abdominal pain, and diarrhea, which suggest inadequate enzyme intake, often lessen in older children and adults.

Low-fat diets were previously the dictum for all cystic fibrosis patients with pancreatic insufficiency. With the improved enzyme preparations and with the recognition of essential fatty acid deficiency (linoleic acid) in cystic fibrosis patients with treated pancreatic insufficiency, the recent trend has been toward no fat restriction in the diet. Patients may vary in their ability to tolerate certain dietary fats even with good enzyme replacement, and diets must be individualized. We aim for 150 per cent of the recommended daily allowance for age of calories and protein. When regular meal intake does not provide adequate calories, or when requirements increase, such as during infection, high-calorie liquid supplements are prescribed. Polycose or medium-chain triglycerides can also be added to regular foods as a source of readily utilizable calories. Enteral supplements administered orally or via nasogastric or gastrostomy tubes are an important adjunct in some patients. In hospitalized children who have *lost* weight and cannot maintain adequate calorie intake, we have found supplemental peripheral hyperalimentation to be an effective and safe way to provide 700 to 1500 extra calories/day over a 2-week period. Solutions of 10 per cent glucose, 1 to 2 gm/kg/day of crystalline amino acids, and 1 to 2 gm/kg/day of 10 per cent Intralipid solution (except in severely hypoxic patients) may be administered by peripheral intravenous infusion. All our patients receive supplemental vitamins containing water-soluble or miscible forms of A, D, and E.

Meconium Ileus. Meconium ileus is a common cause of neonatal intestinal obstruction and occurs in 5 to 10 per cent of all children with cystic fibrosis. Perforation and meconium peritonitis can occur, and this requires immediate surgical intervention. More typically, clinical signs of obstruction develop in the first 24 hours of life, and if cystic fibrosis is not suspected, surgical intervention is usually prompt. In cases in which cystic fibrosis is suspected and the baby is stable, diatrizoate (Gastrografin) enemas with pressure may flush the contrast medium above the area of obstruction. In about 50 per cent of these cases, enough fluid is drawn into the bowel lumen to flush out the inspissated meconium. Diatrizoate is very hypertonic and must be administered only after an intravenous line has been established for fluid and electrolyte replacement. After relief of the obstruction, attention must be directed to achieving adequate nutrition, either orally or with supplemental parenteral alimentation.

Meconium Ileus Equivalent: Intussusception. About 20 per cent of the older cystic fibrosis patients develop episodic (often recurrent) accumulations of bowel contents in the distal ileum and ascending colon. This partial obstruction, often associated with inadequate pancreatic enzyme intake, may lead to intermittent abdominal pain and a decreased number of stools. Adjustment of pancreatic enzyme dosage and saline enemas are often all that is needed. If more complete obstruction develops, the patient should be admitted to the hospital and treated with saline enemas containing N-acetyl-L-cysteine (4 to 5 per cent by volume). If this treatment is not effective, diatrizoate* enemas under fluroscopic control are done in an attempt to flush out the obstructing material. Surgery to relieve the obstruction is occasionally required. A similar clinical presentation may also be observed with intussusception. This occurs with an increased frequency in the infant with cystic fibrosis, and cystic fibrosis is one of the few causes of intussusception in older children and adults. The intussusception is usually ileocolic and may be suspected on a plain film of the abdomen. Reduction by barium enema should be tried, but if it is unsuccessful, surgical reduction is required.

Liver Disease. A small percentage of newborn infants with cystic fibrosis may have prolonged cholestatic jaundice. Frequent monitoring of the transaminases is important, especially in those infants requiring hyperalimentation. This problem usually resolves completely within 6 to 12 months. Prior to diagnosis, some older infants may develop fatty infiltration of the liver secondary to malnutrition. This resolves promptly with the institution of appropriate diet and pancreatic enzymes. At least 25 per cent of the patients develop a focal biliary cirrhosis that is characteristic of cystic fibrosis. In most, this is manifested by increased alkaline phosphatase and elevations of the transaminases. About 20 per cent of the patients with focal biliary cirrhosis progress to a more severe multinodular cirrhosis and portal hypertension. There is no specific treatment for the liver disease, and hepatic function usually remains adequate until late in the course. The complications are managed in the same way as in other types of liver

---

*This use of diatrizoate (Gastrografin) is not listed in the manufacturer's directive.

disease. Ascites is treated with a low-salt diet and at times with diuretics. Esophageal varices may lead to frequent chronic blood loss or massive hemorrhage. Vitamin K should be given to patients with prolongation of their prothrombin times, and salicylates should be avoided. Effective control of acute hemorrhage can be achieved with nasogastric intubation, cold saline lavage, and infusion of vasopressin. If hemorrhage continues, endoscopy may identify the bleeding site, and hemostasis may be achieved by sclerosis of this area. Severe hypersplenism may result from portal hypertension, and when this occurs in association with bleeding varices, splenectomy and a splenorenal shunt are effective treatment. Portacaval anastomosis has been avoided because of the frequency of postoperative hepatic encephalopathy. Liver transplants have been performed successfully in those with mild pulmonary involvement in whom liver failure was imminent.

Gallbladder Disease. Up to 40 per cent of older patients with upper abdominal pain have been found to have gallstones by abdominal ultrasonography or cholecystography. Only an occasional patient has colic or pain typical of cholelithiasis and requires surgical treatment.

Pancreatitis. The 10 to 15 per cent of patients without clinically significant pancreatic insufficiency at an early age often develop acute or recurrent pancreatitis as young adults. The symptoms often are mild and may be similar to those of cholelithiasis. Patients with severe symptoms and elevated amylase levels are best treated with nasogastric drainage, intravenous fluids, and analgesics.

Rectal Prolapse. In the untreated cystic fibrosis patient who has frequent loose stools, the rectal mucosa may prolapse at the time of defecation. Similarly, prolapse may occur in patients with known cystic fibrosis taking insufficient pancreatic enzymes to control steatorrhea. In either instance, the prolapse often can be spontaneously reduced by placing the patient in the knee-chest position. If not, the rectal mucosa may be replaced manually. Prolapse ceases as steatorrhea is controlled by pancreatic enzymes. Surgical treatment is rarely indicated.

Gastroesophageal Reflux. In some infants the finding of gastroesophageal reflux has been used to explain recurrent pulmonary infiltrates, thereby resulting in a delay in the diagnosis of cystic fibrosis. Appropriate diagnosis followed by treatment of the cystic fibrosis lung disease with chest physiotherapy and antibiotics usually decreases the severity of the cough and eliminates the need for antireflux measures. A small percentage of older patients have been found to have significant reflux with or without hiatal hernia. These symptoms usually improve with medical reflux management and measures to minimize paroxysmal coughing. Bethanechol should be avoided in patients with symptomatic pulmonary disease.

MISCELLANEOUS PROBLEMS

Salt Depletion. During the warmer months, infants with cystic fibrosis may present with a characteristic hyponatremic, hypochloremic dehydration with alkalosis secondary to excessive losses of electrolytes in the sweat. Maintenance of adequate salt and fluid intake during hot weather may prevent the development of such problems. Intravenous fluid and electrolyte correction have been necessary in some infants. Older children and adults may develop a similar state of dehydration if they work or exercise vigorously in hot weather. This can be controlled by giving salt supplements (500-mg tablets once or twice daily) in addition to the liberal use of dietary salt.

Hyperglycemia. In older patients fibrosis of the pancreas may be severe, and encroachment on the pancreatic islets may occur, with resulting carbohydrate intolerance. In 3 to 5 per cent of patients, polyuria, polydipsia, and weight loss occur, and insulin is required. Ketoacidosis rarely develops, but during periods of stress (infection) increased amounts of insulin may be required.

Otolaryngologic Complications. Young children with cystic fibrosis may develop chronic serous otitis media and persistent rhinitis. Ventilation with polyethylene tubes may be required if hearing loss develops. Sinus opacification is radiographically evident in over 90 per cent of the patients but is rarely associated with fever, pain, and purulent drainage. If repeated courses of antibiotics and decongestants are ineffective in the symptomatic patient, surgical drainage may be required. Nasal polyps also occur in a very high percentage of patients with cystic fibrosis. When very large, the polyps can obstruct one or both nares. Beclomethasone nasal spray may result in temporary relief. Surgical removal is sometimes needed, and postoperative recurrence is common.

Surgery. When surgical therapy is indicated in patients with cystic fibrosis, careful attention to pulmonary toilet will reduce the risk. Five to 10 days of maximized pulmonary therapy, including antibiotics, is given in the hospital prior to surgery. Every effort to use local or spinal anesthesia should be made. If this is not possible, general anesthesia time should be kept to a minimum. After surgery, postural drainage and coughing, with support of surgical wounds, are reinstituted as soon as feasible. A common surgical problem in older patients is inguinal hernia. This presents a particularly difficult situation during the postoperative period. Coughing is indicated for the pulmonary disease but even with support of the wound may have a detrimental effect on the healing surgical reconstruction.

Reproductive Problems. Ninety-eight per cent of males with cystic fibrosis are infertile. This is due to azoospermia resulting from obstruction of the vas deferens. Females with cystic fibrosis have a reduced fertility rate, possibly due to abnormal cervical mucus. Significant lung disease may make pregnancy an undesirable medical risk, and birth control measures should be advised appropriately. These problems should be discussed with the patients, and alternatives (such as artificial insemination of the spouses of males with cystic fibrosis) should be offered on an individual basis.

A MAJOR BREAKTHROUGH: THE FINDING OF THE CYSTIC FIBROSIS GENE

The localization of the CF gene to chromosome 7 in 1985, and the advances in DNA technology that followed, led to the availability of prenatal testing and carrier detection in known CF-affected families. In August 1989, the CF gene was further isolated and characterized, and proposals for the structure and function of the resultant "CF-protein" followed. Work is ongoing to characterize the multiple deletions that will likely explain clinical differences in disease severity. Gene-based therapy or therapy to replace the defective CF protein is a distinct possibility for the future.

CHRONIC DIARRHEA AND MALABSORPTION SYNDROMES

MARTIN H. ULSHEN, M.D.,
and MITCHELL D. SHUB, M.D.

Diarrheal illnesses are common in childhood but are most often acute and self-limited. An episode of diarrhea is considered chronic when a stool pattern of increased frequency and water content persists for more than 2 weeks in early infancy or 1 month in the older child. Stool volume normally varies with the size of the child. Daily stool weight is less than 5 to 10 gm/kg for infants under 10 kg of body weight; older children and adults may have up to 100 to 250 gm of stool per day. In infancy, bowel movements tend to occur at more frequent intervals than later in life. Loose stools are seen commonly in infants who nurse or take elemental formula.

Chronic diarrhea occurs most commonly in infancy. There are a large number of potential causes of chronic diarrhea in infancy and childhood (Table 1). The findings of weight loss or inadequate weight gain, recurrent dehydration, and nocturnal stools tend to suggest a more serious etiology. However, dietary restrictions can cause a child with no underlying organic disorder to fail to gain or to lose weight because of inadequate nutrient intake.

Diarrhea results from malabsorption or secretion of osmotically active solutes. In the gastrointestinal tract, water moves passively across the mucosa following these solutes. Pathophysiologic mechanisms of diarrhea fall into three basic categories: (1) poor absorption of an osmotic load, (2) secretion or diminished absorption of electrolytes, and (3) abnormal gastrointestinal motility. This classification can be the basis for a rational approach to diagnosis and treatment of diarrheal diseases. For example, the diarrhea associated with a disaccharidase deficiency would be expected to resolve with removal of the offending sugar from the diet, whereas this treatment would be unsuccessful for the diarrhea associated with a neuroblastoma (i.e., a secretory diarrhea). Often, more than one mechanism is involved.

Two classes of solutes can cause osmotic diarrhea: (1) Normal dietary components (e.g., lactose) under certain circumstances may be incompletely absorbed, transiently or permanently. (2) Solutes that are normally transported across the intestinal mucosa in limited amounts may cause diarrhea when ingested in quantities that surpass the absorptive capacity (e.g., magnesium and phosphate); as a result, these substances are useful as cathartics.

It is now recognized that a large number of infectious agents are capable of producing a secretory diarrhea. Furthermore, malabsorbed bile acids or long-chain fats stimulate colonic secretion. Prostaglandins released during an inflammatory response (e.g., in ulcerative colitis) may produce intestinal secretion as well. Diarrheal disorders mediated by gastrointestinal hormones, such as vasoactive intestinal polypeptide in neuroblastoma, are also secretory in nature.

Increased motility causes diarrhea by allowing less time for contact between intraluminal contents and the absorptive surface. In disorders with compromised bowel function, such as short bowel syndrome, the duration of contact of luminal contents with bowel surface may be a critical factor. In contrast, slowed transit or disordered motility may lead to intraluminal stasis. Stasis can result from an anatomic obstruction (e.g., blind loop or bowel stenosis) as well. Progressive movement of bowel contents through the small intestine is one of the protective mechanisms preventing bacterial colonization, whereas stasis encourages overgrowth. Bacterial overgrowth in the small bowel may lead to deconjugation of bile acids and mucosal damage resulting in fat malabsorption.

CHRONIC NONSPECIFIC DIARRHEA SYNDROME

Chronic nonspecific diarrhea syndrome, also known as toddler's diarrhea or irritable colon of infancy, is the most common cause of a pattern of persistent loose stools in young children. Symptoms, which generally begin between 6 and 36 months of age, are characterized by persistent or intermittent passage of three or more runny to mushy stools per day. Children with this stool pattern are typically active, healthy-appearing, and thriving. On examination, these children appear well with no suggestion of malabsorption. A child with a stool pattern suggesting toddler's diarrhea requires little or no medical evaluation beyond a history and physical examination. Treatment includes reassurance, adjustment of the dietary pattern to reduce gastrocolic stimulation, and restriction of the volume of dietary liquids. When simpler measures fail, other approaches that have been used, although less clearly beneficial, include an increase in dietary fat (especially in children receiving fat-restricted diets), an increase in dietary fiber, and a short course of oral cholestyramine. Prolonged use of highly restrictive elimination diets is common but can place a child at risk for growth failure from calorie deprivation and should be avoided. The stool pattern may improve at the time of toilet training, and acquisition of this developmental skill need not be delayed.

MALABSORPTION STATES

Carbohydrate intolerance is a common cause for chronic diarrhea, especially in infancy. Symptoms are

TABLE 1. Treatment of Chronic Diarrhea and Malabsorption

Condition	Treatment
Chronic nonspecific diarrhea (toddler's diarrhea)	Reassurance Avoid frequent feedings Limit dietary liquid frequency and volume Avoid fluids with high carbohydrate content (e.g., fruit juices)
Protracted diarrhea of infancy	
Infectious etiologies	
Bacterial (*Campylobacter, Yersinia, Salmonella, Clostridium difficile, Escherichia coli,* etc.)	Antibiotics only when indicated
Parasites (*Giardia,* ameba, etc.)	Specific antimicrobials
Parenteral diarrhea (i.e., urinary tract infection, otitis media, etc.)	Treat underlying infection with antibiotics
Malabsorption states	
Carbohydrate intolerance	Remove offending carbohydrate from diet
Primary: sucrase-isomaltase deficiency lactase deficiency (congenital or adult-onset) congenital glucose-galactose malabsorption	Remove sucrose from diet Restriction of starch intake may be necessary Remove lactose from diet or add commercial lactase to milk Replace glucose and lactose with fructose
Secondary monosaccharide and/or disaccharide intolerance	Treat as above
Fructose-induced diarrhea	Avoid excessive fructose intake
Cystic fibrosis	Pancreatic replacement (use enteric-coated microspheres and/or H_2 blockers as necessary) Fat-soluble vitamin supplementation Protein-calorie supplements
Celiac disease	Strict gluten-free diet When necessary, avoid lactose early in treatment
Bile salt malabsorption (without insufficiency)	Cholestyramine
Bile salt insufficiency (e.g., cholestasis, terminal ileal dysfunction)	Low-fat diet Medium-chain triglyceride and fat-soluble vitamin supplementation
Shwachman syndrome	Gastrointestinal treatment as for cystic fibrosis
Intestinal lymphangiectasia	Low-fat diet Medium-chain triglyceride and fat-soluble vitamin supplementation
Abetalipoproteinemia	Treatment as for intestinal lymphangiectasia Parenteral vitamin E usually necessary
Acrodermatitis enteropathica	Zinc
Immune deficiencies—diarrhea may be associated with secondary infection	Treat underlying deficiency when possible Evaluate for secondary infection and treat when possible (e.g., giardiasis)
Food allergy/eosinophilic gastroenteritis	Avoid antigens causing symptoms Cromolyn disodium or steroids may occasionally be necessary
Inflammatory bowel disease (Crohn's disease and ulcerative colitis)	
Anatomic anomalies of the gastrointestinal tract (partial small bowel obstruction, short bowel, blind loop syndrome, etc.)	Surgical correction Treatment of bacterial overgrowth with antibiotics Nutritional management of malabsorption
Chronic idiopathic intestinal pseudo-obstruction	Nutritional management Trial of prokinetic drugs Antibiotic treatment of bacterial overgrowth
Hormone-associated diarrhea	
Neuroblastoma, ganglioneuroma, VIP-secreting tumor	Surgical resection of tumor Pharmacologic treatment (e.g., somatostatin analogue)
Zollinger-Ellison syndrome	Pharmacologic control of acid secretion Surgery
Adrenal insufficiency	Adrenal hormone replacement
Hyperthyroidism	Pharmacologic or surgical treatment
Systemic mastocytosis	Antihistamines, H_2 blockers
Hirschsprung's disease with secondary enterocolitis	Temporary decompression with rectal tube prn Surgical decompression
Malnutrition and micronutrient deficiency—zinc, iron, etc.	Nutritional repletion
Habit constipation with overflow "diarrhea"	Evacuate colon and begin chronic treatment
Sorbitol-induced diarrhea	Reduce intake of sorbitol-containing products (e.g., sugar-free gum, apple juice)
Factitious diarrhea	Removal of toxic agent and psychosocial intervention

usually transient, often resulting from a secondary disaccharidase deficiency. Secondary lactose intolerance following a viral gastroenteritis is common and should be considered whenever an infant develops diarrhea upon reintroduction of a lactose-containing formula. Late-onset lactose intolerance typically presents after the first 5 years of life and is common in adults. Congenital sucrase-isomaltase deficiency is much less

common but can mimic chronic nonspecific diarrhea. Congenital lactase deficiency is extremely rare. Treatment of carbohydrate intolerance is aimed at removal of the offending carbohydrate from the diet. A commercial lactase product may be added to cow's milk to hydrolyze lactose. Typically, it is possible to digest 80 to 90 per cent of the lactose with this treatment. Individuals with lactose intolerance often are able to eat live-culture yogurt without symptoms. The bacteria in yogurt produce a lactase enzyme that survives passage through the stomach and is active at body temperature and duodenal pH. In addition to lactose-free formulas, carbohydrate-free formulas are available for infants with carbohydrate intolerance. The latter formulas should not be used without providing a carbohydrate source orally or intravenously.

Cystic fibrosis is one of the most common causes of fat malabsorption in childhood. The combination of hypoproteinemia and diarrhea in early infancy should always make one think of cystic fibrosis. Rectal prolapse or a salty taste also suggests this diagnosis. Treatment includes the use of pancreatic enzyme replacement (unless the child has no evidence of pancreatic insufficiency) and nutritional supplementation. The efficacy of pancreatic replacement may be improved by administration as enteric-coated microspheres or by decreasing gastric acid secretion with H_2 blockers. Fat-soluble vitamin intake should be supplemented as described below.

Celiac disease is a lifelong condition requiring a gluten-free diet. It is important to avoid not only food products containing wheat, oats, rye, and barley but also medications and beverages that contain gluten as well. Extensive lists of gluten-free foods are available through regional celiac organizations. Gluten-free substitutes for wheat products are available commercially as well. A transient lactose intolerance may be symptomatic at the time of presentation of celiac disease. This condition can be treated by removal of lactose from the diet or lactase treatment of milk and should gradually resolve with use of a gluten-free diet.

Other causes of marked steatorrhea include Shwachman syndrome, intestinal lymphangiectasia, and abetalipoproteinemia. Pancreatic insufficiency in Shwachman syndrome is treated in a similar fashion to that for cystic fibrosis. However, the steatorrhea in this condition appears to become milder with age. Avoidance of dietary fat and supplementation of diet with medium-chain triglycerides and fat-soluble vitamins are the major treatments of intestinal lymphangiectasia and abetalipoproteinemia.

NUTRITIONAL TREATMENT OF MALABSORPTION SYNDROMES

Conditions associated with malabsorption result from a wide range of conditions (Table 1). Although specific treatments are available for some of these disorders, supportive nutritional therapy is necessary for most. However, nutrient requirements vary among these disorders. Nutritional deprivation is a frequent consequence of malabsorption states; severe malnutrition secondary to malabsorption may be unresponsive to enteral feedings and may require the use of parenteral nutrition. This approach is indicated for individuals with persistent weight loss or a lack of adequate growth despite optimal enteral feedings. Total parenteral nutrition may be necessary, although parenteral supplementation of oral feedings may be adequate for some individuals. Home parenteral nutrition programs are now a routine form of treatment. A permanent large central venous catheter can be placed surgically and used safely at home following a formal training program. The best care for children in home programs is provided under the supervision of an experienced center with adequate support services, including trained physicians, nutritionists, pharmacists, and TPN nurses. The growth of a number of national and regional companies that provide home enteral and parenteral services has greatly simplified the distribution of formulas and other supplies. In addition, these companies often provide home nursing evaluation and support. Many children receive their entire parenteral requirement overnight and attend regular activities with their peers during the day. Some children who do not absorb an adequate quantity of nutrient by mouth may do well with continuous overnight nasogastric (or gastrostomy) tube feedings. For these children, this method is preferred over parenteral feedings because it is associated with a lower risk of complications and is simpler to administer as well as less expensive.

Fat malabsorption is the most common clinical consequence of the malabsorption syndromes and is usually most pronounced in conditions associated with pancreatic insufficiency or bile salt depletion. For infants, the use of a formula in which a portion or all of the fat is in the form of medium-chain triglyceride (MCT) may improve fat absorption. Older children can benefit from the use of MCT or carbohydrate supplements. Short-chain glucose polymers are often used because they are relatively tasteless but are easier to digest than complex starch. In addition, it may be necessary to provide supplements of the fat-soluble vitamins A, D, E, and K. Patterns of fat-soluble vitamin deficiency vary among individuals with fat malabsorption. Vitamin E deficiency is most pronounced in children with liver disease and cholestasis as well as abetalipoproteinemia. Children with cystic fibrosis and secondary cholestatic liver disease can develop a severe deficiency. Vitamin E deficiency leads to a syndrome of progressive, severe neuromuscular dysfunction. The same children also may have either vitamin D or K deficiency. Often it is possible to maintain adequate vitamin levels with oral replacement using the water-soluble formulations of these vitamins. Vitamin E replacement is most difficult. High-dose oral replacement of vitamin E (i.e., 100 to 150 U/kg) should be tried first, but if it is unsuccessful, parenteral supplementation from once a week to every other day may be necessary. A water-soluble preparation of vitamin E, alpha-tocopherol polyethylene glycol 1000 succinate, is currently under investigation and appears to be well absorbed by individuals who do not absorb other oral preparations. The liquid preparation of vitamin D, ergocalciferol, can be given at 1000 to 2000 units/day. If signs of vitamin D deficiency persist, the more potent 25 and 1,25 hydroxyvitamin D_3 products, calcifediol and calcitriol, respectively, can be tried. However, these formulations are also poorly soluble in water. Menadiol is a water-soluble preparation of vitamin K that is available in 5-mg tablets. For an infant, one-half tablet crushed in feedings every other day may be adequate. Phytonadione, the other oral preparation of vitamin K, is not water-soluble and therefore is less useful in the treatment of fat malabsorption. Measurement of the prothrombin time can be used as a indicator of adequacy of vitamin K repletion. Of the fat-soluble vitamin deficiencies, vitamin A deficiency is the most difficult to recognize clinically but can be confirmed by measuring serum levels. Deficiency of vitamin A may be treated adequately with oral doses of 5,000 to 10,000 U/day.

Other deficiencies that occur in generalized malabsorption states include deficiencies of zinc, iron, calcium, magnesium, folate, biotin, L-carnitine, and vitamin B_{12}. Maintenance of zinc homeostasis is a special problem because of the large losses of zinc in diarrheal fluid. Oral supplementation is usually initiated at 1 to 2 mg/kg of body weight of elemental zinc (a 220-mg tablet of zinc sulfate contains 50 mg elemental zinc). If iron supplementation by mouth (5 to 10 mg elemental iron per kg) does not correct iron deficiency, systemic administration is necessary. In the past, systemic replacement was done largely by intramuscular injection. This injection is painful and may stain the skin. Iron dextran can be added to TPN solutions and administered safely. Although a maintenance dose can be added daily, it is probably simplest to give this drug once a month. A test dose is given on the first day and, if tolerated without evidence of anaphylaxis or hypotension, replacement with standard quantities of iron dextran as recommended by the drug manufacturer can be provided subsequently. This approach appears to be very safe when the iron is administered slowly. A standard intravenous maintenance dose has not yet been established. Calcium malabsorption may be the result of both vitamin D deficiency and steatorrhea. The recommended normal daily dietary allowance for calcium varies from 360 mg in the first 6 months of life to 1200 mg at puberty. Oral supplementation for steatorrhea may require two to three times this dose. Generally, the dose of calcium is titrated until an adequate response is observed. Folic acid is available in a 1-mg tablet, which is more than adequate for daily oral supplementation. L-Carnitine is now available in 250-mg capsules, and adults may require up to three capsules a day. The pediatric dose should be scaled down appropriately for size. For all of these vitamins and trace elements, if oral replacement is unsuccessful, parenteral preparations are available (however, at the time of this writing the intravenous preparation of L-carnitine is an investigational drug). If vitamin B_{12} supplementation proves necessary, this vitamin can be administered in an intramuscular injection of 300 to 1000 μg every 2 to 3 months. For individuals receiving home TPN, daily doses of vitamins and trace elements, including vitamin B_{12}, can be provided in the TPN solution.

DISORDERS OF THE ANUS AND RECTUM

JOHN H. SEASHORE, M.D.

ANORECTAL MALFORMATIONS

Imperforate anus is a complex spectrum of malformations resulting from arrested development at any stage of embryogenesis of the hindgut. Clinically, these anomalies can be divided into three main categories depending on the relationship of the rectum to the puborectalis muscle. In *low* anomalies, the rectum has descended normally through the puborectalis muscle, there is no connection to the genitorinary tract, and meconium is usually discharged from an external perineal fistula. In *intermediate* anomalies, the rectum is at or below the level of the puborectalis muscle but is often displaced anteriorly, and there may be a persistent connection to the genitourinary tract. In *high* anomalies, the rectum ends above the puborectalis muscle, frequently as a fistula to the urinary tract or vagina. These distinctions are important in planning treatment and determining prognosis, since the puborectalis muscle is essential to achieve continence.

Renal ultrasonography is performed prior to discharge in all children who have anorectal malformations to search for major structural abnormalities of the urinary tract. Further evaluation is indicated if there is evidence of urinary tract infection, neurogenic bladder, or other symptoms. Ultrasound examination of the spine is also indicated to evaluate the infant for cord anomalies, particularly tethered cord, which have been identified with increasing frequency. If this study is not done in the neonatal period, magnetic resonance imaging is performed later.

Low Anorectal Malformations. *Imperforate anal membrane* is ruptured with a probe or small dilator and the accompanying anal stenosis is treated by serial dilations over several weeks until the anus accepts a 12-mm Hegar dilator without difficulty. *Anal stenosis* without an obstructing membrane may not be diagnosed until later in infancy and is also treated by serial dilatation. In *anterior ectopic anus* the anus is perfectly normal but is displaced anteriorly. These children have severe constipation and straining because of the sharp angulation of the anorectal canal. Generous doses of mineral oil usually relieve the symptoms, but if constipation persists, a posterior anoplasty is indicated. *Covered anus*, with or without *anocutaneous or anovestibular fistula*, is treated by perineal anoplasty. A cruciate incision through the anal dimple opens directly into the rectum, which is sutured to the skin. The anus is dilated for several weeks postoperatively to prevent stricture.

Intermediate Anomalies. In *ectopic perineal anus* the anal dimple and external sphincter are in the normal position, but the anal opening is located anteriorly in the perineum. The anus is stenotic and is treated initially by dilatation. At about 6 months of age an anal transposition is performed. The rectum is dissected from the surrounding soft tissues for several centimeters and then tunneled posteriorly and sutured to a cruciate incision in the anal dimple. The treatment of *rectovestibular fistula* in girls is the same, but special care is taken to avoid injury to the posterior vaginal wall. Boys who have the rare *rectourethral fistula* to the membranous urethra are treated by colostomy at birth. Sacroperineal reconstruction and division of the fistula are performed at 6 months.

High Anomalies. All high anomalies are treated by double-barreled transverse colostomy at birth. Barium studies through the distal limb of the colostomy are helpful to define the anatomy. Imaging of the pelvic muscles by magnetic resonance or computed tomography may be helpful to define the anatomy and plan surgery. Anorectal reconstruction is performed at 6 months of age. The anomaly is first approached posteriorly through a midline incision from the distal sacrum down through the anal dimple, which can be identified with a muscle stimulator if necessary. The levator muscles and the deep and superficial external sphincter muscles are divided in the midline. The coccyx is removed to facilitate identification of the distal rectum in the presacral space. The anterior wall of the rectum is carefully dissected to look for a fistula to the urethra or vagina. If a fistula is present, it is divided and both ends are oversewn. The rectum is mobilized circumferentially up to the peritoneal reflection, taking care to keep the dissection right on the rectal wall. In most patients, the rectum will then reach the perineum without tension. The distal end is opened and sutured to the skin at the inferior part of the incision. Moderate tapering of the distal 2 cm of rectum may be necessary to make it fit inside the external sphincter, but the bulbous nature of the rectum is preserved above this level to create an ampulla. The various components of the external sphincter and levator ani muscles are individually sutured together posterior to the rectum to complete reconstruction. The skin incision is closed with subcuticular sutures. If the rectum cannot be located easily in the presacral space or if the mobilized rectum does not reach the perineum, the wound is loosely closed and the infant is turned to the supine position. Laparotomy is performed and the rectosigmoid and sigmoid colon are mobilized to allow the rectum to reach the perineum without tension. The abdomen is closed, the patient is turned back to the prone position, the incision is reopened, and the operation is completed as described above. Girls who have a single perineal orifice have a *cloacal anomaly*. There are many anatomic variations of cloacal anomalies, and reconstruction can be very complex. In general, one-stage rectal and vaginal pull-through is preferred. The urogenital sinus is preserved as a urethra. Reflux of urine through large fistulas into the colon or vagina may lead to persistent urinary tract infection or hyperchloremic acidosis; early definitive surgery or division of the fistula may be necessary.

Long-term follow-up of children with high anorectal malformations is essential. Toilet training is difficult, and complete continence by age 3 or 4 is the exception. Bowel control slowly improves with time, but many children do not achieve an optimal result until the teenage years. Habit toilet training, dietary modification, and stool softeners are often helpful. Many of these children have sensory and motor deficits that make it difficult to achieve continence, but it appears that they gradually become aware of alternative sensory pathways and develop the perineal muscles to aid in bowel control. Coercive toilet training is discouraged. Ultimately, about 80 per cent of these children achieve normal or at least socially acceptable continence. Permanent colostomy may be the best solution for a few patients who have total failure of bowel control.

ANAL FISSURES

Fissures are treated by warm baths and liberal doses of mineral oil to soften and lubricate the stool. The dose of mineral oil ranges from 1 to 2 teaspoons a day in infants to 3 to 4 tablespoons a day in older children. For infants under 6 months of age, corn syrup or molasses extract accomplishes the same purpose and may be safer than mineral oil because of the risk of aspiration. The dose is adjusted to keep stools soft but not to the point of oozing. Treatment is continued for 1 to 2 weeks after the fissure heals. Vigorous treatment of fissures is indicated, since inadequately treated anal fissure is a common cause of chronic constipation and encopresis.

PERIANAL AND PERIRECTAL ABSCESS AND FISTULA

Superficial abscesses are incised and drained in the office, but deep abscesses should be opened under general anesthesia to allow adequate drainage. Anal fistulas, manifested by persistent drainage or recurrent abscess, are unroofed. Proctoscopy is helpful to identify the internal end of the fistula, which is opened in continuity with the incision. This may require cutting the external sphincter, but most fistulas in children are superficial to the sphincter. The lining of the sinus tract is curetted and the wound is packed open. Complete healing in 7 to 10 days is expected. Persistent perianal disease in an older child may be a manifestation of Crohn's disease.

RECTAL PROLAPSE

Rectal prolapse is most common in toddlers and is usually caused by straining to pass a large hard stool that overstretches the sphincter. The lax sphincter then allows prolapse to occur even without straining, and this prevents the sphincter from regaining its normal tone. Thus, treatment is directed toward preventing prolapse until tone is restored. Generous doses of mineral oil may be sufficient. Tight strapping of the buttocks with tape is also effective. Children who are toilet trained should use an appropriately sized potty chair to prevent spreading of the buttocks and to provide a firm platform for their feet. As long as the prolapse is easily reducible, persistence in these simple measures is indicated, since they almost always work. If the condition is progressive or does not resolve, several operations are available, but none is totally satisfactory.

TRAUMA

Most *foreign bodies* in the rectum pass spontaneously. The most common foreign body encountered in children is a broken rectal thermometer. More harm may be done by vigorous rectal examination or proctoscopy than by the foreign body itself. Careful observation and administration of mineral oil by mouth to facilitate passage are indicated. Large impacted foreign bodies should be removed; general anesthesia may be necessary to achieve adequate relaxation and dilatation of the anus.

Careful observation after any kind of rectal trauma is indicated, since initial examination may fail to reveal the full extent of the injury. The rectum is so short, especially in infants, that thermometers, sticks, and other pointed objects may cause intraperitoneal *perforation*. Unrecognized extraperitoneal perforations may also have serious consequences. The urinary tract and the vagina may be involved. If a more serious injury is suspected, examination under general anesthesia is performed. If gross or microscopic hematuria is present, a retrograde urethrogram and voiding cystourethrogram are performed preoperatively. Rectal perforations and lacerations are repaired as accurately as possible, and the perirectal space is drained. Most patients who have major rectal injuries require a temporary loop colostomy to divert the fecal stream while the wound heals. Urinary tract injuries are repaired, and suprapubic urinary drainage is established.

7

Blood

ANEMIA OF IRON DEFICIENCY AND CHRONIC DISEASE

NATHAN FISCHEL-GHODSIAN, M.D.

The anemias of iron deficiency and chronic disease are linked by a common lack in the availability of iron for heme synthesis. Whereas in iron deficiency anemia total body iron is depleted, in anemia of chronic disease iron stores are increased but the iron is not transferred to the red blood cell precursors where heme synthesis occurs.

IRON DEFICIENCY ANEMIA

Iron deficiency anemia results from inadequate dietary intake of iron, defective absorption through the intestinal mucosa, or blood loss. Frequently, especially in developing countries, a combination of these factors coexists. The laboratory diagnosis usually depends on a microcytic, hypochromic blood smear, a decreased serum iron, an increased iron-binding capacity, and a less than 15 per cent saturation of the iron-binding protein (transferrin). A quick and usually reliable bedside test is to look at the patient's plasma in a spun hematocrit tube, which in iron deficiency is strikingly pale.

Food Iron

The best therapy for most cases of iron deficiency anemia is dietary prevention. A growing child needs to absorb approximately 1 to 2 mg of iron per day. A mixed western diet of 1000 kilocalories contains 5 to 10 mg of iron, but only a fraction of this is absorbed. Each food therefore needs to be considered not only for the amount of iron it contains but, more importantly, for the availability of its iron for absorption. Heme iron from hemoglobin and myoglobin in meat, poultry, and fish is well absorbed but represents usually only a small fraction of the total iron in the diet. Nonheme iron, on the other hand, which represents over 90 per cent of iron in most diets, is poorly absorbed, and its absorption depends on the type of food and presence of other foods eaten at the same time. In general, the absorption of nonheme iron from foods of animal origin is much greater than from foods of vegetable origin. In addition, iron from meat and fish is better absorbed than iron from eggs and cheese. The presence of ascorbic acid and meat in the diet increases nonheme iron absorption significantly, whereas tea and fiber inhibit absorption. For infants it is important to realize that breast milk not only contains slightly more iron than cow's milk or formula not supplemented with iron (1.5 mg/L versus 0.5 to 1 mg/L) but is also much better absorbed (50 per cent versus 10 per cent or less).

In addition, cow's milk causes microinjuries to the intestinal mucosa in infants, leading to small bleeds and additional iron losses. It should also be noted that the absorption of iron from breast milk can be significantly inhibited by solid foods given near the time of breast feeding. Vegetarians should be advised to eat ascorbic acid–containing vegetables (e.g., cauliflower, citrus fruit) or supplement their meals with ascorbic acid. They should also avoid tea during or after meals.

Blood Loss

Iron deficiency due to blood loss is usually caused by recurrent bleeding from the gastrointestinal tract, although occasionally recurrent nose bleeds, soft tissue bleeds in hemophiliacs, or uterine bleeding can be responsible. Gastrointestinal blood loss is most frequently due to cow's milk in infancy, infectious or inflammatory bowel disease, ulcers, or Meckel's diverticulum. Usually the bleeding is chronic and therefore even at extremely low hemoglobin levels there is often no cardiovascular compromise. Iron replacement therapy (see below) can be started, the cause for the blood loss evaluated and treated, and blood transfusions avoided. The patient needs, however, to be observed very closely, since the response to iron takes a few days and if the cause for bleeding is, for example, a Meckel's diverticulum, a further bleed may cause cardiovascular decompensation. If there is cardiovascular compromise or the risk for recurrent bleeding at very low hemoglobin levels is high, a blood transfusion should be given. Since most patients are normovolemic, a partial exchange transfusion with 5 to 10 ml/kg of packed red blood cells is recommended. This is done most easily by taking out 20 to 40 ml of the very dilute patient blood, infusing the same amount of packed red blood cells, and repeating the procedure as required. Alternatively, a very slow infusion of initially not more than 3 ml/kg of packed red blood cells can be given. Whole blood should be avoided because of the danger of volume overload. It should be stressed that transfusions are only very rarely required in iron deficiency anemia, and therefore I recommend the involvement of a hematologist if a transfusion is considered.

Iron Replacement

The treatment of choice for iron replenishment in almost all cases is oral administration of ferrous sulfate. Ferrous gluconate and ferrous fumarate are as effective but slightly more expensive. Numerous other iron preparations are promoted with claims of improved palatability, enhanced absorption, or fewer side effects. Most of these preparations are therapeutically inferior to ferrous sulfate, and all are more expensive. Practically it is important to be aware that if ferrous sulfate is prescribed generically, the choice of preparation is left to the pharmacist, many of whom will dispense enteric-coated or sustained-release tablets. Those release iron only after passage through the duodenum, and therefore absorption is much less efficient. This may be the cause for failure to respond to iron therapy. Although ascorbic acid, succinate, and fructose have been shown to enhance iron absorption, there is no advantage to using iron preparations containing them. They potentiate the side effects of oral iron and are more expensive, and the same therapeutic effect can be achieved by a small increase in the dose of ferrous sulfate alone.

The elemental iron content of the ferrous salt is used for dosage calculation. For ferrous sulfate the elemental iron content is 20 per cent by weight. An optimal therapeutic response is obtained with 3 to 6 mg/kg/day of elemental iron (15 to 30 mg/kg/day of ferrous sulfate) with a maximum dose of 180 mg/day of elemental iron. Ferrous sulfate can be given in different forms to children of different ages. Infants and small children can use a calibrated dropper with a solution containing 15 mg elemental iron per 0.6 ml. Toddlers can use syrup or elixir containing 30 or 45 mg of elemental iron per 5 ml, and older children can use tablets or capsules containing 40 or 60 mg of elemental iron. The total dose is usually divided into 2 to 4 portions and given either before meals or with meals. Absorption is about twice as good when the medication is given on an empty stomach than with a variety of different meals, but the frequency of side effects is slightly higher. Younger children and infants usually have fewer side effects and therefore can, in most cases, tolerate two doses 30 to 60 minutes before meals per day. Infants can even be given a single dose of 3 mg/kg/day of elemental iron before breakfast. The simplicity of these regimens increases compliance.

Side effects of oral iron therapy occur only rarely in children and include mainly constipation, abdominal cramps, and nausea. If they occur, smaller, more frequent doses should be given with meals. If side effects persist, a different preparation may be tried, and if that fails dosage should be reduced by 50 per cent. Stools usually become black, which must be differentiated from melena. The stool guaiac test should remain negative, since it reacts with heme rather than iron. Iron staining of the teeth may occur with liquid preparations. However, such staining is not permanent and can be minimized by administering the drops on the back of the tongue or by letting the child take the medication with a straw. Accidental iron poisoning should be avoided by using bottles equipped with safety caps and having parents dispense the medication.

The first improvement after starting therapy is a subjective feeling of having more energy, better appetite, and better mood. A reticulocytosis can at the earliest be noted after 3 to 4 days and reaches maximal levels of up to 10 per cent during the second week. At this time the hemoglobin concentration starts to rise, reaches a level midway between the initial value and that which is normal within 3 to 4 weeks, and normalizes within 2 to 3 months. Therapy should be continued for 2 months after correction of the anemia to replenish iron reserves, but should not be extended beyond that time in order to avoid iron overload.

Treatment failure or suboptimal response to iron is most frequently due to failure to administer the iron, inadequate dosage, use of an iron preparation that is poorly absorbed, or ongoing blood losses. Less frequently it is due to coexistent chronic disease that compromises iron utilization in the marrow or to iron malabsorption.

Intramuscular or intravenous iron in the form of iron-dextran (Imferon) is indicated only when compliance with oral therapy cannot be obtained or if significant iron malabsorption is present. The rate of the hemoglobin rise is not greater than with oral therapy. Imferon is marketed as a dark brown solution containing 50 mg/ml of elemental iron. The total dose can be calculated as follows: 2.5 mg/kg of elemental iron raises the hemoglobin concentration by 1 gm/dl and an additional 10 mg/kg is given to replenish the iron stores. The dose per day should not exceed 0.1 ml/kg with a maximum of 2.0 ml. Intramuscular injections are given into the upper outer quadrant of the buttock. They tend to stain superficial tissue, and therefore a separate needle should be used for injection as well as retracting the skin and subcutaneous tissue laterally prior to insertion of the needle. This reduces but does not eliminate the risk of staining. Local pain and systemic symptoms ranging from fever to anaphylaxis can occur. Intravenous injections do not have the local pain and staining problem but can cause thrombophlebitis and all of the systemic complications. Anaphylaxis occurs in less than 1 per cent of patients, is dose-independent, and necessitates close observation after each parenteral administration of iron. Deaths from anaphylaxis after Imferon have been reported.

ANEMIA OF CHRONIC DISEASE

A wide variety of chronic infectious, inflammatory, metabolic, and malignant diseases are associated with a defect in the transfer of iron from the macrophages into the red blood cell precursors in the marrow. The resultant anemia is usually mild to moderate with a hemoglobin concentration of 7 to 11 gm/dl. The red blood cells are sometimes normochromic and normocytic but more frequently mildly hypochromic and microcytic. Plasma iron as well as iron-binding capacity are low, serum ferritin is normal or high, and macrophage iron in the bone marrow is increased. The anemia can be aggravated or obscured by the primary disease, such as chronic blood loss or iron malabsorption in gastrointestinal disease, bone marrow replacement in malignancies, absent erythropoietin in chronic renal failure, and drug-induced bone marrow suppression or hemolysis. The significance of the anemia is its disclosure of a primary disease, and therapeutic efforts should be focused on the underlying disease.

In patients with chronic renal failure, recombinant human erythropoietin, if available, can be used to increase the hemoglobin concentration and in most cases to avoid transfusions. In addition, these patients' subjective well-being improves significantly. However, caution must be exercised to control the side effects of an increased red cell mass such as hypertension and increased viscosity. For this reason the hematocrit is not allowed to increase over 35 and the rate of rise should not exceed 1 gm/dl/week. The usual starting dose is 250 mg/kg subcutaneously three times a week.

APLASTIC ANEMIA

CARL LENARSKY, M.D.,
and ROBERT L. BAEHNER, M.D.

Aplastic anemia is characterized by absent or defective hematopoiesis. Although drugs, chemicals, viral infections, and radiation may be implicated, the etiology is, in most cases, unknown. Aplastic anemia encompasses a spectrum of pathogenic processes with the common clinical features of anemia, granulocytopenia, thrombocytopenia, and a hypocellular bone marrow. Potential pathogenic mechanisms include direct injury to hematopoietic stem cells, abnormalities of marrow microenvironment, and immune-mediated suppression of hematopoiesis. Most cases of aplastic anemia are acquired forms of the disease, although congenital forms of aplastic anemia do exist. Patients with severe aplastic anemia are usually defined as having at least two of the following: granulocyte count below 500/mm³, platelet count below 20,000/mm³, and reticulocyte count below 1 per cent after correction for hematocrit. In addition, the bone marrow biopsy is hypocellular. In severe aplastic anemia (SAA), a specific therapeutic protocol must be instituted.

1. The treatment of choice for children with SAA is histocompatible allogeneic bone marrow transplantation. Therefore, once the diagnosis of SAA is established, the patient and immediate family members should have HLA typing performed. If an HLA-MLC–compatible family member is identified (usually a sibling), arrangements should be made for bone marrow

transplantation. The cost for the procedure is usually between $100,000 and $200,000, but cure rates for children now exceed 80 per cent.

2. Transfusion of blood products should be minimized to reduce the risk of alloimmunization, especially for patients who are eligible for marrow transplantation. If possible, red cells transfused should be washed and leukocyte depleted. The hemoglobin level should be maintained above 7.0 gm/dl. Platelet transfusions are rarely needed if the platelet count exceeds 20,000/mm³. Indications for transfusion of platelets include life-threatening bleeding (usually gastrointestinal or neurologic) and petechial hemorrhages in the fundi. The expected increment from a platelet transfusion is 10,000/mm³ per square meter of body surface area for each unit. A simple calculation for determining the number of units of platelets to administer is 4 units/m² or 1 unit/13 lb. Procedures are now available to prepare leukocyte-poor platelets; these should be utilized when possible. Bleeding in thrombocytopenic patients may be decreased by administration of epsilon-aminocaproic acid (Amicar) 100 mg/kg every 6 hours. Prophylactic granulocyte transfusions have not been shown to be useful despite low absolute granulocyte counts. Granulocyte transfusions may be useful for the treatment of documented sepsis not responding to appropriate antibiotic therapy when the absolute granulocyte count falls below 500/mm³. HLA-matched unrelated donors and single donors are ideal for platelet and granulocyte transfusions in these patients. Patients who are candidates for bone marrow transplantation should not receive transfusion of blood products from family members, since such transfusions may increase the risk of graft rejection.

3. Since the majority of patients with SAA do not have an HLA-matched sibling donor for a marrow transplant, alternative therapies for SAA have been developed. Antithymocyte globulin (ATG) is effective in improving hematopoiesis in some patients with SAA, with an overall response rate, including partial as well as complete remissions, of 50 per cent. The mechanism of action is unknown. ATG may be given 20 mg/kg/day for 7 to 10 days. ATG should not be given to patients with known sensitivity to horse serum. An ATG skin test should be done before systemic administration. If a patient has a systemic reaction to the skin test, further administration of ATG is contraindicated. The side effects of ATG include fever, chills, skin rash, arthralgias, abdominal pain, and liver dysfunction. Prednisone (2 mg/kg/day) is administered for 1 to 2 weeks to reduce the symptoms of serum sickness. Platelet levels should be maintained above 20,000/mm³ during ATG therapy. An improvement in hematopoiesis following ATG therapy generally requires 1 to 3 months.

4. Patients with SAA who are unresponsive to ATG may respond to a trial of high-dose bolus corticosteroids. Methylprednisolone is given in doses of 20 mg/kg/day intravenously for 3 days, then 10 mg/kg/day for 4 days, then 5 mg/kg/day for 4 days, then 2 mg/kg/day for 9 days, then 1 mg/kg/day for 10 days.

5. Androgen therapy is generally ineffective for patients with SAA. However, patients with acquired aplas-

tic anemia of moderate severity or with congenital forms of aplastic anemia may respond to androgens. A rise in the reticulocyte count, with a subsequent rise in the level of hemoglobin, occurs within 6 to 12 weeks in the responsive patient. Platelet and granulocyte levels are slower to respond to therapy. The choice of androgens is important. Some patients may respond to one agent and then relapse and require a different one. We have employed nandrolone decanoate, 1.0 to 1.5 mg/kg IM weekly or twice monthly, since liver dysfunction is rarer with this preparation. Oral androgen preparations include oxymethalone (dihydrotestosterone), 2.0 to 6.5 mg/kg/day, and methandrostenolone (Dianabol), 0.25 to 0.5 mg/kg/day. Other parenteral preparations include testosterone enanthate in oil, 4 mg/kg IM weekly. If there is no response in 4 months, androgen therapy should be discontinued. Side effects of androgen therapy include hirsutism, deepening of the voice, acne, flushing of the skin, nausea, and sodium and fluid retention. Liver function (SGOT, SGPT, bilirubin, alkaline phosphatase) should be monitored closely; abnormalities usually cease when the drug is stopped. Most responsive patients can be weaned from the drug or given it intermittently to maintain hemoglobin levels above 9.0 gm/dl.

6. Cyclosporin A has been utilized with success in a small number of patients with SAA unresponsive to ATG and/or methylprednisolone. The optimal dose and regimen have not been determined. Doses of 10 to 15 mg/kg/day PO for several months have been administered. Side effects include hypertrichosis, gingival hyperplasia, and mild reversible nephrotoxicity.

7. Current investigative trials include the use of various hematopoietic growth factors produced with recombinant DNA technology. Granulocyte-macrophage colony–stimulating factor (GM-CSF) is one such growth factor currently undergoing clinical trials for patients with SAA. Other experimental options include bone marrow transplantation utilizing an unrelated HLA-matched donor located via the National Marrow Donor Program. Families and patients with SAA may obtain more information about this disease from the Aplastic Anemia Foundation of America (telephone number: 301-955-2803).

MEGALOBLASTIC ANEMIA

PHILIP LANZKOWSKY, M.D.

Megaloblastic anemias in children are relatively uncommon and usually are due to folate or vitamine B_{12} deficiency. Most cases are due to folate deficiency. The causes of folate deficiency include inadequate diet, decreased absorption, which may be congenital or acquired (malabsorption syndrome), drug-induced inhibition of dietary folate absorption (phenytoin, phenobarbital), increased folate utilization (growth, malignant disease, hemolytic anemias), and drug-induced inhibition of folate metabolism (methotrexate, pyrimethamine, trimethoprim). The causes of vitamin B_{12} deficiency include dietary insufficiency (rare), absence or abnormality of gastric intrinsic factor, abnormal absorption of the vitamin B_{12} intrinsic factor complex due to previous small intestinal surgery or lack of intestinal receptors (rare), and inherited abnormalities of vitamin B_{12} transport protein.

Rarer metabolic causes of a macrocytic anemia, that is, thiamine deficiency, have occurred in products of consanguineous marriages who have presented neurologic abnormalities. The anemia was responsive to 25 mg of thiamine daily. Inborn errors of pyrimidine and purine metabolism (e.g., orotic aciduria and Lesch-Nyhan syndrome) can be treated with uridine and adenine, respectively. These conditions are unresponsive to folate and cobalamin.

The metabolism of folic acid and vitamin B_{12} is interrelated, however, and this must be considered when therapy is instituted. Large doses of vitamin B_{12} may correct the hematologic problems due to folate deficiency. Conversely, large doses of folate may correct the hematologic disturbances due to lack of vitamin B_{12}. Folate, however, will not correct the neurologic problem associated with vitamin B_{12} deficiency, and large doses of folate should not be given until vitamin B_{12} deficiency has been excluded.

Successful treatment of patients with *folate deficiency* involves (1) correction of the folate deficiency; (2) amelioration of the underlying disorder, if possible; (3) improvement of the diet by increased folate intake; (4) follow-up evaluations at intervals to monitor the patient's clinical status.

In cases of suspected folate deficiency, a therapeutic trial can be instituted with 50 to 100 µg of folate per day orally. This dose produces a prompt reticulocytosis in cases of folate deficiency but is without effect in patients with vitamin B_{12} deficiency. An optimal response occurs in most patients with 100 to 200 µg folic acid daily. Nevertheless, it is usual to treat deficient patients with 0.5 mg to 1.0 mg daily orally. Commercially available preparations include a tablet (0.3 to 1.0 mg) and an elixir (1.0 mg/ml). To reduce the folate content would not significantly reduce the cost, and since pteroylmonoglutamic acid rarely produces side effects except in patients with vitamin B_{12} deficiency, there is little reason to reduce the dose. Further, a smaller oral dose might not always be effective in patients with folate malabsorption. In most patients, 5 mg of folic acid given orally daily for 7 to 14 days induces a maximal hematologic response and significant replenishment of body stores. This may be given orally, since even in those with severe malabsorption, sufficient folate is absorbed from this dose to replenish stores. Before folic acid is given (in these large doses) it is always necessary to ensure that vitamin B_{12} deficiency is not present.

The clinical and hematologic response to folic acid is prompt. Within 1 to 2 days the patient's appetite improves (often becoming voracious) and a sense of well-being returns, with increased energy and interest in surroundings. There is a fall in serum iron (often to low levels) in 24 to 48 hours, a rise in reticulocytes in 2 to 4 days reaching a peak at 4 to 7 days, followed by a return of hemoglobin levels to normal in 2 to 6 weeks. The leukocytes and platelets increase with the reticulocytes, the megaloblastic changes in the marrow diminish within 24 to 48 hours, but large myelocytes, metamyelocytes, and band forms may be present for several days.

The duration of therapy depends upon the underlying pathology, but usually folic acid is given for several months until a new population of red cells has been formed. It is often possible to correct the cause of the deficiency and prevent recurrence of the deficiency, e.g., by an improved diet, a gluten-free diet in celiac disease, or treatment of an inflammatory disease such as tuberculosis or Crohn's disease. In these cases, there is no need to continue folic acid for life. In other situations, however, it is advisable to give folic acid continually to prevent recurrence of the deficiency, e.g., chronic hemolytic anemia such as thalassemia or in patients with malabsorption who do not respond to a gluten-free diet.

Patients receiving drugs that are folic acid antagonists (methotrexate, pyrimethamine) occasionally develop megaloblastic anemia. Trimethoprim, a pyrimidine analogue, inhibits the enzyme that reduces dihydrofolate to tetrahydrofolate. In some cases folate deficiency can be severe, especially in patients with marginal or depleted folate stores. In these cases the antagonism can be overcome by folinic acid, one 5-mg tablet daily.

In cases of a functional deficiency of folate or cobalamin such as occur in an inborn error of metabolism or transport, only massive doses of vitamin may be helpful. These cases are diagnosed only by appropriate biochemical tests, often on cultured fibroblasts obtained by skin biopsy. Inborn errors are rare and patients often show mental deficiency, aminoacidemia, and growth failure rather than simple cases of anemia.

In conditions in which there is a risk of developing *vitamin B$_{12}$ deficiency*, e.g. total gastrectomy or ileal resection, prophylactic administration of vitamin B$_{12}$ should be prescribed.

Patients with suspected vitamin B$_{12}$ deficiency are given a therapeutic trial with 25 to 100 µg of vitamin B$_{12}$. This dose corrects the hematologic problem due to this vitamin deficiency but does not correct the defect in folate-deficient patients. The reticulocyte response to this therapy is similar to that noted in folate deficiency.

Optimal doses for children are not as well defined as those for adults. When the diagnosis is firmly established, several daily doses of 25 to 100 µg may be used to initiate therapy. Alternatively, in view of the ability of the body to store vitamin B$_{12}$ for long periods, maintenance therapy can be started with monthly intramuscular injections in doses between 200 and 1000 µg. Most cases of vitamin B$_{12}$ deficiency require treatment throughout life.

Patients with defects affecting the intestinal absorption of vitamin B$_{12}$, either because of abnormalities of intrinsic factor or of ileal uptake, respond to parenteral vitamin B$_{12}$. Such a therapeutic maneuver completely bypasses the defective step and is the chief means by which these two groups of patients are managed currently.

Patients with complete transcobalamin II deficiency respond only to large amounts of B$_{12}$ (1 mg intramuscularly twice or three times weekly). The exact mechanism of this response remains to be defined.

Patients with methylmalonic aciduria with defects in the synthesis of vitamin B$_{12}$ coenzymes are likely to be benefited by massive doses of vitamin B$_{12}$ (1 to 2 mg vitamin B$_{12}$ parenterally daily). However, not all patients in this group are benefited by vitamin B$_{12}$.

In vitamin B$_{12}$–responsive megaloblastic anemia, the reticulocytes begin to increase on the third to fourth day, rise to a maximum on the sixth to eighth day, and fall gradually to normal on about the twentieth day. The height of the reticulocyte count is inversely proportional to the degree of anemia. Beginning bone marrow reversal from megaloblastic to normoblastic cells is obvious within 6 hours and is completely normoblastic in 72 hours.

Prompt hematologic responses are also obtained with the use of oral folic acid. Folic acid, is, however, contraindicated, since it has no effect on neurologic manifestations and has been known to precipitate or accelerate their development. Indeed, megaloblastic anemia should never be treated before a serum folic acid or vitamin B$_{12}$ assay has determined the precise cause so that correct treatment can be administered. Iron is occasionally required when a generally inadequate diet has been given that is deficient in this mineral.

The indications for red blood cell transfusions are infection or incipient heart failure. For unknown reasons the bone marrow frequently is refractory to hematinic therapy during infections. When transfusions are indicated, packed red blood cells should be given at a very slow rate (2 ml/kg/hr).

HEMOLYTIC ANEMIA

CATHERINE S. MANNO, M.D.,
and FRANCES M. GILL, M.D.

Appropriate therapy for the hemolytic anemias can best be planned once the etiology of the hemolysis has been determined. The premature destruction of red cells in this diverse group of disorders is due to defects that are intrinsic (membrane defects, enzyme deficiencies, or hemoglobin disorders) or extrinsic to the cell. Hemolytic anemias can be congenital or acquired. Red cell destruction occurs in the intravascular space or in the reticuloendothelial system. Hemolysis results in reticulocytosis, elevation of the serum indirect bilirubin level, and a decrease in the serum haptoglobin level. Hemoglobinemia, hemoglobinuria, and an elevated serum lactic dehydrogenase level are characteristic of intravascular hemolysis.

Therapy depends upon the severity of the hemolysis as well as on the etiology. Since increased red cell production, with a consequent increase in nucleic acid production, occurs in all hemolytic disorders, folic acid requirements are increased. Supplementation with 1 mg folic acid daily meets the increased need.

Red cell transfusion therapy is necessary most often in the acute hemolytic anemias but may be necessary in chronic hemolytic states if the anemia suddenly worsens. This happens most frequently during aplastic crises when the bone marrow temporarily stops making red cells. Aplastic crises are usually due to parvovirus infections. In disorders with brisk hemolysis, the hemoglobin level will drop dramatically after only a few days of aplasia. If the hemoglobin level drops low enough to result in cardiovascular compromise, a small transfusion of red cells (usually 5 ml/kg of packed red blood cells) given carefully is necessary. One transfusion is usually sufficient.

In some of the disorders chronic hemolysis is severe enough to require regular transfusions with red cells. These should be given on a regular schedule to maintain a hemoglobin in the range of 10 to 12 gm/dl. Prior to the first transfusion, complete red cell antigen typing should be performed. Candidates for chronic transfusion therapy should be immunized against hepatitis B. If chronic transfusions are necessary over a period of years, accumulation of excessive iron occurs. For patients who no longer need red cell transfusions, excessive iron is best removed by therapeutic phlebotomies. If the need for transfusions continues, iron chelation with deferoxamine therapy is used.

Splenectomy is indicated in some patients. Destruction of damaged and antibody-coated red cells occurs in the reticuloendothelial system, primarily in the spleen. Splenectomy stops hemolysis in hereditary spherocytosis and significantly lessens red cell destruction in some of the other disorders. Patients undergoing splenectomy for red cell disorders appear at higher risk for fulminant bacteremia (due to *S. pneumoniae, N. meningitidis,* and *H. influenzae*) than those whose spleen is removed because of trauma. This risk of splenectomy appears to be higher in younger children, and elective splenectomy should be deferred until the child is at least 5 years old. Polyvalent pneumococcal vaccine, *H. influenzae* b conjugate vaccine, and quadrivalent meningococcal vaccine should be given prior to surgery, and prophylactic penicillin (250 mg of penicillin V orally twice a day) should be used daily after surgery. Careful evaluation of fever is mandatory in any patient who has undergone splenectomy.

MEMBRANE DISORDERS

Hereditary Spherocytosis. Hereditary spherocytosis is the most common hemolytic anemia among Northern Europeans. Since the degree of hemolysis ranges from barely detectable to severe, therapy must be determined on an individual basis. Splenectomy is curative, preventing future aplastic crises and stopping further formation of pigment gallstones, but is not necessary for all patients. Children often feel better with folic acid supplementation. If the patient develops fatigue or increased pallor, the hemoglobin and reticulocyte levels should be determined to see if an aplastic crisis is occurring.

Some infants have increased hemolysis during the first year of life, with a hemoglobin level as low as 7 to 8 gm/dl. If the child is growing and developing normally, red cell transfusions are not necessary. The hemoglobin level usually rises to 9 gm/dl or more after the first year. Occasionally the hemolysis may be so severe as to require regular or frequent red cell transfusions. These patients will benefit from splenectomy, which should be postponed until the patient is at least 2 years of age.

Pigmented gallstones have been reported in 23 per cent of patients with hereditary spherocytosis between the ages of 10 and 20 years. Despite the high incidence of gallstone formation, it is not known how many patients will develop cholecystitis. Although splenectomy will prevent future pigment gallstone formation, its performance solely for this purpose is controversial.

Hereditary Elliptocytosis. Hereditary elliptocytosis is less common than hereditary spherocytosis, and chronic hemolysis occurs in only about 12 per cent of patients. As in hereditary spherocytosis, some infants have marked hemolysis, which usually lessens after the first year. Treatment is similar to that for hereditary spherocytosis. Although splenectomy is not curative, the severity of the anemia almost always decreases after the procedure. The risk of pigment gallstone formation continues, however.

Other Membrane Disorders. The other congenital hemolytic disorders are much rarer. The forms of hereditary stomatocytosis can be managed like hereditary spherocytosis. In hereditary pyropoikilocytosis hemolysis may be severe from birth, and the infants often require regular red cell transfusions. In these cases it has been our practice to support the patient with chronic transfusions until the age of 2 or 3 years, when splenectomy is performed. Although hemolysis persists thereafter, regular transfusions usually are no longer needed. The severity of anemia is variable in congenital dyserythropoietic anemia, type II (known by the acronym HEMPAS). Some patients require transfusions from birth and early splenectomy. Others may be managed as patients with hereditary spherocytosis are managed. In HEMPAS iron overload is very common, and the patient must be monitored carefully for this.

ENZYME DEFICIENCIES

Energy requirements of the erythrocyte are met by production of ATP through glycolysis. Hemolysis results if red cell metabolism is altered by a deficiency of any of several enzymes in the glycolytic pathway, including those of the hexose monophosphate shunt. Deficiencies that cause chronic hemolysis have been called the congenital nonspherocytic hemolytic anemias.

G-6-PD Deficiency. The most common enzyme deficiency is that of glucose-6-phosphate dehydrogenase (G-6-PD). The two most common forms of this X-linked recessive disorder are the African and Mediterranean (Gd and Gd Mediterranean, respectively). The African deficiency occurs in about 10 per cent of American black males. Females are affected less frequently. Hemolysis is limited to acute episodes, beginning hours to days after oxidant stress to the red cells. The patients are well between episodes. Hemolysis is usually precipitated by drug or chemical exposure but occasionally by infection (e.g., hepatitis) or a severe metabolic disorder (e.g., diabetic acidosis). Since young red cells do contain some enzyme activity, hemolysis is usually self-limited. Red cell transfusions may occasionally be necessary. Avoidance of the inciting agents (see Table 1) will prevent almost all episodes of hemolysis.

Hemolysis in Gd Mediterranean deficiency may be severe, and exposure to oxidants produces hemolysis that may be fatal in a matter of hours. Since even young red cells are enzyme deficient, all red cells are susceptible to hemolysis. Transfusions are necessary in severe episodes. Neonatal hemolysis with hyperbilirubinemia can occur in this form. Exchange transfusions may be necessary. Oxidant drugs should be avoided.

In rare forms of G-6-PD deficiency hemolysis is chronic, resulting in anemia and hyperbilirubinemia. Acute exacerbations may require red cell transfusions, and aplastic crises can occur. Response to splenectomy is unpredictable. Vitamin E administration was not found to be helpful.

Other Enzyme Deficiencies. Deficiency of pyruvate kinase results in chronic hemolysis. The clinical spectrum ranges from mild anemia to severe anemia that requires regular transfusions. Splenectomy generally reduces or eliminates the transfusion requirement but does not eliminate hemolysis. Patients previously requiring regular transfusions may need phlebotomy therapy to remove excessive iron. Other enzyme deficiencies have been described but are rare.

HEMOGLOBIN DISORDERS

Sickle cell disease and the thalassemic disorders are discussed elsewhere. Hereditary alterations in the primary structure of hemoglobin can result in instability of the hemoglobin tetramer. The most common unstable hemoglobin is hemoglobin Köln. The severity of hemolysis in the unstable hemoglobin disorders ranges from mild to severe. Most patients require only folic acid supplementation and avoidance of exposure to oxidant drugs, which can exacerbate hemolysis. Rarely, patients require chronic transfusion therapy. Splenectomy may be beneficial in patients with severe, chronic anemia and in those who develop hypersplenism.

AUTOIMMUNE HEMOLYTIC ANEMIA

In most children autoimmune hemolytic anemia is an acute, self-limited disease. The onset of the anemia is usually very rapid, with an acute fall in the hemoglobin level over hours to days. The direct antiglobulin test (also called Coombs' test) result is positive in about 95 per cent of the cases, establishing the diagnosis. In

TABLE 1. Agents to be Avoided in G-6-PD–Deficient Patients

Acetanilid
Chloramphenicol
Chloroquine, pamaquine, primaquine, quinacrine
Fava beans
Methylene blue
Nalidixic acid
Naphthalene (moth balls)
Nitrofurantoin
Phenacetin
Phenylhydralazine
Sulfonamides (sulfanilamide, sulfacetamide, sulfapyridine)

children the disease is usually idiopathic or associated with transient infections. The hemolysis is due either to warm-reacting antibodies (usually IgG) or to cold-reacting agglutinins (usually IgH) or hemolysins.

Most cases in childhood are caused by warm-reacting antibodies and respond to corticosteroid therapy. Treatment should be started immediately in an attempt to prevent worsening of the anemia. The standard dose of 2 mg/kg/day of prednisone in two divided doses is used initially. If the child is severely ill, the equivalent dose of intravenous corticosteroid, usually hydrocortisone, is given. Response, which may be evident within 1 to 2 days, is heralded by clearing of hemoglobinemia and hemoglobinuria and stabilization of the hemoglobin level. Corticosteroid therapy is continued at the full dose until the hemoglobin level reaches about 10 gm/dl. A slow taper over many weeks can then be started. Too rapid a taper may result in an acute exacerbation. Hemolysis usually stops within 2 weeks, but the direct antiglobulin test may remain positive for several months. Most children have only one episode of autoimmune hemolytic anemia. The child who is markedly anemic and does not respond to the standard dose may benefit from a 5- to 7-day course of prednisone at 5 to 10 mg/kg/day. The dosage should be tapered after this short course.

Cold-reacting agglutinin disease is most frequently associated with infections, particularly those due to *Mycoplasma pneumoniae* and infectious mononucleosis. Hemolysis is usually mild and stops as the infection clears. Although most cases do not respond to prednisone, the disorder is usually so mild and transient that no other therapy is needed.

Red cell transfusions are not needed in most patients, even when the anemia is marked. The children should be placed at bed rest and observed carefully. Attention should be given to hydration. If signs of hypoxia or congestive heart failure develop or the hemoglobin falls to extremely low levels, a packed red cell transfusion is necessary. When cold-reacting antibodies are present, the blood must be warmed to body temperature by passage through a blood warmer before transfusion. It is often impossible to find a unit of blood that is compatible by routine blood bank techniques. Every effort should be made to identify the autoantibody, if it has red cell antigen specificity, and to use blood that lacks the antigen. Although transfusion of incompatible blood may increase the rate of hemolysis, it is often necessary to use the most compatible unit of packed cells available. A slow infusion of 5 ml of the unit is given. The patient's plasma should then be checked to see if the level of hemoglobin in the plasma has increased. The human eye can see even small amounts of hemoglobin, and visual inspection of plasma in a spun hematocrit tube is usually satisfactory to detect increased amounts of free hemoglobin. If there is no increase after the test dose, the transfusion may proceed slowly. One or two transfusions of 3 to 5 ml/kg each are usually sufficient to relieve symptoms. The hemoglobin level need not be raised to normal levels. If there is increased hemolysis, another unit should be tried with the same precautions.

Transfusions in the severely affected child may not produce a rise in the hemoglobin level. In these patients, a two-volume exchange transfusion or plasmapheresis with replacement by donor red cells is frequently effective in slowing hemolysis and obtaining a higher hemoglobin level. This may need to be repeated daily until the severe hemolysis abates. These forms of transfusion may also be beneficial to the child with severe hemolysis from cold-agglutinin or cold-hemolysin disease in whom prednisone is not effective.

Children who have slower onset of hemolysis or who have moderate anemia may report only fatigue. Prednisone therapy and bedrest until the hemoglobin level rises may be sufficient treatment. Patients who have a rapid fall of hemoglobin to very low levels may be gravely ill, requiring close observation and intensive care until their condition stabilizes. Patients with hemoglobinuria should receive intravenous hydration in an attempt to prevent renal tubular damage. Rarely, anuria results from the tubular damage, and the child will need temporary dialysis support.

The severely ill child with marked anemia who does not respond rapidly to prednisone may require other treatment. Although there is little experience to date, some patients have responded to high doses of intravenous immunoglobulin (1 gm/kg/day) to slow hemolysis and may require maintenance booster doses. Treatment with immunosuppressive agents should be reserved for the child with refractory acute anemia or for those with chronic or relapsing disease. Splenectomy may also be of benefit but is rarely necessary in acute autoimmune hemolytic anemia.

Acute autoimmune hemolytic anemia is sometimes accompanied by thrombocytopenia and less frequently by neutropenia. These usually resolve as the hemolysis improves. However, since some deaths result from hemorrhage, severe thrombocytopenia with bleeding should be managed aggressively with plasmapheresis, intravenous gamma globulin, or splenectomy.

In some children the course of the disease is chronic, lasting for more than 5 months, or relapsing. These children more frequently have an underlying disorder, such as collagen-vascular disease or immunodeficiency, and more frequently have associated thrombocytopenia or neutropenia. Acute relapses often respond to prednisone therapy, particularly those in patients with systemic lupus erythematosus. Chronic autoimmune hemolytic anemia is a difficult disease best managed by hematologists experienced in this disorder.

THALASSEMIA

CAROL B. HYMAN, M.D.

SPECIFIC TREATMENT

No specific treatment of the thalassemias is available. Bone marrow transplantation, primarily for young infants, is being tried. However, even if the transplant procedure is successful, it must be considered investigational, as the long-term risks from preparatory chemotherapy and/or radiation are not known. We do know that under present day management, most patients can expect to live to at least the third or fourth decade. Also, it can be anticipated that in the future drugs to increase hemoglobin synthesis and/or genetic engineering procedures will be effective in treating the basic abnormality.

SUPPORTIVE CARE

Transfusion Therapy. Patients who cannot maintain a hemoglobin level of approximately 7 gm/dl should be on a regular transfusion program to prevent chronic hypoxia and suppress ineffective erythropoiesis. A transfusion program to maintain the hemoglobin level at 10.5 gm/dl or greater will enable patients to feel well and carry out most age-appropriate activities. Young adults, especially those who are active, may feel better with a pretransfusion hemoglobin level of 12 to 13 gm/dl. This transfusion program will diminish or prevent development of the bony abnormalities usually associated with the thalassemias, decrease spleen size, and, to a lesser extent, improve growth and development. Dietary iron absorption is also decreased. It should be noted that once patients have become accustomed to a high hemoglobin level, symptoms may occur if the level is allowed to drop. For this reason, and because fluctuation in hemoglobin level is not physiologic, our patients are transfused at 2- to 3-week intervals. In fact, some patients require less blood on a biweekly than a triweekly schedule. Leukocyte-poor, i.e., filtered, frozen, or washed red cells less than a week old, should be used to avoid febrile reactions. Neocytes, the most recently produced red cells from a unit of blood, are being used at some centers. Given with partial exchange transfusion, the intertransfusion interval can be increased and total red cell requirement decreased by as much as one third. However, these procedures are costly and wasteful of blood, since only part of each unit is used. Caution should be observed with the rate of infusion of blood or other fluids in iron-loaded patients to prevent fluid overload or heart failure. The older the patient, the less tolerant he or she will be of fluctuations in blood volume. Our patients receive each unit over 3 to 4 hours and wait at least 2 to 4 hours between units. Adults may require 12 to 24 hours between units.

Nonimmune patients should receive hepatitis B vaccine.

Splenectomy. Splenectomy should be considered for correction of hypersplenism with a red cell transfusion requirement above expected (greater than 250 ml/kg/year), for leukopenia or thrombocytopenia, and for massive splenomegaly. Prior to determining whether the procedure should be done, the degree of hypersplenism and the risks of rupture from trauma or discomfort from spleen size should be weighed against the benefits of leaving the spleen in situ. The spleen's protective effect against severe overwhelming infection, especially from pneumococcus and *Haemophilus influenzae*, is well known. The role of the spleen as an innocuous storage site for excess iron is not well understood. The author feels it may offer a greater protective effect for the heart and other organs than has been previously appreciated, and this may be enough to counteract some of the risks of the higher transfusion requirement.

If splenectomy is necessary, consideration should be given to performing a partial splenectomy. At this time, partial splenectomy is not "standard procedure" for thalassemia, as data on its effectiveness are not available. If partial or complete splenectomy is planned, Pneumovax, a vaccine that provides partial immunity to some strains of pneumococci, should be given at least 2 weeks prior to the procedure. Patients and their parents should be educated about the risks of postsplenectomy infection, and this education should be reinforced repeatedly over the following years and for the lifetime of the patient. This education is more valuable than prophylactic antibiotics. However, prophylactic penicillin, 250 mg bid, should be prescribed and patients instructed to call WITHOUT DELAY if they develop fever of 101.5°F or above. Patients who live a distance from the medical center may be given a supply of ampicillin if they can be depended upon to call the physician and complete a course of therapy if needed.

Management of Chronic Iron Overload. Deferoxamine (DF) is the best iron-chelating agent available for clinical use. Its effectiveness depends on dose, time in blood stream, total body iron, and the chelatable iron pool. DF is expensive and 20 mg/kg per day is the most cost-effective dose, but higher doses increase iron excretion. DF must be given parenterally, as oral absorption is minimal. Daily intramuscular (IM) DF removes only one third of iron intake by transfusion, and subcutaneous (SQ) DF is inadequate to prevent continued iron accumulation. Therefore, we use a combined SQ-IV treatment program. SQ DF, 40 to 60 mg/kg over 8 to 10 hours, for 5 to 6 days per week is recommended. For SQ therapy, each 500 mg vial of DF is dissolved in 1.5 ml distilled water without preservative and the total volume increased to 7 ml, with distilled water or normal saline in a 10-ml syringe attached to a 25 G or a 27 G long tube butterfly needle. The needle is inserted in the thigh or lower abdominal wall, and the drug is administered by continuous infusion, using a mechanical pump. The maximum intravenous dose, 15 mg/kg per hour, is infused at the time of transfusion and, if possible, for 24 hours post transfusion or for as many hours as practical thereafter, as it has been found that there is greater iron excretion after than during transfusion. If this is not possible, intravenous pulse therapy for approximately 48 hours at regular intervals should be considered to prevent continued iron accumulation, or in older patients to lower the total body iron load. For infants and young children too small to use the pump, IM DF can be used. Although there is no consensus of opinion, the author believes that chelation therapy should begin when the patient is as young as possible to prevent the chelatable iron from being transported to the heart or other parenchymal organs. With DF, iron is excreted in the urine, coloring it orange-red, and in the stool in variable amounts. Toxicity is minimal, and side effects include abdominal discomfort, mild diarrhea, itching at the injection site and, with rapid intravenous infusions, possible lowering of the blood pressure. Cataracts may occur but are very rare. Therefore, the patient should be seen by an ophthalmologist at 6-month intervals. To ensure the availability of chelatable iron, ascorbic acid, 50 mg, should be given after the daily dose of DF is started. Vitamin C without DF or in large doses is contraindicated, as it can increase iron toxicity, especially to the heart and, if given with meals, can increase food iron absorption.

Hearing should be monitored because sensorineural hearing loss has been reported, especially in young children on high-dose Desferal therapy.

Diet. Patients should be advised to avoid citrus and other high vitamin C containing foods with meals. Tea and cocoa are excellent mealtime beverages, as they interfere with dietary iron absorption. Vitamin E supplements are necessary to counteract the oxidant effects of iron. Infants should receive 100 units, young children 200 units, and older children and adults 400 units per day. Folic acid, 1 mg per day, should be given to all patients.

Iron overload patients should avoid all raw seafood because of the possibility of contamination with organisms, which can cause overwhelming sepsis.

COMPLICATIONS OF THALASSEMIA AND CHRONIC IRON OVERLOAD

Cardiac. The primary cause of death in thalassemia is cardiac disorders. Congestive heart failure, arrhythmias, and pericarditis should be aggressively treated, preferably by a cardiologist familiar with cardiac problems due to chronic iron overload.

Diabetes and Other Endocrine Abnormalities. These should be managed as indicated. Patients who do not go through puberty or develop secondary sex characteristics should be given replacement therapy. Hypoparathyroidism with low serum calcium levels may occur and require treatment with calcium supplements or 1,25 vitamin D or both.

Magnesium Depletion. Magnesium depletion is a frequent problem and may manifest with increased neuromuscular irritability or with cardiac arrhythmias, eyelid twitching, generalized muscle aches, neck pain, and changes in affect. Hypomagnesemia must be corrected, as it may significantly increase cardiac arrhythmias from chronic iron overload. The serum magnesium level should be observed at regular intervals beginning in early childhood and, if low, oral magnesium supplements given. If oral magnesium supplements are insufficient to maintain the serum magnesium level, intravenous infusions of magnesium sulfate may be required.

THALASSEMIA INTERMEDIA

This clinical term includes those patients with beta-thalassemia syndromes who can maintain a hemoglobin level of 6 to 7 gm/dl or greater without regular transfusions. Each patient should be individually evaluated to determine if transfusion therapy and/or splenectomy is indicated, as symptoms may be severe and crippling. The long-term risks of chronic hypoxia and erythroid hyperplasia with osteoporosis, bony deformities, energy wastage, retardation of growth and development, and marked splenomegaly must be weighed against the problems associated with a chronic transfusion program. Severe hemosiderosis, from increased oral iron absorption, can be a significant problem and requires diet modification, including folic acid and vitamin E supplements as outlined above, and sometimes chelation therapy. After considering the factors discussed above, splenectomy or partial splenectomy may be necessary.

THALASSEMIA TRAIT

The diagnosis of beta-thalassemia trait (thalassemia minor) is important for three reasons: (1) to differentiate it from iron deficiency anemia and avoid the chronic use of hematinics. The exception is during pregnancy, when folic acid may prevent the hemoglobin from falling as low as would otherwise occur. (2) To reassure the affected individual that this is not a disease and will not cause illness or affect longevity. (3) For genetic counseling. Screening of family members who are potential parents should be carried out.

HEMOGLOBIN H DISEASE

This is a moderately severe form of alpha-thalassemia and manifests as thalassemia intermedia, with a hemoglobin level of approximately 7 to 10 gm/dl. Symptoms are usually less severe than those of beta-thalassemia intermedia, as ineffective erythropoiesis is less marked. Although these patients do not require regular transfusions, sporadic transfusions may be necessary. The red cells are susceptible to oxidant stress, so drugs such as sulfonamides, antimalarials, and high doses of salicylates should be avoided. Cholelithiasis, hypersplenism, and hemosiderosis from increased absorption of dietary iron may be problems. Splenectomy or partial splenectomy should be considered (as discussed above) for correction of severe hypersplenism. Diet modification and vitamin E supplements as outlined are advisable.

ADVERSE REACTIONS TO BLOOD TRANSFUSION

SAMUEL H. PEPKOWITZ, M.D.,
and DENNIS GOLDFINGER, M.D.

The transfusion of blood components carries with it many potential risks. Patients may experience adverse reactions to the cellular or noncellular constituents of blood; many such reactions are immunologically mediated. Many infectious diseases harbored by a donor can be transmitted to the recipient. Infection also may be transmitted to the recipient by contamination of the blood during collection or storage. The anticoagulants and preservatives, as well as the accumulated products of cellular metabolism and breakdown, can cause undesired effects. Whenever the decision is made to transfuse a blood component, the relative hazards of the transfusion should be balanced against the possible benefits to the recipient. Only when the patient is clearly

in need of transfusion, and the potential value outweighs the risk, should the component be transfused.

Transfusion reactions often are totally avoidable; therefore, the key to safe transfusion therapy is prevention of reactions rather than treatment. When transfusion is necessary, the likelihood of adverse effects can be minimized by careful selection of the proper blood component. Close clinical monitoring of patients receiving transfusions can result in early detection of adverse reactions and prevention of serious complications, should such reactions ensue. By discontinuing transfusion at the onset of a reaction, thereby limiting the quantity of blood product transfused, serious complications can often be avoided.

REACTIONS TO RED BLOOD CELLS

Acute Hemolytic Transfusion Reactions. Red blood cells may be transfused to treat either acute or chronic anemia and may be administered as packed, washed, frozen deglycerolized, leukocyte-poor filtered red blood cells, or as whole blood. The most feared complication of such transfusion is the acute hemolytic transfusion reaction. This reaction may result when the patient possesses antibodies directed against the transfused red blood cells. Usually, the most severe reactions are caused by ABO incompatibility, although equally dangerous reactions may result from antibodies to other (minor) red blood cell antigens. The most common cause for ABO-incompatible transfusion is clerical error (i.e., the patient is given the wrong unit of blood). Occasionally passively acquired anti-A or anti-B antibodies present in incompatible plasma, if of high enough titer, may cause acute reactions.

Acute hemolytic transfusion reactions must be prevented rather than treated. Sophisticated serologic techniques have been developed for the detection of abnormal red blood cell antibodies that may be directed against one or more of the minor red blood cell antigens. Therefore, the danger of acute hemolytic transfusion reactions in alloimmunized recipients has been reduced significantly. Reactions due to ABO incompatibility can be avoided effectively by paying meticulous attention to positive identification of the unit of blood to be infused and the intended recipient. The process that ensures that errors in identification do not occur begins with proper collection of the pretransfusion blood specimen for typing and cross-matching, extends to careful handling of the patient blood sample and units of blood in the blood bank, and ends with positive identification of the patient and the unit of donor blood prior to the start of transfusion.

If a patient receives incompatible red blood cells and develops an acute hemolytic transfusion reaction, two significant complications may ensue—acute renal failure and disseminated intravascular coagulation (DIC). Appropriately, treatment is directed toward preventing these complications. The most important therapeutic consideration is to minimize the volume of incompatible red blood cells transfused. Therefore, as soon as a transfusion reaction is suspected, the infusion of red blood cells should be stopped and the situation analyzed. Often acutely ill patients with suspected transfusion reactions are subsequently found to have coincidental sepsis or hypotension. This should be clarified as soon as possible so that additional transfusions can be given when needed. Usually, if only a small volume of red blood cells has been transfused, specific therapy is unnecessary even if an acute hemolytic reaction did occur (the designation of a "small" volume of red blood cells depends on the size of the recipient, but might be defined as an amount less than 5 to 10 per cent of the patient's blood volume). Additional red blood cell transfusion should be avoided until the cause for the hemolytic reaction has been identified and compatible blood can be provided safely.

Patients who receive relatively large volumes of incompatible red blood cells may develop hypotension, shock, and DIC. These complications, in turn, may lead to acute renal failure. It is now clear that renal failure is not caused by the action of hemoglobin on the kidney. Free hemoglobin is not directly toxic to renal tubular epithelium, nor does it precipitate in the tubules, causing blockage of urine excretion. Instead, renal failure, if it occurs, appears to be due to ischemic damage to the tubules, resulting from decreased renal cortical blood flow, either as a direct effect of systemic hypotension or a local effect due to organ-specific response to vasoactive substances. The widely held belief, therefore, that prevention of acute renal failure can be achieved by the use of diuretics to "flush out" the kidneys makes little sense. Instead, treatment should be aimed at restoration of normal blood circulation. Blood pressure should be maintained by the infusion of fluids (either colloids or crystalloids) and by the use of appropriate drugs. Those drugs that help restore systemic blood pressure, as well as improve renal cortical blood flow, probably are most useful. Dopamine would seem to be the most logical pharmacologic agent for achieving these objectives. However, this drug has not been used extensively in the specific treatment of acute hemolytic transfusion reactions, so its value cannot be stated with certainty.

The development of DIC is a significant risk for patients who receive large quantities of incompatible red blood cells. Early institution of anticoagulation with heparin might be of benefit in preventing this complication and should be considered on an individual basis (the potential benefits of heparinization must be weighed against the possible risks). Although "prophylactic" heparinization has never been evaluated as a treatment modality in patients suffering acute hemolytic transfusion reactions, it is a logical therapeutic intervention for preventing the often fatal complication of DIC, provided that it is instituted before significant activation of the clotting system has occurred. If prophylactic heparinization is deemed appropriate, fully anticoagulating doses should be used, unless relative contraindications exist. In this case, minidoses must suffice. Anticoagulation probably need be maintained only so long as the stimulus for DIC exists (perhaps 6 to 24 hours). This short course of therapy also serves to minimize the likelihood of hemorrhagic complications from heparin.

Delayed Hemolytic Transfusion Reactions. Patients receiving transfusions may become alloimmunized to red blood cell antigens. Months or years later, the concentrations of these antibodies present in the patient's plasma may decline to such low levels that they are undetectable by routine pretransfusion tests. If, under these circumstances, the patient again is transfused with red blood cells that possess an antigen to which sensitization has occurred previously, the patient may develop an anamnestic response, generating large quantities of antibody within days of transfusion. This may result in a delayed hemolytic transfusion reaction, with rapid destruction of the transfused red blood cells. The patient's hematocrit may fall and jaundice may develop. Although renal failure may be precipitated by a delayed hemolytic transfusion reaction, this is an extremely rare occurrence. Specific therapy usually is not indicated for patients suffering such delayed reactions. Instead, the most important factors are to recognize that a delayed hemolytic transfusion reaction has occurred, to avoid transfusion of additional incompatible red blood cells, and to identify the antigen(s) involved. As soon as the specificity of the offending antibody can be determined, it usually is possible to provide safe, compatible blood for further transfusion.

REACTIONS TO LEUKOCYTES OR PLATELETS

Febrile, Nonhemolytic Transfusion Reactions. Fever and chills are the most frequent adverse effects encountered in recipients of blood transfusions. While such signs and symptoms may result from the transfusion of incompatible red blood cells, their most common cause is from a reaction to transfused leukocytes, predominantly granulocytes. If fever or chills develop, the transfusion should be stopped immediately and an investigation begun to determine whether a hemolytic transfusion reaction has occurred. If there is no evidence of a hemolytic reaction, it can be assumed that fever has resulted from a reaction to leukocytes. No specific therapy is indicated for the fever, although antipyretics (e.g., acetaminophen) may be administered.

Patients who have suffered febrile, nonhemolytic transfusion reactions usually can be transfused safely with leukocyte-poor red blood cells. Further transfusion, therefore, should be accomplished with either saline-washed or deglycerolized frozen red blood cells, or red blood cells passed through leukocyte-absorbing filters. All these products are leukocyte-poor, but filters currently provide the most efficient removal. Filters to remove white cells from platelet concentrates are also available.

Alloimmunization to Leukocyte and Platelet Antigens. Transfusions of whole blood or packed red blood cells expose the recipient to large numbers of leukocytes and platelets. This could result in alloimmunization to leukocyte and platelet antigens. If it is desirable to prevent such sensitization, because of possible compromise of future granulocyte or platelet transfusions or because the patient may be a candidate for organ transplantation, red blood cell transfusions may be accomplished with leukocyte-poor blood components. Such products are less likely to sensitize the patient, owing to their reduced content of leukocytes and platelets.

Graft-Versus-Host Disease. Many blood components contain significant numbers of viable lymphocytes. If such immunocompetent lymphocytes are transfused to immunodeficient patients, the cells may survive, replicate, and initiate an immune response to the "foreign" appearing tissues of the recipient, producing the syndrome of graft-versus-host disease, a complication that is frequently fatal. Treatment of this reaction may be ineffective, so prevention is most important. The administration of 1500 to 3000 rads of radiation to lymphocyte-containing blood components (whole blood, red blood cells, platelet concentrates, granulocyte concentrates) renders the lymphocytes incapable of replication and prevents graft-versus-host disease. Therefore, severely immunoincompetent patients may be transfused safely with irradiated blood products. Patients requiring such irradiated products may include premature infants, those with certain congenital immunodeficiency syndromes, certain patients undergoing chemotherapy for malignancies, and perhaps HIV-infected individuals.

Post-traumatic Pulmonary Insufficiency. During the storage of units of blood, large numbers of microaggregates form, consisting of degenerated leukocytes and platelets and possibly fibrin. These particles may be small enough to pass through the standard 170-μ filter used for blood administration. Therefore, large amounts of particulate debris, ranging in size from approximately 20 to 150 μ, may be transfused to the patient. Since the first capillary bed encountered by the blood following intravenous infusion is in the lungs, the microaggregates become trapped at this point. It has been suggested that occlusion of the pulmonary microcirculation by transfused particulate debris may contribute to the development of post-traumatic pulmonary insufficiency, or "shock lung." The possible dangers of microaggregates in stored blood are greatest for patients receiving massive transfusion. Avoidance of infusion of microaggregates to patients receiving large amounts of blood can be achieved by transfusion of relatively fresh blood (less than 7 days old), by the use of special microaggregate filters, or by washing stored blood prior to transfusion. Saline-washed red blood cells have an additional advantage for patients receiving massive transfusion, in that the undesirable products of red blood cell metabolism, which accumulate in stored blood, also are eliminated during the washing procedure (see below).

REACTIONS TO SUBSTANCES CONTAINED IN PLASMA

Urticarial Transfusion Reactions. The development of hives during or shortly after transfusion is the second most frequently encountered transfusion reaction. These reactions are not dangerous and need not be investigated as possible hemolytic reactions unless other signs and symptoms suggestive of possible hemolytic reaction (e.g., chills or fever) also occur. Urticarial transfusion reactions can be treated with antihistamines (e.g., diphenhydramine [Benadryl]). Patients who have experienced repeated urticarial transfusion reactions should be treated with an antihistamine 30 minutes prior to transfusions or should receive washed or frozen red blood cells that are nearly devoid of plasma.

Anaphylactic Transfusion Reactions. Patients who are totally deficient in immunoglobulin A (IgA) proteins may develop severe anaphylactic reactions to transfusions of blood components containing IgA. These reactions can be prevented by transfusing washed or frozen red blood cells that are devoid of most plasma (and devoid of IgA proteins). If transfusions of platelet concentrates or fresh frozen plasma are required, these components must be collected from IgA-deficient blood donors. Registries of IgA-deficient blood donors are maintained by the American Red Cross and by several other blood banking institutions.

If a patient develops an anaphylactic transfusion reaction, treatment should be similar to that used for other forms of anaphylaxis. Treatment is aimed at combating respiratory distress and circulatory collapse. Epinephrine probably is the most useful drug to be used in this situation, as it is in other forms of anaphylactic shock.

Circulatory Overload. Patients who receive too much blood too quickly may develop acute volume overload. This can be an extremely severe, possibly lethal complication that could result in acute pulmonary edema or sudden death. In the case of red blood cell transfusion, circulatory overload is entirely preventable by following two simple rules: Nonbleeding, anemic patients should be transfused with packed red blood cells rather than whole blood; and they should receive no more than 15 ml of packed red blood cells per kilogram of body weight per day. This amount of red cells (having a hematocrit of approximately 75 per cent) should raise the patient's post-transfusion hematocrit by about 12 points, or 4 gm/dl of hemoglobin. Even severely anemic patients who are not bleeding seldom require immediate elevation of their hemoglobin concentration by more than 2 to 3 gm/dl/day.

The only time that volume overload should be risked is in the management of patients with coagulation factor deficiencies. For those deficiencies in which concentrates of the required coagulation factors are not available, it is necessary to administer the missing factor by transfusions of fresh frozen plasma. Relatively large amounts of fresh frozen plasma may be required in order to raise the concentration of a particular coagulation factor to hemostatic levels. Under these circumstances, diuretics can be administered in an effort to reduce the immediate circulatory overload. Alternatively, plasma exchange can be performed. Patients who show signs of cardiac failure from excessive transfusion should be treated in the same manner used to treat heart failure from other causes (e.g., diuretics, morphine, phlebotomy, and so on).

Transfusion of Antibodies to Red Blood Cells. Patients who receive plasma containing antibodies that react with their own red blood cells may develop hemolytic transfusion reactions. The most common cause for these reactions is the administration of ABO-incompatible plasma. This could result from transfusion of ABO-incompatible platelet concentrates (since each unit of platelets contains approximately 50 ml of plasma). The patient may develop a positive direct Coombs' test and evidence of mild hemolysis. Very rarely does a more severe, acute hemolytic transfusion reaction occur. This complication should be prevented by avoiding transfusion of excessive quantities of ABO-incompatible plasma.

Citrate Toxicity. Patients who receive large quantities of blood components may develop signs and symptoms of hypocalcemia, resulting from the infusion of citrate anticoagulant. This is rarely a significant problem, except for patients receiving massive amounts of blood (as in the case of exchange transfusion). To prevent or treat this complication, such patients may be given supplemental calcium solutions intravenously through a separate intravenous line. However, care must be taken not to give too much calcium, because iatrogenic hypercalcemia probably is a greater hazard than citrate-induced hypocalcemia.

Transfusion of Blood Cell Metabolites. During storage of blood components, there may be an accumulation of large quantities of lactic acid and ammonia from the metabolic activity of the various cellular constituents. In addition, significant amounts of potassium may leach out of the blood cells, resulting in concentrations of potassium as high as 75 mEq/L in the supernatant plasma. Complications from the infusion of these substances are likely to be a problem only in patients receiving massive transfusions or exchange transfusions. The risk of complications from these substances can be avoided best by transfusing relatively fresh blood products (less than 7 days old) to patients receiving massive transfusions. If relatively fresh blood is unavailable, saline-washed red blood cells may be substituted for packed red blood cells, since the washing procedure rids the red blood cells of unwanted contaminants.

INFECTIOUS COMPLICATIONS

Post-transfusion Hepatitis. Hepatitis remains the most frequent serious complication of blood transfusion. Studies conducted in the 1970s estimated that as many as 20 per cent of transfused patients acquired non-A, non-B hepatitis, and many such patients developed severe, chronic liver disease. Recently instituted surrogate tests for non-A, non-B hepatitis (i.e., alanine aminotransferase levels and testing for antibody to hepatitis B core antigen) are expected to drop this incidence to about 1 per cent per unit exposure. A specific test for the major agent of non-A, non-B hepatitis (hepatitis C) has been developed but is not yet ready for routine donor testing. The only sure means available for preventing post-transfusion hepatitis is by avoiding transfusions whenever possible and using only autologous products. In addition, products prepared from pooled plasma (e.g., lyophilized Factor VIII and Factor IX concentrates) should be avoided, if single donor blood components can be substituted safely. Repeated use of the same dedicated blood donor for the collection of multiple blood components can limit donor exposure and reduce the risk of disease transmission. Although it has been suggested that administration of immune serum globulin to recipients of transfusions may prevent some cases of hepatitis, studies of the efficacy of such prophylaxis are inconclusive, and routine administration of immune serum globulin to transfusion recipients currently is not recommended.

Cytomegalovirus Infection. There is substantial evidence that cytomegalovirus infection may be transmitted by blood transfusion. The risk appears to be greatest for relatively immunodeficient patients, especially neonates and recipients of organ transplants. Prevention may be possible by selecting blood from donors without cytomegalovirus antibodies (such "CMV-negative" donors are less likely to be cytomegalovirus carriers), or possibly by transfusing leukocyte-poor blood components, since the cytomegalovirus appears to be carried in peripheral blood leukocytes. Leukocyte-poor red blood cells may be supplied most efficiently by transfusing filtered or saline-washed red blood cells, since these products also may avoid many of the hazards of red blood cell transfusion therapy.

Human Immunodeficiency Virus. Careful donor screening by history and testing are used effectively to reduce the risk of transfusing HIV-infected blood. The current incidence of infective units is estimated at approximately 1 in 40,000. If such a unit is transfused, over 90 per cent of recipients will become infected with the virus. Red blood cells, platelet concentrates, fresh frozen plasma, and cryoprecipitate are all capable of transmitting HIV infection. Currently, the best means of prevention is through limiting donor exposure either by collecting autologous blood or by repeated bleedings of dedicated donors.

Human T-Cell Lymphotrophic Virus Type I. HTLV-I is also known to be transmissible by blood transfusion. Recently, HTLV-I antibody testing of blood donations was instituted to reduce such transmission. This program should be successful in preventing significant spread of this disease via transfusion.

Malaria. Transfusion-transmitted malaria is a known hazard of red blood cell transfusion, although its occurrence is extremely uncommon. Prevention is by excluding blood donors who are likely to be carriers of malarial parasites. Consideration of the rare complication of transfusion-transmitted malaria should be given to transfused patients who subsequently develop unexplained fever.

Transfusion of Contaminated Blood. Transfusion of blood that has been contaminated in vitro with bacteria can result in an extremely severe reaction, manifested by chills, fever, and circulatory collapse. The risk of blood contamination has been reduced to minimal levels by the development of blood collection systems that utilize sterile, disposable plastic bags instead of reusable glass containers. In the event that heavily contaminated blood is transfused, the patient will develop severe septic shock, and this must be treated with circulatory support and antibiotics.

MEASURES TO PREVENT REACTIONS

Autologous Blood. The use of autologous blood (the patient's own blood) for transfusion is certainly the best and safest method to prevent transfusion reactions. The technique of autologous blood transfusion is most often used for patients scheduled for elective surgical procedures. Patients may donate blood prior to surgery, and the blood can be stored either in the liquid or frozen state for subsequent reinfusion during surgery or postoperatively. Even relatively small children can donate blood safely, simply by removing a small volume of blood (e.g., one-half pint instead of a full pint) at each donation. These small volume collections can be pooled into volumes of approximately 1 pint and stored in the frozen state for up to 10 years until the time of surgery. Autologous transfusion eliminates almost all of the hazards of blood transfusion therapy, especially the risk of post-transfusion hepatitis and HIV transmission. Intraoperative salvage and reinfusion of shed blood is another technique that can limit exposure to allogeneic blood.

Directed Donor Blood. Directed donations are reserved for use only by a specific patient; if unused by this patient, they may be released into the general blood supply by the hospital blood bank. The safety of directed donations relative to the general blood supply varies; randomly asking a person's co-workers to donate for him or her may yield no added safety. But donations by parents and close friends and family members committed to a child's well-being may provide added safety, especially if repetitive donations are able to limit the number of allogeneic exposures. We especially find this to be valuable for neonates and cardiac surgery patients for whom red cells, platelets, and plasma can be provided from one donor. A type of graft-versus-host disease can occur even in immunocompetent recipients when donor and recipient HLA phenotypes allow engraftment. Therefore, cellular products from directed donors who are first-degree relatives of the recipient should be irradiated.

SICKLE CELL DISEASE

ROLAND B. SCOTT, M.D.,
and JOY H. SAMUELS-REID, M.D.

Rational therapy of this disease is based upon recognition that the syndrome consists of a number of clinical hemoglobinopathies of variable occurrence and morbidity. The most frequently encountered types in the United States are homozygous sickle cell disease (sickle cell anemia), sickle cell–hemoglobin C disease, and the sickle cell beta-thalassemia syndromes. The course of the disease is usually characterized by periods of remission (steady state) and exacerbation (crises). The approach to treatment is generally based upon the nature of the crises and the presence of complications.

PERIOD OF REMISSION

Anemia is usually not present at birth owing to the high concentration of fetal hemoglobin in the red blood cells of neonates. However, it characteristically appears 4 to 6 months postnatally and is persistent, in variable degree, for the remainder of life. In the absence of infections and complications, patients with this disorder tend to compensate reasonably well for the anemia during the steady state, and blood transfusions are not necessary when the patient is active and comfortable. In the periods between crises, opportunity should be taken to determine and record the physical and hematologic status of the patient. This is also an appropriate time to perform elective surgical and dental procedures. Folic acid in dosage of 1.0 mg/day is recommended to supply the need created by the hyperplasia and increased activity of the bone marrow in this disease.

Neonatal detection of sickle cell disease by hemoglobin electrophoresis on cord blood samples taken in the delivery room is now feasible. This offers an opportunity to place infants with sickle cell disease under parental and medical supervision and surveillance for the prevention and early detection of life-threatening infections such as sepsis, pneumonia, and meningitis. Inasmuch as *Streptococcus pneumoniae* is a common and virulent offender, some clinicians are now employing a preventive regimen of prophylactic penicillin administered orally daily or intramuscularly at monthly intervals during infancy. Pneumococcal vaccine (Pneumovac or Pnulmmune) is recommended for infants and children at ages 1 to 2 years or older.

ACUTE CRISES

Vaso-occlusive or Pain Crisis

Vaso-occlusive crises are the most frequently observed variety. They vary considerably in frequency, duration, and degree of intensity. Analgesics and adequate hydration are the two most dependable agents for the control of acute pain. Mild forms with bearable pain and lassitude can often be treated in the home with bed rest and water or other fluids orally (20 ml per kg of body weight per 24 hours divided into four or more portions). Acetaminophen is recommended in single doses of 60 mg for infants under 1 year and as follows for other ages: children 1 to 4 years: 60 to 120 mg; 4 to 8 years: 120 to 240 mg; 8 to 12 years: 240 mg.

If persistent pain is not relieved by the above drugs, then codeine phosphate alone or in combination with Empirin or Tylenol may be used. The dose of codeine for children 12 years and younger is about 3 mg/kg/24 hr divided into six doses. The elixir of Tylenol with codeine (12 mg codeine phosphate per teaspoonful) is a convenient analgesic for administration to small children. In patients 12 years of age or older the following agents are often effective in relieving moderate to severe pain associated with vaso-occlusive crises:

Codeine phosphate—15 to 30 mg, often prescribed orally in such compounds as Tylenol or Empirin.
Meperidine—usually administered intramuscularly in doses of 30 to 70 mg every 3 or 4 hours. The main adverse effect of meperidine is respiratory depression. This drug should be used with caution because long-term administration can be associated with drug/psychic dependence.
Papaverine hydrochloride—usually given orally (tablets) in dosage of 30 to 60 mg three to five times daily for local pain associated with vascular spasm.
Pentazocine hydrochloride (Talwin)—oral dose: 25 to 50 mg repeated in 3 or 4 hours; intramuscular: 15 to 30 mg every 3 or 4 hours.
Talwin compound—supplied in caplets each containing pentazocine hydrochloride 12.5 mg equivalent

and aspirin 325 mg. Dose for older child is 1 caplet three or four times daily.

Morphine sulfate—reserved for treatment of severe pain. Administer subcutaneously or intramuscularly in single dose of 0.1 to 0.2 mg/kg and repeat every 3 to 5 hours until pain is controlled.

Indomethacin (Indocin)—useful for short-term (2 weeks or less) administration in adolescents when pain is combined with local tenderness and swelling of soft tissues, especially in joints and extremities, in dosages of 1 mg/kg given orally every 6 to 8 hours. (This drug has not been officially approved for use in persons under 14 years of age.)

For pain of moderate to severe intensity in children, codeine is often effective and perhaps should be the drug of first choice, as it has the advantage of long duration of action (4 to 5 hours), oral medication is effective in pain control, and the hazard of dependency is less common than for the other narcotics in common use. Morphine is a more effective analgesic and sedative; however, it must be given parenterally to achieve maximum efficacy, and repeated use has a higher addiction risk; therefore its use in children should be reserved for the control of severe painful episodes. Meperidine has the disadvantage of a relatively short duration of action (2 to 4 hours), and patients who frequently receive this agent often exhibit physical drug dependency. Seizures have also been reported after its administration. Adjuvant agents such as hydroxyzine and phenergan are popular with the house staff in many hospitals; however, their value as potentiators of narcotic analgesics is questionable, although they may have some value as sedatives. Vaso-occlusive crises in children usually last 4 to 14 days, with a mean of about 5 or 6 days, followed by an asymptomatic steady state of variable duration.

Occasionally analgesics and parenterally administered fluids are not adequate to control severe pain in the hospitalized patient. In such cases partial exchange blood transfusions may bring relief by reducing the mass of sickled cells in the circulation. The goal of this method is to reduce the Hb S–containing cells to less than 45 per cent. Once this objective has been achieved, small transfusions of packed red blood cells can be administered every 3 to 4 weeks to keep the Hb S less than 45 per cent in patients when vaso-occlusive crises are refractory to conservative medical management. The chief hazards of prolonged or frequently repeated blood transfusions are alloimmunization, hepatitis, and iron overload. Supplemental oxygen is recommended for hypoxic patients with low PO_2.

Painful crises in children are often associated with anorexia, febrile illness, and other conditions that contribute to dehydration; hence parenteral administration of fluid is important. We recommend 5 per cent dextrose in one-fourth strength saline infused at the rate of 2000 to 2500 ml/m²/day. Sodium bicarbonate should be reserved for patients with documented acidosis. Intravenously administered fluids should be carefully monitored to avoid overloading the circulatory system in these children, who often exhibit cardiomegaly associated with varying degrees of anemia. Children should be encouraged to take fluids orally whenever it is feasible to do so. Conditions that have frequently been associated with the onset of pain crises should be avoided. In children and adolescents factors such as infections, dehydration, physical exertion, emotional stress, trauma, and exposure to chilling and inclement weather have been identified as precipitating agents.

In addition to the typical vaso-occlusive crisis, children with sickle cell disease may also exhibit pain associated with the following: hand-foot syndrome, joint effusions (arthropathy), osteomyelitis, ankle ulcers, acute chest syndrome, gallbladder disease, biliary tract obstruction, hepatic infarcts, priapism, avascular necrosis of bone especially involving the femur or humerus, cardiovascular manifestations, musculosketetal crises, and abdominal distention with transient adynamic ileus. These conditions require appropriate therapeutic measures, which should be individualized for the particular patient.

HEMATOLOGIC CRISES

The aplastic crisis is the most frequently observed hematologic crisis in the United States. The transient depression of hematopoiesis in often associated with acute infections, particularly of the viral type. The degree of anemia is variable and on occasion is sufficiently severe to warrant a transfusion of packed red blood cells. Recovery is usually prompt and is heralded by a significant increase in the reticulocyte count.

The so-called hyperhemolytic crisis is uncommon in my experience and is associated with an increase in bilirubin and a reticulocytosis. It can be confused with G-6-PD deficiency in a patient with sickle cell anemia, especially during a febrile illness when antipyretic agents are being administered. Transfusion of packed red blood cells is indicated for significant anemia (Hb less than 5 gm).

Megaloblastic crisis may occur in sickle cell disease owing to folic acid deficiency. This type is more frequently observed in African inhabitants, especially during pregnancy. It can be prevented by folic acid prophylaxis but if the anemia is severe, blood transfusion should be administered with due care to avoid cardiopulmonary overload.

The sequestration crisis involving the collection of large pools of blood in viscera, especially the spleen, can be life-threatening. This type of crisis is most commonly observed during infancy and early childhood. Sudden death may occur from hypovolemic shock. Treatment consists of the administration of whole blood and saline solution to restore circulatory volume; however, overloading the cardiopulmonary circulation is to be avoided. Splenectomy may be necessary in selected cases to prevent repetitive crises. This type of crisis should not be confused, however, with splenomegaly due to chronic and longstanding splenic infarction.

INFECTIONS

Many patients with sickle cell anemia exhibit an immunodeficiency that makes them particularly susceptible to a number of infectious agents. Infants and young children are quite vulnerable to certain micro-organisms, particularly *Streptococcus pneumoniae* and *Haemophilus influenzae*, which are frequently identified with sepsis, bacteremia, meningitis, and pneumonia. In view of the occurrence of sudden death in patients with sickle cell anemia due to these two pathogens, initial therapy for suspected septicemia in children should be ampicillin. When ampicillin-resistant *H. influenzae* infection is encountered, chloramphenicol or an antibiotic such as cefamandole may be a suitable alternative. *Salmonella* and *Staphylococcus aureus* are major pathogens that can cause osteomyelitis in these patients. This complication requires a combination of vigorous antibiotic therapy and orthopedic consultation. Pneumonia caused by the *Mycoplasma* organism often presents a protracted course with delayed resolution. Erythromycin is recommended for this infection. In general antibiotic therapy should be given parenterally without delay at the onset of febrile illness, particularly in children with homozygous sickle cell disease.

TRANSFUSION THERAPY

Blood transfusions are of value in treating certain complications of sickle cell disease. However, the risk:benefit ratio should be carefully evaluated whenever the decision is made to use this therapy in a particular patient. The common risks are iron overload, hepatitis, alloimmunization, and the induction of hyperviscosity. Currently transfusions are used to prepare patients with sickle cell disease for anesthesia and surgery. For elective surgery, packed erythrocytes in dosage of 10 ml/kg body weight can be given to maintain the hemoglobin at 12 gm/dl. It may be advantageous to space the transfusions over several days prior to surgery. When simple transfusions are employed in preparing patients for elective surgery, it is important to keep the hematocrit below 35 per cent in order to avoid hyperviscosity. Partial exchange transfusion is recommended for major operations and emergency surgery in order to provide a hematocrit of 30 to 35 per cent and sickle hemoglobin less than 25 per cent. Following transfusion, the preoperative administration of intravenous fluids prevents dehydration due to an increase in blood viscosity. Following surgery oxygen should be administered until the effects of anesthesia and sedatives have abated.

Partial exchange transfusions have been used in some medical centers for a variety of clinical conditions, including the following: prevention of recurrence of cerebrovascular accidents, prevention of crises and complications in pregnancy, prevention of severe and frequently recurring vaso-occlusive crises, treatment of chronic nonhealing leg ulcers, and treatment of protracted priapism. Usually an attempt is made to keep the level of sickle hemoglobin below 40 to 50 per cent. Once a patient has been brought to an acceptable level of hematocrit and percentage of sickle hemoglobin, maintenance at these levels can be achieved by simple transfusions of packed erythrocytes given every 3 to 4 weeks. This causes suppression of the patient's own erythropoiesis. Chronic transfusion regimens predispose patients to iron overload and hemochromatosis, which may warrant the use of chelation therapy. Selective transfusion frequency may reduce iron deposits in patients who require chronic transfusion therapy. The use of expensive cell separators, however, is required for this procedure.

The frequent use of blood transfusion for the management of patients with sickle cell disease is resulting in an increasing incidence of alloimmunization reaction. This has been attributed in part to the caucasian origin of much of the donor blood, which results in sickle cell anemia patients becoming isoimmunized to blood antigens such as the Duffy system, which is largely absent in people of African descent. Other offending blood group antibodies include the Rh, Kell, and Kidd systems. Some patients with sickle cell disease have become isoimmunized to so many antigens or to such common blood groups that transfusion becomes almost impossible. Therefore, complete genotyping before transfusion has been suggested for patients who will be on a transfusion regimen for a long period of time, because the typing will be difficult to obtain if they prove to be immunologic responders later on. An alternative plan of management for the prevention of transfusion reactions is the use of autologous blood for transfusion. For example, patients who are scheduled for elective surgery may donate blood prior to the surgical operation for cryopreservation and storage for subsequent reinfusion during surgery or postoperatively. This procedure eliminates most of the hazards of blood transfusion, including isoimmunization and hepatitis.

SUMMARY

Although there is no cure for sickle cell disease, there is much that the physician can do to provide symptomatic and supportive care for patients. A team approach is usually required to provide comprehensive medical, psychosocial, and rehabilitative services for patients who have to contend with a chronic painful incurable illness. A major role of the patient's family physician is to provide continuity of medical service, counseling, and integration of the various professional procedures that may be required.

Bone marrow transplants have been performed infrequently for the treatment of selected cases of severe sickle cell anemia.

LEUKOPENIA, NEUTROPENIA, AND AGRANULOCYTOSIS

PHILIP A. PIZZO, M.D.

Children with low white blood cell counts share in common an increased risk of serious infection. The incidence of these infections is directly related to the depth and duration of the neutropenia and inversely related to the degree of preservation of other phagocytic host defenses. Neutropenias may be transient (such as those associated with drug-induced bone marrow suppression, viral infections, or immune medicated events) or prolonged in duration (such as those associated with congenital deficiencies of myelopoiesis or acquired bone marrow failure states). Less frequently, neutropenias can be cyclic and intermittent.

One of the major difficulties in the management of the neutropenic patient is the inability to distinguish a fever that portends a potentially life-threatening infection from a less serious complication. In our prospective assessment of 300 neutropenic children who developed fever, we were unable to ascertain any clinical or laboratory parameters that could distinguish a patient with a bacteremia from one whose cultures were entirely negative. Thus, when faced with a neutropenic child who has become febrile, a potentially life-threatening infection must be assumed until proven otherwise. For this reason, children with a neutrophil count of less than 500/mm^3 who become febrile (we have defined fever as a single oral temperature elevation above 38.5°C or three oral temperatures above 38.0°C during a 24-hour period) require admission to the hospital for examination, a chest radiograph, urinalysis, cultures of throat and urine, and at least two preantibiotic blood cultures. The initial evaluation should be performed promptly and expeditiously, and as soon as possible after its completion (ideally within 2 to 3 hours after the onset of fever) the patient should be started on an empiric antimicrobial regimen.

EMPIRICAL ANTIBIOTIC THERAPY

The goal of empiric antibiotic therapy is to prevent rapid clinical deterioration and early mortality related to an undiagnosed and untreated bacterial infection. Because both gram-positive and gram-negative bacteria can cause such infections, it is imperative that the empiric antimicrobial regimen instituted effectively cover the predominant potential pathogens at a particular institution. In approximately 10 per cent of cases, bacteremias may be polymicrobial, which further underscores the need for effective broad-spectrum coverage. Indeed, perhaps more than any other aspect of management, the practice of promptly instituting empiric broad-spectrum antimicrobial coverage when the granulocytopenic patient becomes febrile has accounted for a significant reduction in the incidence of fatal infectious complications. Until recently, it has been possible to achieve such broad-spectrum coverage only by the use of combination antimicrobial therapy. In most centers, this has included the combination of a beta-lactam (e.g., a cephalosporin or antipseudomonal penicillin) with an aminoglycoside. A variety of two- and three-drug combinations have been effectively utilized, and since no particular regimen has shown itself to be singularly effective, the choice of agents should be based upon the pattern of infection observed at a given treatment center. When an aminoglycoside is included in the drug regimen, it is imperative that serum levels be monitored within 24 hours after the start of therapy and then serially to assure that effective drug levels are being obtained and that potential oto- and nephrotoxicity is minimized.

During the last several years, a number of new beta-lactam antibiotics have been introduced, particularly the third-generation cephalosporins and the ureido- and piperazine penicillins. The third-generation cephalosporins are unique in having a very broad spectrum of activity that in some cases includes not only the enterobacteriaceae but also *Pseudomonas aeruginosa*, gram-positive isolates, and anaerobes. The extended-spectrum penicillins offer increased effectiveness against *P. aeruginosa*, *Klebsiella* sp., and a variety of anaerobes. Additional new agents include the carbapenems (which have perhaps the broadest spectrum of activity of any antibiotic), the monobactams, and the quinolones. The role that each of these new antibiotics will play in the management of the neutropenic cancer patient is evolving. Antibiotic combinations (e.g., a third-generation cephalosporin plus an aminoglycoside or a third-generation cephalosporin plus an extended-spectrum penicillin) are the regimens most frequently used. On the other hand, the unique spectrum of some of the third-generation cephalosporins and carbapenems raises the possibility that one of these drugs might be used as monotherapy for the initial empiric management of the febrile neutropenic patient. Several studies have evaluated monotherapy and suggest that it is a viable option, particularly during the initial treatment of the neutropenic patient who becomes febrile. Regardless of whether a single broad-spectrum antibiotic or a combination of antibiotics is employed, it is imperative that patients be clearly monitored. Indeed, neutropenic patients are subject to second or even multiple infectious complications. In particular, patients with prolonged granulocytopenia (i.e., more than 7 days) or whose preantibiotic evaluation revealed a clinically or microbiologically defined site of infection (see below) are likely to require additions to or modifications of the initial empiric regimen. These may include the addition of other antibiotics as well as antifungal, antiviral, or antiparasitic agents. Such additions or modifications of the initial antibiotic regimen can best be viewed as adjuncts that help assure the successful treatment and survival of the patient.

It is also notable that the changing pattern of infection has led to the reintroduction of an older antibiotic, vancomycin. This drug is particularly effective in the treatment of infections by coagulase-negative staphylococci, methicillin-resistant *Staphylococcus aureus*, and the multiply resistant JK-corynebacteria. Indeed, vancomycin is increasingly used in centers where indwelling intravenous catheters are employed but also been advocated by some investigators as a component of the initial empiric regimen. Even though gram-positive regimens have increased in prevalence, they are generally less virulent than gram-negatives and, in most centers, vancomycin can be withheld until there is microbiologic confirmation of a gram-positive infection. Exceptions to this are centers with a high incidence of methicillin-resistant *S. aureus*.

Because its spectrum of activity is restricted solely to gram-negative aerobes, aztreonam cannot be used alone in the febrile neutropenic patient. However, it does offer, for the first time, a bactericidal antibiotic that can be used in the penicillin- or cephalosporin-allergic patient, particularly if combined with an agent with activity against gram-positive aerobes (e.g., vancomycin).

Although the quinolones represent a promising new class of antibiotics and offer the prospect of agents that can be administered orally, they are not yet available for children less than 18 years of age. They do, however, deserve careful study to assess their potential safety for pediatric patients.

MANAGEMENT OF NEUTROPENIC PATIENTS WITH DEFINED SITES OF INFECTION

Following the initial evaluation and institution of empiric antibiotic therapy, clinical and microbiologic findings that clarify the etiology of the child's fever may become available. Under any circumstance, it is imperative that each patient be examined daily until the resolution of the granulocytopenic episode, since both evolving infections and the emergence of second or superinfections are not infrequent. Additions to or modifications of the initial empiric regimen are frequently necessary, particularly in patients who remain neutropenic for protracted periods. Some examples are considered in the following paragraphs.

Bacteremia. Positive blood cultures are surprisingly infrequent in the granulocytopenic patient with cancer, accounting for only 10 to 20 per cent of the infectious complications. This low incidence may reflect the fact that patients are evaluated and treated early (the improved survival of these patients justifies this approach to management). When the initial preantibiotic blood cultures are positive, it may be necessary to modify the antimicrobial regimen. When coagulase-negative staphylococci are isolated, the addition of vancomycin (40 mg/kg/day in four divided doses) is usually necessary, since these organisms are frequently resistant to beta-lactam antibiotics. Although it has usually been felt to be necessary to remove a foreign body when a site of infection has been defined, nearly 90 per cent of catheter-associated bacteremias (particularly with *Staphylococcus epidermidis*) can be effectively treated with antibiotics alone, without catheter removal. However, if the patient remains bacteremic after 48 hours of appropriate therapy, or if the infection recurs when the antibiotic course is completed (generally 10 to 14 days), catheter removal is necessary.

Another question that commonly arises when a gram-positive organism has been isolated is whether the spectrum of the antimicrobial regimen can be narrowed to control the pathogen specifically. Our results from a retrospective analysis suggested that patients remaining neutropenic for longer than a week had an increased risk of developing a subsequent infection with gram-negative bacteria when they were treated with a narrow-spectrum antibiotic (e.g., oxacillin, nafcillin). In our current prospective study, however, it appears that a narrow spectrum of therapy can be effective as long as the clinician is cognizant that second infections or superinfections might arise during the course of treatment.

The current standard of practice for treating gram-negative bacillary infections in granulocytopenic patients is to utilize a two-drug combination. When such therapy is instituted early, current data suggest that nearly 90 per cent of granulocytopenic patients will survive the episode. The duration of therapy is generally 10 to 14 days. However, if the patient remains neutropenic when treatment is completed (even though all sites of infection have cleared), recurrent infection may occur and the patient should be appropriately monitored. Should a residual focus of infection remain in the neutropenic patient, even at the completion of a standard 14-day trial of therapy, antibiotics should be continued until either the resolution of the granulocytopenia or the disappearance of all signs of infection.

In addition to antibiotics, adjunctive therapies are frequently considered in the neutropenic patient who has a positive blood culture. Foremost among these have been white blood cell transfusions. While this mode of therapy was popularly employed during the mid-1970s, current data suggest that leukocyte transfusions are largely ineffective in the supportive management of granulocytopenic patients, even when patients have a documented gram-negative bacteremia. Most probably this reflects the inability to transfuse adequate numbers of qualitatively normal neutrophils to overcome the quantitative impairment. At present, leukocyte transfusions seem best restricted to neonates with sepsis and perhaps to patients with chronic granulomatous disease. As an alternative to cell component therapy, consideration has been given to antibody replacement by passive immunization. Observations have suggested that patients receiving cytotoxic therapy may have decreased titers of antibody to the core glycolipid of the Enterobacteriaceae. Studies have shown that the passive infusion of antisera with increased core glycolipid titers (so-called J5 antisera) may decrease mortality in patients with proven or putative sepsis. However, our studies with both J5 antisera and pooled immunoglobulins have failed to demonstrate a reduction in the incidence of fever or infection in patients becoming neutropenic. Nor does their administration change the patterns or outcome of secondary infections in patients with persistent neutropenia.

Head and Neck Infections. The oral cavity is a frequent site of primary or secondary infection in the neutropenic patient. Aphthous ulcers frequently occur when the neutrophil count is lowered (e.g., in cyclic neutropenia). Drug-induced stomatotoxicity can result in ulcerations that become secondarily infected by endogenous oral bacteria, thus providing a nidus for local infection and a portal to systemic invasion. We have observed that approximately 20 per cent of patients who receive antibiotics while neutropenic develop a marginal gingivitis characterized by a red periapical line of gingival necrosis. The addition of a specific antianaerobic antibiotic (e.g., clindamycin, 30 mg/kg/day in four divided doses) has appeared to improve this process and can result in the defervescence of the patient who had been febrile on standard antibiotic therapy.

Infection of the oral cavity with *Candida* sp. is common and is characterized by the presence of white mucosal plaques. The diagnosis can be confirmed by scraping and examining the material under wet mount for pseudohyphae and budding yeasts or by culture. Although many centers routinely utilize nystatin for both prophylaxis and therapy, our experience has been that this agent is relatively ineffective. Alternatively, clotrimazole oral troches can be effective. Ketoconazole has been shown to be effective for the oral thrush that occurs in patients with AIDS, but we have found that children with oral mucositis frequently have difficulty in swallowing the tablets. If the mucositis due to *Candida* becomes particularly severe, a short course of intravenous amphotericin B (0.1 to 0.5 mg/kg/day for 5 days) has the highest likelihood of success.

Gingivostomatitis can also be the result of infection with *Herpes simplex*, and a severe necrotizing mucositis may ensue. This infection can be treated with parenteral acyclovir (750 mg/m^2/day in three divided doses). In particularly high-risk groups (patients undergoing intensive chemotherapy or bone marrow transplantation), prophylactic administration of acyclovir may prevent herpetic gingivostomatitis.

While sinus infection in the neutropenic child might be due to aerobic or anaerobic bacteria, consideration should be given to the possibility that the process might be fungal (particularly *Aspergillus* or *Mucor*). Fungal sinusitis may result in the rhinocerebral syndrome with subsequent invasion of the cranial vault. Diagnosis requires histologic demonstration of invading hyphae, and treatment includes both surgical debridement and parenteral amphotericin B (1.0 to 1.5 mg/kg/day). These infections may require protracted courses of amphotericin, usually over 2 or more months. Patients developing the rhinocerebral syndrome should also be carefully monitored for the development of pulmonary aspergillosis, which worsens the clinical outlook.

It is also important to note that middle ear infections in the neutropenic child may be due to gram-negative bacteria as well as to the usual respiratory pathogens. Hence, we institute broad-spectrum antibiotic therapy for neutropenic children who develop otitis media, particularly if a specific diagnosis cannot be made by tympanocentesis.

Respiratory Tract Infections. The lung is the single most common site of infection in the granulocytopenic patient. Presumably, the majority of these infections are the result of aspiration, although they may also occur as part of a hematogenous infection. Indeed, when a gram-negative bacteremia occurs in concert with a pneumonitis, the prognosis is particularly ominous. It should be underscored that the usual signs and symptoms and even the radiographic manifestations of pneumonia may be muted in the granulocytopenic patient. It is, therefore, imperative to monitor serially and even to repeat chest radiographs in neutropenic patients who have persistent fever, since an infiltrate may not be apparent at the time of initial evaluation but may become evident later in the treatment course. A particular difficulty posed by pulmonary infections is their general inaccessibility to direct microbiologic evaluation. Sputum is usually not a reliable diagnostic specimen and is rarely produced in children anyway. Because these patients are not infrequently thrombocytopenic as well, the performance of more direct diagnostic procedures is often fraught with danger.

For the child who presents with a localized pneumonic process and who is febrile and neutropenic, gram-negative pneumonia must be assumed, although gram-positive bacteria, legionellae, mycoplasmas, viruses, and even drugs must also be considered. Our general policy is to start the neutropenic patient who has a localized pulmonary infiltrate on broad-spectrum antibiotics, following standard preantibiotic evaluation as outlined earlier. The patient is carefully monitored, and if improvement is observed within 48 to 72 hours after the initiation of antibiotics, a full course of therapy (at least 2 weeks) is administered. If, however, the patient has failed to improve or is deteriorating after an adequate 48- to 72-hour antibiotic trial, attempts to make a more specific diagnosis by bronchoscopy or open lung biopsy are then pursued.

Another perplexing problem is the finding of a new pulmonary infiltrate in the patient already on antibiotics. This is not an uncommon problem, since nearly one third of all the pulmonary infiltrates we have observed in pediatric granulocytopenic patients during the last 10 years have occurred in this setting. We have observed that when the infiltrate occurred together with a rise in the patient's granulocyte count, the outcome was nearly always favorable and the infiltrate probably reflected the "lighting up" of a prior site of infection by the recovering neutrophils. However, when the infiltrate occurred in a patient who was persistently granulocytopenic, and particularly when it progressed over 2 or 3 days, the most likely diagnosis was a fungal pneumonia (particularly *Aspergillus* or *Candida*). Ideally, it is preferable to establish a microbiologic diagnosis in these patients so that the need for and duration of antifungal therapy can be clearly delineated. Recent studies suggest that the finding of *Aspergillus* in sputum or bronchoalveolar lavage fluid in a febrile neutropenic patient with a new or evolving pulmonary infiltrate is highly associated with *Aspergillus* pneumonia. If the patient's clinical course prohibits the performance of an appropriate diagnostic procedure (such as an open lung biopsy) even if sputum or BAL cultures are nondiagnostic, empiric antifungal therapy with amphotericin B should be promptly instituted.

Diffuse interstitial infiltrates are not unique to the granulocytopenic patient. When they occur in patients receiving immunosuppressive therapy (particularly steroids), *Pneumocystis carinii* pneumonia should be considered. However, bacteria, fungi, and viruses can also present as interstitial infiltrates, raising the question of how aggressively the diagnosis should be pursued. Numerous investigations suggest that the open lung biopsy is the most reliable diagnostic technique, although not without hazard in the patient who is neutropenic and thrombocytopenic. Recent experience with bronchoalveolar lavage suggests that this procedure may have a role in the diagnostic repertoire, but further evaluation is clearly necessary. Alternatively, a trial of antimicrobial therapy might be adequate. We observed in a recent randomized trial that empiric antibiotic therapy with trimethoprim-sulfamethoxazole and erythromycin was an effective alternative to an invasive diagnostic procedure in non-neutropenic cancer patients with diffuse pulmonary infiltrates, although improvement may not be observed for 4 to 5 days. It is not yet established whether similar recommendations can be drawn for neutropenic patients, but if empiric antimicrobial therapy is to be utilized in the neutropenic patient with diffuse infiltrates, it is important to include broad-spectrum antibiotics in addition to coverage for *Pneumocystis* and *Legionella*. Moreover, if the patient was already on antibiotic therapy at the time of onset of the pulmonary lesions, the addition of antifungal therapy appears warranted.

Cardiovascular Infections. Primary or secondary cardiovascular infections are surprisingly infrequent in the neutropenic child. Although endocarditis has been described with gram-negative as well as gram-positive bacteria and fungi, this is a rare complication, even in patients who have had bacteremias and fungemias. Thus, unless there is evidence of persistent bacteremia in the patient on antibiotic therapy, we do not recommend protracted courses of antibiotics. Myocardial abscesses can occur with bacteria as well as fungi, and myocarditis may be a manifestation of toxoplasmosis in the compromised host.

Gastrointestinal Infections. The onset of retrosternal burning pain aggravated by swallowing in the patient who is already receiving broad-spectrum antibiotics suggests the presence of esophagitis. Although esophagitis can rarely be due to bacteria, it is more likely the result of infection with *Candida* or *Herpes simplex*. Since esophagoscopy can be associated with bleeding or a bacteremia in neutropenic patients, we prefer to establish a tentative diagnosis by looking for cobblestoning with a barium swallow. If evident, we initiate either oral clotrimazole or a short course of amphotericin B, with the expectation that if the process is due to *Candida* sp. symptomatic improvement should be observed within 48 hours. If improvement does not occur, the addition of acyclovir or esophagoscopy and biopsy should be considered.

Although the gastrointestinal tract is a major reservoir of potential pathogens, primary gastrointestinal sites of infection are less common in neutropenic patients. A syndrome worthy of note is typhlitis. Patients generally present with right lower quadrant abdominal pain and rebound, mimicking an acute abdomen or a perforated appendicitis. Patients are usually already receiving broad-spectrum antibiotics. Although it is possible that some patients may be treated with supportive care alone, several reports suggest that surgical intervention and removal of the necrotic cecum is essential for effective control.

Diarrhea in the neutropenic patient, particularly when there has been exposure to antibiotics or chemotherapeutic agents, may be due to *Clostridium difficile*. The diagnosis can be established by examining the stool for cytotoxins. The presence of toxin-associated diarrhea warrants the initiation of either oral vancomycin or metronidazole.

Hepatitis due to type B virus has decreased in recent years, but infection with non-A, non-B virus continues to be a problem for patients receiving cytotoxic therapy and blood transfusions. Using abdominal computed tomography scanning or ultrasonography, we have recently observed a series of neutropenic patients who developed "bull's-eye" lesions in their livers; these have been shown by biopsy to be due to hepatic candidiasis. This process has required protracted courses of amphotericin B therapy. Indeed, our most recent experience suggests that the best response is likely to occur with the combination of amphotericin B and 5-fluorocytosine.

The incidence of perianal cellulitis in neutropenic patients has decreased during the last decade, perhaps because of the more aggressive and earlier use of antibiotics in these patients. Although it is commonly assumed that the major cause of perianal cellulitis is gram-negative bacilli, our recent review of patients treated at the National Cancer Institute suggests that mixed infections (i.e., gram-negative rods and anaerobes) are most common. Whether patients developing evidence of perianal cellulitis should be managed conservatively or treated with surgical debridement remains controversial. We have observed that the early addition of a specific antianaerobic antibiotic (e.g., clindamycin or metronidazole) to standard gram-negative coverage when the patient first begins complaining of perianal tenderness may avoid the need for an invasive surgical procedure.

Genitourinary Tract. Except in patients with primary genitourinary malignancies or those who have indwelling catheters, infections of the genitourinary tract are infrequent, even in neutropenic cancer patients.

Rarely, the syndrome of bladder thrush may occur, hallmarked by the presence of *Candida* in urine cultures and cytoscopic evidence of superficial invasion. Treatment of this process generally requires the instillation of amphotericin B into the bladder on a daily basis or a trial of systemically administered amphotericin B.

Central Nervous System Infections. Surprisingly, bacterial meningitis remains uncommon in the neutropenic patient, even in patients with bacteremia. When evidence of meningitis is present, particularly in children with leukemia, careful examination of the cerebrospinal fluid for gram-positive rods should be made, since *Listeria monocytogenes* can be a noteworthy pathogen in this patient population.

UNEXPLAINED FEVER IN NEUTROPENIC PATIENTS

Nearly two thirds of the children who present with fever and neutropenia fail to have a clinically or microbiologically defined site of infection. Nonetheless, it is probable that many of these children have an occult site of infection and that the diagnosis has simply been masked by the early institution of empiric antimicrobial therapy. In the absence of overt infection, however, the duration of antibiotic treatment can be a real problem. We have found that patients can be stratified into low- and high-risk groups. Low-risk patients with unexplained fever have periods of neutropenia lasting a week or less. When the antibiotics are continued in these patients until the resolution of granulocytopenia and then are stopped, the patients appear to do quite well. On the other hand, high-risk patients have neutropenia for longer than a week. Stopping antibiotics in these patients while they remain neutropenic, particularly if they are also still febrile, appears to be associated with recrudescent infection and in some cases with clinical deterioration. Our studies suggest that patients with prolonged granulocytopenia who defervesce after the initiation of empiric antibiotic therapy should be treated for 2 weeks unless the granulocytopenia resolves before then. While stopping antibiotics at 2 weeks in the persistently neutropenic patient is still associated with recurrent fever in one third of patients, careful and expectant observation can usually prevent serious sequelae. However, stopping antibiotics in patients who are persistently febrile and neutropenic is associated with serious sequelae in more than half. Simply continuing antibiotics alone is not a solution, since many of these patients develop evidence of invasive fungal disease. Therefore, our recommendation for patients with persistent fever and neutropenia is that they be continued on broad-spectrum antibiotics and that an antifungal agent be added until the eventual resolution of the granulocytopenia.

While these cases are challenging, it is clear that a high degree of success can be achieved in the management of infectious complications in granulocytopenic patients if treatment is started early and appropriate additions to and modifications of therapy are carefully employed.

PEDIATRIC HEMOSTASIS AND THROMBOSIS

DONNA DiMICHELE, M.D., ERIC LARSEN, M.D., *and* BRUCE FURIE, M.D.

Hemostasis is a host defense mechanism that involves the complex interaction between platelets, endothelial cells, and coagulation proteins. This intricate system undergoes well-defined changes during human maturation and development, providing an additional degree of complexity to pediatric hemostasis. The management of bleeding disorders in children requires a thorough understanding of the underlying defect. A careful medical history and physical examination combined with essential laboratory tests usually establish the nature of the hemostatic defect and allow the clinician to institute appropriate therapy.

GENERAL APPROACH TO BLEEDING DISORDERS

The medical history and physical examination should result in a provisional diagnosis that can then be confirmed by specific laboratory tests. The history should focus on the type of bleeding, the onset and duration of bleeding, and the relationship of bleeding to a hemostatic challenge, such as trauma, tooth extraction, circumcision, surgery, and menstruation. Frequently, the use of specific closed-ended questions are revealing: "Exactly how long did he bleed following the tooth extraction?" or "How many sanitary pads do you use during your menstrual period?" Taking the extra time to review specific points in the history often reveals minor but significant bleeding disorders. Additional aspects of the history should include previous or con-

current illnesses and medications. A complete family history is essential. It is often useful to develop the actual pedigree rather than simply asking if anyone in the family has a bleeding problem.

The primary goal of the physical examination is to assess the type of bleeding. The skin should be carefully inspected for petechiae and purpura. The distribution of the lesions is important. Ecchymoses limited to areas of frequent trauma such as the lower legs in an active toddler are probably normal. However, an ecchymotic lesion in an area not usually subject to trauma is suggestive of easy bruisability. The nasal and oral mucosa should be carefully examined for petechiae and for evidence of bleeding. The extremities should be examined for the presence of hematomas and hemarthroses.

The combination of history and physical examination should lead to a tentative classification of the patient's bleeding disorder. Hemostatic defects involving the platelet, vessel wall, or the interaction between the platelet and the vessel wall are characterized by petechiae, ecchymoses, and mucosal bleeding that occur spontaneously or following hemostatic challenge. Alternatively, deficiencies of the clotting proteins commonly result in deep tissue hematomas or hemarthroses, which may be spontaneous or have a delayed presentation following trauma.

The laboratory evaluation of a suspected bleeding disorder includes screening tests and specific assays to define the defect. Basic screening tests include a platelet count, bleeding time, prothrombin time, and PTT (partial thromboplastin time). In some clinical situations the thrombin time and the fibrinogen level should be included in the initial screen. The platelet count is usually measured as part of an automated complete blood count. The principle of this method is to count particles on the basis of size. When platelets aggregate they form large clumps that escape detection in this system, leading to the false impression of thrombocytopenia. Therefore, a low platelet count obtained by automated instrumentation should be confirmed by examination of the peripheral smear. The causes of thrombocytopenia are outlined below. The bleeding time is the best screening test for the platelet–vessel wall interaction, but it remains a crude assay that only loosely correlates with a bleeding tendency. The test should be performed consistently by the same method and by the same well-experienced individual, especially when repeated observations on a single patient are required. The template method is the most widely used and involves making a standardized incision on the arm distal to a blood pressure cuff inflated to 40 mm Hg. In infants and premature newborns, cuff pressures of 30 and 20 mm Hg, respectively, should be used. Platelet counts below 100,000/mm^3 prolong the bleeding time to a degree inversely proportional to the platelet count. A prolonged bleeding time in the setting of a normal platelet count suggests a qualitative platelet defect, von Willebrand's disease, or a vascular abnormality. Whereas the platelet count and bleeding time screen for platelet and vascular causes of bleeding, the prothrombin time and PTT screen for coagulation factor abnormalities. The prothrombin time is a measure of the extrinsic coagulation pathway, which includes Factors VII, X, and V, prothrombin, and fibrinogen. Causes of a prolonged prothrombin time include congenital deficiencies of these factors, liver disease, and vitamin K deficiency. The PTT assesses the intrinsic system, which includes prekallikrein, high molecular weight kininogen, Factors XII, XI, IX, and VIII, and the components of the final common pathway: Factors X and V, prothrombin, and fibrinogen. A quantitative or functional deficiency of any of these factors results in a prolonged PTT. The thrombin time measures the conversion of fibrinogen to fibrin by thrombin, thus evaluating the presence and function of fibrinogen. A fibrinogen activity level is determined concurrently to complete this evaluation.

The results of these basic screening tests should allow the clinician to develop a presumptive diagnosis, which can then be confirmed with specific tests. There are conditions, however, in which the screening tests are abnormal and the patient is at no risk for excessive bleeding. These conditions include deficiencies of Factor XII, prekallikrein, or high molecular weight kininogen and the presence of a lupus anticoagulant. There are also rare patients at risk for serious bleeding who have normal screening tests. Factor XIII deficiency and abnormalities of the fibrinolytic system are associated with significant bleeding, but patients with these disorders have normal screening tests, and the condition must be diagnosed using specific assays. Therefore, it is essential to systematically investigate the child with a significant bleeding history even if the initial screening tests are normal.

The sophisticated laboratory offers a large number of assays to further evaluate hemostatic function. In vitro platelet aggregation tests determine the ability of a patient's platelets to aggregate in response to various agonists. Specific coagulation factors can be assayed immunologically and functionally. Electrophoresis can be used to determine the qualitative defects in quantitatively normal coagulant proteins that can render them dysfunctional. Inhibitors of coagulation can be detected by mixing the patient's plasma with normal plasma and performing specific assays. The diagnosis of disseminated intravascular coagulation is facilitated by the detection of fibrin degradation products or the presence of D-dimers. Bone marrow aspiration and biopsy may be necessary to investigate fully cellular abnormalities leading to hemostatic disturbances. Assays of clot stability and of the fibrinolytic system can define defects in coagulation that are not detectable by routine screening tests.

PLATELET–VESSEL WALL ABNORMALITIES

Quantitative Platelet Disorders

Thrombocytopenia is defined as a platelet count of less than 150,000/mm³. Patients with platelet counts between 100,000 and 150,000/mm³ are not at risk for bleeding due to a deficient number of platelets. Platelet counts between 20,000 and 100,000/mm³ are rarely associated with spontaneous bleeding, but may be associated with bleeding after surgery or trauma. Patients with platelet counts of less than 20,000/mm³ are at risk

for spontaneous bleeding, usually characterized by petechiae, purpura, mucosal bleeding, menorrhagia, and, less commonly, by gastrointestinal or genitourinary hemorrhage. The most serious type of bleeding that occurs in severely thrombocytopenic patients is intracranial hemorrhage.

Patients with thrombocytopenia should be carefully questioned with regard to intercurrent illnesses, ingestion of medications, and bleeding manifestations. The physical examination should include a search for petechiae, purpura, mucosal bleeding, lymphadenopathy, splenomegaly, and limb deformity. The laboratory evaluation should begin with a complete blood count to establish whether or not an isolated thrombocytopenia exists. The low platelet count should be confirmed by a careful inspection of the peripheral blood smear to rule out platelet clumping as an artifactual cause of reported thrombocytopenia. The examination of the peripheral blood smear will also reveal abnormal platelet morphology as well as immature blood cells and signs of bone marrow infiltration.

The management of the thrombocytopenic patient should be individualized and depends on the etiology of the thrombocytopenia and the need for therapy. The stable patient without life-threatening hemorrhage should undergo a careful evaluation to determine the underlying cause of the low platelet count. The rare patient with life-threatening hemorrhage should immediately be treated empirically and then given a timely diagnostic evaluation.

Thrombocytopenia may be due to increased peripheral destruction, decreased bone marrow production, or splenic sequestration. Destructive processes are usually limited to platelets, whereas the white cell count and red cell count usually remain normal. In contrast, most disorders involving platelet hypoproduction also affect the other two cell lines. Exceptions to this are rare congenital disorders of platelet production which have characteristic findings. Examination of the bone marrow may help to distinguish between decreased production and increased destruction but this is not always necessary. The third general cause of thrombocytopenia is platelet sequestration due to hypersplenism. Hypersplenism is usually characterized by splenomegaly and frequently by concomitant decreases in the white and red cell counts.

Increased Platelet Destruction

The increased destruction of platelets may be due either to immune or nonimmune processes. The prototype of immune-mediated destructive thrombocytopenia in childhood is immune thrombocytopenic purpura (ITP). ITP usually affects young children, with the peak incidence in the 2 to 5 year age group. The typical patient is a healthy child with a history of a recent viral illness who presents with a petechiae, bruises, and/or epistaxis. Less commonly, affected children experience hematuria or mucosal or gastrointestinal bleeding. Mild splenomegaly is present in 5 to 10 per cent of children. Marked splenomegaly should alert the clinician to alternative diagnoses. A complete blood count reveals isolated thrombocytopenia. Platelet size in

ITP may be increased, as assessed by the review of the peripheral blood smear or the mean platelet volume calculated by most automated cell counters. Abnormalities in platelet, white cell, or red cell morphology suggest an alternative diagnosis. The bone marrow, when examined, is normocellular with normal erythroid and myeloid precursors and normal to increased megakaryocytes. A bone marrow examination is only necessary to rule out bone marrow pathology secondary to aplastic anemia or leukemia when either of these diagnoses is highly suspect or prior to corticosteroid therapy for presumed ITP. Some laboratories have the capacity of measuring platelet-associated IgG (PAIgG). Most patients with ITP will test positive for PAIgG. However, this finding is nonspecific; it supports but does not confirm the diagnosis of ITP.

The treatment of ITP consists of general measures and specific therapy. Contact sports and activities involving a high risk of trauma should be avoided until the platelet count has risen to a safe range, conservatively estimated as greater than 100,000/mm^3. The child should avoid all medications affecting platelet function including aspirin, antihistamines, and phenothiazines. Consideration should be given to the wearing of a helmet in the case of the active toddler with a particularly low platelet count. Whether to add specific therapy to these general measures varies with the individual case. Approximately 90 per cent of children with ITP achieve a complete and permanent recovery of their platelet count. Over half of these patients recover within a month of diagnosis and nearly all children who recover do so within six months from the time of diagnosis. Specific therapy for ITP frequently increases the platelet count but does not influence the likelihood of recovery or the time to recovery. The rationale for treating ITP is to reduce the morbidity and mortality from bleeding by raising the platelet count more rapidly than would otherwise occur naturally. The major source of morbidity and mortality in ITP is spontaneous intracranial hemorrhage, a rare event occurring in less than 1 per cent of all patients. No clinical studies have demonstrated that therapy reduces the incidence of or mortality from intracranial hemorrhage.

Important factors regarding treatment include patient age, platelet count, and bleeding manifestations. Younger patients, particularly active toddlers, children with platelet counts less than 20,000/mm^3, and patients with significant mucosal bleeding or fundal hemorrhage may be at greater risk for serious hemorrhage. There exist two basic forms of specific therapy for ITP; corticosteroids and intravenous gamma globulin. The standard steroid therapy for ITP is oral prednisone, 2 mg/kg/day, for two weeks followed by a taper over the third week. Patients should be evaluated for any contraindications to steroid therapy such as a concurrent varicella infection. Most patients on prednisone experience an increase in the platelet count which usually occurs over several days. Alternatively, parenteral corticosteroids have been effectively employed in the initial therapy of ITP. The advantages of this form of treatment include a more rapid rise in the platelet count and assurance of patient compliance. A typical regimen is methylpred-nisolone 30 mg/kg intravenously every day for three days. It is very common for the platelet count to decrease upon cessation of steroid treatment but generally to a level above that measured at diagnosis. This drop in the platelet count is usually accompanied by anxiety on the part of the family and the clinician. At this stage of the illness, the clinician should focus on the clinical condition of the child rather than on the platelet count. Except in the rare patient who resumes significant bleeding, or the patient at high risk for bleeding from trauma whose platelet count decreases below 20,000/mm^3, reinstitution of steroid therapy is usually not necessary. An alternative therapy to corticosteroids is gamma globulin. Gamma globulin is effective in raising the platelet count in ITP and acts more rapidly than steroids, particularly oral prednisone. However, the overall response rate is comparable. Gamma globulin is administered intravenously in two comparable dosage regimens; 400 mg/kg for 5 days or 1 gm/kg for 2 days. The major advantage of gamma globulin is the rapidity of the response, a characteristic which is particularly desirable in emergency situations. Nonetheless, splenectomy remains the standard emergency treatment for the child with ITP who has a life-threatening complication such as an intracranial hemorrhage. This remains the most rapid method of elevating a patient's platelet count. It should be emphasized that children with intracranial hemorrhage should receive additional therapy such as platelet transfusion, corticosteroids, and possibly gamma globulin as they are being prepared for surgery. The side effects of gamma globulin include headache, nausea, fever, and anaphylaxis. The major disadvantage of gamma globulin use in situations that are not life-threatening is its high cost. A typical course of gamma globulin for a small child may cost $5,000 as compared to $10 for a course of prednisone.

Chronic ITP is defined as the persistence of a low platelet count for greater than six months. This occurs in approximately 10 per cent of children with acute ITP. Increasing age is associated with an increased risk of developing chronic ITP, but it is not possible to accurately predict which patients will go on to the chronic form of the disease using current diagnostic methods. In addition, about 20 per cent of those patients with chronic ITP will ultimately have spontaneous remission. The treatment of chronic ITP should be individualized. Patients who do not have bleeding manifestations and have a platelet count over 20,000/mm^3 may not need therapy. If treatment is indicated, various options exist. The classic approach to the treatment of chronic ITP has been splenectomy, which is effective in elevating the platelet count in a majority of patients. The decision to perform splenectomy needs to be carefully assessed, especially in the young child. Patients undergoing splenectomy should preoperatively receive pneumococcal, meningococcal, and *Haemophilus influenzae* vaccines. After splenectomy, patients should receive daily penicillin prophylaxis, and the family should be alerted to the need for prompt medical evaluation of fever. Alternatives to splenectomy in the management of chronic ITP include gamma globulin, steroids, and danazol. Treatment with gamma globulin results only in temporary increases in the platelet count and must be readministered every 3 to 6 weeks. Long-term corticosteroid therapy has serious side effects in the pediatric age group. However, some patients can be maintained on low-dose alternate-day prednisone with minimal side effects and an acceptable platelet count. Danazol, a synthetic androgen, may lead to significant increases in the platelet count in up to 50 per cent of patients but has serious adverse effects, including delayed bone age and hirsutism.

There are a number of other disorders associated with a shortened platelet life span due to immune-mediated destruction. Most of these conditions are associated with a concurrent process such as bacterial infection, drug ingestion, anaphylaxis, or organ rejection. In these situations, platelet destruction is controlled by the recognition and appropriate management of the underlying disorder.

Thrombocytopenia in the neonate may be due to any of the processes that cause thrombocytopenia in the older child. However, the neonate may also be affected by two forms of immunologic destructive thrombocytopenia, resulting from the transfer of antiplatelet antibodies across the placenta. In one form platelet auto-antibodies cross the placenta (maternal ITP) and in the other form there is transfer of an antiplatelet alloantibody directed specifically against the platelets of the fetus (neonatal alloimmune thrombocytopenia). The hallmark of these two conditions is that aside from manifestations of bleeding, these infants are usually healthy and thriving.

Infants born to mothers with active ITP or ITP in remission are at risk to develop thrombocytopenia. This risk of significant thrombocytopenia in the neonate (platelet count <50,000/mm³) is approximately 20 per cent, so the majority of newborns are unaffected. The determination of those infants who will be affected is difficult. The maternal platelet count at delivery does not predict the platelet count of the newborn. Furthermore, there is no current technique that accurately and safely measures the fetal platelet count to allow the clinician to individualize therapy. Affected infants who have very low platelet counts frequently develop generalized petechiae. The greatest danger of this condition is the development of intracranial hemorrhage, which fortunately occurs in less than 2 per cent of cases. Aside from the presence of a low platelet count in the fetus and newborn, the precise risk factors for intracranial hemorrhage have not been clearly identified. Although treating the mother with either steroids or gamma globulin may increase the maternal platelet count, this therapy has no clear benefit for the infant. Furthermore, the strategy of performing cesarean section to prevent birth trauma during vaginal delivery, although frequently used, has not been demonstrated to result in a better outcome for the newborn. Once the infant is born, it is important to recognize that thrombocytopenia may worsen in the first week of life. The platelet count should therefore be followed. Those infants with low platelet counts who do have significant bleeding may be treated with gamma globulin or corticosteroids. Life-threatening hemorrhage should be managed with exchange transfusion and random donor platelet transfusion. Since the origin of the offending antibody in these cases is maternal, this condition invariably resolves within the first few weeks to months of life.

The second type of immune platelet destruction in neonates is neonatal alloimmune thrombocytopenia (NAITP). In this situation the maternal platelet count is normal and the thrombocytopenia results from placental transfer of antibodies that are specific for the infant's platelets. This is due to the presence of a particular antigen on the infant's platelets which is lacking on maternal platelets. Half of all cases occur in first pregnancies, and there is no accurate method to detect which pregnancies will be affected. Unlike infants born to mothers with ITP, there is a significant incidence of thrombocytopenia and serious hemorrhage in infants with NAITP. The incidence of intracranial hemorrhage is 10 to 20 per cent and may occur antenatally. The affected infant with a low platelet count or significant bleeding should be managed with gamma globulin. Since maternal platelets lack the antigen against which the antibody is directed, the transfusion of maternal platelets serves as both a diagnostic test and effective therapy, especially in the case of a life-threatening hemorrhage. In clinical practice, however, this form of therapy involves a time delay and may not be necessary. Since serious hemorrhage is thought to occur before birth, in many cases it is critical to clearly identify cases of NAITP so that future pregnancies may be appropriately managed. Prenatal treatment of the mother with a history of bearing a child with NAITP should include corticosteroids or gamma globulin and consideration of cesarean section to avoid head trauma secondary to vaginal delivery.

Increased platelet destruction is also observed in microangiopathic processes, hemolytic-uremic syndrome, disseminated intravascular coagulation, and the Kasabach-Merritt syndrome. The diagnosis of these conditions is usually straightforward owing to the presence of the associated features of these syndromes. Evaluation for azotemia, an active urinary sediment, intravascular hemolysis, and disseminated intravascular coagulation is usually abnormal in these disorders. The treatment of thrombocytopenia in these cases is directed at the underlying process. Treatment of bleeding manifestations due to thrombocytopenia is with platelet transfusion, although the half-life of the transfused platelets will be shortened because of platelet destruction. The management of disseminated intravascular coagulation is discussed later in this chapter.

Decreased Platelet Production

Thrombocytopenia secondary to decreased production may be congenital or acquired. Congenital causes of hypoproductive thrombocytopenia are commonly associated with easily recognizable physical or laboratory findings. Thrombocytopenia absent radii (TAR) syndrome and Fanconi's aplastic anemia are characterized by typical physical stigmata. Bernard-Soulier syndrome, May-Hegglin anomaly, and Wiskott-Aldrich syndrome all display characteristic platelet morphology. More commonly, however, hypoproductive thrombocytopenia is acquired. Severe aplastic anemia, myelosuppression secondary to chemotherapy, and bone marrow infiltration by malignancy or storage disease are the usual causes of decreased platelet production. These conditions usually result in pancytopenia rather than isolated thrombocytopenia. The major mode of therapy in these disorders is supportive platelet transfusion and treatment of the primary process. Since platelet transfusion carries certain risks, the need for this treatment must be carefully assessed in each patient. Patients with decreased platelet production who have significant bleeding manifestations are candidates for platelet transfusion. Alternatively, those patients with low platelet counts but without bleeding manifestations raise controversy. Many medical centers have adopted the guideline that patients with platelet counts under 20,000/mm³ should receive prophylactic transfusion during temporary periods of thrombocytopenia. This is a reasonable guide, but the individual patient needs to be evaluated. Patients with chronic thrombocytopenia can be safely followed with platelet counts less than 20,000/mm³ if they are free of active bleeding. The management of patients with chemotherapy-related thrombocytopenia must address the expected duration of myelosuppression.

Platelet concentrates are prepared from units of whole blood or from the pheresis of a single donor. A dose of one unit per 10 kg will result in an estimated increase in the platelet count of 40,000/mm³. Platelets are administered through a 170 μm blood filter and can be given as rapidly as the patient's tolerance for volume will allow. Platelet transfusion reactions are quite common and are generally characterized by fever with or without chills starting any time during or soon after the transfusion. These reactions are typically self-limiting and are due to contaminating white blood cells in the transfusion. Patients who have received several platelet transfusions may become alloimmunized such that they no longer experience the expected rise in their platelet counts following transfusion. HLA-matched platelets from single donors may result in better increments in these patients, but this therapy is costly. It is unclear whether the prophylactic administration of HLA-matched platelets delays the development of alloimmunization. In addition to transfusion reactions and alloimmunization, platelet transfusions, like other blood products, may transmit viral diseases like hepatitis B, non-A, non-B hepatitis, and HIV. Furthermore, since platelet concentrates are contaminated with lymphocytes, there is the possibility of causing severe graft-versus-host disease in an immunocompromised host if the concentrate is not irradiated.

Platelet Sequestration

Splenomegaly of any etiology may be accompanied by moderate thrombocytopenia, usually in the 50,000 to 100,000/mm³ range, and rarely results in clinical hemorrhage. Patients are readily identified by significant splenomegaly and often by decreases in the hematocrit and white blood cell count. In rare situations in which the diagnosis is not clear, the administration

of ⁵¹Cr-labeled autologous platelets demonstrates excessive localization in the spleen. Patients rarely require treatment for the thrombocytopenia. Although splenectomy normalizes the platelet count, this procedure is usually undertaken for reasons other than the thrombocytopenia.

Qualitative Platelet Disorders

In addition to disorders of platelet number, there is a group of conditions in which platelet function is altered. Qualitative platelet disorders are characterized clinically by spontaneous or trauma-induced skin and mucosal bleeding in a patient whose platelet count is usually normal. The family history is often positive for similar bleeding manifestations. These patients are identified by a prolongation of the bleeding time. Further evaluation may include studies of platelet aggregation and adhesion, and other platelet assays that evaluate specific platelet functions.

Qualitative platelet disorders may be congenital or acquired. The congenital disorders of platelet function include membrane receptor deficiencies (Bernard-Soulier syndrome and Glanzmann's thrombasthenia), deficiencies of platelet granules (gray platelet syndrome and dense granule deficiency), and metabolic defects (enzyme deficiencies and secretion defects).

Patients with qualitative platelet disorders manifest the same signs and symptoms as a mildly to moderately thrombocytopenic patient. Drugs should be eliminated as the cause of the platelet dysfunction. The laboratory evaluation should include a complete blood count, review of the peripheral smear, bleeding time, as well as von Willebrand factor assays. The platelet count usually is normal, the smear may show characteristic platelet morphology in some cases, the bleeding time will be prolonged, and a normal von Willebrand factor will rule out von Willebrand's disease as an alternative cause of the prolonged bleeding time. The bleeding time should be repeated to confirm the initial result. Platelet aggregation tests may provide information as to the nature of the defect. The diagnostic evaluation should be performed on symptomatic parents and siblings, since many of these disorders are hereditary.

The general therapeutic approach to the child with dysfunctional platelets is a combination of general defensive measures combined with platelet transfusion or DDAVP (1-desamino-8-D-arginine vasopressin), if such therapy is indicated. Most patients do not have problems with spontaneous bleeding but do suffer from extensive hemorrhage following surgery or trauma. Patients should avoid all antiplatelet medications, be counseled with regard to the risk of bleeding, and practice good dental care. Girls with menorrhagia may be considered candidates for anovulatory medication. Specific therapy for the treatment and prevention includes DDAVP and platelet transfusion. Common side effects of DDAVP include facial warmth and flushing, headache, and nausea which occur at the time of administration. Hypertension and hyponatremia are less common side effects. In addition, patients frequently experience tachyphylaxis characterized by a diminution of therapeutic response with repeated doses. DDAVP is administered in a dose of 0.3 μg/kg in 30 cc of normal saline intravenously over 15 to 20 minutes. The response is rapid, within 30 to 60 minutes, and persists for at least several hours. All patients considered for this treatment should first undergo a DDAVP challenge in which they are administered the drug and the effect on the bleeding time is evaluated. Patients who demonstrate a shortening of the bleeding time into the normal range are candidates to receive DDAVP either prophylactically for surgery and dental procedures or for minor hemorrhagic complications. Patients should be monitored for the aforementioned side effects, of which hyponatremia is the most serious. Repeat doses of DDAVP may be given every 12 hours, but extreme caution should be exercised in the younger child, who is at high risk for developing hyponatremia. Platelet transfusion (10 ml/kg) is effective therapy for patients with qualitative platelet defects. Since this treatment is associated with the risk of viral transmission and of alloimmunization, platelet transfusion should be used judiciously in these patients.

Platelet function may also be altered by certain diseases and medications. The most common cause of qualitative platelet disorders in childhood is the ingestion of drugs that affect platelet function. Drug-induced platelet dysfunction alone rarely causes spontaneous hemorrhage but may contribute significantly to postoperative or post-traumatic bleeding and will cause abnormal platelet function tests. Aspirin is the traditional offender, causing a mildly prolonged bleeding time and a minor bleeding tendency that persists for the entire 7- to 10-day life span of the platelet. Trisalicylates, however, do not inhibit platelet function. Other medications used commonly in children which may adversely affect platelet function include certain antibiotics, antihistamines, phenothiazines, and nonsteroidal anti-inflammatory agents. The diagnosis of drug-induced platelet dysfunction is considered in the patient with a recent history of mild bleeding or a prolonged bleeding time without another explanation. The diagnosis is confirmed and the condition treated by discontinuing the drug and documenting clinical improvement or the shortening of the bleeding time. In nearly all cases, discontinuation of the medication is sufficient. Platelet transfusion may occasionally be needed to temporarily restore effective hemostasis.

Platelet function may also be altered in renal, hepatic, cardiac, and neoplastic disease. Patients with uremia may experience bleeding due to a combination of coagulation abnormalities, thrombocytopenia, and platelet dysfunction. The hemostatic defect in this disorder may improve following dialysis or alternatively with the administration of DDAVP. The platelet dysfunction associated with liver disease may also respond to DDAVP. A number of platelet abnormalities have been characterized in children with cardiac defects, myeloproliferative disorders, and leukemia. Although few data are available regarding the specific therapy of these abnormalities, in general platelet function normalizes as the underlying disease is effectively treated. Significant bleeding can usually be controlled with platelet transfusion.

Von Willebrand's Disease

Von Willebrand's disease is a bleeding disorder characterized by a quantitative and/or qualitative defect of von Willebrand factor (vWf). This disease is the most common hereditary disorder of hemostasis. The two major hemostatic functions of vWf are to promote the adhesion of platelets to the subendothelium via the platelet glycoprotein Ib receptor and to act as a carrier molecule for Factor VIII. Moderate deficiencies in vWf are characterized by skin and mucosal bleeding, whereas severe deficiencies are associated with manifestations of deep tissue bleeding. There are three major types of von Willebrand's disease based on the underlying defect. Type I von Willebrand's disease is characterized by quantitatively low levels of normal vWf. Type II is characterized by normal or slightly decreased amounts of abnormal vWf. This qualitative defect in vWf is due to an absence of the largest, most biologically active multimers. Type III von Willebrand's disease is the most severe form, in which homozygous patients exhibit low to undetectable levels of vWf.

Patients with von Willebrand's disease often have a positive family history. However, the history of bleeding in the family may be mild enough to escape detection. The common manifestations of this disorder are those of a platelet-vessel wall interaction defect and include easy bruising, epistaxis, oral mucosal bleeding, and menorrhagia. Patients will often be initially identified after excessive bleeding following surgery or dental extraction. Persons with severe type III disease also develop deep tissue hematomas and hemarthroses due to associated low levels of Factor VIII. The essential laboratory evaluation of the child with suspected von Willebrand's disease should include a platelet count, a bleeding time, a Factor VIII level, a von Willebrand factor antigen determination (vWf:Ag), and a ristocetin cofactor assay, a measure of vWf functional activity. Patients characteristically display a normal platelet count, a prolonged bleeding time, and decreased levels of Factor VIII, vWf:Ag, and ristocetin cofactor activity. Typically the decreases in Factor VIII parallel those of vWf:Ag, since vWf acts as a carrier molecule for Factor VIII. These determinations may vary with time, since both physiologic stress and high circulating levels of estrogen may elevate vWf levels. Therefore, a single normal laboratory screen does not eliminate the diagnosis of this disorder in a patient with bleeding symptoms. Furthermore, it may not be possible to make the diagnosis during pregnancy or while a patient is taking oral contraceptives. Once the diagnosis of von Willebrand's disease is established, it is important to distinguish type I from type II disease, since this will have therapeutic implications. In type I disease, there is a comparable decrease in Factor VIII, vWf, and ristocetin cofactor activity. In type II disease, the ristocetin cofactor activity is further decreased with respect to the levels of Factor VIII and vWf:Ag owing to the functional defect caused by abnormalities of multimer formation. Multimeric analysis is an important diagnostic tool in further elucidating type II disease.

Therapy for von Willebrand's disease involves both general measures and specific treatments. Local measures like pressure, cold packs, and nasal packing may be sufficient for many cases with minor bleeding. Patients with more severe hemorrhage or patients undergoing surgery will often require more specific therapy. The traditional treatment for this disorder has been cryoprecipitate. Cryoprecipitate contains the entire Factor VIII/vWf complex, in contrast to most intermediate-purity or monoclonal antibody–purified Factor VIII concentrates, which lack sufficient amounts of functional vWf. However, certain concentrates, such as Humate-P, do contain significant amounts of functional vWf and are frequently administered as a substitute to cryoprecipitate. The standard dose of cryoprecipitate is one bag per 5 kg of body weight. Humate-P is administered at a dosage of 20 units/kg. The half-life of vWf in plasma is 24 hours. The frequency of administration of these products varies with the treatment situation. Cryoprecipitate and factor concentrates carry all the side effects and risks involved in the administration of blood products. The advent of DDAVP has revolutionized therapy for children with mild or moderate von Willebrand's disease. The administration of DDAVP to patients usually results in a two- to threefold increase in vWf levels owing to the temporary release of endogenous stores from endothelial cells. DDAVP is indicated for patients with type I disease for mild to moderate bleeding manifestations or as prophylaxis prior to surgery or dental procedures. It is administered at a dosage of 0.3 μg/kg intravenously in 30 cc normal saline over 15 to 20 minutes. In general, DDAVP is less useful in type II disease and is contraindicated in the IIb subtype of the disease because of the risk of developing concomitant severe thrombocytopenia. The administration and adverse effects of DDAVP are detailed above. All patients who are candidates to receive DDAVP should undergo a DDAVP challenge to document a response prior to its use during a bleeding episode. This involves the administration of a single standard dose of DDAVP and documentation of both the correction of the bleeding time and the expected rise in the Factor VIII level, vWf:Ag, and ristocetin cofactor activity. The responsiveness to DDAVP is generally consistent within affected families.

COAGULATION ABNORMALITIES

Hereditary bleeding disorders due to clotting factor abnormalities commonly present outside of the newborn period but within the first year of life. In contrast to abnormalities of platelet-vessel interaction, bleeding associated with coagulation factor deficiencies is characterized by deep tissue hematomas and hemarthroses. Oral mucosal bleeding, however, does occur with regularity. Bleeding episodes occur with greater frequency in children after the age of 1 year, corresponding to a period of increased mobility and susceptibility to minor trauma. In the medical history, the presence or absence of an antecedent event helps to determine the severity of the defect. In severe deficiency states, bleeding is often spontaneous. In less severely affected children, the degree of trauma necessary to cause bleeding usually correlates with the extent of the clotting factor abnormality. Whereas the nature of the bleeding episode and the inciting event suggest a clotting factor defect and provide important information as to its severity, a careful family history determines the pattern of inheritance and gives an important clue to the specific diagnosis. Clotting factor defects may be initially suspected by a prolongation of one or a combination of laboratory screening tests which include the prothrombin time, PTT, thrombin time, and fibrinogen assays. They are specifically diagnosed using immunologic and functional assays for the individual factor in question. A specific diagnosis allows for specific replacement therapy.

Hemophilia A and B

Classic hemophilia (hemophilia A), the most common of the inherited coagulation factor deficiencies, is a bleeding disorder characterized by decreased plasma levels of Factor VIII and is seen with a prevalence of 1:10,000. Christmas disease (hemophilia B) is characterized by decreased plasma levels of Factor IX. Although it is the second most common of the inherited factor deficiencies, it is only one tenth as common as hemophilia A. Both are inherited as X-linked recessive disorders, thereby affecting males almost exclusively. The diagnosis is suspected on the basis of the patient's bleeding history, a family history of bleeding in two thirds of cases, and a prolonged PTT in all but those patients with very mild disease. The diagnosis is confirmed on the basis of decreased Factor VIII or IX coagulant activity. Mild hemophilia B may be difficult to diagnose in the newborn, since adult levels of Factor IX are not achieved until the age of 5 to 6 months. Hemophilia A can be distinguished from von Willebrand's disease, in which low levels of Factor VIII are also present, by the family history, the type of bleeding manifestations, a normal bleeding time and normal levels of von Willebrand factor antigen and ristocetin cofactor activity. The clinical presentation of hemophilia A and B are indistinguishable and vary with the severity of the disease. Severe hemophilia (Factor VIII or IX levels less than 1 per cent) is characterized by frequent and often spontaneous bleeding involving muscles, joints, skin, mucous membranes, and viscera. Mild hemophiliacs (Factor VIII or IX levels of 6 to 35 per cent) can exhibit the same type of tissue bleeding, but usually only after significant trauma or surgery. In the absence of a positive family history, they are frequently first diagnosed under these circumstances. Moderate hemophilia (Factor VIII or IX levels of 1 to 5 per cent) is characterized by symptomatology in between that of mild and severe disease. Bleeding is occasionally spontaneous, but is more frequently induced by trauma or surgery. When hemophilia does present in the newborn period, it does so most frequently with postcircumcisional or umbilical cord stump bleeding, oozing from heel stick puncture, or cephalohematoma. In both hemophilia A and B, the factor levels and the corresponding degree of clinical severity tend to remain constant both through the life of the individual and within affected families.

Treatment of Hemophilia

There are two aspects to the optimal treatment of hemophilia: long-term comprehensive care of the physical, psychosocial, emotional, reproductive, and educational concerns of the hemophiliac patient and his family and semiacute therapy of the bleeding episode and possible ensuing complications.

COMPREHENSIVE CARE

Since hemophilia is a chronic, life-long disease affecting all aspects of the lives of those afflicted as well as their families, comprehensive care is an important component of the total care of the hemophiliac. Optimally, it is delivered semiannually or annually through a team approach that coordinates the efforts of the primary caregiver, the hematologist, the hemophilia nurse, the orthopedist, the physical therapist, the dentist, the infectious disease specialist, the psychologist, the social worker, and the genetic counselor. The services of a blood bank and a special coagulation laboratory are also necessary.

ACUTE CARE

The basis of treatment of an acute bleeding episode in hemophilia is factor replacement to a level at which hemostasis is achieved. For moderate to severe hemophilia A and severe hemophilia B, the mainstay of replacement therapy at the present time is concentrated Factor VIII or IX that is commercially prepared from the plasma of 2000 to 30,000 donors who undergo screening for hepatitis B, HIV, and to some extent, non-A, non-B hepatitis. The concentrates are purified lyophilized products that are easily stored and administered, thus allowing for the early treatment of bleeding, often at home by the patient or his family. Major technologic advances in the manufacture of Factor VIII products have resulted in a current generation of concentrate that is safer through the use of both effective viral inactivation and better product purification. This progress has not been made, however, without significant increases in the unit cost of replacement factor. The currently available Factor IX concentrates also undergo viral inactivation. These intermediate-purity products also contain prothrombin, Factor VII, Factor X, and protein C. More highly purified Factor IX concentrates have recently been developed and may soon be available.

For mild to moderate hemophilia B or severe hemophilia B in the very young child, when bleeding episodes are infrequent or the quantity of factor needed to achieve hemostatic levels is low, fresh frozen plasma is used preferentially to minimize blood donor contact. Factor IX concentrates are primarily used in the case of major surgery or life-threatening bleeding when large quantities of replacement factor are needed. For the infant with severe hemophilia A, high purity factor concentrate or single-donor cryoprecipitate is currently used.

Treatment of the patient with mild hemophilia A deserves special consideration and is discussed later in this section.

Dosage. Calculation of the Factor VIII or IX replacement dose is based on the assumption that a child has 50 ml of plasma volume per kilogram of body weight. Furthermore, by international standardization, 1 ml of normal plasma contains 1 unit of Factor VIII or IX, which is equivalent to a 100 per cent level of coagulant activity. Since exogenous Factor VIII is confined to the intravascular space, the administration of 50 units/kg will restore 100 per cent clotting activity in a severely deficient hemophiliac child. Otherwise stated, the infusion of 1 unit/kg of Factor VIII correlates with the 2 per cent rise in the plasma factor level. Factor IX, however, diffuses into the extravascular space making an exact calculation of plasma levels difficult. Approximately twice the calculated dose of Factor VIII is used. Therefore, the administration of 100 units/kg is needed to restore 100 per cent of clotting activity and the administration of 1 unit/kg of Factor IX correlates with a 1 per cent rise in plasma factor levels. The half-life of infused Factor VIII in plasma is 12 to 17 hours and that of Factor IX is 18 to 24 hours. Factor VIII and IX concentrates are supplied in vials containing 500 to 1000 units of factor. One unit of fresh frozen plasma contains 200 to 250 units of Factors IX and VIII. One unit of cryoprecipitate contains about 100 units of Factor VIII.

The goal of therapy in treating hemorrhage in hemophilia is to achieve a plasma level of Factor VIII or IX at which hemostasis can occur. The minimal hemostatic level is 20 to 30 per cent, but the actual level at which hemostasis occurs and the duration of time during which effective hemostasis is needed depends both on the site and the severity of the bleeding episode and on the timing of therapy relative to its occurrence.

Musculoskeletal Bleeding. Bleeding into joints, soft tissue, and muscle is the most frequent complication of hemophilia. If not treated promptly and completely, bleeding can be recurrent, resulting in joint deformity, muscle atrophy, flexion contracture, and chronic disability. In early childhood, hemophiliacs begin to recognize an early bleed by a peculiar sensation felt within the joint before the typical signs of bleeding, i.e., pain, swelling, warmth, and restricted motion, occur. Ideally this is when replacement therapy to a factor level of 30 to 40 per cent should be initiated. Early infusion should be accompanied by the application of ice to the site of injury and by rest for 12 to 24 hours followed by gradual remobilization. Analgesic therapy is rarely needed. If analgesics are used, acetaminophen will usually suffice. Splinting is not necessary under these circumstances, since a child automatically self-splints as long as there is discomfort and remobilizes the limb as the discomfort disappears. Symptomatic improvement is seen within 24 to 48 hours. If a hemarthrosis is severe or treated at an advanced stage when there is already pain, swelling, and restricted mobility, several transfusions to a factor level of 40 per cent may be necessary. In this case, immobilization of the joint in a splint for 2 to 5 days may be indicated. When the splint is removed and the joint remobilized, it is often with the assistance of physical therapy and under transfusion coverage because the risk of rebleeding at this time is high. In rare instances in which there is a large accumulation of blood in a joint as a result of a severe bleed, joint aspiration may be performed by an experienced orthopedist immediately following an infusion to a factor level of 40 per cent. However, this procedure is usually unnecessary.

In the case of a severe or advanced hemarthrosis, the control of pain is important. Since pain is due to the accumulation of blood under pressure within a joint space, effecting hemostasis greatly facilitates the treatment of pain. When analgesia is used, it is important to avoid the use of drugs such as aspirin or indomethacin which, because of their effect on platelet function, could exacerbate bleeding. Although the severity of the pain associated with severe hemarthrosis can exceed the effectiveness of acetaminophen alone, narcotics should be used with caution in the outpatient setting. This is because of the propensity for addiction and misuse, especially in the older hemophiliac. In the rare case in which there is severe pain that does not require hospitalization, drugs such as oxycodone, codeine, or propoxyphene can be used with careful monitoring. In circumstances in which severe pain from hemorrhage requires hospitalization or following orthopedic surgery, however, narcotics should not be withheld. It is at these times that morphine, meperidine, and hydromorphone are most useful.

In a large majority of severe hemophiliacs, one or more target joints may develop. A target joint is defined as a site of recurrent hemarthrosis accounting for the majority of the patient's transfusions. The pathophysiology of recurrent hemarthrosis in a target joint includes two major factors: (1) the toxic effect of proteolytic enzymes released from the breakdown of red cells and hemoglobin on the cartilage matrix and (2) the propensity of hypertrophied synovium to extend into weight-bearing areas of the joint with subsequent rebleeding. This vicious circle may be stopped by the institution of a prophylactic transfusion program for a period of 2 to 6 weeks. In cases in which severe synovial inflammation is suspected, a 1- to 2-week course of prednisone (1 to 2 mg/kg) is often added to the regimen. Rehabilitative management should stress muscle strengthening to increase joint stability and prevent injury. The control of chronic pain in hemophilic arthropathy is often difficult. Trisalicylates, which have low gastric irritability and no effect on platelet function, can be used. In some hemophiliacs relaxation, self-hypnosis, and biofeedback techniques may be efficacious.

Since joint disease is an important cause of chronic morbidity, the prevention of hemarthrosis is one of the most important aspects of the care of the hemophiliac. Currently this is accomplished through the encouragement of general physical fitness to promote the muscle tone and strength that lead to joint stability. Recreational activities should avoid excessive body contact or joint stress. Long-term prophylactic transfusion regimens currently used in Europe are limited in their potential benefit by both the cost and the infectious complications of factor therapy. Future advances in transfusion safety may create new options in the therapy of hemarthrosis.

Bleeding into soft tissue and superficial muscles presents as a painful, expanding mass. Treatment is best accomplished by early replacement therapy to a level of 30 to 40 per cent, accompanied by rest for 12 to 24 hours, and followed by early remobilization to prevent muscle flexion and contraction. Bleeding into the muscles of the calf and forearm merit early therapy and special attention by the physician since hematoma expansion is restricted by the fascial compartment and can produce tense swelling with neurovascular compromise.

Deep muscle hematomas should be treated with early replacement therapy to a level of 40 to 60 per cent for several days. Retroperitoneal bleeding usually presents with hip flexion and pain and the diagnosis is confirmed by ultrasound or CT scan. Because considerable blood loss can occur into the iliopsoas muscle, these bleeding episodes should be monitored carefully, frequently under close hospital supervision. Initial rest followed by mobilization as soon as symptoms abate is important in preventing muscle contractures and chronic disability. Careful analgesic management is critical.

A rare complication of recurrent muscle bleeds is hemophilic pseudotumor, defined as a progressive, destructive, cystic swelling of muscle or bone. Treatment of this lesion is difficult and initially includes replacement therapy and immobilization. If this is unsuccessful, radiation therapy is sometimes employed and surgery may be necessary. Prevention of recurrent muscle bleeds is important and may be accomplished through a regular fitness program.

Undue trauma to the muscle should be prevented. Immunizations should not be withheld from the hemophiliac child but should be administered carefully using a 25-gauge needle with firm pressure applied to the injection site for 10 minutes. The vastus lateralis muscle in infants and small children can be used as the site of injection, but in older children with sufficient muscle mass, the deltoid, where early hemorrhage is easily visible, is preferred. Alternatively, immunizations can be administered subcutaneously, but this route is less effective in producing immunity. Intramuscular injections should otherwise be avoided.

Oral Mucosal Bleeding. Early manifestations of hemophilia occurring in the first year of life usually involve bleeding from the mouth secondary to tooth eruptions as well as minor trauma to gums, frenula, tongue, and oral mucosa. Later in childhood, bleeding occurs with the traumatic loss of a tooth or tooth extraction. Treatment of oral bleeding includes a one-time correction of the Factor VIII or IX level to 40 to 50 per cent and the oral administration of an antifibrinolytic agent such as epsilon-amino caproic acid which inhibits the action of fibrinolytic enzymes present in saliva and retards clot dissolution. The use of epsilon-amino caproic acid effectively diminishes the factor requirement but cannot totally replace it. It is given initially at the time of factor infusion at a dose of 200 mg/kg and then every 6 hours at a dose of 100 mg/kg for 2 to 5 days until complete healing occurs. Gastrointestinal disturbance is common with this medication. Dental restoration in the hemophiliac patient involves the use of special techniques designed to reduce the potential for hemorrhage. The prophylactic infusion of factor and the oral administration of epsilon-amino caproic acid is usually recommended.

Visceral Bleeding. Visceral hemorrhage in the hemophiliac, although less common than musculoskeletal bleeding, does occur. Renal bleeding in the form of microscopic or gross hematuria occurs in the severe hemophiliac. If it is severe or complicated by fever or flank or abdominal pain, the child should be evaluated for genitourinary infection or pathology. Mild uncomplicated bleeding is often treated with bed rest and a 5- to 7-day course of prednisone at a dose of 2 mg/kg/day. Although daily transfusion therapy to factor levels of 40 per cent is sometimes used, it is frequently not efficacious. The use of epsilon-amino caproic acid is contraindicated in this setting. Gastrointestinal bleeding must be evaluated with respect to a possible anatomic abnormality. With significant bleeding, factor replacement to a level of 40 per cent is indicated.

Trauma. Minor trauma in a hemophiliac, as in any child, happens frequently. In the event of a significant laceration, the patient should be transfused to a factor level of 40 per cent every day or other day until wound healing is complete. If sutures are necessary, retransfusion following suture removal is indicated. Major trauma is a life-threatening emergency for the hemophiliac. Intracranial hemorrhage, in particular, carries with it a high mortality rate. Accordingly, all hemophiliacs with a history of head trauma should be treated rapidly and empirically to a factor level of 80 to 100 per cent and maintained at that level for a minimum of 10 days if an intracranial bleed is confirmed.

Surgery. Major surgery can be safely performed in any hemophiliac patient without an inhibitor if proper medical expertise and support services are available. The risks and benefits must be weighed for each procedure and performed on an elective basis whenever possible. A preoperative evaluation should establish baseline factor levels, confirm the absence of an inhibitor, and determine the half-life of infused factor for that particular patient. At the time of surgery, the patient should be infused to a level of 100 per cent. Postoperatively, he should be maintained at a factor level of 50 per cent or greater until wound healing is evident, and at a level of at least 30 per cent until wound healing is complete. Frequent monitoring of factor levels is extremely important in the postoperative period.

Mild Hemophilia A

Mild hemophilia A differs significantly from the more severe forms of the disease. Frequently the patient bleeds only after trauma and during dental extraction or surgery. Consequently, he may experience long intervals between bleeding episodes, particularly if he avoids activities that predispose him to injury. When a mild hemophiliac does bleed, however, the signs and symptoms are similar to those described for severe disease and treatment should be prompt to avoid chronic morbidity. The decision to treat with blood products must be a judicious one, balancing the risk of transfusion-related complications against the risk of complications associated with hemorrhage. When factor infusion is absolutely necessary, high-purity concentrates are used to minimize the risk of transmission of

viral disease. Alternatively, cryoprecipitate, a single donor product, can be used, particularly in regions of the country where the risk of viral contamination of blood products is low.

The patient with mild hemophilia A who has baseline Factor VIII levels of greater than 10 per cent may be preferentially treated with DDAVP (1-desamino-8-D-arginine vasopressin). This synthetic analogue of vasopressin transiently raises endogenous plasma levels of Factor VIII an average of fourfold when administered intravenously. Patients should undergo a DDAVP challenge to document their response to the drug prior to its use in the treatment or prevention of bleeding. Once established, the response in an individual patient continues to be predictable. DDAVP is administered at a dose of 0.3 µg/kg in 30 ml normal saline intravenously over 15 to 20 minutes. Depending on the patient's baseline factor level and the hemostatic level required, DDAVP can be used alone to achieve hemostasis or as adjunctive therapy to reduce the patient's total transfusion needs. The drug does not raise endogenous levels of Factor IX and thus has no application in hemophilia B.

Complications of Replacement Therapy

The complications associated with therapy include the development of inhibitors to Factor VIII and less commonly to Factor IX, the transmission of viral disease, allergic and hemolytic transfusion reactions, and, with the use of Factor IX concentrates, thrombosis and DIC.

THE DEVELOPMENT OF INHIBITORS

Inhibitors to Factor VIII occur in about 10 per cent of patients with severe hemophilia A owing to the development of antibodies against the exogenous protein. This phenomenon can develop unpredictably at any point in the life of the hemophiliac, so regular testing is essential, particularly before surgery. The development of an inhibitor can often present as a failure of the bleeding patient to respond promptly to replacement therapy. The treatment of inhibitor patients remains challenging. Conservative therapy for minor bleeds is often indicated and includes rest and immobilization of the affected joint or muscle. Some inhibitors are present in low titers (less than 3 to 5 Bethesda units), and are not inducible upon re-exposure to Factor VIII. During a bleeding episode, these antibodies can be neutralized with large replacement doses of Factor VIII. The inhibitor titer must still be closely followed at 6-month intervals. Low-titer inhibitors that are inducible can also be treated with large doses of Factor VIII until the anamnestic response occurs within 3 to 7 days and the plasma recovery and half-life of infused factor are greatly reduced. Because these inhibitors are inducible to high titers that can no longer be overcome with Factor VIII replacement, this therapy is reserved for life-threatening bleeding or surgery. For significant bleeds that are not life-threatening, Factor IX concentrates can effect hemostasis in these patients without the requirement for Factor VIII. Both Factor IX concentrates and activated prothrombin complex concentrates (Autoplex, FEIBA) can be used, although the judicious use of the latter is appropriate owing to their expense and thrombotic potential. Both agents appear to be are equally effective. Severe or life-threatening hemorrhage in a high titer inhibitor patient is often treated immediately with Factor IX concentrate at a dose of 100 units/kg or activated prothrombin complex at a dose of 50 to 100 units/kg followed by the use of porcine Factor VIII in patients without cross-reacting antibodies. Alternatively, plasmapheresis can reduce the inhibitor titer and allow for the use of high doses of human plasma-derived or porcine Factor VIII. The therapy of Factor IX inhibitors is more problematic, but these occur infrequently. Recombinant Factor VIIa is now in clinical evaluation for the treatment of both Factor VIII and Factor IX inhibitors. Immunosuppressive therapy, involving immunoabsorption of the inhibiting antibody and the administration of intravenous gamma globulin and high-dose Factor VIII, may be of some value in lowering the inhibitor titer. Long-term therapy is required to establish a response and is costly.

The Transmission of Viral Disease

Hepatitis. Transfusion-related viral hepatitis is often a subclinical disease manifested by transient changes of liver function tests. Although the risk of acquiring the hepatitis B virus through transfusion has been greatly reduced through blood donor screening and improved methods of viral inactivation, occasional new cases of hepatitis B infection do occur in non-immunized patients. It remains important, therefore, that newly diagnosed hemophiliacs receive the hepatitis B vaccine. In the infant, immunizations are begun soon after birth. Five to 10 per cent of previously infected patients are carriers for HBsAg and should be followed for the development of chronic liver disease, liver tumors, and coinfection with delta hepatitis.

Transfusion-related infection with the non-A, non-B hepatitis (NANBH) virus, otherwise known as hepatitis C, is suspected on the basis of persistently or intermittently elevated liver transaminases in the majority of transfused hemophiliacs. Since about 20 per cent of these patients will develop chronic liver disease, NANBH is a major cause of transfusion-related morbidity. Currently, the screening of blood donors for the presence of hepatitis B core antibody and an elevated ALT has reduced NANBH transmission by 60 per cent. A new antibody test that is specific for hepatitis C will be introduced shortly. Furthermore, the newer viral inactivation techniques of monoclonal antibody purification and wet heat or solvent/detergent treatment of Factor VIII concentrates show great promise, decreasing even further the transmission rate of NANBH. Currently available Factor IX preparations are not approved to undergo wet heat or solvent/detergent treatment for viral inactivation. The less effective dry heat processing that they do undergo does not eliminate NANBH transmission. Although no satisfactory therapy exists for the chronic active hepatitis resulting from NANBH infection, afflicted patients should be followed carefully for progression of liver disease.

Infection with EBV, CMV, and parvovirus remains a problem, since no satisfactory method of inactivation of these viruses in blood products yet exists.

Human Immunodeficiency Virus (HIV-1). The viral transmission of HIV-1 through the use of blood products occurred predominantly between 1979 and 1983. Greater than 50 per cent of all hemophiliacs and 90 per cent of severe hemophiliacs are estimated to have been infected as adults. It has been recently demonstrated that 13 per cent of hemophiliacs under 18 years of age infected with HIV-1 for a period of 8 years develop AIDS. As of 1989, 1300 cases of AIDS have been confirmed in the hemophiliac population. Therefore, testing for HIV seropositivity is generally recommended in any patient who has had blood product exposure prior to 1985. Monitoring of the absolute numbers of CD4+ cells (T helper/inducer lymphocytes) at least every 6 months is also indicated. A decline in the absolute number of CD4+ cells may signal progression from exposure to disease. However, a decrease in the absolute number of CD4+ cells as well as abnormal T cell function are also seen in HIV-seronegative individuals owing to the exposure to large amounts of exogenous protein present in factor concentrates.

Currently, azidothymidine (AZT) must be considered for the treatment of HIV-seropositive hemophiliacs with an absolute CD4+ cell number of less than 500/μl. The benefit of therapy must be weighed against the drug's substantial bone marrow suppressive effect.

Currently, AZT is FDA-approved only for children over 12 years of age. The dosage schedule for AZT administration in this population is under re-evaluation, but 100 mg taken orally 5 times daily has been shown to be as effective in the delay of progression of disease in HIV-positive asymptomatic patients as the standard higher dose, but with reduced toxicity. A safe dosing schedule for children under the age of 12 years is currently being investigated. Aerosolized pentamidine therapy for the prevention of *Pneumocystis carinii* pneumonia must also be considered in HIV-seropositive individuals with CD4+ cell counts of 200/μl or less. The currently recommended regimen is 300 mg delivered by jet nebulizer every 4 weeks.

Prevention of HIV infection, however, remains the most effective approach to the problem of AIDS in hemophilia. Since 1985, blood donors have been tested for HIV-seropositivity, thus reducing the risk of HIV-contaminated blood to one in 50,000 to 100,000 units. Furthermore, factor concentrates treated with wet heat or solvent and detergent and subjected to monoclonal antibody purification have produced no documented cases of HIV seroconversion in previously untreated hemophiliacs.

Transfusion Reactions. Two types of transfusion reactions can occur. The more frequent type of reaction is allergic and occurs more often with the use of single donor products than with concentrate. The patient may exhibit a febrile reaction, chills, itching, hives, and respiratory compromise. Mild reactions are treated by slowing or stopping the transfusion. More serious reactions can be treated with diphenhydramine, corticosteroids, or epinephrine.

A less frequent complication is the hemolytic transfusion reaction that can occur in blood type A or B patients receiving a large amount of factor concentrate, since low levels of anti-A and anti-B antibodies contaminate these products. This does not occur in blood type O patients or in those receiving type-specific single donor units of cryoprecipitate or fresh frozen plasma. Management of a hemolytic transfusion reaction is indicated. If severe, the patient should be transfused with type O red cells.

Thrombosis and Disseminated Intravascular Coagulation. Thrombosis and disseminated intravascular coagulation are complications associated with the treatment of Factor IX–deficient patients and of Factor VIII–deficient patients with inhibitors when Factor IX concentrate or activated prothrombin complex concentrate is used. This complication is less frequently observed in children than in adults. The particular combination of postoperative immobility and the large quantities of Factor IX concentrate needed with surgery puts the surgical patient at a particularly high risk for this complication. The concurrent use of heparin is sometimes employed to minimize these risks. Higher purity Factor IX concentrate, when available, may minimize this complication.

Prenatal Screening

The prenatal diagnosis of hemophilia A or B involves the identification of both the obligate carrier and the affected fetus. Both can be reliably performed using DNA restriction enzyme analysis to identify restriction fragment length polymorphisms in the Factor VIII or IX genes.

Inherited Abnormalities of Other Coagulation Factors

Deficiencies of coagulant proteins other than Factor VIII or IX are less common and may not always be associated with a bleeding tendency. When the tendency does occur, deep tissue bleeding is observed. The severity of symptoms usually correlates with the severity of the factor deficiency.

Deficiency of the Contact Phase Factors

The contact phase factors include Factor XII, prekallikrein, and high molecular weight kininogen. Deficiencies of these factors are inherited in an autosomal recessive manner. These defects in both the homozygote and the heterozygote are associated with a prolongation of the PTT but are not associated with a bleeding tendency. If a contact factor defect is determined to be responsible for a prolonged PTT, no therapy is necessary.

Deficiency of Factor XI

Factor XI deficiency, inherited in an autosomal recessive manner, is significantly less common than Factor IX deficiency. It is most commonly observed in the Jewish population. The bleeding tendency is absent in heterozygotes. In homozygotes it is variable and does not correlate specifically with the degree of the defect. When bleeding does occur, it usually does so at Factor XI levels below 15 per cent and is often mild. Treatment

may be necessary for significant trauma or at the time of surgery and is accomplished through the infusion of 10 to 15 ml/kg of fresh frozen plasma, which will raise the plasma level to 20 per cent. The half-life of infused Factor XI is 60 hours.

Deficiency of the Vitamin K–Dependent Factors

The vitamin K–dependent proteins, Factors VII, IX, X, and prothrombin require vitamin K during biosynthesis. Deficiencies in Factors VII and X, as well as hypo- and dysprothrombinemia, are rare. The diagnosis of these disorders may be difficult in the newborn before adult plasma factor levels are achieved. All are inherited as autosomal recessive disorders (except for Factor IX deficiency), and bleeding manifestations occur only in the homozygote. Bleeding tends to be of moderate severity, but severe hemorrhage can be seen in Factor VII deficiency. Furthermore, hypoprothrombinemia and Factor VII deficiency have been known to present in the newborn period. Deficiencies of Factors VII, X, and prothrombin cause a prolongation of the prothrombin time. Significantly low levels of Factor X or prothrombin will also cause a prolongation of the PTT. The treatment of Factor VII deficiency with replacement therapy is complicated by its short half-life of 4 to 6 hours. Moreover, Factor IX concentrates contain variable amounts of Factor VII. Nonetheless, they are currently the product of choice, infused at a dose of 20 to 40 units/kg. Prothrombin defects are also treated with Factor IX concentrates. Twenty units per kilogram achieves a hemostatic level of 20 per cent and the half-life of infused protein is 60 hours. Factor X deficiency is often treated to a hemostatic level of 15 per cent with 10 to 15 ml/kg of fresh frozen plasma, although Factor IX concentrates can also be used. The half-life of this factor is 42 hours. The risks associated with the use of single or multiple donor blood products must be considered in the treatment plan for patients with these disorders.

Deficiency of Factor V

Factor V deficiency is also inherited in an autosomal recessive manner. Homozygotes display a moderate bleeding tendency and present with a prolongation of both the prothrombin time and the PTT. Bleeding in the newborn has been reported. Treatment of bleeding is with 10 to 15 ml/kg of fresh frozen plasma, which will raise factor levels to 20 to 25 per cent, an adequate hemostatic level. The plasma half-life of infused Factor V is 24 to 36 hours. Because of the occasional finding of combined Factor VIII–Factor V deficiency, all patients diagnosed with Factor V deficiency should undergo determination of their Factor VIII level.

Abnormalities in Fibrinogen

Hereditary quantitative abnormalities in fibrinogen are rare. Homozygotes present with afibrinogenemia and heterozygotes with hypofibrinogenemia. The bleeding tendency is usually not severe, although umbilical cord bleeding, ecchymoses, and intracranial hemorrhage have been reported in the newborn period secondary to afibrinogenemia. The dysfibrinogenemias, a group of disorders characterized by qualitative defects in fibrinogen, also occur rarely. They are inherited in an autosomal dominant manner and are associated with a variable bleeding tendency. Paradoxically, some patients develop thrombosis. Screening tests for these disorders include a reptilase time, which is prolonged with qualitative and quantitative abnormalities in fibrinogen, and the thrombin time, which is also prolonged in the presence of a dysfibrinogenemia and fibrinogen levels below 100 mg/dl. The clotting assay for fibrinogen usually provides the definitive diagnosis, although an immunologic measurement may be necessary to document a dysfibrinogenemia. When it is necessary to treat bleeding associated with these abnormalities, it is best accomplished with an infusion of cryoprecipitate which contains 250 mg of fibrinogen in each unit. An infusion of 40 to 50 mg/kg of fibrinogen will raise the plasma level by 80 to 100 mg/dl and provide adequate hemostasis for several days, since the half-life of this protein is 80 hours.

Deficiency of Factor XIII

The function of Factor XIII is to crosslink fibrin and thus stabilize a formed clot. A deficiency in this factor is rare and is inherited as an autosomal recessive disorder. Heterozygotes are asymptomatic, but hemorrhage in the homozygote can be severe. The pattern of bleeding is characteristically delayed in onset from the time of injury. Factor XIII often presents in the newborn with persistent bleeding from the umbilical cord. Because of the less frequent but significant incidence of intracranial hemorrhage, and because of the long half-life of infused Factor XIII of 100 to 150 hours, the prophylactic transfusion of fresh frozen plasma is often recommended in the neonatal period. An infusion of 1 to 2 ml/kg will raise the level of Factor XIII in plasma to 2 to 3 per cent, sufficient for hemostasis. An infusion of 10 ml/kg, however, provides prophylaxis for 10 to 14 days, thereby minimizing trauma to the infant and the total number of blood product exposures. Routine coagulation tests will not detect Factor XIII deficiency, which is diagnosed by the clot solubility assay.

Acquired Abnormalities in Coagulation

Vitamin K Deficiency

Vitamin K is an important cofactor in the carboxylation of certain coagulant and anticoagulant factors that are made almost exclusively in the liver. These vitamin K–dependent proteins include prothrombin and Factors VII, IX, and X, as well as proteins C and S. In the absence of vitamin K, these proteins circulate in the blood in an inactive form. The causes of vitamin K deficiency include a diminished bioavailability in utero, decreased oral intake, prolonged diarrhea, antibiotic suppression of normal gut flora, and malabsorption, as well as the ingestion of warfarin, a vitamin K antagonist, either by accident or as prescribed for the therapy of thrombosis. The resulting coagulopathy is manifested by a significantly prolonged prothrombin time and PTT in the face of a normal thrombin time and fibrinogen and platelet counts. The tissue-type bleeding manifes-

tations are dependent on the extent of the coagulopathy. The treatment of choice in most cases is the intramuscular administration of vitamin K. The dose in a newborn is 0.5 to 1 mg and for an older child is in the range of 5 to 10 mg. If malabsorption is not present, vitamin K can be given orally at a dose of 5 to 10 mg in newborns and older children. Vitamin K can be administered intravenously if no other route is possible. Since rare anaphylactic reactions do occur with this route of administration, the drug must be given cautiously at a maximum rate of 1 mg/min and with epinephrine available. The effect of vitamin K therapy in restoring normal hemostasis is fairly rapid, occurring within hours. In the face of severe hemorrhage, however, immediate replacement of the vitamin K–dependent coagulation proteins is necessary, justifying the use of fresh frozen plasma at a dose of 10 to 15 ml/kg.

Hemorrhagic Disease of the Newborn

Hemorrhagic disease of the newborn (HDN) presents as generalized bleeding occurring in otherwise healthy babies during the first week of life and is due to vitamin K deficiency. Three distinct syndromes have been described depending on the time of manifestation: (1) early HDN, occurring in the first 24 hours of life, (2) classic HDN, occurring in the first week of life, and (3) late HDN, occurring in the infant aged 1 to 3 months. In early and classic HDN, maternal vitamin K deficiency may be implicated. The etiology of this deficiency is unclear in those mothers who have not been on anticonvulsant or antituberculous chemotherapy but may relate to diet. In classic HDN, vitamin K deficiency may be further exacerbated by breast feeding, since breast milk contains approximately 60 per cent less vitamin K than cow's milk. The reported bleeding manifestations have included cephalohematoma and intracranial, intrathoracic, intraabdominal, skin, and mucosal bleeds. A prolonged prothrombin time and PTT are observed.

Vitamin K deficiency can always be treated and bleeding almost always prevented with the intramuscular injection of 0.5 to 1 mg of vitamin K immediately at delivery. The deficiency is corrected within hours. When intramuscular injections are contraindicated and malabsorption is not a problem, 5 mg of vitamin K can be given orally. Life-threatening bleeding is treated with the concomitant infusion of 10 to 15 ml/kg of fresh frozen plasma. The syndrome of late HDN, manifested often by intracranial bleeding in an otherwise normal young infant, has been related to malabsorption syndromes. Other cases are associated with the exclusive use of breast feeding, sometimes exacerbated by antibiotic administration. Late HDN occurs very rarely in babies given 1 mg of vitamin K intramuscularly at birth. Treatment is with vitamin K or with vitamin K and fresh frozen plasma given as described in the previous section. In infants at continued risk owing to malabsorption or parenteral feeding, vitamin K should be readministered empirically every 2 to 4 weeks.

Severe Liver Disease

The coagulopathy of severe hepatic parenchymal disease is due to a combination of decreased synthesis of blood-clotting proteins; increased consumption of coagulant proteins and platelets due to tissue and endothelial cell damage, DIC, and increased fibrinolysis; and hypersplenism. The severity of each of these components can be assessed in the laboratory. Determinations of the platelet count, prothrombin time, PTT, thrombin time, fibrinogen, fibrin split products, and D-dimer allow assessment of the contribution of DIC and fibrinolysis. A level of Factor VII, with its short plasma half-life of 4 to 6 hours, is an indicator of hepatic synthetic function. Treatment consists of replacement therapy with platelet concentrate for thrombocytopenia, fresh frozen plasma for factor replacement, and cryoprecipitate for the replacement of fibrinogen. Major hemostatic abnormalities sometimes respond only to exchange transfusion with fresh whole blood or fresh frozen plasma–reconstituted packed red cells, followed by platelet transfusion. The neonate with severe congenital or acquired liver disease is treated similarly.

Disseminated Intravascular Coagulation

Disseminated intravascular coagulation (DIC) is characterized by a generalized pathologic activation and consumption of clotting factors and platelets. Fibrin deposition throughout the microvasculature and subsequent development of microthrombi accompany this disorder. A microangiopathic hemolytic anemia and organ failure can be the result of this pathologic process. The ill child may thus exhibit both generalized hemorrhage and thrombosis. However, DIC is always a secondary phenomenon, triggered by primary events which include infection, hypoxia and acidosis, tissue injury with the release of tissue factor, malignancy, severe liver disease, giant hemangiomas, major vessel thrombosis including purpura fulminans, and, in the neonate specifically, respiratory distress syndrome. The laboratory manifestations of DIC include thrombocytopenia, a prolongation of the prothrombin time and PTT, and a decrease in fibrinogen, all of which reflect consumption of clotting proteins. The presence of D-dimer and fibrin split products correlates with fibrinolysis and fibrinogenolysis. A prolonged thrombin time reflects a low fibrinogen level and elevated fibrin split products. Anemia with fragmented red blood cells and schistocytes on blood smear reflects microangiopathic shearing and destruction.

Since DIC is triggered by a primary event, the first rule of therapy is aggressive treatment of the primary disease process with careful monitoring of the hematologic status. In many instances specific hematologic therapy is not necessary. Replacement therapy is indicated, however, when the triggering primary event cannot be adequately treated, when the child presents with significant or life-threatening bleeding manifestations or the potential for such exists, as with the need for imminent surgery, or when there is development of purpura fulminans. In these cases, fresh frozen plasma at 10 to 15 ml/kg, platelets at 10 ml/kg, and cryoprecipitate at 20 ml/kg as needed for the replacement of fibrinogen should be administered to partially correct abnormal coagulation parameters and to treat bleeding. Infusion of packed red blood cells may be required for

anemia. An exchange transfusion may be required when the amount of replacement product needed begins to exceed fluid volumes that can be safely infused.

The use of heparin, which can otherwise worsen the bleeding diathesis, is reserved for (1) the DIC associated with acute promyelocytic or monocytic leukemia, (2) major vessel thrombosis including purpura fulminans, and (3) impending tissue necrosis. Full-dose heparin should be used with a loading dose of 50 units/kg followed by a continuous infusion rate of 20 units/kg/hr. This rate can be adjusted to yield a PTT in the range of two times the upper limit of normal. Effective therapy can be monitored by the cessation of clinically significant hemorrhage or thrombosis and the correction of the prothrombin time, PTT, and fibrinogen.

DIC in the sick newborn can be particularly severe because of a decreased capacity for clearance of activated clotting factors and fibrin split products by the immature reticuloendothelial system and because of decreased compensatory factor synthesis due to liver immaturity. Furthermore, the neonate is particularly susceptible to any of the primary triggers of DIC. In the neonate, the laboratory can also be used to diagnose and monitor the severity of DIC. The PTT tends not to be as useful in the premature infant since it is usually already significantly prolonged in the well baby. One must remember that DIC and purpura fulminans in the newborn may represent homozygous protein C deficiency. The indications for the use of replacement therapy and heparin in neonates remain the same as in older children. Increased tolerance to heparin occurs in the neonate, and larger maintenance doses in the range of 25 to 30 U/kg/hr may be required. Adequate heparinization may be achieved by maintaining the Laidlaw microclotting time in the range of 100 to 180 seconds in preterm infants and the PTT at twice the normal value in term babies.

THROMBOTIC DISORDERS

Neonatal Thrombosis

The newborn exhibits physiologically low levels of the contact and vitamin K-dependent factors, normal adult levels of Factors V and VIII, fibrinogen, and von Willebrand factor, and low circulating levels of all the known major anticoagulants and their cofactors, i.e., antithrombin III, heparin cofactor II, protein C, and protein S. This results in a tendency toward hypercoagulability. The newborn does not present with thrombosis, however, unless stressed by illness, subjected to catheter placement, or genetically predisposed through an inherited deficiency of one of the anticoagulant proteins. When thrombosis does occur under these circumstances, it can be life-threatening and requires prompt intervention.

Hereditary Predisposition to Thrombosis

Heterozygous anticoagulant deficiencies, in their autosomal dominant forms, tend to present in late childhood and early adulthood. Homozygous deficiency usually manifests in the newborn but is extremely rare. Homozygous protein C deficiency, of which fewer than

20 cases have been described, is the most common. The principal manifestation of this disorder, severe purpura fulminans, usually develops within hours to days after birth and can result in severe scarring or partial loss of an extremity. CNS thrombosis with permanent neurologic sequelae and retinal artery thrombosis resulting in blindness also occur and may represent intrauterine events. Screening laboratory studies often reveal DIC. The diagnosis is made on the basis of undetectable levels of protein C activity in the newborn's plasma. Both parents often exhibit about 50 per cent levels of protein C, but are clinically asymptomatic. The recommended initial therapy for both the purpura and DIC is fresh frozen plasma, infused at a dose of 10 ml/kg every 12 hours. These infusions result in peak protein C plasma levels of 15 to 30 per cent within 30 minutes. Trough levels at 12 hours of 4 to 10 per cent are still protective against thrombosis. Fresh frozen plasma infusions are usually maintained from 4 to 8 weeks until purpuric lesions are healed. The addition of heparin to this regimen is not beneficial. Long-term therapy is most often accomplished through the use of oral anticoagulation with warfarin. The doses range from 0.15 to 0.4 mg/kg/day but must be individually regulated to maintain the prothrombin time at 1.5 to 2 times the normal value. Long-term therapy with oral anticoagulants is complicated by unpredictable absorption and compliance leading to the possibility of overdosage and bleeding, or underdosage and the redevelopment of thrombosis. For this reason, fresh frozen plasma should be continued during the initial regulation of the anticoagulant dose. Once it is in the desired range, the prothrombin time must be carefully monitored every 2 to 4 weeks. Since the long-term effect of warfarin use in early childhood is unknown, it is recommended that bone growth and development be assessed every 6 to 12 months.

One case of severe homozygous protein S deficiency has been recently reported presenting at the age of 2 weeks. Management is similar to that described for homozygous protein C deficiency. Homozygous antithrombin III deficiency has not been described.

Acquired Predisposition to Thrombosis

Thrombosis can be a significant cause of morbidity in the sick newborn. Complicating factors associated with an increased risk of thrombosis include physiologic states and medical interventions that alter blood flow and the vessel wall such as polycythemia, hyperviscosity, and catheter placement. Infants born to diabetic mothers and to narcotic addicts are also prone to thrombosis, as are babies born small for gestational age.

The diagnosis of thrombosis is made using noninvasive technology if possible. Depending on the site of the lesion, Doppler ultrasonography, computed tomography scan, echocardiography, renal and pulmonary scans, and venography have all been helpful both in diagnosis and in following the effect of therapy. The mainstay of therapy for neonatal arterial and venous thrombosis is heparin. At the first sign of the thrombosis, which in the extremity may be decreased pulses or color changes, heparin therapy should be begun with a loading dose of 50 U/kg followed by a continuous infusion of 20 to 30 U/kg/hr. Neonates often require higher doses of heparin because of an accelerated metabolism of the drug. The dose should be monitored 4 hours into the infusion and daily thereafter by the Laidlaw time in preterm infants (desired range of 100 to 180 seconds) or the PTT in the term infant (desired range of two times the normal value). Prior to heparinization, baseline values for these parameters should be obtained. Proteins C and S as well as antithrombin III levels may also be measured to rule out a possible underlying inherited deficiency. Heparinization is maintained until thrombosis is almost resolved. This may take only 48 to 72 hours for early catheter-related arterial thrombosis or as long as 10 to 14 days for a major renal vein thrombosis. When used in this manner, heparin does not place the sick infant at an increased risk for bleeding.

For a very extensive or life-threatening thrombosis, surgical removal of the clot may be considered. If this is not possible and the lesion is not resolving with heparin therapy alone, a trial of fibrinolytic therapy is indicated. The agent most frequently used is urokinase with a loading dose of 4400 U/kg/hr followed by a continuous infusion of 4400 U/kg/hr. Fresh frozen plasma may also be necessary to raise plasminogen levels that are physiologically low in the newborn. The fibrinolytic state is measured by a decrease in baseline fibrinogen and plasminogen levels and an increase in fibrin split products. Once the fibrinolytic state is attained, thrombolysis, if it is to occur, will do so within 48 to 72 hours.

Thrombosis Outside the Neonatal Period

Isolated thrombosis in pediatric patients outside the neonatal period is distinctly rare. Most cases of thrombosis in children are secondary events. Not infrequently thrombosis may complicate vascular instrumentation. Less commonly it may occur during certain infections, purpura fulminans secondary to meningococcemia being the classic example, or in association with nephrotic syndrome, homocystinuria, Kawasaki syndrome, or pregnancy. In these cases of secondary thrombosis the proper management of the underlying condition and routine anticoagulation is generally sufficient. Patients should receive a heparin bolus of 50 U/kg followed by a continuous infusion of 20 U/kg/hr, which should be titrated to maintain the PTT at approximately two times the normal value. Since extensive tissue damage with necrosis is common in purpura fulminans, there is continuous production of tissue factor, which serves to augment the thrombotic process. Therefore, it is essential that anticoagulation be maintained for an extended period of time and, optimally, until the process has resolved.

Thrombosis may also occur in children due to a genetic predisposition. Homozygous deficiencies of the naturally occurring anticoagulants generally present in the neonatal period with the severe manifestations of thrombosis. Individuals who are heterozygous for antithrombin III, protein C, and protein S have a propensity to develop thrombosis, but this generally occurs later in life. These patients usually have levels that are approximately 50 per cent of normal for the affected protein. There are occasional patients who have a qualitative defect in these anticoagulant factors, requiring specialized function assays for detection. Affected individuals generally do not experience thrombotic problems until the second or third decade of life and sometimes even later. Commonly, thrombotic events are triggered by additional prothrombotic factors such as pregnancy, trauma, surgery, inflammation, or bed rest in addition to the underlying tendency. Patients who develop thrombosis at a young age in the absence of an underlying clinical condition that would promote thrombosis should be screened for these deficiencies. Since these disorders are inherited in mendelian fashion other members of the family may be affected. Therefore, a careful family history is an important part of the evaluation. This should include specific questions regarding sudden unexpected deaths, episodes of deep venous thrombosis or pulmonary embolism at an early age, infant deaths, or stillbirths.

The management of the acute thrombotic event in these patients should include appropriate anticoagulation with heparin. If a homozygous deficiency of one of the regulatory proteins is detected, the administration of fresh frozen plasma will partially restore plasma levels. Antithrombin III concentrate is being developed for treatment of heterozygous antithrombin III deficiency and may be useful in the management of patients with antithrombin III deficiency. Beyond the acute event, chronic maintenance oral anticoagulation with warfarin is recommended.

ACUTE LEUKEMIA

DONALD PINKEL, M.D.

Acute leukemia is a curable disease. The cure rate depends not only on the species of acute leukemia but also on the skill of treatment. For this reason, every child with acute leukemia should be referred to a pediatric hematology/oncology research and treatment center where the best-honed skills are available to the child.

Treatment of acute leukemia is continuously evolving, so that methods outlined here may be more or less obsolete when they are published. This is an additional reason for referral to a center where the latest and often yet unpublished information about treatment is known.

After initial evaluation of the child and planning of treatment are completed in a research and treatment center, much of the week-to-week care of the child can be managed by the child's community pediatrician, with periodic consultation and monitoring by the center.

Chemotherapy of acute leukemia varies with biologic species (Table 1). Supportive measures are similar for all types.

Chemotherapy of Acute Lymphoid Leukemia

Morphology, cytochemical stains, immunologic markers, and cytogenetic findings are used to classify acute lymphoid leukemia (ALL), which constitutes about 80 per cent of all childhood acute leukemia. Antileukemia drugs are chosen and scheduled according to immunophenotypic and genotypic properties. This allows administration of maximum dosage of more effective drugs while avoiding the immediate and delayed side effects of minimally effective or ineffective drugs. Experience to date suggests that anthracycline compounds and alkylating agents carry the greatest long-term risk in children. Excessive adrenocorticosteroid usage also has serious sequelae. Largely because of its growth-inhibitory and carcinogenic effects in children, the use of irradiation is highly restricted.

The most frequent immunophenotype of acute lymphoid leukemia in children is early pre-B (common). Next is pre-B, T-cell, early pre-B/monocytoid or myeloid (null), and the rare B-cell ("Burkitt cell") form. Hyperdiploidy is frequently associated with early pre-B ALL. Pseudodiploidy of leukemia cells is often detected in pre-B and T-cell ALL and is usually present in early pre-B/monocytoid or myeloid and in B-cell ALL.

Remission Induction. For early pre-B, pre-B, and early pre-B/monocytoid or myeloid ALL we administer prednisone, vincristine, and asparaginase in order to produce clinical and laboratory disappearance of leukemia and to allow regeneration of normal hematopoiesis. Most patients experience a complete clinical and hematologic remission after 4 weeks of this treatment. For children with T-cell ALL we add daunorubicin as a fourth drug. Children with B-cell ALL receive high-dosage cyclophosphamide and cytarabine in addition to the three primary drugs.

Preventive Meningeal Chemotherapy. In order to destroy leukemia cells in the arachnoid meninges and thus prevent meningeal relapse, intrathecal chemotherapy is administered four times during the first 6 weeks of treatment and periodically thereafter. I recommend 8-week intervals for 2 years for those with early pre-B and pre-B ALL, 4- to 6-week intervals for 18 months for those with T-cell ALL, and 2-week intervals for 6 months for those with B-cell ALL. We use an age-related dosage schedule of methotrexate, cytarabine, and hydrocortisone. All three drugs are dissolved in Elliott's B solution or preservative-free buffered normal saline in concentrations of 1.5 mg/ml for methotrexate and hydrocortisone, and 3 mg/ml for cytarabine. The three-drug solution is passed through a millipore filter prior to administration, or a millipore filter is attached to the syringe during injection. The lumbar puncture is atraumatic and the cerebrospinal fluid is flowing freely by gravity prior to injection. No other drugs, particularly vincristine, are allowed in the vicinity. The patient is maintained in a lateral recumbent position during administration and in a semi-inverted (head low, hips high) prone position for a half hour afterward.

Continuation Chemotherapy. Once clinical and hematologic remission is achieved, children with early pre-B, pre-B, and early pre-B/monocytoid or myeloid ALL receive mercaptopurine daily and methotrexate weekly

TABLE 1. Drugs Used in Children with Acute Leukemia*

Drug	Usual Dosage	Route	Principal Side Effects
Asparaginase†	10,000–20,000 units/m² once weekly or 6,000 units/m² 3× weekly	IM	Local and systemic allergic reactions, anaphylaxis, pancreatitis, coagulopathy, hyperglycemia, fatty liver, ketosis, azotemia, emesis, cerebral dysfunction, alopecia, immunosuppression
Azacytidine‡	150 mg/m²/day for 5 days by continuous infusion	IV	Hematosuppression, emesis, mucositis
Cyclophosphamide	(1) 100–150 mg/m² daily for 7 days (2) 300–600 mg/m² once weekly	IV or Oral	Hematosuppression, immunosuppression, emesis, alopecia, hemorrhagic cystitis, hyponatremia with seizures, bladder fibrosis, bladder carcinoma, oligospermia, amenorrhea, permanent sterility, cardiac toxicity
	(3) 1000 mg/m² by continuous 24-hr infusion	IV or Oral	
Cytarabine	(1) 100–200 mg/m² daily by continuous infusion for 3 to 10 days	IV or SC	Hematosuppression, immunosuppression, mucositis, fever, alopecia, emesis, diarrhea, conjunctivitis
	(2) 1 gm/m² by continuous 24-hr infusion	IV or SC	
	(3) 10–50 mg (age related)	Intrathecal	Headache, backache, emesis, arachnoiditis, seizures, encephalopathy, paraparesis
Daunorubicin	25–35 mg/m² once weekly or daily for 2 to 3 days (maximum total cumulative dose = 250 mg/m²)	IV	Hematosuppression, immunosuppression, mucosal ulcers, emesis, diarrhea, cardiomyopathy, aggravation of radiation reaction, alopecia, phlebitis, paravascular tissue necrosis
Etoposide (VP-16)	(1) 150–300 mg/m² once or twice weekly	IV	Hematosuppression, emesis, diarrhea, alopecia, hypotension, allergic reactions
	(2) 100 mg/m² daily for 5 days		
	(3) 200 mg/m² daily for 2 to 3 days		
Mercaptopurine	(1) 50–75 mg/m² daily	Oral	Hematosuppression, immunosuppression, hepatic dysfunction, alopecia, mucositis
	(2) 1000 mg/m² continuous infusion over 8 hours	IV	
Methotrexate	(1) 20–30 mg/m² once weekly	IM or Oral	Mucosal ulceration, megaloblastosis, abdominal cramps and diarrhea, malabsorption, cerebral dysfunction, hematosuppression, seizures, immunosuppression, leukoencephalopathy, hepatic dysfunction, hepatic fibrosis, photosensitivity, alopecia, dermatitis, conjunctivitis, pneumonitis
	(2) 1 gm/m² by continuous 24-hr infusion followed by leucovorin rescue	IV	
	(3) 5–15 mg (age related)	Intrathecal	Headache, backache, leg pain, arachnoiditis, emesis, oral ulcers, encephalopathy, myelopathy, paraparesis
Prednisone, prednisolone	40 mg/m² daily in two to four divided doses	Oral or IV	Hypertension, hyperglycemia, edema, polyphagia, potassium deficit, acne, obesity, behavior change, muscle atrophy, striae, immunosuppression, ketosis, cataracts, osteonecrosis
Teniposide (VM-26)‡	100–200 mg/m² once or twice weekly	IV	Hematosuppression, emesis, diarrhea, alopecia, hypotension, allergic reactions
Thioguanine	40–60 mg/m² daily	Oral	Hematosuppression, immunosuppression, hepatic dysfunction, alopecia, mucositis
Vincristine	1.5 mg/m² weekly (maximum 2 mg)	IV	Peripheral neuropathy, constipation, inappropriate ADH secretion, alopecia, ineffective erythropoiesis, seizures, immunosuppression, paravascular tissue necrosis

*Special precautions are needed in the preparation and administration of antileukemic drugs. For example, parenteral injections and infusions must be prepared in a vertical laminar flow hood. Patients must meet certain criteria of renal, hepatic, and hematopoietic function. High-dose methotrexate requires concurrent hydration and alkalinization.

†When local or systemic allergic reactions to *E. coli* asparaginase develop, *Erwinia* asparaginase can be obtained from the National Cancer Institute as a substitute.

‡Available from the National Cancer Institute.

for 2½ to 3 years. It is important to monitor these patients closely, at least once every 2 weeks, with assessment for infection, nutrition, growth, compliance, emotional and social adjustment, and hematologic status. On the one hand, it is important to avoid life-threatening toxicity. On the other hand, it is necessary to assure that the child is receiving maximum tolerated dosage in order to have optimal benefit of the drugs. I adjust the dosage of mercaptopurine to keep the white blood cell count between 1000 and 3000/μl with 500/μl or more phagocytes (granulocytes + monocytes) and 500/μl or more lymphocytes. I adjust the methotrexate dosage to maintain macrocytosis of the red blood cells and hypersegmentation of the granulocytes while avoiding oral ulcerations, sprue-like symptoms, or evidence of persistent cerebral dysfunction. Methotrexate polyglutamate can be measured in the patient's red blood cells to monitor adequacy of dosage and compliance.

In addition to the conventional daily mercaptopurine and weekly methotrexate, brief courses of intravenous chemotherapy are administered intermittently. For early pre-B and pre-B ALL, high-dosage methotrexate is given in 24-hour continuous intravenous infusions followed by its antidote, leucovorin. High-dosage intravenous or oral mercaptopurine is often given concurrently. For pre-B ALL the periodic administration of intravenous high-dosage methotrexate and cytarabine may have merit. For early pre-B/monocytoid or myeloid ALL the addition of etoposide and cytarabine infusions appears to be reasonable. Finally, many treatment protocols include "pulses" of reinduction chemotherapy with prednisone, vincristine, and asparaginase.

Continuation chemotherapy for T-cell ALL differs considerably. Cytarabine, cyclophosphamide, etoposide, daunorubicin, and asparaginase appear to be the drugs of choice rather than methotrexate and mercaptopurine. For B-cell ALL highly intensive intravenous multiple drug chemotherapy is used with primary emphasis on cyclophosphamide.

Continuation chemotherapy is usually terminated after 2 to 3 years of continuous complete remission for children with early pre-B or pre-B ALL, 18 months for early pre-B/monocytoid or myeloid and T-cell ALL, and 6 months for B-cell ALL.

Since ALL is a curable disease, careful consideration must be given to the immediate and long-term hazards of each component of treatment in relationship to its benefits. To reiterate, current evidence suggests that irradiation, anthracycline drugs such as daunorubicin and doxorubicin, alkylating agents such as cyclophosphamide, and prolonged corticosteroid regimens carry the greatest risk of long-term serious sequelae of leukemia therapy.

Cure of ALL is defined as continuous complete freedom from all clinical and laboratory evidence of leukemia for 7 years and cessation of leukemia therapy for 4 years. Approximately 50 per cent of children with ALL are currently cured, with expectation of a rising cure rate in the future.

Chemotherapy of Acute Nonlymphoid Leukemia

Acute myeloid, myelomonocytoid, and monocytoid leukemias are the most frequent varieties of acute nonlymphoid leukemia (ANLL) in children. Acute promyeloid leukemia occurs largely in adolescents and acute megakaryocytoid in infants, especially those with trisomy 21. Clinical features, light and electron microscopy studies, cytochemical stains, and cytogenetics are used to classify the leukemia and to select therapy. With modern chemotherapy and supportive measures, approximately 20 to 30 per cent of children with ANLL are experiencing lengthy leukemia-free survival and possibly cure.

Conventional chemotherapy of ANLL consists of cytarabine by continuous infusion for 7 to 10 days and daunorubicin by daily injection for 3 days. This treatment results in a hazardous period of mucositis, neutropenia, and thrombocytopenia lasting about 2 weeks which is often followed by hematologic remission. For patients with persistent leukemia in the bone marrow after 3 weeks, the initial course of chemotherapy is repeated.

For acute promyeloid leukemia a *low-dosage* heparin infusion is often initiated prior to chemotherapy and continued for 7 to 10 days to help control the consumptive coagulopathy characteristic of this type of leukemia. However, administration of fresh frozen plasma (10 ml/kg) and fresh platelets (4 units/m²) on a regular every 8- or 12-hour schedule to maintain fibrinogen levels over 100 mg/dl and platelet levels over 50,000/µl is the mainstay.

For acute monocytoid and myelomonocytoid leukemias, intravenous etoposide appears to be highly effective. Etoposide and vincristine may be a useful drug combination in megakaryocytoid leukemia.

Achievement of complete remission tends to take longer and pose more life-threatening hazards in patients with ANLL than in those with ALL. Coagulation abnormalities, leukostatic and hypoperfusion phenomena, and serious bacterial and fungal infections are more frequent. In promyeloid leukemia the neoplastic promyelocytes may persist for several weeks, or normal regenerating promyelocytes may be mistaken for the neoplastic variety. Megakaryocytoid leukemia is often associated with marrow fibrosis, so that regeneration of normal hematopoiesis can be delayed. It is important to avoid overtreatment when only time is needed for remission to develop, not more intensive hematosuppressive chemotherapy.

Preventive meningeal therapy is utilized as in acute lymphoid leukemia. Continuation chemotherapy consists of cytarabine, daunomycin, etoposide, and thioguanine or mercaptopurine. High-dosage cytarabine and azacytidine are included in many treatment regimens, and methotrexate, vincristine, and prednisone in some. The optimal duration of continuation chemotherapy is uncertain.

Lethal total body irradiation and chemotherapy followed by allogeneic or autologous bone marrow transplantation is currently used by many hematologists for ANLL in first remission. There is no proof that this approach is more efficacious than modern combination chemotherapy. On the other hand, the immediate and delayed sequelae of this method in children are considerable. All surviving children exhibit complete growth failure, and many have chronic graft-versus-host disease. Multiple endocrinopathies, irreversible pulmonary disease, leukoencephalopathy, renal disorders, and secondary cancers also contribute to the current unacceptably high risk-benefit ratio. I believe that marrow ablation and transplant procedures remain experimental studies to be conducted only in major leukemia research centers.

EVALUATION STUDIES

Since acute leukemia involves all tissues and organs and has profound influence on the life of the child and his family and friends, extensive evaluation is required. The following studies are carried out routinely.

At Diagnosis. Complete blood cell count, differential, reticulocyte count; SMA-18 panel; prothrombin, partial thromboplastin times; fibrinogen and fibrin split products; urinalysis; chest roentgenogram; tuberculin skin test; serology for varicella-zoster, cytomegalovirus, and herpes simplex I; hepatitis panel; bone marrow aspiration with differential count, special cytochemical stains, cell surface markers, cytogenetic analysis with banding, electron microscopy, flow cytometry; cerebrospinal fluid examination with cytospin preparation; dental evaluation and care; oral hygiene instruction; nutritional evaluation; neuropsychological assessment; social service evaluation.

During Treatment. Periodic blood cell counts, spinal fluid cytology, SMA-18 panel, urinalysis; growth charting and reassessments of nutrition and psychosocial status.

At Cessation of Therapy. Physical examination; blood cell counts, SMA-18 panel, urinalysis; bone marrow morphology; spinal fluid cytology; ultrasonogram of testes or ovaries.

Following Treatment. Periodic blood cell counts; growth charting; psychosocial and vocational evaluation and counseling; endocrinologic assessments by physical examinations and measurements of T_3, T_4, TSH, FSH, LH, and testosterone or estrogen levels.

SUPPORTIVE CARE

Excellent supportive care is an important determinant of survival.

Metabolic Disorders. Children with rapidly evolving leukemia, high initial white blood cell counts, and large masses of tumor often have hyperuricemia initially or after treatment is started. Consequently, these children receive intravenous hydration with 3 liters/m²/24 hours of 5 per cent glucose and one-fourth normal saline containing 40 mEq/L of $NaHCO_3$ and allopurinol 100 mg/m² orally every 8 hours for the first 3 to 4 days of treatment. An initial infusion of 500 ml/m² of 5 per cent glucose and one-third normal saline is sometimes administered in the first 2 hours. *No potassium is given!* Urinary output, specific gravity, and pH are monitored to ensure appropriate volume, pH, and dilution. A pH of 6.0 to 7.0 and specific gravity of 1.004 to 1.010 are desirable.

Hyperkalemia, hypercalcemia or hypocalcemia, hyperphosphatemia, azotemia, and lactic acidemia are other metabolic disturbances seen in children with leukemia at diagnosis or relapse. They often require prompt corrective measures such as aluminum hydroxide for hyperphosphatemia, sodium polystyrene sulfonate for hyperkalemia, calcium gluconate for hypocalcemia, and prednisone and furosemide for hypercalcemia.

Prednisone and/or asparaginase can cause hyperglycemia and ketosis to the point of demanding therapy with insulin, intravenous fluids, and sodium bicarbonate.

Infections. The hematosuppression, immunosuppression, and mucosal damage resulting from chemotherapy as well as the leukemia itself make children with leukemia highly susceptible to serious infections. Preventive measures include minimal hospitalization; avoidance of instrumentation, intubation, catheterization, and rectal examination; scrupulous handwashing by physicians, nurses, and technologists; and removal of infectious foci such as dental abscesses. Venipuncture sites are changed every 2 to 3 days, and all skin puncture sites are prepared and dressed with povidone-iodine. We try to maintain the absolute phagocyte count (granulocytes + monocytes) at or above 500/μl and the absolute lymphocyte count at or above 500/μl. The child and his family are instructed about personal hygiene and control of infectious hazards such as questionable food and drink, animals, insect bites, paronychia, and persons with contagious diseases. Cotrimoxazole, 5 mg/kg of trimethoprim and 25 mg/kg sulfamethoxazole, is administered 3 days a week to prevent *Pneumocystis carinii* pneumonia.

Fever in the child with leukemia is assumed to be the result of infection. Physical examination and blood, urine, and other indicated cultures are generally followed by prompt intravenous bactericidal antibiotic therapy if the child has granulocytopenia. For the child in relapse, suspect organisms are *Staphylococcus, Haemophilus influenzae,* and enteric bacteria, but fungal infections can appear after prolonged antibiotic treatment. *Staphylococcus epidermidis* is a threat to children with central venous lines.

Varicella-zoster can be a catastrophic infection in susceptible children with leukemia. Varicella-zoster vaccine is a useful preventive measure for varicella but is not generally available. Varicella-zoster immune globulin (125 units/10 kg) given within 48 hours of varicella exposure provides partial passive immunity. The decision whether to interrupt chemotherapy during the incubation period, especially full-dose prednisone, is individualized. Most important, acyclovir 500 mg/m² intravenously every 8 hours is initiated at the *first* sign of clinical infection.

Measles, another serious infection in these patients, can manifest as giant cell pneumonia without cutaneous expression. Susceptible patients exposed to measles receive immune serum globulin 0.5 ml/kg (15 ml maximum) for prevention.

Emergencies. In addition to serious infections, profuse bleeding, and acute metabolic disorders, two other emergency situations deserve mention. One is T-cell ALL/lymphoma and a mediastinal mass with or without leukemic leukocytosis. Fatal airway obstruction, superior vena cava syndrome, or hyperkalemia can occur suddenly with little warning. Rapid hydration, intravenous hydrocortisone or methylprednisolone, and cardiac monitoring can be life-saving.

The second situation is leukemic leukocytosis above 100,000/μl, particularly with monocytoid or myelomonocytoid ANLL, and evidence of pulmonary and/or cerebral hypoperfusion. Generous hydration, chemotherapy, and leukapheresis are among the measures promptly introduced.

Blood Component Support. Red blood cell transfusions, 10 ml/kg, are used to maintain hemoglobin levels above 7 gm/dl, or higher if the patient has pneumonia or sepsis. In children with very high white blood cell levels, the hemoglobin is raised above 6 gm/dl only as the white cell count is reduced and good hydration is established. Platelet transfusions, 4 to 6 units/m², are administered for significant bleeding associated with platelet counts less than 30,000/mm³. To avoid risk of graft-versus-host disease, red cells and platelets are irradiated before transfusion.

Granulocytes obtained by single-donor leukapheresis are used in some centers for patients with granulocytopenia and proven bacterial sepsis or cellulitis that fails to respond to several days of appropriate antibiotic therapy.

Nutrition. Adequate nutrition is essential to recovery from leukemia and tolerance to chemotherapy. Because of mucosal impairment by chemotherapy, the diet is simple and bland with limitation of fat and salt and restriction of spices, peppers, nuts, popcorn, and other possible irritants. Use of nasogastric and parenteral alimentation is minimized.

Psychosocial Support. Every child with leukemia needs his or her own personal physician to provide continuous comprehensive care, advocacy, and counsel. The child needs to know the diagnosis and to be consulted as feasible along with parents about management decisions. Families need the help of nurses, social workers, and psychologists in learning how to cope with the numerous challenges of caring for the child with leukemia. However, the child's personal physician retains primary responsibility.

Home health service is an integral component of treatment. Home visits are important for social assessment, reinforcement of medication schedules, family instruction, and care of the dying child.

RELAPSE

Hematologic relapse of acute leukemia during combination chemotherapy usually signifies drug-resistant leukemia. Although second and third remissions can be induced, the outlook for cure is sharply reduced. However, continuation chemotherapy with drugs, drug combinations, or drug schedules not previously used is administered in a renewed attempt to cure. In some centers, patients with hematologic relapse while on therapy are considered for bone marrow ablation and transplantation if they have histocompatible donors. Autologous and mismatched donor transplantations are other experimental possibilities. There is no proof at this time that any type of marrow transplant procedure is superior to intensive combination chemotherapy for these children.

Hematologic relapse 6 months or more after cessation of therapy may signify inadequate duration of treatment. Remission induction and continuation chemotherapy utilizing both previously administered and additional drugs often result in lengthy second remissions and sometimes cures.

Isolated meningeal relapse at any time can be effectively treated with intrathecal chemotherapy followed by craniospinal irradiation. Approximately one fourth of these patients become long-term survivors.

Clinically isolated testicular relapse is treated by testicular irradiation, modification of chemotherapy, and an additional 2 years of drug treatment. Prognosis is better when the relapse occurs after cessation of chemotherapy than during chemotherapy.

NEUROBLASTOMA

JAMES FEUSNER, M.D.

Neuroblastoma is a tumor of the sympathetic nervous system. It is the fourth most frequent pediatric solid tumor overall and the most common such tumor in young children. Its incidence is estimated at 9 per million children per year.

There are several features of this tumor (such as spontaneous regression or maturation) that favor survival, but in its disseminated form it has remained difficult to treat. Unfortunately, in two thirds of children, the tumor is disseminated at diagnosis.

In order to better understand and treat this tumor,

it is important to fully estimate the extent of disease at diagnosis. We routinely stage our patients according to the system of Evans (Table 1). Patients with completely resected disease (stage I) have an excellent chance (greater than 90 per cent) for long-term survival. On the other hand, children older than 1 year with stage IV disease have had a very poor prognosis (10 per cent 2-year survival) until recently. Age is next most important in estimating prognosis. Survival for all infants is approximately 74 per cent as compared with 12 per cent for children over 2 years of age at diagnosis. Other factors considered to indicate a more favorable prognosis include urinary vanillylmandelic acid (VMA) to homovanillic acid (HVA) ratio of greater than 1, serum neuron specific enolase (NSE) of less than 100 ng/dl, serum ferritin of less than 150 mg/dl, thoracic or cervical site of primary tumor, and presence of some ganglionic differentiation in the primary tumor. More recently, amplification in tumor cells of the oncogene n-myc and unfavorable histologic features (Shimada classification) are emerging as powerful prognostic indicators.

TREATMENT MODALITIES

Surgical. Surgery may involve biopsy only, radical attempts at complete excision of huge tumors, or "second look" operations attempting complete resection of tumors initially felt to be unresectable. Most recently the surgeon has been called upon to attempt "debulking" of tumors before bone marrow transplantation is performed.

There is no question of the vital role of surgery in stage I and II neuroblastoma. Recently several studies have suggested a survival advantage in children with stage III neuroblastoma rendered disease-free with either initial or delayed primary surgery. However, it has not been clearly demonstrated that primary tumor resection has altered the ultimate outcome for children with stage IV neuroblastoma. The importance and timing of surgery before marrow transplantation remain to be determined in future studies.

TABLE 1. Staging Criteria for Children with Neuroblastoma (System of Evans)

Stage	Criteria
Stage I	Tumor confined to the organ or structure of origin
Stage II	Tumor extending in continuity beyond the organ or structure of origin but not crossing the midline
	Regional lymph nodes on the ipsilateral side may be involved
Stage III	Tumor extending and infiltrating beyond the midline
	Regional lymph nodes may be involved bilaterally
Stage IV	Remote disease involving the skeleton, organs, soft tissue, and distant lymph node groups
Stage IV-S	(Special category) Patients who would otherwise be Stage I or II but who have remote disease confined to liver, skin, or bone marrow and who have no radiographic evidence of bone metastases on complete skeletal survey or bone scan

Radiotherapy. Neuroblastoma is a radiosensitive but not often radiocurable disease. Most centers utilize radiotherapy for treatment of emergencies involving organ compromise (e.g., spinal cord compression), for palliation of pain, or as an adjunct in treating stage III patients. It clearly is not necessary for stage I patients or for many stage II patients.

Total body irradiation has been attempted as the primary treatment of advanced neuroblastoma. It has not improved upon the results of contemporary radiotherapy and chemotherapy protocols. Its use in higher dosage in conjunction with high-dose chemotherapy and bone marrow transplantation may be improving the outcome for high-risk advanced neuroblastoma (see below). Use of radioactive isotopes for treatment by coupling iodine 131 or iodine 125 to the guanethidine analog benzylguanidine (called MIBG) has proved effective in some patients with recurrent neuroblastoma.

Chemotherapy. In the last 20 years many chemotherapeutic agents have been used in the treatment of neuroblastoma. Those that have proven activity include vincristine, cyclophosphamide, doxorubicin (Adriamycin), DTIC, nitrogen mustard, VM-26, VM-16, cisplatinum, and melphalan. Past studies have not demonstrated improved survival for patients of stage I or II treated with chemotherapy. In stage III and IV patients, the median disease-free survival *has* been improved but not (until recently) the ultimate survival. Some recent protocols utilizing high-dose cisplatinum or the agents in bone marrow transplant preparative regimens at near the doses used in bone marrow transplantation appear to be providing better initial disease-free survival. In fact, some of these aggressive, rationally sequenced chemotherapy protocols are providing such good disease control that plans are under way (by the Children's Cancer Study Group) to initiate a randomized treatment study of bone marrow transplantation versus high-dose chemotherapy alone. In addition, agents with completely different mechanisms of action are being evaluated in patients who have relapsed: for example, IL-2, gamma interferon, and Desferal.

Bone Marrow Transplantation. In the last 10 years several centers in the U.S. and Europe have begun utilizing bone marrow transplantation in treating patients with relapsed neuroblastoma. Good initial responses to this treatment have led to use of transplantation for patients initially rather than only at relapse. The exact preparative regimens have varied, but most have included high-dose chemotherapy (VM-26, doxorubicin, cyclophosphamide, cisplatinum, and melphalan) followed by total body irradiation. Both allogeneic and autologous transplants have been used. This treatment regimen appears to be providing some patients longer disease-free periods than would otherwise be expected. For children with advanced neuroblastoma having transplantation while they are still showing response to initial chemotherapy treatment, 25 to 55 per cent 2-year relapse-free survivals have been reported.

Other. Several other more novel approaches to treatment are being investigated. One is based on the infrequent but well-known occurrence of maturation of neuroblastoma. Laboratory studies have shown that several drugs can induce maturation of neuroblastoma cell lines. Vitamin E and retinoic acid are two such agents being studied in certain patients who have recurrent disease, especially those with minimal residual disease.

Another approach stems from monoclonal antibody technology. Either chemotherapy (daunomycin) or radioisotopic therapy is being administered to some patients by coupling the treatment "agent" to monoclonal antibodies raised to neuroblastoma. The advantage of this therapy would be lessened toxicity to the patient, since the therapy would be directed primarily to the tumor(s) and not to normal tissue.

Although these approaches are based on sound observations, it is too early at this time to predict how successful they will be in the clinic.

SPECIFIC THERAPY RECOMMENDATIONS

Stage I. These children require only a careful surgical resection. In several reported series 90 to 100 per cent of these children survive. Even those who have not had a complete excision of their tumor almost always do well without further therapy.

Stage II. The same approach for stage I patients applies to most children with stage II disease. There is some controversy regarding treatment for certain stage II patients: those 2 years or older at diagnosis, those with involved regional lymph nodes, those with amplification of the oncogene n-myc, and those with unfavorable histologic features.

It is our practice to treat stage II patients with n-myc amplification and/or unfavorable histology as advanced neuroblastoma (see below). If the child is over 2 years or has involved regional nodes, but without n-myc amplification or unfavorable histology, we utilize aggressive surgery alone, but with close follow-up to detect any signs of disease progression.

Stage III. In some respects this stage is arbitrary; not many children fit in this category. According to Evans' original criteria, such children have had a 50 to 60 per cent 2-year survival, with therapy consisting of surgery, radiation, and combination chemotherapy. Recently, the CCSG has re-examined this group of patients and redefined them according to age at diagnosis and three biologic factors: n-myc amplification, tumor histology, and serum ferritin. Those children more than 1 year are considered very high risk if they have unfavorable histology, n-myc amplification, or elevated serum ferritin (>150 mg/dl). These types of stage III patients have had less than 20 per cent relapse-free survival with prior treatments, and should be treated currently with protocols for advanced stage neuroblastoma. If the child with stage III disease is less than 1 year and has at least one of the three aforementioned unfavorable factors, or is more than 1 year old with no other unfavorable factors, we would utilize moderately intense combination chemotherapy (cyclophosphamide, cisplatinum, doxorubicin, and VP-16) with delayed surgery(s) to attempt to remove all of the primary tumor. With this approach we estimate the disease-free survival should be improved to 70 per cent or better for these "better-risk" stage III patients.

Stage IV. Because of the uniformly dismal outcome for these patients when using standard chemotherapy and irradiation, we explore the possibility of bone marrow transplantation for these children. Currently, autologous bone marrow transplantation appears to be giving superior overall survival results compared with allogeneic transplantation. Thus, we prepare our patients with combination chemotherapy (cisplatinum, doxorubicin, VP-16, cyclophosphamide) for 8 to 10 weeks. At that time if their disease is still responding to therapy and their bone marrow is free of neuroblastoma (as assessed by sensitive monoclonal antibody techniques), we store their marrow for future reinfusion. At approximately week 16 the patients are fully re-evaluated and have a second surgery with or without local radiotherapy to render them as disease-free as possible before autologous transplantation. The dosages and fields for this radiation must be coordinated carefully with the transplant center to avoid excess toxicity with the transplantation therapy to follow.

For patients not having their marrow free of neuroblastoma and not having an HLA-matched donor, we continue the same four-drug chemotherapy for 12 months total treatment time. In the event of disease progression, we consider use of investigational agents immediately.

Stage IV-S. Children with this stage of neuroblastoma (Table 1) have an excellent prognosis (80 to 90 per cent 2-year survival) with minimal therapy. Unless there is a life-threatening problem with compression of a vital organ (e.g., respiratory compromise due to massive hepatomegaly), we take an expectant stance on treatment. Low-dose (400 to 600 cGy) radiation, delivered via lateral ports, may be utilized to decrease liver size, if needed. Otherwise, we provide full supportive care to allow time for these children to outgrow their tumors. Whether some of these infants can be predicted to be at high risk based on n-myc amplification of their tumors remains to be seen.

SUPPORTIVE CARE

As the therapy has intensified for neuroblastoma, so has the need for supportive care. This is a tumor that demands the expertise of a comprehensive pediatric facility. Chemotherapy and radiotherapy will produce nausea and vomiting, which deserve treatment with the newest antiemetics, singly or in combination. We usually start with metoclopramide (1 mg/kg IV) plus diphenhydramine (0.75 mg/kg IV). If these fail, we increase the doses, up to 2 mg/kg and 1 to 1.25 mg/kg, respectively. Other agents that may help include dexamethasone and lorazepam.

Weight loss and poor nutritional state can occur during treatment or prior to it in some aggressive stage IV cases. There is a growing body of data suggesting that nutritional deficiencies may be harmful to these children by prolonging the myelosuppression following therapy or even possibly by affecting the patient's response to chemotherapy. We generally institute supplemental alimentation when the patient has lost 5 to 10 per cent of his initial lean mass, has a weight for height less than the 5th percentile, or a serum albumin of <3.2 gm/dl.

Graft-versus-host disease (GVHD) has been reported in patients transfused with nonirradiated blood products. In fact, one of the earlier reports involved a neuroblastoma patient from our institution. It is our policy to irradiate (1500 cGy) *all* blood products given to patients with neuroblastoma. To our knowledge there has never been a case of graft-versus-host disease in a patient transfused with blood so irradiated.

Interstitial pneumonia due to *Pneumocystis carinii* is a well-known potential complication of immunosuppressive therapy. This complication can affect neuroblastoma patients as well. Therefore, it is our policy to use trimethoprim/sulfamethoxazole (Bactrim) prophylactically (5 mg/kg/day trimethoprim, 25 mg/kg/day sulfamethoxazole) in all patients for three consecutive days per week.

Other infections are occurring more frequently than in the past, reflecting the greater degree and duration of myelo- and immunosuppression effected by new treatment regimens. The prompt institution of broad-spectrum intravenous antibiotics is mandatory in any child with fever (38.5°C or 101.3°F) and neutropenia (absolute granulocyte count of less than 500/μl). In addition, amphotericin B for presumed systemic fungal infection is often added in children who remain febrile for 4 to 7 days on antibiotics. We utilize granulocyte transfusions only in patients with proven sepsis or soft tissue infection who are severely neutropenic (absolute neutrophil count less than 200 μl) and not responding to appropriate antibiotic therapy.

A rare but recently emphasized potential complication is hypertension. Some children may present with serious systolic and diastolic hypertension, while others will manifest it during surgery or chemotherapy. This problem may be serious enough to warrant short-term use of alpha-adrenergic blocking agents.

Finally, the nature of neuroblastoma makes the child who is affected a classic example of the patient who needs comprehensive psychosocial support. There can be tremendous financial, social, and psychological stresses on the patient and family. The effective delivery of appropriate and thorough care to these children requires a multidisciplinary team approach that includes the skills of a social worker, child-life worker, psychiatrist, and compassionate physician.

8

Spleen and Lymphatic System

POSTSPLENECTOMY SYNDROME

JERRY A. WINKELSTEIN, M.D.

Although the spleen was once considered to be of relatively little value to the host, in recent years there has been a growing appreciation that it plays a critical role in defense against infection. The spleen is composed of two distinct but interrelated immunologic compartments. Fixed phagocytes of the reticuloendothelial system line the sinusoids of the red pulp and are important in the clearance of hematogenously borne bacteria in the nonimmune host. Lymphoid tissue found in the follicles and periarteriolar sheaths of the white pulp apparently plays an important role in producing early antibody in response to particulate antigens in the blood.

Since 1952 when the first report on postsplenectomy sepsis appeared, it has become clear that the risk for developing sepsis after splenectomy is not the same for all patients, but rather is related to a number of different variables. The age of the patient at the time of splenectomy is one such variable; the younger the patient at the time of splenectomy, the greater the risk of sepsis. The interval since splenectomy is another important variable; the risk is greater in the first few years after splenectomy and diminishes somewhat thereafter. Finally, the reason for which the splenectomy was performed influences the risk considerably; the risk is greater if splenectomy was performed because of some underlying disease that involves the reticuloendothelial system or the immune system than if splenectomy was performed because of trauma. Thus, the risk of developing postsplenectomy sepsis is much greater for the 3-year-old child with histiocytosis within the first few years after splenectomy than it is for the 50-year-old adult who had a traumatic splenectomy 20 years previously. Nevertheless, although the risk varies, it is clear that *any* patient who is missing his/her spleen carries some risk for postsplenectomy sepsis.

One reason so much attention has been focused on patients with postsplenectomy syndrome is the nature of their infections. As one would expect, patients without a spleen do well when infections are confined to mucosal surfaces or soft tissues. If bacteria invade the blood, however, a fulminant sepsis may develop. The episode of sepsis is usually characterized by subtle early clinical findings, a rapidly progressive course, and a high rate of mortality, even when treated with appropriate antibiotics. Pneumococci are responsible in one-half to two-thirds of cases. Meningococci, *Escherichia coli*, *Haemophilus influenzae*, and *Streptococcus pyogenes* account for most of the additional cases.

The physician who cares for the asplenic patient must be concerned with both preventing blood-borne bacterial infections and treating the episodes of sepsis once they occur.

Indications for Splenectomy. Splenectomy should be performed only when clearly indicated and with the knowledge that any patient who has had a splenectomy will have some finite future risk for postsplenectomy sepsis.

Conservative Management of Splenic Trauma. Although traditional therapy for traumatic injury to the spleen has been splenectomy, in recent years more conservative management aimed at preserving the spleen has been advocated. If possible, lacerations of the spleen are repaired. In some instances, if repair is not possible, partial splenectomy with preservation of the vascular pedicle is performed. Only when repair or partial splenectomy is not possible is total splenectomy for trauma indicated.

Immunization. Patients without a spleen should receive polyvalent pneumococcal vaccine and the *H. influenzae*, type b conjugate vaccine. The current pneumococcal vaccine contains the polysaccharide capsules from the 23 pneumococcal serotypes most commonly responsible for bacteremic disease. Unfortunately, like most polysaccharide antigens, the pneumococcal vaccine is poorly immunogenic in children under the age of 2, the very ones with the greatest age-related risk for postsplenectomy sepsis. Nevertheless, pneumococcal vaccine should be given to all asplenic individuals over the age of 2. The current *H. influenzae* vaccine is composed of the polysaccharide capsule from the type b organism conjugated to protein antigens in order to increase its immunogenicity in young children 18 months of age and older.

Prophylactic Antibiotics. The question of whether to use prophylactic antibiotics, such as penicillin, in asplenic patients is difficult to answer, since not all splenectomized patients have the same likelihood of developing sepsis and, therefore, the risk-benefit ratio of prophylactic antibiotics is not easy to establish for the group as a whole. In addition, there have been no controlled studies performed to assess the effectiveness of antibiotic prophylaxis in these patients. Finally, once antibiotics are initiated, it is difficult to know when to discontinue their use.

Most physicians would agree that prophylactic oral penicillin (200,000 units bid) or oral ampicillin (50 mg/kg/day) is indicated for all asplenic children under the age of 5 regardless of the indication for splenectomy or the interval since splenectomy. A case can also be made for penicillin prophylaxis (400,000 units bid) in older children through adolescence, especially those patients in whom the splenectomy was performed for an underlying disorder involving the reticuloendothelial system, the immune system, or a malignancy and especially in the first few years after splenectomy.

Patient and Family Education. Neither immunization, prophylactic antibiotics, or both used together guarantee protection from postsplenectomy sepsis. For example, even though the patient may have received the pneumococcal vaccine, he may be challenged with pneumococcal serotypes not contained in the vaccine. Similarly, the patient may not respond normally to either vaccine because of the underlying hematologic or immunologic condition for which the splenectomy was performed. Finally, even though the patient may be on prophylactic antibiotics, the possibility of infection with resistant bacteria, or bacteria for which the antibiotic may not be appropriate, still exists.

Thus, one of the most important elements in the care of the asplenic host is to counsel the patient and his family as to the role of the spleen in host defense and the relative risk that the given patient will develop sepsis. Armed with that information and with the knowledge that postsplenectomy sepsis is rapidly progressive and has an extremely high mortality rate, both the patient and the physician will be in a better position to assess any febrile episode and initiate early and intensive antibiotic therapy.

Treatment of Suspected Sepsis. It is difficult to recommend specific conditions under which the asplenic host should be admitted to the hospital and treated for sepsis. Each patient's risk is different, response to immunization will vary, compliance with prophylactic antibiotic regimens may not be known, and clinical symptoms and signs will necessarily be highly individual. Nevertheless, if there is any question that the asplenic child may be in the early stages of bacterial sepsis, he

should be promptly treated and admitted to the hospital. It is hoped that as rapid diagnostic tests for bacterial pathogens become more widely available, they will offer help in deciding when to treat for sepsis.

The treatment for sepsis in the asplenic host is generally the same as for any other patient with sepsis. Special consideration should be given to the kinds of organisms responsible for postsplenectomy sepsis and to the fulminant nature of the sepsis and the high incidence of disseminated intravascular coagulation.

INDICATIONS FOR SPLENECTOMY

WILLIAM H. ZINKHAM, M.D.

Over the years thousands of splenectomies have been performed for a variety of reasons. From this vast experience several important facts have emerged. First, the mortality associated with the procedure is extremely low. Second, splenectomy has been and continues to be the only effective form of therapy for certain medical and surgical disorders. And third, the benefits of the procedure should outweigh the risks of the patient developing the postsplenectomy syndrome. Medical and surgical conditions for which splenectomy may be indicated are the following.

Congenital Spherocytic Hemolytic Anemia. This entity comprises a heterogeneous group of disorders in which an abnormality of spectrin and possibly other membrane proteins causes selective sequestration of red cells in the spleen. The spectrum of clinical severity is quite broad. Splenectomy is indicated in children with severe anemia requiring frequent transfusions. Whether and when to do a splenectomy in children with mild to moderate anemia is less clear. Splenectomy prevents the formation of gallstones, aplastic and sequestrative crises, and the development of leg ulcers. However, the risks of splenectomy and the postsplenectomy syndrome may exceed those associated with these complications.

Other Hemolytic Disorders. A variety of inherited red cell membranopathies (e.g., elliptocytosis) and enzymopathies (e.g., involving pyruvate kinase or hexokinase) may be associated with severe hemolysis. The decision to do a splenectomy should be based on transfusion requirements, the effect of the anemia on growth and development, and the frequency of aplastic or sequestrative crises.

Immunohematologic Disorders. The majority of children with idiopathic thrombocytopenic purpura or autoimmune hemolytic anemia recover spontaneously. However, life-threatening situations may arise, including serious bleeding or severe, recurrent anemia. If the patient fails to respond or cannot tolerate the dose of medication necessary to maintain remission, splenectomy should be performed. Splenectomy, therefore, is indicated only after medical management fails. A rare exception to this rule is the child with idiopathic thrombocytopenic purpura who early in the course of the disease develops signs of an intracranial hemorrhage.

Under these circumstances, an emergency splenectomy may be life-saving and may also prevent crippling neurologic disturbances.

Hypersplenism. This term is applied to a heterogeneous group of disorders characterized by varying degrees of cytopenia in the peripheral blood, a large spleen, and normal bone marrow. The blood abnormalities may be corrected by splenectomy or a shunting procedure in patients with portal hypertension. Rarely is the degree of anemia, thrombocytopenia, or leukopenia of sufficient severity to justify a splenectomy. Two major candidates for splenectomy are transfusion-dependent patients who have developed red cell antibodies—e.g., children with Cooley's anemia—and patients with splenic gigantism.

Malignant Tumors of the Spleen. Laparotomy with splenectomy remains the standard procedure for defining abdominal and pelvic malignant disease in patients with Hodgkin's disease. Alternative approaches under review are subtotal splenectomy for staging and irradiation of the spleen without splenectomy. Both procedures have inherent risks; the first may fail to define malignant cells, and splenic atrophy may occur after splenic irradiation.

Splenic Gigantism. In some patients the spleen is enormous, occupying a large portion of the abdominal cavity. An appropriate description of this clinical situation is "splenomegalopolis." Splenic gigantism may occur in children with lysosomal storage diseases (e.g., Gaucher's disease, sea-blue histiocyte syndrome), thalassemia major, hemangiomas, lymphangiomas, cysts, and hamartomas. In these patients the movement of the diaphragm is compromised, there is postprandial abdominal discomfort, and the risk of splenic rupture is great. In addition, most of these conditions are associated with a moderate to marked degree of pancytopenia. Thus, splenectomy may be beneficial for a variety of reasons.

Traumatic Rupture of the Spleen. In the past, traumatic rupture was a major indication for splenectomy. The risk of postsplenectomy infection in subjects splenectomized after trauma is relatively low. Even so, alternative forms of therapy should be considered: nonoperative management of splenic injury, suturing of lacerated surfaces, and subtotal splenectomy or hemisplenectomy.

LYMPHANGITIS

MAX L. RAMENOFSKY, M.D.

Lymphangitis is an inflammation of the lymphatic channels due to a local spreading distal infection. This was referred to in the past as "blood poisoning." Clinically lymphangitis is manifested as painful red streaks starting distally and moving proximally from the site of an infection. Regional lymph nodes are also usually affected.

In children, erysipelas is the most common cause, although deep puncture wounds are often incriminated.

The most common organism is the group A beta-hemolytic *Streptococcus*, and consequently any bacterial therapy is directed at eradicating this organism. Other occasionally involved organisms are *Staphylococcus* and the gram-negative organisms.

Treatment. The infection at the site of entry must be cleaned, cultured, drained (if indicated), and appropriately dressed. Initial antimicrobial therapy is penicillin, and the route of administration is dictated by the severity of the illness. Usually, oral penicillin V, 250 mg every 6 hours, is adequate for the child under 10 years of age. For the older child, 500 mg every 6 hours is a reasonable dosage. The child who is septic and toxic and whose disease process is rapidly progressing should receive parenteral penicillin G, 100,000 U/kg/day. Should the child be allergic to penicillin, erythromycin, 50 mg/kg/day in four divided doses, is effective therapy. Antibiotics should be continued for 10 days and the physician should be alert for complications of streptococcal infection. Should *Staphylococcus* be the offending organism, dicloxacillin, 50 mg/kg/day in four divided doses orally, or penicillinase-resistant beta-lactam antibiotic, 100 mg/kg/day IV, for severe infections should be used.

Puncture wounds deserve special attention when they result in lymphangitis. The puncture may have resulted in the inoculation of *Clostridium tetani*, which in the unimmunized child may be catastrophic. The puncture should be opened in a sterile fashion, irrigated, and dressed. If tetanus prophylaxis is not adequate, tetanus toxoid, 0.5 ml, or tetanus immune globulin, 250 units IM, should be given.

Patients at special risk for the development of lymphangitis as well as lymphadenitis are those in whom there is an abnormality of the lymphatic drainage system, such as lymphedema. The group A beta-hemolytic *Streptococcus* is a common offending organism in this situation, although gram-negative organisms are more frequently cultured than in patients who do not have lymphedema. The appropriate antimicrobial drug should be started depending on the results of the culture. Oral penicillin V at doses described previously should be the drug of choice until the cultures return.

LYMPH NODE INFECTIONS
(Lymphadenitis)

MAX L. RAMENOFSKY, M.D.

Lymph node enlargement is common in childhood and adolescence but quite rare in the newborn. The most common cause of a mass in the neck during childhood is an enlarged lymph node, and it must be differentiated from other congenital cystic cervical masses such as branchial cleft cyst, thyroglossal duct cyst, and cystic hygroma. Infectious causes should be differentiated from noninfectious causes such as hyperplasia or neoplasia. Lymph node infections are either acute, developing over a period of 2 to 3 days, or chronic, developing over weeks to months.

Lymph nodes anywhere in the body provide drainage from other more peripheral areas. The location of the node(s) gives one an indication of where to look for the primary infection. The most common inflammatory lesion of a cervical lymph node is suppurative lymphadenitis, which is generally an acute process. The most common chronic cervical lymph node infections are atypical mycobacterial lymphadenitis, tuberculous lymphadenitis, and cat-scratch disease.

ACUTE SUPPURATIVE CERVICAL LYMPHADENITIS

Acute suppurative lymphadenitis is generally thought to be secondary to bacterial entry at some distal site. In the child it is most common from the first to the eighth year. Prior to the penicillin era, the most common offending organism was group A beta-hemolytic *Streptococcus*. At present, the most common organism is *Staphyloccus aureus*, with *Streptococcus* occupying the second position, and gram-negative organisms and anaerobes being found with increasing frequency.

There is a sudden onset of a rapidly growing painful, red swelling in the neck, 2 to 3 days after an upper respiratory infection. The patient may be febrile and appear toxic. A leukocytosis is usual, with a left shift. At this point, unless the mass is fluctuant, needle aspiration or drainage is not recommended. A diligent search for the primary organ of entry should be done. In cervical lymphadenitis, sites to be carefully examined are the ears, the pharynx for tonsillitis or pharyngitis, and the oral cavity, particularly for dental caries and dental abscess. Therapy is started with an antistaphylococcal drug such as dicloxacillin sodium, 25 mg/kg/day orally, or a parenteral beta-lactamase–resistant semisynthetic penicillin, 100 mg/kg/day IV in four divided doses for 10 days. At these dosages both staphylococci and streptococci are adequately covered. The use of the antibiotics for greater than the prescribed interval is to be discouraged, as prolonged use often results in a chronic granulomatous lymphadenitis that will neither resolve nor fluctuate.

The lesions should be followed at frequent intervals and the antibiotics continued for 10 days. If, however, the lesion softens and becomes fluctuant, incision and drainage are mandatory and should be carried out following the principles of adequate drainage with optimal cosmesis. The incision should be along Langer's lines in the neck, with insertion of a soft rubber drain and a collecting dressing. At the time of drainage an adequate culture and Gram's stain should be done to identify the offending organism. Anaerobic cultures should be included in the examination. The antibiotic may be discontinued 24 hours after a lesion has been drained unless there is evidence of a spreading cellulitis. The drain should be removed when there is adequate saucerization of the wound.

On occasion organisms other than staphylococci and streptococci have been identified. Of particular note is the plague-causing organism *Yersinia pestis*. Tularemia is another cause of cervical lymphadenitis but is usually associated with an eye infection or skin ulceration. The treatment for *Yersinia pestis* is streptomycin, 30 mg/kg/day, or chloramphenicol sodium succinate, 50 mg/kg/day IV, in four divided doses for 10 days if the child is less than 8 years of age. For older children, tetracycline, 25 to 50 mg/kg/day in four divided doses, is effective therapy. Occasionally the involved nodes from plague or tularemia require incision and drainage, but these nodes should not be drained until after 24 hours of antibiotic therapy.

CHRONIC LYMPHADENITIS

Most patients with chronic lymphadenitis have enlarged, nontender, asymptomatic cervical masses.

Mycobacterial Lymphadenitis. Most cases of mycobacterial cervical lymphadenitis are no longer due to *Mycobacterium tuberculosis* but to nontuberculous mycobacteria (MOTT, mycobacteria other than tuberculosis). Cervical lymphadenitis due to *M. tuberculosis* is usually an extension of a primary pulmonary infection and thus involves the supraclavicular nodes. Cervical lymphadenitis due to atypical mycobacteria is thought to be a primary infection gaining entrance through the pharynx or tonsils and thus involves higher cervical nodes such as the submandibular group.

The nodes of the child with tuberculous lymphadenitis are generally large, matted, and asymptomatic. Evidence of pulmonary tuberculosis is frequently found when the cervical lymphadenopathy is encountered, but progress of the disease from lymphadenitis to pulmonary tuberculosis is rare. Central necrolysis of the involved nodes with the development of sinus tracts is uncommon but may occur if the nodes have not been aspirated or were incompletely excised at biopsy.

MOTT infection occurs in high cervical lymph nodes, generally the submandibular group. Very rarely is there extranodal involvement and then only in the child who is immunosuppressed either primarily or secondarily. The involved nodes are usually large, matted, fixed, and nontender. The nodes of MOTT are likely to break down spontaneously and drain externally with the development of sinus tracts.

Diagnosis. The diagnosis of *M. tuberculosis* can be aided by identification of pulmonary tuberculosis on chest films. Skin testing will identify most children with mycobacterial infections. Most of these children have a positive skin test to PPD-S, first strength. In children having atypical mycobacterial lymphadenitis this is not so. Use of first strength PPD-S in MOTT infections yields negative or questionable results in over half of children tested. Second strength PPD-S may confirm infection due to MOTT.

Treatment. The treatment of tuberculous lymphadenitis is antituberculous chemotherapy. Regardless of how the diagnosis is made, antituberculous chemotherapy should be instituted and continued for 2 years unless a rifampin-containing regimen is utilized. In this situation, 9 months of therapy are usually adequate to eradicate the infection. Complete resolution of the disease is to be expected, including cutaneous sinus tracts. Chemotherapeutic agents for tuberculous lymphadenitis are isoniazid, 10 to 20 mg/kg/day up to 300 mg daily, and rifampin, 10 to 20 mg/kg/day up to 600 mg daily.

The treatment of lymphadenopathy due to atypical mycobacteria is complete excision of the involved nodes including culture. Antituberculous chemotherapy is neither indicated nor necessary. The vast majority of these children are cured if all the involved nodes are removed.

CAT-SCRATCH DISEASE

Although the etiology of cat-scratch disease has never been proven, the infectious agent is thought to be a bacillus of the *Chlamydia* genus, other members of which cause lymphogranuloma venereum and psittacosis. Cat-scratch disease is the most common cause of chronic, nonbacterial lymphadenopathy.

The disease is generally transmitted by the scratch of a kitten, but monkeys and dogs as well as a thorny plant have been implicated in transmission. The animal carrier is not affected by the disease, nor does it react with the antigen of cat-scratch disease.

Patients, when closely questioned, give a history of a minor scratch by a kitten 2 to 4 weeks before the onset of the lymphadenopathy. The inoculation site generally reveals a papule or blister. The most common sites of lymphadenopathy, corresponding to a distal inoculation site, are, in order of decreasing frequency, axillary, cervical, preauricular, submandibular, and epitrochlear.

Diagnosis. The diagnosis can be confirmed by a positive reaction to a skin test antigen prepared from the purulent aspirate of an involved node. As the antigen is not commercially available and is difficult to obtain, the appropriate history with the findings of a chronic lymphadenitis allows a presumptive diagnosis of cat-scratch disease. Occasionally the diagnosis can be suspected from stains on involved lymph nodes which reveal gram-variable organisms.

Treatment. There is no chemotherapy available for this disease. Excision of the involved node is generally curative, but on occasion aspiration will allow the node to heal. However, observation alone will see the gradual subsidence of symptoms in most cases. Culture and histologic evaluation of the aspirated or excised material will exclude other causes of chronic lymphadenopathy. Supportive care for such symptoms as headache, malaise, fever, and vomiting is indicated.

Cat-scratch disease is self-limited, and complete resolution is to be expected.

LYMPHEDEMA

PETER S. SMITH, M.D.

The accumulation of lymph in the extremities, the genitalia, or both, lymphedema in children is usually congenital, sometimes familial (Milroy's disease). Repeated infestation by filariasis in childhood can cause lymphedema in later years. In either case, lymphedematous swelling is typically nonpitting and results from hypoplasia or obstruction of microscopic lymphatic channels.

The management of lymphedema depends upon its cause and the stage of evolution. In instances of acquired lymphedema, early treatment minimizes or prevents microlymphatic obstruction. Hence filariasis is best treated early to prevent the often grotesque deformity called elephantiasis. Larvae of the tropical parasite *Wuchereria bancrofti* are transmitted by mosquitoes to man, in whom they reach maturity. The adult settles in the lymph nodes and lymphatics of the legs and genitalia, where it causes obliterating allergic and inflammatory reactions. At the microfilarial stage, administration of diethyl carbamazine (DEC) has significantly decreased the lymphangitis and subsequent elephantiasis rate. When inflammation predominates, a trial of anti-inflammatory drugs and steroids, in addition to specific treatment, is warranted. In one study corticosteroids were infused directly into the lymphatics with good results.

In congenital and late stages of acquired lymphedema, surgery and physical measures are the mainstay of treatment. Use of an elastic stocking, special massage techniques, and wrapping the extremities with Ace bandages have sufficiently reduced swelling to allow good function. In others, particularly with massive limb distention, surgery yields better functional results, such as improved motion, less discomfort, and the possibility of wearing shoes. The appearance is modestly improved but nevertheless socially more acceptable. Preoperative evaluation by lymphangiography is often recommended, enabling the surgeon to decide which patients are most likely to benefit and which procedure to perform. These range from anastomosing lymph nodes or channels to veins (lymphovenous shunts), burying a dermal flap to drain the superficial lymphatics into the muscular compartment (Thompson procedure), to the staged subcutaneous excision of a large pannus of swollen tissue. None of the procedures is curative.

Infections such as lymphangitis and cellulitis easily develop in a lymphedematous limb, frequently from minor skin lesions. Affected children must maintain consistent cleanliness, and their physician should consider warmth and tenderness of the distended limb a sign of bacterial infection to be treated accordingly.

LYMPHANGIOMA

LUIS A. CLAVELL, M.D.

Lymphangiomas are uncommon congenital benign malformations of the lymphatic system. Forty per cent are present in the newborn period, 50 per cent by the end of the first year, and 75 per cent by the end of the second year. The most common site of involvement is the head and neck, with a 45 per cent occurrence rate.

Therapy should be directed toward (1) relief of life-threatening complications due to pressure by the tumor such as airway obstruction and dysphagia; (2) removal of the entire tumor when possible (the degree to which this is possible may be determined by the location and extent of the lymphangioma and the involvement of important neural, vascular, and skeletal structures); (3) return and preservation of function of the involved structures; (4) obtaining the best possible cosmetic results; and (5) relief and stabilization of emotional consequences of this formidable benign pathologic entity.

Observation or patiently awaiting spontaneous resolution may be hazardous and unrewarding, since spontaneous resolution rarely if ever occurs. Surgery should be as complete as possible, yet not excessive, and staged surgery may be necessary to prevent life-threatening intraoperative and postoperative complications. The lesion is radioresistant, and its use is associated with inconsistent results and severe complications. Incision and drainage or needle aspiration, with the exception of emergencies, should be discouraged because of infection and the possibility of sepsis.

Cyclophosphamide has been proposed as a therapeutic modality for life-threatening lesions when other therapies are not feasible or have failed. Patients with airway lesions benefit from perioperatively administered steroids, which help protect the airway and reduce traumatic edema. Steroids as single modality therapy have demonstrated no role in the management of lymphangiomas. Early antibiotic implementation is essential for the patient's safety in an effort to prevent the often frightening febrile course following surgical removal of cystic hygromas.

MALIGNANT LYMPHOMA

SHIAO Y. WOO, M.D.

Lymphomas in children are generally divided into Hodgkin's disease and non-Hodgkin's lymphoma. These two heterogeneous disease categories have different biology and natural history and are therefore treated differently.

HODGKIN'S DISEASE

After a diagnosis of Hodgkin's disease is established, a careful staging work-up is essential for optimal treatment planning. The Ann Arbor Staging System is shown in Table 1. The staging work-up should include a careful history and physical examination, routine blood counts and chemistry, erythrocyte sedimentation rate, serum copper, chest radiography, computed tomography of chest, abdomen, and pelvis, and bipedal lymphangiography. The necessity for a routine staging laparotomy remains controversial, although the staging laparotomy can generally provide the most accurate information regarding the presence or absence and the extent of infradiaphragmatic disease. The procedure includes a splenectomy, biopsy of the liver, bone marrow biopsy, and biopsy of lymph nodes at the splenic hilum, porta hepatis, and celiac, para-aortic, and pelvic regions. In girls an oophoropexy is usually performed at the same time, so that the ovaries can be easily shielded from the future radiotherapy fields.

Stage I and Stage II Hodgkin's Disease

Early-stage Hodgkin's disease is highly curable by extended-field high-dose (35 to 40 Gy) radiotherapy. However, subtotal or total nodal irradiation can pro-

TABLE 1. Ann Arbor Staging for Hodgkin's Lymphoma*

Stage I	Involvement of single lymph node regions (I) or single extralymphatic sites (I^e).
Stage II	Involvement of two or more lymph node regions on one side of the diaphragm (II) or localized involvement of extralymphatic organs or sites and one or more nodal regions on the same side of the diaphragm (IIe).
Stage III	Involvement of lymph node regions on both sides of the diaphragm, which also may be accompanied by localized involvement of extralymphatic organs or sites (IIIe) or, for example, spleen (III^s), or both (III^{s,e}).
Stage IV	Diffuse or disseminated involvement of one or more extralymphatic organs or tissues, with or without lymph node involvement.

*Each stage is subclassified into A or B according to the presence or absence of constitutional symptoms. These are unexplained fever of 38°C or more, night sweats, and unexplained weight loss of more than 10 per cent of body weight. Superscripts, after laparotomy, are applied to indicate sites of involvement, e.g., liver, spleen, lung, bone marrow, pleura, bone, and skin, respectively.

duce significant long-term morbidity in children such as decreased bone and soft-tissue growth, hypothyroidism, and secondary solid tumors. Therefore, although primary radiotherapy is still appropriate for adolescents who have completed their growth, the treatment approach now for most children is either with combined-modality treatment using multiagent chemotherapy and low-dose (15 to 30 Gy) involved field radiotherapy, or with primary chemotherapy, reserving radiotherapy for sites of incomplete response or salvage. The commonly used chemotherapy combinations are MOPP (nitrogen mustard, vincristine, procarbazine, prednisone), CVPP (CCNU, vinblastine, procarbazine, prednisone), and ABVD (adriamycin, bleomycin, vinblastine, DTIC) (Table 2). A regimen consisting of four to six cycles of chemotherapy and low-dose involved field radiotherapy can produce a 5-year survival rate of 90 to 95 per cent in children. Besides acute side effects, chemotherapy can also produce long-term morbidity, including infertility, increased risk of leukemia, and cardiac and pulmonary dysfunction. Studies are under way to test the ability of reduced cycles of chemotherapy and low-dose radiotherapy to produce equal cure rate with decreased long-term morbidity.

TABLE 2. Chemotherapy Regimen for Hodgkin's Disease

MOPP
  Nitrogen mustard, 6 mg/m², IV, days 1 and 8
  Vincristine, 1.4 mg/m², IV, days 1 and 8
  Procarbazine, 100 mg/m², PO, days 1–14
  Prednisone, 40 mg/m²/day, PO, days 1–14
  Rest, days 15–27
  Repeat cycle every 4 weeks
CVPP
  CCNU, 7 mg/m², PO, day 1
  Vinblastine, 4.0 mg/m², IV, days 1 and 8
  Procarbazine, 100 mg/m², PO, days 1–14
  Prednisone, 40 mg/m²/day, PO, days 1–14
  Rest, days 15–27
  Repeat cycle every 4 weeks
ABVD
  Adriamycin (doxorubicin), 25 mg/m², IV, days 1 and 15
  Bleomycin, 10 mg/m², IV, days 1 and 15
  Vinblastine, 6 mg/m², IV, days 1 and 15
  DTIC, 375 mg/m², IV, days 1 and 15
  Repeat cycle every 4 weeks

Stage III and Stage IV Hodgkin's Disease

Combination chemotherapy is the mainstay of treatment for advanced Hodgkin's disease in children, although radiotherapy is again frequently added to sites of bulky disease or incomplete response. Patients with a large mediastinal mass regardless of the stage have a significant local-regional recurrence rate if treated with either chemotherapy alone or radiation alone. A combined-modality approach is generally needed to control the disease. Six to 12 courses of chemotherapy have been used in these patients. With optimal treatment, 80 to 90 per cent of children with stage III Hodgkin's disease and up to 80 per cent of children with stage IV Hodgkin's disease can be expected to survive five years.

Treatment of Relapse

Many children who suffer a relapse of Hodgkin's disease can be salvaged by further chemotherapy and/or radiotherapy. Some of the aforementioned chemotherapy combinations or agents such as VP-16 and Ara-C can be effective in salvage therapy. About 90 per cent of children can achieve a complete remission after their first relapse of Hodgkin's disease. In selected patients in whom the usual salvage therapy fails, bone marrow transplantation can be considered.

NON-HODGKIN'S LYMPHOMA

The non-Hodgkin's lymphomas are a group of diseases with different histopathologic features and clinical behaviors. In children, follicular lymphomas are extremely rare. The most common histologic subtypes encountered are diffuse undifferentiated lymphomas (Burkitt's or non-Burkitt's type), lymphoblastic lymphoma, and diffuse large cell lymphoma. Burkitt's lymphoma will be discussed in a separate section. The staging work-up is similar to that of Hodgkin's disease, although the staging laparotomy is generally not recommended. The St. Jude Children's Research Hospital

TABLE 3. St. Jude Children's Research Hospital Staging Scheme for Non-Hodgkin's Lymphoma

Stage I	A single tumor (extranodal) or single anatomic area (nodal), with the exclusion of mediastinum or abdomen
Stage II	A single tumor (extranodal) with regional node involvement
	Two or more nodal areas on the same side of the diaphragm
	Two single (extranodal) tumors with or without regional node involvement on the same side of the diaphragm
	A primary gastrointestinal tract tumor, usually in the ileocecal area, with or without involvement of associated mesenteric nodes only
Stage III	Two single tumors (extranodal) on opposite sides of the diaphragm
	Two or more nodal areas above and below the diaphragm
	All the primary intrathoracic tumors (mediastinal, pleural, thymic)
	All extensive primary intra-abdominal disease
	All paraspinal or epidural tumors, regardless of other tumor sites
Stage IV	Any of the above with initial CNS or bone marrow involvement

TABLE 4. Chemotherapy for Lymphoblastic Lymphoma

LSA2 = L2

Induction

Cyclophosphamide	Daunomycin
Vincristine	Intrathecal methotrexate ±
Prednisone	radiotherapy to bulky primary site

Consolidation
  Cytosine arabinoside
  6-Thioguanine
  L-Asparaginase
  Intrathecal methotrexate

Maintenance

6-Thioguanine	Vincristine
Cyclophosphamide	Daunomycin
Hydroxyurea	Methotrexate
Cytosine arabinoside	BCNU

APO

Induction and consolidation

Adriamycin	L-Asparaginase
Vincristine	Intrathecal methotrexate ±
Prednisone	radiotherapy

Maintenance

Adriamycin	6-Mercaptopurine
Vincristine	Methotrexate
Prednisone	

staging system for non-Hodgkin's lymphoma has gained popularity and is commonly used (Table 3).

Lymphoblastic Lymphoma

Lymphoblastic lymphoma is probably in the same spectrum of malignancies as T-cell acute lymphoblastic leukemia. In general, children with bulky adenopathy and less than 25 per cent blast in the bone marrow are considered to have stage IV non-Hodgkin's lymphoma, whereas those with greater than 25 per cent blast in the bone marrow are considered to have acute lymphoblastic leukemia. The primary treatment for lymphoblastic lymphoma is chemotherapy. Two regimens of proven value are LSA2-L2 and APO (Table 4). Routine radiotherapy to sites of bulky primaries and prophylactic cranial irradiation have not significantly improved survival. Radiotherapy, however, is effective in relieving airway obstruction from bulky disease in an emergency situation and in the treatment of established central nervous system involvement by lymphoma.

Nonlymphoblastic Lymphoma (Excluding Burkitt's Lymphoma)

Chemotherapy regimens such as APO, COMP (cyclophosphamide, vincristine, methotrexate, prednisone), or CHOP (cyclophosphamide, Adriamycin, vincristine, prednisone) are effective. The usual duration of therapy is about 1 year. The role of radiotherapy is again limited but may convert a partial response of localized bulky disease after chemotherapy to a complete remission state. In the case of primary lymphoma of bone, radiotherapy can decrease the risk of local recurrence. For localized lymphoma of the bowel such as the terminal ileum, surgical resection followed by chemotherapy is the preferred treatment. Primary lymphoma of the central nervous system is rare, but tends to occur in children with inherited or acquired immune deficiency syndrome and in children receiving immunosuppressive therapy. The histology is usually diffuse large cell lymphoma. Primary radiotherapy with or without chemotherapy is given, but the prognosis is generally poor.

Most children with early-stage non-Hodgkin's lymphoma can be cured with modern therapy. The prognosis of children with advanced non-Hodgkin's lymphoma is less favorable. Nevertheless, about 60 to 80 per cent of children with advanced-stage non-Hodgkin's lymphoma may still be cured with intensive therapy. As in the case of Hodgkin's disease, studies are under way to test the ability to reduce the intensity of therapy for children with favorable early-stage non-Hodgkin's lymphoma, and new approaches such as bone marrow transplantation are continually being sought for children with very advanced stage non-Hodgkin's lymphoma.

BURKITT'S LYMPHOMA

MOLLY R. SCHWENN, M.D.

The majority of Burkitt's lymphoma patients present with a rapidly enlarging abdominal mass involving bowel, retroperitoneum, ovaries, kidneys, etc., without extra-abdominal involvement. The treatment of diffuse undifferentiated lymphoma, both Burkitt's and non-Burkitt's, is challenging because of the tumor's high growth fraction and fast doubling time. These features explain its exquisite sensitivity to chemotherapy, as well as its often explosive presentation.

Diagnosis must be made quickly, with minimal time for staging procedures, and then appropriate therapy (both specific and supportive) should be initiated promptly, preferably within 48 hours of presentation and within 24 hours of surgery. Cytologic examination of fluid (pleural, ascitic, or CSF) or touch imprint of a biopsy specimen (bone marrow or mass) may aid in rapid diagnosis.

PREPARATION FOR TREATMENT

Rapid staging should include abdominal ultrasonography and/or computed tomography scan, chest radiography, lumbar puncture, bone marrow, and the following blood tests: CBC, smear, creatinine, electrolytes, uric acid, and LDH. LDH elevation correlates well with total tumor burden.

Simultaneous with staging tests, preparation for definitive treatment should be undertaken with allopurinol (200 to 500 mg/m²/day), fluids, and sodium bicarbonate (70 mEq/L) to raise urine pH to 7. These maneuvers may prevent uric acid nephropathy from developing or becoming severe. Rarely, hemodialysis is necessary at presentation; some patients have renal failure secondary to kidney infiltration or ureteral obstruction. More often, dialysis becomes necessary with initiation of treatment because of tumor lysis. Dialysis should be considered when phosphorus rises to 10 mg/dl or higher, creatinine approaches 10 mg/dl or is rapidly rising, potassium is greater than 6 mEq/L, hy-

pocalcemia becomes symptomatic, or anuria or volume overload develops.

Close monitoring is essential before, during, and for the first few days following treatment and should include total input/output, hourly urine output, at least daily weight, and frequent measurement of calcium, phosphorus, potassium, uric acid, and creatinine. Definitive treatment should be undertaken only in a cancer center where pediatric intensive care and dialysis facilities are available. Otherwise, transfer should be planned as soon as possible.

Acute tumor lysis is unlikely to develop in patients with small tumor burdens (stage I or II by the Murphy system and A, B, or AR by the Ziegler system). These patients do not require monitoring as frequently as patients with large tumor burdens (stage III or IV and C or D).

ROLE OF SURGERY

Surgery is indicated in patients with abdominal tumors when there is a possibility of 90 per cent or greater tumor reduction. Partial resection is not useful and should not delay chemotherapy. At times, a "second look" laparotomy is undertaken when complete response to induction chemotherapy is uncertain.

ROLE OF RADIATION THERAPY

There is no demonstrated benefit of radiation therapy in Burkitt's lymphoma. It may be used in an emergency for symptomatic neurologic involvement but has not been helpful for CNS prophylaxis. A randomized Pediatric Oncology Group (POG) study has shown no benefit from radiation for treating localized Burkitt's lymphoma. Other trials have shown that abdominal radiation is not indicated. Radiation should never delay beginning or continuing chemotherapy.

SPECIFIC THERAPY

Chemotherapy alone can be curative for Burkitt's lymphoma in both early and advanced stages. Cyclophosphamide is the most effective drug and in Africa has been used alone with success in some patients. It is the mainstay of all effective regimens.

In the United States, one of the best drug combinations developed and tested in the 1970s at NCI and by the Children's Cancer Study Group (CCSG) is COM or COMP: cyclophosphamide, vincristine (Oncovin), methotrexate, with or without prednisone. Survival for patients of all stages together is approximately 60 per cent with COM(P) regimens and 90 per cent for patients with limited disease, such as those with resected abdominal tumors. Patients who are free of disease for 1 year after diagnosis rarely relapse and can be considered cured.

In the late 1970s, the necessity of including central nervous system (CNS) prophylaxis in Burkitt's treatment was recognized. Intrathecal cytosine arabinoside (ara-C) and methotrexate are effective in preventing CNS relapse for the majority of patients. The addition of high-dose systemic drugs—methotrexate and ara-C—may also improve the rate of CNS relapse–free survival. The optimal method is yet to be determined.

As mentioned earlier in this chapter, CNS radiation does not appear to be necessary or beneficial.

RECENT ADVANCES

In the 1980s, centers in the United States and Europe have attempted to improve treatment for patients with advanced-stage disease (stage III/IV, C/D) in order to increase survival above 50 per cent. Regimens have become more intensive: Methotrexate has been given at high doses with leucovorin rescue; cyclophosphamide has been given in high fractionated doses by some investigators. In some trials, drugs have been added: doxorubicin, ara-C (standard and high dose), the podophyllotoxins (VP-16 and VM-26), 6-thioguanine, and CCNU. Many of these intensive regimens have been successful, with survival rates of patients with advanced disease now approaching 75 per cent. The most aggressive regimens are also suitable for treating B-cell ALL successfully.

Despite these advances, patients with CNS involvement at diagnosis and those who do not respond fully to induction therapy or who relapse continue to have a poor prognosis. Current therapeutic trials are addressing even more intensive treatment for these patients with autologous bone marrow rescue. Marrow is sometimes purged with antibodies directed against antigens on the surface of B cells.

Duration of therapy is another area of investigation. Regimens of 12 to 18 months are still being utilized by some research groups (e.g., CCSG), but others have reduced therapy to 6 months or less, even for advanced-stage Burkitt's lymphoma and B-cell ALL. In Boston, we have successfully piloted a 60-day protocol with similar probability of survival (75 per cent) as regimens of longer duration.

Because these intensive regimens are both myelosuppressive and immunosuppressive, patients are very susceptible to infection, both during treatment and in the months following treatment. Trimethoprim-sulfamethoxazole prophylaxis is recommended. Some patients may also benefit from intravenous gamma-globulin support.

FUTURE DIRECTIONS

As the treatment of Burkitt's lymphoma has advanced, a fascinating series of laboratory discoveries has unfolded in the past 15 years. The characteristic (8,14) and variant (2,8 and 8,22) reciprocal translocations were described. Next, the breakpoints of these translocations were reported to coincide with the location of the c-myc proto-oncogene (on chromosome 8) and with the loci of the immunoglobulin heavy-chain gene (on 14), kappa light chain (on 2), and lambda light chain (on 22). Other revelations have followed. Eventually, understanding the mechanisms of oncogenesis in Burkitt's lymphoma will impact on prevention, especially in Africa, where the tumor is endemic, and on treatment strategies.

9

Endocrine System

HYPOPITUITARISM AND GROWTH HORMONE THERAPY

LOUIS E. UNDERWOOD, M.D.

DECIDING WHICH CHILDREN ARE GROWTH HORMONE DEFICIENT

Now that growth hormone (GH) is plentiful and decisions about whether a patient will be treated are not made on the basis of availability, physicians must wrestle with the problem of which short children should be treated. This decision is sometimes difficult because results of diagnostic tests of GH secretion are not completely reliable indicators of endogenous GH secretion and often are imprecise predictors of GH responsiveness. Even when good short-term growth responses to GH injections are observed, the long-term response and the impact on adult stature are not foreseeable.

Diagnosis is easy in patients who have severe GH deficiency. Such children have slow growth (usually 3.5 to 4.0 cm/yr), diminished muscle mass, increased body fat, absent or very poor serum GH responses to provocative stimuli, and low serum IGF-I values. Diagnosis is more problematic in less severe cases because the capacity of short children to secrete GH and to respond to exogenous GH forms a continuum. At one end of this spectrum are patients that all agree are GH deficient. As one proceeds along the spectrum of GH responses and responsiveness, however, one encounters patients in whom secretory bursts differ among various stimuli and vary in magnitude from one day to another. Compared to those who have severe deficiency, exogenous GH may produce less growth acceleration in these children.

Our inability to define GH secretory capacity in these children is due in large part to our inability to define normal GH secretion by available methods. There is growing acceptance that the tests we use now are too imprecise to differentiate between short children who will benefit from therapy and those who will not. Investigators debate which provocative tests (e.g., insulin hypoglycemia, arginine, clonidine) are the most useful in diagnosis and whether provocative tests are as informative as measurements of GH on serum sampled frequently or continuously over prolonged periods. In many instances, none of the studies of GH secretion gives clear answers, and the physician is forced to make decisions about treatment on other grounds.

DECIDING WHICH SHORT CHILDREN TO TREAT WITH GH

Physicians making decisions about who to treat with GH must rely on clinical judgments as well as on measurements of GH secretion. Reasonable effort must be made to determine the cause of the child's short stature and to exclude the possibility that the growth failure is due to a disease not related to GH secretion. Following this, factors that might favor the use of GH treatment include extreme short stature without evidence of catch-up growth, slow growth rate, a tendency toward adiposity and diminished muscle mass, low serum IGF-I despite good nutrition and absence of chronic illness, equivocal GH values, and evidence that the child might benefit psychologically if growth is accelerated. Before a therapeutic trial is begun, the family should be informed about the possibility of treatment failure, and the criteria for an acceptable increase in growth rate over a finite period of time should be defined. Such goals should be agreed to by the family and used as the basis for discontinuing treatment if they are not met.

TREATMENT OF GH-DEFICIENT CHILDREN

Since the discovery in 1985 that a few children who had been treated years earlier with pituitary GH had contracted Creutzfeldt-Jakob disease, the GH used in North America and most other countries has been derived by recombinant DNA techniques. Typically, a dose of 0.1 mg/kg is given every other day. Growth rates are better, however, if treatment is given daily at a dose of 0.05 mg/kg. Although GH usually has been given intramuscularly, subcutaneous injections work just as well and permit the use of smaller needles. GH-deficient children typically increase their growth rate from 3.5 to 4.0 cm/yr before treatment to 8.0 to 10.0 cm/yr during the first year of treatment. Young children usually respond better than adolescents, and the obese respond better than the thin. As treatment continues, the rapid growth that occurs early in therapy declines, so that after 2 to 4 years the growth velocity is average for age and developmental status.

If the growth response to GH therapy is inadequate, several possible causes should be considered. These include incorrect diagnosis, failure to administer the GH properly, formation of growth-attenuating antibodies to GH, development of hypothyroidism, and intercurrent illness or poor nutrition. The frequency with which GH antibodies develop during therapy depends on the GH preparation used. With high-quality preparations, it is as low as 5 per cent. Such antibodies only rarely reach high enough concentrations to attenuate growth. If attenuation occurs, growth is usually restored by using another GH preparation.

Most children with hypopituitarism are not clinically *hypothyroid*, but some may have serum thyroxine levels below the normal range. Modest doses of L-thyroxine (2 to 3 µg/kg) are given to children with subnormal serum thyroxine concentrations. Approximately 5 to 10 per cent of patients receiving GH develop hypothyroidism, which will attenuate the response to GH.

Symptoms of *hypoadrenalism* are uncommon in older children with hypopituitarism. Therefore, we usually do not prescribe glucocorticoids unless the patient has syncope, postural hypotension, attacks of hypoglycemia, or laboratory evidence of loss of pituitary-adrenal axis function, which may occur as a result of pituitary-hypothalamic surgery or radiation therapy. Because excessive doses attenuate the growth response to GH, we administer glucocorticoids cautiously (approximately 10 mg/m²/day). Pharmacologic doses of glucocorticoids (approximately 50 mg/m²/day) are given during periods of stress to any child with hypopituitarism who shows evidence of impaired pituitary-adrenal axis function (i.e., impaired response to metyrapone or injections of ACTH).

Deficiency of *antidiuretic hormone* is uncommon in children with idiopathic hypopituitarism but occurs frequently after pituitary region surgery. It is treated by administering desmopressin (DDAVP) intranasally in a dosage of 0.05 to 0.1 ml one to two times daily. The dosage schedule of this agent must be individualized.

In boys with hypopituitarism who fail to undergo puberty by 14 years of age, we prefer to use long-acting testosterone enanthate intramuscularly. We begin treatment with 25 to 50 mg every 2 weeks and gradually increase the dosage over several years to 150 to 200 mg every 2 weeks.

In girls requiring estrogen replacement, we begin treatment with conjugated estrogen (0.3 to 0.6 mg/day) or ethinyl estradiol (0.05 mg/day). After 9 to 12 months of continuous estrogen therapy, cycling with a progestational agent is begun.

OUTCOME OF THERAPY

If GH treatment for GH deficiency is begun in the first 2 to 3 years of life or before prolonged growth failure is evident, an adult height within the normal range can be anticipated. Delayed diagnosis and sub-

optimal therapy will compromise final adult height. Delayed emotional development and problems in coping are common in GH-deficient children. These result from infantilization and low expectations on the part of those who come into contact with these children. Counseling of parents and patients is usually beneficial and sometimes essential.

SHORT STATURE
MITCHELL E. GEFFNER, M.D.

TREATMENT OF CLASSIC GH DEFICIENCY
Growth Hormone

On a purely statistical basis, 2.5 per cent of all children would be considered to have short stature. True growth hormone (GH) deficiency occurs in about 1 in 5000 children, so that less than 1 per cent of all short children are actually GH deficient. The treatment of true GH deficiency remains crystal clear: Replace the missing hormone. Of course, associated central hormone deficiencies (if any) must be identified and appropriately treated.

Since 1985, all GH used to treat children with GH deficiency in the United States has been manufactured by recombinant DNA technology. Until that time, since the first patient was treated with GH in 1958 by Raben, GH had been extracted from human pituitary glands, purified by various processes, and distributed either by the National Hormone and Pituitary Program (previously called National Pituitary Agency) or by several commercial sources. Because of the identification of the very rare slow viral disease, Creutzfeldt-Jakob disease (CJD), in a total of seven patients in the world who had received pituitary GH, the possibility of viral contamination of one or more batches of pituitary-derived GH had to be seriously entertained. Since this frequency of CJD far exceeded the expected incidence rate, use of pituitary GH was terminated.

Perhaps fortuitously, the gene for GH had been cloned in the late 1970s, and the recombinant product was already being tested when the CJD association was noted. The FDA approval of recombinant GH in 1985 was obviously timely and has ultimately allowed a greater availability of product for use in GH-deficient children. Additionally, it has allowed endocrinologists to challenge traditional dogma about routes of administration and dosing regimens for GH.

The first issue that was examined was the need for intramuscular (IM) administration for GH. Because of early reports of development of growth-attenuating antibodies with the use of subcutaneously administered pituitary GH, the intramuscular route was uniformly recommended. However, with recombinant GH this has not been a problem, and patients have expressed preference for the subcutaneous (SQ) route, which should foster increased compliance. In fact, approximately 50 per cent of patients treated with recombinant GH by pediatric endocrinologists now receive it by the SQ route, and the Food and Drug Administration has recently approved this route of administration.

The second break with traditional dogma involved the dose of GH to be prescribed. For many years dosage was based on availability of pituitary product so that the dose was limited in this country to 0.18 to 0.3 unit/kg/week. Studies in the United States and Great Britain, performed before the availability of recombinant GH, already suggested better linear growth responses with doses of 0.3 unit/kg/week than with lower doses. Newer studies suggest that doses as high as 0.6 unit/kg/week are even more efficacious. A dose of recombinant GH greater than 0.55 unit/kg/week is now being used by approximately two thirds of GH-deficient patients in the United States. Although higher doses appear to be associated with better height responses, the proportional difference in growth rate is not nearly as much as the increase in dose. One must also be cautious about possible side effects at higher doses (see below).

The last change in the practice of GH delivery is its schedule of administration. Historically, a thrice-weekly program of administration was devised as a result of short supply of pituitary GH. This intermittent schedule is obviously nonphysiologic, since normally GH is secreted on a daily (predominantly nocturnal) basis. Thus, a number of studies were conducted comparing patients with established GH deficiency, half of whom received GH on their existing thrice-weekly schedule and the other half of whom received the same weekly dose divided into daily injections. In each study, the daily-dose group had a step-up in velocity compared to the group receiving three doses per week. These findings have now been extended to newly diagnosed patients. Preliminary findings from a national collaborative study in the United States suggest better height velocity for GH-deficient children during the first year of treatment with daily versus thrice-weekly administration. At the current time, however, about 25 per cent of all GH-deficient patients in the United States receive their GH on a daily basis.

Thus, in clinical practice, the following guidelines for GH administration appear most practical and efficacious: (1) subcutaneous administration, (2) a dosage of 0.3 to 0.6 unit/kg/week,* and (3) daily administration.

Side effects of growth hormone have been remarkably infrequent. Although about 5 per cent of newly started patients and 30 per cent of patients previously treated with pituitary GH develop antibodies to recombinant GH, these have only rarely affected the growth response. Issues concerning induction of insulin resistance with resultant derangements of carbohydrate tolerance, even at higher doses of GH, do not appear to be clinically relevant. With any form of GH treatment, induction of central hypothyroidism within the first few months of therapy needs to be identified and treated

---

*For younger children, the dosage should be at the high end to avoid wastage of GH. Diluted vials of GH have guaranteed stability for only 14 days. Routine use of maximal doses, while probably most efficacious, must be weighed against cost differences of approximately 100 per cent versus minimum dosage, with consideration of higher doses after evaluation of initial response.

with thyroid hormone replacement. A possible association between GH treatment and slipped femoral capital epiphysis has been suggested, although more recent data suggest that this is not due to the treatment. Development of acral enlargement, particularly at higher doses of GH, needs careful consideration. The author has seen one patient who developed facial changes of acromegaly which resolved with cessation of treatment. Anecdotally, foot size appears to increase faster (although not to unusual dimensions) than linear growth. Lastly, in 1988, a possible relationship between GH treatment and induction of leukemia surfaced. Fifteen cases of leukemia were identified worldwide in patients who had previously been treated with either pituitary and/or recombinant GH. A government committee was convened which concluded that, while the association was higher than would have been predicted based on the incidence of leukemia in the general population, the largest cluster was limited to Japan; and, in the other cases, most were associated with extenuating circumstances, such as radiation exposure or diseases with higher cancer risks, which limited the significance of any possible connection. Subsequently, the only two new cases were also from Japan. Overall, outside of Japan, there appears to be a very limited association between GH and leukemia. Furthermore, GH therapy has not been linked to recurrence of leukemia or solid tumors in patients who had received radiation therapy that inadvertently led to their GH deficiency. It would appear thus far that recombinant GH is quite safe.

Growth Hormone–Releasing Hormone

It is now recognized that most causes of GH deficiency (idiopathic, radiation-induced, anatomic, etc.) have a hypothalamic basis. In 1982, the structure of the hypothalamic-releasing hormone (RH) for pituitary GH (GHRH) was determined, followed by the preparation of synthetic, biologically active fragments. At this time, there has been limited experimental administration of GHRH to GH-deficient children. Although this approach is potentially attractive because it might be considered a more physiologic form of replacement than GH itself, the optimal dose, frequency of administration, and route of administration remain unclear, and, hence, height responses to date have been variable. Based on the better-understood physiology of other hypothalamic-releasing factors, it is conceivable that multiple daily doses of GHRH would be required, necessitating some form of pump administration. On the other hand, the much smaller size of the GHRH molecule would make its synthesis by recombinant DNA technology much less intricate and expensive (compared to GH). Issues related to possible side effects, including hyperplastic changes in the pituitary and induction of GHRH antibodies, require further study. At this time, the use of GHRH to treat GH deficiency remains investigational, with studies ongoing to determine its future application(s).

TREATMENT OF OTHER CAUSES OF SHORT STATURE
Constitutional Short Stature

This common condition, associated with short stature and delayed puberty, represents a variation of normal growth. Children with this condition are born with lengths in the expected genetic percentile range and show diminished height velocity beginning sometime between 6 months and 3 years of age, with a concomitant delay in epiphyseal maturation. This is followed by resumption of a nearly normal height velocity thereafter with heights less than, but parallel to, a given child's genetically predicted percentile line. Pubertal changes usually develop later than normal, commensurate with the observed delay in bone age. Ultimate height is usually within 5 cm (2 inches) of the predicted height. A similar growth pattern in one of the two parents occurs about 50 per cent of the time.

The frequency of occurrence of this growth pattern is unknown, since not all cases are necessarily referred to endocrinologists. Whether it occurs more commonly in boys or girls is unknown, but, since short boys seek referrals for growth delay much more often than short girls, there is a male preponderance of patients with this diagnosis. The author would hope, in the future, that if this represents an ascertainment bias, it is recognized by physicians and avoided (girls have less time for therapy than boys and should be identified). Thus, most current treatment recommendations are targeted to males. Historically, treatment has been equated with the use of male sex hormones, their administration usually beginning after the onset of puberty to appropriately avoid prepubertal masculinization.

The decision to intervene should be made only after documentation of associated problems with psychosocial adjustment related to body image perception. The expectations related to therapy must be clearly understood from the beginning by both adolescent and parents. Specifically, treatment is low-dose androgen, given short term (usually not more than 6 months and certainly not longer than 1 year), and carefully monitored (with height and weight measurements and physical examinations every 3 months and bone age radiographs every 3 to 6 months). Most importantly, families must understand that this treatment regimen does not increase the expected adult height, but rather helps the child reach that height sooner, a goal that is designed to help the adolescent cope better with height-related psychosocial issues. For cases with major behavioral problems, concomitant psychological counseling may be indicated.

Reported treatment regimens vary somewhat, but, generally, parenterally administered, long-acting testosterone esters are given every 3 to 4 weeks. For example, testosterone enanthate, 50 to 100 mg, can be given every 3 weeks (four injections every 3 months). The injections may be given by the patient himself or by a parent or through a physician's office. Because these testosterone preparations are oil-based, a 22-gauge (or larger) needle must be used and a deep muscular injection site chosen.

With the use of low-dose, short-term regimens, side effects are rare. In particular, undue advancement of bone age with rapid growth initially, followed by ultimate shortening of the total growth period with resultant loss of adult stature, is minimized with protocols as outlined above. Liver toxicity is almost completely eliminated with parenteral administration, which avoids the first-pass, nonphysiologic hepatic exposure that follows administration of oral anabolic steroids. "Side effects" of increased muscle bulk, voice deepening, and advancement of puberty are well-appreciated by the patients.

Other nontraditional therapies have been attempted or are under study in children with constitutional short stature. Although a few studies have suggested that children with constitutional short stature have a relative GH deficiency, most have shown normal GH secretion in this population. Short-term trials (less than 1 year) with agents ordinarily used to acutely stimulate GH secretion, including clonidine and L-dopa, have been used. Reported results have been variable, suggesting differences in patient populations studied. At this time, these therapies cannot be routinely recommended. Additionally, controlled trials using recombinant GH itself to treat prepubertal children with constitutional short stature are currently in progress. Although preliminary 1-year data show an acceleration in height velocity by about 75 per cent in children with constitutional short stature treated with GH, it is unknown whether this will be sustained and if ultimate height will be affected. Therefore, at this time, GH therapy cannot be considered standard of care for these children.

Turner's Syndrome

The average adult height of women with Turner's syndrome, either untreated or after "traditional" growth-promoting treatment with anabolic steroids and/or low-dose estrogen, is only about 143 cm (56 inches). Although it is believed that most girls with Turner's syndrome do not have GH deficiency,* treatment trials with recombinant GH with or without anabolic steroids were initiated almost 6 years ago. Unlike any previously attempted growth-promoting strategy, there appears to be, on average, an improvement in predicted adult height by over 8.2 cm (3.2 inches) after the first 3 years of combined growth hormone/anabolic steroid therapy. The dose of GH used (0.75 unit/kg/week) is higher than that used to treat GH deficiency. The incidence of side effects appears to be no different than with lower doses. There have been no reports of acromegaloid changes despite the higher GH doses employed. Careful, repeated evaluations for abnormalities in carbohydrate tolerance and insulin resistance are necessary considering the heightened risk of these problems which are part of Turner's syndrome itself.

The anabolic steroid used in the studies has been oxandrolone (currently in doses of 0.0625 mg/kg/day). However, this product is being discontinued by its manufacturer. Alternatively, fluoxymesterone at a dose of 0.05 mg/kg/day can be used. To avoid androgenic side effects in these girls, whose ages range between 5 and 10 years, such low doses of oral anabolic steroids are recommended. These agents tend to promote

---

*When girls with Turner's syndrome who are older than 10 years of age undergo routine GH testing, they often have low GH levels because of lack of endogenous estrogen secretion secondary to their ovarian failure. This should not be construed as true GH deficiency.

growth rather than to virilize. At the currently recommended dosage of oxandrolone, evidence of virilization, such as clitoromegaly, has been rare. Anabolic steroids themselves may heighten the risk for insulin resistance, so that patients treated with these agents alone or in conjunction with GH need to be followed closely.

Many girls in the United States with Turner's syndrome are being treated with GH outside of research protocols. For most patients, treatment is probably instituted after age 10 years, since that is when these girls frequently seek medical attention and thus when the diagnosis of Turner's syndrome is usually made. Based on observed efficacy of GH in GH-deficient children, the use of GH at the earliest age possible appears to result in the best ultimate height outcome. For those girls who are diagnosed with Turner's syndrome at a young age, usually because of associated physical stigmata, if GH is to be considered, it should be prescribed as soon as height velocity starts to slow down.

Other Conditions Associated with Short Stature

In the last few years, there has been described a possible new form of GH deficiency, in which spontaneous GH secretion (e.g., measured every 20 minutes during sleep) appears to be abnormal, yet that following standard pharmacologic provocation is normal. It is rationalized that the pharmacologic stimuli are unnatural and induce a false sense of GH sufficiency, whereas without such drugs in the body, the neuroendocrinologic control of GH secretion is deficient for facilitation of normal growth (hence, the term GH neurosecretory deficiency). The most clearly documented association of this growth pattern and a neurosecretory GH deficiency is seen in children following radiotherapy for central nervous system tumors. Until more normative, age-stratified data are available, it remains unclear whether this entity exists to any significant degree in otherwise normal short children.

If the decision to initiate GH treatment is made, the same guidelines used for administration of GH to classically GH-deficient children would apply. It should be underscored that when contemplating GH therapy in this setting, the growth of such children should be carefully monitored for at least 1 year prior to treatment using a well-counted measuring system (stadiometer) to avoid confusion by seasonal variations in growth rate and/or physiologic variants of normal growth. If such stringent criteria are not applied, the plentiful availability of GH could lead to its misapplication. The only exception to this long duration of observation would be children who have previously received head irradiation and who are medically stable. Since there is a known high risk of hypothalamic hypopituitarism in this population, the observation period could be reduced to 6 months prior to initiating GH treatment. However, if, after a 6-month therapy trial, the observed height velocity, does not increase by at least 50 per cent above baseline, the GH should be discontinued. Careful observation for possible side effects is even more imperative in this setting, in which the GH deficiency may be only partial.

Growth delay may result from many other causes for which there is no clear-cut pathophysiologic explanation. Familial short stature is the prototype for this category. Defective cartilage may be responsible for significant short stature in conditions such as achondroplastic dwarfism. Poor growth may also occur in children born with intrauterine growth retardation and in those who develop chronic diseases, such as renal failure. In all these situations, there have been no effective growth-promoting treatments.

Investigational use of GH is being attempted or planned in many of these conditions. Renal failure patients are being treated in experimental GH protocols. Experimental bone-lengthening surgical techniques are also being explored, particularly in achondroplastic dwarfs. The characterization and synthesis of the GH-dependent growth factor, somatomedin-C (also called insulin-like growth factor I, or IGF-I), may open up new horizons for treatment of short children. Its obvious application would be in children who are resistant to the growth-promoting actions of GH (Laron-type dwarfs). This product has only recently been administered to humans; there is as yet no information concerning its efficacy to promote human growth.

TALL STATURE

MITCHELL E. GEFFNER, M.D.

The "definition" of tall stature depends on cultural background, sex, and family height patterns. In the United States, it is rare for boys to seek evaluation for isolated tall stature. With greater acceptance of tall females in our society, referrals for evaluation of tall girls are dwindling. In clinical practice, girls are considered to be tall if their adult height projects to greater than 183 cm (72 inches). Analogous to the role of short parental heights in contributing to a short adult height of a child, tall parental stature plays a pivotal role in leading to tall stature of a child. Before concluding that tall stature is due to familial factors, however, certain organic disorders associated with excessive and/or rapid height growth should be considered, at least on clinical grounds. Excessive height frequently occurs in boys with Klinefelter's syndrome and may occur in either sex in association with Marfan's syndrome or homocystinuria. Rapid growth, reflected by crossing of height percentiles and advancement of bone age, prior to age 10 years, occurs in association with sexual precocity, untreated thyrotoxicosis, and perhaps exogenous obesity.

ESTROGEN THERAPY FOR FEMALES

The only effective pharmacologic therapy for girls with familial tall stature is high-dose estrogen. Sex steroids promote rapid osseous maturation, during which time height growth per year is less than expected for each year of bone age advancement. Although administration of estrogens to limit the height of tall girls has been practiced for 50 years, its current use has been limited because of concern about serious side effects as well as greater acceptance of tall women in our society (as mentioned above). Various forms of estrogen have been employed and at various dosing schedules. These include ethinyl estradiol, 0.06 to 0.5 mg/day; premarin (conjugated estrogens), 10 mg/day; and estradiol valerate, 6 to 8 mg/day. In some studies, the estrogen was given on days 1 to 23 of each month and combined with a progestational agent (such as Provera, 5 to 10 mg) from day 10 or 14 to day 23 of each month. The addition of the progestational agent is reserved for those girls who are at least 1 year into puberty to provide cyclic withdrawal bleeding, which markedly diminishes the likelihood of estrogen-induced uterine neoplasia. Initiation of menses in younger subjects would not be appropriate for psychodevelopmental reasons.

In most females, the greatest efficacy of estrogen treatment is seen when begun between 10 and 12 years and continued until growth ceases (bone age 15 years). It has recently been confirmed in a controlled study which followed tall girls until growth cessation that ethinyl estradiol at a dose of 0.1 mg/day was as effective as a dose of 0.3 mg/day, in both cases resulting in approximately a 40 per cent decrement in predicted adult height. This occurred regardless of whether the initial bone age was less than or greater than 12.5 years. However, the estrogen resulted in a diminution in adult height prediction which, in absolute terms, was greater in those girls with younger bone age (7.4 cm, or about 3 inches) than in those girls with older bone age (3.6 cm, or about 1.5 inches).

Because the doses of estrogen employed for height reduction are at least three times the normal "replacement" dose, and the dosage may be employed for as long as 5 years, concern about untoward effects must be registered. The actual risk of estrogen-mediated side effects, such as suppression of the hypothalamic-pituitary-ovarian axis, endometrial carcinoma, thrombophlebitis, and hypertension, is unknown. Clinical but mostly anecdotal experience suggests that side effects are minimal or transient and usually consist of nausea, weight gain, and anemia secondary to excessive uterine bleeding. Use of progestational withdrawal should prevent development of endometrial neoplasia and hypermenorrhagia.

Although the author still has reluctance to prescribe estrogen, some endocrinologists may consider estrogen use for the girl who, by analysis of growth velocity and bone age, is likely to exceed 183 cm in adult height and who, along with her parents, has significant psychosocial concerns about this prediction. Initiation of treatment as early as age 10 years appears most efficacious and is not associated with untimely pubertal development. Ethinyl estradiol at a dose of 0.1 mg/day for 1 year, followed by cycling with Provera beginning in the second year, appears both efficacious and reasonably safe. Treatment efficacy should be evaluated by measurement of height, weight, and blood pressure every 3 months, with semiannual determination of bone age and hepatic function.

TESTOSTERONE TREATMENT FOR BOYS

Analogous to the use of estrogens to limit growth of the tall female child, high-dose testosterone has been employed in boys whose adult heights project to greater than 200 cm (79 inches). As already mentioned, it is extremely rare that any pharmacologic approach is requested by male patients. However, if there are overriding psychosocial concerns, treatment may be indicated. The regimen that is most commonly recommended is a long-acting (oil-based) testosterone ester (e.g., enanthate) given at a dose of 500 mg/m² as monthly intramuscular injections. This dose extrapolates to greater than four times the normal adult testosterone production rate when viewed on a daily basis. Its use should be restricted to boys who are at least 1 year into puberty. As with high-dose estrogens, the efficacy of testosterone is best in boys in whom treatment is commenced earlier than later. For boys started between the bone ages of 12 and 14, greater than 14 to 15, and greater than 15 years, the adult height predictions are reduced by approximately 8 cm (slightly greater than 3 inches), 5.7 cm (slightly greater than 2 inches), and 3 cm (slightly greater than 1 inch), respectively (mean duration of treatment, 1 to 2 years). However, a recent study suggests a similar reduction in projected adult height with only a 6-month course of testosterone enanthate given as 50 mg intramuscularly every 2 weeks.

An increased risk of side effects needs to be considered with such supraphysiologic doses of testosterone. These include suppression of the hypothalamic-pituitary-testicular axis, which occurs frequently, as manifested by decreased testicular size. Such suppression appears fully reversible but may take more than 1 year from the time of discontinuation of treatment. Sperm counts also normalize in this time frame. Advancement of pubertal changes also occurs, but no other significant side effects have been noted during follow-up.

OTHER APPROACHES

Low-dose estrogens have been employed on occasion to treat tall males, with at least short-term success. It has recently been noted that tall adolescents have mild elevations in serum GH concentrations and paradoxically increased responses of the serum GH concentration following stimulation with thyrotropin-releasing hormone and/or oral glucose. This has led to trials of bromocriptine therapy, analogous to its use in some patients with acromegaly. Reported results, using daily doses as high as 7.5 mg for up to 8 months, have been variable, although most studies suggest a reduction in predicted adult height similar to that seen with high-dose sex steroid therapy. Cholinergic muscarinic blockers, under experimental conditions, have been used to induce partial suppression of GH secretion in tall children, but without significantly reducing short-term height velocity. Development of other similarly acting but more efficacious drugs may add to our pharmacologic armamentarium to treat familial tall stature.

THYROID DISEASE

DENNIS M. STYNE, M.D.

The absence or excess of thyroxine can have profound effects upon the entire organism, including growth, mentation, and reproduction. Thus, the diagnosis of thyroid disease is essential, especially in the neonate. The knowledge gained in the physiology of the hypothalamic-pituitary-thyroid axis in the last three decades has allowed the development of straightforward diagnostic maneuvers in acquired thyroid disease, while advances in assays have provided us with methods of virtually eliminating the retardation caused by untreated congenital hypothyroidism. This section will review normal thyroid physiology and standard diagnostic techniques before turning to disorders of thyroid function and their treatment.

NORMAL THYROID PHYSIOLOGY

Thyroxine is synthesized in sequential steps: (a) plasma iodide is trapped by the thyroid follicular cell; (b) iodide is oxidized to iodine; (c) tyrosine molecules (attached to the thyroglobulin molecule) are organified by the addition of one iodine at the 3 position (causing the formation of monoiodotyrosine [MIT]) or two iodines at the 3 and 5 positions (forming diiodotyrosine [DIT]); (d) DIT is coupled with DIT to form $3,5,3',5'$ tetraiodothyronine (T_4) or one DIT is coupled with one MIT to produce $3,5,3'$ triiodothyronine (T_3).

T_4 and T_3 are released from the thyroid gland, but most of the circulating T_3 is derived from peripheral deiodination of the beta-ring of T_4. Reverse T_3 (RT_3), or $3,3',5'$ triiodothyronine, is a metabolically inert product of the peripheral deiodination of the alpha-ring of T_4.

Circulating T_4 is predominantly bound by serum proteins; 75 per cent is bound to thyroid-binding globulin (TBG), 20 per cent to thyroxine-binding prealbumin (TBPA), and 5 per cent to albumin with only 0.20 to 0.60 per cent present in the circulation as free thyroxine (FT_4); less than 1 per cent of T_3 circulates as free T_3 (FT_3). FT_4 is monodeiodinated to form FT_3, which is the metabolically active form of thyroid hormone.

The thyroid gland is controlled by the hypothalamic-pituitary unit. Hypothalamic thyrotropin-releasing hormone (TRF) is released from the median eminence into the pituitary portal circulation to stimulate the pituitary gland, which in turn releases thyrotropin-stimulating hormone (TSH) into the general circulation. TSH reaches the thyroid gland and stimulates the production and release of thyroid hormones. In the absence of adequate thyroid hormone (primary hypothyroidism), TSH rises to very high levels, whereas in the presence of autonomous and excessive production or administration of thyroid hormone, TSH is suppressed.

Laboratory Diagnosis of Thyroid Function

Total serum T_4 and T_3 as well as FT_4, FT_3, and TSH are measured by radioimmunoassay (RIA). Direct measurement of TBG by RIA is available, but most laboratories still offer an indirect indication of protein binding, such as the resin T_3 uptake (RT_3U). The values reported in the RT_3U are inversely proportional to available protein-binding sites in a patient's serum sample. One commonly used method to correct the T_4 for protein binding is to multiply the T_4 by the RT_3U, with the result called the free thyroxine index (FTI), or the T_7. Thus, with decreased TBG the total T_4 and T_3 are low, the RT_3U is high, and the FTI is normal, as are the FT_4 and FT_3. In true hypothyroidism the T_4 is low, and with reduced T_4 the protein-binding sites are more available, thereby lowering the RT_3U as well; the FTI is low, as are the total T_4 and total T_3. In TBG excess, T_4 and T_3 are high, but with increased protein-binding sites, the RT_3U is low and the resulting FTI is normal. In true hyperthyroidism, the T_4 is high, causing decreased available thyroid-binding sites so that the RT_3U also is elevated; as a result of high T_4 and RT_3U, the FTI, the FT_4, and the FT_3 are high. As a rule of thumb, if the T_4 varies from normal and RT_3U varies in the opposite direction, the patient likely is euthyroid with an abnormality of thyroid-binding protein; if the T_4 deviates from normal and the RT_3U varies in the same direction, it is likely that a disorder of thyroid function is present. Thus, every patient with a low T_4 is not hypothyroid and does not necessarily require therapy, just as every patient with a high T_4 does not have hyperthyroidism.

Normally, TSH is less than 5 to 7 mIU/ml (depending upon the laboratory standards), so that there is no effective difference between a normal value and a "low" value. New ultrasensitive TSH assays are becoming widely available to measure TSH accurately down to 0.5 mIU/ml. Thus a patient with Graves' disease will have a value less than 0.5 mIU/ml, and a normal patient will have a value between 0.5 and 5 mIU/ml. To differentiate between secondary hypothyroidism and tertiary hypothyroidism, however, requires a dynamic TRF test. A dose of 200 μg of TRF is given intravenously, and TSH is measured at 0, 10, 15, 30, 60, 90, 120, and 180 minutes. A normal response is a rise in TSH to at least 10 mIU/ml about 15 minutes after TRF; in secondary hypothyroidism, there is no rise in TSH, and in tertiary hypothyroidism the rise is often delayed until 60 to 120 minutes and the TSH may continue to rise during the 180-minute period. The TRF test is also useful in the diagnosis of hyperthyroidism, as there is no rise in TSH with the autonomous thyroxine secretion characteristic of Graves' disease.

Thyroid scanning and radioactive iodine uptake have a limited role in pediatric diagnosis. Imaging of a thyroid gland is essential for diagnosis in the presence of nodules of the thyroid gland (to determine if they are functional or "cold" and therefore nonfunctional) or for the localization of an ectopic thyroid gland. However, in a clear case of Hashimoto's thyroiditis or Graves' disease, little is added by thyroid scan, although it often has been (uselessly) performed in children. The scanning of a neonate or infant presents particular problems; the radioactive tracer, which is administered orally, may be spit up by the infant and leave tracks on the skin, falsely suggesting thyroid tissue. Further, a neonate with primary hypothyroidism may have no detectable gland on scan just after birth, but after months to years a normal gland may be detected; in several cases, this has been traced to the transient presence of thyroid-binding inhibitory immunoglobulin (TBII) in the neonatal circulation which was passed from the mother (who may herself have symptomatic autoimmune thyroid disease) to the fetus. Other cases of transient hypothyroidism are due to the use of iodine-containing cleaning compounds on the skin of the neonate. A congenital iodine-trapping defect can lead to a lack of thyroidal iodine uptake that is not reversible. The demonstration of an ectopic gland in a neonate, however, is good evidence that the child has a permanent defect. In the differential diagnosis of goiter, a perchlorate discharge test may be used in which a thyroid uptake is performed and then repeated with the administration of potassium perchlorate, which causes the discharge of nonorganified iodine; if the turnover of iodine is much higher with perchlorate than without, an enzyme deficiency causing an organification defect is present. An important consideration in performing thyroid uptake determinations is to measure the uptake early, such as at 4 to 6 hours, as well as at 24 hours. A quick turnover of radioactive iodine, as may occur in Graves' disease, may lead to a low uptake at 24 hours but a very high uptake at 4 to 6 hours. Scanning is done with ^{123}I or ^{99m}Tc-pertechnetate.

Ultrasonographic scanning of the thyroid gland is useful to differentiate cystic from solid masses and determine the relationship of the mass to neck structures. If a mass is solid, it is more likely to be carcinoma than if it is cystic, and recent studies suggest improved accuracy in the diagnosis of thyroid carcinoma by ultrasonography. Ultrasonography is also used to guide a biopsy needle.

DISORDERS OF THE THYROID GLAND

Goiter

An enlargement of the thyroid gland from any cause is a goiter. Palpation of the older child usually is accomplished with the examiner's fingers directed anteriorly around the neck while the examiner stands behind the patient. If the patient swallows water during the examination, the mobile nature of the thyroid gland may be appreciated as it rises and falls on swallowing. Hashimoto's thyroiditis may be accompanied by a midline, pea-sized Delphian node located 0.5 to 1 cm above the isthmus; the Delphian node does not move with swallowing.

Most goiters in early childhood or infancy are diagnosed by the newborn screening programs and are due to maternal ingestion of goitrogen or an inborn error of thyroid biosynthesis. The majority of goiters in the late childhood and adolescent years are due to euthyroid or hypothyroid Hashimoto's thyroiditis, followed by a lower incidence of Graves' disease or hyperthyroidism. There remain a minority of indeterminate goiters of mild degree which may persist for years; these may be colloid goiters, a diagnosis established only after all other diagnoses are eliminated.

A solitary nodule in childhood is unusual and worthy of careful attention. A thyroid scan is indicated to determine whether the nodule is hot and functional or cold and nonfunctional. A cold nodule is particularly worrisome, as it may indicate neoplasia.

Hypothyroidism

Neonatal Hypothyroidism

If therapy is not begun soon after birth, mental retardation will result from congenital hypothyroidism. Neonatal hypothyroidism has an incidence close to 1 in 4000 live births. Routine neonatal screening is used owing to the difficulty in making the diagnosis early enough on clinical grounds alone. Heelstick samples of blood are collected on a filter paper and sent to a centralized laboratory, where blood is eluted from the paper and analyzed for T_4 and TSH. If the T_4 is low and the TSH high, the diagnosis is presumptive primary hypothyroidism. If the T_4 and the TSH are both low, the patient may be referred for further evaluation to rule out secondary or tertiary hypothyroidism. Screening program results are usually available within 2 weeks of birth, but if a suspicion exists about a patient, an on-site T_4 and TSH determination should be requested immediately.

TSH quickly rises after delivery and peaks at 30 minutes, T_4 is secreted in response and peaks at 24 to 72 hours, and T_3 exhibits a primary rise in the hours after birth owing to increased beta-ring deiodination. A normal term child has serum T_4 concentrations in the adult hyperthyroid range during the 24 to 72 hours after birth, whereas a bona fide hypothyroid child has T_4 either below or in the normal adult range. Healthy premature babies have a lower concentration of the thyroid hormones, and premature babies with respiratory distress syndrome have values lower still. Small-for-gestational-age infants likewise have lower thyroid hormone concentrations than do normal children. The majority of false-positive tests reported from a screening center are due to premature babies or small-for-gestational-age infants with low T_4 concentrations and normally low TSH. The present practice of releasing term babies from hospital at 12 to 24 hours of age makes a false-positive result more likely, as the serum T_4 will not have reached its postnatal peak and TSH will not have reached its postnatal nadir by that age.

The classic signs and symptoms of congenital hypothyroidism include large tongue, coarse facies, umbilical hernia, a combination of lethargy and irritability, poor growth and weight gain, short extremities with a delayed or high upper-to-lower segment ratio, persistently open posterior fontanelle, large anterior fontanelle, and coarse voice. Further, pericardial effusion can be noted on ultrasound study in infants untreated for a prolonged time. These signs and symptoms take weeks to months to develop, and by then irreversible mental changes are already established. More subtle signs of congenital hypothyroidism include prolonged gestation with large birth weight, persistent jaundice, temperature instability, lag in the time of the initial stool to more than 20 hours after birth, edema, and hypoactivity and poor feeding in the neonatal period.

The etiology of congenital hypothyroidism is usually athyreosis, hypoplasia of the thyroid gland, or a lack of descent of the thyroid gland from its initial site of formation at the back of the tongue at the foramen cecum to its normal mature location (thyroid ectopy or "cryptothyroidism"). A thyroid scan can correctly demonstrate thyroid ectopy, but the diagnosis of athyreosis is more difficult. Absence of uptake of ^{123}I on scan may be due to maternal blocking antibodies, which cross the placenta, and may falsely suggest a permanent anatomic abnormality when in fact a transient condition is present.

Biochemical abnormalities of the thyroid gland are usually hereditary and often involve the appearance of a goiter. These conditions include dyshormonogenesis, such as peroxidase defects (organification defects), iodotyrosine deiodinase defect, and thyroglobulin defects (causing lack of coupling of MIT and DIT). A defect in TSH receptors and a defect in the transport of iodine into the gland have been described and do not lead to goiter; there is no ^{123}I uptake on scan. Several families are described with peripheral resistance to thyroid hormone; thyroid hormone and TSH concentrations are high, and the patients are clinically euthyroid but may have deaf-mutism, skeletal abnormalities, and goiter. Maternal TSH-binding inhibitory immunoglobulin (TBII) or thyroid growth-blocking immunoglobulins may be transplacentally transferred from the mother and cause congenital hyperthyroidism. With the passage of time as TBII decreases, the apparently athyreotic newborn may become euthyroid in these rare cases.

Congenital hypopituitarism may include secondary or tertiary hypothyroidism as a feature, but there may be other pituitary hormone deficiencies present as well as a midline defect. Rarely (less than 1 in 100,000 live births), isolated TSH deficiency is seen.

Radioactive iodine mistakenly given to a pregnant woman with Graves' disease (if, for example, she denied being pregnant) crosses the placenta and damages the developing gland. Propylthiouracil (PTU) given to a pregnant woman with hyperthyroidism crosses the placenta and can cause profound hypothyroidism; when the PTU is cleared post partum, the baby recovers from the hypothyroidism, and the thyroid-stimulating immunoglobulin that was passed from the mother begins to exert its effect, causing transient hyperthyroidism. Paradoxically, excessive iodine given to the mother can suppress thyroid gland formation just as a deficiency of iodine can.

Decreased thyroid-binding globulin, or TBG deficiency, occurs in 1 in 10,000 live births in a sex-linked pattern. The serum T_4 and T_3 are decreased, and the child will be identified by the newborn screening program but requires no therapy. Familial dysalbuminemic hyperthyroxinemia (FDH) leads to increased T_4 but a normal serum T_3; the free forms of both hormones are normal, and the patient is asymptomatic and requires no therapy.

With the receipt of a screening test suggesting congenital hypothyroidism, another set of serum samples for confirmatory T_4 and TSH should be drawn. The decision of whether to perform a thyroid scan is con-troversial owing to the false positives, as noted above. A bone age determination of the knee and foot in a patient with a positive screen is quite useful: The distal femoral epiphysis calcifies at 36 weeks of gestation, the proximal tibial at 38 weeks, and the cuboid at term. A delayed bone age suggests that true hypothyroidism was present in utero.

In transient hyperthyrotropinemia, a child has a perfectly normal T_4 concentration for age but a slightly elevated TSH (often in the range of 20 to 30 mIU/ml.) Usually TSH decreases to normal by 1 to 2 years of age in the absence of treatment. Children with laboratory values characteristic of transient hyperthyrotropinemia should be watched for evidence of decreasing thyroid function in case they have an ectopic or hypoplastic thyroid gland that decompensates with time. Such patients may maintain a normal T_4 concentration at the time of the newborn screening at the expense of an elevated TSH.

Treatment of congenital hypothyroidism should begin when the diagnosis is established; confirmatory serum T_4 and TSH should be obtained before therapy starts. If there is an extremely low T_4 and high TSH, treatment can be started before the confirmatory results are available, to save time as the diagnosis is clear. At present, recommended dosage of synthetic thyroxine is 10 μg/kg/day for the newborn (a dose of 25 μg is the usual daily dose in most term newborns) and 2 to 5 μg/kg/day after 1 year of age, with an eventual maximal dose of 100 to 150 μg in a teen-ager. Thyroxine is most widely available in tablets and is crushed and administered in a small amount of formula or applesauce. Liquid thyroxine is available for parenteral use but is quite expensive; it has been used for patients who are unable to take medications orally. It is totally inappropriate to make a bottle of a slurry of crushed thyroxine tablets to use for multiple doses: The dose is likely to vary from day to day even if the bottle is shaken.

Neonates with congenital hypothyroidism may continue to have elevated TSH concentrations for months or years after the onset of therapy even if T_4 is raised to normal. The goal of therapy should be to maintain a normal serum thyroxine concentration for age rather than to suppress the TSH to normal values for age. Nonetheless, the TSH should not rise during treatment. A rising TSH may indicate that the child is outgrowing the T_4 dose (elevated TSH may also indicate lack of compliance). The half-life of thyroxine is 5 days, so the serum T_4 is not likely to stabilize until at least 1 week after a change in dose. Thus T_4 and TSH determination should be obtained 1 and 2 weeks after onset of therapy to assure compliance, absorption, and the correct dose and then T_4 is measured monthly times three, then every 3 months until 2 years of age, and every 6 to 12 months thereafter. Overtreatment with thyroxine will cause advancement of the bone age and can lead to craniosynostosis as well as poor weight gain, jitteriness, disturbed sleeping, diarrhea, and diaphoresis. The administration of normal doses of thyroxine to infants with congenital hypothyroidism who have been untreated for months may trigger congestive heart failure due to the rapid mobilization of fluid accumulated during the myxedematous state; pericardial effusions can be noted in such children. In cases of late onset of therapy, it is preferable to work up to the full dose over a period of 7 to 14 days. Patients treated early and appropriately with thyroxine are likely to have normal intelligence, according to follow-up studies. It is becoming more common to test patients who do not have proven ectopic thyroid glands, athyreosis, or neonatal goiters at 3 years of age to see if they have permanent hypothyroidism or one of the transient defects. In those patients who have reliable families and can be counted upon to return for follow-up, thyroxine can be discontinued for 2 to 4 weeks with T_4 and TSH measured at 2 and 4 weeks to determine function. Most brain growth is completed at 3 years, so that the test is safe, but it is not advisable to leave a child off thyroxine for any longer interval if thyroid function appears impaired.

Acquired Hypothyroidism

Classic symptoms of acquired hypothyroidism in childhood include poor weight gain, poor growth, delayed puberty, apathy, and decreased activity level. Mental retardation, however, does not occur in hypothyroidism acquired after infancy. Physical signs include decreased pulse rate, reduced relaxation time of reflexes, and, in severe cases, myxedema. Skeletal maturation is delayed and limb length reduced, leading to an increased upper to lower segment ratio.

Hashimoto's, or chronic lymphocytic, thyroiditis is responsible for the majority of cases of acquired hypothyroidism. This autoimmune disorder is found on a continuum with Graves' disease, and both disorders may coexist or one may be followed by the other. Both disorders occur frequently in a family pattern. Hashimoto's thyroiditis frequently is associated with diabetes mellitus and Turner's syndrome, so that patients with either condition should undergo surveillance for the development of this condition. Clinical characteristics include goiter, a Delphian node, minimally to severely elevated TSH concentrations, a positive titer of antimicrosomal antibodies or antithyroglobulin antibodies, and frequently a family history of thyroid disease. Euthyroid goiter or compensated hypothyroidism is diagnosed if TSH concentrations are normal to slightly elevated with normal T_4I or FT_4. Elevated TSH and decreased total T_4 or FT_4 indicate obvious primary hypothyroidism. Thyroxine is administered until the TSH is suppressed to normal and the serum T_4 is normal if primary hypothyroidism is found. If the TSH is not elevated and the goiter is minimal, the patient may be watched for further deterioration in thyroid function. If an obvious goiter causes cosmetic deformation, thyroxine may be given for a period of 3 months to see if the goiter will shrink; if the small goiter does not change, thyroxine is stopped and the patient is followed clinically.

A thyroglossal duct cyst in the midline of the neck may contain all of the functioning thyroid tissue available to the patient; if any midline congenital defect of the neck is removed surgically, the patient must be followed for the development of hypothyroidism. Some children are born with only one lobe of thyroid gland, and it is usually located on the left. This tissue may undergo compensatory hypertrophy; in a susceptible person Hashimoto's thyroiditis may develop in such a lobe, causing hypothyroidism and unilateral goiter.

Acquired hypothyroidism is treated with thyroxine in a dose of approximately 3 to 5 μg/kg to a maximum of 100 to 150 μg. Unlike neonates with congenital hypothyroidism, older children can have their dose titrated to suppress the TSH to normal. Long-term cases that have not been treated should receive low doses of thyroxine at first with a gradual increase. Remarkably, children appropriately treated with thyroxine have a shortening of their attention span and an increase in their activity levels, which in some cases may reduce their cooperation in school and cause their grades to drop. This probably should be considered a reversion to their appropriate behavior state had they not developed hypothyroidism, but the parents may not see it that way and may resist treatment. Often a child demonstrates a remarkable increase in growth (catch-up growth) with the onset of therapy; the bone age also advances with this growth. If a child has been hypothyroid for many years, final height will probably be reduced in spite of catch-up growth.

Acquired increased TBG binding of thyroid hormones occurs with estrogen treatment or pregnancy or due to an inherited condition; androgen therapy, protein-losing conditions, and phenytoin therapy cause acquired decreased TBG binding or thyroid hormones.

Hyperthyroidism

Graves' disease is an autoimmune disease that may coexist with Hashimoto's thyroiditis in the same person or the same family. Thyroid stimulatory IgG (often called TSI or a host of other abbreviations) antibodies are directed toward the TSH receptor, leading to autonomous thyroid function and hyperthyroidism. T_4 and T_3 exceed the TBG capacity so that FT_4 and FT_3 rise. In some cases, the T_4 is normal but the T_3 is elevated. Weakness, increased pulse, emotional lability to the point of apparent psychiatric disease, hyperactivity and short attention span, weight loss, and diarrhea are characteristic findings. These excess thyroid hormones cause heightened autonomic tone and can cause lid retraction and "stare." Exophthalmos may occur owing to infiltration of glycoprotein in the posterior orbit; mild cases may require only the use of artificial tears at night, but an ophthalmology consultation is recommended for more severe cases. Pretibial myxedema is found in some patients, more rarely in children than adults.

Thyroid storm is rare in childhood but consists of an acute onset of hyperthermia and tachycardia in a patient with underlying hyperthyroidism. Surgery, infection, and diabetic ketoacidosis may precipitate an attack. Symptoms of thyroid storm include high fever, sweating, tachycardia, and reduced mental state ranging from confusion to coma.

Propranolol (1 to 2 mg/kg/day given orally every 6 to 12 hours) can control some symptoms of thyroid storm. In extreme cases, propranolol can be given intravenously at a dose of 0.1 mg/kg up to a total of 5 mg, but an intra-atrial pacing catheter is a recommended precaution. Dexamethasone in a dose of 1 to 2 mg every 6 hours can lower serum T_3. Intravenous NaI in a dose of 1 to 2 gm/day may temporarily decrease the release of thyroid hormone from the thyroid gland; Lugol's solution can be given orally if the patient is conscious. A cooling blanket can help control the hyperemia. Fluid management must be watched and, if tachycardia causes heart failure, digitalis may be necessary. Propylthiouracil will not take effect for several days, but to plan for the possibly extended course of the disorder, 200 to 300 mg can be given every 6 hours by slurry, if necessary.

Hyperthyroidism is diagnosed by elevated total and FT_4 and T_3, nondetectable TSH, positive thyroid-stimulating immunoglobulin titer, and often low positive titers of antithyroglobulin and antimicrosomal antibodies. Elevation of antimicrosomal and antithyroglobulin antibodies in hyperthyroidism may indicate the combination of Graves' disease and Hashimoto's thyroiditis. A thyroid scan is not necessary in a classic case of Graves' disease. The white blood cell count may be decreased in hyperthyroidism and may be decreased further by medical therapy for hyperthyroidism; WBC should be measured. An ANA and SMA20 should be determined if propylthiouracil is to be used as treatment.

The three types of treatment for hyperthyroidism include medication, surgery, and radiation therapy. Propylthiouracil (PTU) and methimazole are the medical therapies available in the United States; in Europe, carbamazole is also available. PTU blocks organification and decreases T_4 to T_3 conversion and may inhibit the formation of the offending IgG, whereas methimazole demonstrates only the first activity. PTU is administered in doses of 150 to 450 mg/day divided every 8 hours (and methimazole in doses of 15 to 50 mg/day). Enough PTU is given to provide a sufficient block to cause hypothyroidism, and then replacement thyroxin is added to allow a euthyroid state. An alternative treatment regimen requires tapering the PTU dose to achieve euthyroid status. The gland is examined regularly for a decrease in the goiter; every 2 years that patients are followed with medical therapy there is an incidence of remission of hyperthyroidism of 25 per cent. Thus, after 11 years of therapy 75 per cent of patients in one series achieved remission. Lupus-like syndromes, rashes, granulocytopenia or agranulocytosis, and hepatitis (possibly leading to cirrhosis) can occur and are generally idiosyncratic, occurring early in the course of therapy with PTU or methimazole. These drugs should be stopped if such side effects are found and alternative methods of therapy used; many of the side effects are reversible. If a patient demonstrates lack of compliance, alternate therapy is indicated.

Propranolol (1 to 2 mg/kg/day divided into two to four doses per day, with 5 to 10 mg q6h as a starting dose in larger children) can control symptoms of hyperthyroidism and is useful in preparation for surgery; side effects of propranolol upon respiratory or circulatory function are possible. Propranolol has not generally been used long term in children.

Surgical management is another possible therapy. An experienced thyroid surgeon should perform the subtotal thyroidectomy. Recurrent laryngeal nerve paralysis is an unusual but possible complication. Hypocalcemia can follow thyroidectomy transiently owing to postoperative edema of the parathyroid glands, or permanently if the parathyroid glands are removed with the thyroid tissue. Medical management should be invoked to control the hyperthyroid state in preparation for surgery. Supersaturated iodine (Lugol's solution) is used for the 10 days prior to surgery to harden the gland and reduce the blood supply to the gland. Escape from iodine usually occurs after 2 to 4 weeks. No matter how accurate the surgery, the patient will usually be hypothyroid by 10 years after surgery.

Radioactive iodine (^{131}I) therapy has proved safe in studies of children and adolescents with Graves' disease. However, some consider it inappropriate to give radioactive iodine to children; it has been suggested that the younger the child receives the radioactive iodine, the more likely is the development of thyroid carcinoma and that there are as yet inadequate data to state that this form of therapy is safe in childhood. Further, one dose of radioactive iodine may not cure the patient, and another dose may be necessary. After the treatment, some patients may be euthyroid, but as in surgical treatment, by 10 years post-therapy almost all will be hypothyroid owing to continued scarring of the gland.

Neonates with hyperthyroidism usually have transplacentally acquired thyroid-stimulating immunoglobulin (TSI). As the mother who has Graves' disease is usually on therapy with PTU, and PTU freely crosses the placenta, the child will have been exposed to PTU. The child may be born profoundly hypothyroid and the statewide screening program will report the child's test as positive with a low T_4 and a high TSH. After the PTU leaves the circulation over 3 to 6 days, the child develops nervousness, diarrhea, shakiness, and tachycardia owing to rising T_4 and T_3. Treatment can include Lugol's solution of iodine (1 drop every 8 hours) to suppress thyroid hormone output, propranolol (2 mg/kg/day divided into two to four doses/day) temporarily to counter the effects of hyperthyroidism, and PTU (5 to 10 mg/kg/day) or methimazole (0.5 to 1.0 mg/kg/day) if the condition is severe. The dose should be adjusted to the severity of the disease and the response. The condition usually lasts for 6 weeks. Monitoring thyroid hormone levels while slowly tapering therapy determines the correct time to stop treatment.

Neoplasms

Carcinomas of the thyroid gland are rare in childhood but should be suspected in certain situations. A history of prior irradiation of the thyroid gland (radiation was used three decades ago for acne, enlarged thymus, or ringworm) is significant, and if the irradiation was done for the therapy of another cancer (e.g., for head and neck cancer or at the time of bone marrow transplant), the risk is higher.

A single firm nodule is more ominous in childhood than multiple nodular goiter. The majority of solitary nodules in several series have been benign. Lack of concentration of ^{123}I on thyroid scan (a cold nodule) increases the likelihood of carcinoma more than does a functioning nodule (warm or hot nodule); however, autonomous functioning thyroid nodules in children have an 11 per cent incidence of carcinoma. Ultrasonographic evidence that the nodule is a cyst makes it less likely to be malignant, but carcinomas have been found in the walls of thyroid cysts. The presence of enlarged anterior cervical lymph nodes, metastases on chest radiograph, or hoarseness all make the likelihood greater that the single thyroid nodule is malignant. A patient with a family or personal history of multiple endocrine neoplasia syndrome has a great likelihood of having medullary carcinoma of the thyroid gland. Medullary carcinoma of the thyroid is often evaluated by elevated calcitonin concentrations in the basal state or after pentagastrin or calcium stimulation. Pentagastrin (0.5 µg/kg) can be given as a intravenous bolus over 5 to 10 seconds and calcitonin measured at 0, 2, and 3 minutes. Elemental calcium at 2 mg/kg has been infused intravenously over 50 to 60 seconds before the pentagastrin to decrease the incidence of false negatives.

In the presence of a solitary nodule, either a needle biopsy or an open surgical biopsy can be performed. Needle biopsy is safe and has a low level of false-negative results if the pathologist is experienced. In the absence of experienced clinical help in the procedure of needle biopsy or in a situation heavily suggestive of a malignant diagnosis, open biopsy seems best.

Painful Thyroid Glands

Tenderness of the thyroid gland may indicate a viral infection (subacute thyroiditis), which is uncommon in childhood, or a bacterial infection (suppurative or acute thyroiditis), which is even less frequent. Suppurative thyroiditis presents with severe localized pain over the thyroid gland, erythema, and signs of infection, including fever, tachycardia, and diaphoresis. Subacute thyroiditis may also present with localized tenderness, but not the rest of the picture. Both of these conditions are accompanied by an elevated sedimentation rate. Unless an abscess is palpable or visible on ultrasound examination, a needle biopsy for culture may be necessary to differentiate between the two. Bacterial infections are treated with appropriate antibiotics and viral infections with pain control medications and anti-inflammatory drugs.

PARATHYROID DISEASE

KEVIN E. HALBERT, M.D., *and* REGINALD C. TSANG, M.B.B.S.

Vitamin D and Metabolites

The mainstay of treatment for hypoparathyroidism and pseudohypoparathyroidism is vitamin D and its analogues. Ergocalciferol (vitamin D_2), which is of plant origin, traditionally has been the principal agent used. It has a prolonged onset of action, from 7 to 14 days after therapy has begun. Furthermore, because of a long half-life of 2 to 4 weeks, prolonged hypercalcemia (20 to 40 days) easily occurs if vitamin D intoxication occurs. Doses of ergocalciferol have ranged from 8,000 to 1,200,000 IU per day, with the usual range being 50,000 to 100,000 IU/day or 1,000 to 2,600 IU/kg/day. Individual responsiveness to ergocalciferol can be variable and can change after a period of prolonged control with a fixed dose. In addition, ergocalciferol has a very narrow therapeutic index, thus making undertreatment and intoxication real possibilities. Because of these problems ergocalciferol is no longer considered the primary agent for management of hypoparathyroidism or pseudohypoparathyroidism, and vitamin D analogues have moved to the forefront.

Dihydrotachysterol (DHT) is an alternative agent to ergocalciferol. This agent is an ultraviolet irradiation product of ergocalciferol and is marketed in a crystalline form. Because of its structural conformation it does not require 1α-hydroxylation by the kidney before it is biologically active. Its onset of action of 1 to 2 weeks is still relatively long. Usual doses range from 0.2 to 3.0 mg/day, or 8 to 22 µg/kg/day (1 mg DHT equals 120,000 IU of ergocalciferol). Because of its relatively long onset of action, dose adjustments should not be made more often than every 2 to 3 weeks.

25-Hydroxycholecalciferol (25-hydroxyvitamin D_3) is also effective in the management of hypoparathyroidism and pseudohypoparathyroidism. At high serum concentrations 25-hydroxycholecalciferol may have similar actions on intestine and bone as does 1,25-dihydroxycholecalciferol, the naturally occurring active vitamin D metabolite; i.e., 25-hydroxycholecalciferol will increase intestinal absorption of calcium and phosphate and increase mobilization of bone calcium and phosphate. Peak serum concentrations of 25-hydroxycholecalciferol are reached about 4 hours after an oral dose, and an onset of action is seen in less than 1 week after therapy is begun. Doses that have been effective in controlling the hypocalcemia of hypoparathyroidism and pseudohypoparathyroidism have ranged from 20 to 50 µg/day or 3 to 6 µg/kg/day.

Another vitamin D analogue that has recently become available is 1α-hydroxycholecalciferol (1α-hydroxyvitamin D_3). This agent requires 25-hydroxylation by the liver before becoming a biologically active form but avoids the necessity of 1α-hydroxylation by the kidney, which can be impaired with decreased serum parathyroid hormone concentration or hyperphosphatemia. Initial starting doses range from 0.5 to 1.0 µg/day, with maintenance requirements between 0.5 and 3.0 µg/day, or 0.03 to 0.08 µg/kg/day. The major advantages of 1α-hydroxycholecalciferol are rapid onset of action and short serum half-life, which allow for rapid resolution of hypercalcemia (usually within 1 to 5 days of discontinuation) when inadvertent intoxication occurs.

The metabolite that has the most utility in management of hypoparathyroidism and pseudohypoparathyroidism is 1,25-dihydroxycholecalciferol (1,25-dihydroxyvitamin D_3). This is the most active naturally occurring metabolite of vitamin D, being the product of 1α-hydroxylation of 25-hydroxycholecalciferol in the kidney. Once ingested, 1,25-dihydroxycholecalciferol requires no further biochemical conversions for bioactivity. Rapid onset of action enables rapid correction of hypocalcemia, usually within 1 to 4 days. Because of the serum half-life of less than 24 hours, discontinuation of the agent in the event of hypercalcemia during therapy results in return to normocalcemia in 1 to 2 days. Biologic activity, as manifested by continued increased intestinal calcium absorption, may persist for several days after 1,25-dihydroxycholecalciferol has been cleared from the blood. Therapy is usually begun at 0.25 μg/day (0.03 μg/kg/day) and increased daily by 0.25 μg in older children, or 0.015 μg/kg in infants, until normocalcemia is obtained. Usual maintenance doses range from 0.5 to 1.25 μg/day or 0.03 to 0.08 μg/kg/day.

Goals of Therapy

The main objective in treatment of hypoparathyroidism and pseudohypoparathyroidism is maintenance of normocalcemia and normophosphatemia with minimal complications. Whichever form of vitamin D is chosen for treatment, the initial dose should be at the low range of usual therapeutic efficacy and gradually increased while monitoring the serum calcium concentration carefully. For example, with 1,25-dihydroxycholecalciferol, serum calcium concentration should be measured once or twice daily once therapy is begun. For the slower-acting vitamin D metabolites, serum calcium measurements need to be begun as one approaches the time of onset of action (e.g., since ergocalciferol has an onset of action of 7 to 14 days, serum calcium measurements need to begin near the end of the first week of therapy).

Increases in the doses of vitamin D metabolites should be made cautiously, taking into consideration the onset of action as well as half-life of the metabolites, each of which will affect the steady state. The target serum calcium concentration should be maintained in the 8.5 to 9.0 mg/dl range. Once stability has been obtained, serum calcium, magnesium, and phosphate values can be checked every 3 to 6 months. In addition, renal function should be assessed at least once every 6 to 12 months. Examination of serum concentrations of 1,25-dihydroxycholecalciferol have not proved to be of value, in that maintenance of normal serum concentrations are associated with a high incidence of hypercalcemia. Serum phosphate concentrations require much longer to correct than serum calcium concentrations. Phosphate concentrations are usually corrected within 2 to 3 months after serum calcium concentrations are normalized. Larger doses of vitamin D may result in faster correction of serum phosphate concentrations, but they also greatly increase the risk of vitamin D intoxication.

Dose requirements of vitamin D in pseudohypoparathyroidism tend to be lower than in hypoparathyroidism. Dose requirements for either hypoparathyroid condition also can change with time, even after years of stability on a single dose, resulting in either hypocalcemia or hypercalcemia. Thus, consistent long-term follow-up examinations are required. Finally, continuous anticonvulsant therapy can increase vitamin D metabolism, thus leading to increased maintenance vitamin D requirements.

Adjunctive Therapy. Although vitamin D is the primary agent in the management of these conditions, several adjunctive therapies have been utilized. The principal among these is oral calcium supplementation. Although not necessary in the patient who has a normal calcium intake, this can add a little additional margin of safety in the difficult-to-control patient. Usually 50 mg of elemental calcium per kg of body weight or 530 mg calcium gluconate per kg is given in three or four divided doses over the course of a day. Maximum doses are 1 gm and 10 gm, respectively, for elemental calcium and calcium gluconate. Doses greater than 75 mg of elemental calcium per kg of body weight or 750 mg of calcium gluconate per kg of body weight may result in diarrhea. Milk is not a desirable source of calcium supplementation because of its relatively high phosphate content.

A few patients resistant to vitamin D therapy will respond after magnesium supplementation. These individuals are usually hypomagnesemic (serum concentrations less than 1.5 mg/dl), and once this problem is corrected their condition becomes easier to control. Giving 7 to 15 mg of elemental magnesium or 70 to 150 mg magnesium sulfate per kg body weight per day is usually adequate therapy.

Chlorthalidone, a thiazide-like diuretic, plus sodium restriction has been suggested as a means of managing hypocalcemia secondary to hypoparathyroidism and pseudohypoparathyroidism without the use of vitamin D. It is thought to work by decreasing urinary calcium losses and contraction of extracellular water. There is no experience with the use of this regimen in children, and it cannot be recommended as an alternative to standard therapy.

Complications of Therapy

There are principally two complications of vitamin D therapy: vitamin D intoxication with resultant hypercalcemia, and hypocalcemia that can progress to tetany. Vitamin D intoxication is characterized by weakness, fatigue, lassitude, headache, nausea, and vomiting. Polyuria and polydipsia are usually present. On laboratory examination an elevated serum calcium concentration and possibly elevation of serum blood urea nitrogen and creatinine concentrations will be noted. Treatment of this disorder requires the discontinuation of vitamin D and any calcium supplements, which may be the only necessary therapy when the faster-acting vitamin D metabolites are used. Institution of a low calcium diet is advisable. Intravenous isotonic saline at 200 to 250 ml/kg/day should be given to increase urinary calcium losses. Furosemide diuretics 1 mg/kg three to four times daily should also be given to increase urinary losses of calcium. Careful evaluation of serum electrolyte concentrations is essential with furosemide therapy. Calcitonin (4 to 10 MRC units/kg every 3 to 4 hours IM with a maximal initial dose of 100 units) or prednisone (1 to 2 mg/kg/day) can also be given to lower serum calcium but usually is not necessary. If either 1α-hydroxycholecalciferol or 1,25-dihydroxycholecalciferol is used, discontinuation of these agents will result in reduction of serum calcium concentration to normal levels in 1 to 5 days. On the other hand, when ergocalciferol is used, normocalcemia usually returns by 4 to 6 weeks; it is possible to have a 20-week period before normocalcemia is attained. If hypercalcemia is prolonged, nephrocalcinosis can develop, resulting in renal failure. Other areas of ectopic calcification may also be noted. One probable long-term sequela of moderately severe hypercalcemia is growth arrest. This can last for 6 months or more after the onset of hypercalcemia. The resulting deficit in height is sometimes not recovered once growth resumes.

Hypocalcemic tetany is readily corrected with 2 ml of 10 per cent calcium gluconate per kg of body weight given via a slow intravenous infusion. While calcium is being given, the heart rate (via electrocardiographic monitoring) and blood pressure need to be measured. Rapid administration of calcium can result in cardiac arrhythmias or hypertension. After the acute episode of hypocalcemia is corrected, calcium should be continued at 50 to 70 mg of elemental calcium per kg of body weight per day to assure maintenance of normocalcemia. Until serum calcium concentrations are stabilized, serum calcium concentrations should be examined once or twice daily.

Hypocalcemia may occur during a febrile illness. The hypocalcemia may be effectively managed by temporarily increasing the dose of rapid-acting vitamin D metabolites or calcium supplements. Parents and patients need to be aware of the association of fever and hypocalcemia and to seek medical care at the first sign of illness.

Associated Conditions

Chronic mucocutaneous candidiasis will be encountered in a small number of patients with hypoparathyroidism. Nystatin can be used to control the infections, but currently no satisfactory therapy is available for complete eradication.

Many patients with pseudohypoparathyroidism will also have associated hypothyroidism. This is usually mild but occasionally will require thyroid replacement. There are also patients with autoimmune hypoparathyroidism who have associated malabsorption and steatorrhea. As a result they may have difficulty absorbing fat-soluble vitamins such as vitamin D and may seem resistant to therapy. Usually with large doses of vitamin D and oral calcium supplements these patients can be adequately managed. Occasionally patients will not respond until placed on a diet containing a significant proportion of fat as medium-chain triglycerides.

DISORDERS OF THE ADRENAL GLAND
GEORGE E. BACON, M.D.

CONGENITAL ADRENAL HYPERPLASIA (CAH) DUE TO 21-HYDROXYLASE DEFICIENCY

Initial Therapy

Salt-losing infants often present with hyperchloremic acidosis and require rehydration with intravenous normal saline or one-half normal saline with sodium bicarbonate. Initially, mineralocorticoid is usually provided as desoxycorticosterone acetate (DOCA), 1 to 3 mg/day IM. When oral medication is tolerated, fludrocortisone (Florinef), 0.1 to 0.3 mg/day, is suitable. Supplemental sodium chloride, 0.5 to 2 gm/day, may be necessary in some cases, particularly if the lower dose of mineralocorticoid is selected.

After blood has been drawn for appropriate laboratory studies, both salt losers (SL) and non-salt losers (NSL) are treated with hydrocortisone, either intravenously, intramuscularly, or orally, depending upon the condition of the patient. A typical initial dose is 20 to 25 mg/m²/day in three or four divided doses. (Note that 0.1 mg of fludrocortisone also has the glucocorticoid activity of approximately 1.5 mg of hydrocortisone, which should be considered in these calculations in order to avoid overtreatment in the very young infant.)

Chronic Therapy

Chronic medical management for SL patients consists of fludrocortisone; average dose for all ages beyond infancy is 0.1 mg/day (typical range: 0.05 to 0.2 mg/day). It is usually possible for older children to obtain additional table salt when necessary. However, dietary sodium chloride should not be considered a substitute for mineralocorticoid replacement, since susceptibility to adrenal crisis appears to be increased in these circumstances. In fact, some patients diagnosed as having the NSL type of CAH on the basis of normal serum sodium and potassium concentrations have been found to have elevated plasma renin activity (PRA), leading to the practice by some endocrinologists of recommending mineralocorticoid treatment for these children as well.

Glucocorticoid therapy for both types of CAH in the growing child consists of oral hydrocortisone, usually given three times daily, as close to 8 hours apart as conveniently possible. Although the normal cortisol production rate (CPR) is about 12 mg/m²/day, approximately 20 to 25 mg/m²/day is typically required in CAH (with considerable individual variation) because of the need to suppress ACTH as well as to replace cortisol. Presumably, supraphysiologic doses are necessary because the hypertrophic adrenal gland is highly sensitive to ACTH. Rather than administering hydrocortisone in three equally divided doses, there may be some advantage in providing a larger amount h.s. to more effectively suppress the early morning rise of ACTH.

Use of an equivalent dose of a longer-acting preparation such as prednisone, which is also about 3.5 times as potent as hydrocortisone, has the advantage of requiring twice-a-day rather than three-times-a-day administration in most patients. However, there is some evidence that this and similar analogues are more likely to retard growth than is hydrocortisone; therefore, it is prudent to withhold these preparations until the patient is fully grown.

Patients are usually followed at 6-month intervals but more frequently during infancy or if response to therapy is not optimal. Important parameters are growth velocity, bone age (may be obtained at yearly intervals, but frequency depends on the clinical course), serum androstenedione and 17-hydroxyprogesterone. (Note that 17-OHP concentrations in particular depend somewhat on the timing of medication; e.g., satisfactory adrenal suppression may be documented within 1 or 2 hours after administration, but levels can rise significantly prior to the next dose.) Measurement of serum testosterone may also be useful for monitoring control in girls and prepubertal boys. These serum determinations have now essentially eliminated the need for urinary 17-ketosteroid and pregnanetriol assays.

It is not always possible to achieve entirely normal hormone concentrations without overtreating to the extent that undesirable side effects of glucocorticoid occur. Therefore, some elevation is generally considered acceptable as long as growth velocity is appropriate and skeletal maturation is not advanced.

It is usually not necessary to obtain serum electrolytes in SL patients on a routine basis. Hypertension is a sign of excessive administration of mineralocorticoid. Undertreated infants may fail to gain weight and be prone to episodes of dehydration, and older children demonstrate increased salt craving. Under these conditions, serum sodium and potassium concentrations are indicated, and measurement of PRA may also be helpful.

Emergency Treatment

Empirically, patients with otitis media, strep throat, and other similar febrile conditions should increase their dose of glucocorticoid two- or threefold during the duration of the illness. This recommendation does not apply to children with minimal signs and symptoms (e.g., mild upper respiratory infections) but primarily to those who are sufficiently ill to miss school and/or consult their physician. An exception is the child with a viral exanthem, particularly varicella, since high doses of glucocorticoid encourage spread of the disease and fatalities have occurred. Therefore, in these circumstances, it is suggested that steroid therapy be maintained at about 1.5 to 2 times physiologic level.

Patients undergoing more severe physical stress (e.g., meningitis, major surgical procedures) should receive hydrocortisone, up to 100 mg/m²/day IM or IV in four to six divided doses, the rationale being that a normal adrenal gland is able to respond to maximal stress by increasing cortisol secretion in the neighborhood of tenfold. Ideally, parents should be taught to administer intramuscular hydrocortisone when oral medication is not tolerated because of vomiting, particularly if medical attention is not readily available.

Surgical Management

Guidelines for surgical intervention vary from center to center. Clitorectomy in girls can sometimes be avoided if the enlargement is minimal, since further growth may not be a problem if medical management is adequate. However, psychological trauma is probably minimized if clitorectomy or relocation and recession are performed in the newborn period. Widening of the introitus in patients with a urogenital sinus can also be accomplished at this time, to decrease the chance of urinary tract disorders secondary to retention. Definitive vaginoplasty is probably best postponed until pu-

bertal development is complete. Pelvic ultrasonography is helpful in determining when the uterus has reached mature size.

CAH DUE TO OTHER ENZYMATIC DEFICIENCIES

The other forms of CAH occur much less frequently than 21-OHD, but principles of management (i.e., replacement and suppression of ACTH with glucocorticoid, and treatment with mineralocorticoid in the salt-losing types) remain the same. In the very rare genetic males with CAH and ambiguous genitalia due to a block in the androgen pathway, options include a trial of testosterone or phallic amputation, gonadectomy, surgical creation of a vaginal vault, and eventual estrogen therapy.

ADRENAL INSUFFICIENCY

Addison's Disease

Children with Addison's disease are treated with glucocorticoid and mineralocorticoid, similar to those with congenital adrenal hyperplasia. However, unlike CAH, the adrenal gland is not hypersensitive and it is not critical that ACTH be completely suppressed; therefore, replacement of hydrocortisone in doses similar to the physiologic production rate, approximately 12 mg/m²/day, is often adequate. Also, although administration in equally divided doses (typically three times a day) is generally satisfactory, there may be some theoretical advantage in providing the largest dose in the morning in order to mimic the normal circadian rhythm.

Laboratory monitoring of these patients can be held to a minimum as long as the clinical course is normal. Features such as unsatisfactory growth velocity, poor or excess weight gain, abnormal blood pressure, frequent episodes of vomiting and diarrhea, or apparent hypoglycemic episodes indicate the need for more aggressive laboratory evaluation (e.g., serum electrolytes and glucose, bone age radiographs). These patients may experience mild delay of growth and maturation because of lack of adrenal androgen. However, treatment is rarely necessary, since testicular production of male hormone is unimpaired.

Other Forms of Adrenal Insufficiency

Other types of hypoadrenalism include those due to ACTH deficiency (usually associated with lack of other anterior pituitary hormones) and hereditary adrenocortical unresponsiveness to ACTH. Both conditions are treated with glucocorticoid as in classic Addison's disease, but mineralocorticoid replacement is not necessary, since adequate production of these hormones is not dependent upon ACTH stimulation. Patients with hereditary adrenal hypoplasia, however, require treatment with both types of steroid.

CUSHING'S SYNDROME

Treatment of Cushing's syndrome depends upon the underlying cause and even then is often controversial and not entirely satisfactory. Adrenal tumors (the most common etiology, other than iatrogenic, up to the age of about 7 years) are surgically removed, and adrenalectomy is also an option for patients with hyperplasia due to increased ACTH (Cushing's disease). However, chronic hormonal replacement will be necessary, and evidence of pituitary tumor (Nelson's syndrome) may develop postoperatively. If pituitary microadenomas are identified as the probable cause of adrenal hyperplasia, transsphenoidal resection in the hands of an experienced neurosurgeon is the treatment of choice. Glucocorticoid is required in the postoperative period, but usually not indefinitely.

Other alternatives for patients with Cushing's disease include high-voltage pituitary irradiation and neurotransmitter inhibitors such as cyproheptadine; however, results are not uniformly satisfactory and undesirable side effects occur. Drugs that interfere with adrenal function, such as ketoconazole, have also been tried successfully but should be reserved for patients in whom more conventional therapy has failed.

PHEOCHROMOCYTOMA

Pheochromocytoma, often arising from the adrenal medulla, is encountered rarely but requires delicate medical and surgical management by experienced specialists. Preoperative administration of the alpha-adrenergic blocker phenoxybenzamine, which has reduced mortality significantly, is indicated for at least 1 week prior to surgery or any invasive diagnostic procedure, to control hypertension. Typical dose ranges from 0.25 to 1.0 mg/kg/day, administered twice daily. Lower doses are employed initially, with stepwise increases until the desired results are achieved. High salt intake during this time helps to restore plasma volume. Acute hypertensive crises can be treated with phentolamine; 1 mg IV or IM is usually satisfactory. Propranolol is a useful adjunct but, because a paradoxical increase in blood pressure can occur, should not be used until after phenoxybenzamine therapy has been initiated.

Patients must be observed closely for acute elevation of blood pressure during and immediately after surgery, and the possibility of significant hypotension thereafter. If surgery is successful, urinary catecholamines and metabolites should subsequently return to normal.

OTHER ADRENAL DISORDERS

Feminizing and masculinizing tumors of the adrenal gland ideally are treated surgically. Postoperatively, patients are monitored with serum estrogens (estradiol) and/or androgens (DHEAS, testosterone).

Surgical intervention is indicated for hyperaldosteronism due to adenoma. Dexamethasone is effective in the hereditary glucocorticoid-suppressible type, and antihypertensives such as spironolactone often suffice in patients with idiopathic hyperplasia. Isolated hypoaldosteronism is treated with fludrocortisone.

Benign premature adrenarche (pubarche) requires no treatment, since bone age usually is only mildly advanced and the remaining secondary sexual characteristics generally occur at the appropriate time.

ENDOCRINE DISORDERS OF THE TESTIS
ROBERT L. ROSENFIELD, M.D.

HYPOANDROGENISM

Indications

Microphallus. Microphallus occurs as part of the spectrum of intersex (with hypospadias) if intrauterine hypoandrogenism is severe, or it occurs as an isolated phenomenon (with a penile urethra) if the androgen deficiency is less severe. It may occur as part of the congenital hypopituitarism syndrome in association with hypoglycemia and hyperbilirubinemia. In older children it must be distinguished from pseudomicrophallus, in which the penile shaft is buried in the suprapubic fat pad in obese subjects.

Androgen therapy is indicated to facilitate hypospadias repair or for psychological reasons. Low-dose testosterone stimulates growth of the penis, provided that the child does not have androgen resistance. The optimum age for treatment is within the first 6 months of life when the minipuberty of the newborn normally stimulates a surge in testosterone secretion and penile growth. However, there is no evidence that the ultimate size of the penis will become normal. A 3-month course of topical testosterone or depot testosterone (25 mg intramuscularly every 3 weeks × 4) will stimulate penile growth without virilizing the child. A second or third course of treatment as the child grows tends to normalize penis size for age. Reassurance as to the adequacy of a small penis for sexual satisfaction of the partner is usually indicated. Extreme microphallus is an indication for sex reversal in early infancy.

Sexual Infantilism. In patients in whom the diagnosis of primary or secondary hypogonadism can be established early (as when gonadotropins are elevated or anorchia or anosmia are present), physiologic androgen replacement therapy can be begun at about 12 years of age. Typically, the bone age is 11 to 12 years and the linear growth rate begins to fall at this time. In such cases therapy can commence with an anabolic dose of depot testosterone, 50 mg/m^2 intramuscularly monthly for 1 year. In the long-term treatment of hypogonadal boys, we advise subsequently advancing virilization with depot testosterone 100 mg intramuscularly monthly for 1 year, followed by 200 mg monthly for 1 year, followed by the adult maintenance dose of 200 mg every 2 weeks. If short stature is a major problem, we advise advancing these doses according to a slower schedule. Once clinical virilization is complete in the late teen-age years, oral androgen analogues may be substituted for testosterone injections. In hypogonadal patients, associated hormone deficiencies, particularly those of thyroid or growth hormone, should be concurrently replaced in order for the full expression of the androgen treatment to be manifest. Whatever underlying disease may be the cause of the hypogonadism should be treated appropriately. Hypogonadal patients can be reassured that they will experience normal sexual development and sexual function in response to androgen therapy, without compromising growth potential. Patients with infertility often have feelings of "incompleteness" about not being able to father children, and these feelings must be recognized and discussed when they surface. In patients with anorchia, testicular prostheses can be placed surgically during the teen-age years.

In constitutional delay of puberty, detection and explanation of the subtle early signs of puberty which may be present, together with agreement to monitor progress, are helpful in allaying anxiety and may obviate treatment. However, in boys who are emotionally upset because of the lack of pubertal development or short stature, we recommend depot testosterone treatment commencing as early as 14 years of age. The aim of such treatment is to provide enough short-term pubertal change to bridge the gap in physical growth and maturity to boost the boy's self-image. A 6-month course of 50 mg/month (if the main problem is short stature) or 100 mg/month (if the main problem is pubertal delay) for 6 months is prescribed. Children with constitutional delay of puberty usually spontaneously enter the normal pubertal process within the subsequent 6 months and go on to progress in their masculinization. However, some patients whose daytime plasma testosterone levels have not reached the adult range will benefit from a repeat 6-month course of treatment, provided that height potential remains acceptable (see Adverse Effects). Systemic illnesses mimicking constitutional delay should be ruled out. In counseling children and parents about the place of androgen treatment for delayed puberty, it should be noted that although no deleterious effects of such treatments are known, the state of knowledge about long-term outcome is meager. Psychotherapy may be needed for unusually severe problems of adjusting to or focusing upon the delayed puberty.

Klinefelter's Syndrome. Approximately half of these patients are mildly hypoandrogenic. Androgen replacement therapy is indicated for these patients. Gynecomastia may be aggravated by virilizing doses of testosterone. When gynecomastia is severe, reduction mammoplasty is the only available treatment. The infertility in Klinefelter's syndrome is irreversible.

Androgens and Anabolic Agents

Topical Androgens. Crystalline testosterone in 1 per cent hydrophilic petrolatum (nonformulary) may be prescribed with thin application twice daily as one to three 3-month courses for microphallus.

Parenteral Androgens. Depot forms of testosterone are the preferable agents to induce full sexual development in sexually infantile males. Intramuscular injection of depot forms of testosterone results in peak blood levels within a few days which decline to baseline levels by approximately 3 weeks. The depot forms of testosterone available for intramuscular use are the cypionate (Depo-Testosterone) and enanthate (Delatestryl) esters in cottonseed and sesame oil, respectively. The former is available in a concentration of 50 mg/ml, and both are available in concentrations of 200 mg/ml in 10-ml containers.

Oral Androgens. Methyltestosterone (17α-methyltestosterone) is short-acting, with a half-life of about 2.5 hours. The usual oral dose for maintaining secondary sexual characteristics in hypoandrogenic patients is 5 to 20 mg bid. This agent is available generically in 10- and 25-mg tablets.

Fluoxymesterone (9α-fluoro-11β-hydroxy-17α-methyltestosterone; Halotestin) has a half-life of about 10 hours. The usual doses for maintenance of secondary sexual characteristics in hypogonadal males is 10 to 20 mg/day. It is available in tablets of 2, 5, and 10 mg.

Anabolic Steroids. Anabolic steroids are synthetic modifications of the testosterone molecule which have been claimed to exhibit partial separation of anabolic from androgenic effects according to bioassays in animals. They are used for the treatment of short stature which is associated with hypogonadism syndromes. The most widely used for this purpose is oxandrolone (17α-methyl-2-oxo-dihydrotestosterone; Anavar). The usual dose for growth stimulation in children is 0.1 mg/kg/day. It is available in 2.5-mg tablets and is given in one to two daily doses. It is likely to be withdrawn soon from the market as government restrictions are placed on the dispensation of anabolic steroids because of concern about their abuse by athletes.

Gonadotropin Therapy. Gonadotropin therapy has no place in the treatment of hypogonadal teen-agers. Human chorionic gonadotropin has a place only as a diagnostic agent. Gonadotropin or pulsatile gonadotropin-releasing hormone therapy is indicated only in hypogonadotropic patients at an age when they desire spermatogenesis for fertility in adult life. The gonadotropin effect on spermatogenesis continues for only as long as the treatment is given.

Adverse Effects

Androgen treatment of children carries the risk of compromising adult height through premature epiphyseal closure. This is a time- and dose-related effect. The risk can be avoided by use of the physiologic treatment regimen outlined above. Androgen therapy is not generally appropriate until a bone age of approximately 11 years has been achieved. Height prediction should be made from an evaluation of height and bone age before treatment and at 6-month intervals during treatment. The parenteral (depot) forms of testosterone have several advantages over orally active androgens. They provide the natural form of testosterone itself. This is the only form of androgen available which is potent enough to bring about full virilization. Furthermore, the 17α-methyl–substituted steroids are unique in their ability to cause intrahepatic cholestasis (causing nausea, often in the absence of jaundice, and usually reversible when the drug is discontinued), hepatic cellular carcinoma, and peliosis hepatis.

Acne and gynecomastia are side effects of all androgens. If a full androgen replacement is begun suddenly in eunuchoid individuals, the frequency of erections may be very disturbing psychologically. Sodium and fluid retention is an inherent effect of androgens and may present problems in patients with a pre-existent tendency to develop edema.

PRECOCIOUS PUBERTY

Indications

True sexual precocity results from premature activation of pituitary gonadotropin secretion by hypothalamic pulsatile gonadotropin-releasing hormone (GnRH) release. About 50 per cent of boys with complete isosexual precocity have a central nervous system disorder. Even in the absence of other symptoms or signs of hypothalamic disturbance, a thorough search for a hypothalamic tumor should be made and, if negative, repeated in 6 months. Pseudoprecocity, virilization without symmetric pubertal testicular enlargement, can be caused by chorionic gonadotropin–producing tumors and a variety of primary testicular disorders, such as Leydig cell tumors, familial Leydig cell hyperplasia ("testotoxicosis"), and the syndrome of familial hypersecretion of LH, as well as adrenal virilizing disorders. Testicular enlargement without virilization, on the other hand, may be a clue to the fragile X syndrome.

Medical treatment is indicated to control the embarrassing frequent erections and secondary sexual maturation for psychosocial reasons. In addition, treatment is indicated in an attempt to minimize the amount of premature epiphyseal maturation, which may compromise adult height and result in short stature if untreated. Treatment is not indicated if the child and family are not disturbed by the pubertal changes and there is not a severe or progressive deleterious effect on predicted adult height.

Agents

No agent is marketed for the indication of treating sexual precocity. However, a variety of agents may be prescribed for this purpose, since no approved treatment exists for these disorders.

The best form of treatment for true sexual precocity appears to be with gonadotropin-releasing hormone agonist, the *repeated* administration of which desensitizes the pituitary to the endogenous pulsatile secretion of GnRH, thereby causing a state of functional gonadotropin deficiency. Leuprolide (Lupron) is marketed for the purpose of treating metastatic prostate cancer, and nafarelin (Synarelin) may well be on the market in 1990. Treatment should commence with an adult dose, that is, approximately 1 mg of Lupron intramuscularly or 800 µg bid of nafarelin as an intranasal spray. Adequate treatment will reduce plasma testosterone to prepubertal levels (below 40 ng/dl) by 1 month, and dosage should be adjusted upward accordingly if this goal is not met. Later the child may be cautiously weaned to a lower maintenance dose with monitoring at 1- to 3-month intervals.

Medroxyprogesterone acetate (Depo-Provera) in intramuscular doses of 50 to 200 mg every 2 to 4 weeks has been used for the treatment of sexual precocity.

Androgen antagonists may be used for the treatment of primary testicular oversecretion of testosterone which cannot otherwise be controlled. In patients with pubertal bone ages, blockade of androgen action may disinhibit gonadotropin release and gonadotropins rise to overcome the blockade; this problem can be circumvented by instituting GnRH agonist therapy. Cyproterone acetate is available in Canada, Mexico, and Europe. It is effective when given orally in a dose of 70 to 150 mg/m²/day. Spironolactone in high doses has an antiandrogenic effect. Two to 4 mg/kg in two divided daily doses are required for this effect. Recently the pure antiandrogen flutamide has become available in the United States for the treatment of metastatic prostate cancer. It is used in a dose of 50 mg PO tid.

Antiandrogen treatment may not be as effective as anticipated because the estrogenic androgen metabolites may play an important role in the pubertal growth spurt of these children. Consequently, testolactone (Teslac), a competitive inhibitor of the enzyme aromatase which converts androgens to estrogens, has been investigated. An apparently effective regimen consists of beginning at a dose of 20 mg/kg/day in four divided doses and increasing to 30 mg/kg and 40 mg/kg at 2-week intervals thereafter. Teslac is available in tablets of 50 mg.

Ketoconazole, an antifungal drug, has recently been reported to be effective in the management of gonadotropin-independent precocious puberty. This imidazole derivative in high doses inhibits testosterone synthesis at multiple sites, particularly at the step between 17-hydroxyprogesterone and androstenedione. Treatment is initiated with 8 to 10.5 mg/kg every 12 hours; treatment every 8 hours may be required. Ketoconazole is supplied in tablets of 200 mg.

The physician must help the family and child cope with the psychological problems that come with premature puberty. The physician can help the family by explaining that even though their child looks older and more mature than other children the same age, the child's behavior is age-appropriate. Such children neither feel nor act more mature. These children tend to be moody and to have psychosocial adjustment problems. Most children with precocity tend to be withdrawn because of shyness and bewilderment. Friendship with children 1 to 2 years older should be encouraged to help shorten the time affected children spend in social limbo. The family and child need to be reminded that in a few years the child will not be unique from the standpoint of physical development. The libido of these children is not increased. In idiopathic cases one should not forget to include reassurance that the child is simply going through a normal process early. Sex education books may be helpful in explaining precocious puberty to parents and children. To parents we recommend *Sex Errors of the Body* by John Money (Johns Hopkins University Press, 1969). For children we recommend *What's Happening to Me?* by Peter Mayle (Lyle Stuart Inc., 1973).

Adverse Effects

The major problem with the use of a GnRH agonist is that undertreatment aggravates the sexual precocity. This is because the agonistic effect of the analogue predominates, and the desensitization effect that one desires does not come into play. This is particularly important because central precocity may not be reversed until doses substantially greater than those required to suppress the pituitary function of adults are reached. Prolonged use of these agents in adults is known to lead to bone demineralization. No side effects are known other than those related to the hypogonadism that is induced.

Medroxyprogesterone has been suspected to cause infertility, prolactinomas, and breast tumors, but there is no clear-cut evidence that these are truly the result of treatment. The lowest effective dose should be used, keeping in mind that it has weak androgenic effects on bone maturation itself and is a weak glucocorticoid.

Both cyproterone acetate and spironolactone in antiandrogenic doses are progestational. Children on spironolactone should be monitored for possible electrolyte disturbances and hepatotoxicity. Mild gynecomastia also may result from spironolactone treatment. Ketoconazole is potentially hepatotoxic.

GYNECOMASTIA

WILLIAM W. CLEVELAND, M.D.

Breast enlargement in the male, gynecomastia, occurs in three groups, with different significance in each. Neonatal breast enlargement in the male infant is common and requires no diagnostic or therapeutic intervention.

Breast enlargement in the prepubertal boy is comparatively uncommon and deserves careful consideration. Investigation of exposure to estrogen or drugs is important. It should be recalled that certain adult vitamin preparations contain sex steroids. Clinical evaluation and hormonal measurements should be undertaken to exclude endogenous production of steroids by a tumor of either the adrenals or the gonads. Virilization due to sexual precocity may result in gynecomastia just as it does in normal adolescent development. Investigation ordinarily does not reveal any abnormality, however, and the condition is considered idiopathic. No medical treatment is available. Although the condition spontaneously disappears, it may persist for many months or a few years. Tumors of the breast in prepubertal boys are very rare and have included carcinoma along with lipomas, neurofibromas, and hemangiomas. Surgical removal may be indicated if the patient manifests sufficient concern or if a tissue diagnosis appears warranted.

Gynecomastia occurs commonly in adolescent boys. In most there is coin-sized enlargement involving one or both breasts. In others obvious enlargement reaching diameters of 6 to 10 cm may be found. Significant gynecomastia occurs more commonly in males who are undergoing rapid pubertal development. The mechanism is not clearly understood but may reflect conversion of androgen to estrogen in a ratio that results in stimulation of mammary tissue. Adolescent breast enlargement may also occur in pathologic situations, including Klinefelter's syndrome; if the gonads are unusually small or abnormalities of mental development are present, karyotyping may be indicated. Measure-

ment of testosterone, estrogen, and prolactin concentrations in serum is helpful in excluding rare aberrations in hormonal function such as adrenal or gonadal tumors.

A particular problem is presented by the obese adolescent boy who has apparent breast enlargement. Differentiating mammary and adipose tissue by palpation may be difficult. In most instances the enlargement represents accumulation of adipose tissue in the area; this assumes importance in considering treatment.

No satisfactory medical treatment for gynecomastia has been established. Treatment with testosterone in an effort to bring about a more favorable androgen:estrogen ratio is not effective and is contraindicated. Clomiphene, a drug that has antiestrogenic action, has been used with equivocal results and its use at this time should be considered experimental. The only satisfactory treatment is surgical removal of mammary tissue. This relatively simple operation, involving a circumareolar incision, gives generally good results with minimal apparent scar. What are the indications for mammoplasty? Although breast enlargement tends to diminish with time, it may take months or years to disappear. Meanwhile many young men experience much embarrassment from the condition, resulting in considerable alteration of lifestyle. Given the simplicity of the operation and its good results, it should be offered to patients with significant gynecomastia who are concerned to the point of being enthusiastic about treatment. Caution should be exercised, however, in management of the obese male with apparent breast enlargement, which is largely due to accumulation of adipose tissue in the area. In this case surgical treatment is more difficult and less apt to yield satisfactory results. Obviously the best approach in this instance would be to treat the obesity in order to achieve a reduction in the enlargement of the area, however difficult this may be.

AMBIGUOUS GENITALIA

SELWYN B. LEVITT, M.D.,
STANLEY J. KOGAN, M.D.,
and EDWARD F. REDA, M.D.

The most cogent caveat in the management of the newborn with ambiguous genitalia is avoidance of the impulse to prematurely announce the sex assignment based upon a first impression of the external genital appearance. The pressure on the clinician to do so is enormous. Parental anxiety, the guilt of having conceived a child with abnormal genitalia, family concerns, and social expectations all contribute to this sense of urgency, and the clinician must exercise special caution. Improper sex assignment without due consideration of all of the factors that are involved in such a monumental decision can be catastrophic psychosocially and lead indirectly to suicide in later years in the involved individual as well as cause major social disruption to the family. Families have actually been pressured into moving from their homes and familiar neighborhoods and resigning from their occupations in order to escape the social stigma and ridicule associated with sexual reassignment when an improper announcement was prematurely made. Factors that contribute to appropriate sex assignment include the following, in order of their importance: (1) The feasibility of genital reconstruction and its complexity in accordance with the proposed sex assignment. (2) Gonadal potential with respect to hormone production and the avoidance of life-long administration of exogenous hormones. (3) Malignant gonadal predisposition, which varies in different syndromes and may be life-threatening. Depending upon the underlying condition, the dysgenetic gonad may have a predilection to developing a gonadoblastoma (or dysgerminoma), a tumor with a low malignant potential, as opposed to the more life-threatening gonadal tumors that develop in phenotypic females with Y chromosomes. The syndromes that pose an increased risk include XY "pure" gonadal dysgenesis and testicular feminization syndrome, for which gonadectomy should be undertaken at the first opportunity; gonadoblastomas generally occur in patients with mixed gonadal dysgenesis and in dysgenetic male pseudohermaphrodites. (4) Fertility, which is the rule in female pseudohermaphrodites whether due to congenital adrenal hyperplasia, exposure in utero to exogenous maternal masculinizing hormones or endogenous androgens elaborated by maternal ovarian arrhenoblastomas or adrenal tumors. Additionally, fertility is possible in rare instances of true hermaphrodites in either a male or a female role. Fertility has also been recorded in occasional patients with the syndrome of hernia uteri inguinalis, a condition due to isolated Müllerian inhibiting factor deficiency. (5) Moreover, when sex assignment is "negotiable," as in some cases of true hermaphroditism in which both a well-formed phallus, a vagina and uterus, and complete lateralization of ovarian and testicular tissue is present, it may be possible and even advantageous to acquiesce to the family's wishes, particularly if they have a strong inclination about the child's sex. (6) The potential for attainment of adequate height in a male sex role needs serious consideration, particularly in the syndrome of mixed gonadal dysgenesis. Short stature, often less than 5 feet, is frequent in this syndrome. One additional factor favoring the assignment of a female sex role in this syndrome is the significantly increased proclivity toward malignant transformation of the retained gonad with development of a gonadoblastoma.

The many and widely divergent factors requiring consideration and the profound implications of inappropriate sex assignment have resulted in a team approach involving a panel of experts, which usually includes a pediatric urologist, geneticist, endocrinologist, radiologist, and in some centers, a clergyman, all of whom are important in the final decision for optimum sex assignment.

Sex assignment, for obvious reasons, is an urgent matter, and due consideration must be given to prompt assessment of the aforementioned factors as well as the tests that form the basis for sex assignment. Consider-

able diplomacy and sensitivity are required in dealing with the anxious parents while awaiting the results of the laboratory determinations, which include a buccal smear, karyotype, urogenital sinogram, pelvic ultrasonogram, serum electrolytes, 17-hydroxyprogesterone, dehydroepiandrosterone (DHA), and renin levels in suspected cases of congenital adrenal hyperplasia. It is important during this waiting period, before sex assignment can be made with confidence, to reassure the family of the intrinsic health of the baby. Moreover, the explanation for being unable to assign a sex role should be blamed on the baby's immature sexual development at the time rather than on the concept of a malformation of the genitalia which conjures up the image of a "freak." Furthermore, the family should be informed that once the sexual identity is confirmed with certainty, the genital appearance and function with respect to sexual performance will be normal, albeit with some type of surgical intervention.

Specific medical treatment in neonates with the various forms of congenital adrenogenital syndrome should be initiated as soon as the diagnosis is clear. Hydrocortisone and, in salt-losing states due to 21-hydroxylase and especially 3 beta-ol-dehydrogenase deficiency, mineralocorticoids as well must be administered within the first 7 to 10 days of life to prevent vascular collapse.

Definitive surgical treatment of the genital ambiguity in children with congenital adrenal hyperplasia is best deferred until the child is endocrinologically stable. A stable state is generally achieved between 6 weeks and 3 months. Surgical reconstruction of the genitalia should be directed as early as possible toward removing the prominent hypertrophied phallic shaft, since this is the feature most challenging to a female gender role. Viewing a phallic structure in a baby assigned to a female gender role at every diaper change certainly must add to the anxiety, guilt, and embarrassment of the parents and produce further doubts as to the child's real sex. In cases of clitoral enlargement other than that secondary to the adrenogenital syndrome, the clitoroplasty is best done even earlier, preferably prior to discharge from the hospital, provided that the neonate is full term and otherwise healthy. Despite clinical studies that indicate that orgasm is possible without a clitoris, the operation of total clitorodectomy has generally been abandoned. Most pediatric urologists favor preserving the clitoris either by clitoral recession without resection of the corporal bodies or by excision of the corporal tissue, preserving the dorsal neurovascular bundle and glans in order to maintain clitoral sensation. Clitoral recession without resection of the corporal bodies is applicable only to the mildly hypertrophied case. Even advocates of this procedure admit that on long-term observation a number of girls subsequently develop an unsightly enlarged appearance to the clitoris, particularly at puberty, and, in addition, many complain of painful erections. A number of different surgical techniques have been developed which preserve the clitoris and retain its sensation. They all involve reducing the size of the glans clitoris, excising the corporal tissue, and preserving the neurovascular supply. The shaft skin is mobilized and used to bury the reduced clitoral shaft as well as to form labia minora.

We perform flap vaginoplasty simultaneously with the clitoroplasty in most instances of low confluence of the vagina with the urogenital sinus, viz., when the vagina enters the urethra distal to the external urinary sphincter. Cystoscopic examination at the time of the surgery, as well as a good urogenital sinogram, delineates the exact site of junction of the vagina and the urogenital sinus. Some surgeons prefer to defer the vaginoplasty until puberty because some of these patients develop vaginal stenosis when vaginoplasty is done in infancy, necessitating periodic vaginal dilatations. However, we believe that a minor revision of the introitus at puberty is a less formidable procedure and poses less of a psychological problem for the teen-ager than the anxiety of knowing that she lacks an entry to the vagina and requires a primary vaginal reconstruction. In the relatively rare instance of high convergence of the vagina with the urogenital sinus, at or proximal to the external urethral sphincter, a pull-through vaginoplasty is required. This is a difficult surgical endeavor and should be deferred until the baby is 18 months to 2 years old.

Laparoscopy for more complete identification of the internal duct and gonadal structures in cases other than the adrenogenital syndrome can be carried out simultaneously with clitoroplasty and vaginoplasty. Laparotomy and excision of discordant gonadal and ductal tissue are generally best deferred for a few months. However, if the baby is stable and the genital reconstruction can be accomplished expeditiously, the laparotomy could be done simultaneously.

Finally, the sex-assigned girl who lacks a vagina must have one constructed. A nonoperative technique has been described in which a vagina is created by pressing tube dilators against the perineum to produce invagination, which is gradually enlarged to the appropriate size. Generally this requires that there be at least a 1- to 2-cm perineal sinus present. In addition, it calls for tremendous self-control on the part of the teen-ager. Most surgeons prefer to construct the vagina in these girls using split-thickness grafts sutured around a form. This is fashioned when the girl reaches maturity and expresses the desire for sexual activity. Small and large bowel segments are also quite satisfactory for constructing a vagina, although they tend to produce a fair amount of vaginal mucous discharge. This technique for vaginal construction is generally reserved for those cases of genital ambiguity associated with cloacal anomalies.

Reconstruction of the genitalia in sex-assigned males is usually deferred until 6 months of age. Orchidopexy, gonadal biopsy, excision of discordant internal duct structures and gonadal tissue, and hysterectomy and vaginectomy are performed simultaneously. Care must be taken to avoid injuring the posterior urethra. Hypospadias repair and scrotal recession if required may be done simultaneously, although in most instances the hypospadias is of the more severe variety with significant chordee and is best done at a separate time, generally between 12 and 15 months of age. This may be accomplished as a single-stage procedure or in two stages, depending upon the specific circumstances. Most pediatric urologists prefer single-stage total reconstruction whenever possible; however, considerable judgment is necessary in assessing individual cases.

10

Metabolic Disorders

INFANTS BORN TO DIABETIC MOTHERS

JOHN P. CLOHERTY, M.D.

The recent reduction in perinatal mortality and morbidity in infants of diabetic mothers (IDMs) has been due to improvements in medical and obstetric care of mothers and advances in the care of the newborn. One of the major causes of this improvement has been the prolongation of pregnancy, and the ability to assess pulmonary maturity in the fetus has reduced the incidence of respiratory distress syndrome (RDS) in IDMs. Infants of mothers with severe renal and vascular disease are often delivered because of maternal problems (hypertension, renal failure) or fetal distress. These infants are more likely to have complications such as asphyxia, respiratory distress syndrome, jaundice, and poor feeding. Before the delivery of the IDM there should be clear communication between specialists in medicine, obstetrics, and pediatrics so that problems can be anticipated.

CLASSIFICATION

Mothers with diabetes are classified according to White's classification (Table 1). There is a relationship between perinatal outcome and White's class. The risk of complications is minimal in gestational diabetes. Macrosomia and neonatal hypoglycemia are sometimes seen. The most difficult maternal, fetal, and neonatal problems occur in women with renal, cardiac, or retinal disease. Class F disease (renal) has an adverse affect on fetal outcome. It is associated with the necessity for early delivery. Class H (cardiac disease) is associated with maternal death. Retinopathy may progress during pregnancy.

MATERNAL-FETAL PROBLEMS

Fertility

Diabetic women appear to have normal fertility.

TABLE 1. White's Classification of Maternal Diabetes (Revised*)

Gestational Diabetes (GD)	Diabetes not known to be present before pregnancy
	Abnormal glucose tolerance test in pregnancy
GD diet	Euglycemia maintained by diet alone
GD insulin	Diet alone insufficient—insulin required
Class A	Chemical diabetes: glucose intolerance prior to pregnancy; treated by diet alone; rarely seen
	Prediabetes: history of large babies more than 4 kg or unexplained stillbirths after 28 weeks
Class B	Insulin-dependent: onset after 20 years of age; duration less than 10 years
Class C	C_1: Onset between 10 and 19 years of age
Class D	C_2: Duration 10 to 19 years
	D_1: Onset before 10 years of age
	D_2: Duration 20 years or more
	D_3: Calcification of vessels of the leg (macrovascular disease)
	D_4: Benign retinopathy (microvascular disease)
	D_5: Hypertension (not preeclampsia)
Class F	Nephropathy with over 500 mg/day of proteinuria
Class R	Proliferative retinopathy or vitreous hemorrhage
Class RF	Criteria for both classes R and F coexist
Class G	Many reproductive failures
Class H	Clinical evidence of arteriosclerotic heart disease
*Class T	Prior renal transplantation

All classes below A require insulin. Classes R, F, RF, H, and T have no criteria for age of onset or duration of disease but usually occur in long-term diabetes.

Abortions

There is no increase in the spontaneous abortion rate in early pregnancy in *well-controlled* diabetic pregnancies as compared with nondiabetic pregnancies. The spontaneous abortion rate in nondiabetic pregnancy is 16 per cent. Women with poor diabetic control in pregnancy had a significantly increased incidence of spontaneous abortion.

Problems During Pregnancy and Delivery

In the first half of pregnancy hypoglycemia and ketonuria are common. The nausea and vomiting seen in any pregnancy may make control difficult. Moderate hypoglycemia not associated with hypotension may not be harmful to the fetus.

In the second trimester, the *insulin requirement* increases. This increased requirement is sometimes associated with *ketoacidosis*, which may result in high fetal mortality.

In the third trimester, a major problem is *sudden, unexpected fetal death*. Such deaths are sometimes associated with ketoacidosis, pre-eclampsia, or maternal vascular disease of the decidua and myometrium, but many are unexplained. The incidence of this problem has decreased during the past 10 years with the use of tests of fetal well-being, but it still occurs occasionally.

In the third trimester, class F mothers may have anemia, hypertension, and decreased renal function. Women with class H disease have a great risk of myocardial failure with infarction. Women with class R disease have a risk of neovascularization, vitreous hemorrhage, or retinal detachment; their infants are usually delivered by cesarean section.

Fetal macrosomia and enlargement of the cord and placenta may be seen in gestational diabetics and in classes A, B, C, and some D diabetic pregnancies. Macrosomia increases the potential for difficult delivery, obstetric trauma, or primary cesarean section.

In diabetic women with vascular disease (especially class F), there is an increased risk of in utero growth retardation (20 per cent). This growth retardation is associated with a small infarcted placenta, decreased uteroplacental perfusion, decreased urinary estriols, and increased incidence of in utero fetal death, fetal distress, neonatal complications, and poor outcome. Hypertension in pregnancy is the largest cause of premature delivery and thus of respiratory distress syndrome in our patient population.

Many diabetic pregnancies are associated with *polyhydramnios*. Although this is usually not a sign of significant fetal anomaly (as it is in the nondiabetic pregnancy), it may be associated with premature rupture of membranes, early cord prolapse, or abruptio placentae. Women with the best metabolic control have the least polyhydraminos.

PREGNANCY MANAGEMENT

Diabetic women should be educated about the need to gain metabolic control of their diabetes before conception. This control may decrease the incidence of major congenital anomalies. Good control throughout the pregnancy improves the perinatal outcome. All pregnant patients should have a screening test for gestational diabetes (GD). If they have GD or class A diabetes, they should be managed by diet to keep their fasting plasma glucose below 105 and their postprandial plasma glucose below 120 mg/dl. If these goals are not reached by dietary therapy, then insulin should be used. Oral agents should not be used, since they cross the placenta and may be associated with severe neonatal hypoglycemia if used near the time of birth. Gestational diabetics who can maintain fasting plasma glucose under 105 mg/dl and 2-hour postprandial blood sugars under 120 mg/ml on a diabetic diet should be followed with weekly blood sugars because 15 per cent of them eventually require insulin in pregnancy. If they are maintained on diet alone, they do not appear to be at risk for stillbirth. If they develop an insulin requirement, required insulin in the past, or have pre-eclampsia or a history of stillbirth, they should be treated as any other insulin-requiring diabetic. Diabetics who require insulin should maintain fasting plasma glucose levels as in gestational diabetes. Hemoglobin A_1 (HbA_1) is measured to assess control over a longer period of time.

At the first prenatal visit a thorough medical history and physical examination are done. The estimated date of conception is determined by history of last menstrual period and ultrasonography. Besides the usual prenatal tests, the following studies are done: glycosylated hemoglobin (Hb_{A1}), thyroid function studies, a 24-hour urine for total protein and creatinine clearance, and an ophthalmologic evaluation. The mother should begin a comprehensive diabetes education program stressing the importance of good glycemic control to reduce perinatal morbidity and mortality. Mothers in poor metabolic control at this visit or at any time should be admitted for regulation.

At the next visit the mother's situation is reviewed and her diabetic control is assessed. She is informed about the risks of congenital malformations in diabetic women in relationship to her glycemic control as measured by her level of glycosylated hemoglobin. A repeat ultrasound examination is done at 18 weeks if there is significant risk of fetal anomaly. This examination, when performed by experienced personnel, diagnoses most (95 per cent) major anomalies of the central nervous system, heart, skeleton, gastrointestinal tract, and urinary tract.

In the second trimester, anticipate an increasing insulin requirement to avoid ketoacidosis, which is associated with fetal death. Measure maternal serum alpha-fetoprotein at 16 to 18 weeks. Diabetic pregnancies are associated with a lower maternal serum alpha-fetoprotein than nondiabetic pregnancies. Do fetal ultrasonography at 18 weeks to rule out anomalies and to confirm the duration of the pregnancy. Monitor hematocrit, renal function, blood pressure, diabetic control, and fetal growth.

In the third trimester there is usually a rise in insulin requirement until 34 to 36 weeks. The problems in this trimester are fetal demise, premature delivery, and macrosomia. The mother must be monitored for glycemic control, polyhydramnios, pre-eclampsia, premature labor, and decreasing renal function. The fetus must be monitored for well-being, size, and pulmonary maturity. Repeat ultrasonography at 26 to 28 weeks, and start weekly nonstress tests (NSTs) or oxytocin challenge test (OCT). Mothers with problems may need to start this monitoring at 26 weeks. Before 30 weeks the OCT is probably more reliable than the NST. In the Joslin Pregnancy Clinic, with careful maternal care and fetal monitoring, there were only two unexplained, unanticipated fetal deaths after a normal nonstress test or oxytocin challenge test since 1976 (about 1000 patients). This is still a significant problem, and results such as these can be obtained only with much meticulous effort.

Amniocentesis is performed at 38 weeks for measurement of the lecithin-sphingomyelin (L/S) ratio and saturated phosphatidylcholine (SPC), unless there are fetal or maternal reasons to deliver earlier. In our laboratory, in nondiabetic pregnancies with an L/S ratio greater than 2:1, there is a 5 per cent incidence of hyaline membrane disease (HMD); with an SPC greater than 500 μg/dl, there is a 1 per cent incidence. The levels of L/S and SPC considered "mature" in an IDM should depend on the experience of the local laboratory. In our hospital, 10 per cent of IDMs with L/S between 2.0 and 3.5:1.0 have HMD, and 1 per cent of IDMs with L/S greater than 3.5:1.0 have HMD. An SPC of 500 μg/dl is usually considered mature in non-IDMs; in our hospital, however, 11 per cent of IDMs with SPC between 501 and 1000 had HMD, and 1 per cent of IDMs with SPC over 1000 had HMD. In the 244 diabetic pregnancies from which these data are taken, none had HMD if both the SPC was greater than 1000 μg/dl and the L/S was over 3.5:1.0. We thus consider a fetus of a diabetic mother to have mature indices when the L/S is over 3.5 and the SPC is over 1000.

Diabetic pregnancies requiring insulin should continue to 38 to 39 weeks as long as (1) there are no maternal contraindications and (2) there is evidence of fetal growth and well-being. This practice results in more vaginal deliveries, more mature babies, and a lower perinatal mortality and morbidity, because the increased incidence of HMD in IDMs is not seen at term but rather in the premature. The time of delivery is decided in each case by an assessment of maternal health and of the relative fetal and neonatal risks as judged by gestational age, pulmonary maturity, and tests of fetal growth and well-being. Mothers with vascular complications (e.g., White's class F) who have proteinuria of more than 400 mg/day in the first half of pregnancy without a urinary tract infection and who have elevated blood pressure and a creatinine clearance of less than 90 ml/min often require hospitalization at 26 weeks' gestation for bed rest and antihypertensive medication. They are the group at greatest risk for uncontrollable hypertension and decreasing renal function and are most likely to have fetuses with intrauterine growth retardation and fetal distress, leading to early delivery. The perinatal survival (after 24 weeks' gestation) in this group is about 85 to 90 per cent. More recent data (after 24 weeks' gestation) from the Joslin Clinic show no increased mortality but more prematurity and low birth weight. There are still fetal losses in the second trimester. These mothers have an increased risk of intrapartum fetal distress, cesarean section, perinatal asphyxia, and HMD. Insulin-requiring diabetics are delivered at 38 to 39 weeks' gestation after pulmonary maturity is documented.

Emergency delivery may be necessary even in the face of pulmonary immaturity because of maternal problems such as hypertension, decreasing renal function, and pre-eclampsia or because of poor fetal growth or evidence of fetal distress. Because of the difficulty in controlling the maternal diabetes while waiting for an effect, we usually do not use steroids to accelerate fetal pulmonary maturity unless the L/S ratio is less than 2:1 and the SPC is less than 500 μg/dl and the patient is at very high risk to deliver in the following 7 days. This policy is usually followed at Boston Hospital for Women, but other centers may not follow it. The route of delivery selected is based on the usual obstetric indications. If the infant appears large based on clinical and ultrasonographic examination (greater than 4000 gm), cesarean section is usually indicated because of the risk of shoulder dystocia. Prolongation of gestation beyond 38 weeks does not increase the incidence of dystocia and birth trauma. In labor the maternal blood glucose is kept around 120 mg/dl, and fetal well-being is assessed by electronic monitoring and measurement of fetal scalp pH. About 25 per cent of diabetic women undergo primary cesarean section because of fetal distress in labor. Because of failure of induction, dystocia, or fetal distress in labor in our insulin-requiring diabetics, 47 per cent undergo primary cesarean section. Twenty-five per cent have repeat cesarean section and 28 per cent vaginal delivery.

EVALUATION OF THE INFANT

The evaluation of the infant in the delivery room begins prior to the actual delivery. Immediately before opening the amniotic sac at the time of cesarean section, the obstetrician can obtain a sterile sample of amniotic fluid for culture, Gram's stain, L/S ratio, shake test, or SPC when indicated.

Once the baby has been delivered, a careful assessment made on the basis of the Apgar score should indicate the need for any resuscitative efforts. The infant should be dried well and placed under a heat source, with careful attention paid to clearing the airway of mucus. The stomach is not suctioned at this point, because of the risk of reflex bradycardia and apnea with pharyngeal stimulation. In the delivery room, a screening physical examination for major congenital anomalies should be performed, and the placenta should also be examined. A specimen of cord blood should be obtained for glucose determination in anticipation of the reactive hypoglycemia associated with hyperglycemia at delivery. Cord pH should also be measured.

TABLE 2. Lecithin-Sphingomyelin Ratio, Saturated Phosphatidylcholine, and Respiratory Distress Syndrome in IDMs at the Boston Hospital for Women 1977–1980

SPC μg/dl	<2.0:1.0	2.0–3.4:1.0	≥3.5:1.0	Mild, moderate, or severe RDS/total
Not done	0/1	0/12	0/13	0/26 (0%)
≤500	6/6	1/9	1/2	8/17 (47%)
501–1000	0/2	3/20	1/15	4/37 (11%)
>1000	0/0	2/22	0/142	2/164 (1.2%)
Total (RDS)	6/9 (67%)	6/63 (10%)	2/172 (1.2%)	14/244 (5.7%)

Key: SPC = saturated phosphatidylcholine; L/S = lecithin/sphingomyelin; RDS = respiratory distress syndrome.

TABLE 3. Lecithin:Sphingomyelin (L:S) Ratio and Saturated Phosphatidylcholine (SPC) and RDS in Infants of Mothers with Insulin-Requiring Diabetes Mellitus Antedating Pregnancy at the Brigham & Women's Hospital, Jan. 1, 1983 to June 30, 1988

| | | Insulin Dependent Diabetics L/S to Delivery Interval ≤ 72 Hours | | | |
L/S		SPC	No RDS	RDS	%
≥3.5		≥1000	255	0	0
—		≥1000	288	1	0.3
≥3.5		—	285	1	0.3
2.0–3.4	and	≥1000	31	1	3.1
2.0–3.4	and	500–999	25	4	13.8
—		500–999	52	7	11.9
2.0–3.4		—	57	5	8.1

Samples were all obtained within 72 hours of delivery.
From Green, M.F., Torday, J., Wilson, M., and Richardson, D.: Abstract presented at the Meeting of the Society of Perinatal Obstetricians, New Orleans, LA, February, 1989.

In the nursery, the initial care involves the simultaneous provision of what is needed to support the baby and continuous evaluation of the infant. This includes providing warmth, suction, and oxygen as needed, while checking vital signs (heart rate, temperature, respiratory rate, perfusion, color, and blood pressure). The presence of cyanosis should make one consider cardiac disease, respiratory distress syndrome (RDS), transient tachypnea of the newborn (TTN), or polycythemia. A careful examination should be done for the presence of anomalies because of the 6 to 9 per cent incidence of major congenital anomalies in IDMs. Special attention should be paid to the brain, heart, kidneys, and skeletal system. Reports indicate that IDMs have a 35 per cent risk of significant hypoglycemia, a 22 per cent risk of hypocalcemia, a 19 per cent risk of hyperbilirubinemia, and a 34 per cent risk of polycythemia; therefore, the following studies are performed:

1. *Blood glucose* levels are checked at 1, 2, 3, 6, 12, 24, 36, and 48 hours.
2. *Hematocrit* levels are checked at 1 hour and 24 hours.
3. *Calcium* levels are checked if the baby appears jittery or is sick for any reason.
4. *Bilirubin* levels are checked if the baby appears jaundiced.

The baby is fed oral or intravenous glucose by 1 hour of age (see Hypoglycemia below). Every effort is made to involve the parents in the care of the baby as soon as possible.

SPECIFIC PROBLEMS FREQUENTLY OBSERVED IN IDMs
Respiratory Distress

In studies from the 1960s, IDMs had an approximately sixfold increased risk of HMD compared to infants of nondiabetic mothers of the same gestational age, independent of the method of delivery. With changes in the management of pregnant diabetics resulting in longer gestations and more vaginal deliveries, the incidence of RDS in IDMs has fallen from 28 per cent in 1950–1960 to 8 per cent in 1975–1976 to 5.7 per cent in 1983–1984. Since the major difference in the incidence of RDS between diabetics and nondiabetics is in infants before 37 weeks of gestation, the longer

gestations allowed by better in utero surveillance and the more accurate prediction of pulmonary maturity have had a marked influence on the reduction of RDS in the IDM. Most of the deaths are in infants under 37 weeks' gestation who were delivered by cesarean section because of fetal distress or maternal indications. Delayed lung maturation in IDMs occurs because hyperinsulinemia may block cortisol induction of lung maturation. Other causes of respiratory distress that may be present in IDM are cardiac or pulmonary anomalies (4 per cent), hypertrophic cardiomyopathy (1 per cent), transient tachypnea of the newborn, and polycythemia. Pneumonia, pneumothorax, meconium aspiration and diaphragmatic hernia should be considered in the differential diagnosis. The following studies should be done in infants with respiratory distress: *Gastric aspirate* should be obtained during the first hour of life, after the baby has been stabilized. The gastric aspirate is used for *Gram's stain* for polymorphonuclear leukocytes and bacteria and *gastric aspirate shake test* to assess the amount of pulmonary surfactant in the newborn's lungs. *Chest roentgenogram, blood gases, electrocardiogram,* and blood pressure measurements should be done. If hypertrophic cardiomyopathy or a cardiac anomaly is thought to be present, an *echocardiogram* should be done. *Cultures* should be taken from gastric aspirate, urine, and blood. Spinal fluid examination and culture should be included if the infant's condition allows. The differential diagnosis and management of respiratory disorders are discussed elsewhere in this book.

Hypoglycemia

Hypoglycemia is defined as a blood glucose level less than 30 mg/dl in any infant, regardless of gestational age and whether associated with symptoms or not.

Incidence. The incidence of hypoglycemia in IDMs is 30 to 40 per cent. The onset is frequently within 1 to 2 hours of birth and is most common in macrosomic infants.

Pathogenesis. The pathogenesis of the neonatal hypoglycemia of the IDM is explained by the maternal hyperglycemia–fetal hyperinsulinism hypothesis of Pederson. The correlation between fetal macrosomia, elevated HbA_1 in maternal and cord blood and neonatal hypoglycemia, and also between elevated cord blood c-peptide or immunoreactive insulin levels and hypoglycemia, suggests that control of maternal blood sugar in the last trimester may decrease the incidence of neonatal hypoglycemia in IDMs. Some studies have shown less neonatal hypoglycemia if the maternal blood sugar is in the normal range at delivery. Mothers should not receive large doses of glucose before or at delivery because this may stimulate an insulin response in the hyperinsulinemic offspring. We attempt to keep the maternal blood sugar at delivery around 120 mg/dl. Hypoglycemia in small-for-gestational-age infants born to mothers with vascular disease may be due to inadequate glycogen stores; it may present later (e.g., 12 to 24 hours of age). Other factors that may cause hypoglycemia in IDMs are decreased catecholamine and glycogen secretion as well as inadequate substrate mobilization (diminished hepatic glucose production and decreased oxygenation of fatty acids).

Symptoms. If IDMs have symptoms from hypoglycemia, they usually are quiet and lethargic rather than jittery. Other symptoms such as apnea, tachypnea, respiratory distress, hypotonia, shock, cyanosis, and seizures may occur. If symptoms are present, the infant is probably at greater risk for sequelae than if asymptomatic. The significance of hypoglycemia without symptoms is unclear, but conservative management to maintain the blood sugar in the normal range appears to be indicated.

Diagnosis. Blood glucose is measured at birth and at 1, 2, 3, 6, 12, 24, 36, and 48 hours. It is measured more often if the infant is symptomatic, if the infant has had low blood glucose, and to check the response to therapy.

Treatment

ASYMPTOMATIC INFANTS WITH NORMAL BLOOD GLUCOSE. In our nursery, we begin to feed "well" IDMs by bottle or gavage with dextrose 10 per cent (5 ml/kg body weight) at or before 1 hour of age. Infants less than 2 kg should not be given oral feedings; they should have parenteral dextrose starting in the first hour of life. Larger infants can be fed hourly for three or four feedings until the blood sugars are stable. The feedings can then be given every 2 hours and later every 3 hours; as the interval between feedings increases, the volume is increased.

If the infant feeds successfully by 12 hours of age and the blood sugar is normal, he or she should be given 20 cal/30 ml formula, with extra dextrose added as needed. This method of rapid oral feeding prevents or corrects the hypoglycemia in most "well" IDMs.

If by 2 hours of age the blood glucose is low (under 30 mg/dl) in spite of feeding or if feedings are not tolerated, as indicated by large volumes retained in the stomach, parenteral treatment is indicated to raise the blood glucose.

SYMPTOMATIC INFANTS. These include infants with a low blood glucose after an enteral feed, sick infants, and infants less than 2 kg in weight. The basic element in treatment is *intravenous glucose administration*. This must be done through a reliable route.

Administration of intravenous glucose is usually by peripheral veins. These sites are free of the infectious and thrombotic complications of central catheters. Peripheral lines may be difficult to place in obese IDMs, and sudden interruption of the infusion may cause a reactive hypoglycemia in these hyperinsulinemic infants. Use of an indwelling peripheral venous catheter eliminates the latter problem. In emergency situations with symptomatic babies, we have utilized umbilical venous catheters placed in the inferior vena cava until a stable peripheral line is placed.

Specific treatment is determined by the baby's condition. If the infant is in distress (e.g., seizure or respiratory compromise), 0.5 to 1.0 gm glucose/kg body weight is given by an IV push of 2 to 4 ml/kg of 25 per cent dextrose in water (D/W) at a rate of 1 ml/min. For example, a 4-kg infant would receive 8 to 16 ml of 25 per cent D/W over 8 to 16 minutes. This is followed by a continuous infusion of dextrose at a rate of 4 to 8 mg/kg/min of glucose.

The concentration of dextrose in the intravenous fluid depends on the total daily fluid requirement. For example, on day 1 the usual fluid intake is 65 ml/kg, or 0.045 ml/kg/min. Therefore, 10 per cent D/W would provide 4.5 mg/kg/min of glucose, and 15 per cent D/W would provide 6.75 mg/kg/minute. In other words, 10 per cent D/W at a standard intravenous fluid maintenance rate usually supplies sufficient glucose to raise the blood glucose level above 30 mg/dl. The concentration of dextrose and the infusion rates, however, are increased as necessary to maintain the blood glucose in the normal range.

Another method is to give 200 mg/kg of glucose (2 ml/kg of 10 per cent dextrose) over 2 to 3 minutes. This is followed by a maintenance drip of 6 to 8 mg/kg/min of glucose (10 per cent dextrose at 80 to 120 ml/kg/day).

If the infant does not have symptoms but has a blood glucose level in the hypoglycemic range, an initial push of concentrated sugar should not be given. (This is to avoid a hyperinsulinemic response.) Rather, an initial infusion of 5 to 10 ml of 10 per cent D/W at 1 ml/min is followed by the continuous infusion of glucose at 4 to 8 mg/kg/min. Blood glucose levels must be carefully monitored at frequent intervals after beginning intravenous glucose infusions, to be certain of adequate treatment of the hypoglycemia as well as to avoid hyperglycemia and the risk of osmotic diuresis and dehydration.

Parenteral sugar should never be abruptly discontinued because of the risk of a reactive hypoglycemia. As oral feeding progresses, the rate of the infusion can be decreased gradually, and the concentration of glucose infused can be reduced by using 5 per cent D/W. It is particularly important to measure blood glucose levels during this process of tapering the intravenous infusion.

Since the hypoglycemia of most IDMs responds to the above treatment, unresponsiveness or persistence (over 48 hours) should cause a search for the other problems (e.g., infection, islet cell tumor). Hydrocortisone (5 mg/kg/day IM in two divided doses) has occasionally been helpful. In our experience, other drugs (epinephrine, diazoxide, or growth hormone) have not been necessary in the treatment of the hypoglycemia of IDMs.

In a hypoglycemic infant, if difficulty is experienced in achieving vascular access, we have administered crystalline glycogen IM or SQ (300 µg/kg to a maximum dose of 1.0 mg). This causes a rapid rise in blood glucose in large IDMs who have good glycogen stores, although it is not reliable in the smaller infants of maternal classes D, E, F, and others. This rise in blood glucose may last 2 to 3 hours and is useful until parenteral glucose can be administered.

Hypocalcemia

Hypocalcemia (calcium less than 7 mg/dl) is found in 22 per cent of IDMs. It is not related to hypoglycemia. Hypocalcemia may be caused by a delay in the usual postnatal rise of parathyroid hormone (PTH). Other factors in IDMs may be vitamin D antagonism at the intestine from elevated cortisol and hyperphosphatemia from tissue catabolism. There is no evidence of elevated serum calcitonin concentration in these infants in the absence of prematurity or asphyxia. Other causes of hypocalcemia such as asphyxia and prematurity may be seen in IDMs. The nadir in calcium levels occurs between 24 and 72 hours, and 30 to 50 per cent of IDMs become hypocalcemic as defined by a total serum calcium under 7 mg/dl. Hypocalcemia in "well" IDMs usually resolves without treatment. We do not routinely measure serum calcium in "well" asymptomatic IDMs. Infants who are sick for any reason such as prematurity, asphyxia, infection, or respiratory distress, or IDMs with symptoms of lethargy, jitteriness, or seizures should have serum calcium measured. If the infant has symptoms that coexist with a low calcium level, has an illness that will delay onset of calcium regulation, or is unable to feed, treatment with calcium may be necessary. Hypomagnesemia should be considered as a cause of hypocalcemia in IDMs, since the hypocalcemia may not respond until the hypomagnesemia is treated.

Polycythemia

Polycythemia is common in IDMs. In infants who are small for gestational age, polycythemia may be related to placental insufficiency, causing hypoxia and increased erythropoietin. In IDMs it may also be due to reduced oxygen delivery secondary to elevated glycosylated hemoglobin in both maternal and fetal serum. If there was fetal distress, there may be a shift of blood from the placenta to the fetus.

Jaundice

Hyperbilirubinemia (bilirubin greater than 15) is seen with increased frequency in IDMs. Bilirubin levels over 16 were seen in 19 per cent of IDMs at Boston Hospital for Women. Bilirubin production is increased in IDMs as compared to infants of nondiabetic mothers. Insulin causes increased erythropoietin. When measurement of carboxyhemoglobin production is used as an indicator of increased heme turnover, IDMs are found to have increased production compared to controls. There may be decreased red blood cell life span because of fewer deformable red blood cell membranes, possibly related to glycosylation of the red blood cell membrane. This mild hemolysis is compensated for but may result in increased bilirubin production. Other factors that may account for the increased jaundice are prematurity, impairment of the hepatic conjugation of bilirubin, and an increased enterohepatic circulation of bilirubin. Infants born to well-controlled diabetic mothers have fewer problems with hyperbilirubinemia. The increasing gestational age of IDMs at delivery has contributed to the decreased incidence of hyperbilirubinemia. Hyperbilirubinemia in IDMs is diagnosed and treated as in any other infant.

Congenital Anomalies

Congenital anomalies are found more frequently in IDMs than in infants of nondiabetic mothers.

Incidence. In a series of 150 IDMs in 1976 and 1977 from the Boston Hospital for Women, 9 per cent had major anomalies, and anomalies accounted for 50 per cent of the perinatal mortality. As mortality from other causes such as prematurity, stillbirth, asphyxia, and RDS falls, malformations become the major cause of perinatal mortality in the IDMs. Infants of diabetic fathers showed the same incidence of anomalies as the normal population; consequently, the maternal environment may be the important factor. Most studies show a 6 to 9 per cent incidence of major anomalies in IDMs. This is three- to fivefold greater than the rate of major congenital malformations in the general population. The usual major anomaly rate for the general population is 2 per cent. Anomalies seen in IDMs are central nervous system (anencephaly, meningocele syndrome, holoprosencephaly), cardiac, vertebral, skeletal, and renal, as well as situs inversus and the caudal regression syndrome (sacral agenesis). The central nervous system and cardiac anomalies make up two thirds of the malformations seen in IDMs. Although there is a general increase in the anomaly rate in IDMs, no anomaly is specific for IDMs, although half of all cases of caudal regression syndrome are seen in IDMs.

Pathophysiology. In a study of 116 IDMs at Boston Hospital for Women in 1981, there was a positive correlation between poor control of diabetes in early pregnancy (as measured by maternal HbA_{1c} levels) and major congenital anomalies in offspring of these pregnancies. This finding suggests that good metabolic control before conception and in the first 3 months of pregnancy may decrease the incidence of major congenital anomalies. There have been several other studies correlating good metabolic control of diabetes, as measured by maternal glycohemoglobin values in early pregnancy, with decreased incidence of anomalies in offspring. A recent multicenter study of IDMs compared outcomes in 347 diabetics who were full participants in a rigid control program from early pregnancy, 279 diabetics coming for care in late pregnancy, and 389 nondiabetic pregnancies. Major malformation rates were 4.9 per cent in the full participants, 9.0 per cent in the late entrants, and 2.1 per cent in the controls. There were no significant differences in the home glucose results from weeks 5 to 12 in the mothers of the malformed and normal infants. Nor were there any significant differences in levels of glycosylated hemoglobin or frequency of hypoglycemic episodes in the mothers of the malformed and normal infants. Of note, diabetic women coming for early care had fewer infants with malformations than those coming late for care. This study could not show a correlation between hyperglycemia, elevated glycosylated hemoglobin levels, and malformations in women who prospectively opted for rigorous control of diabetes. The authors believe that some but not all malformations can be prevented by good control of blood sugar and that more subtle means are needed to identify the teratogenic mechanisms in IDMs. There were only a few diabetic women in both the full participant and late entry group who had glycosylated hemoglobin levels as high as those seen in some studies. Thus, most of the women in this study had rather good control of diabetes in pregnancy. A more recent study measured the relationship between hemoglobin A_1 in the first trimester and spontaneous abortions and major malformations in 303 insulin-requiring ground diabetics. The range of diabetic control was broader than in the above study. The risk for spontaneous abortion was 12.4 per cent with first trimester Hb_{A1} under 9.3 per cent and 37.5 with Hb_{A1} over 14.3 per cent. The risk for major malformations was 3 per cent with Hb_{A1} under 9.3 per cent and 40 per cent with Hb_{A1} over 14.4 per cent. The risks were high with poor control in the first trimester but reasonable (4 per cent) with "acceptable control."

Detection. Because of the high incidence of malformations in IDMs, ultrasonography should be performed in early pregnancy. Maternal alpha-fetoprotein (AFP) should also be measured. The newborn should have a careful physical examination to diagnose any anomalies that were missed by intrauterine surveillance.

Poor Feeding

Poor feeding is a major problem in these infants. It occurred in 37 per cent of a series of 150 IDMs at the Boston Hospital for Women. Sometimes poor feeding is related to prematurity, respiratory distress, or other problems; however, it often occurs in the absence of other problems. In our more recent experience (unpublished), it was found in 17 per cent of classes B to D IDMs and in 31 per cent of class F. Infants born to class F diabetic mothers are often premature. There was no difference in the incidence of poor feeding in large-for-gestational-age infants versus appropriate-for-gestational-age infants and no relation to polyhydramnios. Poor feeding is a major reason for prolongation of hospital stay and parent-infant separation.

Macrosomia

Macrosomia, defined as a birth weight over the 90th percentile or over 4000 gm, may be associated with an increased incidence of primary cesarean section or obstetric trauma such as fractured clavicle, Erb's palsy, or phrenic nerve palsy due to shoulder dystocia. It was 28 per cent at the Brigham & Women's Hospital between 1983 and 1984. An association was found between elevated maternal blood sugars in the last trimester and macrosomia. There also was an association between hyperinsulinemia in IDMs and macrosomia and between macrosomia and hypoglycemia. Macrosomia is not usually seen in infants born to mothers with class F diabetes. Better control of maternal diabetes in the third trimester should be associated with less macrosomia, resulting in less trauma and a lower primary cesarean section rate.

Myocardial Dysfunction

Transient hypertrophic subaortic stenosis resulting from ventricular septal hypertrophy in IDMs has been frequently reported. The infants may present with congestive heart failure, poor cardiac output, and cardiomegaly. This cardiomyopathy may complicate the management of other illnesses such as RDS. The diagnosis is made by echocardiography, which shows hypertrophy of the ventricular septum, the right ventricular anterior wall, and the left ventricular posterior wall in the absence of chamber dilation. Cardiac output decreases with increasing septal thickness.

Most symptoms resolve by 2 weeks of age. The septal hypertrophy resolves by 4 months of age. Most infants respond to supportive care. Digitalis and other inotropic drugs are contraindicated unless myocardial dysfunction is seen on echocardiography. Propranolol is the most useful drug.

The differential diagnosis of myocardial dysfunction due to diabetic cardiomyopathy of the newborn includes (1) postasphyxial cardiomyopathy, (2) myocarditis, (3) endocardial fibroelastosis, (4) glycogen storage disease of the heart, and (5) aberrant left coronary artery coming off the pulmonary artery. There is some evidence that good control of diabetes in pregnancy may reduce the severity of hypertrophic cardiomyopathy.

Renal Vein Thrombosis

Renal vein thrombosis may occur in utero or post partum. Intrauterine and postnatal diagnosis may be made by ultrasonography. Postnatal presentation may be as hematuria, flank mass, hypertension, or embolic phenomena. Most renal vein thrombosis can be managed conservatively (nonsurgically) with fluid and electrolyte therapy as well as heparin, allowing preservation of renal tissue.

Small Left Colon Syndrome

Small left colon syndrome presents as generalized abdominal distention because of inability to pass meconium. Meconium is obtained by passage of a rectal catheter. An enema performed with meglumine diatrizoate (Gastrografin) is diagnostic and often results in evacuation of the colon. The infant should be well hydrated before Gastrografin is used. The infant may have some problems with passage of a stool in the first week of life, but this usually resolves after treatment with half-normal saline enemas (5 ml/kg) and glycerine suppositories.

Perinatal Survival

Despite all these problems, the diabetic woman has a 95 per cent chance of having a healthy child if she is willing to participate in a program of pregnancy management and surveillance in a modern perinatal center. In 147 IDMs over 24 weeks of gestation born to mothers who required insulin at the Boston Hospital for Women in 1976 and 1977, the perinatal mortality was 34 per 1000. Between 1977 and 1980 at the same center the perinatal mortality of infants born to women with class B, C, D, H, or R diabetes was 20 per 1000. In the earlier series 24 infants born to class F diabetic women had a perinatal mortality of 125 per 1000. More recent data at the Brigham & Women's Hospital do not show an increased perinatal mortality in pregnancies complicated by class F diabetes as compared to other insulin-requiring diabetics. However, there is increased morbidity.

In a more recent series of 215 IDMs at the Brigham & Women's Hospital from 1983 to 1984, the total perinatal mortality from 24 weeks of gestation to 28 days post partum was 28 per 1000. There was one intrauterine demise of a singleton near term. Thus, perinatal survival is encouragingly good and results from advances in medical, obstetric, and neonatal treatment. More infants are born healthy than ever before, and, if ill, more survive.

Risk of Insulin-Dependent Diabetes in Offspring of Diabetic Parents

Infants born to an insulin-dependent diabetic father have a 6 per cent risk of having insulin-dependent diabetes by age 20. In infants born to an insulin-dependent mother, the risk is 1.3 per cent. This difference may be due to some effect on the fetal immune system which makes the offspring of the diabetic mother more resistant to the development of diabetes.

POLYCYTHEMIA

SHELLY C. BERNSTEIN, M.D., Ph.D.

During the first week of life, hemoglobin values above 22.0 gm/dl or hematocrit values of more than 65 per cent should be considered evidence of polycythemia. In childhood and adolescence, hemoglobin values above 17.0 gm/dl or hematocrit values of more than 50 per cent are significant. The diagnosis should be verified by venipuncture; capillary blood samples should not be used. Hemoconcentration due to dehydration must be excluded as a cause.

NEONATAL POLYCYTHEMIA

Polycythemia in the neonate may be due to twin-to-twin transfusion, maternal-fetal transfusion, delayed cord clamping, placental insufficiency, congenital adrenal hyperplasia, maternal diabetes mellitus, Down's syndrome, or Beckwith's syndrome. The signs and symptoms may consist of lethargy, plethora, cyanosis, jaundice, respiratory distress, congestive heart failure, seizures, priapism, thrombocytopenia, renal vein thrombosis, necrotizing enterocolitis, hypoglycemia, and hypocalcemia. Many infants with polycythemia are, however, asymptomatic. Prophylactic treatment is not recommended. However, all infants with polycythemia should be monitored carefully, and treatment should be instituted at the first sign of symptoms. Treatment should be designed to reduce the venous hematocrit value to approximately 60 per cent, accomplished by partial exchange transfusion using fresh frozen plasma to reduce the hematocrit value while maintaining the blood volume. The volume of exchange may be estimated from the following formula:

$$\text{Volume of exchange (ml)} = \frac{\text{Blood volume} \times (\text{Observed Hct} - \text{Desired Hct})}{\text{Observed Hct}}$$

The infant's blood should be removed in volumes of 10 ml for full-term (and smaller volumes for low-birth-weight) infants and replaced with an equal volume of fresh frozen plasma. A blood volume of 80 ml/kg may be estimated for newborn infants. The procedure is usually performed through an umbilical venous line.

Simple phlebotomy should not be performed unless the infant is hypervolemic.

CHILDHOOD POLYCYTHEMIA

Primary Polycythemia

Polycythemia Vera. This disorder consists of an increase in red cell mass of unknown etiology, often accompanied by thrombocytosis, and is rarely seen in childhood. The Polycythemia Vera Study Group recommends phlebotomy for patients under the age of 40 years. Erythropheresis with isovolemic exchange of fresh frozen plasma or Ringer's lactate, rather than simple phlebotomy, should be performed to maintain the hematocrit between 40 and 45 per cent. Patients with complications (such as massive splenomegaly, vascular obstruction, or symptoms associated with hypermetabolism) or with extreme thrombocytosis (platelet counts greater than 10^{12}/L) should be treated with myelosuppressive agents. Hydroxyurea, 30 mg/kg orally in three divided doses per day, is given until the platelet count falls to 10^{11}/L. At that time, busulfan, 0.12 mg/kg (maximum dose of 6 mg) orally per day for 7 days, is given. This dose may be repeated for another 7 days if significant myelosuppression does not occur. Periodic pulses of busulfan may be required to control thrombocytosis and may need to be given on a regular basis. Repeated erythropheresis leads to iron deficiency, causing an increase in whole blood viscosity related to decreased erythrocyte deformability, as well as thrombocytosis. Therefore, iron deficiency should be avoided by oral iron supplementation.

Benign Familial Polycythemia. This term is used to describe familial cases with increased red cell mass that are otherwise normal, with no other recognizable etiology. Therapy is not required unless the patient has symptoms related to hyperviscosity. Erythropheresis or phlebotomy may then afford symptomatic relief.

Secondary Polycythemia

These conditions refer to an increase in red cell mass secondary to a recognizable cause and may result from tissue hypoxia, leading to a compensatory response of erythropoietin, or from increased production of erythropoietin despite normal tissue oxygenation.

Cyanotic Congenital Heart Disease. Children with cyanotic congenital heart disease with a right-to-left shunt develop polycythemia in response to chronic systemic arterial desaturation. Symptoms are headaches, irritability, anorexia, and dyspnea. In addition, polycythemia, when accompanied by iron deficiency, may be associated with an increased incidence of intravascular thrombosis and a consumptive coagulopathy. Arterial saturation should be surgically corrected, if possible. If the patient has symptoms, reduction of hematocrit values should be attempted cautiously by partial exchange transfusion or erythropheresis. Since acute phlebotomy in these patients may result in vascular collapse, cyanotic spells, cerebrovascular accidents, or seizures, sudden hemodynamic alterations should be avoided. Erythropheresis should be performed, removing aliquots of blood (5 ml for infants and 30 ml for older children) and infusing equal volumes of fresh frozen plasma, estimating the total exchange volume from the above formula. The hematocrit should be reduced to 60 to 65 per cent over 30 to 60 minutes. Strict adherence to critical blood volume maintenance must be maintained. Because of the complications associated with iron deficiency and polycythemia, iron deficiency should always be corrected. These measures have led to reduced coagulation abnormalities, decreased operative mortality, and symptomatic improvement in polycythemic patients with cyanotic congenital heart disease.

Abnormal Hemoglobins. A number of hemoglobin variants have been described with a marked increase in oxygen affinity and compensatory polycythemia via increased production of erythropoietin. Affected individuals have minimal clinical manifestations, other than erythrocytosis, with the exception of one reported family with Hb Malmö, the children of which were reported to have cardiovascular symptoms. Hematocrit values rarely are high enough to necessitate treatment.

Congenital methemoglobinemia due to NADH-diaphorase I deficiency and acquired methemoglobinemia due to exposure to various agents capable of oxidizing heme iron to the ferric state may produce cyanosis and polycythemia. Treatment of methemoglobinemia, regardless of the etiology, is dictated by the severity of the hypoxia. Most patients with hereditary disease require no therapy. Severe methemoglobinemia can be treated initially by methylene blue in a dose of 1 to 2 mg/kg administered intravenously as a 1 per cent solution. Further treatment is accomplished with daily oral doses of methylene blue, 1 to 2 mg/kg.

Inappropriate Erythrocytosis. Polycythemia has been associated with a number of tumors in which erythropoietin secretion is elevated, such as Wilms' tumor, hepatoma, cerebellar hemangioblastoma, and benign lesions of the kidney such as cysts and hydronephrosis. Endocrine disorders such as pheochromocytoma, aldosterone-producing adenoma, and Cushing's syndrome, as well as exogenous administration of testosterone or growth hormone, may also cause increased red cell mass. Correction of the underlying condition results in elimination of the polycythemia.

DIABETES MELLITUS

JOSEPH I. WOLFSDORF, M.D.

The diverse needs of the child with diabetes can seldom be adequately met by a physician working in isolation. Therefore, whenever possible, care should be provided by a team consisting of health care professionals with complementary roles who are knowledgeable about the physical and emotional growth and development of children and experienced in the management of type I or insulin-dependent diabetes (IDDM). The multidisciplinary team should include a pediatrician, a diabetes educator, a mental health professional, and a nutritionist, whose role is to provide nutrition education and assist with the details of individual meal planning.

The members of the team should communicate with the important individuals in the child's life, for example, teacher, school nurse, school guidance counselor, and team coach. To provide optimal care for children with diabetes, it is necessary to involve the entire family unit. The efforts of the diabetes team are aimed at ensuring that children and their families acquire the knowledge and skills necessary to cope successfully with this lifelong disease. The diabetes treatment team provides not only medical and nutritional care for the child, but of equal importance, continuing diabetes education, family guidance, and psychological support.

EDUCATION

Patient education is the foundation of successful diabetes management. Few diseases demand so much day-to-day participation by the patient; consequently, the patient must possess extensive knowledge and understanding of all aspects of diabetes. Education involves more than just imparting facts and teaching skills; one of the most important aspects of a comprehensive patient education program is the promotion of desirable health beliefs and attitudes in the person who has to live with a chronic incurable disease. This applies particularly to adolescents with diabetes.

The educational curriculum for children must be concordant with each child's level of cognitive development, and in order to be meaningful, the process must be specifically adapted to the individual child. Parents should be fully involved, because delegating complete responsibility to the child is likely to have disastrous consequences. The educational program should be designed to gradually transfer the responsibility for diabetes care from the parents to the child so as not to impede the normal process of separation and attainment of independence that occurs during adolescence.

The process of educating the child and his family begins soon after the diagnosis has been made and evolves over a period of several years. The aim is to impart the fundamental knowledge and to teach the practical skills that enable the patient and his family to competently and confidently assume complete responsibility for self-care.

The grief reaction that follows the diagnosis of a serious disease leaves parents and patients too upset and anxious to assimilate an extensive body of largely abstract information; therefore, the initial educational goals should be limited. During the first several days the child and family should learn what diabetes is and how it is treated and acquire the survival skills necessary to care for the child at home and to permit his early return to school. During the next few weeks the child's metabolic status is stabilized, and the basic aspects of diabetes care are consolidated by practical experience at home and frequent contact with the diabetes educator and physician. Once the grief reaction has subsided, the family is more ready to learn the sophisticated details of management necessary to achieve near-normal blood glucose levels and to cope with intercurrent illnesses and other variations in the child's daily routine. Many patients find it necessary and should be encouraged to periodically review and update their knowledge of diabetes self-care during the ensuing several years.

INSULIN

Replacement of insulin is the cornerstone of treatment of insulin-dependent diabetes. It is important to appreciate, however, that conventional insulin replacement therapy does not mimic normal insulin physiology. The healthy pancreas secretes insulin at a low basal rate upon which are superimposed bursts of increased insulin secretion that coincide with eating. Accordingly, insulin levels in the blood increase and decrease in concert with the rises and falls in blood glucose levels. Furthermore, insulin is secreted into the portal circulation, so that the liver, which is the chief site of glucose production and is also important in glucose disposal, is the target organ normally exposed to the highest concentration of insulin. In contrast, injection of insulin into the subcutaneous tissue results in absorption of insulin into the systemic circulation, so that the concentration of insulin to which the liver is exposed is reduced by dilution in the systemic circulation. Given these inherent limitations, conventional daily or twice-daily insulin regimens can seldom restore normal carbohydrate metabolism. Even programs of intensive insulin therapy that include injections of quick-acting insulin (regular) before each meal cannot always restore the normal pattern, although the wide fluctuations in blood glucose concentration that typically occur with a single injection of intermediate-acting insulin or even two injections per day can be significantly improved.

Most children with total diabetes (patients without significant residual insulin secretion) can be satisfactorily controlled with a twice-daily insulin regimen consisting of a mixture of rapid-acting (regular) and intermediate-acting (NPH or Lente) insulins drawn up into the same syringe and given before breakfast and again before the evening meal. The amount of rapid-acting insulin needed before breakfast is determined by the results of late morning and early afternoon (before lunch) blood glucose tests. Similarly, the decision to provide quick-acting insulin before supper is determined by the results of blood glucose tests at bedtime; if high at this time, regular insulin is added to the presupper dose of intermediate-acting insulin. When presupper regular insulin is not necessary, better glycemic control during the night and early morning and avoidance of nocturnal hypoglycemia are achieved when the intermediate-acting insulin is given at bedtime.

There is no way of predicting the precise dose of insulin that is necessary. Therefore, the insulin program must be empirically worked out for each patient. On an average, about 60 to 75 per cent of the total daily dose is given before breakfast and approximately 25 to 40 per cent before the evening meal. Usually about one third of each dose consists of quick-acting insulin; however, the optimal ratio of quick- to intermediate-acting insulin for each patient must be determined by trial and error based on the results of blood glucose monitoring. Shortly after starting insulin therapy, many children can be well-controlled using intermediate-acting insulin alone. Children's insulin requirements are not fixed; they change during growth and development. It is, therefore, necessary to periodically reevaluate and adjust each child's insulin regimen. Also, most children are considerably more active during the spring and summer months and usually require less insulin during this part of the year. The insulin dose should be changed by approximately 10 per cent at any one time, and one should allow a minimum of 3 days to elapse after each change before further adjustments are made.

Whenever possible, regular insulin should be given at least 30 minutes before meals. This interval allows sufficient time for the quick-acting insulin to be absorbed; and when this is done, the rise in blood glucose after meals is significantly less than when the meal is eaten immediately after receiving the injection.

Early in the course of diabetes, some children achieve satisfactory glycemic control with a single daily injection of insulin. Persistent nocturnal hyperglycemia, manifested as nocturia or enuresis, or significant fasting hyperglycemia with or without ketonuria, usually signifies the need to give a second dose of intermediate-acting insulin, either before supper or at bedtime. If the morning dose of intermediate-acting insulin is substantially increased in an attempt to prolong its activity through the night and early morning hours, this may cause hypoglycemia or intense hunger and overeating during the period of maximum insulin activity, which is usually in the late afternoon and evening.

The technique of drawing up and injecting insulin should be taught to the patient when appropriate as well as to both parents. The average child of 12 or older can and should be encouraged to learn to give his own insulin injections. Although even younger children can also master this skill, they should not be coerced into giving their own shots. If a young child does wish to give his own injections, it is important to ensure that this always is done under close parental supervision. Young children should never be hurried into accepting full responsibility for their own injections until they are psychologically mature enough to fully appreciate the consequences of omitting insulin. Careful rotation of the injection sites (using the arms, thighs, buttocks, and anterior abdominal wall) prevents lipohypertrophy. Lipoatrophy is rarely if ever seen with the use of highly purified insulin (pure pork or human).

The total daily insulin dose in prepubertal children is usually in the range of 0.5 to 1 unit/kg; in pubertal individuals, the usual range is 0.8 to 1.5 units/kg. Less insulin is needed during the phase of partial remission (less than 0.5 units/kg). When the dose of insulin exceeds the above ranges, one should consider the possibility that the patient may be receiving more insulin than is actually necessary and is experiencing intermittent hypoglycemia followed by rebound hyperglycemia; this is a well-recognized cause of unstable glycemic control.

During the remission period ("honeymoon"), the insulin requirement may decrease to a negligible amount, so that one may be tempted to eliminate it completely. Most physicians experienced in the care of diabetes in children insist that insulin should not be eliminated, even if only one or two units are given each day. The remission phase in children usually lasts a few weeks or at most a few months, and larger amounts of insulin will be required when it ends. Thus, by continuing to give insulin each day, one avoids fostering false hopes that the child no longer has diabetes or no longer requires insulin injections. Furthermore, it has been suggested that discontinuing insulin may lead to sensitization, which could cause an allergic response to occur upon restarting the insulin.

DIET THERAPY

Principles. When insulin is given subcutaneously, it is absorbed from the injection site in a more or less predictable fashion that depends on the type of insulin or combination of insulins used. Each type of insulin has a characteristic time of onset, peak effect, and total duration of action. Food consumption must be matched to the time and course of action of injected insulin. Meals and snacks have to be eaten at the same times each day, and the total consumption of calories and the proportions of carbohydrate, protein, and fat in each meal and snack must be consistent from day to day.

Because insulin is absorbed continuously from the injection site, hypoglycemia, exacerbated by exercise, may occur if snacks are not eaten between the main meals. Hence, most children receiving twice-daily injections of insulin have a snack between each meal and at bedtime. A snack should always precede strenuous exercise unless the blood glucose is known to be very high.

The nutritional needs of children with diabetes do not differ from those of healthy children. They do not require special foods, nor do they need different amounts of vitamins or minerals. The total intake of calories and nutrients must be sufficient to balance the daily expenditure of energy and satisfy the requirements for normal growth. The American Diabetes Association currently recommends that carbohydrate provide 50 to 60 per cent of the total calories, protein 15 to 20 per cent and fat no more than 30 per cent. The diet prescription has to be adjusted periodically to maintain a normal rate of physical growth and maturation. The main objective of dietary therapy in obese non–insulin-dependent patients is to lose weight initially and then maintain a desirable body weight.

Exchange System. The meal plan is formulated in consultation with a clinical nutritionist and is individualized to meet the ethnic, religious, and economic circumstances of each family and the food preferences of the individual child. The exchange system is based on six food groups: milk, fruit, vegetable, bread (starch), meat (protein), and fat. Individual food choices (exchanges) included in the list of foods in a particular category contain approximately the same amount of carbohydrate, fat, and protein. The portion size of each exchange is given by either weight or volume. Thus, the meal plan is prescribed in terms of the number of exchanges from each food group that should be included in each meal and snack. This method provides a means of ensuring day-to-day consistency of total calories, carbohydrate, protein, and fat while allowing the patient to choose from a wide variety of foods.

Prudent Fat. Because individuals with diabetes are predisposed to atherosclerosis, the amount of fat should not exceed 30 per cent of the total daily calories, and dietary cholesterol should not exceed 300 mg/day. Saturated, monounsaturated, and polyunsaturated fat should constitute less than 10 per cent, 10 to 15 per cent, and up to 10 per cent, respectively, of the total calories. Fat intake is reduced by consuming less beef and pork and more lean meat, chicken, turkey, fish, low fat milk, and vegetable proteins.

Fiber. Dietary fiber may benefit the diabetic patient by blunting the rise in blood glucose after meals. Soluble fiber can also reduce serum cholesterol and triglyceride levels. Unrefined or minimally processed foods such as grains, legumes, whole fruits, nuts, and vegetables should replace highly refined carbohydrates. To avoid abrupt increases in blood glucose, children should eat fruit whole and avoid fruit juices, which should be reserved for treating episodes of hypoglycemia.

The clinical nutritionist or dietitian has the important task of educating the patient and family in the basic principles of nutrition and the application of these principles to the formulation of an individualized meal plan. The aim is to lay a foundation for a life-long change in eating habits. A single instructional session is totally inadequate; nutrition education, like all aspects of diabetes education, has to be an ongoing process, with periodic review of the meal plan and assessment of the child's and parent's levels of comprehension.

EXERCISE

The effects of exercise on diabetes are complex. Exercise acutely lowers the blood glucose concentration to an extent that depends on the intensity and duration of the physical activity and the concurrent level of insulinemia. Acute vigorous exercise in the child with poorly controlled diabetes can aggravate hyperglycemia and stimulate ketoacid production. Therefore, the child whose diabetes is out of control (pronounced hyperglycemia with ketonuria) should be discouraged from exercising until satisfactory control has been restored. Exercising the limb into which insulin has been injected accelerates the rate of insulin absorption as a result of the massaging effect of contracting muscles and increased regional blood flow. Therefore, if exercise is planned, it is recommended that the preceding insulin injection be given in a site least likely to be affected by exercise. For example, the insulin might be injected into the anterior abdominal wall on the morning preceding a sports event or other variety of physical activity.

Children's activities tend to be spontaneous, making this advice difficult, if not impossible, to implement consistently. Consequently, bursts of increased energy expenditure should be "covered" by providing an extra snack before and, if the exercise is prolonged, during the activity. A rule of thumb is to provide one bread or fruit exchange (15 gm carbohydrate) per 30 minutes of vigorous physical activity. Physical training increases tissue sensitivity to insulin. Consequently, when the frequency and duration of physical activity increases consistently, as occurs during the summer vacation, a reduction in the total daily insulin dose is necessary to avoid hypoglycemia. Youngsters who participate in organized sports are advised to adjust their insulin dose in anticipation of sustained physical activity during a specific period of the day, e.g., reduction in the morning dose of NPH or Lente insulin on certain days of the week for the youth who engages in an after-school sports program. The precise amounts of such adjustments are determined by trial and error.

Exercise helps to maintain ideal body weight and, in combination with an optimal insulin regimen and adherence to the meal plan, may be a useful adjunct in achieving good glycemic control. It has beneficial effects on mental health, cardiovascular function, and blood lipids. A program of regular exercise allows young people with diabetes more leeway with food and enables them occasionally to have "forbidden" foods, which can be used judiciously as sources of quickly absorbed carbohydrate to combat hypoglycemic reactions.

MONITORING

Blood Glucose. Self blood glucose monitoring (SBGM) is the preferred method of metabolic monitoring. The technique should be routinely taught to all patients with IDDM, and the ability of patients to obtain accurate results must be confirmed. A variety of glucose meters are available which enable the user to obtain measurements of glucose concentration on a single drop of capillary blood within 10 per cent of the value obtained in a clinical chemistry laboratory. When insulin therapy is started, during periods of unstable control requiring adjustments to the insulin dose, and for patients using intensive insulin therapy regimens (insulin infusion pumps or multiple daily injections) aimed at achieving near normoglycemia, blood glucose concentration should be measured before each meal and at bedtime. For most children, this frequency of testing is impractical or intolerable. A satisfactory compromise is to perform SBGM before each dose of insulin, with additional tests before lunch and at bedtime at least twice each week and at 2 to 3 A.M. once or twice each month. Alternatively, for patients who cannot tolerate such frequent monitoring or who cannot afford the cost of the reagent strips, a period of intensive monitoring before each meal, at bedtime, and between 2 and 3 A.M. for several consecutive days before an office visit often provides sufficient information to confirm satisfactory control or indicate a trend so that appropriate adjustments can be made to the insulin regimen.

Frequent SBGM (every 3 to 4 hours throughout the day and night) in conjunction with urine tests for ketones is essential to manage intercurrent illnesses and prevent ketoacidosis. SBGM is of great value to parents uncertain of the cause of their child's crankiness or unusual behavior when the question frequently arises, "Is this child's behavior due to hypoglycemia?" Children and adolescents not infrequently fabricate results to please their parents or physician and avoid criticism for "bad blood sugars." Inaccurate test results are common and usually the result of poor technique. Frequent problems include obtaining an inadequate drop of blood to cover the reagent strip, failure to time the reaction carefully, and wiping or blotting the reagent strip too vigorously. Some of these technical problems have been eliminated by the newer glucose meters.

Urine Testing. Urine glucose testing has many limitations as a means of optimally monitoring the control of diabetes, and urine glucose concentration correlates poorly with blood glucose concentration. With a normal renal threshold, a negative urine test cannot distinguish between a blood glucose level in the hypoglycemic range and one that is normal or even slightly or moderately increased. Therefore, parents, fearful of a hypoglycemic reaction when their young child's urine contains no sugar, often deliberately undertreat the child to ensure that "there is always a little sugar in the urine."

The urine should always be tested for the presence of ketones whenever the child is sick, when the blood glucose level exceeds 250 mg/dl, and when blood glucose levels are high before breakfast and the possibility of nocturnal hypoglycemia with rebound hyperglycemia (the Somogyi phenomenon) is considered.

Glycosylated Hemoglobin (Hemoglobin A$_1$ or A$_{1c}$)

Diabetes in children is characterized by blood glucose levels that constantly fluctuate over the course of a single day as well as from day to day. Assessment of glycemic control based on symptoms, urine tests, or infrequently performed blood glucose measurements at home or in the office is inaccurate; therefore, quarterly determinations of glycosylated hemoglobin should be used to provide an objective measure of average glycemia during the intervening period. The level of glycosylated hemoglobin, formed when glucose is bound nonenzymatically to the N-terminal valine of the beta chain of the hemoglobin molecule, is directly proportional to the time-integrated mean blood glucose concentration over the preceding 2 to 3 months. This test is objective and is independent of the patient's cooperation and time elapsed since the last meal. There are several different methods of measuring glycosylated hemoglobin; therefore, to be able to make meaningful comparisons of results from one evaluation to the next, it is advisable to perform the assay in the same laboratory.

ACUTE COMPLICATIONS

Hypoglycemia

Occasional episodes of hypoglycemia are virtually an inevitable consequence of insulin therapy. The aim of therapy should be to achieve the best possible glycemic control while minimizing the frequency and severity of hypoglycemia. The most common reasons that hypoglycemia occurs are bursts of physical activity without a preceding snack; meals or snacks that are delayed, omitted, or incompletely consumed; inadvertent errors in insulin dosage; and inappropriate insulin regimens. Occasionally, severe reactions occur unexpectedly and inexplicably; one suspects that some of these are due to an inadvertent error in the insulin dose, e.g., giving the morning dose in the evening or reversing the amounts of short-acting and intermediate-acting insulins. It should be noted that hypoglycemia after periods of sustained physical exercise may occur several hours after the activity has ended, the "lag effect of exercise." The child with diabetes who participates in prolonged physical activity should consume additional carbohydrate and protein before as well as during the exercise. It may also be necessary to reduce the dose of insulin. The precise amount of extra food and the reduction in insulin dose have to be determined empirically for each individual and adjusted according to the duration and intensity of the exercise.

The symptoms and signs of hypoglycemia are due to both increased adrenergic activity and impaired brain function resulting from glucose deprivation (neuroglycopenia). Enhanced activity of the adrenergic nervous system and increased catecholamine levels account for nervousness, pallor, tremulousness, sweating, hunger, and palpitations. Weakness, dizziness, headache, blurry vision, drowsiness, irritability, loss of coordination, confusion, convulsions, and coma are due to altered central nervous system function resulting from cerebral glucose deprivation. If the patient is unable to perceive the onset of hypoglycemia (hypoglycemia unawareness) for any reason, is too young to treat himself, or has impaired counter-regulatory mechanisms, the physician should be cautious and avoid attempting to achieve "tight" glycemic control. These circumstances place the child at a considerably greater risk of having hypoglycemia-induced coma and seizures.

Patients and family members must be taught to recognize the early signs of hypoglycemia and treat it promptly with a suitable form of rapidly absorbed carbohydrate. Depending on the size of the child and the severity of the hypoglycemia, most episodes of hypoglycemia are satisfactorily treated with 5 to 20 gm of glucose, provided in the form of glucose tablets (each contains 5 gm of glucose), 3 to 7 small pieces of hard candy, granulated table sugar, or orange or apple juice (4 ounces contain 15 gm of carbohydrate). Family members are taught to use glucagon, which should be available at home, to treat severe hypoglycemia when the child is unconscious or unable to swallow or retain ingested carbohydrate. Glucagon (0.02 mg/kg, maximum dose 1.0 mg) is injected IM or SC and raises the blood glucose level within 5 to 15 minutes. Nausea and vomiting often follow the administration of glucagon. A carbohydrate-containing snack to prevent hypoglycemia from recurring should be given when consciousness has been regained after treating a severe insulin reaction with glucagon.

If the patient cannot take or retain sugar-containing solutions orally, an equivalent amount of glucose should be given intravenously followed by a continuous infusion of glucose at a rate of at least 10 mg/kg/min, with frequent blood glucose monitoring to ensure that a satisfactory blood glucose concentration has been achieved and is maintained.

A Medicalert bracelet or necklace should always be worn identifying the patient as having diabetes mellitus.

Recurrent hypoglycemia itself can be a cause of poor glycemic control, since the counter-regulatory hormone responses to hypoglycemia stimulate hepatic glucose production and induce a state of relative insulin resistance that persists for 12 to 24 hours. This phenomenon, referred to as the Somogyi phenomenon or rebound hyperglycemia, together with excessive consumption of carbohydrate and other calories to treat hypoglycemia, should be suspected in any child who is gaining weight rapidly, with blood or urine glucose levels that fluctuate wildly associated with intermittent ketonuria, and whose insulin dose appears to be high (in excess of 1 to 1.5 U/kg/day) and/or is increasing steadily. More frequent blood glucose monitoring, especially at times of anticipated peak insulin action and during the night (2 to 3 A.M.) usually helps to confirm that hypoglycemia is the cause of the glycemic instability. Alternatively, one can empirically reduce the insulin dose; subsequent improved glycemic control is presumptive evidence that the patient was experiencing episodes of hypoglycemia, which are especially likely to occur during the night.

ASSOCIATED DISORDERS

Autoimmune thyroid disease is commonly associated with type 1 diabetes. About one in every five white children and young adults with IDDM have thyroid antimicrosomal antibodies (TMA) in their serum. The prevalence of TMA in black children with diabetes is lower. A goiter without any evidence of thyroid dysfunction may be the only clinical evidence of thyroiditis; however, either hyperthyroidism or hypothyroidism may develop. The latter occurs more commonly; therefore, it is important to carefully monitor the diabetic child's rate of linear growth with the aid of a growth chart and look for other signs of hypothyroidism. It has been recommended that all children with diabetes be screened for TMA; those found to have antibodies should have thyroid function tests performed annually. Because immediate family members are also at increased risk of developing autoimmune thyroid disease, examination of the neck for a goiter and screening for thyroiditis, especially in female relatives, has been recommended.

Adrenal autoantibodies have been found in nearly 2 per cent of white children and young adults with IDDM; about 25 per cent of those with antiadrenal antibodies have overt adrenal insufficiency. Patients with type 1 diabetes also have an increased risk of developing other autoimmune diseases such as atrophic gastritis and pernicious anemia; however, these disorders rarely appear in childhood. If antiadrenal antibodies are detected, the patient must be carefully followed for the possible development of adrenal insufficiency, which may first manifest as a progressive decrease in insulin requirement due to increased sensitivity to insulin.

PSYCHOLOGICAL ASPECTS

Diabetes management is not simply a matter of insulin administration, meal planning, and testing. It also involves a child's emotional and social development and the impact on the family of a chronic incurable disease in a child. The child's diabetes involves the whole family and frequently places a considerable strain on the family; some parents, perhaps already struggling with other issues, give up and leave the child to get on with diabetes care as best he can. This often results in dreadful glycemic control and numerous episodes of ketoacidosis.

The diagnosis of a chronic disease usually stirs emotions that are similar to those experienced by the bereaved: shock, disbelief, denial, anger, and depression. The emotional upheaval that follows the diagnosis may temporarily limit a family's ability to learn; therefore, the initial educational goals should be to teach survival skills.

The major psychological task of the adolescent is to develop increasing autonomy, and this often leads to turmoil. Growth toward independence is complicated for the teen-ager with diabetes for a variety of reasons. The need for closer medical intervention occurs at just the time that the teen-ager is striving for less dependence on adult guidance. Adolescence normally involves a struggle for self-identity and a temporary rejection of the values of parents or other authority figures. Diabetes care often becomes the battleground for this struggle. Some adolescents want to find out whether they really have diabetes; this may take the form of omitting insulin injections, overeating, or refusing to monitor. This is a period of rapid physical growth and sexual maturation, and both physical as well as psychological factors presumably lead to more erratic diabetes control during the adolescent years than during childhood. The teen-ager with diabetes, already vulnerable to feeling different, may wish to prove to his friends that "nothing is wrong"; this may lead to omitting insulin injections and eating haphazardly. Numerous emergency room visits due to recurrent episodes of ketoacidosis signal the need for intensive psychosocial intervention and support.

Caring for the young person with diabetes is not solely a medical problem. Emotional and behavioral issues inevitably arise and must be identified and dealt with. In this regard the mental health worker, psychiatric social worker, or clinical psychologist plays an extremely important role as a member of the diabetes treatment team.

DIABETIC KETOACIDOSIS (DKA)
Initial Evaluation of the Patient

1. Rapidly perform a clinical evaluation to confirm the diagnosis and determine its cause (look especially for any evidence of infection). Weigh the patient and measure height or length. Make a clinical assessment of the patient's degree of dehydration. Most patients are between 5 and 10 per cent dehydrated.

2. Determine the blood glucose concentration with a reagent strip method (e.g., Chemstrip bG) and plasma ketones (Acetest tablet method) at the bedside.

3. Obtain a blood sample for the laboratory measurement of glucose, electrolytes, total CO_2, BUN, pH, PCO_2, PO_2, hemoglobin, hematocrit, white blood cell count and differential, calcium, and phosphorus.

4. Perform a urinalysis and obtain appropriate specimens for culture (blood, urine, throat).

5. Perform an electrocardiogram for baseline evaluation of potassium status.

6. Record clinical and biochemical data on a flow sheet.

TABLE 1. Potassium Replacement in Diabetic Ketoacidosis

Serum Potassium (mEq/L)	Infusate Potassium Concentration (mEq/L)
<3	40–60
3–4	30
4–5	20
5–6	10
>6	0

Supportive Measures

1. To prevent the possibility of pulmonary aspiration, empty the stomach by continuous nasogastric suction in the unconscious or semiconscious patient.

2. Antibiotics should be given to febrile patients after obtaining appropriate specimens of body fluids for culture.

3. Supplementary oxygen is given to cyanotic patients, those in shock, and when the PaO_2 is less than 80 mm Hg.

4. Catheterization of the bladder is usually not necessary; bag collection or condom drainage suffices to permit an accurate assessment of urine output in most patients who are unable to void on demand.

5. Some of the details concerning the treatment of diabetic ketoacidosis are still controversial. However, successful management of diabetic ketoacidosis requires meticulous monitoring of the patient's clinical and biochemical response to treatment so that timely adjustments in the treatment regimen can be made when necessary. The physician is aided considerably in his task by maintaining an accurate flow chart that records the patient's clinical and laboratory data, details of fluid and electrolyte therapy, administered insulin, and urine output.

6. Ideally, the severely ill child should be treated in an intensive care unit or other facility where intensive clinical and metabolic monitoring can be performed.

Fluid and Electrolyte Therapy

All patients with DKA are dehydrated and suffer total body depletion of sodium, potassium, chloride, phosphate, and magnesium. With severe DKA, the extent of dehydration is usually between 5 and 10 per cent. Prompt and adequate rehydration restores tissue perfusion and renal blood flow and suppresses the elevated levels of stress hormones. The top priority of treatment is to start an intravenous infusion using a large-bore cannula inserted into the largest accessible vein and to infuse 10 to 20 ml/kg or 500 ml/m² of isotonic saline (0.9 per cent sodium chloride) in 60 minutes. If hypotension or shock persists, an additional 10 ml/kg of isotonic saline (or an equal amount of colloid) is given over 60 minutes. Once the circulation has been stabilized, change to half-normal saline (0.45 per cent sodium chloride) and aim to replace the calculated fluid deficit at an even rate over 24 to 36 hours. When the blood glucose concentration reaches 300 mg/dl, 5 per cent dextrose is added to half-normal saline. The concentration of dextrose may have to be increased to 10 per cent to avert hypoglycemia in patients whose acidosis corrects slowly but in whom blood glucose concentration falls briskly.

Early in the course of therapy, osmotic diuresis may contribute significantly to ongoing fluid losses and consideration should be given to replacing those ongoing losses with half-normal saline and added potassium. When the osmotic diuresis subsides, maintenance fluid is given at a rate of 1500 to 2000 ml/m²/day.

Insulin

Because it is simple to use, safe, and effective, we use low-dose continuous intravenous insulin administration controlled by an infusion pump or drip. Regular (short-acting, soluble) insulin is diluted in saline (50 U regular insulin in 50 ml saline) and is given intravenously at a rate of 0.1 U/kg/hour after an intravenous priming dose of 0.1 to 0.25 U/kg. This rate of insulin infusion is sufficient to reverse DKA in the majority of patients; however, if the response is inadequate (failure of blood glucose level to fall, pH and bicarbonate to rise, or anion gap to decrease) owing to severe insulin resistance, the rate of insulin infusion should be increased until a satisfactory response is achieved. A minority of patients with severe insulin resistance do not respond satisfactorily to low-dose insulin infusion and require two or three times the usual dose. Therefore, it is essential to monitor the blood glucose, pH, serum bicarbonate, and anion gap in response to insulin therapy and increase the dose of insulin until a satisfactory rate of fall of blood glucose and increase in blood pH and serum bicarbonate are obtained. When the blood glucose level reaches 250 mg/dl, the rate of insulin infusion may have to be reduced to 0.05 U/kg/hr but must not be stopped until the acidosis is completely reversed. This method of administering insulin allows the rate of insulin infusion to be finely controlled and reduces the risk of hypoglycemia and hypokalemia. A potential disadvantage of low-dose continuous insulin infusion is that inadequate insulinization rapidly occurs if the infusion infiltrates or stops for any reason. Therefore, low-dose insulin therapy should not be used unless it can be closely supervised.

When DKA has resolved and a change to subcutaneous insulin is anticipated, the first subcutaneous injection should be given at least 60 to 120 minutes before stopping the infusion to allow sufficient time for the injected insulin to be absorbed.

Potassium Replacement

Although the initial serum potassium concentration may be normal or even increased, all patients with DKA are potassium-depleted (3 to 10 mEq/kg). Patients whose initial level of potassium is low are the most severely depleted and should receive early (after the patient has voided and insulin has begun) and vigorous potassium replacement. The administration of fluid and insulin may cause a rapid decrease of the serum potassium concentration and induce a cardiac arrhythmia. The serum potassium level should be maintained in the range of 4 to 5 mEq/L. If the laboratory has not reported the pretreatment level within an hour, potassium should not be withheld if insulin has been given and the patient has urinated. Table 1 is a guide to initial potassium administration based on the serum concen-

tration. Use the electrocardiogram as a guide to therapy by following the configuration of the T waves in standard lead 2 and V_2 at 30- to 60-minute intervals. Flattening of the T wave, widening of the QT interval, and the appearance of U waves indicate hypokalemia. Tall peaked symmetrical T waves and shortening of the QT interval are signs of hyperkalemia.

Half the potassium is given as potassium chloride and the other half as potassium phosphate, thus reducing the total amount of chloride administered and partially replacing the phosphate deficit.

Bicarbonate

Substantial evidence now indicates that administration of sodium bicarbonate neither hastens resolution of the acidosis nor improves survival. It may impair tissue oxygenation by increasing the affinity of hemoglobin for oxygen, i.e., shifting the hemoglobin-oxygen dissociation curve to the left. Because it has been shown to improve myocardial contractility and enhance peripheral vascular responsiveness to catecholamines, bicarbonate is indicated in the patient in shock or whose circulation is unstable. In these circumstances, 1 to 2 mEq/kg or 40 to 80 mEq/m² of sodium bicarbonate is infused over 1 to 2 hours.

HYPOGLYCEMIA
BORIS SENIOR, M.D.

If a report of a low blood sugar is correct and not attributable to a mishandled sample or other laboratory error, there are both immediate and long-term therapeutic objectives. Because of the danger of irreparable brain damage, particularly if hypoglycemia is severe, symptomatic, and prolonged, the immediate aim is to restore the level of glucose. In addition to prompt corrective action, one attempts to identify the underlying disorder. However, measures taken to correct the hypoglycemia often alter the metabolic profile and make diagnosis more difficult. Thus, if the cause of the hypoglycemia is not known, before any corrective action, one should first draw a blood sample for assay of free fatty acids, ketones, lactate, insulin, cortisol, and growth hormone.

IMMEDIATE THERAPY

Whatever the cause, intravenous administration of a solution of glucose, 0.5 gm/kg as a 25 per cent solution (2 ml/kg), effectively raises the level of glucose. If hypoglycemia is unquestionably attributable to insulin, as in the child who is treated for type I diabetes mellitus, it is often easier and just as effective to administer an intramuscular injection of glucagon, 30 μg/kg. This should be followed by a carbohydrate-rich meal. Further management then depends on the cause and is directed at preventing recurrence of the hypoglycemia.

LONG-TERM THERAPY

Here the approach depends on the underlying disorder. We divide these into two broad functional categories—those that cause hypoglycemia primarily by reducing the release of glucose from the liver and those that give rise to hypoglycemia because of enhanced utilization of glucose.

Decreased Release of Glucose from the Liver

Glycogenosis Types Ia and Ib. The constraint on the release of glucose from the liver caused by inactivity of the enzyme glucose-6-phosphatase in type Ia or of the translocase in type Ib results in severe postabsorptive hypoglycemia. What glucose is produced by the liver is generated by an alternating flow between lactate and glycogen which replenishes the 1,6 branch points. These are released as glucose through the action of amylo-1,6-glucosidase. Therapy is aimed at putting the liver at rest in terms of need to produce glucose by providing a constant supply of exogenous glucose. In infancy this is achieved by feeds at regular intervals during the day of a formula providing approximately 60 to 70 per cent of the calories as carbohydrates. Fructose and galactose should be avoided, as these can only give rise to glucose after undergoing the same shuttle process.

The interval between feeds is determined by monitoring the level of glucose just prior to a feed. During the night a continuous infusion of Vivonex, Polycose, or other glucose polymer, given through a fine nasogastric tube to provide 6 to 10 mg/kg/min of glucose should sustain the levels of glucose. Adequacy of the delivery of glucose may be ascertained by monitoring the level of glucose.

It is important that the infusion not be interrupted and, again to avoid symptomatic hypoglycemia, that the first morning feed after discontinuation of the infusion be given without delay. Beyond infancy, intervals between feeds can be lengthened to about 6 hours by administering the glucose in the form of a suspension of uncooked corn starch, between 1.5 and 3 gm/kg/dose. Monitoring glucose levels just prior to feeding enables one to determine the precise interval between feeds.

Glycogenosis Type III; Amylo-1,6-Glucosidase Inactivity. The liver glycogen proximal to the outermost 1,6 branch points constitutes the major part of the total liver glycogen and is unavailable for release as glucose. In younger patients hypoglycemia occurs if breakfast is omitted or if, because of an intercurrent infection, caloric intake is reduced. Management is to ensure that breakfast is not unduly delayed nor feeding neglected during an illness.

Fructose-1,6-Diphosphatase Deficiency. In this rare disorder glucose can be released from glycogen and formed from galactose, but the pathways from lactate, glycerol, and fructose to glucose are blocked. Fasting results in severe hypoglycemia. Therapy consists of the provision of carbohydrate-containing meals at regular intervals. The duration between feeds is determined by measurement of the glucose levels prior to a feed. Fructose should be excluded from the diet. The corn starch regimen may also be employed in these patients.

Fructosemia (Fructose-1-Phosphate Aldolase Deficiency) and Galactosemia (Galactose-1-Phosphate Uridyl Transferase Deficiency). In each case ingestion of the offending sugar results in impaired release of glu-

cose from the liver and hypoglycemia. Management consists of avoiding the particular sugar. Simply omitting milk in the case of galactosemia or sugar and fruit in fructosemia is not enough, as both milk and sugar are commonly added to a large array of foods. Kosher breads and cookies are free of milk and are useful in managing the child with galactosemia. In fructosemia dietary management is complicated not only by the ubiquitous presence of sugar in so many prepared foods and drinks but also by its existence in a variety of vegetables. One needs close involvement of a knowledgeable nutritionist in both cases. The parents are also urged to read the content label of any prepared food that is given.

Pyruvate Carboxylase Inactivity. In these patients the conversion of glycerol, fructose, and galactose to glucose is unimpeded, as is the release of glucose from glycogen, but recycling of lactate to glucose is hindered and hypoglycemia occurs on fasting. Here, too, feeds should be given regularly and promptly. The use of uncooked corn starch also has a place by allowing a longer interval between feeds. As in the other hypoglycemic disorders, it is especially important to maintain carbohydrate intake during intercurrent illnesses.

Hyperinsulinemia

Hyperinsulinemia results in hypoglycemia by suppressing hepatic release of glucose as well as by increasing glucose use. The two major forms of hyperinsulinemia in children are the hypoglycemia occurring in patients with type I diabetes mellitus and the hypoglycemia of nesidioblastosis.

Hypoglycemia in children with diabetes mellitus requires prompt intervention. If the child is conscious and able to swallow, a sweetened drink may be given. If the patient is unable to swallow, administration of glucagon, 30 μg/kg IM, should not be delayed. Parents should be familiar with and comfortable with the use of glucagon, which also should be available for use, if needed, by the school nurse. Total prevention of hypoglycemia may not be attainable in the most tightly regulated patients, but the incidence can be lessened by not omitting meals and by the intake of a carbohydrate-containing snack just before participating in any vigorous or prolonged physical activity.

Nesidioblastosis is the most devastating form of hypoglycemia in infancy and also the most difficult to manage. Once it is diagnosed, therapy should begin promptly. A central line is placed to facilitate uninterrupted infusion of a solution of glucose to provide glucose at a rate of 12 mg/kg/min or more. The line permits use of a more concentrated solution, 10 to 20 per cent, than can be administered for prolonged periods through a peripheral vein. The concentrated solution also avoids the excessive volumes of fluid that must be given if a more dilute solution of glucose is used.

In addition to the administration of intravenous glucose, treatment consists of the use of diazoxide 8 to 15 mg/kg/24 hours in three equally divided doses at 8-hour intervals. Glucose levels should be monitored at regular intervals. If glucose levels are sustained for several days, attempts are made to gradually reduce the rate of infusion.

In milder cases it is possible, with continued use of diazoxide, to discontinue the intravenous glucose. However, the need for diazoxide persists and its use should be continued, sometimes for years. Side effects include water retention, excessive hair growth, and hyperuricemia.

In these patients, too, meals must be given regularly and every effort made to maintain intake during periods of illness. The use of uncooked corn starch is also of help in sustaining the levels of glucose.

In more severely affected subjects any slowing of the delivery of glucose causes glucose levels to decline. Just how long one can wait is uncertain, but if after 2 weeks the needed rate of infusion of glucose has not decreased, the next step is a subtotal pancreatectomy. In the most severe cases, initial removal of as much as 90 per cent of the pancreas may be inadequate, and excision of even more becomes necessary. Diabetes mellitus, temporary or permanent, is a complication.

Several recent reports describe benefit from the use of SMS201-995, a long-acting somatostatin analogue that is effective in suppressing the secretion of insulin. At present this form of therapy is still considered investigational.

Increased Utilization of Glucose

Impaired ability to generate or use ketones results in greater use of glucose and hypoglycemia. Disorders in this category include palmitoyl-CoA transferase deficiency, long-chain acyl-CoA dehydrogenase deficiency, medium-chain acyl-CoA dehydrogenase deficiency, multiple acyl-CoA dehydrogenase deficiencies, and hydroxymethylglutaryl-CoA lyase deficiency. Of these disorders, medium-chain acyl-CoA dehydrogenase deficiency, which mimics and may be mistaken for Reye syndrome, occurs most frequently.

In all of these the ability to generate ketones is impaired. Hypoglycemia occurs at the times that ketones would normally be produced and used—when fasting and when caloric intake is diminished during illness.

Therapy consists of the intravenous administration of a solution of glucose in amounts sufficient to raise the level of glucose to the normal range. The precise amount should be ascertained by careful monitoring of the levels of glucose. The appropriate therapy, in theory, would be to provide ketones, but in practice, with two possible exceptions, the mainstay of treatment is to administer glucose. The possible exceptions are inactivity of long-chain palmitoyl-CoA transferase I and of long-chain acyl-CoA dehydrogenase. In these two rare disorders, supplements of medium-chain triglyceride should be beneficial by giving rise to ketones. The medium-chain fatty acids enter into the mitochondria directly, bypassing the need for transferase activity, and are oxidized without the mediation of long-chain dehydrogenase activity. However, even in these two disorders it may be easier to proceed directly with the provision of glucose.

Once liver glycogen is depleted, in the virtual absence of ketones, the sole fuel for the brain is intravenously administered glucose. Until recovery occurs and nourishment can be taken by mouth, glucose infusion should be uninterrupted and in sufficient quantity to maintain glucose levels in the normal range.

Beta-ketothiolase and succinyl CoA-transferase deficiencies affect the ability to utilize rather than to generate ketones. Once again, hypoglycemia occurs during fasting. Prevention of recurrences depends on ensuring that carbohydrate intake is maintained, particularly during illness.

HORMONAL DEFICIENCIES

Hypoglycemia is often the presenting feature of hypopituitarism in the newborn. It can also be caused by adrenal insufficiency and by isolated growth hormone lack. Once the hormonal deficiency(ies) is identified, replacement therapy is given. In the case of growth hormone deficiency, conventional therapy consists of injections of growth hormone three times a week. However, in some cases so treated hypoglycemia has been noted approximately 48 hours after the last injection. Should this occur, the same total weekly dose divided and given daily has prevented the appearance of hypoglycemia. Replacement therapy if cortisol is lacking consists of 10 to 15 mg/m^2 of hydrocortisone divided into two doses.

Finally, it should be stressed that young children as a group are prone to become hypoglycemic if fasted (ketotic hypoglycemia) or if caloric intake is severely compromised during an illness. Because of this particular vulnerability of children, care should always be taken to prevent any prolonged interruption to the nutritional needs of the child.

DIABETES INSIPIDUS

SHARON E. OBERFIELD, M.D.

Diabetes insipidus (DI) is a disorder in the ability of the body to conserve water. *Central* diabetes insipidus results from an inadequate secretion of antidiuretic hormone (ADH) for a given state of hyperosmolality. *Nephrogenic* diabetes insipidus is due to an impaired renal response to appropriate levels of ADH. The clinical hallmarks of DI are marked polyuria and compensatory polydipsia. In infancy, growth failure and fever of unknown origin can be the presenting signs of DI. If patients have both an intact thirst mechanism and free access to water, most are able to maintain a normal state of hydration by simply drinking large amounts of water. Practically, this is unacceptable, as frequent urination and excessive thirst are not usually compatible with the performance of normal daytime activities. Further, the excessive urination frequently results in the disruption of normal sleep patterns. In childhood, a reduction of urinary flow to acceptable levels and relief of nocturia with return to a normal sleep pattern are the major goals of treatment.

TREATMENT

DDAVP (1-Deamino-8-D-Arginine Vasopressin). This synthetic compound is degraded more slowly and has enhanced antidiuretic activity and decreased pressor activity compared with native vasopressin. There are intranasal and injectable preparations. The intranasal preparation is administered by a soft flexible plastic tube that has dose marks at 0.2, 0.15, 0.1, and 0.05 ml. Each milliliter is equivalent to 0.1 mg. In a young child or an infant, an adult will need to blow the solution into the child's nose using the provided rhinyle. The usual starting dose is 5 μg (0.05 ml) at night. This may provide satisfactory control or may need to be repeated every 12 or every 8 hours. Alternatively, the evening dose may be increased and allow for a greater duration of action. Most children can be controlled on 2.5 to 10 μg (0.025 to 0.1 ml) of DDAVP once or twice daily. Doses in premature infants of 1 to 2 μg/kg have provided effective antidiuresis. Dilution of the DDAVP 1:10 in normal saline allows for administration of these very small doses. In the very young infant, care should be taken not to overload the child with fluid during treatment. Nasal congestion and/or rhinitis may interfere with administration of the drug and cause erratic absorption. DDAVP should be kept refrigerated, but closed sterile bottles maintain stability for 3 weeks at room temperature.

Intravenous or subcutaneous DDAVP is useful when a patient is undergoing transsphenoidal surgery with postoperative nasal packing or has had major head trauma that may have obliterated access of the nasal passages. In this preparation 1 ml provides 4 μg of DDAVP. In adults, the recommended daily dose is 2 to 4 μg (0.5 to 1.0 ml). In infants and children, 0.5 μg or 0.125 ml subcutaneously can be used as a starting dose and the effects can last 12 hours or more.

Recently, DDAVP was given sublingually as a single daily dose of 2 μg to a child who had a marked facial deformity. In Europe, DDAVP has also been given orally in tablet form. The tablet was most effective if given three times a day in a dose that was 10 to 40 times greater than that used by the nasal route (100 to 400 μg three times a day). The duration of action appears to be shorter than by the intranasal route of administration. It is possible that this will be a preferred route of administration in the future, especially in the visually impaired child. However, this is not yet available in the United States.

Aqueous Pitressin. This compound has a short duration of action and can be given by intramuscular or subcutaneous injection every 3 to 4 hours. In adults, 5 to 10 units (0.25 to 0.5 ml) is usually an appropriate starting dose. In children, starting doses should be proportionately reduced. Use of continuous intravenous vasopressin is limited to the ICU setting. The dose is variable and has been reported as 0.5 mU/kg/min. The effects are reversed promptly with discontinuation of the infusion. Inasmuch as the intravenous infusion results in prompt reversal of diuresis, extreme care, especially in the comatose patient, must be taken to prevent water intoxication.

Synthetic-8-Lysine Vasopressin (Diapid). Until the introduction of DDAVP, this had been the most useful nasal preparation. It has a short duration of action. The dose is variable, one to two sniffs in one or both nostrils. The action lasts 4 to 6 hours. A combination of Diapid with a dose of DDAVP at night may be efficacious in some children.

Pitressin Tannate in Oil. Currently this preparation is rarely used in children because of prolonged action and inherent risk of water intoxication. The dose is 0.25 to 1 ml per dose.

Chlorpropamide. This is an oral hypoglycemic agent that is believed to enhance the renal response to vasopressin. Because of its hypoglycemic effects, it is not routinely recommended for use in children, although it can be an effective adjunct to therapy with vasopressin preparations. A dose of 150 mg/m^2 can be given daily.

Thiazide Diuretics. These agents act paradoxically to reduce urinary output in patients with nephrogenic diabetes insipidus. They aid in water retention by inducing a sodium diuresis that is associated with an increase in the reabsorption of fluid from the proximal tubule. In children, use of diluted formula should accompany this regimen as well.

SPECIAL CONSIDERATIONS IN THE MANAGEMENT OF INFANTS AND CHILDREN WITH DISORDERS OF WATER BALANCE

Most pediatric patients with DI can be maintained chronically on relatively constant doses of medication without major problems. Indeed, even if there is a change in the duration of action of the prescribed medication, as long as the child has intact thirst, water balance is maintained. Parents must be advised to be alert to changes in urinary output. If a child has not voided for more than 24 hours, then families should be instructed to contact the physician for evaluation and to avoid excessive fluid intake until the child starts to urinate again. The urine output of children who are diapered with the new "super-absorbent" diapers may be difficult to ascertain and thus use of "old-fashioned" paper or cloth diapers should be considered in these children. Frequent colds may interfere with nasal absorption of DDAVP and cause unpredictability of the onset and duration of action of the antidiuretic effects of this preparation. In the past, initiation of treatment often required hospitalization. Most parents can be taught to measure urine output and to identify concentrated versus nonconcentrated urine by visual inspection, and thus treatment may be initiated without hospitalization of the child in a compliant and cooperative family setting.

RICKETS

SUSAN M. SCOTT, M.D.

Rickets, a disease of the growing bones, came under control in the early 20th century with the discovery that vitamin D prevents this disease. It became a health problem once again with the advent of neonatal intensive care units. Defined as a decrease in the mineral/osteoid ratio of bone, rickets becomes evident in a prematurely delivered neonate only when good linear growth is obtained. Only then do the poor mineral/osteoid ratios of infants born early in the third trimester of pregnancy and our inability to mimic intrauterine calcium to phosphorus (Ca/P) accretion rates become limiting factors in normal bony development. This usually becomes evident only after a premature infant is returned to a secondary care center for growth before discharge. Beyond the newborn period, rickets is usually linked to genetic causes (discussed later), although infants exposed to little sunlight and abnormal diets may present with nutritional rickets.

NEONATAL PERIOD

In premature infants being fed the newer generation, especially adapted formulas, inadequate Ca/P accretion leading to rickets is not a problem. There are, however, large numbers of premature infants who have as their sources of calories breast milk, full-term formulas, and/or TPN (total parental nutrition) for whom rickets is a potential disease. The pediatrician should strive for a goal of supplying 400 IU of vitamin D a day. Yet with the frequent combinations of different caloric sources used, it may be impossible to calculate the amounts of Ca/P being given. A few warnings will help at least to anticipate the infants who are at risk. Breast milk from mothers who have delivered low birth weight infants is inadequate in Ca/P for their infants. There are breast milk fortifiers (1 packet per 25 cc or 50 cc), which add calories, sodium, and Ca/P and can be used to compensate for the inadequacies of such breast milk. Soy formulas, which are not recommended for long-term use in premature infants, have decreased bioavailable Ca/P. TPN not particularly designed for premature infants may also be deficient in Ca/P. Finally, diuretics, such as furosemide, when used chronically in premature infants, may be a significant cause of urinary calcium loss.

Surveillance for signs of osteopenia or rickets includes bimonthly ionized calcium (1.1 to 1.4 mmol/L) and phosphorus (5 to 10 mg/dl) measurements and alkaline phosphatase levels. This should begin when adequate calories and good linear growth have been established for several weeks. A normal range for alkaline phosphatase is more difficult to define, since active growth will increase alkaline phosphatase three to five times the normal adult values. Rising alkaline phosphatase over two or three measurements is probably an indication of inadequate Ca/P or vitamin D nutrition. If measurements are done only after good growth has been established, the normal increase in alkaline phosphatase will not be confusing. Vitamin D metabolites are not easy to measure or interpret, and radiographs are usually helpful only when an experienced neonatal radiologist is available.

The signs and symptoms of rickets, which include frontal bossing, rachitic rosary, and limb and rib deformities, as well as apathy, hypotonia, and weakness, should alert the practitioner to potential rickets in an infant or child but should be anticipated and prevented in the premature infant. In infants who may become chronic lung patients, hypotonia and rib deformities leading to a worsening of their pulmonary status must be prevented, since the limb and rib deformities of rickets will take months to years to correct.

VITAMIN D–DEPENDENT AND VITAMIN D–RESISTANT RICKETS

The genetic forms of rickets present as growth failure frequently because of an increasingly inadequate mineral:osteoid ratio, which slows linear growth outside of the newborn period. The two forms most frequently seen, vitamin D–dependent and vitamin D–resistant rickets, are both poorly descriptive names for these disorders. Vitamin D–dependent rickets (autosomal recessive), probably secondary to a deficiency of the 1α-hydroxylase enzyme for the production of 1,25-dihydroxyvitamin D (calcitriol), presents with tetany/convulsions and growth failure. It responds well to large doses of vitamin D (10,000 to 100,000 IU/day) or to 1 to 2 μg of calcitriol daily. Vitamin D–resistant rickets (also called X-linked hypophosphatemic rickets) is caused by a renal leak of phosphate of unclear etiology. This type of rickets causes growth failure, and although convulsions are uncommon and successful treatment of the rickets with vitamin D (10,000 to 50,000 IU/day) and oral phosphate (Neutra-Phos 450 to 600 ml/day) can be obtained, this therapy does not prevent short stature. As can be seen by the dosage ranges given and the real complication of hypercalcemia with overdosage, it is recommended that the care of these children be undertaken with the assistance of a pediatric endocrinologist.

RICKETS WITH ANTICONVULSANT THERAPY

This form of rickets, thought to be secondary to increased production of inactive vitamin D metabolites in the liver, is treated with 50 to 100 μg/day of 25-hydroxyvitamin D.

RICKETS AND FANCONI'S SYNDROME AND RENAL TUBULAR ACIDOSIS

Although the causes of Fanconi's syndrome are multiple, phosphaturia and vitamin D deficiency are commonly associated findings. Replacement of phosphate, correction of acidosis, and the addition of up to 25,000 to 50,000 IU of vitamin D are often required to treat the bone disease. Rickets associated with renal tubular acidosis usually responds to correction of the acidosis.

TETANY

SUSAN M. SCOTT, M.D.

The possible etiologies and therapies for tetany are dependent on the age of onset as well as on the ion involved (calcium, magnesium, or hydrogen). The end result is a hyperexcitable state of the peripheral and central nervous systems leading to muscular spasms and seizures.

NEONATAL PERIOD

Symptoms presenting within the first weeks of life are usually related to the hypocalcemia of prematurity, the various forms of hypoparathyroidism, or hypomagnesemia of a nutritional source.

Tetany is rarely seen or recognized in a premature infant but is readily treated with calcium gluconate, 200 mg/kg (2 ml/kg) given by intravenous injection at 1 ml/minute while observing the heart rate for signs of bradycardia. With the institution of feedings, this problem will resolve.

Hypoparathyroidism. The causes of hypoparathyroidism include a transient form of unknown etiology, maternal hyperparathyroidism, and a permament, but usually incomplete, absence of parathyroid function in isolated disease or as a component of DiGeorge's syndrome. The net result of each cause is hypocalcemia with hyperphosphatemia. Treatment is with enrichment of calcium and/or decrease in phosphorus in the diet, usually by the addition of calcium gluconate to the formula. This will continue usually for several days to months.

Transient Hypoparathyroidism. This hypocalcemia used to be described only in infants on cow's milk feedings because of its high phosphorus content. Since this is probably due to a relative dysfunction in PTH secretion, it can be seen with normal phosphorus load formulas. The result of PTH dysfunction is a retention of phosphorus that inhibits the production of 1,25-dihydroxyvitamin D and thus decreases the absorption of calcium.

Maternal Hyperparathyroidism. A search for maternal disease must be considered when an infant presents with signs of hypoparathyroidism. Most patients with true hyperparathyroidism will have calcium concentrations within the normal ranges but consistently high-normal on repeat measurements. If maternal disease is found, the infant may require weeks of therapy, but parathyroid function will usually return to normal.

Congenital (Permanent) Hypoparathyroidism. This cause of hypocalcemia does not respond to calcium alone and requires large doses of vitamin D. In DiGeorge's syndrome, the low-set ears and cardiac anomalies, such as interrupted aortic arch, may be the presenting features. Also, immunologic abnormalities secondary to thymic aplasia or dysfunction are usually more life threatening than the parathyroid dysfunction leading to tetany.

For treatment in the neonate, the calcium gluconate preparation used for intravenous therapy can be given by mouth and will avoid the hyperosmolar insult of high concentrations of sucrose in the oral preparations, which will cause diarrhea in the dosages necessary for therapy.

Hypomagnesemic Tetany. The neonate with this cause of tetany will often have a mother with diabetes mellitus or with a poor diet, particularly as seen in alcoholism. Intramuscular injection of 50 per cent solution of $MgSO_4$ in a dosage of 0.1 to 0.2 ml/kg will correct both the magnesium and the hypocalcemia that accompany this disorder.

INFANCY AND CHILDHOOD

Tetany beginning outside of the neonatal period may be related to vitamin D disorders, primary hypomagnesemia of infancy, and alkalosis.

The vitamin D disorders described under rickets may have tetany associated with them. They are treated acutely with intravenous calcium (as above) and large doses of vitamin D (500,000 units over 24 hours).

Primary hypomagnesemia is usually secondary to an intestinal absorption abnormality and requires 500 to 2000 mg of magnesium per day in divided doses.

Tetany of alkalosis is usually due to hyperventilation and can be treated by rebreathing into a paper bag.

IDIOPATHIC HYPERCALCEMIA

F. BRUDER STAPLETON, M.D.

Hypercalcemia is defined as a total serum calcium concentration greater than 11.0 mg/dl. Severe idiopathic hypercalcemia may present in early infancy as a component of the Williams "elfin facies" syndrome.

In Williams syndrome, and in most instances of idiopathic hypercalcemia, increased gastrointestinal absorption of calcium appears to be responsible for elevation of the serum calcium concentration. Therefore, dietary calcium should be minimized and any source of exogenous vitamin D intake should be avoided. Frequently, corticosteroid therapy with prednisone (1 to 2 mg/kg/day) must also be given to reduce dietary calcium absorption. Owing to the adverse effects of corticosteroids, chronic daily prednisone therapy should be avoided. A further reduction in gastrointestinal calcium absorption may be accomplished with cellulose phosphate (Calcibind, Mission Pharmaceutical, San Antonio, TX) at a dose of 10 to 15 gm/1.73 m^2/day administered with meals. Finally, increased bone resorption may contribute to hypercalcemia in some patients. Therapy with subcutaneous calcitonin at a dose of 1 to 5 units/kg every 12 hours may be beneficial. Since idiopathic hypercalcemia may be a "self-limited" condition, periodic attempts to discontinue therapy are warranted.

Neonatal hypercalcemia from parathyroid hyperplasia may occur in infants born to mothers with familial hypocalciuric hypercalcemia. Frequently, such infants are asymptomatic and no therapy is required; however, in selected infants, parathyroidectomy may be necessary.

MAGNESIUM DEFICIENCY

SE MO SUH, M.D., Ph.D.

Magnesium deficiency manifests with hypomagnesemia and clinical symptoms of neuromuscular irritability such as tremor, tetany, convulsions, cardiac arrhythmia, and mental disorientation. Frequently, hypocalcemia or hypokalemia, which are usually refractory to treatment with calcium or potassium unless magnesium therapy is added, may also occur. Normal ranges of serum magnesium levels in infants and children are 1.5 to 1.8 mEq/liter. Some of the clinical symptoms of magnesium deficiency may be manifest without obvious reduction in serum magnesium level but with tissue depletion of magnesium, particularly in patients with diminished renal glomerular filtration rate.

In acute episodes of hypomagnesemic tetany and convulsions, magnesium may be administered intravenously as 10 per cent solution of $MgSO_4$ at the dose of 0.8 mEq of Mg per kg body weight (1.0 ml/kg of 10 per cent $MgSO_4$) up to 20 ml. The infusion rate should not exceed 1.5 ml of 10 per cent $MgSO_4$ per min. This may be followed by a continuous drip of Mg at the dose of 1 mEq/kg/day up to 40 mEq/day (10 ml of 50 per cent $MgSO_4$) diluted in 5 per cent dextrose or normal saline to make up less than 10 per cent of $MgSO_4$ concentration for the first 24 hours. In severe convulsions, in addition to the initial intravenous dose, an equal dose of magnesium (0.8 to 1 mEq/kg) may be injected intramuscularly as 20 per cent (0.5 ml/kg) or 25 per cent $MgSO_4$ solution (0.5 ml/kg). The effect of a bolus dose of intravenous injection of magnesium takes place immediately and lasts about 30 minutes, whereas following intramuscular injection the onset of action occurs in about 1 hour and lasts about 3 to 4 hours. If an intravenous route is not readily available, intramuscular injection of $MgSO_4$ at the dose of 1 mEq/kg (0.5 ml/kg of 25 per cent $MgSO_4$) may be repeated every 4 to 6 hours for the first 24 hours.

Parenteral administration of magnesium solution may be continued 3 to 5 more days in one-half the dose of the first 24 hours; then the patient may be switched to oral therapy. Any form of magnesium salts shown in Table 1 may be used for this purpose. All magnesium salts in large doses tend to induce diarrhea. One should start with a smaller dose initially and increase gradually up to 2 to 3 mEq/kg/day in three to four doses.

TABLE 1. Magnesium Salt Preparations

	Amount of Salt to Make Up 100-ml Solution	Amount of Mg
Oral Solution		
Mg chloride	4 gm of $MgCl_2$ $6H_2O$	2 mEq/5 ml
Mg citrate	6 gm of $MgHC_6H_5O_7$ $5H_2O$	2 mEq/5 ml
Mg chloride and citrate	4 gm of $MgCl_2$ $6H_2O$ & 6 gm of $HgHC_6H_5O_7$ $5H_2O$	4 mEq/5 ml
Mg gluconate	4.2 gm of $MgC_{12}H_{24}O$	2 mEq/5 ml
Milk of magnesia	7 gm of $Mg(OH)_2$ (in suspension)	12 mEq/5 ml
Tablet		
Mg hydroxide		13.8 mEq/400 mg
Mg gluconate		4.8 mEq/500 mg
Parenteral Solution		
Mg SO_4 $7H_2O$	10%	0.8 mEq/ml
	20%	1.6 mEq/ml
	25%	2.0 mEq/ml
	50%	4.0 mEq/ml

Patients who waste magnesium in urine or stool require a larger dose, and patients with imparied renal glomerular filtration require as low as one-fourth the normal dose. Progress should be checked by repeated serum magnesium determinations.

ZINC DEFICIENCY

K. MICHAEL HAMBIDGE, M.D.

The occurrence of mild nutritional zinc deficiency has been documented in some infants, preschool children, and pre-adolescent children in North America. These growth-limiting zinc deficiency states can be treated with Zn^{++} 0.5 to 1.0 mg/kg/day up to a maximum of 20 mg/day for an initial period of 3 months. Secondary zinc deficiency has been reported to occur in association with a variety of conditions and disease states. The quantity of zinc required depends on the circumstances and especially on the extent of malabsorption or of excessive losses. In general, it is reasonable to start therapy with Zn^{++} 1.0 mg/kg/day, but this may need to be increased to 2.0 mg/kg/day during rapid catch-up growth or if ongoing losses are severe.

Severe acquired zinc deficiency states with acro-orificial skin lesions and other features of severe zinc deficiency are quite rare in enterally fed subjects. One circumstance in which these occur is the lethal milk syndrome, in which the mother fails to secrete a normal quantity of zinc into her milk. With only one exception, the reported cases of this syndrome have been breast-fed premature infants. Recommended initial treatment is with Zn^{++} 10 mg/day. This can be modified as necessary depending on the speed of the clinical response and the changes in plasma zinc concentrations. Once normal zinc status has been restored, continue to provide a supplement of 2 mg/day of Zn^{++} until weaning.

The autosomal recessively inherited disorder acrodermatitis enteropathica is attributable to an inherited defect in the major pathway of zinc absorption functioning at normal dietary zinc concentrations in the lumen of the gastrointestinal tract. Oral zinc therapy in quantities sufficient to compensate for the effects of this inherited molecular defect results in a rapid and complete clinical and biochemical remission, which is also sustained by zinc therapy on a life-long basis. The quantities of Zn^{++} required usually range from 30 to 50 mg/day. This dose is not related to age or size, but a smaller quantity (starting with 3 mg/kg/day) is recommended for infants.

Recommendations for maintenance intravenous zinc during total parenteral nutrition are 400 µg/kg/day of Zn^{++} for premature infants; 200 µg/kg/day for term infants aged 0 to 3 months; 100 µg/kg/day for older infants, and 50 µg/kg/day for children. In the presence of excessive losses, especially via the gastrointestinal tract, larger quantities may be needed. Plasma zinc concentrations should be monitored. For treatment of severe zinc deficiency states in patients fed intravenously, give 300 to 500 μg/kg/day of Zn^{++} until skin lesions resolve and normal plasma zinc concentrations are restored.

Copper deficiency can be induced by excessive zinc therapy. This has occurred with as little as 50 mg/day of Zn^{++} given to adults and 25 mg given to an infant for several weeks. Depression of HDL cholesterol levels may also occur with excessive zinc therapy.

Monitoring zinc therapy is important, particularly in the treatment of severe zinc deficiency states. Plasma zinc determinations in samples collected with scrupulous care to avoid contamination are reasonably adequate for this purpose in most cases.

Zinc absorption appears to be influenced very little by the choice of inorganic zinc salt. The sulfate and acetate, both of which are soluble, are among those most frequently used. A commercial preparation of zinc chloride is available for intravenous use. There is no evidence that expensive commercial preparations of zinc that are liganded to proteins or amino acids are absorbed any better. Foods have a major although variable effect on the absorption of pharmacologic quantities of zinc. Hence, for maximal absorption, zinc should be administered 1 to 2 hours before meals.

HEPATOLENTICULAR DEGENERATION
(Wilson's Disease)
OWEN M. RENNERT, M.D.

Wilson's disease may present in the pediatric patient without the classic clinical triad of Kayser-Fleischer corneal rings, hepatic cirrhosis, and neurologic dysfunction. Early diagnosis is paramount, since effective treatment may prevent irreversible organ damage and progression of the disease. Symptoms occur as early as 4 years of age, although the second and third decades are the usual ages of onset. The mode of presentation is variable, but the hepatic form is most common in childhood. Presenting symptoms may include hand tremors, slurred speech, spasticity, decreased academic performance, and behavioral disturbances. Two neurologic variants have been identified: dystonic (predominantly seen in young patients) and pseudosclerotic; the dystonic variant appears to be less responsive to therapy.

It is important to stress the wide variability of expression of Wilson's disease. This extends to age of onset, mode of presentation, severity of organ system involvement, and response to therapy. The less common manifestations, such as renal, skeletal, hematologic, and psychiatric disturbances, may occur at any time during the disease course and usually are preceded by hepatic or neurologic manifestations.

The liver is the *central* homeostatic organ for copper metabolism. Wilson's disease is characterized by a congenital inability to maintain normal copper homeostasis, with resultant accumulation in the liver and other viscera. Impaired secretion of copper via ceruloplasmin and diminished lysosomal biliary copper excretion are associated with saturation of hepatic binding capacity

and subsequent release of copper into the circulation, leading to hemolytic crisis and diffusion into the central nervous system and kidneys, giving rise to the distinctive clinical manifestations.

Therapeutic Rationale

Excessive storage of copper in viscera leads to organ system failure because the organism is unable to mobilize, utilize, and detoxify this trace metal. The principles of therapy are based upon enhancing the mobilization and excretion of copper, limiting copper intake, and monitoring the function of copper-toxic target organs. Successful therapy requires early recognition and diagnosis.

Chemotherapy is the central approach for achieving negative copper balance in patients. Penicillamine is the most effective agent utilized in the treatment of these patients.

Therapy

Penicillamine. The dosage of penicillamine used in children is related to the age of the patient. Children under 10 years of age are treated with 0.5 to 0.75 gm/day—in adults the dose is 1.0 to 1.5 gm/day. Initial dosage may be calculated as 0.02 gm/kg/day, divided into two to four doses/day. *Treatment is life-long.* Following initiation of therapy, cupruresis of 1000 to 5000 μg/24 hours may occur. Over a 4- to 6-month period, following initiation of therapy, the degree of cupruria gradually falls to approximately 1000 μg/24 hours. Because penicillamine inhibits pyridoxine-dependent enzymes, patients should be given daily supplements of 12.5 to 25.0 mg/day of vitamin B$_6$. In patients with far-advanced neurologic disease L-dopa has been proposed as adjunctive therapy. Published data identify variable success of this therapeutic maneuver.

During the life-long therapy, patients should be monitored regularly, not only for toxic side effects but also for assessment and maintenance of negative copper balance and clinical improvement. Improvement of symptomatology defines successful therapy, and demonstration on physical examination of symptom reversal usually postdates chemical laboratory evidence of betterment.

An adjunct to penicillamine therapy that has recently been proposed is the treatment of patients with orally administered zinc acetate. Zinc acetate is administered to patients at a dose of 25 to 50 mg given three times a day. This therapeutic maneuver is based on the following observations: (1) intake of supplemental zinc (zinc/copper ratio greater than 8:1 in diet) results in negative copper balance, (2) oral zinc therapy of patients with Wilson's disease leads to enhanced excretion of copper, and (3) oral zinc treatment results in induction of intestinal metallothionein, which in turn blocks absorption of copper. Since zinc therapy also competes with iron absorption, patients treated with zinc sulfate should be monitored for iron deficiency.

Patient evaluation includes regular assessment of serum copper and ceruloplasmin concentration, as well as 24-hour urinary copper excretion. Improvement of hepatic function is documented by measurement of prothrombin time, serum transaminases, and bilirubin determination. Renal function may be sequentially evaluated by measurement of serum BUN and creatinine; additionally, examination of the urine for the characteristic aminoaciduria and glycosuria seen as evidence of heavy metal intoxication (Fanconi's syndrome) is a valuable adjunct. Recent clinical studies have documented hypercalciuria as a component of the renal dysfunction seen in Wilson's disease.

Successful therapy can be confirmed by regular slit-lamp ophthalmoscopy to document disappearance or absence of the Kayser-Fleischer corneal rings, as well as absence of the "sunflower cataracts" seen in some untreated patients. Recent reports document the potential usefulness of computed tomography to evaluate central nervous system anatomy prior to and during therapy.

Hematologic manifestations occur as a consequence of the pathologic processes of Wilson's disease itself and also as a cytotoxicity of penicillamine therapy. The hemolytic crises seen have been ascribed to a variety of pathophysiologic mechanisms, including copper inhibition of erythrocyte glycolytic enzymes, direct erythrocyte membrane damage, and oxidative denaturation of hemoglobin. During hemolytic crises, patients show marked cupriuria and elevated serum copper concentrations. Thrombocytopenia and leukopenia have been reported to occur as a consequence of hypersplenism.

Thrombocytopenia may be an early sign of penicillamine cytotoxicity. Anemia or granulocytopenia may also occur. Regular evaluation of hematologic status is required. Anemia may develop during therapy as a consequence of red cell aplasia secondary to penicillamine toxicity. The toxic hematologic sequelae of penicillamine therapy are reversed by discontinuation of the drug. Early hypersensitivity reactions have occurred in one third of treated patients; however, these usually respond to gradual desensitization under steroid therapy, usually accomplished by a 2-week discontinuation of penicillamine. Subsequently, the patient is started on half the calculated penicillamine dose in addition to 20 mg/day of prednisone. The steroid therapy is continued for 2 weeks; then the penicillamine dosage is gradually increased. In certain instances penicillamine dosage may have to be reduced to 50 mg/day for 7 days, rather than the simple 50 per cent reduction, and then gradually increased.

In the past decade clinical reports have identified undesirable side effects of penicillamine therapy. These toxicities are seen infrequently; however, the nature of the reactions is diverse. Descriptions in the literature include nephrotic syndrome, immunocomplex nephritis, immune system alterations (including lupus erythematosus–like syndrome, alterations in T-cell and B-cell function), lymphadenitis, dermatologic manifestations (including elastosis perforans serpiginosa, papular eruptions, and cutis hyperelastica), myasthenia-like syndrome, defects in retinal pigmentary epithelium, and Goodpasture's syndrome. These have remitted following discontinuation of penicillamine therapy.

Alternate chemotherapy is available for the patient who develops toxic side reactions to penicillamine and who cannot be desensitized to this drug. The newly developed copper-chelator triene-2 HCl (triethylene tetramine dihydrochloride)* has been shown to be a safe alternative for the treatment of Wilson's disease.

Other Considerations

To minimize copper deposition, dietary restriction of copper should be advocated. Foods high in copper that should be limited or excluded from the diet are liver, nuts, chocolate, cocoa, mushrooms, brain, shellfish, and broccoli. The average American ingests approximately 3.5 to 5.0 mg of copper per day; the patient with Wilson's disease should ingest no more than 1.5 mg per day.

Because of successful therapy of patients with Wilson's disease, it has become necessary to recognize the potential teratogenic action of penicillamine when used during the reproductive period. Penicillamine crosses the placental barrier. Considerations relating to its potential detrimental effect on the fetus are based upon three factors: (1) the drug's capacity to increase solubility of collagen and decrease intramolecular cross-linking, (2) its ability to chelate copper (and potentially other trace metals) and make it unavailable to the fetus, and (3) its structural antagonism to pyridoxine-dependent enzymes. Thus, penicillamine dosage should be kept as low as possible when used in the pregnant woman.

Supportive therapy is directed at palliation and minimization of the handicaps that are a consequence of irreparable damage from copper toxicosis. These relate to treatment and rehabilitation of the neurologic sequelae and management of hepatic damage and cirrhosis. Treatment of the agitation and emotional instability has involved use of benzodiazepine and phenothiazine derivatives. Treatment of movement disorders has consisted of use of trihexyphenidyl and related drugs. In the past few years two patients have been treated with liver transplantation. This is consistent with the premise that the central metabolic defect of Wilson's disease is expressed in the liver. This therapeutic maneuver is reserved for the patient with irreversible cirrhosis as a consequence of copper toxicosis.

---

*Investigational drug, not commercially available in the United States.

HYPERPHENYLALANINEMIAS

STANLEY BERLOW, M.D.,
and VIRGINIA E. SCHUETT, M.S.

The hyperphenylalaninemias are a heterogeneous group of autosomal recessive hereditary metabolic diseases that should be identified by newborn screening. Persistent hyperphenylalaninemia, without elevation of other plasma amino acids, is most commonly secondary to a deficiency of phenylalanine hydroxylase. Multiple allelic mutations in the gene for phenylalanine hydroxylase (PH) and compound heterozygosity probably account for the range of decreased phenylalanine activity and the degree of hyperphenylalaninemia. For therapeutic purposes, Table 1 is an operational classification of these defects in phenylalanine hydroxylase. The incidence of these types of PH deficiency vary. In populations of North European ancestry about 1:10,000 newborn infants who are screened for PKU will require treatment, i.e., will have classic or variant PKU.

During the past 10 years, hyperphenylalaninemia secondary to dihydropteridine reductase deficiency and biopterin synthesis defects has been recognized. Much lower than that of phenylalanine hydroxylase deficiency, the exact incidence of these disorders is not known but has been estimated to be 1 to 3 per cent of all hyperphenylalaninemic infants. Treatment for these two groups of conditions is quite different from hyperphenylalaninemia secondary to phenylalanine hydroxylase deficiency.

PHENYLALANINE HYDROXYLASE DEFICIENCY

Principles of Nutritional Management

Although other possible modes of treating phenylketonuria (PKU) have been suggested, there is currently no effective alternative to dietary manipulation.

Since phenylalanine is an essential amino acid, the primary goals of PKU therapy are to restrict dietary phenylalanine intake to the minimum required for growth and to avoid any excess that could compromise development. This balance of phenylalanine must be maintained, and at the same time an adequate intake of essential amino acids, protein, energy, and other nutrients must be assured. Needs of persons with PKU are presumed to be approximately the same as for normal individuals for all dietary components.

Following a decision to initiate diet therapy, whether the child has classic PKU or a variant form, the immediate goal is to lower the serum phenylalanine level to a therapeutic range as quickly as possible. Age at initial treatment is a strong predictor of the child's eventual I.Q.; infants treated within the first several weeks of life will have the best chance of achieving their expected intellectual potential.

Because of the variability in expression of the disease, the necessity for tailoring the diet to each infant's individual needs, the importance of frequent monitoring, and the ongoing need for family counseling, PKU can best be managed by experienced clinicians. In order for optimal therapy to be started immediately, prompt referral to one of over 100 specialized treatment centers in the United States should be made for any infant with an elevated blood phenylalanine level.*

A therapeutic range for serum phenylalanine levels is generally considered to be 2 to 8 mg/dl in young infants, and up to 10 mg/dl for older children. There is evidence from the National Collaborative Study of Children Treated for PKU (1967 to 1984) that loss of dietary control at young ages is related to a deficit in the intellectual performance of the PKU child compared with the performance of siblings or parents. Children who maintain good control have I.Q. and school achievement scores that are no different from those of their normal siblings. Maintaining blood phenylalanine levels of children with PKU in the normal range of 1 to 2 mg/dl can result in severe phenylalanine deficiency and lead to poor growth, dermatitis, brain damage, and death. Frequent monitoring of blood phenylalanine levels is essential to avoid a deficient or toxic intake of phenylalanine.

Phenylalanine constitutes approximately 3 to 5 per cent of all protein, and it is not possible to design a diet based only on natural foods that is sufficiently limited in total phenylalanine yet nutritionally adequate. Formulas very low in, or free of, phenylalanine are available to substitute nutritionally for those foods that must be eliminated owing to their high protein/phenylalanine content (including milk, meat, fish, eggs, cheese, nuts, and legumes).

Formulas available in the United States now include Lofenalac* (a casein hydrolysate containing a small amount of phenylalanine), and Phenyl-Free,* PKU 1,† PKU 2, Maxamaid XP,‡ and Maxamum XP‡ (all synthetic amino acid preparations devoid of phenylalanine). Lofenalac and Phenyl-Free are currently the most commonly used formulas for infants and older children, respectively. They provide 80 to 90 per cent or more of the child's requirement for protein, vitamins, and minerals and up to 75 per cent or more of energy needs. PKU 1 (for infants) and PKU 2, Maxamaid XP, and Maxamum XP (for older children) are primarily protein supplements with added vitamins and minerals, with insignificant amounts of carbohydrate and fat. The amino acid pattern in PKU 1 corresponds more closely to that of human milk than Lofenalac. When prescribing PKU 1, PKU 2, Maxamaid XP, or Maxamum XP, great care must be taken to ensure that adequate calories are provided by low phenylalanine dietary sources of fat and carbohydrate. For young infants, fat in the form of corn oil and carbohydrate as dextrose, dextrimaltose, cornstarch, or preparations of glucose polymers (such as Polycose or Dietary Specialties Caloric Supplement) should be added directly to the formula powder.

Use of PKU 2, Maxamaid XP, or Maxamum XP for the older child allows flexibility in adjusting caloric intake for those who are gaining weight too rapidly; for

TABLE 1. Classifications of Defects in Phenylalanine Hydroxylase

	Phenylalanine Level (mg/dl)	Risk of Mental Retardation	Need for Treatment
Classical PKU	>20	High	All
Variant PKU	10–20	Low–Moderate	Most
Benign hyperphenyl-alaninemia	<10	0	0

---

*Treatment Programs for PKU and Selected Other Metabolic Diseases in the United States: A Survey. DHHS Publication No. (HRSA) 83-5296, 1983.

*Mead Johnson Company, Nutritional Division, Evansville, Indiana 47721.

†Milupa Corporation, 397 Old Post Road, Darien, Connecticut 06820.

‡Scientific Hospital Supplies, Inc., P.O. Box 117, Gaithersburg, Maryland 20877.

children who dislike formula, protein, vitamin, and mineral needs can be met by a much smaller volume than with either Lofenalac or Phenyl-Free.

All six formulas are expensive, costing from $1000 to $7000 per year depending on the child's age and consumption. Some states still provide formula free of charge. In many states they are available only through PKU treatment centers. When reconstituted with water, the formulas look much like regular milk or infant formula. These formulas have a very objectionable flavor for the unaccustomed, but for children begun on formula in infancy, acceptance is generally good to excellent given competent parental management in the home.

Because any of the PKU formulas alone will not provide a child with adequate phenylalanine in infancy, natural protein is added to the formula as measured quantities of milk or infant formula. Solid foods are introduced at normal ages (4 to 6 months) and gradually substituted for the added milk or infant formula. Low phenylalanine foods are allowed in small weighed and measured amounts, including fruits, vegetables, small cereal and grain products, and a variety of special low-protein products. Phenylalanine-free foods such as carbonated beverages and Popsicles are allowed as needed for energy and at parental discretion. Any food or drug containing the sweetener NutraSweet (aspartame) should be carefully avoided by children with PKU owing to the high phenylalanine content. There are cookbooks and food lists of phenylalanine content available to families from PKU treatment centers.

A PKU diet prescription will include recommendations for phenylalanine intake from foods, formula preparation instructions, and a minimum average formula intake. Formula is fed at the normal dilution (20 kcal/oz) during infancy, but is gradually concentrated to 30 to 45 kcal/oz as the child's protein and energy needs increase.

In recent years, partial breast-feeding of infants supplemented by PKU formula has been successfully carried out by a growing number of motivated mothers. Mature human breast milk is significantly lower in phenylalanine (mean 41 mg/dl) compared with infant formulas (mean 75 mg/dl) or cow's milk (159 mg/dl), and it may be used to provide the additional phenylalanine traditionally provided by milk or infant formula. Individual variability in breast milk phenylalanine content is great, however, and content decreases gradually with duration of lactation. Breast milk analysis for phenylalanine at intervals and more frequent analysis of the child's blood phenylalanine levels may be necessary. The infant's intake of phenylalanine can be estimated from the mother's breast milk phenylalanine content and by weighing the infant before and after feeding. Alternatively, a specified number of breast feedings may be prescribed. Usually two to four breast feedings are possible, with supplemental formula feedings. A guide to breast-feeding infants with PKU is available.

Serum phenylalanine levels in the newborn period are typically lowered to the therapeutic range within 2 to 7 days when formula without an added source of natural protein is fed. On such a phenylalanine-deficient regimen, the blood level will fall at a rate of approximately 7 to 9 mg/dl/24 hr. In the past, initial therapy has often been instituted in the hospital. More recently, many centers manage the neonate as an outpatient. This requires intensive parental education, counseling, and cooperation plus the utilization of frequent, mailed capillary blood samples for phenylalanine analysis.

After the serum phenylalanine level has dropped below 8 mg/dl, the infant's individual tolerance of phenylalanine must be established through weekly monitoring, in combination with diet intake records. Optimal dietary phenylalanine intake can sometimes be quickly determined, but in some infants this can take weeks or months of minor dietary phenylalanine adjustments. Individual phenylalanine needs are extremely variable, depending on factors such as residual enzyme activity, growth rate, and age.

Infants, including those with PKU, generally require phenylalanine at 60 to 90 mg/kg in the newborn period, with a rapid drop to less than 20 mg/kg by 1 year of age, and by late childhood to less than 10 mg/kg. Milk supplements and food intake must be frequently adjusted, especially during the first year of life, when growth is most rapid. As a toddler, the child with "classic" PKU will be able to consume no more than approximately 10 per cent of the average amount of phenylalanine consumed by normal children of the same age, and formula will continue to supply up to 90 per cent of total nutritional needs. Children with a variant form of PKU may tolerate a somewhat more liberal diet.

Even with good parental management of the diet and appropriate recommendations from specialized health care professionals, many factors can adversely influence serum phenylalanine levels. Fluctuations in appetite or formula refusal, leading to inadequate energy, protein, or essential amino acid intake; physical trauma; and even minor illness can cause elevations in phenylalanine levels. Prompt attention to ear infections and other common childhood illnesses is essential to avoid prolonged high blood levels.

Despite the severe dietary restrictions and requirements of the diet, children with PKU fall within growth norms for age, suggesting that protein and energy intakes meet acceptable levels when the diet is properly managed. Further, vitamin and mineral supplements are unnecessary when formula consumption is adequate to meet protein needs. There are indications that for some trace minerals, intake or utilization of children on the diet may be lower than that of normal children, but the clinical significance of these findings has not been proven. No nutritional deficiencies have been documented in children on these formulas during the past 15 years.

Duration of Nutritional Management

In the past, the routine practice of most clinicians in the United States was to discontinue diet at early school age (5 to 8 years). In recent years, an increasing accumulation of follow-up data on children who discontinued diet at these ages has documented the risk of terminating diet. Problems reported post discontinuation, when blood phenylalanine levels typically range from 20 to 40 mg/dl, have included significant drops in I.Q., poor school performance, mood and behavior changes, EEG abnormalities, and eczema. Data from 119 children enrolled in the National Collaborative Study of Children Treated for PKU confirm that deficits in intellectual performance and on school achievement tests are more likely to occur in children whose levels are consistently above 15 mg/dl before the age of 8 years. Data on children beyond age 8 is incomplete. Levels somewhat lower than 15 mg/dl, especially if these occur early in life, may also place the child at greater risk.

A number of clinics have attempted to reinstitute diet, and significant improvement has been noted in some children. However, few patients have been able to achieve mean blood phenylalanine levels of 10 mg/dl or less, and many have not been able to tolerate returning to diet at all.

In a 1983 survey of diet termination practices, two-thirds of 90 clinics treating PKU recommended indefinite maintenance of diet, a growing trend both nationwide and worldwide. Experience with on-diet older children and teenagers points to the difficulty but also the feasibility of following a phenylalanine-restricted diet into adulthood.

Education

For the difficult PKU diet regimen to be successful, parents and the entire family (including grandparents) need to understand and accept restrictions and requirements of the diet. Ongoing counseling by an experienced team of professionals can help diminish chronic anxiety, the frequency of elevated blood phenylalanine levels, and behavior problems revolving around food and facilitate a positive family attitude toward indefinite diet maintenance.

Any amount of cheating on the diet can result in significant elevations of serum phenylalanine levels. It is crucial that the children themselves learn about their diets and gain self-control at an early age. Booklets designed to teach children as young as age 3 are available through treatment centers. By the teenage years, self-management is a goal that can be achieved by many.

DEFECTS IN THE METABOLISM OF TETRAHYDROBIOPTERIN

Tetrahydrobiopterin (BH_4) is the cofactor for the hydroxylation of phenylalanine, tyrosine, and tryptophan. Either a defect in the regeneration of BH_4, due to a deficiency of dihydropteridine reductase, or a biopterin synthesis defect will cause defective production of the neurotransmitters DOPA, serotonin, epinephrine, and norepinephrine. Thus, the defect in neural transmission must be the major focus of treatment in these disorders, although hyperphenylalaninemia is generally the first phenotypic marker that is recognized. All newborn infants with persistent hyper-

phenylalaninemia should be screened for these defects.* Total reported cases worldwide number about 50, and the majority are either dihydropteridine reductase deficiency or a biopterin synthesis defect.

The enzyme required in the first step in BH_4 synthesis from guanosine triposphate (GTP) has been identified. But the synthetic pathway consists of at least two other enzymes that have not been unequivocally defined. At present the remainder of the biopterin synthesis defects are a heterogeneous group, which have only been generically described as complete or partial ("leaky" mutants), transient (in the neonate), and "peripheral" which do not involve the brain. In the latter two conditions, therapy is probably not necessary.

Patients with a complete or partial biopterin synthesis defect have been treated with a low phenylalanine diet and neurotransmitter replacement (DOPA, 5-hydroxytryptophan, and a decarboxylase inhibitor), with BH_4 alone, or with a combination of BH_4 and neurotransmitter replacement. It is reasonable to begin BH_4 alone. Small doses of 2.5 mg/kg/day have been used and often lower phenylalanine blood levels without markedly increasing CSF neurotransmitter metabolite concentrations. Moderate (10 mg/kg/day) and high (20 mg/kg/day) doses of BH_4 have been employed with better clinical and CSF neurotransmitter response. Some patients do not respond even to high BH_4 doses and require neurotransmitter therapy. The doses that have been employed alone or in combination are DOPA, 5 to 10 mg/kg/day; 5-hydroxytryptophan, 2.5 to 10 mg/kg/day; and decarboxylase inhibitor, 1.0 to 2.5 mg/kg/day. Optimal management requires monitoring CSF neurotransmitter metabolites, since their determination in blood or urine may not accurately reflect CNS concentrations. However, this caveat is issued with the recognition of the need for more age-related data on major and minor neurotransmitter metabolites in the CSF.

The efficacy of treatment has been difficult to measure, since most patients have been identified because of severe neurologic manifestations. There is little doubt that some patients have been helped by therapy, which has by no means reversed all of the neurologic impairment. With earlier diagnosis based on neonatal screening for biopterin metabolic defects in all infants with hyperphenylalaninemia, and treatment in the asymptomatic period, it is hoped that these poor results will be improved.

It is important to emphasize the limitations of neurotransmitter replacement which circumvents regulatory mechanisms. BH_4 is probably more physiologic but certainly more expensive. In addition, complications of DOPA therapy similar to those reported in the treatment of Parkinson's disease have been noted. On the other hand, experience with BH_4 is so limited that knowledge of its complications is meager.

In dihydropteridine reductase deficiency, it has been

---

*The following screen for defects in biopterin metabolism: Dr. Edwin Naylor, Department of Reproductive Genetics, Magee-Women's Hospital, Forbes Avenue and Hackett Street, Pittsburgh, PA 15213 (412–647–4168) and Dr. Reuben Matalon, Genetics Section, University of Illinois, 840 S. Wood Street, Chicago, IL 60612 (312–996–6714).

estimated that the theoretical requirement for BH_4 of about 1 gm/day for a 10-kg child would cost over $40,000 per year. This may explain why there are only a few—and conflicting—reports of short trials of BH_4 in this deficiency. In almost all of the reported cases to date, neurotransmitter replacement has been generally used in the doses described above. Higher doses occasionally have been employed, i.e., DOPA to 20 mg/kg/day, 5-hydroxytryptophan to 20 mg/kg/day, and carbidopa to 4 mg/kg/day. Although the higher doses may be more effective at raising neurotransmitter metabolite levels in the CSF, they are also associated with an increased incidence of vomiting and dyskinesia. Neurotransmitter replacement therapy should be employed in conjunction with a low phenylalanine diet if blood phenylalanine levels are over 15 mg/dl. Finally, it has been demonstrated that patients with dihydropteridine reductase deficiency can become folate depleted and will respond to folinic acid administration.

MATERNAL PKU

Infants who are born to women with classic or variant PKU can suffer intrauterine growth retardation, microcephaly, congenital heart malformations, and mental retardation. For mothers with phenylalanine levels over 20 mg/dl, the risk of the maternal PKU syndrome is over 90 per cent. In other hyperphenylalaninemic pregnancies, paucity of data precludes risk estimates. It has been estimated that by 1990, the incidence of mental retardation from untreated maternal PKU would equal the incidence of mental retardation secondary to PH deficiency were affected infants not identified in newborn screening and treated.

Counseling about maternal PKU should be included in parental interviews that discuss the genetics and course of the disease. Parents should be encouraged to discuss maternal PKU with their daughters during adolescence. The options of birth control, adoption, and dietary management should be introduced and reviewed in family counseling sessions.

Fewer than 50 case reports on the dietary management of maternal PKU have appeared. At present it is considered that the best results will be obtained for women on diet prior to conception. This is a compelling reason for a young woman to remain on diet during the childbearing period in order to preserve her option to carry her own child. The published case reports on treatment of maternal PKU cannot substitute for a controlled study and a national collaborative study has been established. This research effort will employ a low phenylalanine regimen adapted for pregnancy, frequent plasma phenylalanine and amino acid measurement, nutritional analysis, and routine ultrasound examinations.

DISORDERS OF AMINO ACID METABOLISM

MARY G. AMPOLA, M.D.

Disorders of amino acid degradation may be divided into three major groups. If the enzyme defect involves the conversion of an amino acid to its ketoacid derivative (with release of ammonia), a classic amino acid disorder results. If there is a defect in degradation of one of these ketoacid derivatives, an acidic compound accumulates, leading to the designation of the disorder as an organic acid disease. Finally, if the disorder involves an abnormality in the detoxifying of ammonia via the urea cycle, the disorder is a hyperammonemia disease. With the notable exception of one urea cycle disease, all are inherited in an autosomal recessive manner.

AMINO ACID DISORDERS

Large excesses of certain amino acids have serious toxic effects on many organs, particularly the developing central nervous system. The liver and kidneys are often also involved. Numerous mechanisms by which this damage occurs are known and vary with the particular disorder involved. Frequently, large excesses of an amino acid inhibit movement of other amino acids that must depend on the same membrane transport system. This is especially notable when a large neutral amino acid is involved, since most amino acids are in this category. There may be direct toxicity of an amino acid such as phenylalanine on the neurons, with a lowering of the seizure threshold. Key central nervous system and other enzymes may be saturated with the accumulating amino acid, preventing them from utilizing their usual substrate. Sequelae may also be the result of deficiency of an essential substance that is normally produced beyond the point of the defect.

Clinical features are variable, depending upon the tissues involved. Progressive mental-motor retardation, seizures, coma, and even death may occur. Progressive liver failure may be seen if this organ is involved. Often there is also failure to thrive.

The diagnosis may be made by paper or thin-layer chromotography followed by ninhydrin staining. Attention is paid to excess of a normally occurring amino acid or to the presence of an intermediary metabolite not normally seen. To rule out amino acid abnormalities, it is essential to test both blood and urine, since some diseases are best detected in blood and some in urine. Further identification and quantitation of the accumulating compound is done using an amino acid analyzer. Finally, definitive diagnosis is made by enzyme assay in an appropriate tissue. Since some of the amino acid disorders are detectable by routine screening in the newborn period, certain treatable diseases are identifiable early, before irreversible damage has occurred.

Treatment of these disorders is based on the principle of limiting the dietary intake of the unmetabolizable amino acid. Clearly, this is most effective when an essential amino acid is involved, and fortunately most clinically significant disorders are in this category. Further, if there is an essential substance that is normally produced beyond the block, this should be provided whenever possible.

The mainstay of dietary treatment is to limit the intake of the offending amino acid while providing all other essential amino acids, as well as enough nonessential amino acids to meet nitrogen needs. In addition, other nutrients such as vitamins, minerals, essential fats, and a carbohydrate source are included. For many of these disorders it would be impossible, using normal foods, to provide sufficient protein for growth without greatly exceeding tolerance for the unmetabolizable amino acid. Special formulas are available that have little or none of the offending amino acid(s) for a number of amino acid diseases and are invaluable in the care of these children. In infancy, a small amount of normal formula or evaporated milk is used to meet growth requirements. After infancy low-protein foods such as fruits, vegetables, and grain products are given in measured amounts to provide the optimal amount of the amino acid in question; the major source of other essential amino acids continues to be the formula. The amount of normal foods or of formula which is given depends upon the results of frequent blood or urine tests. An optimal amino acid range has been established for each disorder, which is above the normal range to assure that there is no deficiency. On the other hand, the ideal range is geared low enough so as not to approach the known toxic level for the amino acid. At times, pharmacologic doses of a vitamin are effective if the disorder is a vitamin-responsive one. This usually is given in conjunction with the low-protein diet. Occasionally, specific medications may be helpful in certain disorders.

Ideally, children with amino acid disorders are identified before irreversible damage has occurred. If they are not detected by screening, treatment is often delayed until after clinical features have become apparent. Some irreversible damage may already have occurred, and the goal in this instance is to prevent any further detrimental effect.

These children should be treated in a center experienced in caring for these disorders. A specialty clinician and pediatric nutritionist should be available. A well-qualified analytic laboratory is essential to monitor the blood or urine levels of the accumulating amino acid accurately. Once a diagnosis is made, intensive educational efforts are directed to the family, including careful genetic counseling. Often it is very helpful to arrange for the family to talk with the parents of another child with the same disorder. Social workers or psychologists should be available if needed at any point in the course.

At the time of each clinic visit, the family brings a carefully detailed three-day dietary record, which is analyzed by the nutritionist for the intake of the unmetabolizable amino acid, calories, and protein. These are expressed per kilogram of body weight. An interval history is taken to assess the overall progress, the health, and the general issues of adjustment by the family and the child. The child's height and weight as well as head circumference are carefully followed and plotted. Developmental landmarks are recorded. A fasting blood sample (or at least a sample taken at the same time with each visit) is collected. Alternatively, if the disorder is best monitored by a urine sample, this is collected. The amino acid analysis is run and the result reported to the clinician. The clinician and the nutritionist discuss the results of the total assessment and make decisions concerning dietary or other changes that are needed.

The family is called with follow-up instructions (usually within 2 or 3 days), and a return appointment is made. Children are seen very frequently at first, often once or twice a week. The intervals are gradually increased as the child is stabilized and as the growth rate slows with time. Periodic neuropsychometric and neurologic testing is done if the central nervous system is potentially affected by the disorder.

With some amino acid diseases, early diagnosis and treatment should result in essentially normal growth and development. The situation with others is that health and metabolic stability are improved, but some permanent sequelae result.

ORGANIC ACID DISORDERS

These disorders are caused by an enzyme defect in the degradation of an alpha-ketoacid derived from protein. Clinical symptoms begin as early as 2 or 3 days of life. There is lethargy, poor feeding, vomiting, and dehydration, which may progress to coma or death. Severe ketoacidosis is present, often accompanied by hypoglycemia and elevated blood ammonia levels. It is important to note that the hyperammonemia is often so severe that it can be more threatening to life and brain function than the acidosis. Bone marrow suppression, when present, may be profound and can lead to sepsis and coagulation problems in addition to anemia.

These acidic products do not stain with ninhydrin. Thus, they cannot be detected on routine amino acid screening, although nonspecific elevations of glycine and/or glutamine may be seen. It is necessary to have the urinary organic acids quantitated as soon as possible when one of these diseases is suspected. This is done using gas chromatography with mass spectrometry. Serum lactic acid and pyruvic acid levels should also be measured, since enzyme disorders causing lactic acidosis are best detected by this means.

The acute episodes of ketoacidosis must be treated rapidly. Intravenous fluids containing bicarbonate and glucose are used. Initially, sodium bicarbonate is given in a dose of 1 to 2 mEq/kg by rapid intravenous infusion over 5 to 10 minutes, followed by continuous drip in a 10 per cent glucose solution, calculated to provide at least 1 mEq/kg/hour of bicarbonate. The basic solution should be given as glucose in water rather than in saline, since the large amount of sodium being given as bicarbonate often causes the serum sodium to rise dramatically. The 10 per cent glucose is given both to correct any tendency to hypoglycemia and to minimize protein catabolism. Temporary elevation of serum glucose to 200 or 300 mg/dl is not detrimental and thus is not a reason to reduce glucose administration. Potassium is added as needed.

Since many of these children are already septic when they present, it is prudent to take a wide range of cultures, and to begin broad-spectrum antibiotic therapy immediately. If cultures prove negative, the drugs may of course be discontinued.

In any severely ill child, it is often necessary to remove the accumulating acids more rapidly than is possible with intravenous therapy and renal excretion. This is done by initiating some form of therapy that allows continuous removal of the acid, which is present in very high concentration throughout body fluids. Either hemodialysis or the often more readily available peritoneal dialysis can be used; exchange transfusion is of little value because it cannot be continued for any length of time.

Dialysis accomplishes three goals. First, large amounts of the offending acid can be removed rapidly. Second, any ammonia that has accumulated is removed simultaneously; indeed, the hyperammonia is often far more difficult to correct than the ketoacidosis. Finally, excesses of sodium are removed, allowing continuation of the needed intravenous bicarbonate therapy to correct the acidosis. A standard peritoneal dialysis solution is used, containing 1.5 per cent glucose with electrolytes to which potassium is added as needed. The fluid is administered through the dialysis catheter in an amount sufficient to distend the abdomen without interfering with respiration. For a neonate, about 20 ml/kg/cycle is used at first and gradually increased if tolerated without interfering with respiration to 30 to 50 ml/kg/cycle. The solution is left in the abdomen for about 1 hour (as little as 1/2 hour if the situation is critical), after which it is drained by gravity and fresh solution is instilled. Careful records are kept of dialysis intake and output, as well as intravenous intake and urinary output. Blood electrolytes and gases are frequently monitored, as are blood ammonia levels. The dialysis is discontinued when the acid-base balance and the blood ammonia are at or close to the normal range. It is notable that improvement in the level of consciousness often lags about a day behind improvement in biochemical parameters, because of slow clearing of ammonia across the blood-brain barrier.

Since a number of the organic acid disorders are responsive to pharmacologic doses of vitamins, it is recommended that the following vitamins be given immediately if the child is in critical condition. Daily doses of 2 mg of vitamin B_{12} intramuscularly and 10 mg of biotin by nasogastric tube are recommended. The former is often effective in methylmalonic acidemia, which is the most common of these disorders, and biotin is useful in the treatment of biotinidase and holocarboxylase synthetase deficiencies.

After the acute crisis has ended, enteral therapy should begin as soon as possible to minimize protein catabolism. This is given orally if the child is able to suck well or by slow nasogastric drip otherwise. The initial formula should be a normal formula diluted to provide about 1 gm/kg/day of protein. To this should be added additional sources of calories to provide a total of 125 to 140 kcal/kg/day; about half of the calories may be given as a fat such as MCT oil (Mead-Johnson) and half as carbohydrate such as Polycose powder (Ross). If such a formula is tolerated without metabolic decompensation, the protein content may gradually and incrementally be increased to about 1.5 gm/kg/day of protein.

Long-term therapy involves a low-protein diet, with added vitamin therapy if appropriate. For many of these diseases, special formulas are available which are devoid of the unmetabolizable amino acid(s). Growth requirements for these amino acids are met by adding appropriate amounts of normal formula for infants and later by use of low-protein foods. The latter include vegetables, fruits, and cereals, all in carefully controlled amounts. Caloric intake is kept at about 120 cal/kg/day to promote growth, while sparing the small amount of protein being given.

Chronic mild acidosis, despite these measures, is common and should be prevented to avoid problems such as failure to thrive and osteoporosis. A supplement of alkali (e.g., Polycitra, Willen) is given in daily divided doses sufficient to keep the serum bicarbonate level well within the normal range.

It is now well known that patients with organic acid diseases have low blood levels of carnitine, a substance necessary for fatty acid transport into mitochondria. Depletion results because accumulating acids form complexes with carnitine which are excreted into the urine. Both free and total serum carnitine levels are reduced, with the former being most affected. Failure to grow and poor muscle tone can result if supplementation is not provided. An initial dose of 100 mg/kg/day orally is suggested. Therapy results in a rise of both free and total carnitine, although the ratio of the two never fully corrects. Adjustments of the carnitine dosage are made to keep the free carnitine level as close to normal as possible.

Children with these disorders are prone to periodic bouts of ketoacidosis precipitated by intercurrent infections, trauma, or excessive protein intake. Since any one of these episodes may be life-threatening or may lead to some loss of brain function, each must be treated as soon and as vigorously as possible. A very useful scheme is to have the family double the usual Bicitra intake at the first sign of any illness. If the child is not taking alkali chronically and the urine is ketone-positive, Bicitra is given in a dose of 0.5 to 1 mEq/kg every 4 hours in a small amount of juice or water. Protein intake is cut to an absolute minimum. If hospitalization is required, it should be done as early in the course as possible. Usually, intravenous fluid and bicarbonate therapy, as described previously, suffice; occasionally dialysis may be necessary. Vitamin supplements are continued if the disorder is responsive to a particular vitamin. If the episode continues more than 2 or 3 days, it is important to provide carnitine supplements orally or by nasogastric tube; intravenous carnitine is currently under clinical investigation by Kendell-McGraw. Death caused by cardiomyopathy after a period of hospitalization in several patients may have been associated with severe depletion of carnitine.

Children with organic acid diseases must be closely followed by an experienced metabolic specialist and a nutritionist. Growth, development, and acid-base status are monitored frequently. Frequent amino acid analysis of plasma is done to ensure that normal levels of all amino acids are being provided.

For many of these children, this regimen helps prevent the repeated crises that formerly led to death or to progressive mental retardation. Indeed, many of these children now are able to lead an essentially normal life.

THE HYPERAMMONEMIAS

There are five disorders involving the urea cycle. Each corresponds to a deficiency of one of the five enzymes responsible for converting ammonia to urea. These disorders include carbamyl phosphate (CPS) deficiency and ornithine transcarbamylase (OTC) deficiency, which involve steps 1 and 2, respectively. Citrullinemia, caused by argininosuccinic acid synthetase (AS) deficiency, and argininosuccinic aciduria, which results from argininosuccinic acid lyase (AL) deficiency, correspond to steps 3 and 4. Finally, there is argininemia or arginase (ARG'ase) deficiency at step 5. Four of the five diseases are inherited in an autosomal recessive manner; the exception is the OTC deficiency, which follows an X-linked recessive pattern.

Complete enzyme deficiency of one of the first four enzymes usually manifests itself as a fulminant disorder in the newborn period; argininemia appears later. Partial enzyme deficiency for any of the disorders results in clinical illness in later months or even years.

Babies with a neonatal crisis become ill between 1 and 3 days of life, presenting with lethargy, poor feeding, and vomiting when the blood ammonia level reaches at least two to three times the normal concentration. If untreated, seizures appear and eventually the child lapses into a coma and may die when the quantity of ammonia exceeds 10 times the normal level. Even with treatment many die, and the survivors have significant neurologic deficits.

Children with urea cycle enzyme defects are at risk for repeated hyperammonemic crises, with symptoms similar to those described and generally precipitated by infection, trauma, or excess protein intake.

Argininemia does not cause symptoms in the neonatal period. Rather, at some point, usually during the first or second year, there is gradual onset of vomiting, failure to thrive, seizures, progressive spastic diplegia, and psychomotor retardation. In this disorder, the hyperammonemia may not be the sole detrimental factor. Arginine excess and possibly also partial deficiency of ornithine and lysine may be contributory.

Diagnostically, the most critical factor in suspecting a urea cycle defect is determination of the blood ammonia level. If the child is acutely ill, the sample can be drawn at any time. If the condition has stabilized and the child is alert, or after a period of intravenous therapy, a normal ammonia level may be present. A single high-protein feeding equivalent to 1.5 to 2 gm/kg of protein is given, and 2 hours later blood is drawn for an ammonia level determination. Elevation of two or more times above normal is significant. Amino acid studies are diagnostic for the last three disorders of the cycle—citrulline, argininosuccinic acid, and arginine accumulate, respectively. In any of the disorders, glutamine may be elevated secondary to the ammonia excess. Urinary orotic acid elevation is found if the defect is OTC (step 2) deficiency, distinguishing this disorder from CPS (step 1) deficiency, after amino acid determination has ruled out diseases at steps 3 through 5 of the urea cycle. Orotic acid is one of the pyrimidines formed when accumulating carbamyl phosphate excesses cross into the cytosol. Final confirmation of the diagnosis may be made by doing enzyme assay in an appropriate tissue.

In the instance of a newborn with hyperammonemia, organic acid diseases and transient hyperammonemia of the newborn (THAN) must be ruled out. The organic acidemias cause severe ketoacidosis in addition to hyperammonemia. The body fluids in urea cycle diseases and in THAN do not involve serious disturbance of acid-base balance, although mild alkalosis or acidosis is not uncommon.

Any child with a hyperammonemic crisis must be treated as rapidly and as vigorously as possible. As soon as blood and urine samples have been collected for diagnostic purposes, high-calorie, non-nitrogenous intravenous solutions are administered. Respiratory support may be necessary.

Dialysis (preferably hemodialysis but peritoneal dialysis if hemodialysis is not available) should be instituted immediately if there is a significant hyperammonemia. When the ammonia level reaches about four times upper normal, the child's sensorium is usually altered and there may be seizures. Short-term efforts such as exchange transfusion are not particularly effective.

In conjunction with the dialysis, three medications have been found to be useful for promoting ammonia excretion and should be given in conjunction with the dialysis. Arginine, given as arginine hydrochloride, is a mainstay of therapy for any of these patients with an acute neonatal crisis. This amino acid stimulates step 1 of the urea cycle and thus enhances excretion of ammonia via pyrimidines (and also via argininosuccinic acid if the step 4 enzyme is lacking). In addition, whenever there is a urea cycle defect at steps 1 through 4, arginine becomes an essential amino acid and must be provided for protein synthesis. The second useful medication is sodium benzoate, which conjugates with glycine to form hippuric acid. Each glycine molecule excreted eliminates one nitrogen atom. Further glycine synthesis from ammonia and bicarbonate is thus stimulated; supplemental pyridoxine and folic acid should be given to optimize glycine formation. Finally, sodium phenylacetate is effective because it conjugates with glutamine and is excreted as phenylacetylglutamine. This removes two nitrogen atoms per molecule. Detailed protocols describing the medication dosage are readily available.

Dialysis is usually successful in lowering ammonia levels to nearly normal within 2 to 4 days. As with dialysis for organic acid disorders, improvement in mental status lags about a day behind that expected for the given ammonia level, because of slow clearing of ammonia across the blood-brain barrier.

After about 2 days of dialysis, alimentation via nasogastric tube should begin if bowel sounds are present. Diluted infant formula, to provide about 1 gm/kg/day of protein is used as a base. For disorders at steps 1 or 2, the formula can be designed so that much of the protein is given as an essential L-amino acid mixture, further minimizing the ammonia burden. The formula should contain a high calorie content of 125 to 140 kcal/kg/day, the caloric deficit in the formula being made up by a fat source such as MCT oil (Mead-Johnson) to provide about half the calories and a glucose polymer such as Polycose (Ross) for the remainder.

On the first day of alimentation, about one third of the planned formula is given by continuous drip, together with one third of the medications; the remainder of the latter is given with the intravenous fluids, which are continued at reduced volume. If tolerated, the amount of formula and medications is increased to two thirds the next day, and finally to full amounts. In the meantime, peritoneal dialysis will have been terminated, allowing for the increased volume to be presented. As the child's condition allows, intermittent oral feedings are substituted for the continuous nasogastric mode of administration.

Chronic care of patients with urea cycle disorders is based on the principle of providing sufficient protein for growth without precipitating significant hyperammonemia. Diluted formula (often with addition of an essential amino acid mixture for defects at steps 1 and 2) is used. A nonprotein base (Product 80056, Mead-Johnson) provides additional calories, vitamins, and minerals. Caloric content should be kept in the range of 120 kcal/kg/day. Smaller, more frequent feedings than for most children help reduce the tendency to postprandial hyperammonemia. In terms of medications, arginine supplements, geared to keep the serum arginine level in the high normal range, is useful for AS and AL deficiencies, whereas sodium benzoate and sodium phenylacetate may be needed on a continuing basis for CPS, OTC, and AS defects. Added citrulline compensates for failure to produce this amino acid in the CPS and OTC disorders. Protocols are available which provide details of the long-term therapies.

The results of therapy in children with urea cycle defects are variable. Infants who suffer a severe neonatal crisis frequently die in this early period. If they survive, there is invariably brain damage, the extent depending on the degree and duration of the hyperammonemia. If a neonatal episode is avoided, the outlook is brighter. The children are always at risk for repeated hyperammonemic crises, and indeed many die within the first few years. Prompt and careful treatment of each episode is essential to maximize chances for survival and preservation of intellect, as well as prevention of other neurologic sequelae such as cerebral palsy.

HYPERLIPOPROTEINEMIA

PETER O. KWITEROVICH, Jr., M.D.

The diagnosis and treatment of inherited disorders of plasma lipid and lipoprotein metabolism are important in order to prevent their two major complications, namely, atherosclerosis and pancreatitis. The hyperlipoproteinemias may be broadly classified into disorders of the major cholesterol-carrying lipoproteins, low density (beta) lipoproteins (LDL), or of those associated with increases in one or more of the triglyceride-rich lipoproteins, namely, chylomicrons, very low density (pre-beta) lipoproteins (VLDL), and the remnants of their metabolism, chylomicron remnants and intermediate density lipoproteins (IDL). In certain children at risk for atherosclerosis, hyperlipoproteinemia may not be present; such children may have a very low level of high density (alpha) lipoproteins (HDL).

Dietary Management

For most children with hyperlipoproteinemia, the unified dietary approach currently developed by the Nutrition Committee of the American Heart Association can be used. This diet is used for disorders of both LDL cholesterol and triglyceride metabolism. It is divided into three phases of progressive stringency (Table 1). Many children will need a phase 2 diet to effect a significant lowering of their hyperlipidemia. In those with a disorder of LDL metabolism, a lowering of 10 to 15 per cent in plasma total and LDL cholesterol level is often observed. For the hypertriglyceridemics, such a diet, often combined with suitable reduction in weight, often lowers and maintains the triglyceride level in the normal range.

The principles of the diet include a reduction in total fat, which will decrease both chylomicrons (and their remnants) and LDL cholesterol (Table 1). The decrease in the percentage of calories as saturated fat will lower LDL cholesterol, and a reduction in dietary cholesterol and calorie control will lower VLDL, IDL, and LDL cholesterol. Restrictions of simple sugars (with an increase in complex carbohydrates) will decrease VLDL cholesterol. The major reductions include meat, dairy products, and eggs. Skim or 1 per cent milk is substituted for whole milk, low fat cheeses are recommended, and only one to two eggs per week are permitted. Commercially baked goods and desserts, chocolate, fatty snacks, and fast foods are eliminated. Lean meat, fish, and poultry in limited amounts (3 to 5 oz/day) are recommended. This unified dietary approach to treatment of hyperlipidemia may be obtained in a booklet from the American Heart Association, National Headquarters, Dallas, Texas.

For the unusual child with severe hypertriglyceridemia associated with increased chylomicrons, a more stringent restriction in dietary fat (at least phase 3) will be necessary. Medium chain triglycerides, which go directly to the liver via the portal vein and do not require chylomicron formation for absorption, can be

TABLE 1. Unified Approach to Dietary Treatment of Hyperlipoproteinemia

Nutrients as Percentage of Total Calories*	Phase 1	Phase 2	Phase 3
Fat	30–35%	<30%	20–25%
Saturated fat	<10%	8%	6%
Polyunsaturated fat	10%	10%	8%
Monounsaturated fat	10–12%	10%	8%
P/S	1.2–1.4	1.1–1.5	1.1–1.5
Cholesterol (mg/day)	<300	<200	100
Carbohydrate	45–50%	50%	55–60%
Protein	20%	20%	20%

*Approximate averages are provided; the percentage of nutrient intake will vary depending on the total daily caloric intake (e.g., 1200 to 2300 calories/day).

used as an oil substitute, at up to 15 per cent of the total caloric intake.

For the child with hypoalphalipoproteinemia, a phase 1 diet is recommended. Reduction to ideal body weight, regular aerobic exercise, and cessation of cigarette smoking may raise the HDL cholesterol level 5 to 10 mg/dl.

Drug Treatment

Familial Hypercholesterolemia. The majority of pediatric patients with hyperlipoproteinemia can be managed by diet alone. The primary need for therapy with drugs in the pediatric age group will be the child with heterozygous familial hypercholesterolemia. The drug of choice is a bile acid sequestrant, either cholestyramine (Questran) or colestipol (Colestid). These anion exchange resins bind bile acids in the intestine and prevent their reabsorption, and the complex is eliminated in the feces. Such an interruption of the enterohepatic circulation perturbs cholesterol metabolism in the liver. More hepatic cholesterol is converted to bile acid, prompting an increase in the production of LDL receptors, which mediate the uptake and catabolism of LDL from blood.

The decision to use a bile acid sequestrant must be individualized. We usually reserve the use of these agents for children at least 10 years of age who also have a family history of premature coronary atherosclerosis and who have not lowered their total and LDL cholesterol levels into the normal range with diet. The medication is dispensed either in a packet (cholestyramine 9 gm, 4 gm active ingredient; colestipol, 5 gm active ingredient), or in bulk form (1 scoop equals 1 packet). The dose-response relationship for children and young adults with familial hypercholesterolemia (FH) is summarized in Table 2. In general, heterozygous FH children will require a lower dose of bile acid sequestrant to lower their total and LDL cholesterol levels into the normal range than will adults. The dry powder must be mixed in a liquid, such as water or orange juice, before ingestion. The medicine is most effective when given just before, during, or after a meal. The primary side effects include constipation, abdominal bloating, and a feeling of fullness. Rarely, steatorrhea has been observed when the medicine is given in very high doses (6 packets or more/day). Potential side effects include malabsorption of fat-soluble vitamins and folic acid. A multivitamin containing vitamins, minerals, iron, and folic acid can be given when the child is being treated with the resin. Often, low plasma serum levels of folate will be observed

during therapy, but it is rare for the folate content of the erythrocytes to be affected; consequently, anemia due to folic acid deficiency rarely occurs. The medication can also interfere with the absorption of other medicines, particularly digoxin, warfarin, and thyroxine, and consequently should be given at a time when other medications are not given.

Other medications have been used to lower the LDL cholesterol level in FH heterozygotes. These include D-thyroxine (Choloxin), in a dose of 0.05 mg/kg up to a maximum of 4 mg/day, and paraaminosalicylic acid. Such therapy is not routinely recommended for the pediatric age group.

The rare FH homozygote requires therapy with diet, bile sequestrant (6 to 8 packets/day) and nicotinic acid (up to 3 gm/day), but more aggressive measures such as plasmapheresis, portacaval shunt, and liver transplantation will usually be required. Partial ileal bypass is not effective in the FH homozygote.

Hypertriglyceridemia. Almost all hypertriglyceridemias are very responsive to weight reduction and diet (see Table 1) and will not require the use of drug therapy in the pediatric age group. In the rare patient with dysbetalipoproteinemia (type III hyperlipoproteinemia), clofibrate (Atromid-S),* 1 to 2 gm/day, is most effective.

Summary

In summary, the diagnosis and treatment of hyperlipoproteinemia in the pediatric age group are an important part of the traditional preventive approach taken by pediatricians. The recent results of the Lipid Research Clinics Coronary Primary Prevention Trial indicate that the treatment of patients with elevated LDL cholesterol levels is associated with significant reduction in morbidity and mortality from coronary artery disease. Such data, combined with the growing literature on the expression of hyperlipoproteinemia in children, the tendency of the hyperlipoproteinemias to persist into adulthood, and the strong association with coronary atherosclerosis, provide a strong rationale for appropriate diagnosis and treatment of these conditions. Finally, the rare child with profound hypertriglyceridemia needs to be treated to prevent life-threatening pancreatitis.

*Manufacturer's warning: Safety and efficacy for use in children have not been established.

TABLE 2. Dosage Schedule for Treatment of Familial Hypercholesterolemic Children and Young Adults with a Bile Sequestrant

Daily Doses of Bile Sequestrant	Postdietary Plasma Levels	
	Total Cholesterol (mg/dl)	*Low Density Lipoprotein Cholesterol (mg/dl)*
1	<245	<195
2	245–300	195–235
3	301–345	236–280
4	>345	>280

GALACTOSEMIAS

GEORGE N. DONNELL, M.D.

Diseases caused by inborn errors of the three enzymes involved in the major pathway of galactose metabolism have been described. Galactose-1-phosphate uridyltransferase deficiency galactosemia is the most frequently encountered. General use of newborn screening for galactosemia has significantly altered the pattern of its presentation. Most affected individuals are initially asymptomatic if treatment is instituted promptly. Symptomatic patients may still be encountered owing either to delays in diagnosis of the disease or to institution of therapy. Patients, whether symptomatic or not, require the same approach to management (see below).

DIETARY THERAPY

Treatment for infants and children with galactosemia is the elimination of lactose (galactose) from the diet. This is accomplished in infancy by the use of milk substitutes free of lactose (soya preparations, casein hydrolysates). It is recommended that older children remain on milk-free diets indefinitely. Patients and their families require the guidance of a nutritionist to ensure that the diet is nutritionally adequate. Since milk solid is a common additive to many foods, and lactose is a common filler in medicinal tablets and capsules, close attention to product labels is necessary to avoid intake of lactose. Compliance with the diet is monitored by interim dietary histories and by periodic measurement of erythrocyte galactose-1-phosphate. It should be recognized that even in well-managed patients, galactose-1-phosphate is detectable in erythrocytes. This is believed to be due to endogenous metabolism of galactose.

GENETIC COUNSELING

Counseling is an important part of disease prevention. Galactosemia is inherited as an autosomal recessive trait. The genetic risks to the offspring of carriers and the prognosis for affected individuals should be clearly presented to families.

PRENATAL DIAGNOSIS

Prenatal diagnosis is available through direct enzyme determination on chorionic villi sampling or first trimester amniocentesis. Mothers at risk for having an affected child should be placed on a lactose-free diet during pregnancy in order to diminish the galactose load to the fetus.

PREGNANCY

Despite the high incidence of ovarian failure, some galactosemic females have borne children. In contrast to PKU, the offspring are not adversely affected. Restriction of galactose during pregnancy is advisable.

COMPLICATIONS

Early Complications. Fluid and electrolyte disturbances, jaundice, infection, and cataracts are common manifestations in untreated patients. The indications for fluid and electrolyte replacement are the same as those in other disorders. Infection, particularly with gram-negative organisms, in untreated neonates with galactosemia is extremely common, and the choice of antimicrobial drugs should take this into consideration.

Jaundice usually clears rapidly after removal of galactose from the diet. Occasionally the bilirubin is sufficiently elevated to warrant exchange transfusions.

Late Complications. Recently it has been recognized that despite adequate dietary management the child with galactosemia may develop one or more of the following complications: (1) Learning disabilities and

behavioral problems are commonly encountered, and early intervention is recommended. (2) Speech and language difficulties have been reported in many. Early recognition is helpful in preventing disability from these complications. (3) Ovarian failure is very common in female patients with galactosemia, presumably due to the abnormal galactose metabolism. Gonadal function in males appears to be unaffected. Treatment of the gonadal failure in females follows the currently accepted approaches for the disorder. (4) Neurologic sequelae characterized by progressive mental retardation, tremor, and ataxia have been described in some treated patients. Only supportive treatment is currently available.

GALACTOKINASE DEFICIENCY

A second disorder of galactose metabolism is due to a deficiency of the enzyme galactokinase, which catalyzes the first step in the galactose metabolic pathway. Galactose accumulates in blood and urine and galactitol accumulates in urine, ocular lenses, and brain, but galactose-1-phosphate is not generated. The major clinical manifestations include lenticular cataracts and pseudotumor cerebri. Dietary restriction of lactose is as described for transferase deficiency.

EPIMERASE DEFICIENCY

A third disorder, epimerase deficiency, may be found in two forms: benign and severe. The benign form is more common and is not associated with any known clinical manifestations. The decrease in epimerase activity is confined to the red cells. The mode of inheritance is autosomal recessive. The erythrocyte galactose-1-phosphate concentration in early infancy may be elevated and as a consequence may be confused with galactosemia on newborn screening when the microbiologic assay is used. No treatment is required. Epimerase deficiency associated with severe clinical manifestations is extremely rare. The symptoms are similar to those of galactosemia due to the transferase deficiency. In this situation dietary treatment with *limitation*, but not exclusion, of galactose intake has been recommended. The outcome is still uncertain.

DISORDERS OF PORPHYRIN, PURINE, AND PYRIMIDINE METABOLISM

PHILIP ROSENTHAL, M.D., *and* M. MICHAEL THALER, M.D.

THE PORPHYRIAS

The porphyrias are a group of disorders characterized by defects in heme synthesis resulting in excessive accumulation of heme precursors in the tissues. Most fatalities are caused by delays in diagnosis and treatment. Awareness of the clinical patterns associated with these disorders and investigation of family members of patients with porphyria will accelerate the diagnostic process and may prevent unnecessary surgery. Appropriate therapy will bring about relief from acute attacks and ensure a favorable long-term outcome.

Congenital Erythropoietic Porphyria (Günther's Disease). For this, one of the rarest inborn errors of metabolism, treatment includes avoidance of sunlight, screening window light, use of special light bulbs, protective clothing, avoidance of minor trauma to the skin, barrier skin creams, and appropriate topical and systemic antibiotics. Photosensitivity in some patients has been reduced with beta-carotene (30 to 150 mg/24 hr orally). Beta-carotene capsules may be opened and contents mixed in orange or tomato juice to aid administration in children. Recently, canthaxanthin (4,4-diketo-beta-carotene) has been utilized in doses of 25 to 100 mg/24 hr with good results. Instead of a yellow hue from beta-carotene, canthaxanthin causes a brownish discoloration of the palms and a pleasant suntanned appearance to the face.

Blood transfusions frequently are necessary to treat the hemolytic anemia. Splenectomy may reduce transfusion requirements and decrease formation of porphyrins responsible for photosensitivity. However, the increased risks of sepsis in children susceptible to repeated skin infections should be considered in the decision for splenectomy.

Erythrodontia, a pinkish-brown discoloration of teeth due to porphyrin deposition, may be improved cosmetically with dental crowns. Patients with such crowns should receive careful dental surveillance, since gingivitis may develop, forcing removal of the crowns.

Congenital Erythropoietic Protoporphyria. Congenital erythropoietic protoporphyria occurs more commonly than erythropoietic porphyria. Treatment consists of avoidance of sunlight by screening window light and by using special wavelength light bulbs (not in the 400 nm range), protective clothing, and barrier skin creams. Oral administration of beta-carotene at a dose of 30 to 150 mg/24 hr, maintaining serum carotene concentrations above 500 µg/dl over a period of months, has been found to dampen photosensitivity. Hemolytic anemia is a rare complication that may require splenectomy. Formation of porphyrin gallstones has been reported, which has been treated by cholecystectomy.

Acute Intermittent Porphyria (Swedish Type). Treatment of acute attacks includes provision of 450 to 600 gm of glucose/24 hr, infused through a central vein as 10 to 15 per cent solution in water. Pain is treated effectively with chlorpromazine or chloral hydrate. Hyponatremia secondary to inappropriate secretion of antidiuretic hormone (ADH) often develops during an acute attack and should be managed with fluid restriction. Careful replacement of the sodium deficit with hypertonic saline may be necessary. Severe hypertension is an occasional complication and should be treated as primary malignant hypertension. Paralysis of intercostal muscles with respiratory insufficiency may develop in patients with acute intermittent porphyria in the acute phase. Paresis is often reversible with aggressive management in an intensive care unit. Treatment includes tracheal intubation or tracheostomy and mechanical respiratory support with frequent blood gas monitoring.

A recently introduced therapeutic strategy intended to reduce porphyrin production by means of intravenously administered hemin for injection (Panhematin, Abbott Laboratories, North Chicago, IL) appears to be extremely effective. An intravenous line running normal saline is used to inject hemin as a bolus over a period of 15 minutes at a dose of 1 to 4 mg/kg body weight. The tubing is then flushed with normal saline (0.9 per cent NaCl). Hemin for injection adminstration may be repeated with 12- to 24-hour intervals depending on response, but no more than 6 mg/kg in any 24-hour period. Because Panhematin contains no preservatives and because it undergoes rapid chemical decomposition in solution, it should not be reconstituted until immediately before use. After the first withdrawal from the vial, any solution remaining must be discarded.

Intravenous administration of the carbohydrate levulose* has also been reported to reduce the severity of acute attacks in adults.

In patients whose attacks may be precipitated by menstruation, the use of ovulatory suppressants, androgens, oophorectomy, and oral contraceptives may be indicated.

Porphyria Variegata (Congenital Cutaneous Hepatic Porphyria, South African Type, Mixed Porphyria). Treatment consists of protection from sunlight (see Congenital Erythropoietic Porphyria) and careful avoidance of even trivial trauma. Cholestyramine (note: dosage of cholestyramine resin for infants and children has not been established), 12 gm daily, has proved useful in the management of cutaneous manifestations. The resin binds porphyrins in the intestinal tract, thus preventing their reabsorption. Fat-soluble vitamins (such as vitamins A, D, and K) should be supplemented in patients treated with cholestyramine.

Porphyria Cutanea Tarda. For porphyrias of this type, treatment should be nonaggressive, since the disease is not life-threatening. Dermatologic manifestations should be managed as previously described (see Congenital Erythropoietic Porphyria). When ingestion of toxic chemicals is discovered and discontinued, complete recovery often follows within a few months.

Other modes of therapy include attempts to increase porphyrin excretion by alkalinization of the urine and administration of cholestyramine. The antimalarial agent chloroquine forms complexes with uroporphyrin in the liver, which are readily excreted in urine. However, this form of treatment is potentially dangerous and should be avoided in most cases.

Vitamin E (alpha-tocopherol acetate), 400 IU daily, increased to 1600 IU daily, administered for several months has reduced the dermatologic complications in limited trials with adult patients.

Hereditary Coproporphyria. Treatment of hereditary coproporphyria is as described for acute intermittent porphyria.

DISORDERS OF PURINE AND PYRIMIDINE METABOLISM

Hyperuricemia. Hyperuricemia is rare in childhood. While gout is the major complication of hyperuricemia

---

*Investigational procedure.

in adults, formation of urate renal stones is the most frequently observed manifestation of hyperuricemia in children.

Two categories of drugs are used in treatment: those for control of hyperuricemia and those for acute attacks of gout. Since hyperuricemia is rare in childhood, agents currently employed in treatment of hyperuricemia with or without gout have not been adequately evaluated in children. Recommended doses are the usual adult doses, unless specifically noted as designed for children.

The rapid cell turnover and breakdown of nucleic acids in neoplastic diseases such as leukemia and lymphoma induce hyperuricemia, which may lead to clinical complications, especially in the course of chemotherapy or radiation therapy. As mentioned, the major complication of hyperuricemia in childhood is formation of uric acid stones in the urinary tract. The xanthine oxidase inhibitor allopurinol (hydroxypyrazolo pyrimidine) is indicated in children with hyperuricemia due to malignancy. To ensure maximal inhibition of xanthine oxidase, treatment with allopurinol at 10 to 20 mg/kg/24 hr should be initiated several days prior to chemotherapy. When pretreatment is not possible, allopurinol in doses ranging from 120 to 500 mg/day is used concomitantly with cytotoxic agents. The actual dose of allopurinol is adjusted to body weight, monitored with determinations of serum uric acid, and reduced when renal function is impaired. Side effects of allopurinol include nausea and diarrhea, hepatotoxic manifestations, and skin rashes. Hepatic microsomal enzymes may be partially inactivated by allopurinol, resulting in prolongation of the effective half-life of other drugs metabolized by the liver. When the antileukemic agents mercaptopurine and azathioprine are used in conjunction with allopurinol, their usual doses must be reduced by two thirds to three fourths. Allopurinol and ampicillin should not be administered concomitantly because of an increased risk of serious skin rashes.

An abundant fluid intake and alkalinization of the urine to increase solubility of uric acid are important adjuncts in the treatment of hyperuricemia. This can be accomplished by the use of oral sodium bicarbonate (2 to 6 gm/24 hr) or sodium citrate (20 to 60 ml/24 hr). If renal stone formation occurs in association with diminished renal function, peritoneal dialysis or hemodialysis may be used to remove excess uric acid.

Dietary manipulation includes elimination of purine-rich foods such as organ meats (liver, sweetbreads, kidney), anchovies, sardines, wild game, meat extracts, and meat concentrates (gravies).

Acute attacks of gout are usually treated with colchicine administered orally (0.5 to 0.6 mg once hourly) until objective improvement is obtained. The drug must be discontinued when gastrointestinal complications of colchicine develop (cramping, diarrhea, nausea, vomiting). The maximum daily dose of colchicine is preferably administered intravenously (1 to 3 mg total dose, based on body size and weight, diluted in 20 ml normal saline) to minimize the gastrointestinal side effects. Colchicine is contraindicated in patients with leukopenia or substantial renal or hepatic disease. The drug must

be injected slowly, with care taken not to infiltrate. In addition to gastrointestinal toxicity, side effects include granulocytopenia, alopecia, aplastic anemia, and respiratory depression.

The prostaglandin inhibitor indomethacin* is also effective in acute gouty arthritis at 50 mg orally every 8 hours, continued until symptomatic relief is obtained. The dose should be rapidly tapered after resolution of inflammatory signs. Side effects include anorexia, nausea, abdominal pain, bleeding peptic ulcers, headaches, dizziness, mental confusion, depression, and convulsions. Bone marrow depression has also been described.

Phenylbutazone (contraindicated in children under 14 years of age) is a potent anti-inflammatory agent useful in the treatment of gout. Usual adult dosage for acute gout is 400 mg initially, followed by 100 mg every 4 hours until inflammation subsides, usually within 4 days. The smallest dose possible should be utilized. In general, 600 mg in four divided doses during the first 24 hours of an acute attack is sufficient in adults. Gastrointestinal toxicity is similar to that of indomethacin (see above). Other significant side effects are aplastic anemia and salt retention.

Naproxen, ibuprofen, fenoprofen, and piroxicam have been utilized with moderate success in adults to treat acute attacks of gout but have not been evaluated in children.

Lesch-Nyhan Syndrome. Severe deficiency of hypoxanthine-guanine phosphoribosyl transferase in this disorder causes marked uric acid overproduction associated with choreoathetosis, mental retardation, and self-mutilation. Hyperuricosuria and urate gravel or stone formation are treated with allopurinol* until the serum urate level and urinary urate excretion return to normal. Dosages must be individually titrated, but usually range from 100 to 300 mg daily in divided doses. Prevention of urate stones may be accomplished with increased fluid intake, which stimulates increased renal output of uric acid.

Treatment with allopurinol cannot reverse the neurologic manifestations of Lesch-Nyhan syndrome. Physical restraints (elbow splints and hand bandages) may be used to control self-mutilating behavior of patients. Lip biting may require extraction of teeth, but permanent teeth should be spared, since lip biting usually diminishes with age. Nondestructive behavior should be rewarded when possible, but attempts at self-injury should not be punished. This approach is based on reports which suggest that positive reinforcement is preferable to punishment in controlling self-destructive behavior in children with Lesch-Nyhan syndrome.

Recently, 5-hydroxytryptophan,† a precursor of serotonin, in a dose of 8 mg/kg/24 hr in four equal increments, in conjunction with the peripheral decarboxylase inhibitor carbidopa (safety in children not established), 1 to 10 mg/kg/24 hr in two to four equal portions, has been shown to reduce athetoid movement significantly and to produce a sedative effect without

---

*Manufacturer's Warning: Safe use in children has not been established.
†Investigational drug.

improvement in mood or self-mutilation. Unfortunately, tolerance may develop within 1 month, with permanent loss of efficacy upon retreatment.

Xanthinuria. Xanthine accumulates owing to deficiency of xanthine oxidase, the enzyme that converts xanthine to uric acid. Uric acid levels are low in serum and urine, and xanthine stones form in the urinary tract. Treatment consists of reducing the intake of foods with a high purine content such as organ meats, anchovies, sardines, wild game, meat extracts, and meat concentrates (gravies). Fluid intake should be increased and the urine alkalinized to facilitate renal excretion of xanthine. These measures should be carefully monitored, since continuous alkalinization of urine may induce formation of calcium stones and may enhance susceptibility to infection with organisms that thrive in an alkaline environment. Once formed, xanthine stones may require surgical removal.

Orotic Aciduria. Hereditary orotic aciduria is due to a deficiency of two enzymes, orotidylic pyrophosphorylase and orotidylic decarboxylase. Mixtures of cytidylic and uridylic acid have been reported to produce remissions but have not been well tolerated. Treatment with uridine, the nucleoside of uracil, in divided doses of 150 mg/kg/24 hr is readily tolerated and has resulted in hematologic improvement and diminished urinary orotic acid excretion. A copious intake of fluids assists in dilution of orotic acid in urine and may diminish precipitation of orotic acid crystals.

LYSOSOMAL STORAGE DISEASES

ARTHUR L. BEAUDET, M.D.

The lysosomal storage diseases are due to the genetic deficiency or dysfunction of one or more lysosomal enzymes. This group of disorders includes the lipid storage diseases, the mucopolysaccharidoses, the mucolipidoses, glycoprotein storage diseases, and type II glycogen storage disease (Table 1). The pattern of organ involvement depends on the usual site of degradation of the accumulating macromolecules. Almost all the

TABLE 1. Lysosomal Storage Diseases

G_{M1} gangliosidosis	Sialidosis
G_{M2} gangliosidosis, Tay-Sachs	Aspartylglycosaminuria
G_{M2} gangliosidosis, Sandhoff	Hurler, MPS IH*
Krabbe leukodystrophy	Scheie, MPS IS
Metachromatic leukodystrophy	Hunter, MPS II
Niemann-Pick disease	Sanfilippo A, MPS IIIA
Gaucher disease	Sanfilippo B, MPS IIIB
Fabry disease	Sanfilippo C, MPS IIIC
Wolman disease	Sanfilippo D, MPS IIID
Cholesteryl ester storage disease	Morquio, MPS IV
Farber lipogranulomatosis	Maroteaux-Lamy, MPS VI
Pompe disease, glycogenosis type II	β-Glucuronidase deficiency, MSP VII
Acid phosphatase deficiency	Multiple sulfatase deficiency
Fucosidosis	Mucolipidosis II, I-cell disease
Mannosidosis	Mucolipidosis III
	Mucolipidosis IV

*MPS, mucopolysaccharidosis.

disorders are autosomal recessive defects, although a few are X-linked. Although these diseases are heterogeneous and often have infantile, juvenile, and adult forms associated with the same enzyme defect, the disorders regularly exhibit a progressive course. An enzyme-specific diagnosis is a prerequisite for optimal management.

Medical management of patients with these diseases is largely symptomatic and supportive, but a few specific forms of intervention are important. Hypersplenism develops frequently in adult Gaucher disease, and splenectomy is indicated for correction of significant hematologic abnormalities. The Morquio phenotype is associated with odontoid hypoplasia with instability at the atlantoaxial joint. This joint should be evaluated carefully, even in the absence of symptoms. Prophylactic cervical fusion is indicated during the first decade if instability is significant, since acute and chronic cervical cord damage is likely. Judicious use of corrective orthopedic procedures is appropriate, particularly for the mucopolysaccharidoses such as mild Hunter, Morquio, and Maroteaux-Lamy diseases in which intellectual impairment is minimal or absent. Careful cardiac and opthalmologic follow-up also is needed for the mucopolysaccharidoses and related diseases when these organs are involved.

Myringotomy and polyethylene tubes to prevent recurrent ear infections are very important in the mucopolysaccharidoses, mucolipidoses, and similar phenotypes such as mannosidosis. Hearing can be preserved in intellectually normal patients, and recurrent episodes of fever, irritability, and family stress can be avoided in profoundly impaired children.

Fabry disease has a progressive renal impairment, and renal transplantation and dialysis should be considered according to usual criteria. Renal involvement is usually severe enough to require such intervention in hemizygous males but not in heterozygous females. Painful neuropathy occurs in males and females with Fabry disease, and symptomatic relief often can be obtained with Dilantin in usual therapeutic dosage.

Cardiac and respiratory failure occur in type II glycogen storage disease and are managed symptomatically as for any cardiac and skeletal myopathy. Many of the disorders cause intellectual impairment, and special educational and training support is indicated. At times the possibility of progressive dementia exists, but the child should be given the usual special educational support, since prognosis is never certain.

Unfortunately, many children with these diseases experience progressive and ultimately severe neurologic impairment. Proper emotional and social support for the family is very important. Some of these diseases are most tragic and burdensome for families. The family should be encouraged early to explore local resources for institutional care. This can be of value in the event of family illness and can allow the family vacation time. Eventual long-term institutional care should be at the discretion of the family. Assistance can be provided with some medical problems. Seizures occur in many of the disorders and can be treated routinely. Constipation is frequent and can be managed with stool softeners, laxatives, and enemas in a usual manner. Feeding is progressively difficult and may require blenderized or liquid diets. Behavioral abnormalities, which include emotional outbursts, crying out as if in pain, and failure to sleep at night, are extremely burdensome for the family. Sedative medications may assist a family in managing a child at home, but erratic responses to drugs are not unusual in the face of brain damage. Behavioral difficulties are particularly severe in the Sanfilippo mucopolysaccharidoses but occur with other juvenile disorders. Major tranquilizers such as Mellaril,* in doses up to 3 mg/kg/24 hr may be quite helpful. Finally, there may be many difficult ethical decisions late in the course of these patients. When endless hours are required to feed the patient, tube feeding or gastrostomy may be necessary. Institution of these methods of nutritional support should be discussed with the family as they may prolong the life of a helpless child, a result that may or may not be desired by the family. The family should be involved in deciding when to hospitalize and how to manage pneumonias in terminally ill children.

Specific correction of the enzyme defects in these diseases is a subject of active research. While prenatal diagnosis and other reproductive options can prevent the disease in subsequent siblings, these diseases will continue to occur within families unless heterozygote screening, as applied to Tay-Sachs disease, can be extended to other disorders. For the present, effective therapy is a major need. Enzyme replacement is one research modality. Enzyme activity can be delivered to some organs, such as the liver and spleen. There might be cause for optimism that certain non-CNS manifestations could be treatable by enzyme infusion. To be effective in treating CNS damage, enzyme replacement must overcome the additional obstacle of the blood-brain barrier. At present, enzyme replacement is not of proven effectiveness and is not standard therapy in any lysosomal storage disease. Recent reports have revived interest in bone marrow transplantation or amnion implantation as modes of therapy. Carefully planned research trials are appropriate and are in progress. Some families may wish to explore the opportunities for their children to participate in human studies, but at present there is no proof of effective treatment or prevention of central nervous system symptoms. A variety of physical and biochemical methods for targeting enzyme to affected tissues and for overcoming the blood-brain barrier are being explored. The hope of replacing the defective gene itself is still quite uncertain, although considerably more realistic than at the time of

the last edition of this book. Numerous cDNAs and genomic DNAs for genes encoding lysosomal enzymes are being cloned. Strategies for gene therapy are being formulated, and human trials are expected soon. Lysosomal storage diseases are attractive candidate disorders, since alternative treatment is so limited. On the other hand, there are potential drawbacks, such as the possible need to target genetic material to the central nervous system. Considerable obstacles still remain, and the feasibility of such therapy remains in question.

The final aspect of management of the lysosomal storage diseases is concerned with the family and prevention of future cases. The first step is complete genetic counseling, including a discussion of the risk of the disease, the burden of the disease, and reproductive options. In autosomal recessive conditions, the major risk is for subsequent pregnancies of the parents of the propositus. Occasionally a sibling of the mother will marry a sibling of the father, creating a high-risk situation. Genetic counseling must be extended to maternal relatives in the case of X-linked diseases. Heterozygote detection is feasible for most of the diseases in question and can be offered to aunts, uncles, and unaffected siblings of the patients with autosomal recessive disorders. For reliable heterozygote detection, however, a laboratory should have substantial experience in assaying normal controls and obligate heterozygotes. Samples from the obligate heterozygote parents of the propositus should be assayed simultaneously to assist in family-specific interpretation of unusual laboratory data which may result from rare alleles (mutant forms of the gene) in a family. Heterozygote testing of relatives is most important in disorders in which the carrier frequency is great, such as for Gaucher or Tay-Sachs disease in the Ashkenazi Jewish population. Mass screening for heterozygotes has been applied for the prevention of Tay-Sachs disease but has not been used significantly for other lysosomal storage diseases to date.

As part of the genetic counseling process, contraception, sterilization, adoption, and artificial insemination should be discussed as alternative methods for reducing the risk of disease. Prenatal diagnosis has been accomplished or presumably could be carried out for almost all the lysosomal storage diseases. The enzyme defects routinely are demonstrable in cultured fibroblasts and amniotic fluid cells. The newer diagnostic procedure of chorionic villus biopsy is proving reliable for most or all lysosomal storage diseases. This earlier prenatal test is attractive to many families with these high genetic risks. The vast majority of biochemical prenatal diagnoses in the last decade has involved the lysosomal storage diseases, with Tay-Sachs disease, type II glycogen storage disease, Krabbe leukodystrophy, metachromatic leukodystrophy, and Hurler disease among the most frequently tested.

---

*Manufacturer's precaution: Mellaril is not recommended for children under 2 years of age.

11

Connective Tissue

RHEUMATIC DISEASES OF CHILDHOOD

ILONA S. SZER, M.D.

The rheumatic diseases (collagen vascular diseases) are a diverse group of conditions characterized by inflammation of the connective tissues. Manifestations of this chronic inflammation may include arthritis, fever, and rash, as well as evidence of specific extra-articular organ inflammation, such as nephritis, carditis, and uveitis.

To control the often crippling and sometimes fatal sequelae of inflammation, the management of rheumatic diseases in children calls for a co-ordinated, multidisciplinary approach that not only addresses specific disease manifestations but also assures both child and family function at home, at school, and in the local community.

A high level of expertise is required by professionals experienced in dealing with children and skilled in pediatric rheumatology, nursing, physical, and occupational therapy, nutrition, social services, ophthalmology, and orthopedics. Ideally, this team of experts should be available each and every time the child is seen at the tertiary pediatric rheumatology center to avoid fragmentation of care, miscommunication, and multiple visits.

At the level of the local community, a similar team of consistent providers led by the pediatrician should be identified. All of the health providers must have knowledge of federal and state laws regarding special services for chronically ill children. Through education, the parents become child advocates and, as such, members of the management team. Yearly school meetings should be encouraged, and whenever possible, attended by a member of the health care team to outline the specific education plan for the child and ensure optimal function in the classroom.

JUVENILE RHEUMATOID ARTHRITIS (JRA)

The principles of therapy for children with various types of JRA are largely the same whether the onset of disease is pauciarticular, systemic, or polyarticular, even though these represent distinct clinical entities with the common feature of chronic joint inflammation. The overall prognosis for children with JRA is excellent, although children with pauciarticular-onset juvenile rheumatoid arthritis carry a more favorable prognosis regarding long-term joint function than do those with multiple joint involvement. Because true bony changes are uncommon in children and 80 to 85 per cent achieve remission, maintenance of proper joint function and strength is critical. This is accomplished by anti-inflammatory drugs and physical and/or occupational therapy.

The goal of drug therapy is to reduce the inflammation, which produces pain, swelling, warmth, and tenderness. Once pain control is achieved, children are able to tolerate an individualized exercise program aimed at maintaining normal ambulation, range of motion, and muscle strength and reducing and preventing flexion contractures and muscle atrophy. With daily physical and occupational therapy, children with arthritis are fit to participate in normal recreation and play and are independent in activities of daily living and ambulation. The use of wheelchairs, buggies, and crutches should never be encouraged. These and other assistive devices should be deferred for as long as possible. Above all, positive thinking about an independent and productive future should be taught and practiced.

Drug Therapy

Control of inflammation is the goal of the medical therapy for children with chronic arthritis. In general, the milder the disease, the less medicine is required to achieve control. Approximately 5 per cent of children with juvenile rheumatoid arthritis do not require drug treatment, as they do not experience pain, stiffness, or limitation of motion. Painless swelling that does not interfere with function may be left untreated unless there is muscle atrophy from even minimal favoring or leg length discrepancy develops.

Nonsteroidal Anti-inflammatory Drugs (NSAIDs)

SALICYLATES. Salicylates remain the mainstay of treatment for children with JRA. These come in a variety of sizes and preparations requiring different dosing regimens (Table 1). In general, an anti-inflammatory serum level of approximately 20 mg/dl or 200 mg/L can be achieved within 10 days of administering salicylates at 70 to 100 mg/kg/day for children up to 25 kg and 50 to 70 mg/kg/day for children whose weight exceeds 25 kg. The dose for all patients should be titrated to the desired clinical response, as some children respond to a lower dose and others require a much greater amount. For example, children with systemic-onset JRA often need salicylate doses above 120 mg/kg/day to achieve control. Unfortunately, the rate of intolerance rises when the salicylate level approaches 25 to 30 mg/dl. The most commonly encountered side effects in young children are irritability and personality changes, with concomitant rise in hepatic enzymes. These abnormalities are usually dose-related and disappear when the drug is reduced. Nausea, vomiting, and rapid, heavy breathing, which indicate metabolic acidosis, are clear indicators of salicylism and call for discontinuation of the drug. The risk of Reye syndrome associated with aspirin intake has recently been emphasized. Fortunately, only a handful of case reports describe an association of high-dose, chronic salicylate use with Reye syndrome. In our clinic, we recommend stopping aspirin temporarily for children with chickenpox and a flu-like syndrome with vomiting. In addition, we recommend flu vaccines for children receiving chronic salicylates.

NONSALICYLATED NSAIDs. Tolmetin sodium (Tolectin) and naproxen (Naprosyn) are the only other nonsteroidal anti-inflammatory drugs labeled by the FDA for use in children with chronic arthritis (Table 1). Tolmetin should be tried in those children who either do not respond to salicylates or cannot tolerate a dose required to achieve control. Tolmetin is usually well tolerated, but its effectiveness may not be as great as that of salicylates. A 1-month trial is probably sufficient, although 3 months are often needed, before changing to another agent. Gastrointestinal irritation and, rarely, headaches may limit the utility of Tolmetin administration and necessitate change to another agent. Naproxen is the most recently approved agent for the treatment of childhood arthritis. This drug is often preferred because of its easier, twice-daily dosing schedule. It is also available in liquid form preferred for young children. Similar to tolmetin, naproxen may take weeks to begin to control symptoms, but it is well tolerated and safe. Rarely, gastrointestinal intolerance necessitates discontinuation.

Over the last decade many additional NSAIDs have become available for adults with arthritis; some of these have been tested in children through collaborative multicenter studies. Dosing, efficacy, and side effects are known, but there is no approval from the FDA for use in children. These include ibuprofen, fenoprofen, meclofemate sodium, and indomethacin (Table 1). In our clinic, we start with salicylates, followed by tolmetin or naproxen. Sometimes combining two NSAIDs, while paying close attention to gastric protection, is effective. If any of the approved agents or combinations fail to sufficiently control inflammation, we try a NSAID not approved for children, but one that has been studied for both safety and efficacy in a pediatric setting. All of these medicines should be taken with milk after a meal. It is also appropriate to prescribe antacids such as Maalox and Mylanta.

The total length of treatment varies for each patient. Generally, anti-inflammatory therapy is required for as long as there is active inflammation. For most children with pauciarticular-onset JRA, therapy is continued for 1 to 2 years, using as parameters clinical signs and

TABLE 1. Drug Therapy for Chronic Childhood Arthritis

	Size (mg/tab)	Schedule	Dose (mg/kg/day)	Max Amount (mg/day)
Nonsteroidal Anti-inflammatory Drugs (NSAIDs)				
Salicylate preparations				
Acetylsalicylic acid (aspirin)	81 or 325	qid	75–100 to get	
Zorprin	800	bid	serum level of	
Choline magnesium trisalicylate (Trilisate)	500*	tid	20–25 mg/dl	
Choline salicylate (Arthropan)	650*	tid		
Nonsalicylate NSAIDs approved for children				
Tolmetin sodium (Tolectin)	200 or 400	tid	20–30	2000
Naproxen (Naprosyn)	250,375,500	bid	10–15	750
Naproxen liquid	125*	bid or tid	10–15	750
NSAIDs not approved for use in children				
Indomethacin (Indocin)	25	tid or qid	1–3	200
Ibuprofen (Motrin, Advil)	200,300, or 400	qid	20–50	2400
Fenoprofen calcium (Nalfon)	200,300, or 600	qid	40–50	3200
Meclofenamate sodium (Meclomen)	50,100	tid	4–6	300
Sulindac (Clinoril)†	150,200	bid	4–6	400
Piroxicam (Feldene)†	10,20	od	0.5	20
Slow-Acting Antirheumatic Drugs (SAARDs)				
Gold salts				
Myochrysine, Salgenol		every week (IM)	0.5–1‡	50
Auranofin (Ridaura)	3	every day	0.1	6
Hydroxychloroquine (Plaquenil)	200	every day	7	400
Methotrexate	2.5	every week	5–10§	

*mg/5ml
†not tested in children
‡mg/kg/week
§mg/m²/week

symptoms and weaning the medicine 3 to 4 months after signs of inflammation have subsided. Blood tests are usually of no value in assessing the activity of the disease but may be used for those patients who had abnormal values at the onset of the disease. The antinuclear antibody, often positive in these children, may remain in the serum for many years and does not serve as a guide to drug management.

Children with polyarticular and systemic-onset JRA require treatment for prolonged periods of time, often marked by times of lesser disease activity during which lower doses, or no medicine, may be given. The principle of giving the least medicine sufficient to control inflammation interfering with normal function applies at all times.

Second-Line Agents

The slow-acting antirheumatic drugs (SAARDs), also known as disease-modifying or remittive agents, are reserved for those children with aggressive multijoint disease. These children are adversely affected despite proper use of NSAIDs and are threatened with crippling and the risk of nonambulation. Administration of these agents, which include gold salts, penicillamine, and hydroxychloroquine, must be carried out in a pediatric rheumatology setting because of the high risk of side effects and the absolute need for close follow-up. Gold salts, previously available only in the form of intramuscular injection (Myochrysine or Salganol), are now available in a pill form (Auranofin). Both preparations have been studied in children and shown to be only mildly effective while quite toxic. Up to 30 per cent of children do not tolerate intramuscular gold, necessitating its withdrawal. The incidence of side effects as well as efficacy is somewhat less with the oral preparation. Reasons for discontinuation include allergic rashes and itching, mouth sores, diarrhea, proteinuria, and eosinophilia. Children with systemic-onset JRA are at a serious additional risk for the development of life-threatening disseminated intravascular coagulation (DIC), reported after the second injection of intramuscular gold. This complication has not been reported following administration of Auranofin. Although the potential for inducing remission exists with gold therapy, this event is exceedingly rare. More commonly, there seems to be a modification of disease activity with improved function, less pain and stiffness, and more endurance. It may take up to 6 months for clinically appreciable change to take place, but a positive effect may be noted after the second month. A 6-month trial of one or the other form of gold is usually attempted for selected patients.

Hydroxychloroquine (Plaquenil) is commonly used for adults with arthritis. This agent, whose mechanism of action is not understood, has been studied in children and found no more effective than placebo. However, because of its relative short-term safety, it may be tried for 3 to 6 months if the disease is not too aggressive and time is of no issue. Long-term toxicity of Hydroxychloroquine is limited to the eyes and secondary to accumulation of the drug in the macula. We recommend twice yearly ophthalmologic evaluations and discontinue the drug if there is interference with color or peripheral vision.

The last of the SAARDs, D-penicillamine, is sometimes helpful in adult rheumatoid arthritis but has not been found effective in children when compared to placebo. The rate of side effects is high, making this agent of limited, if any, use in the pediatric rheumatology setting.

Corticosteroids

Systemic and local steroids have a limited, but important, role in the treatment of juvenile rheumatoid arthritis. Their use should be restricted to the pediatric rheumatology clinic and avoided if at all possible. There are, however, several specific criteria for their use: (1) Systemic steroids are often needed to control extra-articular manifestations of systemic-onset JRA, such as hectic fever, anemia, and pericarditis. Steroids should be weaned as soon as control of these parameters is achieved. Although the initial indication for corticosteroids is not arthritis, joint inflammation responds well to steroids, and tapering may result in severe flare of arthritis. Small doses of 1 to 5 mg of prednisone daily or every other day may enable an otherwise bedridden child to function independently. (2) A single local steroid injection into an inflamed and contracted joint may be considered for a child with monoarticular disease unresponsive to medical and physical therapy. Since the risks of this procedure include infection, local osteopenia, and damage to the growing epiphesis, it should not be repeated. (3) The use of steroid drops in the treatment of eye inflammation is reviewed elsewhere.

Although steroids are potent anti-inflammatory agents and offer rapid relief of symptoms, the many risks associated with their use, in addition to osteoporosis, avascular necrosis of bone, and muscle atrophy, should absolutely discourage their use for children with chronic joint inflammation.

Third-Line Agents

Cytotoxic drugs, which include methotrexate, cyclophosphamide (Cytoxan), azathioprine (Imuran), and chlorambucil, are reserved for those children whose disease is crippling and unresponsive to more conventional therapies. A 6-month double-blind placebo-controlled multicenter methotrexate trial for children with severe JRA has recently been completed. This agent promises to be quite effective while not posing a high risk of side effects. In adult trials, methotrexate was effective in 70 per cent of patients, compared with 20 per cent receiving placebo. Recent data from studies of adult patients suggest that the dose of methotrexate may need to be increased with time and that discontinuation of the drug may result in severe, hard-to-control exacerbations. These considerations in children are all the more potent, as we may be committing our young patients to a lifetime of cytotoxic therapy. However, it appears that the drug is well tolerated and not associated with a high rate of side effects. These side effects may include bone marrow, liver, gonadal, and, rarely, renal toxicity. Azathioprine, cyclophosphamide, and chlorambucil have not been studied in children. In our clinic, none of the cytotoxic agents except methotrexate has been tried.

Physical Management

Physical and occupational therapy form a cornerstone in the management of chronic childhood arthritis. Since the potential for remission exists for the majority of children, it is imperative to preserve joint integrity. Bony erosion is rare in JRA, but tendon and ligament shortening and muscle atrophy are common. The goal of a physical therapy program, including passive, active, and resistive exercises, is to preserve full range of motion and muscle strength. This is accomplished by a daily exercise program carried out at home by the parent, at school by a school therapist, or in a hospital or health club setting. Normal play and recreation are always encouraged. The goal of occupational therapy is to preserve independence in activities of daily living and age-appropriate function, often curtailed by arthritis of small joints of the hands and wrists. Daily exercise in addition to specific training in various tasks is prescribed and monitored by the therapist.

Nighttime use of splinting devices and braces is limited to persistent contractures only. The most frequent use of splinting is for flexion contractures of the knee. Removable bivalve casts are fabricated in as much extension as tolerated. These are adjusted as extension improves, and their use is discontinued when the contraction resolves. The other common application in splinting is in wrist arthritis to arrest progressive loss of wrist dorsiflexion (extension) and to prevent hand weakness. Splints are fabricated to encourage as much dorsiflexion and position of function as possible. We do not prescribe resting or day splints. Air splints may sometimes be used for children with elbow flexion contractures or small children with knee contractures, at night only. Small lifts are frequently placed inside shoes or over the soles for children with leg length discrepancy. This is particularly common in young children with pauciarticular-onset JRA with asymmetric knee or ankle inflammation. Leg lengths must be monitored regularly, as with time the discrepancy diminishes and the lift should be removed.

Iridocyclitis

One of the most important and potentially devastating extra-articular complications of JRA is inflammation of the anterior uveal tract. Iritis or iridocyclitis is asymptomatic but diagnosed easily by a slit lamp examination, which reveals cells and flare in the anterior chamber of the eye. Children with pauciarticular-onset JRA are at highest risk for the development of this complication, which may result in blindness if ignored. Ophthalmologic evaluations must be performed quarterly for children with pauciarticular-onset JRA and once or twice per year for all other children with chronic arthritis. The need for slit lamp examination continues for several years after the arthritis has remitted. Treatment is highly successful if initiated early and before any scarring takes place. It consists of local steroid eye drops, often given in conjunction with mydriatic drops. Unfortunately, long-term side effects of local steroid application include cataract formation and, rarely, glaucoma.

SYSTEMIC-ONSET JRA

Extra-articular manifestations of this disease often overshadow the arthritis and require special management. Control of fever may sometimes be accomplished with salicylates alone or in combination with tolmetin or naproxen. As already mentioned, rather high doses of salicylate may be needed, presumably owing to malabsorption, increasing the risk of toxicity as the child improves and begins to absorb the drug. When the illness is complicated by severe anemia and/or pericarditis, systemic steroids are usually required for control. A dosage of 1 to 2 mg/kg/day or 2 to 3 mg/kg every other day achieves response in virtually all children. Since steroids interfere with salicylates, aspirin levels must be monitored carefully and dosage adjusted appropriately. As steroids are weaned, salicylate level rises again.

Pericarditis, if present, is often complicated by a pericardial effusion, which may need surgical drainage. The procedure can be done in the cardiac catheterization laboratory and the drain is left in place for 24 to 48 hours. By this time systemic steroids usually take effect and drains may be removed. Once control is achieved, steroids are weaned to an alternate-day regimen and slowly discontinued while salicylates or other NSAIDs are maintained. Since systemic manifestations abate in the majority of children within 6 to 12 months, long-term management focuses on arthritis and is identical to that discussed previously.

SPONDYLOARTHROPATHY SYNDROMES

Children with spondyloarthritis are treated similarly to children with other forms of chronic arthritis, with additional attention to lumbosacral spine flexibility and chest expansion. The physical therapy program focuses on both range of motion and strengthening of low back and respiratory muscles. It is generally accepted that spondyloarthritis responds better to tolmetin and naproxen than to salicylates, but we have not found this to be uniformly correct. Similarly, gold is thought not to be helpful for this form of arthritis; however, in the occasional patient with severe peripheral joint involvement, it may be of benefit. Gold or other SAARDs have not been studied in patients with spondyloarthritis; neither is there any experience with methotrexate. Eye involvement in spondyloarthritis is usually symptomatic and responds well to local steroid drops.

DERMATOMYOSITIS

The treatment of children with dermatomyositis differs from center to center. Although all pediatric rheumatologists treat this disease with steroids and physical therapy, dosing schedules vary greatly.

In our clinic, the approach to dermatomyositis is aggressive, and results have been extremely satisfying. The course of treatment can be summarized as induction and maintenance therapy that is completed over a 2-year period. The initial dose of prednisone is between 2 and 3 mg/kg/day in a split dose. Physical therapy is initiated early and prescribed twice daily to improve strength and mobility. Gentle stretching of Achilles tendons and hamstrings is imperative. Children are seen weekly or admitted to the hospital if there is any compromise of the palatal or respiratory muscles. Once muscle enzymes return to normal (2 to 4 weeks), the dose is consolidated to once daily and maintained until muscle strength reaches nearly normal level (2 to 3 months). At this time follow-up can be adjusted to monthly visits and the dose tapered every month by 10 per cent, provided that muscle enzymes remain normal and muscle strength continues to improve. Within 12 months the daily dose is usually down to 5 mg/day, at which it is maintained for another 6 to 8 months and then slowly discontinued. With this protocol, most children are well within 2 to 3 months and at decreased risk of late complications of poorly controlled disease such as muscle contractures, persistent weakness, and calcinosis. The rate of complications, except for commonly encountered cushingoid appearance, weight gain, and temporary growth arrest, has been extremely low in our patients. Occasionally, however, the prednisone cannot be tapered because of recurrence of weakness. For those patients, cytotoxic therapy, usually given in the form of methotrexate, either orally or through intramuscular or intravenous injection, at 1 mg/kg/week (maximum 20 to 25 mg weekly) is prescribed. Following the addition of methotrexate, prednisone may usually be tapered to 5 mg/day followed by gradual methotrexate elimination.

Treatment of Skin Manifestations

The rash of dermatomyositis usually begins to fade as muscle strength improves and does not require special treatment. Some children, however, develop severe cutaneous manifestations. Sun screens and other devices protecting skin from ultraviolet light should be tried. Steroid creams usually do not help. Hydroxychloroquine may be of use in some cases. The dose is the same as that for arthritis (Table 1).

Vasculitic ulcers are sometimes early signs of dermatomyositis. These respond to corticosteroid treatment but often become superinfected with skin flora and require local hygiene, frequent soaking, and systemic antibiotics.

SYSTEMIC LUPUS ERYTHEMATOSUS (SLE) AND MIXED CONNECTIVE TISSUE DISEASE (MCTD)

Treatment of SLE and the related disorder, MCTD, must be tailored to the individual child and carried out by physicians experienced in the care of children with lupus. General principles of our management are based on the knowledge of the natural history of this disease in children; it is more severe than in adults, and mild SLE in children occurs only rarely. Our goals are (1) to prevent major flares, which invariably result in organ scarring and shorten organ life span; (2) to control clinical manifestations of the disease and allow normal activity without frequent hospitalizations; and (3) to do the least harm with the therapeutic regimen.

As virtually all children with SLE present with multiorgan disease and severe immune abnormalities, early treatment is focused on rapid control of both clinical and serologic parameters of disease activity accomplished with high-dose (2 to 3 mg/kg/day) prednisone, given three to four times daily. Within 2 to 3 weeks clinical improvement can be expected. The complement and anti–native DNA antibody levels usually normalize within 4 to 8 weeks, at which time the dose may be consolidated to once daily. Provided that there is no exacerbation in either serologic parameters (complement and anti-DNA antibody levels) or organ function, the prednisone is changed to an alternate-day regimen by doubling the daily amount and adding another 20 to 30 per cent. All of the children in our clinic tolerate "the switch" with only minimal feeling of dizziness during the first "off" day, which may be treated with 5 or 10 mg of prednisone. The dose is then tapered monthly by 10 per cent, provided that complement and anti-ds DNA antibodies are normal and there is no clinical evidence of major organ involvement. After several years of monthly follow-up, the prednisone may be discontinued. Those children whose disease flares during the taper, even if the flare is manifested only by immune abnormalities, become candidates for steroid-sparing cytotoxic therapy. Azathioprine is a well-tolerated cytotoxic drug that often controls disease activity at a dose of 2 mg/kg/day and allows steroid withdrawal. Cyclophosphamide is reserved for those children who have major organ disease such as nephritis despite high-dose steroid treatment and those children for whom azathioprine did not allow steroid withdrawal. We have used intravenous cyclophosphamide at a dose of 0.5 to 1 gm/m²/month for 6 months in children with active glomerulonephritis. Several children have reached complete remission, whereas others have continued with every-3-month treatments and have done well. Encouraging results of randomized trials using intravenous cyclophosphamide for patients with severe renal disorder suggest that cytotoxic therapy is superior to prednisone alone in the treatment of lupus nephritis.

It is not clear that other treatment protocols, such as intravenous monthly corticosteroids, combination chemotherapy, or other cytotoxic drugs, offer advantages over any other regimen. These are employed rarely when other interventions fail.

For those few children with SLE whose disease is limited to skin and joints, NSAIDs offer relief of pain and inflammation, and hydroxychloroquine or dapsone may be tried to control rash. Raynaud phenomenon responds well to biofeedback training taught by the occupational therapist.

Prognosis for children with SLE has changed dramatically from nearly 100 per cent mortality to over 90 per cent survival. Earlier recognition and attention to the immune abnormalities as well as aggressive treatment have no doubt had an impact. The next two decades, as our patients are surviving into adulthood, will tell whether the newer treatment regimens are leading to morbidity such as unacceptably high rate of avascular necrosis of bone, cataract formation, atherosclerotic heart disease, gonadal dysfunction, and malignancy.

EOSINOPHILIC FASCIITIS

Children with this rare disorder are treated successfully with moderate (0.5 to 1 mg/kg/day) doses of prednisone. Most children respond quickly and can be weaned off the medication within 1 year. If there is no appreciable response, steroids should be discontinued after a 3-month trial. Physical therapy should always accompany medical management to prevent contractures resulting from soft-tissue scarring. Prognosis is favorable in the majority of patients, although skin changes may persist for years.

EOSINOPHILIC FASCIITIS

NICHOLAS A. PATRONE, M.D.

Most patients with eosinophilic fasciitis respond dramatically to corticosteroids. The dose of prednisone is 20 to 60 mg/day (0.5 mg/kg/24 hr), tapered gradually over 3 to 6 months to an every-other-day dosage. Length of treatment varies; there are no guidelines for total duration of therapy, but lack of response within 3 months should lead to discontinuation of corticosteroid therapy.

Although nonsteroidal anti-inflammatory agents may bring symptomatic relief, they have not been shown to reverse pathologic changes. In refractory cases penicillamine may lead to remission, but practitioners must remain alert for a multitude of possible side effects. In addition, individual case reports describe improvement with hydroxychloroquine, azathioprine, colchicine, and cimetidine; however, large studies showing consistent improvement are lacking.

Delays in diagnosis may lead to irreversible flexion contractures, but a response may occur with the institution of steroid therapy. The long-term natural history of eosinophilic fasciitis is unknown. Although most patients with this disease improve, flexion contractures and skin changes may remain for years after the onset of symptoms. Progression to systemic disease such as scleroderma is unusual. Physical therapy may be indicated for severe flexion contractures and muscle atrophy secondary to disuse.

12

Genitourinary Tract

RENAL HYPOPLASIA AND DYSPLASIA

MAX MAIZELS, M.D.

NORMAL EMBRYOLOGY

Conceptualizing the pathoembryology of the kidney is useful in the treatment of children with renal hypoplasia and dysplasia. Normal kidney development requires a proper and complete interaction between the components of the renal blastema, the ampullae of the ureteral bud branches (formative ureter, pelvis, calyces, and collecting ducts), and the metanephrogenic mesenchyme (formative nephrons and renal capsule). Normally, this interaction occurs over about 30 weeks, from approximately 6 weeks of gestation to term, and creates a newborn's full complement of nephrons.

RENAL HYPOPLASIA

Hypoplasia should refer simply to kidneys with a reduced complement of nephrons induced by the blastema. However, as nephron counting is not clinically feasible, it has come to be common practice to refer to hypoplastic kidneys as those that are seen to be small at surgery or as imaged radiographically.

Most commonly, small kidneys are found in association with vesicoureteral reflux, with or without urinary tract infection. Reflux in such kidneys should be corrected by surgically reimplanting the ureter into the bladder trigone. Less common causes, such as renal artery stenosis or renal lithiasis, should be treated by saphenous vein aortorenal bypass or shock wave lithotripsy, respectively. Small kidneys in association with obstructive uropathy, such as ureteropelvic junction obstruction, primary obstructive megaureter, prune belly syndrome, or posterior urethral valves, should have surgical reconstruction of the obstructed segment. Drainage procedures, such as nephrostomy, ureterostomy, or vesicostomy, should be few and only temporary. Kidneys that are small consequent to renal vein thrombosis require nephrologic management.

RENAL DYSPLASIA

Dysplasia should refer simply to an abnormal interaction of the components of the renal blastema that results in a reduced complement of nephrons. Many of these nephrons may not be normally formed, as indicated grossly by cysts, histologically by the presence of abnormal renal architecture with or without primitive ducts, and on renal scintigraphy by the lack of function. Obstruction commonly accompanies clinical dysplasia but is not required in laboratory models. This pathoembryology may result in a spectrum of clinical renal developments. When obstruction coexists with renal dysplasia and the involved kidney functions, reconstruc-

TABLE 1. Algorithm to Manage Children with Multicystic Kidney

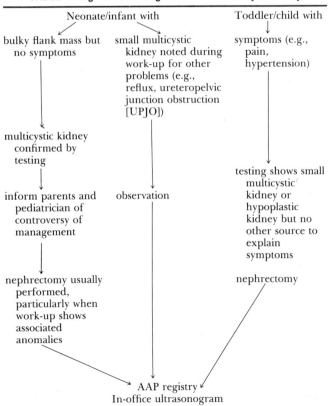

343

tive surgery, rather than nephrectomy, should be attempted (e.g., ipsilateral ureteroureterostomy for ureterocele or ectopic ureter). Maternal-fetal ultrasonography has contributed to early detection of such anomalies and has permitted repair before clinical symptoms appear. This practice of early detection and repair has undoubtedly reversed the old notion that such conditions progress to uremia despite surgical reconstruction.

Less information is available on the appropriate management of children with the classic multicystic kidney because there is little known about the natural history of this condition. The notion that such kidneys may lead to urinary tract infection, hematuria, hypertension, or carcinoma has led to "prophylactic" nephrectomy. However, because these problems were believed to be unusual, observation of selected cases has shown that some kidneys have involuted in 1-year-old children. In recognition of the lack of basic facts upon which to base treatment, an algorithm is presented (Table 1) to aid empiric treatment. Because of the tendency toward infection in the large cysts of a multicystic kidney, nephrectomy is suggested, especially when cysts remain large in infants older than 6 months.

Irrespective of the decision regarding surgery, the contralateral kidney should be surveyed by ultrasonography for hydronephrosis, as about 20 per cent of these kidneys show obstructive uropathy. Similarly, parents and siblings of the index child may be screened for hydronephrosis or solitary kidney simply, using in-office ultrasonography. To further our understanding of the natural history and appropriate treatment of multicystic kidney, diagnosed cases should be reported to the American Academy of Pediatrics (AAP), Section on Urology, Multicystic Kidney Registry.

HYDRONEPHROSIS AND DISORDERS OF THE URETER

EVAN J. KASS, M.D.

"Idiopathic hydronephrosis" is a descriptive term indicating the presence of an enlarged pelvicalyceal system. "Hydroureter," similarly, indicates the presence of a dilated ureter. Until recently, the mere observation of such upper urinary tract dilatation on an excretory urogram was often sufficient evidence to diagnose obstruction and justify corrective surgery. However, considerable evidence now demonstrates that not all dilatation of the upper urinary system is the result of an obstruction, and in such cases progressive loss of renal function is not inevitable. Nonobstructive dilatation may occur as an isolated condition unassociated with any underlying abnormality or in association with prune-belly syndrome, diabetes insipidus, or vesicoureteral reflux. The goal of any evaluation protocol is to determine whether an obstructive lesion is present, determine the location of this obstruction, and assess renal function. Only with all of this information can one decide on the appropriate course of management.

The magnitude of the pelvicalyceal dilatation is not a reliable guide to the presence of obstruction, since similar degrees of enlargement may be observed in both obstructed and unobstructed systems. Although the presence of abdominal pain, hematuria, or urinary tract infection may prompt the initial urologic evaluation, the presence or absence of such symptoms is not an absolute determinant of urinary obstruction. In addition, hydronephrosis is frequently detected incidentally during an evaluation for enuresis or cardiac defects; and more recently, with the use of antenatal ultrasonography, the diagnosis of in-utero hydronephrosis is being made with ever-increasing frequency. Therefore, it is imperative that every child with urinary tract dilatation be objectively evaluated to determine the functional significance of this observed upper tract dilatation. Only then can a rational decision be made as to the best plan of management.

In obstruction the intrapelvic pressure is directly related to the urine flow rate and duration of the diuresis as well as the degree of obstruction. The loss of renal function is proportional to the magnitude and the duration of this rise in intrapelvic pressure. In a complete obstruction for more than 1 week, permanent deterioration of glomerular and tubular function will take place. However, congenital obstruction is rarely complete and the elasticity of the collecting system often serves to cushion the nephron from the full effect of the elevated intrapelvic pressure. Because the intrapelvic pressure remains within the normal physiologic range except when the diuretic load exceeds the transport capacity of the obstructed system, it is not unusual in chronic obstruction for the glomerular filtration rate to be preserved for a long period of time. Systems that are dilated but not obstructed do not demonstrate this rise in intrapelvic pressure, even under maximal diuresis, and therefore are not at risk for progressive renal damage.

This underlying physiologic difference between obstructed and unobstructed systems can be employed to discriminate between true obstruction and nonobstructive dilatation. The pressure perfusion study described by Whitaker is based upon the concept that an unobstructed urinary system is unable to transport urine at a rate of 10 cc/min without a concomitant elevation of intrapelvic hydrostatic pressure. Only an unobstructed system is capable of transporting fluid at this rate without a concomitant pressure rise. The major advantage of this study is that the perfusion medium is introduced directly into the renal pelvis via a percutaneous catheter; therefore, impaired renal function is not a limiting factor. However, since percutaneous puncture of the renal collecting system is required, the study is invasive and frequently requires sedation or general anesthesia.

The diuretic-augmented renal scan is a noninvasive isotope study capable of providing objective criteria for diagnosing urinary obstruction. Interpretation is based upon the concept that prolonged retention of the radionuclide in the dilated, unobstructed collecting system is the result of a reservoir effect. When urine flow is increased by diuretic administration, the urine containing the tracer rapidly leaves the unobstructed collecting system and is replaced by tracer-free urine. In the presence of obstruction the radionuclide leaves the system slowly, even with diuretic stimulation. With the aid of a gamma camera microcomputer system, the tracer activity within the dilated collecting system can be accurately determined and the time required for half the tracer to leave the collecting system measured. When this half-time is less than 15 minutes, no obstruction is present, and when the half-time is over 20 minutes, obstruction is thought to be present. With a half-time between 15 and 20 minutes, or when renal function is significantly compromised, this study is not reliable and other means of assessing urinary obstruction must be employed.

Both the pressure perfusion study and the diuretic augmented renal scan have an accuracy of greater than 90 per cent. Frequently, both studies will be required to completely evaluate a dilated collecting system. At the present time, there is no single study or test that reliably diagnoses obstruction or excludes its presence with 100 per cent accuracy.

The standard excretory urogram, even when combined with retrograde pyelography or ultrasonography, is not a reliable indicator of urinary obstruction. These studies merely depict the anatomy of the collecting system. When hydronephrosis is detected, a diuretic renal scan should be obtained to provide baseline information concerning individual renal function as well as an objective evaluation of obstruction. When the diuretic scan does not adequately define the situation, a pressure perfusion study may be required.

When objective evidence confirms the presence of urinary tract obstruction, surgical correction should be carried out promptly. Nonoperative management is indicated only for those children who show no objective evidence of obstruction; however, until long-term information is available as to the ultimate fate of the child with a dilated, unobstructed system, periodic renal scans are recommended to ensure that asymptomatic renal damage does not occur.

The ureteropelvic junction is the most common site of upper urinary tract obstruction in infants and children. The diagnosis of ureteropelvic junction obstruction requires prompt surgical correction. The most commonly performed surgical procedure is a dismembered Anderson-Hynes pyeloplasty. In this procedure, the abnormal ureteropelvic junction is excised and the normal ureter spatulated and reanastomosed to the renal pelvis. It is not uncommon to find aberrant blood vessels or bands causing angulation of the ureteropelvic junction. Management of these extrinsic abnormalities alone rarely relieves the obstruction, since virtually all children with congenital ureteropelvic junction obstruction have an intrinsic ureteral abnormality responsible for the obstruction.

The second most common site of upper urinary tract obstruction is the ureterovesical junction. In all children with such dilatation a voiding cystourethrogram should be obtained to exclude vesicoureteral reflux and infravesical obstruction. Dilatation of the pelvicalyceal system is a common finding in children with vesicoureteral reflux and can also be seen in children with posterior urethral valves or neuropathic bladder dysfunction. In infants, significant transient ureteropelvic dilatation can be seen following a severe urinary tract infection that resolves with appropriate antimicrobial therapy.

The treatment of primary ureterovesical junction obstruction includes excision of the abnormal ureteral segment and reimplantation of the ureter into the bladder. Since the ureter that is to be reimplanted may be considerably dilated, it is often necessary to tailor it so that a proper ratio of ureteral diameter to submucosal tunnel length can be achieved. The abnormality responsible for a ureterovesical junction obstruction is an intrinsic abnormality of the muscle itself, similar to that seen in a ureteropelvic junction obstruction. Although this entity has been termed "obstructive megaureter," it does not share the aganglionic abnormality associated with congenital megacolon.

The majority of obstructed kidneys are salvageable, and nephrectomy is rarely necessary. In the past the criteria for nephrectomy have been subjective; however, a poorly visualizing kidney on an excretory urogram, or a kidney providing less than 10 per cent of the total renal function on a renal scan, may still be salvageable. The final decision for nephrectomy should always be made at surgery. Since there is little risk to attempted salvage of a hydronephrotic kidney, nephrectomy should be reserved for obviously hopeless cases.

Long-term follow-up of renal function is required in all children with obstructive uropathy, since delayed deterioration has been described in these individuals even when they appear to have maintained stable renal function for years. The diuretic-augmented renal scan provides an objective measure of individual renal function and drainage and, when compared with preoperative studies, gives invaluable information as to the success of corrective surgery.

The prenatal diagnosis of hydronephrosis is being made with ever-increasing frequency. Antenatal intervention strategies for the management of such hydronephrosis are currently being experimented with at some centers; however, extreme caution must be advised about general adoption of these techniques. At this time no objective criteria exist for defining upper urinary tract obstruction in utero, nor are there any data to suggest that in utero decompression of an obstructed kidney is superior to postnatal intervention. Until these data become available, the primary role of prenatal sonography will be to identify those infants with an abnormality who will benefit from early postnatal evaluation of their hydronephrosis. Following delivery, a prompt, thorough evaluation should be carried out, and those individuals found to have obstruction can be appropriately managed before complications occur, thereby maximizing the preservation of renal function. Individuals who do not meet the objective criteria for urinary obstruction do not require surgery but should be monitored for evidence of progressive hydronephrosis or loss of renal function.

MALIGNANT TUMORS OF THE KIDNEY

GEORGE T. KLAUBER, M.D.

Wilms' tumor or nephroblastoma is the most common malignant tumor of the kidney and urinary tract in children, accounting for approximately 95 per cent of all such cancers. Survival rates have improved dramatically in the past 25 years, resulting in "cures" for the majority of affected children. This is due largely to the advent of chemotherapy plus the evolution of referral centers. Collaborative studies, such as the National Wilms' Tumor Study (NWTS), have shared group experience for a tumor that occurs approximately 500 times per year in the USA.

The diagnosis should be suspected in any child with an abdominal mass, hypertension, or hematuria. Radiologic studies, including computed tomography and ultrasonography, if available, should be performed as soon as possible. Surgery should follow within 48 to 72 hours. Prognosis and specific therapy are dependent on accurate surgical staging and histology. Severe anemia, cachexia, or hypertension may need to be corrected or stabilized prior to surgery. Five to 10 per cent of children are misdiagnosed preoperatively so that preoperative chemotherapy should be withheld.

Surgery

Excellent surgical exposure can be obtained with the child supine by elevating the tumor-bearing side. A large transverse incision is made from the tip of the twelfth rib across the midline. Both rectus muscles can be divided, but frequently the contralateral rectus can be retracted laterally after incision of the sheath. This exposure allows access to both renal pedicles, vena cava, liver, spleen, and para-aortic lymph nodes from diaphragm to aortic bifurcation. Very large tumors can be biopsied and shrinkage induced with chemotherapy and radiation, thus making subsequent complete excision feasible. The contralateral kidney should be exposed, if complete ipsilateral excision appears possible, by opening Gerota's fascia and palpating both surfaces. Ligation of the renal artery followed by the vein should be attempted prior to mobilization of the tumor, and tumor spillage by rupture should be avoided. The adrenal gland can usually be spared, unless tumor occupies the upper pole of the kidney. Regional lymph nodes must be sampled for staging purposes, but radical lymphadenectomies are not necessary. En bloc resection of adjacent organs involved with tumor can be performed in some cases; otherwise maximal debulking is indicated, followed by tagging of residual tumor with surgical clips to delineate extent. If available, nonmetallic clips should be used to avoid interference with later CT scanning. Some oncology groups are now advocating "conservative" surgery with excision of tumor only; however, the potential for satellite lesions remains.

Prognostic Factors. NWTS I and II have clearly demonstrated three major prognostic factors in Wilms' tumor. They are presence or absence of favorable (FH) or unfavorable histology (UH), hematogenous metastases, and lymph node involvement. Lesser factors are age, tumor size, intravascular extension beyond the kidney, operative tumor spillage, and direct abdominal extension of tumor. Histology appears to be the single most important prognostic factor, with anaplasia, rhabdoid tumors, and clear cell carcinomas constituting the unfavorable variants (12 per cent). Tumors demonstrating any differentiation, FH, have a much better prognosis than tumors with UH.

Staging of the Wilms' Tumor (NWTS III)
Stage I: Tumor confined to kidney and completely excised
Stage II: Tumor extends beyond kidney but is completely excised
Stage III: Residual nonhematogenous tumor confined to the abdomen
Stage IV: Deposits beyond stage III, including hematogenous metastases
Stage V: Bilateral renal involvement ($\sim 7\%$)

Treatment Protocols for NWTS VI

Treatment is based on histology and stage, following results of NWTS I through III. All children should undergo preliminary surgery, and by stage, the following:

Stage I (FH and UH): No radiation therapy. Randomized actinomycin D (AMD) and vincristine (VCR) for 6 months.

Stage II (FH): Receive no radiation but more intensive AMD plus VCR for 15 months.

Stage III (FH): Triple therapy (TT) AMD, VCR, and doxorubicin plus radiotherapy 1000 to 2000 cGy.

Stage IV (FH): Radiotherapy 1000 cGy plus pulmonary radiation and FT.

UH Stages II–IV: All receive radiation therapy and are randomized to receive TT or quadruple therapy (TT plus cyclophosphamide).

Survival Rate (NWTS). The survival rate for FH is 96 per cent for Stage I, 92 for Stage II, 87 for Stage III, and 83 for Stage IV; versus 68 per cent for Stage I–III and 54 per cent for Stage IV for UH at 4 years. Relapse-free survival rate is 82.6 per cent for patients without metastases at presentation versus 54 per cent with positive nodes. Survival for synchronous bilateral Wilms' tumor is 87 per cent and for metachronous ipsilateral involvement is only 40 per cent. Thus, treatment for bilateral Wilms' tumor should be directed toward preservation of as much normal kidney function as possible, avoiding high doses of irradiation.

Other Tumors

Infants under 6 months of age constitute a special group of patients. The vast majority have mesoblastic nephromas, which should be treated by nephrectomy alone. Chemotherapy is potentially lethal in infancy and should be reserved only for those children with bilateral UH disease and for the rare rhabdoid tumors and sarcomas.

Renal angiomyolipomas can occur in up to 80 per cent of patients with tuberous sclerosis. Tumors are usually benign, although occasional malignant transformation can occur; they are almost invariably bilateral, so that nephrectomy should be avoided when possible. Rupture can cause retroperitoneal hemorrhage, which should be managed with transfusion and/or embolization of bleeding vessels whenever possible. Renal cell carcinomas are exceedingly rare in childhood. Complete surgical removal by means of a radical nephrectomy is the treatment of choice. Transitional cell tumors of the renal pelvis are also exceedingly rare and should be treated by nephroureterectomy. Fibroepithelial polyps are not malignant and should be treated by local excision.

GLOMERULONEPHRITIS

ALFRED J. FISH, M.D.,
and LAURIE S. FOUSER, M.D.

A child presenting with glomerulonephritis may have symptoms of hypertension and renal insufficiency with abnormal findings on urinalysis and electrolyte and acid-base imbalances. After the initial work-up and investigation of the patient it is usually several days before all laboratory data are available and it can be determined whether acute or chronic glomerulonephritis is present.

POSTINFECTIOUS GLOMERULONEPHRITIS

Postinfectious glomerulonephritis in childhood is usually an acute event with an excellent prognosis. Treatment is directed toward management of the consequences of acute glomerular injury with a reduction in glomerular blood flow and glomerular filtration.

Hospitalization. Patients with acute postinfectious glomerulonephritis, when presenting with edema and gross hematuria, are assessed for significant oliguria and hypertension. If these are not present, and if fluid and electrolyte balance is normal, hospitalization is not indicated. Children managed on an outpatient basis are observed carefully at home for oliguria, puffiness, and weight gain and are seen at regular intervals in the office or clinic to be checked for the development of hypertension or electrolyte imbalance.

Fluid Overload. Children with acute loss of glomerular filtration capacity become oliguric and develop edema and hypervolemia. Fluid restriction (to 300 ml/m²) is begun if hypervolemia is present, and sodium intake is reduced. Diuretic therapy is usually helpful if significant edema and fluid overload are present. In most patients there is a response to hydrochlorothiazide, 1 to 2 mg/kg/day. Responsiveness to diuretics depends upon the degree of glomerular capillary injury; in some patients the use of furosemide, 1 to 5 mg/kg/day intravenously or orally, will be more effective. In rare instances, when complete anuria with severe fluid overload is associated with pulmonary edema and congestive heart failure, peritoneal dialysis or hemodialysis may be needed.

In some patients the development of edema is secondary to heavy proteinuria with hypoalbuminemia, decreased colloidal osmotic pressure, and hypovolemia. Management of these problems is outlined in Nephrotic Syndrome, later in this section.

Otherwise, it is important to monitor fluid balance carefully, with daily assessment of weight, total intake, and output. When ongoing oliguria is a problem, fluid intake should be restricted to the urinary output plus 300 ml/m², which replaces insensible losses. Fluids low in sodium and potassium are judiciously administered.

Electrolyte and Acid-Base Abnormalities. Children with severe forms of postinfectious glomerulonephritis may develop electrolyte imbalances due to the loss of glomerular filtration. In addition to the difficulties with water balance already described, hyperkalemia, acidosis, hypocalcemia, and hyperphosphatemia may be present.

Hyperkalemia is a serious complication of postinfectious glomerulonephritis, carrying the risk of cardiac electrical disturbances. Frequently hyperkalemia is associated with acidosis, intracellular shifts of retained hydrogen ions, and subsequent movement of potassium out of the intracellular compartment. Moderately stable degrees of hyperkalemia (5.0 to 6.0 mEq/l) are not associated with electrocardiogram abnormalities and are managed with potassium restriction and hydrochlorothiazide or furosemide, as outlined, to enhance urinary potassium excretion. However, serum potassium levels higher than 6.0 mEq/l indicate treatment with oral or rectal doses of sodium polystyrene sulfonate, 1.0 gm/kg in 20 per cent sorbitol; this may be repeated every 2 to 3 hours until the hyperkalemia is controlled. The management of patients with electrocardiogram T-wave changes or with severe hyperkalemia exceeding 7.0 mEq/l should include the following: 10 per cent calcium gluconate in a dose of 100 to 200 mg/kg IV given slowly over 10 to 15 minutes, which will temporarily diminish the cardiac effects of hyperkalemia, and 25 per cent dextrose in water, 5 ml/kg (1.25 gm/kg) IV given over 30 minutes, followed by crystalline insulin 0.1 to 0.2 unit/kg. Simultaneous correction of acidosis using sodium bicarbonate, 2 to 3 mEq/kg IV, will enhance return of potassium to the intracellular pool.

Acidosis is more completely corrected using the formula of 0.6 × body weight (kg) × base deficit = mEq of sodium bicarbonate required. Ongoing administration of oral sodium bicarbonate, 1 to 2 mEq/kg/day, may be needed to maintain acid-base balance. If hypertension, dilutional hyponatremia, and fluid overload are evident, there may be limits to the amount of sodium-containing salts that can be administered.

Hypocalcemia and *hyperphosphatemia* may be encountered in acute glomerulonephritis. Hypocalcemia may result in tetany and convulsions, complications that may be precipitated by the correction of acidosis as previously outlined. Hypocalcemia is managed with 10 per cent calcium gluconate in a dose of 100 to 200 mg/kg IV given over 3 to 4 hours, followed by elemental oral calcium, 10 to 20 mg/kg/day. Hyperphosphatemia is treated by restriction of phosphorus intake and the administration of aluminum hydroxide orally in a dose of 50 to 150 mg/kg/day.

Hypertension. Hypertension is a frequent and potentially serious complication of acute glomerulonephritis.

Its etiology in this illness is probably related to both vasoconstriction and expanded intravascular volume from reduced glomerular filtration. Activation of the renin-angiotensin system may be affected as well. The goal of therapy is to prevent hypertensive encephalopathy with its sequelae and to avoid overtaxing a cardiovascular system already stressed by an expanded blood volume.

Severe blood pressure elevation in glomerulonephritis may lead to drowsiness, headache, stupor, palsy, or seizure and constitutes a medical emergency. Diazoxide,* a potent vasodilator, is given in a dose of 2 to 5 mg/kg as an intravenous bolus in a peripheral vein; it usually takes effect within minutes, with a duration of 4 to 36 hours. This dose is repeated if there is no response within 20 minutes. Furosemide, 0.5 to 1.0 mg/kg/dose IV, is given concurrently with diazoxide in patients with increased intravascular volume and edema. Both diazoxide and furosemide may be repeated at these doses in 4 to 6 hours if severe blood pressure elevations recur, although multiple doses of diazoxide may be associated with hyperglycemia. Labetalol 1 to 4 mg/kg/hr administered intravenously also may be used to stabilize acute hypertension. The rare patient with persistent severe hypertension who fails to respond to these measures can be stabilized with a continuous intravenous infusion of nitroprusside, beginning at 0.5 µg/kg/min and increasing gradually, as needed, to 2.0 µg/kg/min. This therapy requires very close monitoring of vital signs, as well as measurement of thiocyanate levels to avoid central nervous system (CNS) and bone marrow toxicity. The symptoms of hypertensive encephalopathy usually subside once blood pressures have been controlled, although diazepam or phenytoin may be needed acutely for seizures. The use of reserpine and alpha-methyldopa is discouraged in this clinical setting, since these agents may produce CNS depression that obscures the assessment of neurologic status in a patient at risk for encephalopathy.

Moderately severe, but non–life-threatening, blood pressure elevations are stabilized with hydralazine, 0.4 to 0.8 mg/kg/dose IM or IV, and furosemide IV as often as every 6 to 8 hours. Mild and moderate hypertension are managed with 2 mEq/kg sodium restriction and oral diuretic therapy (hydrochlorothiazide, 1 to 2 mg/kg/day in two divided doses if the glomerular filtration rate [GFR] is greater than 50 per cent of normal; furosemide, 1 to 2 mg/kg/dose every 6 to 12 hours if the GFR is less than 50 per cent of normal), with addition of hydralazine or propranolol if necessary. Propranolol† is instituted at 1 mg/kg/day in two divided oral doses and is increased by 0.5 mg/kg every 1 to 2 days until hypertension is controlled. Hydralazine is initiated at 0.75 mg/kg/day in three divided oral doses and can be increased, as necessary, up to 7.5 mg/kg/day (maximum, 200 mg/day). Use of propranolol is discour-

aged in patients with asthma, heart failure, or diabetes mellitus, and children on this drug are observed for bradycardia. Hydralazine may provoke a reflex tachycardia that can be effectively controlled with the addition of a beta-adrenergic blocking agent such as propranolol. The use of these medications is seldom required for long, since in the majority of cases of postinfectious glomerulonephritis hypertension is transient and resolves during the first week after presentation.

Supportive Care. *Nutrition* is an important consideration during the recovery from renal insufficiency in acute glomerulonephritis. Anorexia; dietary restriction of sodium, potassium, and phosphorus; and the ingestion of unpalatable medication contribute to inadequate total caloric intake. Although protein restriction is usually recommended, an intake of at least 2 gm/kg/24 hours should be offered as the renal insufficiency begins to improve.

Antibiotics (penicillin or erythromycin) are given to treat streptococcal pharyngitis, although they will not alter the established course of glomerulonephritis. Antibiotics are recommended to prevent the transmission of nephritogenic streptococci to other family members.

Dialysis, either peritoneal dialysis or hemodialysis, is recommended if severe oliguria is present in association with pulmonary edema, cardiac failure, hypervolemia, or hypertension that does not respond to the measures described. Similarly, severe hyperkalemia, acidosis, hyponatremia or hypernatremia, seizures, and stupor due to uremia are indications for dialysis.

Follow-up over the coming weeks allows discontinuation of diuretics and antihypertensive agents when the blood pressure is consistently normal and the edema, oliguria, and uremia have resolved. If, after a period of convalescence (about 12 weeks), the serum complement (C3) level has not returned to normal, the glomerular filtration rate remains low, or severe proteinuria is present, a renal biopsy is indicated.

CHRONIC GLOMERULONEPHRITIS

Chronic glomerulonephritis may be a primary disease of the kidney, but it may also develop secondary to systemic disorders. Most primary forms of glomerulonephritis have a variable clinical course, and management is directed toward the avoidance of complications. In some instances, treatment of the systemic illness has a significant effect on the outcome of children with secondary types of glomerulonephritis.

Supportive Care. *Hypertension* accompanies most cases of chronic glomerulonephritis. The initial approach employs sodium restriction and diuretics (hydrochlorothiazide or furosemide) and, if necessary, propranolol in the doses previously outlined. Serum electrolyte levels are monitored in patients taking thiazides or furosemide, since the kaliuresis that occurs with these diuretics may lead to hypokalemia. Thiazides may also cause hypercalcemia or hyperuricemia.

In more severe cases, drugs with different mechanisms of action are sequentially added to the above regimen until hypertension is controlled. Hydralazine, in the doses described, is usually the first drug to be

---

*Manufacturer's precaution: Safety of diazoxide in children is not established.

†Safety and efficacy for use of propranolol have not been established.

added, followed by the alpha-adrenergic blocker prazosin,* 0.05 to 0.04 mg/kg/day, according to age and size, given two or three times daily. The first dose of prazosin may result in sudden loss of consciousness, so the patient should be observed carefully. Another approach in patients refractory to a combination of diuretic and propranolol is the use of the angiotensin I–converting enzyme inhibitor captopril,† starting with 0.5 mg/kg/dose every 6 to 8 hours and increasing gradually to 2.0 mg/kg/dose if necessary. Sudden hypotension may occur after the first dose in rare cases, so the patient should be observed closely. White blood cell counts are monitored during captopril therapy, and the drug dosage should be reduced or discontinued if mild or severe neutropenia occurs. A long-acting converting enzyme inhibitor, enalapril, may be more convenient and can be used at 0.15 to 0.60 mg/kg/day in one or two doses. When these approaches are insufficient to control hypertension, they are replaced by minoxidil, beginning at 0.1 mg/kg/dose (maximum initial dose, 2.5 mg) given every 12 hours. Since minoxidil is a potent vasodilator, reflex tachycardia and marked sodium and water retention may occur if propranolol and furosemide are not used adjunctively. Hypertrichosis is also seen with chronic minoxidil therapy.

Edema due to nephrotic syndrome is managed with sodium restriction, hydrochlorothiazide (2 mg/kg/day), and spironolactone (2 to 3 mg/kg/day). For more severe edema, furosemide (2 to 5 mg/kg/day) is used. Attention to serum potassium levels is important, and supplemental dietary potassium, up to 2 mEq/kg/day, may be required.

The need for *nutrition* to sustain adequate growth in children is balanced against the recommendation of protein restriction to diminish the rate of progression of renal insufficiency. Protein intakes of high biologic value, 2 to 3 gm/kg, are required for growing children. Attention to the consequences of renal osteodystrophy involves the use of supplementary oral calcium, phosphate binders, and vitamin D analogues (dihydrotachysterol and 1,25 cholecalciferol). Either aluminum hydroxide or calcium carbonate (beginning with 1 gm/m²/day of elemental calcium orally) is used as a phosphate binder. Calcium carbonate therapy offers the benefits of simultaneous calcium supplementation and avoidance of aluminum toxicity but carries the risk of producing hypercalcemia as doses are increased to reduce hyperphosphatemia. Use of the vitamin D compounds is outlined in Chronic Renal Failure in this section.

Primary Glomerulonephritis. Type I *membranoproliferative glomerulonephritis* (MPGN) is a variably progressive form of glomerulonephritis. Some investigators have advocated the use of alternate-day steroids in these patients. Type II MPGN, or dense deposit disease, is unresponsive to specific therapy and has a high rate of recurrence in the transplanted kidney.

Idiopathic membranous glomerulopathy is frequently associated with heavy proteinuria. Treatment of edema and nephrotic syndrome is managed with diuretics and spironolactone, as described. There is no convincing evidence to support the use of steroids or immunosuppressive agents in this disorder.

Diffuse crescentic glomerulonephritis may be idiopathic or associated with various etiologies. When this lesion develops secondary to circulating antiglomerular basement membrane antibodies, immunosuppression (prednisone and azathioprine or cyclophosphamide) and plasmapheresis are recommended. When it is part of a systemic vasculitic process (e.g., periarteritis, Wegener's granulomatosis), similar treatment strategies are used.

Secondary Glomerulonephritis. *Systemic lupus erythematosus* (SLE) frequently has associated renal involvement with variable degrees of glomerular injury. Long-term survival studies in SLE have shown that prognosis is closely tied to the extent of renal disease. In mild cases of mesangial lupus nephritis we use prednisone, 2 mg/kg/day in divided doses (maximum, 100 mg/day), to achieve immune suppression, which usually results in the disappearance of circulating antibodies to native DNA and the return of serum complement levels to normal. These parameters, as well as renal function and urinary protein excretion, should be carefully watched; patients are maintained on alternate-day prednisone, 2 mg/kg as a single morning dose. In instances of focal or diffuse proliferative lupus nephritis we use the same regimen of prednisone therapy with the addition of azathioprine,* 2 to 3 mg/kg/day; the latter is continued over several years until the serologic parameters of SLE are controlled, along with reduction of proteinuria and restoration of renal function to normal. In certain selected patients who have a relentless progressive course in SLE, we have also added cyclophosphamide for immunosuppression.

Steroids used on a long-term basis have produced many recognized complications, including cushingoid facies, hirsutism, hypertension, infection, avascular necrosis, and osteoporosis. Similarly, immunosuppressive agents may reduce host defense mechanisms and result in bacterial infections (abscesses, sepsis) and opportunistic infections with fungal, parasitic (*Pneumocystic carinii*), and viral (herpes zoster) agents.

Anaphylactoid purpura nephritis occurs in approximately one-half of children with Henoch-Schönlein purpura. In the majority of patients, renal involvement is mild and does not require specific treatment. Children with severe glomerular injury who have loss of renal function and heavy proteinuria are at risk of permanent renal injury. In these instances we use a combination of prednisone and azathioprine,* as outlined in SLE.

Glomerulonephritis can also occur with *bacterial endocarditis, infection, sepsis, and infected ventriculoatrial shunts.* These patients have continued chronic infection of bacterial origin. The chronic release of bacterial antigen is the source of antigen(s) resulting in immune complex injury of the glomerulus. Treatment with sur-

---

*Manufacturer's warning: Safety of prazosin in children has not been established.

†Manufacturer's warning: Safety and efficacy of captopril have not been established.

---

*This use of azathioprine is not listed in the manufacturer's directive.

gery and antibiotics to eliminate the offending micro-organisms has a marked effect in ameliorating the glomerular injury.

THE NEPHROTIC SYNDROME

PAUL S. KURTIN, M.D.

A diagnosis of the nephrotic syndrome (NS) is based upon the findings of heavy proteinuria, hypoalbuminuria, edema, and hyperlipidemia. When caring for a child with the NS, the following two questions must be answered. Is the NS due to a primary renal disease, or is it part of a systemic illness? Second, is a renal biopsy necessary, or can empiric corticosteroid therapy be instituted without a biopsy?

Secondary causes of the nephrotic syndrome are uncommon in children and represent only approximately 10 per cent of patients. Although unusual, the secondary or systemic causes of the NS to be aware of include systemic lupus erythematosus, Henoch-Schönlein purpura, sickle cell disease, toxins such as gold or penicillamine, and infections such as syphilis or hepatitis B. The majority of these secondary causes can be eliminated on the basis of a careful history and screening laboratory tests.

Once the NS is determined to be of primary renal origin, the need for a renal biopsy versus empiric therapy must be considered. Approximately 75 per cent of children with primary NS will have minimal change disease (MCD), also known as nil disease or lipoid nephrosis. This disease occurs primarily in young children, aged 2 to 6 years, and uncommonly manifests with hypertension, renal insufficiency, or hematuria. Gross hematuria and hypocomplementemia are exceedingly rare and should suggest another etiology of the NS. If MCD is suspected, an initial renal biopsy is not indicated, and a therapeutic trial of steroids should be initiated. MCD is relatively less common in children under 1 year or older than 10 years of age. In addition, the presence of gross hematuria, significant hypertension, renal insufficiency, or hypocomplementemia should suggest another renal lesion, such as focal glomerulosclerosis or membranoproliferative glomerulonephritis. A renal biopsy would therefore be indicated to determine the etiology of the NS, define the patient's prognosis, and design an appropriate therapeutic protocol. A renal biopsy is also indicated in children with presumed MCD who do not respond to an initial 8-week course of steroid therapy.

THERAPY

A number of effective protocols have been utilized for the treatment of the NS secondary to MCD. Initial therapy usually consists of prednisone, 2 mg/kg/day (60 mg/m²/day) in divided doses (maximal dose of 80 mg/day), until the proteinuria has remitted for 3 to 4 consecutive days. The dose of prednisone is then consolidated to a single morning dose given every other day for a total of 1 month. The alternate-day steroid dosage is tapered to 1 mg/kg (40 mg/m²) for a second month and is finally discontinued over the next 2 to 4 weeks. The child's urine must be monitored daily to document the continued absence of proteinuria. On such a regimen, 75 per cent of patients will become free of proteinuria after 2 weeks, and 90 per cent will be in remission after a month. Approximately 5 per cent of patients will continue to have proteinuria after 8 weeks of therapy.

Relapses will occur within the first year in nearly 80 per cent of patients who have become free of proteinuria. Half of these patients will experience more than one relapse. It is therefore important to instruct the family in monitoring the patient. The patient or parents should test the urine with a dipstick daily. A flow sheet consisting of the date, urine protein results (e.g., 1+, 3+), prednisone dosage, and any intercurrent illnesses or problems should be kept and brought to each visit with the physician. A relapse is often indicated by 3 to 4 days of 3+ or 4+ proteinuria, and prednisone therapy (2 mg/kg/day) should be started prior to the onset of clinical edema. The first relapse is treated similarly to the initial course. A second relapse is treated with a similar initial dosage of prednisone; however, the taper from approximately 1 mg/kg on alternate days to no drug at all should be extended up to 6 months. Small amounts of proteinuria (less than 1 gm/day), especially if the child is asymptomatic, need not be suppressed with steroids.

Patients who relapse frequently (three or more relapses within a year) and patients who become steroid dependent (relapse while on tapering dosages of steroids) present difficult therapeutic problems. The challenge is to maintain the health of the child without inducing serious steroid toxicity. Although cytotoxic drugs have clearly been shown to be of benefit for these patients, their use should be reserved for patients with significant steroid toxicity or for those children whose disease cannot be controlled with moderate doses of prednisone (approximately 1 mg/kg on alternate days). Iatrogenic complications from drug therapies must be avoided in a disease with an ultimately good prognosis.

Patients who remain steroid dependent or who frequently relapse may need a renal biopsy prior to the initiation of additional drug therapy. If the biopsy confirms the presence of MCD, and if the patient suffers from unacceptable side effects of the disease or its treatment, a course of cyclophosphamide or chlorambucil may be considered. Cyclosporine A, a drug that has provided great benefit to transplant recipients, has also been used in this setting. Although cyclosporine can induce remissions, patients appear to relapse as soon as the drug is stopped.

Cyclophosphamide is currently the drug of choice and, when given in the dose of 2 to 3 mg/kg/day for 6 to 10 weeks, has been shown to induce prolonged, drug-free remissions. If relapses do occur, the patients appear to be more sensitive to a subsequent course of steroids alone. Similar benefits are obtained with chlorambucil (0.2 mg/kg/day for 8 weeks). The important side effects of a short course of cyclophosphamide in this dosage range include hemorrhagic cystitis and neutropenia.

The long-term side effects of cyclophosphamide, including an increased risk of sterility and late malignancies, as well as hair loss and opportunitistic infections, are rare with this total dose. Hemorrhagic cystitis can be avoided by giving cyclophosphamide in a single dose in the morning and forcing a liberal fluid intake throughout the day. Neutropenia can be lessened by maintaining the patient on 1 to 2 mg/kg of prednisone on alternate days throughout the course of the cyclophosphamide administration. Cyclophosphamide should be withheld if the white blood count falls below 3000 per cubic millimeter.

Two additional classes of drugs have been used in patients with steroid-resistant NS. These are the antihypertensive angiotensin-converting enzyme inhibitors and nonsteroidal anti-inflammatory agents. Both types of medications are able, at times, to reduce proteinuria, but neither has an effect on the underlying disease process.

MANAGEMENT OF COMPLICATIONS OF THE NEPHROTIC SYNDROME

Infections

In the preantibiotic era, infection was the most common cause of death for children with the NS. In addition, infections, even when clinically mild, often precipitate a relapse. Children with the NS are at an increased risk for infections while they are nephrotic or on high doses of steroids or cytotoxic agents. The most common infections are with encapsulated organisms such as *Streptococcus pneumoniae*, *Escherichia coli*, and *Hemophilus influenzae*. Parents need to be made aware of this risk and should call the physician for any febrile episode that may arise. Because of the increased risk of peritonitis, episodes of abdominal pain must be carefully evaluated. Despite the risk of infection, prophylactic antibiotics have not been beneficial, but patients may benefit from polyvalent pneumococcal vaccine. It is generally agreed upon that live virus vaccines should be avoided while the child is on steroid therapy. In addition, because routine immunization may lead to a relapse of the NS, immunizations should be withheld until the child is in a stable, drug-free remission for approximately 6 months. While nephrotic or on steroids or cytotoxic drugs, children exposed to chickenpox should be treated with immunoglobulin G (IgG) prophylaxis.

Hypercoagulable State

Owing to a complex interaction of an increase in the production of coagulation factors, the loss of inhibitors of coagulation in the urine, and changes in platelet function, children with the NS are at increased risk of vascular thrombosis. Both venous and arterial thrombosis can occur. Venous thrombosis is more common, and renal vein thrombosis with subsequent pulmonary emboli presents a particular problem in the NS. There is no proven role for prophylactic anticoagulation. Documented thrombosis should be treated with intravenous heparin, followed by a course of sodium warfarin (Coumadin) therapy.

Edema

Children with the NS frequently present with disabling anasarca. Although true intravascular hypovolemia is rare, diuretics should be used cautiously in these patients. Loop diuretics, such as furosemide, are often required because thiazide and spironolactone diuretics may not be effective in inducing a diuresis. Severe edema can be treated with 0.5 to 1.0 gm/kg of salt-poor albumin, followed 1/2 to 1 hour later with 1 to 2 mg/kg of intravenous furosemide. Some patients, however, may become refractory to furosemide. For those children, metolazone (1 to 2 mg twice a day), in addition to furosemide, may be effective.

Mild degrees of edema need not be treated. Edema will quickly disappear once the proteinuria resolves. To prevent edema while the child has proteinuria or is on high doses of steroids, a mildly salt-restricted diet (tell the patient, "If the food tastes salty, don't eat it") should be instituted. Fluid restrictions are rarely needed, unless the child develops hyponatremia (values less than 130 mEq/L).

Last, diuretics and steroids can induce hypokelemia. Potassium supplements are often poorly tolerated; therefore, potassium-sparing diuretics and foods rich in potassium may be needed.

GROWTH AND NUTRITION

Children with the NS are frequently growth retarded. The etiology of this is multifactorial and includes frequent use of high-dose steroids, poor appetite, intercurrent infections, protein losses, and abnormalities in calcium and vitamin D metabolism. Accelerated growth is frequently seen shortly after the child enters a drug-free remission. In general, children with the NS should be given a diet with a caloric intake appropriate for age. A restricted caloric intake may be needed for children who are gaining too much weight while on steroids. Carbohydrates should make up approximately 55 per cent of caloric intake, while protein and fat contribute 15 per cent and 30 per cent, respectively. There is no benefit to a high-protein intake. High-protein diets can theoretically be harmful to patients with renal disease.

Hyperlipidemia

Patients who frequently relapse, or who are steroid dependent or resistant, develop both hypercholesterolemia and hypertriglyceridemia because of increased production and decreased clearance of lipoproteins. Although not firmly established, these children may be at risk for early or accelerated atherosclerosis. Thus, the total fat intake in the diet should be limited to no more than 30 per cent of calories, and the ratio of polyunsaturated fat to saturated fats should approximate 1.0 to 1.5:1.0. The hyperlipidemia slowly resolves after a sustained remission has been achieved.

GENERAL PRINCIPLES

Children with the NS should be encouraged to maintain as normal an activity level as possible. Massive edema may limit a child's mobility and cause discomfort. In addition, children with low serum albumin level frequently complain of fatigue and may need to nap. These complaints disappear with remission of the NS.

Families need to be reassured that the long-term prognosis of children with MCD is excellent. Renal failure is extremely unusual in this disease. Other forms of renal disease causing the NS do have a higher incidence of eventual renal failure.

The basic management approach should emphasize a good prognosis by minimizing the side effects of therapeutic interventions. Although late relapses are reported, most patients are free of their disease by late adolescence.

RENAL VENOUS THROMBOSIS

THOMAS L. KENNEDY, III, M.D.

Renal venous thrombosis is an unusual condition that varies greatly in signs and symptoms, extent, and clinical severity. Because it may occur at birth or at any age thereafter in a variety of clinical settings, there is no uniform approach to therapy. In fact, treatment may require minimal or very aggressive measures.

Renal venous thrombosis is considered when there are predisposing factors, clinical findings, and results of laboratory studies, including imaging, that support the diagnosis. Although the diagnosis is almost always presumptive, currently the easiest and safest study to confirm renal venous thrombosis is ultrasonography with deep Doppler. This imaging technique should be carried out before invasive therapy is considered.

Treatment initially should be preventive. That is, the infant or child at risk for renal venous thrombosis must be recognized and have the predisposing condition corrected. Risk factors include hyperosmolarity, hypernatremia, hemoconcentration, hypovolemia, septicemia, poor cardiac output, and hypercoagulable states. On the basis of these risk factors, specific groups predisposed to renal venous thrombosis include infants of diabetic mothers; asphyxiated and dehydrated newborns; children receiving angiographic contrast agents; children with serious burns, disseminated intravascular coagulation, septic shock, and the nephrotic syndrome; and teenagers taking oral estrogen contraceptives. There are also several extrarenal associations with renal venous thrombosis to be considered, including distant thromboses and concomitant adrenal hemorrhage in the newborn.

After removing or correcting the initiating cause, treatment is supportive and must be directed at the consequences of renal insufficiency. Acute renal injury may vary from oliguric or anuric renal failure to mild tubular dysfunction. If the renal disturbance is mild (for example, an infant with hematuria, flank mass, and little or no azotemia), treatment need only include maintenance of normal fluid and electrolyte balance and good urine output. Such presentation and treatment constitute the majority of cases of renal venous thrombosis in infancy.

The major dilemma in the treatment of renal venous thrombosis is the approach to the child with a severe presentation, such as anuric renal failure, diffuse systemic thromboses, and hypercoagulable states. The role of antiplatelet, anticoagulant, and thrombolytic agents is unsettled. There is little experience with these drugs in infants and children with renal venous thrombosis, and there are no controlled studies upon which to base firm conclusions. In addition, there is a significant risk of bleeding with their use.

Antiplatelet (e.g., aspirin and dipyridamole) and anticoagulant (heparin, dicumarol, and warfarin) drugs have a role in the treatment of renal venous thrombosis with hypercoagulable states, such as the nephrotic syndrome and inherited thrombotic disorders. Heparinization should be considered in patients (1) in whom there is a history of recurrent thromboses, (2) in whom the risk of thrombus progression or thromboembolism is high, (3) in whom there are multiple thromboses, or (4) in whom there is uncontrolled, severe, disseminated intravascular coagulation with persistent thrombocytopenia and hypofibrinogenemia. If heparin is given, it should be started intravenously with a loading dose of 50 to 75 units/kg and followed with a constant infusion of 25 units/kg/hr for approximately 5 days. The dose is titrated to keep the partial thromboplastin time 1.5 to 2.0 times the normal value.

Thrombolytic agents currently available are streptokinase and urokinase. Either may be used to treat large bilateral renal venous thromboses resulting in severe acute renal failure or other life-threatening thromboses (e.g., pulmonary embolism). If the thrombus is limited to the renal veins and inferior vena cava, direct local infusion of the agent by a radiologist experienced in invasive pediatric procedures is preferred to systemic thrombolytic therapy. Urokinase, a direct plasminogen activator, has the advantage of producing fewer allergic reactions than streptokinase. If thrombolysis is successful, heparin therapy should be instituted for 1 week, followed by oral anticoagulation for several months.

There is now little controversy regarding the role of surgery. In short, nephrectomy has no place in the treatment of acute renal venous thrombosis, and thrombectomy is indicated rarely, if ever.

Follow-up data on infants with renal venous thrombosis are limited. A variety of renal functional and structural abnormalities may result, and these may mimic other conditions. Functional changes may be both glomerular and tubular. Glomerular injury results in a diminished filtration rate, which varies from mild to severe but is usually not progressive. If there is a slowly progressive fall in renal function, the diagnosis of chronic renal venous thrombosis must be considered. The nephrotic state and renal venous thrombosis has long been the source of a cause-and-effect controversy. It is certain that the hypercoagulability of the nephrotic syndrome can lead to renal venous thrombosis. What is uncertain is whether renal venous thrombosis can produce renal injury leading to the nephrotic syndrome. At present, there are few data to support the latter possibility.

Tubular injury may result in impaired concentrating capacity, glucosuria, aminoaciduria, and Type IV renal tubular acidosis. Hypertension may also occur as a late complication of renal venous thrombosis. The elevation of blood pressure is usually not severe and may not be permanent. However, prolonged, severe hypertension in association with a unilateral atrophic kidney is an indication for nephrectomy.

Recurrent or diffuse thromboses or a positive family history of thrombotic events suggests the possibility of an inherited hypercoagulable state. An appropriate work-up should include assays of antithrombin III, protein C, protein S, and the fibrinolytic system, where these tests are available.

Structural changes include focal or generalized atrophy of one or both kidneys, with or without intrarenal calcification. Focal atrophy is usually accompanied by caliectasis and may be mistaken for the focal scar of pyelonephritis or segmental hypoplasia. Generalized atrophy may be indistinguishable radiographically from congenital renal hypoplasia or dysplasia.

CHRONIC RENAL FAILURE

JOHN T. HERRIN, M.B.B.S., F.R.A.C.P.

Chronic renal failure is a slow, inevitably progressive condition in which changes in homeostasis and body compensation gradually lead to disordered growth, abnormal calcium and phosphorus metabolism with renal osteodystrophy, developmental retardation, and delayed sexual maturation. Early treatment is usually nonspecific and is aimed at preventing emergency problems resulting (1) from loss of homeostatic function, such as hyperkalemia, metabolic acidosis, and hypocalcemia, or (2) from a disturbance in the maintenance of fluid and sodium balance, such as edema, hypertension, or, less commonly, dehydration.

The aims of treatment of chronic, progressive renal failure are to maintain linear growth, to prevent renal osteodystrophy or minimize its consequences, and to protect development and maturation, including sexual maturation. Meticulous treatment at an early stage is crucial to maintain normal growth and development.

The increasing efficiency of replacement therapies for end-stage renal disease (dialysis and transplantation) makes it important for the pediatrician to (1) recognize the process in an asymptomatic stage and forecast future deterioration; (2) monitor and maximize growth before replacement therapy by controlling acidosis; supplementing calories, calcium, and vitamin D; and restricting phosphorus and protein if necessary; (3) introduce the patient and family to the end-stage renal failure program so that early integration into the extra psychological, social, and financial resources is possible; and (4) plan for ongoing monitoring so that replacement therapy can be appropriately timed.

Reversible conditions, such as volume depletion, hypokalemia, hypercalcemia, and infection, should be corrected and the patient stabilized before long-term therapy for chronic renal failure is instituted. Chronic, progressive renal failure may be prevented or delayed by appropriate treatment of obstruction, urinary tract infection, certain glomerulonephritides, removal of nephrotoxins, or control of hypertension.

CONDITIONS REQUIRING URGENT THERAPY

Urgent treatment may be required for (1) circulatory collapse or failure, secondary to dehydration or sepsis in the patient with obstructive uropathy; (2) fluid overload manifesting as severe hypertension or pulmonary edema; or (3) metabolic abnormalities, such as severe metabolic acidosis, hyperkalemia, hypocalcemia, or hypokalemia resulting from loss of homeostatic balance with decreasing renal function. Acute dialysis may be required to correct severe fluid overload or metabolic abnormalities before commencing a long-term conservative regimen.

Circulatory Collapse

Isotonic fluid (20 ml/kg body weight) is administered to stabilize the circulation and allow time for full chemical review and more specific correction of deficits. The initial bolus is administered rapidly and may need to be repeated to produce improvement in circulation and blood pressure. Appropriate cultures of blood and urine, as well as others that may be clinically indicated, are obtained. Antibiotics are given in a standard loading dose, with further administration adjusted to monitored renal function and to serum antibiotic levels—peak and through levels to ensure adequacy of therapy and safety.

Hypertension

Prophylactic restriction of salt and water intake—with early and judicious use of potent diuretics, such as furosemide (1 to 5 mg/kg once to four times daily) alone or in combination with metolazone (1.25 to 5.0 mg once to three times daily)—may prevent severe hypertension with pulmonary edema or hypertensive encephalopathy requiring urgent therapy. Sublingual nifedipine (0.1–0.2 mg/kg) or labetalol (1 to 3 mg/kg/hr) intravenously provides effective therapy and has replaced hydralazine and diazoxide in emergency therapy. Sodium nitroprusside (as a constant drip infusion commencing at 0.25 to 0.5 µg/kg/min may be titrated until control is attained, at 1 to 8 µg/kg/min). A potent loop diuretic, such as furosemide, is usually necessary to sustain urine flow as blood pressure is brought under control. If urine flow cannot be adequately sustained with diuretics or pulmonary edema is not improved, hemodialysis or peritoneal dialysis may be necessary to maintain volume control.

After initial control, maintenance treatment for hypertension is commenced with propranolol (1 to 2 mg/kg once to four times daily), hydralazine (0.25 to 1.0 mg/kg orally twice to four times daily), captopril (0.1 to 0.4 mg/kg/day in younger children or 25 to 50 mg twice to four times a day in adolescents), or minoxidil (0.1 to 1.5 mg/kg/day). Diuretic therapy or dialysis is necessary for volume control. A single daily dose of a long-acting beta blocker, such as atenolol (25 to 100 mg), or a single dose of enalapril (2.5 to 20.0 mg) may assist compliance in adolescents.

Pulmonary Edema

In the patient who presents with pulmonary edema and severe hypertension, vigorous antihypertensive treatment (as described previously) is undertaken, concurrent with protection of oxygenation and tissue perfusion. Oxygen is provided by face mask, nasal prongs, or, if necessary, endotracheal intubation to allow use of positive-pressure respiration. Morphine may be used as a sedative, with modification of dosage (clearance is often reduced in these critically ill patients, and the initial dose is reduced and subsequent doses are titrated to response). If urine output cannot be sustained or readily restored, ultrafiltration is instituted using hemodialysis or peritoneal dialysis. Furosemide and metolazone may potentiate or initiate diuresis, allowing stabilization.

Hyperkalemia

Serum potassium levels are maintained within a safe range until very low glomerular clearance rates are present (approximately 5 ml/min/1.73 ml). However, acute changes in serum potassium level may be precipitated by severe acidosis, circulatory failure, and indiscriminate intake of high-potassium foods (potato chips, nuts, fruits such as watermelon, and salt substitutes), particularly in the presence of constipation. Aldosterone antagonist diuretics (spironolactone, triamterene, and amiloride) should be avoided; beta blocker and angiotension-converting enzyme inhibitors should be used with caution and close monitoring.

When an elevated serum potassium level (>6 mEq/L) is found, an immediate rhythm strip electrocardiogram (lead 2) should be obtained. Should there be an increase in the size of T waves, peaked T waves, or changes in the QRS complex suggestive of elevated serum potassium levels (decreased amplitude of the R wave, widening of QRS complex, or fusion of the QRS with the T wave to form a "sine wave" pattern), emergency stabilization of the heart muscle membrane potential with calcium is undertaken. Calcium may be given as calcium gluconate 10 per cent (1 to 3 ml/kg = 0.5 to 1.5 mEq/kg) IV over 10 to 20 minutes, with electrocardiographic monitoring for bradycardia. Calcium chloride (0.5 to 1.5 mEq/kg) may be used but is more irritant to the vein and more concentrated, thus requiring a lower volume to provide the appropriate ionized calcium. The electrocardiogram will usually show rapid reversion to a normal rhythm after calcium administration.

Sodium bicarbonate, in a dose of 1.0 to 2.5 mEq/kg IV over 20 to 30 minutes, will assist potassium movement into cells, producing a fall in the serum potassium level of approximately 1 to 2 mEq/L.

Glucose and insulin may also aid serum potassium control by producing movement into cells. A dose of 0.5 gm/kg of glucose as 50 per cent dextrose in water (1 ml/kg) is used. One unit of regular insulin is added for each 4 gm of dextrose, and the mixture is infused over 10 to 20 minutes. In the very young patient, that is, the infant under approximately 10 kg of weight, the endogenous insulin response to glucose loading is often sufficient to allow treatment without the need for exogenous insulin. These measures provide initial control, but the effect can be negated as potassium leaks, once again from cells, over a period of the first few hours. If urine output can be sustained at greater than 0.5 ml/kg/hr loop diuretics, such as furosemide, may produce a negative potassium balance; otherwise, sodium polystyrene sulfonate resin may be necessary to remove potassium.

Sodium polystyrene sulfonate resin (1 to 2 gm/kg body weight) is administered in a solution of 20 per cent sorbitol to produce mild water and electrolyte flux into the bowel and to produce loose stool, with subsequent elimination of bound potassium. For rapid control, rectal administration is advised; oral administration is preferred for prolonged and more efficient action. Commencing with concurrent doses rectally and orally will provide for better control in the patient with markedly diminished renal function. Rectal administration may require a large Foley catheter with the balloon inflated in the rectum and the buttocks taped together to prevent early loss of the enema with consequent decrease in efficiency.

Since sodium polystyrene sulfonate exchanges sodium for potassium ions, there will be relative sodium loading with potassium exchange. This situation can aggravate hypertension and fluid overload. In patients with persistently low urine output, dialysis may be necessary to balance sodium and potassium exchange while maintaining fluid balance.

Hypokalemia

Hypokalemia is rarely a major problem in the patient with renal disease but may occur following illness characterized by anorexia, vomiting, or diarrhea; long-term diuretic therapy; or aminoglycoside or amphotericin therapy. Slow repletion with potassium is to be preferred. Judicious and carefully monitored concurrent magnesium replacement may be necessary. Intravenous potassium replacement should not exceed 0.5 to 0.75 mEq/kg/hr unless an arrhythmia is already present, when 1 mEq/kg/hr may be used with electrocardiographic and chemical monitoring.

Metabolic Acidosis

Severe metabolic acidosis interferes with many cellular enzyme processes, impairs circulation and tissue perfusion, and potentiates hyperkalemia. Chronic acidosis is a potent cause of growth suppression, and correction should be undertaken early to maximize growth and minimize effects on bone development. Sodium bicarbonate on Shohl's solution (Bicitra) may be used in a dose of 1 to 3 mEq/kg/day (approximately 1 to 3 ml/kg of Bicitra) on a chronic basis. Acute, severe acidosis may follow respiratory infection (pneumonia), sedative or analgesic administration, and thoracic or abdominal surgery, often requires intravenous correction of acidosis based on bicarbonate level; the decrease in alveolar ventilation prevents respiratory compensation, and severe acidosis can potentiate hyperkalemia, impair circulation and tissue perfusion, and lead to sudden death if not corrected. In those patients with renal tubular acidosis, in whom concurrent potassium losses are high, a triple citrate mixture (Polycitra) is often more palatable and reduces the sodium load 1 to 3 ml. Polycitra will usually provide sufficient correction in the patient with chronic renal failure. Close monitoring of serum potassium level is necessary. These bicarbonate replacement solutions are hyperosmolar and can cause significant nausea or diarrhea; dilution in juice, water, or formula is recommended for tolerance and acceptance. Sodium bicarbonate may cause distressing bloating and flatulence. Sodium bicarbonate may be given as liquid (1mEq/1ml); as tablets, 330 mg (3.9 mEq of bicarbonate) or 650 mg (7.8 mEq of bicarbonate); or as powder (44 mEq per teaspoon). A trial of multiple chemical forms and various compounds may be necessary to find the best supplement for each patient.

The large sodium loads necessary to provide adequate bicarbonate replacement make monitoring of volume status necessary. These large loads are a particular problem in the late stages of renal failure, when volume overload, edema, and hypertension make dialysis a preferable therapeutic mode.

DIETARY THERAPY

The aim of dietary therapy is to provide sufficient calories to sustain growth while reducing solute, electrolyte, and protein loads to a level at which homeostasis can be maintained within the limits of remaining renal function. Present clinical trials of a low-protein diet to protect against, or slow the progression of, renal failure await further assessment. In the pediatric patient, a minimum of 0.6 gm of protein of high biologic value (meat, fish, eggs, and cheese) should be provided daily to prevent catabolism. An increase to 1.0 to 1.5 gm/kg daily can be made if growth is occurring. High-protein vegetables are best avoided, since they provide protein of low biologic value and an increased potassium load. Intake of cow's milk should be limited, since it provides a high solute and phosphate load. In infants, human milk substitute formula, such as S.M.A. or Similac PM 60/40, may be used to provide a low-solute, low-phosphate formula. It must be remembered that decreased-protein diets may need supplemental calories in the form of Polycose, Controlyte, or corn oil to maintain adequate caloric levels for growth.

Close monitoring of the child's growth pattern is necessary, particularly if a modified protein diet is used. In the early stages of chronic renal failure, a well-balanced diet without restriction may be used if the blood urea nitrogen (BUN) is not markedly elevated, homeostatic functions are maintained, and the child is growing. Although a decrease in protein load is associated with a concurrent decrease in acid load and potassium intake (100 gm of dietary protein produces approximately 70 mEq of hydrogen ion and 80 to 100 mEq of potassium), consideration of replacement therapy (dialysis or transplantation) should be made if it is necessary to limit dietary intake severely for metabolic control.

Within reason, the highest tolerable quantity of sodium and water should be provided, and growth, blood pressure, and weight should be carefully monitored. In patients with obstructive uropathy or medullary cystic disease, there are sustained obligatory sodium losses. Supplemental sodium and water are mandatory to maintain hydration and sustain urinary function. Sodium restriction (0.2 to 0.5 mEq/kg/day) is indicated in patients with volume overload, hypertension, or extremely low glomerular clearance rates. Dialysis is a better treatment than severe sodium restriction, which renders the diet tasteless and unacceptable to most patients. Low-sodium milk and salt substitutes are high in potassium and should be avoided.

Dietary restriction of potassium and phosphate poses practical problems, since the substances are ubiquitous and the foods high in phosphate, particularly dairy products, are often a relatively inexpensive source of calcium and protein of high biologic value. Moderate restriction of high-potassium and high-phosphate food should be undertaken as serum levels are elevated. Phosphate binders, such as calcium carbonate (10 to 20 mg/kg/day of elemental calcium also provides bicarbonate supplement) or aluminum gels (50 to 150 mg/kg/day of aluminum), are often necessary for full control even if low-phosphate formulas are used. Aluminum gels are not palatable and often cause significant constipation, making a wetting agent, such as Colace, or a softening agent, such as mineral oil, necessary. Aluminum gels should be used for acute binding only, and calcium carbonate should be switched as soon as practical, to prevent aluminum toxicity (neurologic and bone disorders, anemia). As control of the phosphorus levels is obtained, monitoring of serum levels is necessary to prevent severe depletion, which may cause rickets or osteomalacia or may aggravate renal osteodystrophy.

In patients who require both aluminum gel and sodium polystyrene sulfonate resin, an extra dose of 20 per cent sorbitol solution may be given to obtain a softer and more predictable bowel movement and to potentiate potassium removal.

Dietary restrictions are difficult to enforce in childhood and can be a major source of stress between parent and child, as well as highlighting the difference between the child with chronic renal failure and his or her peers. Compliance becomes more difficult as renal disease progresses and restrictions become more stringent. As growth continues, less stringent dietary restriction is necessary. For psychological reasons, modification should be instituted slowly, with mild restriction and a change to protein of high biologic value; earlier dialysis or transplantation, rather than increasingly stringent dietary restrictions, should be considered, particularly if the child cannot maintain growth parallel to normal percentiles.

HYPOCALCEMIA AND BONE DISEASE

Decreased Serum Calcium Levels. Hypocalcemia may produce muscle cramps, weakness, tetany, or seizures. Treatment consists of lowering the serum phosphorus level: low-phosphate diet, aluminum-binding gels, and provision of calcium supplements in the form of calcium lactate or carbonate in a dose of 10 to 20 mg/kg/day of elemental calcium (1 gm of calcium lactate = 130 mg of calcium; 625 mg of calcium carbonate = 250 mg of calcium).

Vitamin D. Vitamin D is hydroxylated in both liver and kidney to produce the active form. With decreasing renal function, supplementation is required, either as 1,25-(OH)$_2$ D$_3$ (Rocaltrol), 0.125 to 2.0 µg/day, or as dihydrotachysterol, 0.125 to 0.75 mg/day. A steady rise in parathyroid hormone occurs as renal function is reduced below 60 per cent of normal and may occur even in the presence of normal serum calcium and phosphorus levels. Doses of vitamin D titrated to effective levels may prevent secondary bone changes. Dosage is adjusted at 4- to 5-day intervals, guided by serum calcium levels. After serum calcium levels have stabilized, monthly chemical monitoring is adequate. Should toxicity occur, the vitamin D dose and calcium supplements are withheld until the serum calcium level returns to normal (usually 2 to 4 days). It is important that vitamin D therapy not be commenced before control of hyperphosphatemia, to prevent painful dystrophic calcification or occasional calcium deposition in vessel walls with subsequent peripheral vascular damage (milligrams per deciliter of calcium × milligrams per deciliter of phosphorus totaling >70 is an absolute contraindication to using vitamin D and an urgent indication for serum phosphate control).

Since renal osteodystrophy leads to inevitable interference with growth and a change in the mechanical shear forces at the joint margins and epiphyseal plate, with potential epiphyseal slip fractures, early orthopedic review and coordinated therapy with bracing are necessary to decrease bone deformity and assist in maintaining straight limbs and functional joints. Osteotomy, bracing, and vigorous chemical control of bone diseases should be undertaken before renal transplantation. Bone healing will occur if chemical control is maintained. The small number of patients whose condition is not chemically controlled on maximal conservative therapy should be considered for parathyroidectomy to allow bone healing and maximize growth.

ANEMIA

Anemia is a common, significant, and progressive symptom of diminishing renal function. Transfusion of packed red blood cells or washed packed red blood cells is justified to maintain an asymptomatic course. Hematocrits of 16 to 20 per cent in the chronic state are well tolerated, provided that the patient is allowed to acclimatize slowly. Transfusion carries the dangers of sensitization, volume overload, hypertension, and the acquisition of infectious diseases, such as hepatitis B, non-A, non-B hepatitis, cytomegalic inclusion disease, and acquired immunodeficiency syndrome (AIDS). These risks should be balanced against the symptomatic changes in the child.

Evidence suggests that blood transfusion may be of value in immune alteration for future transplantation. Donor-specific transfusion and elective transfusion protocols exist, and the management preference and protocol of the local pediatric nephrology-transplantation unit should be considered before transfusion.

Erythropoietin has become established therapy for dialysis patients with large transfusion requirements. Further investigation and consideration are necessary

to define the most appropriate usage in patients prior to dialysis therapy.

EXTRARENAL MANIFESTATIONS OF ADVANCED CHRONIC RENAL FAILURE AND AZOTEMIA

A number of problems have been correlated with marked or prolonged elevations of BUN and creatinine, including serositis (e.g., pericarditis and pleurisy), bleeding disorders, susceptibility to infection, and neurologic abnormalities. Vigorous supportive therapy is carried out, and growth can be maintained with early replacement therapy (dialysis and transplantation) when control is no longer possible.

Pericarditis and Pleurisy with Effusion

Inflammation of the serous membranes and the accompanying effusion occur in the later stages of uremia or in an episode of decompensation with a prolonged elevation of BUN and creatinine. Confirmation of significant pericardial effusion by chest radiograph and echocardiogram is an indication for vigorous dialysis. This treatment usually leads to resolution of the pericarditis. If the pericardial effusion is large, it is probably safer to use peritoneal dialysis to prevent tamponade from bleeding, secondary to heparinization in hemodialysis. Heparin-free hemodialysis may be used as an alternative. Should the effusion not be responsive to vigorous dialysis or if symptoms of tamponade develop, pericardial drainage and the placement of a pericardial drainage catheter for repeated fluid removal (to dryness) and instillation of nonabsorbable steroid into the pericardial space may be used. Surgical drainage either to create an anterior pericardial "window" or to perform pericardial stripping is sometimes necessary for control.

Bleeding Disorders

Bleeding disorders occur with an elevation of the BUN to greater than 100 ml/dl or a creatinine level greater than 6.0 mg/dl. Platelet dysfunction occurs regularly, and bleeding time becomes prolonged by mechanisms that are not fully understood. It is postulated to be a secondary toxic effect of retained nitrogenous products (e.g., guanidinosuccinic acid). Spontaneous bleeding may occur from the gastrointestinal tract, and skin purpura or ecchymosis is often present. Dialysis to maintain lower BUN and creatinine levels is the most effective method of therapy. If emergency surgery is required, 1-deamino-(8-D-arginine)-vasopressin (DDAVP), 0.3 µg/kg, may be given over 30 minutes intravenously and repeated, if necessary, in 2 to 6 hours. Drugs such as aspirin and, to a lesser extent, the nonsteroidal anti-inflammatory agents that produce further platelet inhibition should be avoided. Platelet transfusion is of little benefit, since the platelets transfused into the uremic environment function abnormally.

Infection

There is an increased incidence and severity of infections in uremia. Prophylactic attention to skin, mouth, and perianal areas is necessary, since early diagnosis and vigorous treatment with prompt diagnostic measures are helpful in attaining control of infection. Prophylactic antibiotics are not helpful and often cause more significant side effects by selecting resistant organisms.

Viral and bacterial vaccines should be given in the presymptomatic stage of renal disease rather than in advanced uremia for maximal benefit. Transplantation candidates should have immunization with tetanus and diphtheria-pertussis-tetanus (DPT) updated and pneumococcal vaccine given if indicated. Thus, exogenously administered vaccines may be avoided during the post–renal transplantation period, when immunization may precipitate rejection from consequent immunostimulation.

Neurologic Disorders

With advancing uremia, there is regularly a change in mood and responsiveness. Children show fatigue, malaise, drowsiness, and headache from neurologic as well as psychiatric causes. Organic brain syndrome may be secondary to metabolic abnormalities, such as azotemia, or aluminum retention may produce seizures, asterixis, and peripheral neuropathy. Such organic brain syndromes are responsive to increased dialysis, suggesting that the major problem may be that of retained toxins, either endogenously or exogenously produced. Aluminum-binding gels should be stopped and desferrioxamine therapy considered if plasma levels of aluminum are elevated.

Peripheral neuropathy is common, and paresthesias with tingling, burning, and numbness may be noted in the older child. Loss of vibration sense, pin prick localization, and position sense may be demonstrated, with the symptoms greater in the lower extremities. Additional symptoms include decreased muscle strength and diminished deep tendon reflexes, which can progress to footdrop or paralysis. Early dialysis is prophylactic, and if these conditions are present, vigorous dialysis or transplantation should be undertaken.

Seizures from multiple causes may occur in the clinical course of uremia. Differential diagnosis includes, in addition to the standard etiologies, hypertensive encephalopathy, hypocalcemia, hypoglycemia, hyponatremia, dialysis dysequilibrium (secondary to rapid osmolar changes), cerebral edema, intracranial thrombosis, or intracranial infections. Metabolic abnormality, if detected, should be corrected. Once dialysis treatment has commenced, consideration of using drugs that have limited renal excretion is appropriate, and the dosage is coordinated with dialysis and is adjusted to monitored levels.

PSYCHIATRIC AND FAMILY SUPPORT

In children with chronic illness, a formal psychiatric review of family interactions, an appreciation of chronic renal failure and its effect on development, and a review of the family "defenses" should be undertaken.

A knowledgeable social worker who can assist with financial planning and integration into a future endstage renal disease program can ease the path for the family and assist in building a support system.

Frank discussions of the potential course of chronic renal failure and the need to provide consistency in limit setting and support to the child are held. Normal schooling is continued when possible, and tutorial assistance is provided when needed. The school is apprised of dietary and medication regimens, limitations of activity, and potential effects of therapy on attention and work ability. Integration of schooling into the scheme of future hospitalizations and specialized treatment before and during replacement therapy (dialysis and transplantation) is necessary to maximize rehabilitation.

PERITONEAL DIALYSIS

RICHARD N. FINE, M.D.

HISTORICAL PERSPECTIVE

Studies initiated in the nineteenth century were continued in the early 1920s and established that solute and water could be added to or removed from the body by placing solutions of appropriate compositions in the peritoneum. The peritoneum was initially used to remove uremic substances in humans in 1923, but the widespread clinical use of peritoneal dialysis (PD) awaited the commercial availability of dialysate solutions and disposable tubing sets in the late 1950s. A permanently implantable peritoneal access catheter (Tenckhoff Catheter, Quinton Instrument Company, Seattle, Washington) and automated equipment for dialysate delivery made PD a realistic alternative to hemodialysis (HD) for patients with end-stage renal disease (ESRD) in the late 1960s. However, the actual use of intermittent PD in children was minimal because of its reduced efficacy with respect to solute removal compared with HD.

A renaissance of interest in PD occurred in the mid 1970s, when a "novel portable/wearable equilibrium, peritoneal dialysis technique" (continuous ambulatory peritoneal dialysis, or CAPD) was described. This technique, along with continuous cycling peritoneal dialysis (CCPD), has continued to gain enthusiasm among ESRD patients, and currently more than 17,000 patients in the United States with ESRD utilize these treatment modalities.

INDICATIONS

Acute Renal Failure (ARF)

PD is the most frequently used dialysis technique for infants, children, and adolescents with ARF. Limited expertise is required for percutaneous catheter insertion, and previously inexperienced nursing personnel can be readily instructed in the dialysis procedure.

The indications for initiating PD in pediatric patients with ARF are variable and primarily depend upon the clinical status of the patient. Absolute indications are (1) deteriorating central nervous system function (coma); (2) congestive heart failure unresponsive to diuretics, especially in an anuric patient; and (3) hypertension that is not controllable with antihypertensive medication. Various biochemical parameters are used to indicate the propitious time to commence PD: a blood urea nitrogen (BUN) greater than 150 mg/dl, a serum carbon dioxide content less than 12 mEq/L, a serum potassium level greater than 6.0 mEq/L, and a falling hematocrit (< 20 per cent), necessitating transfusion in the face of hyperkalemia and hypertension. Each of these biochemical abnormalities can be managed without PD; however, the decision to initiate PD should be based on the clinical status of the patient in conjunction with assessment of the biochemical abnormalities.

End-Stage Renal Disease (ESRD)

CAPD and CCPD are currently the therapeutic modalities of choice for infants and children with ESRD. Both techniques provide adequate solute and fluid and can be performed at home without the need for a vascular access, repetitive venipuncture, or the extracorporeal availability of blood. Neonates with ESRD can be managed for protracted periods (>1 year) with either modality until a successful kidney transplantation can be performed. CCPD is less labor intensive in that it requires only one connection to the automatic cycler machine at bedtime and one disconnection in the morning, compared with four to five connections and disconnections (exchanges) daily with CAPD. Therefore, most parents of infants and school-aged children who must undertake the procedures prefer CCPD. Adolescents (>12 years) who perform the procedure themselves also prefer CCPD because it eliminates the need to perform exchanges at school and the potential for scrutiny by peers.

The absolute indication to initiate PD in an infant, child, or adolescent with ESRD is the presence of pericarditis, myocardiopathy, and progressive osteodystrophy with concomitant osseous abnormalities. Uncontrolled hypertension, repetitive episodes of congestive heart failure, or hyperkalemia also indicates the need to commence PD before the development of significant uremic symptomatology. The latter is usually accomplished if a peritoneal access is established once the creatinine clearance (C_{cr}) is between 5 and 10 ml/min/1.73m² and if PD is initiated once the C_{cr} is less than 5 ml/min/1.73m².

When following an infant with chronic renal failure (CRF), growth, increment in head circumference, and neurologic development must be assessed as indicators to initiate PD. Failure to track in the appropriate height, weight, and head circumference percentile curves, as well as failure to demonstrate normal developmental milestones, should be considered clinical manifestations of uremia in the infant and should dictate the need to commence PD.

Intoxication

PD is beneficial in the treatment of accidental poisoning in children.* In general, any substance that is water

---

*For a detailed analysis of the optimal treatment regimen for drug overdose and accidental poisoning, see Winchester JF, Gelfand MC, Knepshield JH, and Schreiner GE: Trans Am Soc Artif Intern Organs 23:762–842, 1977.

soluble is potentially dialyzable. The efficacy of dialysis generally depends on the degree of protein binding. Fat-soluble substances do not lend themselves to removal with PD. The indications for dialysis depend on the poison ingested, the blood level of the poison, and the clinical status of the patient. The routine use of peritoneal dialysis in the management of children with salicylate intoxication is probably superfluous, if adequate diuresis and alkalinization of the urine can be obtained. However, with severe intoxication, dialysis using a 5 per cent human albumin (Albumisol) solution is beneficial.

Electrolyte Disturbances

Severe hypernatremia can lead to irreversible central nervous system damage and is a pediatric emergency. When the serum sodium level approaches 200 mEq/L, dialysis is indicated. More efficient correction of severe hypernatremia can result with the use of PD than with intravenous fluid administration.

Severe hyperkalemia (serum potassium level of 8.5 to 9.0 mEq/L) with significant electrocardiographic (ECG) abnormalities (absence of P waves and arrhythmia) is best handled with the immediate initiation of PD until the ECG abnormalities abate and the primary disease process is controlled.

Severe acidosis associated with inborn errors of amino acid metabolism (maple syrup urine disease and hyperglycinemia) is an indication for PD. Dialysis not only is beneficial in correcting the acidosis but also facilitates removal of the offending amino acid and metabolites until an appropriate treatment regimen can be instituted.

Congenital urea cycle enzymopathies are characterized by a reduced capacity to synthesize urea, which leads to accumulation of ammonium and other nitrogenous urea precursors. The central nervous system manifestations in affected neonates are thought to be related to the increased blood ammonia concentration. PD is the treatment of choice in these disorders and is clinically superior to the use of exchange transfusion.

Fluid Removal

In the child with normal renal function and intractable congestive heart failure unresponsive to digitalis and diuretics, fluid removal may be facilitated with PD. Such circumstances are rare, and temporary improvement has been reported. Similarly, PD will provide temporary improvement by fluid removal in a child with severe anasarca unresponsive to the usual therapeutic regimen. Intraperitoneal albumin is absorbed when added to the dialysate solution and will transiently increase the serum albumin level, thereby promoting a diuresis.

CONTRAINDICATIONS

The only contraindication to the use of PD is intra-abdominal bleeding subsequent to a coagulopathy. Patients with peritonitis and pancreatitis have undergone successful PD. Recent abdominal surgery, even in the presence of drains, is not a contraindication, although the efficiency of the procedure may be decreased in this circumstance.

TECHNIQUES

Percutaneous Catheter Insertion for Acute Dialysis

Prior to initiating the procedure, a well-functioning site for delivery of intravenous solutions should be present, and 1 or 2 units of whole blood should be available in case of hemorrhage induced by the catheter insertion procedure.

If the patient is not comatose, intramuscular or intravenous analgesia is administered approximately one-half hour prior to initiating the catheter insertion procedure. Respiratory depressants should be minimized because elevation of the diaphragm following instillation of intraperitoneal dialysate may compromise the respiratory effects. The bladder is then emptied by catheterization to avoid inadvertent puncture during the catheter insertion procedure. A surgical preparation of the abdomen from the xiphoid to the pubis is then done.

Trocar Insertion Method

A Trocath (Gambro Engstrom, Lincolnshire, Illinois) is available in neonatal, pediatric, and adult sizes. After the abdomen is prepared, a puncture site 1.5 to 3.0 cm from the umbilicus is selected and is anesthetized with a local anesthetic (lidocaine 1 per cent). A long 14-gauge needle is inserted into the peritoneal cavity. Previously warmed dialysate solution containing 1.5 per cent glucose, 0 to 4 mEq/L of potassium, 1 ml of aqueous heparin (1000 USP units/ml), and 125 mg/L of cephalothin is instilled into the peritoneal cavity until the abdomen is tense; the tense abdomen facilitates insertion of the trocar. The needle is then removed, and a 0.5-cm stab wound is made through the skin at the identified puncture site to permit insertion of the trocar and catheter, which are then inserted into the peritoneal cavity with a steady, circular motion. Once the trocar and catheter are in the peritoneal cavity, which will be evident by a significant, sudden reduction in tension, the trocar is removed, and the catheter is guided into either lower quadrant. The fluid in the peritoneal cavity is removed, and dialysis commences. If the catheter does not fit snugly at the puncture site, a purse-string suture is used to prevent leakage of dialysate fluid during the procedure.

Cook Catheter Method

Limited experience is available with this new catheter (Acute Peritoneal Dialysis Catheters, Cook Critical Care, Bloomington, Indiana), but the design of the catheter facilitates an insertion technique that is much less traumatic than the trocar method. The use of this catheter should minimize complications related to catheter insertion and reduce the incidence of peritoneal bleeding with resultant bloody dialysate.

A short 14-gauge needle is inserted into the peritoneal cavity at a site similar to that selected for trocar insertion, and a modest amount (10 ml/kg) of dialysate solution, the composition of which is described in the previous section, is instilled into the peritoneal cavity. It is not necessary for the abdomen to be tense. A guide wire is then inserted into the peritoneal cavity through the 14-gauge needle, and the latter is removed. It is important that the soft, flexible part of the guide wire is inserted into the peritoneal cavity. The Cook peritoneal catheter is inserted into the peritoneal cavity over the guide wire, and the latter is removed. The catheter is then manipulated to the area of the peritoneal cavity desired. Replacement of a malfunctioning catheter is facilitated by reinserting the guide wire, removing the malfunctioning catheter, and inserting a new one.

Permanent Catheter Insertion

Permanent peritoneal access devices are available in four sizes (neonate, pediatric, juvenile adult, and adult) (Quinton Instrument Company, Seattle, Washington). The neonatal catheter is used for infants weighing less than 5 kg, the pediatric catheter for children weighing up to 20 to 25 kg, and the adult catheter for older children and adolescents. Although the permanent catheter can be inserted percutaneously, it has been our policy to have them inserted surgically. The catheter is placed in the pelvic gutter, with the proximal Dacron cuff just proximal to the peritoneal exit site and the distal Dacron cuff about 3 to 4 cm from the catheter exit site. The proximal Dacron cuff is secured by being sutured to the peritoneum. If long-term dialysis is anticipated, a prophylactic omentectomy should be performed to minimize omental obstruction of the catheter. Catheters are available with only the proximal Dacron cuff, and there is currently controversy regarding the benefit of the distal cuff in preventing exit site infections. Two-cuff catheters are currently used at our institution.

Manual Acute Dialysis

Commercially prepared dialysate solutions—Dianeal (Baxter Health Care Corporation), Delflex (National Medical Care), Dialyte (Gambro), and Impersol (Abbott Laboratories)—are available with glucose concentrations of 1.5, 2.5, and 4.25 per cent and contain no potassium. All three glucose concentrations are hypertonic with respect to plasma and therefore will affect fluid removal during dialysis. Depending upon the patient's serum potassium level, 0 to 4.0 mEq/L of potassium is added to the dialysate. It is dangerous to dialyze with a potassium-free solution because of the potential for hypokalemia. Heparin (0.25 ml of aqueous heparin, 1000 USP units/ml) is added to each liter of dialysate. If the spent dialysate is clear after the initial 6 to 12 passes, the heparin can be deleted. An attempt should be made to maintain the dialysate at 37°C prior to instillation to avoid the potential for producing hypothermia. Although there are no unequivocal data that the use of prophylactic antibiotics either prevents or reduces the risk of intraperitoneal infection, it is accepted practice to add 125 mg/L of cephalothin during the initial 48 hours of dialysis.

The volume of dialysate instilled into the peritoneal cavity is 1000 to 1500 ml/m² or 25 to 50 ml/kg. If a hypertonic glucose (4.25 per cent) solution is to be used for rapid ultrafiltration and fluid removal, it is important to reduce the volume instilled to minimize overdistention and respiratory compromise.

Generally, each pass takes 1 hour: 15 minutes for the fluid to flow into the peritoneum, 30 minutes for dialysis, and 15 minutes for removal. Equilibration between the dialysate fluid and plasma (D/P ratio) approaches 100 per cent for small solutes in 3 to 4 hours; however, it is 50 per cent within the initial 30 to 60 minutes of an exchange. Therefore, the removal of small solutes such as urea and potassium is facilitated by frequent short dwell time dialysis. If dialysis is being performed to reduce a toxic substance of larger molecular weight, longer dwell time dialysis is required. Excessive fluid removal is facilitated by using a more hypertonic glucose solution.

With ARF, dialysis should proceed until sufficient renal function returns to lower the blood urea level spontaneously toward normal. If the Trocath is used, the incidence of infection increases after 48 to 72 hours, and if acute dialysis is required for longer periods, plans should be made to insert a permanent peritoneal catheter. It is possible that the Cook catheter can be left in place for a longer time, without increasing the propensity for infection; however, data in pediatric patients are not available at the present time.

Automated Acute Dialysis

The automated peritoneal dialysis delivery systems warm the dialysate and permit adjustments in inflow, diffusion, and outflow time as well as dialysate volume. The currently available systems can deliver dialysate volumes in 100-ml (PAC-X, Baxter Health Care Corporation, Deerfield, Illinois) and 250-ml (AMP 80/20 Del Med, Ogden, Utah) increments; in addition, the PAC-X provides a cumulative record of dialysate volume removed. The PAC-XTRA can deliver volumes in 10 ml increments.

Continuous Ambulatory Peritoneal Dialysis (CAPD)

This technique closely approximates a wearable artificial kidney. Dialysis is continuous 24 hours a day 7 days a week. Dialysate solution (250 ml, 500 ml, 750 ml, 1000 ml, 1500 ml, 2000 ml, 2500 ml, and 3000 ml, Baxter Health Care Corporation, Deerfield, Illinois) is instilled into the peritoneal cavity four to five times a day and remains in the peritoneal cavity for 4 to 5 hours during the day and 8 hours at night. The patient (if >12 years of age) or parent is taught to perform the procedure under sterile conditions in a clean environment, thereby facilitating maximal mobility with this technique. Dialysate with four different glucose concentrations is available: 1.5 per cent, 2.5 per cent, 3.5 per cent, and 4.25 per cent (Baxter Health Care Corporation, Deerfield, Illinois). Use of the solution with higher glucose content yields increased ultrafiltration and fluid removal.

Continuous Cycling Peritoneal Dialysis (CCPD)

This technique is a variant of CAPD and utilizes the equipment described under "Automated Acute Dialysis" to deliver dialysate at night while the patient sleeps.

Typically, five exchanges at 2-hour intervals are delivered by the automatic cycler machine at night, and a one-half volume dwell remains in the peritoneal cavity during the day. The advantage of this technique is that it is less labor intensive, requiring only one connection and disconnection daily instead of 8 to 10 procedures, as with CAPD. In addition, school-aged children and adolescents prefer this technique because it eliminates the need to perform exchanges at school, thereby limiting exposure to scrutiny by peers.

COMPLICATIONS

Trocar Catheter Insertion

Bladder perforation by the trocar will be evident if the returning dialysate solution smells like urine. If the catheter is placed in the bladder via the trocar perforation, the patient will void large amounts shortly after each pass. Insertion of a Foley catheter for 7 to 10 days is generally curative. Dialysis can continue after insertion of the Foley catheter.

Bowel perforation is usually evident by the appearance of fecal material in the returning dialysis solution. If possible, dialysis should be discontinued and the perforation repaired surgically.

Vessel perforation can lead to catastrophic consequences. If an artery is punctured, shock is the initial finding. Shock should be treated with blood replacement, and the perforation should be repaired immediately. With venous perforation, the dialysis fluid is darker, and shock may not occur.

In patients with a coagulopathy, such as the hemolytic-uremic syndrome, generalized peritoneal bleeding may mimic venous perforation. Since it is difficult at times to discern the degree of intraperitoneal bleeding by visual inspection, a hematocrit determination on the dialysis fluid may be helpful. If the hematocrit is greater than 5 ml/dl, significant bleeding has occurred, and the procedure should be discontinued.

After discontinuation of dialysis, when the catheter is removed, the omentum may adhere to its tip and herniate through the skin. The omentum should be replaced surgically into the peritoneal cavity, and the protruding piece should not be amputated.

Medical

The patient may have a seizure related either to the dysequilibrium syndrome or to hypocalcemia. The former is treated with diazepam (Valium), 1 to 2 mg given intravenously (IV), followed by phenobarbital, 3 to 5 mg/kg every 8 to 12 hours. Hypocalcemia is controlled with intravenous calcium gluconate (10 per cent), 1 to 5 ml. Care should be taken not to infiltrate calcium into the subcutaneous tissue because of the potential for severe skin necrosis.

Since the glucose load with PD is significant, it is possible to produce hyperglycemia and hyperosmolar coma. This situation can be avoided by careful monitoring of the serum glucose level and the judicious use of intraperitoneal insulin if hyperglycemia develops.

The major complication of PD, regardless of technique, is peritonitis. The diagnosis is made by the presence of fever, cloudy dialysate fluid, and abdominal pain. More than 50 white blood cells per cubic millimeter of peritoneal fluid is diagnostic of peritonitis, especially if more than 50 per cent of the white blood cells are polymorphonuclear leukocytes. The most common organism is *Staphylococcus epidermidis*, although other gram-positive and gram-negative organisms are frequently implicated. Prior to identifying the offending organism, 125 mg/dl of cephalothin and 6 to 8 mg/L of gentamicin are instilled into the dialysate. If significant systemic symptoms are present, intravenous antibiotics are administered. These must be adjusted for the degree of renal insufficiency.

HEMODIALYSIS

ANTONIA C. NOVELLO, M.D., M.P.H.

Pediatric nephrologists consider renal transplantation the optimal therapeutic modality for children with renal failure; i.e., a successful transplant provides the best opportunity for normal growth and development and for alleviating the psychological distress of chronic renal failure. However, prolonged dialysis may be needed in some children.

Dialysis is a technique for removing metabolites and toxins and for maintaining a satisfactory equilibrium of electrolytes and volume in patients with disordered excretory capabilities. Hemodialysis, simply stated, is a diffusive process in which blood comes into contact with a balanced salt solution (dialysate) across a semipermeable membrane and solutes pass across by diffusion along a concentration gradient, their rate of removal being determined by their physicochemical properties. Isotonic fluid removal is achieved by applying a hydrostatic pressure gradient on the membrane.

Hemodialysis has been performed in children since the early 1960s. The technique has been utilized in preparation for renal transplant while searching for a suitable donor, after a failed renal transplant, and for the treatment of life-threatening clinical complications. Nevertheless, there seems to be limited experience with long-term (longer than 5 years) hemodialysis in children. Despite this, the overall survival is good, with one report indicating a 5-year actuarial patient survival rate of 95 per cent. Several other options for the treatment of children with chronic renal failure (CRF) have become available during the past decade, e.g., continuous ambulatory peritoneal dialysis (CAPD), continuous cycling peritoneal dialysis (CCPD), and chronic intermittent peritoneal dialysis (IPD).

The number of patients in the pediatric age group with end-stage renal disease (ESRD) reportedly varies from 1 to 3.5 per million population per year. Prior to the widespread availability of hemodialysis and the newer peritoneal dialysis techniques (CAPD, CCPD, and IPD), definite treatment was not initiated until severe uremic complications were apparent. Currently, hemodialysis is begun before severe symptomatology occurs. Absolute indications for dialysis are uncontrollable hypertension with hypertensive encephalopathy or congestive heart failure, congestive heart failure unresponsive to loop diuretics, pericarditis, peripheral neuropathy, renal osteodystrophy, and bone marrow depression with either severe anemia, leukopenia, or thrombocytopenia.

In most instances, symptoms arising from involvement of a single organ system predominate and dictate the need for dialysis. In the child without such absolute indications, the decision to institute dialysis should be based upon his or her ability to perform usual daily activities. In these cases, derangements in biochemical parameters can be useful indicators for starting dialysis: i.e., blood urea nitrogen (BUN) greater than 150 mg/dl, carbon dioxide content less than 12 mEq/L, potassium level greater than 6.0 mEq/L, falling hematocrit (less than 20 per cent, necessitating transfusion in the face of hyperkalemia and volume overload), and severe hypocalcemia (calcium level less than 7.0 mg/dl). These biochemical abnormalities in combination with a glomerular filtration rate of less than 5 ml/min/1.73 m^2 indicate the imminent need for dialysis.

Two other situations may require emergency initiation of hemodialysis: accidental poisoning and acute renal failure. As alternatives, hemoperfusion and peritoneal dialysis, respectively, might be considered in such cases. Peritoneal dialysis is widely available and has the advantage of not requiring heparinization.

DIALYSIS PRESCRIPTION FOR CHILDREN

Vascular Access

Patients undergoing hemodialysis require a vascular access that permits high blood flow rates. Three types of access are commonly used: shunts, fistulas, and temporary access. The Thomas femoral shunt is the preferred access for children weighing less than 15 kg or younger than 5 years of age who require hemodialysis. With any type of vascular access, the goal is to use the largest cannula that fits comfortably without compromising the intima of the vessel in which it is inserted. Disadvantages of the shunt include infections, clotting episodes, and, in some children, inhibition of normal activity and anxiety because of the presence of the external cannula. Ischemic damage to the leg where a groin shunt was placed has been reported as a rare complication.

In children with ESRD who will undergo long-term dialysis and whose weight is more than 15 kg, an arteriovenous fistula—a forearm vein anastomosed to a radial artery—is preferred. Fistulas differ from shunts in requiring "maturation." They must be constructed at least 3 weeks before utilization is anticipated. When the anastomosis provides insufficient blood flow, an alternate internal arteriovenous fistula can be created using either a bovine graft or synthetic material. More recently, microsurgical techniques in infants weighing less than 5 kg have been described. A detrimental effect, as with the use of shunts, is thrombosis. At times the high fistula flow demands an excessively high cardia output, resulting in eventual systolic hypertension and heart failure.

For temporary vascular access, percutaneous catheters have been used via femoral, subclavian, or internal jugular veins, even in children weighing as little as 6 kg.

Dialyzers

Because of the low cardiac output and the small vascular volume of children, the extracorporeal volume of the dialyzers, blood flow rates, and blood lines must be kept to a minimum. The ideal is to fill both the dialyzer and blood tubing with less than 10 per cent of the child's blood volume (10 cc/kg body weight). Hollow fiber dialyzers are preferable to flat or coil dialyzers, since their blood compartment is relatively small and rigid.

There are three types of dialyzers available today: parallel plate, hollow fiber, and coil. Children are usually dialyzed with parallel plate or hollow fiber dialyzers. The main consideration in choosing a dialyzer is its ultrafiltration coefficient and blood compartment volume. Pediatric dialyzers are generally designed for children in either the 10 to 20 kg (0.5 to 0.6 m^2) or the 20 to 40 kg (1.0 m^2) weight range. Children weighing more than 40 kg (1.3 to 1.6 m^2) can usually be treated using adult dialyzers. Children weighing less than 10 kg require a 0.25 m^2 dialyzer.

Delivery System

No special modifications of existing delivery systems are required for pediatric patients. The usual dialysate solution has the following composition: calcium, 3.5 mEq/L; potassium, 1.0 or 2.0 mEq/L; sodium, 135 mEq/L; chloride, 100 mEq/L; magnesium, 1.6 mEq/L; acetate, 38 mEq/L; and glucose, 0 to 250 mg/dl. If the child demonstrates intolerance (nausea, vomiting, hypotension) to acetate, as may occur with high-efficiency dialyzers, bicarbonate can be substituted for acetate in the bath. Likewise, the use of dialyzers with inappropriately high clearance values should be avoided in children. Several techniques, such as intravenous infusion of saline, human albumin, vasopressors, or mannitol, can be used to minimize ultrafiltration-induced hypotension. Separate filtration followed by isovolemic hemodialysis may also be employed. In order to minimize the need for these interventions, the ultrafiltration rate should be calculated to remove the desired quantity of fluid evenly during the course of dialysis.

Prescription

Many schemes have been proposed to determine the optimal frequency, duration, and clearance of dialysis in pediatric patients. The most commonly used method to determine the adequacy of dialysis is kinetic modeling. This technique employs urea as a marker of uremic toxicity and allows for the development of treatment options permitting maintenance of BUN within predetermined limits. The goal is to keep a time-averaged concentration of urea within the range of 60 to 70 mg/dl (predialysis BUN level of about 80 to 100 mg/dl and postdialysis level of about 20 to 30 mg/dl).

The dialysis index, which compares and relates dialyzer surface area × weekly hours of dialysis ÷ body surface area, has been formulated according to values derived from adult experiences. In most pediatric centers the initial prescriptions of dialyzer clearance and time schedule depend on the child's weight (surface area), fluid accumulation between dialysis treatments, and the predialysis level of BUN. In most centers dialysis is usually prescribed three times a week for periods ranging between 4 and 6 hours, utilizing standard priming and heparinization techniques described in the literature.

Ultrafiltration

During ultrafiltration, fluid removed from the plasma is replaced with fluid equilibrated from the expanded interstitial space. The degree of ultrafiltration varies according to the desired weight loss. Excessive ultrafiltration (greater than 3 kg for adolescents or 2 kg for younger children) is frequently necessary. This can cause hypotension, nausea, vomiting, headaches, and cramps. When hypoalbuminemia (less than 3 gm/dl) is present and ultrafiltration is required, the albumin level must be raised to improve tolerance of ultrafiltration. Although equilibration is rapid, at times signs of plasma volume depletion occur. In this event, separate ultrafiltration for 1 hour prior to the initiation of dialysis will aid in the removal of fluid without concomitant hypotension.

Nutrition and Diet in Dialyzed Children

Since growth failure and nutritional energy deficiencies are commonly recognized in dialyzed children with ESRD, an effort should be made to maximize the number of calories ingested. This is difficult, inasmuch as caloric intake must be kept high while sodium, potassium, phosphorus, protein, and fluids must be limited. Today, the goal is to strike a fair balance among these needs. The energy and protein content of the diet must be supplemented and not limited, and dietary restrictions must not produce nutrient deficiencies, even if this means a greater dialytic requirement. The goal is to provide 80 to 100 per cent of the recommended daily allowance energy requirements for these children. Daily dietary recommendations are: calories, 2000/m^2; protein 1.5 to 2.5 gm/kg, or 3 to 4 gm/kg in small children (less than 10 to 16 kg); sodium, 40 mEq/m^2; potassium, 30 mEq/m^2; and fluids, 500 ml/m^2 plus an amount equal to urine volume. B complex vitamins and folic acid, 1 mg daily, are also supplemented. Phosphate-binding gels (preferably without aluminum), 1 to 3 capsules three times a day with meals, or calcium carbonate is given to reduce the serum phosphorus level.

In general, therefore, the dietary intake of dialyzed children should include a balanced energy intake and a protein intake of approximately 2 gm/kg/day.

COMPLICATIONS OF HEMODIALYSIS

Hypertension. Virtually all patients undergoing hemodialysis have periods of hypertension. The usual mechanism is volume expansion, which generally responds to dietary fluid and salt restriction. Ultrafiltration to dry weight also controls hypertension in more than 90 per cent of patients. Occasional hypertension episodes are not controlled by dialysis, and these patients may require hypertensive medication. Occasionally, hypertensive medications are ineffective and bilateral nephrectomy is necessary for blood pressure control. This is rare, however, with the availability of captopril and minoxidil. Most of these cases are associated with high levels of renin. Postnephrectomy hypertension is mostly volume-related. If hypertension persists after nephrectomy, it may be due to changes in peripheral resistance or to vasoactive substances produced outside the kidney. Nevertheless, blood pressure control during hemodialysis generally improves once the patient is well dialyzed.

Anemia. Children with CRF have a normochromic, normocytic anemia secondary to deficient erythropoiesis. When they undergo dialysis, this state is complicated by a continuing loss of blood, mostly in the dialyzer and because of frequent sampling for laboratory determinations. Increased hemolysis due to the mechanical trauma of the extracorporeal circulation is a minor additional factor. If the patient has undergone bilateral nephrectomy, the anemia worsens. Most children need transfusions to maintain the hematocrit level above 20 per cent. Complications from frequent transfusion procedures include infection with hepatitis B antigen, tissue iron deposition, and sensitization to HLA antigens. If patients fail to respond to iron (e.g., adolescents with fused epiphyses), benefit may be obtained from nandrolone phenpropionate* (Durabolin), 50 to 100 mg IM every week for boys and every 2 weeks for girls. This is helpful in stimulating erythropoiesis. This treatment should not be used in patients with unfused epiphyses.

Osteodystrophy. Chronic dialysis usually stabilizes existing renal osteodystrophy. Two types of lesions have been recognized by x-ray examination: rickets-like lesions (osteomalacia) and subperiosteal bone resorption (secondary hyperparathyroidism or osteitis fibrosa). Meticulous control of acidosis and calcium and phosphorus balance by pharmacologic agents or dietary maneuvers may alleviate these problems. Controlling secondary hyperparathyroidism prior to dialysis is also important. During dialysis, the dialysate calcium should be high (7.0 mg/dl) to allow the ionized calcium to be transferred to the patient. Parathyroid hyperplasia, however, rarely involutes with the use of a high calcium-containing dialysate alone. Vitamin D analogues and supplemental calcium result in a more dramatic response. Dihydrotachysterol, 0.2 or 0.4 mg daily, and supplemental calcium carbonate, 500 to 2000 mg daily, have been advocated. If hypocalcemia persists, 1,25-dihydroxycholecalciferol (Rocaltrol), 0.25 μg once or twice daily, should be used instead.

Despite dietary restrictions, most children are also hyperphosphatemic, requiring aggressive therapy to maintain serum phosphorus between 4 and 5 mg/dl. This should be accomplished with phosphate-binding gels (not containing aluminum) or calcium carbonate. If by x-ray examination the lesions of hyperparathy-

roidism fail to show evidence of healing, or if they worsen despite correction of calcium and phosphorus parameters, parathyroid gland extirpation (3½) may be indicated. In the presence of rickets, however, parathyroidectomy is not beneficial. Chronic aluminum loading may cause rickets, as is evident on bone biopsy. Aluminum can be chelated by weekly infusions of desferrioxamine.

Cardiovascular Alterations. Left ventricular performance, as measured by systolic time intervals, may be depressed by uremia; this effect has been reported on echocardiography. In children, hemodialysis results in improvement in left ventricular function. Pericarditis develops in 2 to 19 per cent of patients on dialysis—in some, years after the initiation of dialysis and in others within the first 3 months. Echocardiography appears to be the most helpful method for assessment of patients with pericarditis. Major hemodynamic complications occur as a result of cardiac tamponade and constrictive pericarditis. In patients with dialysis-associated pericarditis, intensive dialysis alone (3 to 4 weeks) is usually curative. Heparin dosage in these individuals should be reduced and carefully monitored because hemorrhage may cause cardiac tamponade. Other treatment modalities are peritoneal dialysis, charcoal hemoperfusion, systemic or intrapericardial steroids, and pericardial stripping. Furthermore, hypertriglyceridemia is frequently found in children on dialysis. Hypercholesterolemia and an increased fraction of low-density lipoproteins can also occur.

Psychosocial Problems. In children, dialytic treatments are time consuming, medical complications are common, and loss of schooling is frequent, often leading to poor peer-group interactions. Associated complications are loss of self-esteem, social isolation, and lack of independence. The treatment goal is to allow patients as much responsibility as possible for their daily care; the ultimate goal is rehabilitation and community integration.

Seizures. In most instances a specific etiology cannot be identified, and thus the seizure is attributed to the disequilibrium syndrome. Patients with high BUN, especially those during their first or second dialysis treatment, are at greater risk. Disequilibrium is prevented by using a relatively high dialysate sodium concentration (140 to 145 mEq/L), by decreasing the efficiency of urea clearance to 1.0 to 1.5 ml/min/kg, or by infusing 25 per cent mannitol, 1 gm/kg over the course of dialysis, in order to maintain extracellular fluid osmolality. In some cases prophylactic phenobarbital prior to and/or during dialysis has been advocated.

Hepatitis. Evidence supports the conclusion that infection with hepatitis B virus increases morbidity and mortality. The incidence of hepatitis in children treated with chronic hemodialysis is approximately 10 per cent. Blood parameters to be followed monthly as a precaution are serum glutamic-oxalic transaminase (SGOT), serum glutamic-pyruvic transaminase (SGPT), bilirubin, and hepatitis B antigen levels. Elevation of SGOT and SGPT in the absence of hepatitis B antigen may be due to hepatitis A or hepatitis non-A, non-B. Methods established to decrease the incidence of HBsAG-positive

---

*This use is not listed by the manufacturer.

hepatitis among patients and staff of hemodialysis units include the provision of gowns and gloves, use of disposable equipment, routine screening for hepatitis B virus, dialysis of HBsAg-positive patients in isolation, and possibly utilization of home dialysis. To contain or prevent an epidemic, hyperimmune serum may be given to ESRD patients and staff members recently exposed to hepatitis virus. Hepatitis B vaccine is also an effective prophylaxis. There is a significant incidence of "e" antigenemia in children with persistent hepatitis antigenemia, indicating infectivity of these patients.

RENAL TRANSPLANTATION

ANTONIA C. NOVELLO, M.D., M.P.H.

The annual incidence of chronic renal failure in children requiring dialysis or transplantation approaches 3 per million total population if adolescents older than 15 as well as infants are included. Since 1972, renal transplantation has been the preferred mode of treatment for the alleviation of end-stage renal failure (ESRD) in children in the developed nations. A successful transplant results in physiologic and psychologic benefits unsurpassed by current modes of chronic dialysis.

Factors determining the actuarial survival of both patients and renal grafts include donor age, donor source, underlying renal disorder, age of the recipient, closeness of HLA match, pretransplant blood transfusions, prior history of transplantation, immunosuppressive therapy, and the experience of the transplant center. Although age need not necessarily be a factor when treatment of a child with ESRD is under consideration, conflicting data have emerged regarding the impact of donor age on the outcome following cadaveric kidney transplantation. Patient and graft survival rates are significantly higher in children 10 to 15 years of age than in those 5 to 9 years old or those less than 5 years of age. Survival rates in infants less than 1 year of age are very low; the short-term outcome of cadaver donor transplantation in these infants has been dismal.

Although technical problems are not inherently different, kidneys obtained from infants and newborns may fail to function more commonly than kidneys from older children or adults. Discouraging results have been obtained when anencephalic donors have been used. Recent studies have shown different graft survival in donor groups less than 11 years old when compared with donor groups between 11 and 50 years old (52 per cent and 57 per cent, respectively). Improved graft survival in children receiving adult grafts rather than a pediatric graft (69 per cent and 52 per cent, respectively) has also been reported.

The outcome of renal transplantation in children, as in adults, improves dramatically if living related donor transplantation is utilized, both in young (less than 10 years old) and older (11 to 20 years old) children. Thus if a live related donor is available, transplantation is the best option, since the results of cadaver donor trans-

plantation in young children (1 to 5 years) have been disappointing and are worse in children less than 1 year old. By contrast, since the outcome for the age group of 1 to 5 years using a live related (parental) donor organ has been encouraging, this is an acceptable mode of therapy.

Criteria For Acceptability

1. *Age*: No limit is generally placed.
2. *Mental Status*: It is known that the uremic state depresses cognitive functioning, which may improve with a successful transplant. Noncompliance is a major problem in children with ESRD, as is psychological or emotional instability. Children with severe mental retardation or behavioral or psychiatric problems require far more involvement with the health care team along with appropriate psychoemotional support. If emotional needs are not met, transplant success may be limited. Transplantation should probably then be deferred until the patient's psychoemotional status is improved so that it would be reasonable to assume that the post-transplant therapeutic regimen will be followed.
3. *Pre-existing Malignancy*: Prior malignancy is a real risk factor because of the possibility of recurrence following transplantation. Recurrence of the tumor or distant metastases have been known to occur in children receiving an allograft within 1 year following treatment for Wilms' tumor (47 per cent). No recurrence has been evident when transplantation has been delayed for more than 1 year. Thus transplantation in children with Wilms' tumor should be deferred for at least 1 year following treatment of the tumor.
4. *Generalized Infection*: If unrecognized, infections can disseminate when immunosuppression is started. Therefore, it is of importance to eradicate infection before transplantation is considered.
5. *Bladder Adequacy*: The presence of an abnormal bladder is not a contraindication for transplantation, an encouraging point for pediatric patients with ESRD, in at least one third of whom obstructive uropathy is present. These children often have scarred and contracted bladders related to previous corrective lower urinary tract or bladder surgery. Although post-transplant urologic complications and urinary tract infections occur with increased frequency, allograft function is not adversely affected, since graft survival rate in pediatric patients with previous urologic surgery is comparable to survival in children with normal lower urinary tracts. If the bladder is unsuitable, an ileal or nonrefluxing colon conduit can be utilized. The allograft ureter may also be anastomosed to an existing cutaneous ureterostomy. When a diversionary procedure is not feasible in patients with neurogenic bladders, clean intermittent catheterization can be performed.

Potential for Recurrence of the Primary Disease

The primary renal disease may influence patient and graft survival. Although graft loss is low, potential involvement with a pathologic process similar to that which affected the recipient native kidney is important when considering renal transplantation. The principal diseases for which recurrence is reported are membranoproliferative glomerulonephritis (MPGN), focal glomerulosclerosis (FGS), hemolytic uremic syndrome (HUS), cystinosis, and oxalosis. In MPGN no observed relationships between recurrence of the histologic lesion and alteration of allograft function have been reported. In FGS immediate recurrence in an initial allograft indicates substantial risks for recurrence in subsequent allografts. Despite this potential for graft loss and the variable incidence of recurrence, children with FGS should not be excluded from transplantation. In children with HUS, clinical manifestations of the disease after transplant have rarely been reported. Thus, in patients with HUS, it seems prudent to delay transplantation until all clinical manifestations of the initial episode abate.

Donor Selection—Surgical Procedure and Histocompatibility

As with adults, allografts from living related donors fare better than cadaveric transplants. The 5-year graft survival rates range between 71 and 85 per cent following live related donation, and between 39 and 65 per cent following cadaver donation. The best graft survival rates are obtained when kidneys from monozygotic twins and HLA-identical siblings are used. Children appear to accept kidneys from adult donors as long as they are 2 years of age and at least 10 kg. Parental or sibling donor allografts can be used. Siblings, however, should have expressed willingness to donate and be of age. Kidneys from a pediatric cadaver donor are excellent sources of donation, since anatomic hypertrophy occurs weeks after transplant. In cases in which the allograft is too large, it might be necessary to place the kidney intraperitoneally, anastomosing it to the recipient's aorta and vena cava if it cannot be placed in its usual extraperitoneal iliac-fossa site.

Improved cadaver graft survival rates do occur with better HLA-A and B antigen matching. A 20 per cent difference in survival rate at the end of 2 years for a two-haplotype match is evident when compared with three or four mismatches. It has been shown that survival rates for grafts improve when the donor and the recipient share two DR antigens. Currently, children receiving parental transplants have significantly higher allograft survival than when cadaver transplants well matched for HLA antigens are used.

Blood Transfusions and Allograft Survival

Donor-specific transfusions (DST) have gained acceptance in pediatric renal transplantation, since they appear to improve the graft survival in one haplotype-matched live related donor recipients with a reactive mixed lymphocyte culture. Data show prolonged graft survival when recipients are treated with donor-specific blood (98 per cent 1-year graft survival rate). The major disadvantage of this procedure is the risk of the development of antibodies against donor histocompatibility antigens. This has been known to occur in 15 to 29 per cent of children. The future of DST in pediatric renal transplantation depends on the lowering (perhaps as low as 10 per cent) of the sensitization rate, which may be accomplished with azathioprine therapy immediately before or during DST. The mechanism by which these transfusions protect against rejection is unknown. However, graft survival in first nontransfused cadaver donor recipients is poor (20 to 40 per cent). Graft survival rates are superior in multitransfused patients (more than five transfusions)—85 per cent vs. 57 per cent (less than five transfusions).

Cross-Match

Preformed lymphocytotoxic antibodies against donor antigens, acquired from blood transfusions, are associated with hyperacute rejection of the allograft. A negative cross-match (utilizing donor T lymphocytes and recipient serum) is essential prior to transplantation. The detection of DR antigens on B lymphocytes—a so-called positive B cell cross-match—is not deleterious to the allograft.

Bilateral Nephrectomy

Bilateral nephrectomy is no longer considered a prerequisite for transplantation. Pretransplant nephrectomies are performed for renin-dependent hypertension unresponsive to newer antihypertensive medications (i.e., captopril, minoxidil), persistent massive proteinuria, and persistent pyelonephritis. Reports of decreased allograft survival rate following nephrectomy, plus the importance of erythropoietin production and vitamin D metabolism in residual kidney mass, point to the importance of preserving even minimally functioning renal parenchyma.

Splenectomy

Despite recent controlled studies indicating improved allograft survival in splenectomized recipients receiving antilymphoblast globulin (ALG), this procedure is not generally indicated in pediatric renal recipients. Risk of infection in splenectomized patients is considerable; thus, the risks outweigh the potential gains.

Retransplantation

At 5 years after transplantation the actuarial survival rate for the second and third allograft is similar to the first (±45 per cent). The primary factor influencing allograft survival is recipient sensitization. The survival rate varies, from less than 5 per cent in nonpresensitized patients to 5 to 50 per cent in moderately presensitized patients and to greater than 50 per cent in highly presensitized patients. Thus, although HLA-A, B, and C antigen does not have a statistically significant effect on retransplant outcome, in the highly presensitized patient three or four HLA-A and B antigen-matched allografts should be utilized whenever feasible for retransplantation, since this appears to influence allograft survival.

Immunosuppression

Steroids and Azathioprine. The dosage and indications for corticosteroids and azathioprine in pediatric renal transplants are shown in Table 1. Recently, cyclosporine has been used in pediatric renal recipients. It appears that superior allograft survival can be attained with relatively low corticosteroid doses when cyclosporine is concomitantly administered with steroids. Al-

Table 1. DOSAGE OF IMMUNOSUPPRESSIVE DRUGS FOR RENAL TRANSPLANTATION

Dosage	Post-transplant Period
Prednisone	
3 mg/kg/24 hr	First 2 weeks, taper to—
2 mg/kg/24 hr	3rd week through 5th week
1 mg/kg/24 hr	6th week through 8th week
0.5 mg/kg/24 hr	3rd month through 5th month
*7.5 to 15 mg/day	6th month through 12th month
*15 to 30 mg/day (alternate-day therapy)	After first year
Azathioprine (Imuran)	
3 mg/kg/24 hr	Initially and maintained at that level unless:
0.5 to 1.0 mg/kg/24 hr if any of these conditions are present	oliguria, or leukopenia <4000 mm³, or hepatic dysfunction

*Depending upon adequate allograft function.

though results using cyclosporine in adults are encouraging, results in children are variable. Cyclosporine should be closely monitored in whole blood or serum. In some patients it may be difficult to achieve adequate cyclosporine blood levels and concomitant optimal immunosuppression; in order to maintain desired blood levels, children may require more cyclosporine than adults, calculated on a milligram per kilogram basis. Other investigators prefer kinetic analysis of cyclosporine blood levels in order to achieve optimal dosage intervals. The major side effects are a transient nephrotoxicity that reverses with dose reduction (27 to 50 per cent of children), moderate depression in glomerular filtration rate (this might be a limiting factor in the future use of cyclosporine in children, since diminished glomerular filtration rate may result in growth retardation), recurrence of the hemolytic uremic syndrome in some recipients, neurotoxic side effects (grand mal seizures, hypomagnesemia), facial hirsutism, and worsened cushingoid appearance. Thus, at present, the role of cyclosporine in pediatric renal transplantation needs further evaluation.

Alternate-Day Therapy (ADT). Because growth suppression is known to occur when the daily prednisone dose exceeds 8.5 mg/m², the concept of ADT was introduced in the field of pediatric renal transplantation. With ADT, growth velocity improves and side effects of steroids (without increased evidence of rejection) are known to diminish. The usual dose is 2¼ times the daily corticosteroid dose, given on alternate days. If graft function remains stable, the dose is then reduced to an equivalent of 1½ to 2 times the previous daily dosage. With ADT, the incidence of hypertension has been found to diminish, growth significantly improves (40 to 55 per cent higher in 1 year on ADT), and serum cholesterol values fall. Controlled studies have not found that ADT is associated with increased incidence of rejection or with greater loss of renal function, as compared with patients on daily steroids.

Rejection Episodes. High doses of corticosteroids are the current treatment of choice for acute rejection episodes (methylprednisolone up to 30 mg/kg IV daily

for 3 days), whereas other studies have shown that 3 to 10 mg/kg of methylprednisolone daily IV for 3 days (i.e., "pulses") can be effectively employed. The previous oral prednisone dose, prior to pulsing, is then continued. The pulse treatment is best administered only twice in 3-month spans since the risks (infection and steroid side effects) may outweigh the benefits. Pulse therapy does not seem to significantly improve allograft outcome, and it may predispose the patient to life-threatening infection.

Postoperative Medical Complications

Infection. Infection occurs with increasing frequency and can cause death in transplanted children. The offending agent is often viral (herpes group—cytomegalovirus, herpes virus hominis, and varicella zoster). It is imperative to differentiate the presence of infection from rejection in the early post-transplantation course, since immunosuppressant therapy must be reduced or discontinued so as to protect the patient. Moreover, lower doses of oral prednisone have been found to provide as efficient immunosuppression as that of high doses, with equivalent graft survival. Other offending infectious agents are bacterial (*Staphylococcus, Legionella*), fungal (*Candida, Nocardia*), and parasitic (*Pneumocystis*). In the latter, prophylactic use of trimethoprim sulfa significantly reduces its development. In data collected from six large centers, of 167 deaths, 56 (or 34 per cent) were due to infection. Thus, survival of transplanted patients can be improved by reducing the mortality related to infection.

Hepatic Dysfunction. Liver impairment is mostly related to drug toxicity (cyclosporine, azathioprine), cytomegalovirus, herpes virus hominis (HVH), hepatitis A, B, or non-A non-B, or viral hepatitis. Progressive liver dysfunction has not occurred in pediatric recipients with persistent antigenemia; thus, these children are acceptable transplant candidates.

Hypertension. Hypertension can occur under various circumstances, and may indicate acute or chronic rejection. Hypertension immediately after transplant is usually related to hypervolemia (complicated with acute tubular necrosis or minimal urinary output) or to the administration of corticosteroids, which increase renin substrate and sodium retention. If hypertension develops during the first 3 months after transplant, renal artery stenosis should be considered. Treatment should be tailored to the cause. Antihypertensive therapy achieving adequate control may curtail deteriorating allograft function. Angiography, followed by surgery, transluminal angioplasty, and captopril have been used in renal artery stenosis. Captopril should be cautiously used, since deleterious effects on graft function have been reported. Finally, in the hypertensive child unresponsive to medications after transplantation, embolization of native kidneys may be performed.

Corticosteroid Toxicity. Several signs of toxicity occur when high doses of steroid are administered. Posterior subcapsular lenticular opacities develop in 55 per cent of patients who have functioning allografts for more than 1 year. Hyperlipidemia, with an abnormal lipoprotein electrophoretic pattern (Type II and IV), which correlates with corticosteroid dosage, has been reported in one half to two thirds of pediatric allograft recipients. Aseptic necrosis involving any bone, multiple bones, or localized to the femoral heads or femoral condyles may occur. The incidence varies from 6 to 21 per cent of pediatric renal recipients, and at least one femoral head is involved. Pain, rather than radiographic findings, antedates the diagnostic confirmation. A correlation between steroid dosage and the development of necrosis cannot be documented; however, a decrement in its incidence has been apparent coincident with a reduction in steroid dosage, with concomitant treatment of renal osteodystrophy.

Although malignancies are known to occur in adult transplant patients, their incidence in pediatric allograft recipients is low (1.3 per cent).

Growth and Development

Growth Potential. Children with a bone age greater than 12 years at transplantation grow minimally, if at all, after transplantation. However, newer data suggest that substantial growth may follow transplantation despite a bone age greater than 12 years. Growth at a bone age under 12 is excellent as long as sexual maturation is not completed, since this may advance bone age as much as 4 years in a single year. Sexual maturity results in progressive epiphyseal closure and a declining growth rate. Improved growth follows in children who receive a transplant before 7 years of age and whose daily steroid dose is low. Male recipients grow better and catch up in growth more readily than female recipients, despite comparable graft function and corticosteroid dosage.

Allograft Function. Modest reduction in glomerular filtration rate (less than 60 ml/min/1.73 m²) and modest rises in serum creatinine (1.3 to 2.0 mg/dl) often result in marked deceleration in growth velocity. This degree of renal impairment may reduce somatomedin activity and diminish growth velocity.

Corticosteroid Dosage. The amount, mode of administration, and route used for administering corticosteroids appear to be important in terms of growth potential. Lower daily doses of oral prednisone (0.1 to 0.18 mg/kg/day) may optimize growth, and linear growth can be maximized by maintaining optimal allograft function. Alternate-day steroid therapy has been associated with improved growth velocity. However, not all authors have found a relationship between glomerular filtration rate, ADT dose, and post-transplant growth. Although "catch up" growth rarely occurs, linear growth can be maximized by utilizing ADT and performing transplantation at a younger age.

Puberty

The changes associated with puberty proceed following a successful transplant. In female pubertal recipients, menses return within a year following transplant. In males, genital maturation lags significantly behind chronologic and bone age. The pituitary testicular axis has been found to be normal when good renal function is restored. Androgen production is decreased, possibly owing to corticosteroid administration. Exogenous an-

drogen therapy should be considered in those male recipients with marked pubertal delay so long as bone age is acceptable and epiphyses are not closed.

Long-Term Outcome

In pediatric living related transplantation, 5-year allograft survival rate ranges from 55 to 73 per cent, and 10-year graft survival rate ranges between 55 and 74 per cent. The outcome for cadaveric survival rate, however, is less satisfactory, ranging from 39 to 43 per cent at 5 years and from 31 to 44 per cent at 10 years. Despite adequate function over 5 years, indolent chronic rejection (due to immunologic attack) probably occurs in most pediatric recipients. The results of long-term kidney transplantation, therefore, are as dependent on the outcome of immune factors as they are on the experience of the physician and the transplant center. Similarly, considering the age at which children receive renal transplants, the possibility that more than one renal transplant will be needed in order to achieve prolonged survival is great.

HEMOLYTIC-UREMIC SYNDROME
PAUL S. KURTIN, M.D.

The hemolytic-uremic syndrome (HUS) is characterized by the triad of thrombocytopenia, microangiopathic hemolytic anemia, and renal disease. The renal disease may be limited to hematuria or proteinuria but is more commonly manifested as acute renal failure. Primary HUS, a disease of uncertain etiology that characteristically involves infants and young children, is currently believed to affect endothelial cells primarily, resulting in a thrombotic microangiopathy. Classically, HUS presents as a prodromal gastrointestinal disease consisting of a diarrheal illness, with or without vomiting, of several days' duration, followed by the onset of bloody diarrhea. This condition is followed by the development of thrombocytopenia, anemia, and oliguria. Although the kidney and bowel are the most commonly affected organs, any organ is at risk, and some children present with neurologic findings secondary to central nervous system (CNS) vascular disease. A number of bacterial and viral pathogens have been etiologically linked to HUS. In North America, many cases have been associated with a cytotoxin-producing strain of *Escherichia coli* (0157:H7). Diagnostically, it is important to culture the stool of all patients for pathogens and assay their serum for antibodies to the verotoxin. Antibiotic therapy does not affect the course of the disease.

Although many anecdotal reports suggest the efficacy of a number of therapeutic interventions, none has consistently been shown to be of benefit, and therapy remains primarily supportive. There is currently no indication for the use of heparin, aspirin, dipyridamole (Persantine), prostacyclin infusions, thrombolytic agents, or plasmapheresis. The efficacy of plasma infusions remains unresolved. The risks of infection and volume overload must be weighed when considering the use of plasma infusions.

The single major advance in the treatment of children with HUS is the timely use of dialysis. The acute mortality of HUS has fallen from 40 to 80 per cent, prior to the widespread use of dialysis, down to approximately 5 to 10 per cent. Poor prognostic indicators include older age, the familial form of HUS, nongastrointestinal prodrome (presentation with CNS disease), and prolonged anuria (greater than 3 weeks).

SUPPORTIVE THERAPY

During the early stages of the disease, characterized by diarrhea and vomiting, careful attention must be paid to the volume status of the child. Hypovolemia should be corrected regardless of the child's renal function. However, great care must be used when administering "fluid boluses" to an oliguric patient. If the oliguria is due to intrinsic renal disease, it will not respond to fluid challenges, and dangerous hypervolemia and hypertension may result. Hypokalemia, secondary to stool losses, should not be treated in the presence of renal disease if the serum potassium level is greater than 3 mEq/L. Hyperkalemia, secondary to hemolysis, catabolism, and renal failure, can be treated with sodium polystyrene sulfonate (Kayexalate) 1 gm/kg, up to 40 gm, orally solution or rectally) and sorbitol (1 ml of 70 per cent solution per gram of Kayexalate) if the intestinal tract is functional. Insulin, glucose, and bicarbonate therapy for hyperkalemia are only temporizing interventions and do not remove potassium from the body. Uncontrolled hyperkalemia is an indication for dialysis.

Edematous children often present with hyponatremia secondary to the administration of hyponatremic solutions. These children should be treated with fluid restriction (input = insensible losses + stool and urine losses). Severe hypervolemia, not responsive to high doses of furosemide (4 to 5 mg/kg), especially if complicated by respiratory compromise, is an indication for dialysis. Metabolic acidosis secondary to diarrhea, renal insufficiency, and catabolism can be managed with oral sodium citrate (Bicitra) or intravenous sodium acetate or bicarbonate to raise the serum bicarbonate level to 15 mmol/L. Prolonged and severe acidosis (a serum bicarbonate level less than 15 mmol/L) not reversible with these therapies is an indication for dialysis. Other indications for dialysis include neurologic symptoms of uremia (altered mental status not attributable to HUS alone) and a severe catabolic state characterized by a rapidly rising blood urea nitrogen (BUN) to levels of 80 mg/dl or more. To deliver enteral or parenteral nutrition without inducing fluid overload or extreme elevations in the BUN or potassium levels, dialysis is often required. Peritoneal dialysis is the modality of choice because it is technically easier to perform in small children and because it allows for continuous control of the patient's volume, electrolyte, and metabolic status without the wide fluctuations induced by intermittent hemodialysis. Because these patients often require 2 to 3 weeks of dialysis and because they are usually thrombocytopenic, a dialysis catheter with Dacron cuffs (Tenckhoff Catheter, Quinton Instrument Company, Seattle, Washington) should be surgically placed. The infection rate with this catheter is less than with older, noncuffed, percutaneous catheters. With the early institution of dialysis, the entire care of the patient is made much easier.

Nutritional Support

Children with HUS are frequently hypercatabolic and require as much as 2 to 3 gm/kg/day of protein. This amount of protein intake, however, may not be tolerated without dialysis. In a child with renal disease, but not yet requiring dialysis, Aminade, which contains only essential amino acids and carbohydrates without electrolytes, will help maintain the child's protein status without significantly increasing the BUN. Children should receive, as a minimum, their recommended daily allowance (RDA) for calories. Intravenous lipid solutions deliver a large number of calories in a small volume, thus reducing the risk of fluid overload. If on dialysis, the patient should receive a multivitamin preparation containing folate and other water-soluble vitamins. Hyperphosphatemia is a frequent complication of acute renal failure. It should be treated with a calcium-containing antacid, which will lower phosphate absorption while maintaining the serum calcium level.

HYPERTENSION

Hypertension is usually related to fluid overload or renal ischemia. Hypervolemia can be treated with fluid restriction, diuretics, or dialysis, as needed. Captopril (1 to 4 mg/kg/day in divided doses) is effective in treating the hypertension of renal ischemia. Parenteral hydralazine is useful for patients not taking oral medications.

TRANSFUSIONS

The anemia and thrombocytopenia of HUS can be quite severe. Unless the patient is hemodynamically compromised, red blood cell transfusions are rarely needed for hematocrits greater than 18 per cent. If the patient is not clinically bleeding, and no invasive procedure (placement of a dialysis catheter) is planned, platelet transfusions are rarely needed for a platelet count greater than 25,000 per cubic millimeter. A continuous, daily rise in the platelet count is the earliest sign of recovery. The anemia is slower to resolve, especially in the presence of renal failure. A normal hematocrit is often not reached for several weeks following resolution of the acute renal failure.

PROGNOSIS

Approximately 80 to 85 per cent of patients require dialysis. Ninety to 95 per cent of patients survive their bout with HUS. Of these patients, approximately 10 to 20 per cent will have renal sequelae. A child's ultimate prognosis is determined by the extent of irreversible renal damage. This damage may be manifested as mild renal functional abnormalities, as hypertension, or, in 5 to 10 per cent, as chronic, progressive renal failure.

A kidney biopsy can determine the severity of renal involvement early in the course of HUS. Although prognostically important, the results of a biopsy do not affect therapy. Nuclear renal scans can also give prognostic information. A renal scan consistent with cortical necrosis would indicate a poor prognosis. Although unusual, recurrent HUS is well described, especially in familial forms. It is hoped that newer investigational therapies will provide more specific treatments for HUS and further diminish the mortality and long-term morbidity of this disease.

PERINEPHRIC AND INTRANEPHRIC ABSCESS

STEPHEN R. SHAPIRO, M.D.,
and RAYMOND D. ADELMAN, M.D.

Intranephric and perinephric abscess formation in children is rare. In most cases, early antibiotic therapy probably aborts the process. When suppuration and necrosis have occurred, an abscess is formed. A renal carbuncle represents coalescence of multiple abscesses into a multiloculated cavity. A perirenal abscess occurs when the infection extends beyond the renal capsule but is confined by Gerota's fascia. A pararenal abscess is present if the infection extends beyond Gerota's fascia.

Whereas in the past, most renal abscesses in children were due to *Staphylococcus aureus*, in the past decade, nearly two thirds of the infections have been caused by gram-negative organisms, of which *Escherichia coli* was the most common. Other organisms reported include *Proteus* and *Pseudomonas*.

Renal abscesses can occur in otherwise healthy children. Occasionally, with *Staphylococcus*, a minor remote focus, such as a cutaneous, respiratory, or dental site, is identified as a source of infection. An underlying urinary tract abnormality may exist, particularly with gram-negative organisms, such as vesicoureteral reflux, obstructive uropathy, renal vein thrombosis, renal calculi, or renal trauma. Occasionally, abscesses have been associated with congenital heart disease involving *Staphylococcus* or *Streptococcus viridans*. Children with an abnormal host response to infection such as chronic granulomatous disease, diabetes mellitus, or leukemia, or those treated with immunosuppressive drugs, such as transplant recipients, are predisposed to renal abscesses.

Blood and urine cultures must be obtained after confirmation of the diagnosis by radiographic techniques. Appropriate parenteral doses of antibiotics must be started as soon as cultures have been obtained. Since it may be difficult to distinguish an abscess radiographically from other lesions (Wilms' tumor in the infant and child, renal cell carcinoma in the teenager, renal hamartoma, and lymphoma), and since pathogens isolated from abscess cultures do not always correlate with those from the urine, we recommend fine-needle aspiration and percutaneous drainage of the abscess unless contraindications exist. The aspirated material should be cultured aerobically and anaerobically, and fungal cultures should also be done. Negative cultures are obtained in 5 to 10 per cent of cases, possibly owing to inadequate culture techniques. A Gram stain should also be performed. If necessary, special stains for the various fungi and acid-fast bacilli can be obtained.

Since a spectrum of renal parenchymal inflammatory disease exists, from acute cellulitis to perinephric abscess, if the condition of the child permits, a trial of intensive antibiotic treatment may be warranted before determining a need for percutaneous aspiration and/or surgical drainage.

Currently, percutaneous catheter drainage offers an attractive alternative to open surgical drainage for patients with a renal or perirenal abscess. After needle aspiration of the purulent material, a catheter or multiple catheters can be inserted into the abscess cavity or cavities. In addition, percutaneous drainage of the urine from the kidney can also simultaneously be accomplished if indicated by obstructive uropathy (ureteropelvic junction obstruction, ureteral calculi, and so forth). The abscess cavity can then be irrigated with antibiotic solution, or in some cases, the catheter may be left indwelling without irrigation, combined with antibiotic therapy. Resolution of the abscess occurs in several days to 4 to 6 weeks. Percutaneous abscess drainage duplicates surgical treatment in providing decompression, continual drainage, and evacuation. In most reported cases, adequate drainage of the abscess cavity has been accomplished with a catheter size as small as 8.3 French, using the pigtail variety of catheter.

Indications for removal of the catheter include resolution of fever, cessation of drainage, return of the white blood cell count to normal, and a sinogram showing nearly complete closure of the abscess cavity. Following removal of the catheter, the drainage tract will rapidly close if all infected material has been adequately removed.

Percutaneous drainage of the abscess will fail if the cavity is inadequately drained, if there are multiple pockets of pus that are not recognized, or if there is continuous drainage despite adequate catheter placement. The last situation might suggest enteric fistula from erosion of the abscess into the second portion of the duodenum on the right side or the descending colon on the left side. Percutaneous techniques may be less suitable for the small infant or neonate, in whom renal abscesses fortunately are extremely rare.

Some patients may require operation without percutaneous drainage or subsequent to it. The decision to perform surgery should be based on the patient's general condition, associated pathologic findings, and the condition of the involved kidney. For example, poorly functioning or nonfunctioning kidneys, particularly those with multiple abscesses, would mandate surgical treatment, probably by nephrectomy and drainage. The clinical response is also critical. Percutaneous drainage of an abscess should result in defervescence within 48 to 72 hours. Failure of such a response may suggest inadequate drainage.

Initial antibiotic therapy must include gram-negative coverage (for *E. coli*, *Proteus*, and *Pseudomonas*) and coverage for *Staphylococcus*. Accordingly, an aminoglycoside and an antistaphylococcal agent in combination will be necessary. Tobramycin (6.0 to 7.5 mg/kg/day*) is recommended, since there has been an increasing resistence of *Pseudomonas* to gentamicin in recent years. Ceftazidime (100 to 150 mg/kg/day*) may be substituted for tobramycin. Intravenous doses of cefazolin or nafcillin (100 mg/kg/day*) continue to provide the best coverage for *Staphylococcus*. In patients allergic to penicillin, vancomycin (45 to 60 mg/kg/day*) should be substituted. *Candida* infections will require amphotericin B. Although documentation in the literature does not exist, it is assumed that parenteral therapy should be continued for 14 days, to be followed by oral therapy for an additional 2 to 4 weeks, as indicated by the clinical condition.

---

*Not to exceed recommended adult dosages.

URINARY TRACT INFECTIONS

DAVID T. UEHLING, M.D.

An acute outpatient urinary tract infection (UTI) can be treated with a high likelihood of success with any of the usual antibiotics, so the choice can be made on the basis of palatability, cost, and history of drug allergy. A urine specimen should generally be obtained by the clean-voided method. A Gram stain or methylene blue–stained smear of urinary sediment establishes the diagnosis at the time of the office visit (the latter is easier and more suitable for office practice). Less reliable are dipstick tests for nitrate conversion by gram-negative bacteria and for white blood cell esterases, but both of these can be very useful when the amount of urine obtained on the clean-voided specimen is small (too small to do a stained smear of the urinary sediment). Culture and sensitivity should usually be done to support the initial diagnostic impression but in selected cases can be omitted, since short rods seen on a stained smear in a child coming for a first outpatient visit usually represent *E. coli* with broad sensitivities.

A good first choice for treatment of acute UTI is trimethoprim-sulfamethoxazole (TMP-SMX) suspension because of its palatability and cost. The recommended dosage is 6 to 12 mg/kg/24 hr of TMP and 30 to 60 mg/kg/24 hr of SMX, given twice daily for 5 to 10 days. This usually works out to 0.5 teaspoon twice a day for small children and 1 teaspoon for bigger children, since 1 teaspoon of the oral suspension contains 40 mg of TMP and 200 mg of SMX. Single-dose therapy is not recommended for children. In children allergic to sulfa, TMP suspension alone is usually effective. Nitrofurantoin suspension (25 mg in 5 ml) is also a good choice for an acute UTI (5 to 7 mg/kg/24 hr in four divided doses). Children not liking the oral suspension sometimes can be managed with the macrocrystals; the capsule is opened, and macrocrystals are mixed with apple sauce, cereals, and so forth. Ampicillin, amoxicillin, cephalexin, and others are occasionally needed for UTIs but should be reserved for problem cases with documented sensitivities because of a harmful effect on intrinsic flora. The quinolones are not safe for use in children, and tetracycline should not be given before age 8.

Children with vomiting may need antibiotics administered intramuscularly or intravenously in the hospital or by visits every 6 to 8 hours to a clinic or emergency room. Evaluation of genitourinary anatomy, such as by ultrasonographic examination of the kidneys and bladder, helps determine seriousness, the need for blood cultures, the need for hospitalization, and so on. The necessary duration of parenteral therapy has not been well worked out but usually is needed for 48 to 72 hours. Useful antibiotics for parenteral therapy are ampicillin (100 to 200 mg/kg/24 hr) or gentamicin (3 to 7 mg/kg/24 hr) for gram-negative bacteria and methicillin (100 to 200 mg/kg/24 hr) or vancomycin (20 to 30 mg/kg/24 hr) for gram-positive bacteria. Antibiotic sensitivities are needed to guide therapy in these sicker children. Any problems such as the growth of multiple organisms from the urine specimen obtained by the clean-voided method should be resolved by urethral catheterization or suprapubic urine aspiration.

Newborns and infants with UTI require special care, since there is more likely an anatomic abnormality complicating treatment. Blood cultures should be obtained in the presence of fever. Parenteral antibiotics are usually necessary because of the likelihood of septicemia and erratic oral absorption. Sulfa and nitrofurantoin are contraindicated in newborns. Early evaluation by ultrasonography should be followed by the appropriate genitourinary evaluation and intervention.

Prophylaxis against UTI is indicated in the presence of recurrent infections or anatomic abnormalities, such as vesicoureteral reflux. Prophylaxis is best accomplished with TMP-SMX or nitrofurantoin suspension at one-quarter the usual daily dosage. Breakthrough infections are uncommon, but if they occur, they are more likely due to antibiotic-resistant bacteria. Therefore, changes in antibiotics need to be more carefully based on sensitivities. Although adverse reactions are uncommon and largely reversible with low-dose prophylaxis, leukopenia from TMP-SMX and neuritis and pneumonitis from nitrofurantoin should be considered. How long to keep the child with reflux on prophylaxis is a problem because children with lower grades of reflux may be managed indefinitely without surgery. Individualization is needed, but one regimen is to stop prophylaxis 1 year after the last UTI and thereafter culture at frequent intervals for recurrence. Children with recurrent cystitis and no anatomic abnormality on intravenous pyelogram and voiding cystourethrogram also benefit from prophylaxis. In addition to wellness, development of urinary continence depends on long-term elimination of bacteriuria. Asymptomatic bacteriuria is uncommon in children but requires considerable discretion in treatment when it is encountered. If there is evidence of upper tract involvement, more vigorous elimination of bacteriuria is indicated. Good localization tests for UTI are not generally available, but reflux on the vesicoureterogram suggests upper tract involvement in the presence of bacteriuria. Lower tract asymptomatic bacteriuria in some cases is almost impossible to eliminate, so administration of potentially toxic antibiotics may be counterproductive. European physicians regard asymptomatic bacteriuria as mere colonization, with minimal risk for upper tract deterioration, and not as an indication for treatment. Children with indwelling urethral catheters, nephrostomy tubes, and so on have bacteriuria after several days. Treatment only results in replacement by other, more antibiotic-resistant bacteria, so treatment should be given only for fever, vomiting, and other signs of systemic sepsis.

UROLITHIASIS

HAL C. SCHERZ, M.D.,
and GEORGE W. KAPLAN, M.D.

The treatment of stone disease in general has changed dramatically during the past decade, owing primarily to technologic advances, in that open surgery has been obviated in many cases. The management of urolithiasis in children is often more difficult than in adults, primarily because of size constraints, and has limited the widespread application of newer modalities commonly utilized in adults. On an acute basis, management concerns include pain relief, hydration, infection, and obstruction. Renal colic is often exquisitely painful and frequently can be alleviated only by parenteral narcotics. Morphine, in full therapeutic doses, is, in our opinion, the drug of choice. Severe vomiting and consequent dehydration may accompany renal colic, and because diuresis may assist in stone passage, intravenous fluids may be necessary. If urinary tract infection is present or suspected because of fever or pyuria, a urine culture should be obtained and broad-spectrum antibiotics instituted pending confirmation of infection. Infection occurring concomitantly with urolithiasis is not likely to be eradicated unless the stone is removed, but urine can be sterilized as long as appropriate antibiotics are administered, and every attempt should be made to do so. Urine pH and examination of the urinary sediment for crystals may elucidate the composition of the stone and guide further therapy. Imaging of the urinary tract is essential early in the evaluation of children to rule out obstruction; intravenous urography is preferred, but ultrasonography can also be helpful. The combination of infection and an obstructing stone is a urologic emergency requiring prompt intervention to prevent generalized sepsis as well as rapid renal deterioration.

The next phase of treatment consists of removal or disintegration of the stone. Most small ureteral stones (< 5 mm) will often pass spontaneously, even in small children, so that intervention may not be necessary. Larger stones are addressed in a variety of ways, depending upon factors such as the volume of stones, or "stone burden," the distribution of stones, and the composition of the stone.

Knowledge of stone composition can often yield clues regarding the etiology of the stone, and appropriate therapy can be better directed. Stone density on radio-

graphs may suggest stone composition: Uric acid and xanthine stones are radiolucent, calcium oxalate and phosphate stones are very radiodense, and struvite (magnesium ammonium phosphate) stones are intermediate in density. Retrieval of passed stone fragments is important for chemical and spectrophotometric analysis. Thus, all voided urines should be strained in patients suspected of having stones.

The many surgical options available today allow for creative and individualized management of stones. Open surgical removal of stones is rapid and permits correction of associated problems, such as obstruction. Size limitations in infants and small children may preclude percutaneous or endourologic techniques, while patients with spina bifida and other severe physical deformities may not be good candidates for newer modalities used to treat stones because they do not fit the equipment currently available. Open surgery may be the most expedient way to handle stones in these patients. Extracorporeal shock wave lithotripsy (ESWL) and percutaneous and endoscopic techniques, alone or in combination, have all been used in children as well as in adults. These techniques are especially appealing in children with metabolic stones who are at risk for recurrences. Calculi can be crushed mechanically or disintegrated using ultrasonography, an electric current, or a pulsed laser. Retrograde endoscopic stone manipulation may be impossible in small children, particularly in boys, because the size of the urethra and the size of the ureteral orifice may preclude passage of the necessary instruments. Stones above the pelvic brim can be extracted endoscopically (if technically feasible) or can be treated with ESWL.

ESWL has been used safely in children. There are no specific guidelines for its pediatric application, but concerns have arisen that as yet are unanswered. The maximal number of shocks that can be given, the maximal voltage, and the effects of the shocks on the developing kidney are still unknown. Overexposure to radiation during ESWL is also of concern. Infants and small children are probably not good candidates for ESWL because of technical problems involving positioning in the equipment. Children with severe orthopedic deformities pose a similar problem. Obstruction distal to the stone is a contraindication to ESWL because passage of stone fragments after treatment will be impeded.

Knowledge of the stone composition is important in devising a treatment plan. Certain stones will dissolve more readily using chemolytic agents administered topically or systemically, while other stones will not be amenable to chemolysis at all. Struvite stones caused by *Proteus* species and other urea-splitting organisms can often be dissolved using hemiacidrin or Suby's G solution, but more commonly, a combined approach consisting of antibiotics to sterilize the urine, surgical stone reduction or removal, and subsequent irrigation with these agents is employed. Hemiacidrin is not currently approved by the Food and Drug Administration for this use but has been shown to be safe and efficacious.*

---

*See Nemoy NJ, Stamey TA: Surgical, bacteriological and biochemical management of "infection stones." JAMA 215:1470, 1971.

Acetohydroxamic acid, a urease inhibitor, has also been used successfully to prevent subsequent struvite stone formation.

The etiology of calcium stone formation can be multifactorial; however, the common causes of these stones in adults are rare in children, and metabolic evaluation is seldom warranted. Treatment generally consists of stone fragmentation or removal, as other measures tend to be ineffective. Prevention consists of hydration, thiazide diuretics to decrease hypercalciuria, and administration of inhibitors of crystal aggregation, such as inorganic phosphate and citrate. Other potentially preventable causes of calcium stone formation are found in patients receiving corticosteroids or in those who are immobilized and who may have hypercalciuria from bone demineralization. Children receiving acetazolamide (Diamox), a carbonic anhydrase inhibitor, for seizures or glaucoma may develop a secondary form of renal tubular acidosis and stones. Stones have also been noted in neonates receiving furosemide.

Various metabolic and acquired disorders are associated with metabolic stones, and awareness of this is important because medical treatment is frequently efficacious (and often preferable to surgery) and subsequent stone formation may be prevented. Patients with cystinuria often form stones, and these may be prevented with a high fluid intake and urinary alkalinization (pH ≥8). Alkalinization can be accomplished using sodium bicarbonate or tromethamine E, given orally or topically. Decreasing protein intake increases the solubility of crystal. D-Penicillamine and mercaptopropionylglycine have also been helpful.

Uric acid stones may develop in patients with hyperuricemia resulting from tissue breakdown caused by chemotherapy for malignancy, in patients with myeloproliferative disorders, and in patients with Lesch-Nyhan syndrome. They are also found in patients with inflammatory bowel disease and in those receiving uricosuric agents. Uric acid stones may be prevented by hydration and urinary alkalinization. Allopurinol, by preventing uric acid formation, is also of some benefit. A rare metabolic form of calculous disease is xanthinuria, which is occasionally seen in patients receiving allopurinol. Xanthine stones may be averted by forcing fluids and by alkalinization of the urine, but this approach is usually unsuccessful in treating stones that have already formed.

Hyperoxaluria may occur on a dietary or familial basis or can be seen in short-gut syndrome. Oxalate stones occasionally can be prevented by oxalate-restricted diets and cholestyramine, vitamin B_6, inorganic phosphates, or magnesium. However, once they are formed, removal is the only treatment, as oxalate stones are insoluble.

VESICOURETERAL REFLUX

JOSEPH Y. DWOSKIN, M.D.

What does reflux do to the human kidney? How long does it take to do damage? What degree of reflux causes what amount of damage to the kidney? What are the long-term effects of what degree of reflux on what age of kidney over how long a period?

These are partially unanswered, complex questions that are difficult to explain in simple terms. The oversimplification of answers to these questions has led to extreme positions regarding the therapy for reflux.

The treatment of vesicoureteral reflux must be carefully individualized for each patient. The broad statements that are proposed about the treatment of reflux by its degree are not always accurate. Factors such as age, symptoms with and number of urinary tract infections, voiding problems, somatic growth, caliectasis, ureterectasis, and parenchymal scarring or reflux nephropathy must be considered in each case. In addition, the pathophysiology of the abnormal ureterovesical junction and ureter must be taken into account. The age of the patient is important; that is, neonates and children in the first year of life are significantly more susceptible to the effects of reflux, sterile or infected, than children who are older.

Reflux can also be considered a form of obstruction, as its occurrence prevents the free flow of urine down the ureters and in this way helps increase the degree of ureteral and parenchymal change. The degree of hydration of the patient, as well as the amount of urine coming down the ureter, also affects the degree of reflux seen on a given cystogram. The cystograms done when there is high urine output will show a lower grade of reflux than is actually present. These phenomena are some of the factors in the variability of the degree of reflux seen on sequential cystograms.

The grading of reflux is done from the standard radiographic cystogram, not the radioisotope study, which is very difficult to grade. The grades are described with exactly the same terminology in both of the current grading systems, each of which has five grades.

Reflux affects the medulla of the kidney first and progressively involves the cortex. Various mechanisms have been theorized in the literature, but the bottom line is that the kidney is scarred, and if enough parenchyma is compromised, then the sequela, particularly hypertension, is probable. Renal failure secondary to reflux is infrequent in this country, but untreated reflux is one of the major reasons for end-stage renal disease in the Third World. As larger groups of patients are followed for longer periods, the natural progression of reflux, and reflux nephropathy, both surgically and medically managed, becomes clearer.

With a significant degree of scarring in one kidney and a normal kidney on the opposite side, hypertension is possible, and if both kidneys have only some scarring, the probability of hypertension is increased by the late teens and early twenties. Thus, patients with any scarring in their kidneys must be followed very carefully for many years. All too often, patients are noncompliant and return years later, only to find that significant renal damage has developed.

SIBLING REFLUX

Several authors have clearly shown that from 26 to 35 per cent of the siblings of patients with reflux, although asymptomatic, have significant reflux. Thus, all siblings, male and female, should be evaluated after the index patient has been diagnosed. The amount of damage seems related to the degree of reflux and to the age of the patient. That is, the higher the degree or the older the patient, the more radiographic changes are noted as a percentage of the group. In addition, 9.6 per cent of the siblings are found to have additional uropathology of many types that is often asymptomatic, but significant.

MEDICAL MANAGEMENT

The lower grades of reflux can often be managed without reimplantation, but if there is upper tract deterioration seen on the initial or later studies, reimplantation may be the treatment of choice.

Most cases of lower grade reflux can be managed with long-term suppressive medication to try to prevent the occurrence or recurrence of urinary tract infection. Small changes in the urethra to lower voiding pressure, by doing a meatotomy in the female patient and a dilation in the male patient, in preliminary studies, have decreased the time that it takes for reflux to resolve without surgery. Depending on grade and individual problems, voiding cystourethrograms (VCUGs) are done every 6 to 12 months.

The problems of long-term drug therapy are now surfacing, and it is becoming more urgent to decrease the length of time a child is exposed to these medications, which have side effects. In addition, radiation exposure is a consideration in the long-term follow-up of these children.

When should medication be stopped? It should be stopped after two negative cystograms are done at least 6 months apart. This practice commits the patient to at least 1 year of medication. In many cases, the antibiotics are given once daily, usually at bedtime, as this allows the medication to be in the bladder for the longest time.

During the course of treatment, urine cultures should be obtained every 2 months, if there are no problems. After the medication is stopped, following the two negative cystograms, the urine should be cultured in 3 weeks and then every 2 months for another year. If an infection is to recur, it will usually do so in that time. Care must be taken to look for those with asymptomatic bacilluria, who are a significant threat to themselves.

If an infection recurs in a patient who has had two negative cystograms, an "emergency" cystogram should be performed to determine if the patient refluxes when infected. This cystogram should be done before instituting therapy, if at all possible and if it does not cause problems with sepsis. If the patient has reflux when infected, then reimplantation must be considered in an effort to prevent upper tract damage with recurrent infections.

If reflux is seen on the second VCUG after a negative study, upper tract re-evaluation with a renal scan or an intravenous pyelogram (IVP), or both, is indicated to determine if any scarring has occurred. If there is evidence of scarring, corrective surgery is indicated. If the grade of reflux has increased or is worse than the initial grade seen on the first VCUG, then depending

on the grade change, and the renal re-evaluation, a decision can be made on an individual basis.

The endoscopic appearance of the bladder base and the position of the ureteral orifices "as the bladder fills" during cystoscopy is extremely important in helping decide on the appropriate therapy for a patient. The hypoplastic trigone and very lateral ureteral orifices are not likely to resolve the reflux, especially if the orifices are patulous. The more normal looking the trigone and ureteral orifices that have some support at the end of filling of the bladder, the better the chance of the reflux resolving without surgery.

SURGICAL MANAGEMENT

Higher grade reflux most often has parenchymal or calyceal changes seen on the initial IVP and renal scan. Also common are ureterectasis and intrarenal reflux, both seen on the VCUG. These cases are best treated with reimplantation of the ureters. Older children with reflux should be considered for reimplantation, as their reflux will probably not resolve. This factor is particularly important for female patients, who can be seriously affected when pregnant.

The cases that require the most judgment are the ones with lower grades of reflux producing minimal changes in the kidneys. If noncompliance or breakthrough infections are noted, reimplantation is in the patient's best interest, to protect the upper tracts from further damage.

In the past, the decision to reimplant a patient's ureters has been thought best deferred until there had been scarring and the decision is unequivocal and clearcut. The concept of reimplanting ureters before there is significant scarring is now gaining popularity. If the degree of reflux is Grade IIB or greater on the initial VCUG, and the patient has had significant urinary tract infection, the scarring may not have had time to appear on the relatively crude noninvasive tests that are available at this time. Rather than subject the patient to long-term medication and repeated radiographic examinations, many visits for follow-up cultures, and high cost, it is a reasonable choice to perform a reimplantation.

Successful reimplantation decreases or eliminates the need for medication in more than 80 per cent of patients, who then do not have recurrent urinary tract infections. After reimplantation, somatic and renal growth is often normal. In many cases, the amount of somatic growth in the first year after reimplantation in patients with and without infections is remarkable, especially in the younger age groups.

Reimplantation surgery is, in the lower grades, over 90 per cent successful but is slightly less so in the higher grades owing to the difficulties with managing the dilated, thickened ureter. These ureters often need tapering and shortening, and this additional surgery does have some complications that are often unavoidable, but correctable.

The infant with significant reflux and dilated ureters needs special care, particularly if infection is present. A different sequence of care, which includes temporary drainage, fluid management, and antibiotics, precedes operative intervention in some cases. In others, upper tract temporary diversion with ureterostomies or percutaneous nephrostomies is indicated to help the patient over the initial problem and to preserve renal tissue as much as possible.

There are no shortcuts in the care of refluxing patients. Diligent, persistent follow-up is necessary. The responsibility for the prevention of renal damage rests clearly on the shoulders of the physician who accepts the patient for the care of this problem. The decision to care for the child "medically or surgically" depends on the specifics of each case, not on the general statistics pertaining to that individual's grade of reflux.

The importance of screening siblings of patients with reflux must also be emphasized owing to the high percentage of these children who, though asymptomatic, have significant reflux or other uropathology.

NEUROGENIC BLADDER

KEVIN A. BURBIGE, M.D.,
and TERRY W. HENSLE, M.D.

Neuropathic voiding dysfunction in childhood can be secondary to many different primary etiologies (Table 1); in general, however, myelomeningocele is the most common cause in children. Our treatment approach is based on the myelodysplastic child; however, the general principles are applicable to most forms of neurogenic bladder. Experience has proved that a coordinated multidisciplinary effort by the pediatrician, neurosurgeon, orthopedist, and urologist will provide the best overall care for the myelodysplastic child. Just as critical is the presence of nursing and support personnel specifically skilled in the care of these patients. The goals of urologic treatment of the myelodysplastic child are basically three: preservation of renal function, control of urinary tract infection, and socially acceptable urinary continence.

The bony abnormality of myelomeningocele occurs most commonly in the lumbosacral region (80 per cent), but the level of neurologic impairment may vary. A

TABLE 1. Voiding Dysfunction in Children

Neurological
  Myelomeningocele
  Sacral agenesis
  Spinal cord trauma
  Spinal cord tumors
  CNS tumors
  Spinal dysraphism
  CNS inflammation

Functional
  Enuresis
  Non-neurogenic neurogenic bladder
  Urinary tract infection

Anatomic
  Exstrophy
  Severe epispadias
  Posterior urethral valves
  Lower urinary tract trauma
  Urethral stricture

differential growth rate of the bony somites and developing vertebral arches in relation to the neural tube accounts for the apparent foreshortening of the spinal cord in the developing fetus with myelomeningocele. Nerves at or below the level of the bony defect are generally most affected, but owing to this differential growth rate, proximal nerve root damage may also occur. Most children with myelomeningocele have a lower motor neuron lesion of the bladder (detrusor hyporeflexia), although an upper motor neuron lesion (detrusor hyperreflexia) is seen in almost 30 per cent.

The urologic evaluation of the myelodysplastic child should begin in the neonatal period and should include a urinalysis, urine culture, and renal function studies as well as an excretory urogram or renal ultrasonography. The vast majority of these babies have normal renal function and normal appearing urinary tracts by either imaging technique. Careful follow-up at regular intervals facilitates early detection of renal deterioration; therefore, repeat excretory urography or ultrasonography should be done at 6 months of age and then yearly until age 10 years, when follow-up should be individualized. A voiding cystourethrogram should be part of the evaluation if there is a history of urinary infection, and probably should be performed in all myelodysplastic children along with the annual upper tract studies in order to assess bladder configuration and emptying.

Urodynamic testing may provide important information relative to bladder management in the child with a neurogenic bladder. This testing should include measurement of intravesical pressure during filling and voiding (cystometrogram phase) as well as simultaneous measurement of urinary flow rate (uroflow) and electromyography of the external urinary sphincter. These studies combined with measurement of a urethral pressure profile constitute a full urodynamic evaluation. The goal of urodynamic testing is to identify neuromuscular abnormalities not readily definable by routine neurologic examination or standard radiographic evaluation.

Simply stated, the bladder has two primary functions, urine storage and urine emptying, and both can be adversely affected in myelodysplastic children. In order to facilitate urine emptying, several options are available. In some few infants and young children the Credé maneuver, manual expression of bladder urine by suprapubic pressure, may be effective. Credé, however, has inherent drawbacks, and if post-Credé residuals become elevated or if there are signs of upper tract deterioration, another method should be selected. Credé is definitely contraindicated in the presence of vesicoureteral reflux or if significant outlet resistance is present. Just as outmoded are medications such as bethanechol chloride (Urecholine), which have been used to facilitate bladder emptying and have proved to be of little benefit in the hyporeflexic bladder.

Clean intermittent catheterization is the single most important advance in bladder emptying and has largely altered the treatment of children with neuropathic voiding dysfunction secondary to myelomeningocele. The bladder is emptied at regular intervals by means of a small-caliber catheter, using a clean but not sterile technique. Clean intermittent catheterization is a simple and straightforward procedure easily performed by the parent or child, and urine sterility can be monitored on a routine basis by an inexpensive home culture method.

In terms of urine storage, adjunctive pharmacologic therapy is usually required to facilitate continence, and the use of these drugs should be based on both clinical and urodynamic findings. If uninhibited bladder contractures (hyperreflexia) are producing incontinence, an anticholinergic medicine (Pro-Banthine, Ditropan) may be helpful. When outlet resistance is low, an alpha-adrenergic agent (Ornade, ephedrine) may increase outlet resistance. If continued incontinence is due to poor bladder emptying (overflow) or there is an upper tract dilatation, then clean intermittent catheterization is indicated in association with the use of these drugs. These medications, used alone or in combination with clean intermittent catheterization, will in most cases produce a reasonable degree of continence. Low-dose prophylactic antibiotics are often added to the regimen; however, their use is not universally advocated. Procedures designed to lower bladder outlet resistance, such as transurethral resection of the bladder neck, sphincterotomy, and overdilatation of the urethra, should be avoided, since they may damage whatever continence mechanism is present.

In general, urinary incontinence is no longer an absolute indication for permanent urinary diversion. In selected instances diversion by means of a nonrefluxing color or ileocecal conduit may be required if clean intermittent catheterization is not technically feasible or upper tract deterioration continues despite appropriate conservative therapy. Temporary urinary diversion may be a reasonable alternative in a very young infant until the age of expected continence, when clean intermittent catheterization can be instituted, and cutaneous vesicostomy is probably the best method for this temporary diversion.

In summary, the urologic care of the child with neuropathic bladder dysfunction requires a thorough evaluation including clinical, radiologic, and urodynamic modalities. Follow-up evaluation is lifelong and therapy is directed at the preservation of renal function, the control of urinary infection, and establishing socially acceptable urinary continence.

EXSTROPHY OF THE BLADDER

STEPHEN A. KRAMER, M.D.,
and PANAYOTIS P. KELALIS, M.D.

Bladder exstrophy is essentially always associated with complete epispadias. Surgical reconstruction in both male and female patients requires a planned and multistaged approach. The primary goal of surgical reconstruction in patients with exstrophy is to achieve complete urinary continence. In males, the establishment of a straight penis of adequate length, which is functional for normal sexual intercourse, is equally important. Factors critical to the achievement of complete continence include age of the patient at the time of operation, bladder capacity, and maturation of the prostate at puberty in boys.

Neonatal bladder closure is the preferred treatment of choice. In children seen within the first 48 hours of life, the bladder can be closed primarily without groin flaps or iliac osteotomies. The presence of circulating maternal hormones allows the pelvis to be approximated anteriorly at this early age.

It is desirable to complete the repair of bladder exstrophy before school age. Essentially all patients with exstrophy have vesicoureteral reflux and will require antireflux surgery. This should be accomplished in combination with vesical neck reconstruction in an attempt to produce urinary continence. These procedures are usually performed at 2½ to 3 years of age. Penile elongation with release of dorsal chordee is performed as a separate procedure around 4 years of age. Six to 12 months thereafter, a neourethra is constructed to advance the urinary meatus to the glans tip.

In females, urethroplasty, approximation of the bifid clitoris, and mons plasty are accomplished at the time of the anti-incontinence procedure. Vaginoplasty is deferred until puberty. In both boys and girls, rotational skin flaps are necessary to improve the cosmetic appearance and distribution of hair in the suprapubic area.

In patients seen after the first week of life, bilateral iliac osteotomy is often required to achieve satisfactory bladder closure. Alternatively, if the bladder is not satisfactory for primary closure because of its small size or fibrosis, a temporary urinary diversion should be performed. We prefer a nonrefluxing colon conduit or nonrefluxing ileocecal conduit to prevent the deleterious effects of long-term vesicoureteral reflux. Ureterosigmoidostomy is an excellent choice to avoid a urinary stoma, provided that there is no anal prolapse and that fecal control is normal. It is important to note that the incidence of adenocarcinoma of the colon at the site of the ureterosigmoid anastomosis ranges between 5 and 8 per cent in patients followed long-term. A sigmoidosigmoidostomy (end-to-side) or ileocecal sigmoidostomy avoids the mixing of urine and feces and may prevent the development of colonic cancer.

In selected patients with small bladder capacities, the temporary cutaneous diversion can be "undiverted" using an ileocecal cystoplasty, cecocystoplasty, or colocystoplasty. Even in patients who have undergone prior cystectomy, bladder substitution procedures, particularly with the ileocecal segment, can be used to replace the bladder; urinary continence then often requires placement of an artificial genitourinary sphincter.

It is imperative to follow the integrity of the upper tracts closely, as any deterioration would indicate the need to abandon efforts at achieving continuity of the urinary tract in favor of an antirefluxing intestinal diversion.

PATENT URACHUS AND URACHAL CYSTS

UMESH B. PATIL, M.D.

The developing embryo is initially nourished by a yolk sac. The earliest structure to emerge from the yolk sac is the allantois, the free end of which merges in the umbilical stalk adjacent to the vessels. The proximal portion of the allantois is incorporated into the cloaca, which becomes the urinary bladder, and the remaining segment becomes the urachus. By the fifteenth week of gestation, the urachus is obliterated, leaving a fibrous stalk, which is the medial umbilical ligament.

Persistence of a patent tract leads to urachal deformities, including urachal cysts, sinuses, and vesicoumbilical fistulas.

PATENT URACHUS

When a patent urachus is diagnosed in the newborn, an abdominal ultrasonogram to rule out abnormalities of the urinary tract is performed. A voiding cystourethrography helps in delineating the distal urinary tract and a connection of the patent urachus with the dome of the bladder, if any. In the newborn baby, the continuous urine leakage via the urachus may result in omphalitis and sepsis. Hence artery and vein should be ligated away from the open urachus.

Via a subumbilical transverse incision, the urachus is separated from the rectus fascia and the peritoneum on the dome of the bladder. The opening in the dome of the bladder is closed in two layers with absorbable sutures. The bladder is drained by way of catheter for 4 to 5 days.

URACHAL SINUS

Urachal sinus develops as a result of a patent urachus without communication with the bladder. The umbilicus usually appears moist, with granulation tissue protruding at the umbilicus. The granuloma can sometimes be treated with silver nitrate application. If this treatment fails, the sinus is excised with a transverse infraumbilical incision.

URACHAL CYST

A urachal cyst represents failure of the midportion of the urachus to be obliterated. There is no communication to the bladder. This condition usually manifests as a subumbilical tender mass associated with erythema of the overlying skin. It is an unusual presentation. Occasionally, the cyst may spontaneously drain into the umbilicus, leading to a mistaken diagnosis of omphalitis, or it may cause urinary tract infection.

Treatment. The infected urachal cyst must be opened and widely drained, and systemic antibiotic therapy must be administered. Later, when infection subsides, the cyst is removed through a transverse subumbilical incision and extraperitoneal dissection. During this procedure, care should be taken to avoid injury to the loops of intestine that may be adherent to the friable peritoneum.

DISORDERS OF THE BLADDER AND URETHRA

JOHN W. DUCKETT, M.D.

MALIGNANT TUMORS

Uroepithelial Tumors. These tumors are universally of low grade and stage and rarely recur. They are rare in the second decade and even rarer in the first but have occurred as early as 5 years of age. They may be resected transurethrally, fulgurating the base. They require periodic endoscopic re-evaluation for several years but then have a benign course.

Rhabdomyosarcoma. Genitourinary rhabdomyosarcomas comprise 27 per cent of all rhabdomyosarcomas; the incidence is approximately 1.2/100,000 children/year. There is a 3:1 male to female predominance. Approximately one third of pelvic rhabdomyosarcomas arise in the prostate and bladder, while another 25 per cent arise in the uterus and vagina. The remainder arise from the pelvis and grow intraperitoneally as a mass lesion with no specific site of origin.

By far the most common cell type is *embryonal rhabdomyosarcoma*. The *botryoid sarcoma* is a subtype of embryonal rhabdomyosarcoma that lies submucosally with a papillary component. This is commonly found in the bladder. The *alveolar* type is more common in the older child and carries a poor prognosis. It is decidedly more rare than the embryonal type. The *pleomorphic* type is exceedingly rare in children.

In the past the prognosis for these tumors was most discouraging, and radical extirpation was the primary treatment. In recent years, there has been a more encouraging response to vincristine, actinomycin D, and cyclophosphamide treatment, and primary ablative surgery has taken a secondary role.

Currently a tissue diagnosis is made, and the patient is treated with chemotherapy for approximately 2 months. Response of the tumor is monitored. Radiation therapy is added later if the chemotherapeutic response is not satisfactory. Extirpative surgery is used as a last resort to control local tumor, but it is hoped that such surgery is performed before distant metastasis has occurred.

Under this regimen, there is approximately a 75 per cent tumor-free survival rate, with maintenance of the bladder or vagina in over 50 per cent of cases.

BENIGN TUMORS

The two benign tumors of the bladder are *hemangiomas* and *neurofibromas*. They usually coexist with similar tumors in adjacent organs and may be controlled with local excision if symptomatic but otherwise should be left alone.

Polyps of the urethra are seen as hamartomatous growths arising from the verumontanum. They may protrude down the urethra and cause symptoms of outlet obstruction. The polyps may, in addition, float freely into the bladder as a mass lesion. They may be excised with transurethral manipulation or removed through the bladder. Recurrence has not been reported.

Bladder Diverticula

Diverticula of the bladder are congenital anomalies. Most occur at the hiatus of the ureter and are called *paraureteral diverticula*. These are most commonly associated with vesicoureteral reflux involving a weak musculature adjacent to the hiatus and a laterally placed orifice. Resolution of reflux in this situation is unlikely but has been reported.

Paraureteral detrusor weakness is associated with uninhibited bladder contractions in children with an unstable bladder. These contractions frequently resolve when the bladder is more mature.

Other diverticula may occur in the posterior wall and up to the dome. These may be multiple and generally require excision. They are associated with infection and hematuria. If left until adulthood, they are prone to develop malignancy of a transitional cell type. Bladder diverticula are also associated with outlet obstructions such as posterior and anterior urethral valves.

POSTERIOR URETHRAL VALVES

This is the most common severe obstruction in males. Most instances of this disorder are now being detected in the neonatal period (up to 75 per cent), and early diagnosis is even more likely as prenatal ultrasonography becomes prevalent.

Bilateral hydronephrosis with distended bladder is the typical appearance on ultrasonography. If the fetus does not demonstrate oligohydramnios, there are no indications for intervention in the prenatal period. In the face of oligohydramnios, poor renal development is likely and bilateral pulmonary hypoplasia will prevail. These fetuses have little chance of surviving. Intervention has been accomplished as early as 21 weeks of gestation without altering the ultimate course. Currently there is very rarely a need for prenatal drainage procedures or early delivery.

Babies with posterior urethral valves may have a very weak urinary stream with abdominal masses and, especially, an enlarged bladder. Urinary ascites may be the presenting problem with respiratory distress.

If the diagnosis is delayed, the babies present with azotemia, acidosis, and failure to thrive. Infection may occur, with rapid dehydration and deterioration. If the diagnosis is delayed for several weeks to months, failure to thrive, vomiting, irritability, and dehydration may develop.

A stabilization period follows diagnosis. This entails drainage of the bladder with either a suprapubic cystocath or a No. 8 feeding tube through the urethra, control of infection with parenteral antibiotics, correction of acidosis, and electrolyte stabilization.

The valves should be destroyed either by transurethral electrocautery using miniature instruments or by creating a temporary vesicostomy to divert the urine through a vent in the bladder. The vesicostomy decompresses the upper tracts quite nicely, and it is not necessary to do high ureterostomies in the majority of cases. At a later date, the valves can be ablated and the vesicostomy closed.

If there is still renal failure following either drainage of the bladder or relief of the obstruction in the urethra, it is appropriate to perform a renal biopsy and to bring out a high ureterostomy if there is evidence of inadequate decompression. This is a rare occurrence these days.

This child is then followed carefully with a "wait and see" program. Reimplanting ureters and correcting reflux have been shown to complicate the situation more than improve it. These procedures may be appropriate but are better done at a later date for very specific reasons.

The long-term prognosis with valve patients depends on how much damage was done to the kidneys in utero. If, at the time of diagnosis, the creatinine level drops to below 0.8 mg/dl, the prognosis is generally satisfactory. This represents about 50 per cent of glomerular filtration rate corrected for age.

The long-term prognosis of patients with posterior urethral valves who sustained kidney damage in utero is discouraging despite optimal care in the neonatal period; in later life, a significant number will develop chronic renal failure, and need dialysis and transplant. The outcome for many of these children can be predicted at an early age, and the parents can be well prepared for what lies ahead.

There are other subtle and symptomatic problems associated with posterior urethral valves, such as wetting. This incontinence is not uncommon in the years prior to puberty, but after puberty prostatic growth appears to control it quite satisfactorily. Inadequate bladder emptying is occasionally a problem and may require intermittent catheterization or other means of improving voiding. Some children will carry a full bladder that obstructs the upper tracts and require double and triple voiding at least twice daily to empty their entire systems.

About 20 per cent of patients have a functionless kidney that refluxes, requiring a nephrectomy. Bilateral reflux carries a worse prognosis than unilateral reflux or no reflux at all.

ANTERIOR URETHRAL VALVES

These are more appropriately called a diverticulum of the anterior urethra. This is a defect of the spongiosum that creates a valvelike lip of the diverticulum. The condition requires excision or transurethral ablation of the lip. Some of these children have severe upper tract changes.

Congenital Urethral Membrane. This is a variable obstruction in the membranous proximal bulb that acts as a diaphragmatic obstruction. It has an etiology different from that of posterior urethral valves. It may be considered a congenital urethral stricture, but this term should be abolished. Males with this condition have severe upper tract changes.

Prominent Urethral Folds. These are normal folds coming from the verumontanum that may be quite prominent in little boys. They are similar to urethral valves but do not form a fusion anteriorly with an obstructing web. They should not be considered obstructing.

Posterior Urethral Polyps. These hamartomatous

benign tumors of the verumontanum may obstruct the outlet and may be removed transurethrally.

Megalourethra. This is a rare lesion most often associated with prune-belly syndrome. There are two types: The *scaphoid* type is a deficiency of the corpus spongiosum that allows ballooning of the urethra during voiding and may be repaired with techniques used for the correction of hypospadias. The *fusiform* type involves a deficiency of the corpora cavernosa, as well as the spongiosum, that results in an elongated flaccid penis with redundant skin. This is usually seen in severe forms of the prune-belly syndrome and may be repaired if the patient survives.

HYPOSPADIAS

This anomaly occurs in a wide spectrum of presentations. There are two basic problems: one is the lack of completion of the urethral folding up to the tip of the penis; the second is chordee, a bending of the penis due to a deficiency on the ventrum with a fibrous replacement. The more severe the defect, the more likely it is that chordee is present. Classification should be based on the location of the meatus after the chordee is released. Under these criteria, 75 per cent of hypospadias is a subcoronal situation and can be managed with a simple meatal advancement and glanuloplasty (MAGPI). Another 10 per cent occur on the penis and may be repaired with a more extensive extension of the urethra to the tip. The other 15 per cent are penoscrotal and more proximal, and these require much more extensive reconstruction.

Management. There are numerous techniques available for repair of hypospadias. The most modern include the MAGPI technique used to correct the simple distal subcoronal meatus, which makes up 65 per cent of hypospadias cases. For the more proximally placed urethra, a Mathieu technique may be used with a perimeatal based flap extending the urethra onto the glans. An onlay preputial island flap may be utilized for those without chordee, leaving a distal urethral strip. Finally, the more severe types may be managed with a transverse preputial island flap with vascularized tissue creating the neourethra. Free skin grafts have also been used for this purpose but have more complications.

Complications. A complication rate of about 10 to 15 per cent should be expected for more severe conditions, with an overall rate of 5 per cent. Problems include urethral cutaneous fistulas and strictures that require secondary surgical techniques. Other complications are infections, diverticula, and residual chordee.

The currently accepted techniques are one-stage procedures that may be done with short hospital stays and even as outpatient procedures. The earlier age, 6 to 18 months, is the preferred time for surgery. Microscopic and optical magnification methods with fine, delicate instruments are currently used.

Other Disorders of the Urethra

Urethral Strictures. A midbulbar urethral stricture is most commonly associated with trauma due to instrumentation or a straddle injury. "Congenital urethral strictures" are not a specific entity. Urethral dilation for such a diagnosis is inappropriate. A narrowing of the bulbar urethra should not be considered a congenital stricture; there is a common bulbar spasm during a voiding cystogram that gives the appearance of a stricture.

Meatal Stenosis (Males). A narrowed urethral meatus is very common in the circumcised male and does not require meatotomy. A tight web on the ventrum will deflect the urinary stream upward, and a meatotomy is indicated for improvement in stream direction. Very few meatal stenoses create significant obstruction. These are usually an inflammatory replacement of the meatus with balanitis xerotica obliterans.

Meatal Stenosis (Females). "Lyon's ring" is a collagenous area just inside the meatus that is the narrowest spot in the female urethra. For many years it was considered an obstructing problem, and dilation and fracture were recommended. There are occasional meatal stenoses that require enlargement, but this condition is much rarer than was previously thought.

Prolapse of the Urethra. This occurs predominantly in black girls and causes irritation and bleeding. There is a circumferential eversion of urethral mucosa, which becomes inflamed and should be carefully excised. This condition rarely recurs. Differential diagnoses to be considered are ectopic ureterocele and sarcoma botryoides.

Accessory Urethra. Urethral duplications in boys are usually asymptomatic and appear on the dorsum as an epispadiac extra urethra. More complex channels may be present, and it is necessary to excise the accessory channel to correct chordee or troublesome double voiding.

UNDESCENDED TESTES

MARTIN A. KOYLE, M.D.

Although in the past surgical therapy for an undescended testis in a young boy was recommended at age 5 to 7 or even as late as puberty, this is no longer acceptable. Most testes that are not present in the scrotum at birth will have descended spontaneously by 1 year of age. Histologic data have demonstrated a reduced number of germ cells in the truly undescended testis by age 1, with a marked diminution in their number by age 2. Thus, fertility in the untreated group may be threatened if the testis is not brought down at an early date. The Leydig cells, however, do appear normal, and thus testosterone production should not be affected by delayed surgical therapy. Although carcinoma of the testis, particularly in the intra-abdominal testis, is a potential complication of cryptorchidism, it is uncertain and unlikely as to whether earlier orchiopexy will reduce this risk. However, it will place the testis into such a position that it can be palpated with ease by the patient, and thus any mass, should it arise, could be identified. Treatment of the undescended testis also allows for repair of the omnipresent accompanying hernia and also minimizes the risks of torsion, which occurs more commonly in the cryptorchid testis.

In managing the unilateral undescended testis, it is important to differentiate a true cryptorchid testis from the more common retractile testis. The latter does not require any surgical therapy. We have found ultrasonography to be helpful in locating only those testes that otherwise may be palpated by hand, and thus it does not appear to be valuable in other circumstances. Computed tomography and magnetic resonance imaging scans, gonadal venography, and herniography have been used with varying degrees of success in locating the nonpalpable undescended testes but suffer from being invasive, expensive, and time consuming, as well as requiring sedation, anesthesia, and/or radiation. At this time, our approach to the child with the unilateral undescended testis is to proceed either to direct inguinal exploration, since most nonpalpable testes will indeed be canalicular, or to just above the internal ring and then proceed with the orchiopexy as appropriate. Alternatively, laparoscopy has become a popular technique to locate the impalpable testis to rule out testicular agenesis or a vanishing testis (a testis lost prior to birth because of vascular compromise).

Special attention must be directed to the child with bilateral impalpable testes. Even in a newborn without overt genitourinary anomalies, such as hypospadias, it is important to rule out an intersex state. Thus, appropriate chromosomal studies, endocrinologic data, and radiologic investigation may be indicated in such a child to exclude adrenogenital syndrome and other genetic abnormalities. If such an infant is found to be an otherwise normal karyotypic and phenotypic male, we wait until the child's first birthday before further evaluation. At that age, if testes are indeed not present, because of the negative feedback loop involving the hypothalamic-pituitary-gonadal axis, serum follicle-stimulating hormone (FSH) and luteinizing hormone (LH) levels should be abnormally high. If serum testosterone, FSH, and LH levels are all normal or slightly depressed, we do perform a human chorionic gonadotropin (hCG) stimulation study (2000 I.U. daily × 3 days). A serum testosterone level 10 times that of prestimulation levels indicates that at least one testis is present. In the anorchid state, basal gonadotropin levels are markedly elevated, and there is no response in testosterone levels to exogenous hCG administration.

At this time, there are insufficient data to indicate a role for the use of hCG or gonadotropin-releasing hormones (GnRH) to induce testicular descent in the truly undescended testis. A critical review of the literature suggests that hormonal stimulation probably will promote descent of retractile testes but will unlikely be associated with descent of the cryptorchid testis.

We usually suggest surgical correction of an undescended testis at or around the first birthday because of the previously mentioned histologic data. Palpable testes are best approached via a standard inguinal incision. In the majority of patients, such surgery is performed in the outpatient setting. The location of nonpalpable testes, particularly if bilateral, can be confirmed by preoperative laparoscopy. This will ensure the proper choice of incision and allow the surgeon various choices with regard to the best option of surgery that might be performed. For bilateral cryptorchid testes, a midline transabdominal approach is preferred. If the testes are not seen at the internal ring, the peritoneum is opened. Although the testes begin their descent from a higher lumbar level, it is unusual to locate the impalpable testis as high as the kidney. The surgeon must make an appropriate decision regarding the best technique of bringing the intra-abdominal or high undescended testis into the scrotum without disturbing the collateral blood supply to the testis. The spermatic cord can be divided as described by Fowler and Stephens, relying on vascular supply via collaterals; however, long-term studies have demonstrated the viability of such testes in only 60 to 70 per cent of cases. As an alternative to the Fowler-Stephens approach, a two-stage procedure might be chosen with preliminary clipping of the vessels performed through the laparoscope or by surgically bringing the testis as far down into the inguinal canal as possible and then wrapping it in Silastic; secondary re-exploration is planned for 6 months later. Some groups have found success with autotransplantation of the testes and microvascular reanastomosis of the spermatic vessels to the inferior epigastric vessels. This procedure can be accomplished in conjunction with the Fowler-Stephens technique in an attempt to increase the chances for success. This approach is indeed tedious and probably not worthwhile in a child with a normally descended contralateral testis. Primary orchiectomy is preferable in such a patient.

The diagnosis of a vanishing or absent testis should not be made, and thus surgical exploration is not complete unless blind-ending gonadal vessels are encountered. A testicular prosthesis should be placed for psychological reasons in such cases, even in the young child.

There has been much debate regarding the optimal therapy for the older child with an undescended testis. In the postpubertal male, we discuss the various options available with the family, that is, no surgery versus orchiopexy versus orchiectomy. In general, for the high nonpalpable or intra-abdominal testes, we recommend exploration and orchiectomy if the contralateral testis is normally descended. Until the age of 32 years, the risks of such surgery are less than the risks of developing cancer, and thus surgery appears to be justified. Beyond this age, however, recent data argue against surgery, even orchiectomy. In intersex states, in which the testes may be dysgenetic and prone to malignant degeneration, primary orchiectomy should be considered early.

Early diagnosis and management of the undescended testes should be pursued. Such a practice may lead to attainment of maximal fertility potential. Although such early intervention probably does not reduce the risk of carcinogenesis, it does at least place such a testis in a location where it can be readily palpated.

PENIS, SPERMATIC CORD, AND TESTES

NORMAN B. HODGSON, M.D.,
DONALD K. STRITZKE, M.D.,
and ANTHONY H. BALCOM, M.D.

PENIS

The Uncircumcised Penis

Preputial adhesions are normal in the uncircumcised penis. By 6 months of age, the prepuce cannot be completely retracted in 80 per cent of male babies. Ten per cent will have unretractable foreskins at 3 years of age. Separation of the prepuce from the glans will eventually occur spontaneously. Forced retraction should be discouraged, as it leads to an increased incidence of balanitis and phimosis.

Phimosis and Paraphimosis

Phimosis is the narrowing of the foreskin, so that retraction over the glans penis becomes difficult. This condition is normal in infants and resolves spontaneously by the age of 5 or so. Acquired phimosis is usually the result of premature retraction of the foreskin, which splits the prepuce and results in the formation of a constricting band as it heals. The phimosis can be so tight that urinary obstruction results, with ballooning of the foreskin upon voiding. Circumcision is the treatment of choice.

Paraphimosis occurs when a tight foreskin is retracted over the glans penis and not promptly reduced. Edema develops and can be painful. Urgent treatment is required. Reduction can usually be achieved by compression and traction on the foreskin and simultaneous counterpressure on the glans. Compression applied for 2 to 5 minutes may be required to help resolve some of the edema and facilitate the reduction maneuver. Occasionally, manual reduction is impossible, and a vertical incision, known as a dorsal slit, in the foreskin is necessary. Elective circumcision is the ultimate treatment.

Balanitis

Balanitis is inflammation of the superficial layers of the glans penis. It usually occurs in the uncircumcised boy and is associated with inflammation of the foreskin, which may lead to phimosis. It is often the result of poor hygiene. Secondary bacterial or fungal infections are not uncommon. In most cases, adequate treatment is provided by local wound care. This includes washing the glans and prepuce two or three times a day with mild soap and water and application of topical antibiotic or antifungal ointment. Oral or parenteral antibiotics may be required for patients with significant cellulitis. Circumcision is recommended for the uncircumcised boy with recurrent episodes of balanitis.

Circumcision

Centuries ago, pubertal male inhabitants of the Middle East were beset by the desert sand fly, which was attracted to preputial secretions. Circumcision prevented this annoying problem and was incorporated into every Middle Eastern culture. The need for circumcision today is a controversial topic. Advantages include the prevention of phimosis, paraphimosis, balanitis, and the rare case of penile cancer (which could be prevented by adequate hygiene). In addition, uncircumcised boys experience two to three urinary tract infections during their childhood, compared with one or less in the circumcised boy. Opponents of circumcision cite the small but not insignificant incidence of complication, the possible unfavorable psychological and sexual effects, and the cost of the operation.

Circumcision is clearly an elective procedure and must be presented to parents in an objective fashion. If circumcision is desired, it should be completed during the neonatal period to avoid the need for local or general anesthesia and to minimize possible psychological trauma.

Meatal Stenosis

Congenital meatal stenosis in the uncircumcised boy is rare, although the meatus associated with hypospadias is often pinpointed. Acquired stenosis is due to irritation of the sensitive urethral mucosa by prolonged contact with urine in the diaper. Most cases are mild, not requiring treatment. If a patient has an unusually forceful narrow stream, treatment is indicated. Simple dilation may suffice, although most will require a formal meatotomy, which can usually be performed in the office with the patient under local anesthesia.

Priapism

Priapism is a persistent, painful, unwanted erection. Most cases of pediatric priapism are the result of a disease process that produces stasis of blood in the corpora cavernosa, and treatment should be directed at that disease. Sickle cell disease is the most common etiology. Treatment includes transfusion, hydration, oxygenation, and alkalinization. Epidural anesthesia has also been helpful in the management of priapism. If the hemoglobin is greater than 12 and supportive measures have been unsuccessful, corpora cavernosal–spongiosal shunting is required. Sludging of leukemic cells may also cause priapism and can be treated by supportive measures coupled with chemotherapy or radiation.

Hypospadias

Hypospadias is the ventral (undersurface) ectopia of the urethral meatus. The meatus may be located anywhere between the corona of the glans and the perineum. Associated ventral chordee is common. Numerous techniques are available for repair of the variable degrees of hypospadias. It is mandatory that the surgeon have a working knowledge of the various techniques. The majority of cases can be repaired in one stage on an outpatient basis. A staged repair may be required in some complex cases. Male infants with hypospadias must not be circumcised, as the foreskin is utilized for the repair.

Epispadias

Epispadias is associated with the bladder extrophy complex. Specifically, it is dorsal (top surface) ectopia of the urethral meatus. Surgical reconstruction is required and can be very complex. Multiple operations are usually needed.

Other Abnormalities

Other penile abnormalities include concealed penis, micropenis, webbed penis, torsion, and chordee. Evaluation by an experienced urologist is required, as surgical revision or reconstruction can be indicated.

SPERMATIC CORD AND TESTES

Torsion

Two anatomic types of testicular torsion exist. The age groups affected and clinical presentations are different. Extravaginal torsion occurs in newborns. The infants are remarkably free of distress and present with a firm, painless scrotal mass that does not transluminate. Surgical exploration reveals an infarcted testis, prompting orchiectomy. Contralateral orchiopexy should be performed.

Intravaginal torsion occurs in adolescent boys. It is the result of an anomalous attachment of the tunica vaginalis that allows the testis to lie in a horizontal orientation, known as the "bell-clapper" anomaly. Patients present with acute onset of scrotal pain. Associated abdominal pain and nausea are not uncommon. A spermatic cord block will facilitate the testicular examination. Nuclear isotope scans may be helpful for distinguishing torsion from epididymo-orchitis. To maintain the viability of the testes, prompt surgical intervention is required. This includes detorsion and orchiopexy of the affected side as well as orchiopexy of the contralateral side. Manual detorsion is occasionally successful and avoids the need for emergent exploration; however, elective bilateral orchiopexy is mandatory.

Torsion of intrascrotal appendages, if recognized, requires no treatment, and symptoms will resolve within a few days. However, in many cases, the condition is indistinguishable from testicular torsion, and surgical exploration is required.

Epididymitis and Orchitis

Epididymitis and orchitis are uncommon conditions in childhood that must be distinguished from testicular torsion or testicular malignancy. Most cases of epididymitis have a bacterial etiology, whereas orchitis is usually viral. If the patient is not febrile, he may be managed on an outpatient basis with oral antibiotics that cover the usual urinary pathogens. Parenteral antibiotics are required for the febrile patient. After resolution of the condition, a voiding cystourethrogram is necessary to rule out the presence of urinary obstruction or abnormality.

Varicocele

Varicoceles are, in general, confined to the left side. The associated testis may be smaller than the contralateral testis, in which case ligation of the incompetent spermatic vein is required. Significant growth of the ipsilateral testis after varicocele ligation is common, although improvement of testicular function has not been clearly documented. Symptomatic varicoceles respond to ligation.

Fat Necrosis

Fat necrosis is a rare condition that presents as a painful swelling in prepubertal boys, frequently after exposure to cold. It resolves spontaneously.

Testicular Tumors

Testicular tumors in children generally manifest as painless testicular masses. As many as half are associated with hydroceles. Eighty per cent are germ cell tumors.

When a testicular mass is encountered, radical orchiectomy through an inguinal incision is mandatory. Preoperative laboratory studies should include the tumor marker beta–human chorionic gonadotropin (BhCG) and alpha-fetoprotein (AFP). Computed tomographic scanning of the chest and abdomen completes the metastatic work-up.

Retroperitoneal lymph node dissection (RPLND) is an important diagnostic and therapeutic procedure in adult nonseminomatous germ cell tumors. With the development of effective chemotherapeutic agents, the need for RPLND in pediatric patients has become controversial. The urologist and oncologist must work together with the family to organize a treatment approach that is acceptable to all.

HERNIAS AND HYDROCELES

JEFFREY WACKSMAN, M.D.

ETIOLOGY AND GENERAL INFORMATION

To treat infants and children with either an inguinal hernia or a hydrocele, it is important for the managing physician to understand certain basic facts with regard to the anatomy and embryology of the inguinal region. During the sixth to seventh month of gestation, both testes are located at the level of the internal inguinal region. Over the next 8 weeks, the testes migrate down to the base of the scrotum. During this descent, the testes "carry" with them the lining of the abdominal cavity as well as the abdominal wall. Following testicular descent, the peritoneal lining over the cord structures and testes is usually obliterated. Often during the testicular descent, peritoneal fluid may be trapped around the testis, giving rise to the common finding of a hydrocele at birth. But if the peritoneal lining along the cord structures remains open, this fluid may "come and go," giving rise to the concept of a communicating hydrocele. If the peritoneal lining over the cord remains patent, but there exists no communication with the testes, a typical indirect inguinal hernia usually develops. If the opening or communication with the abdomen is large enough, the contents of the abdominal cavity—the intestines and mesentery—may protrude through this patent processus and give rise to an incarcerating hernia.

The incidence of inguinal hernia varies from 1 to 4 per cent. Boys predominate, with a ratio of 7 to 8:1.

This incidence gradually rises, with the increasing degree of prematurity going as high as 30 per cent in premature infants less than 1000 gm. The right side is involved twice as often as the left, and the familial incidence is between 15 and 20 per cent.

MANAGEMENT OF HERNIAS

The most important step in effecting a correct management is establishing a correct diagnosis. Commonly, parents may notice an intermittent bulge in the inguinal region. Occasionally, the infant or child may present with fluid around the testis that was not present at birth. Fluid may appear at the end of the day but usually disappears when the child awakens the following morning. This is clear evidence for a communicating hydrocele, as the child still has a patent processus vaginalis. Older children may complain of pain in the inguinal or scrotal region during activity.

The physical examination may disclose a thickened cord at the level of the external ring, the presence of a hydrocele of the testes or cord (exclusive of the neonatal period), or a large, widely patent external ring. One may ask children who are not old enough to cooperate to blow up a balloon while standing, to bring out or fill the patent processus.

Once the diagnosis is secure, and the child has been cleared for anesthesia, surgery is the next appropriate step. Over the years, with early diagnosis and treatment, the incidence of incarcerated or strangulated hernias has markedly decreased. Surgery is usually performed on an outpatient basis, except in children less than 6 months of age with a history of prematurity, in which case overnight observation is usually advocated because of the anesthesia. The surgery itself involves a small, transverse "skin crease" incision in the lower abdominal wall. Through this incision, the external oblique aponeurosis is opened, and the testicular cord structures are identified. Lying on top of the cord structures is the hernia sac or patent processus, which is isolated and traced up to the level of the internal inguinal ring, where this is ligated. If a hydrocele accompanies this structure, the distal end is traced down to the testis, where the hydrocele sac is opened widely, and if an appendix testis or appendix epididymis is seen, it is also removed. Next the testis is returned to the scrotum, and if a large hernia is present, the floor of the canal is reconstructed. Closure is usually done subcuticularly, so no skin sutures need be removed, and the incision is either painted with collodion or dressed with Opsite, Tegaderm, or Steri-Strips. Postoperatively, most surgeons require the parents to keep incisions dry for a week (i.e., no tub baths, swimming pools, and so on) and employ frequent diaper changes during the first week. Pain is usually controlled with acetaminophen with codeine elixir in the older child. Some surgeons prefer to inject bupivacaine hydrochloride (Marcaine) (a long-acting local anesthetic) in addition to general anesthesia to aid in the initial postoperative period. Heavy activity, such as climbing or riding toys or bicycles, is to be avoided during this first week. If a hydrocele is opened, there may be some testicular or scrotal swelling postoperatively, which usually resolves over the next 6 weeks and is no cause for concern.

INCARCERATED HERNIAS

As was mentioned earlier, the incidence of incarcerated-strangulated hernias has markedly decreased, but children still present with incarcerated inguinal hernias. This hernia ordinarily manifests as a firm mass in the inguinal and upper scrotal region. Usually, the infant has associated vomiting and occasional abdominal distention with "fussiness." The toddler may present with a firm, tender mass in the scrotal region. Immediate treatment of this condition is mandatory, as the hernia must be reduced as soon as possible. To aid in this treatment, usually some type of parenteral narcotic is given, an ice pack is applied, and 30 to 45 minutes later the hernia should be reduced. After the hernia has been reduced, it is not uncommon to observe infants and small children for 24 to 48 hours to make sure there are no signs of vascular compromise to the portion of the bowel that has been reduced. Surgery is usually performed shortly thereafter to prevent a recurrence.

If the hernia cannot be reduced by either the general physician or the surgeon, emergency surgery is usually undertaken. Since most incarcerated hernias are able to be reduced, emergency surgery is usually not necessary. If a hernia remains incarcerated for several days without treatment, vascular compromise may ensue, which can lead to strangulation of the involved organ (usually intestine), which will require a bowel resection. Owing to early diagnosis and treatment, however, this is usually a rare occurrence.

Occasionally, children develop an acute, firm, tense swelling above the testis that may mimic an incarcerated hernia. But this mass usually transilluminates and in reality is filled with fluid. This mass represents an acute hydrocele of the cord or testis. Sometimes it may be difficult to distinguish from an incarcerated hernia, and occasionally a scrotal ultrasonogram may be helpful. Treatment of this condition is the same as for an inguinal hernia but need not be handled like an emergency, since this is nothing more than some trapped peritoneal fluid in a patent processus, which can be treated electively.

HYDROCELES

Hydroceles found at birth or in the neonatal period are not uncommon. They usually represent peritoneal fluid trapped in a patent processus that is now undergoing obliteration. These hydroceles can be accompanied by a symptomatic hernia but more often are an isolated finding. Usually, these hydroceles resolve by 6 months to 1 year. If they persist beyond this period, or there is a good history for variation in size (signifying a communication via a patent processus), then surgical exploration is usually indicated.

Hydroceles that develop later in life, outside the neonatal period, should be divided into those occurring in the prepubertal period and those occurring in the postpubertal period. The prepubertal hydrocele that develops acutely or has a definite communication usually requires surgery. Surgical repair is similar to an inguinal hernia repair, discussed previously. On the other hand, hydroceles that develop in the adolescent patient should be treated like a hydrocele that occurs in an adult. These hydroceles have a completely different etiology and require surgery through a scrotal approach. It is important to understand this different approach.

HERNIAS IN FEMALE CHILDREN

Hernias in female children, although less common, may still develop. Historically, they may manifest as an intermittent labial bulge seen during bathing or the development of a grape-sized mass in the area of the pubic tubercle. The mass not uncommonly represents an entrapped ovary or fallopian tube. If the ovary becomes entrapped, many times it cannot be reduced until surgery but rarely gives rise to vascular compromise. Most of these hernias can be handled on a semi-emergent basis, except when ovarian strangulation is suspected.

Girls with indirect inguinal hernias should be suspected of having the testicular feminization syndrome. This syndrome can be ruled out at surgery with a rectal examination to palpate the uterus or vaginal inspection with a cotton swab to make sure the upper two thirds of the vagina has developed. Occasionally, an ultrasonogram of the pelvis is indicated to define the uterine anatomy completely.

Female children rarely, if ever, develop a direct hernia because of inguinal floor weakness but can occasionally or rarely develop a femoral hernia. The femoral hernia usually manifests as an intermittent mass or lump along the inner aspect of the thigh rather than in the region of the labia.

THE QUESTION OF BILATERAL EXPLORATION

Whether to explore the opposite side of a patient with a unilateral inguinal hernia is not an easy decision. In children less than 1 year of age or in children with a history of a neonatal hydrocele on the opposite asymptomatic side, most surgeons would explore the asymptomatic side. In children over the age of 1 who have a thickened cord, exploration of the opposite side may also be justified. In addition, female children seem to have a higher incidence of asymptomatic contralateral hernias, and many surgeons routinely explore the opposite side in female children less than 5. Whether to explore the asymptomatic opposite side is definitely an individual decision and is best left to the surgeon.

VULVA AND VAGINA

LOUIS FRIEDLANDER, M.D.

CONGENITAL OR DEVELOPMENTAL DISORDERS

Developmental abnormalities presenting in the newborn period require early recognition, diagnosis, and institution of appropriate medical therapy. Virilization of the female fetus in utero may result in the development of ambiguous genitalia.

Early diagnosis of ambiguous genitalia will lead to a determination of the child's sexual identity and, in turn,

guide parental child-rearing attitudes. Early gender identification will permit reconstructive surgery at the appropriate time to create female genitalia in an infant with a testis.

Isolated clitorimegaly, when present at birth, is often the result of prenatal exposure to virilizing steroids of maternal or fetal origin. This condition may require plastic repair. Clitoral recession, with preservation of innervation and anatomic configuration, can be deferred to 18 months of age. Clitorectomy is rarely, if ever, indicated.

ACQUIRED HORMONAL DISORDERS

The white vaginal discharge of the neonate, which results from maternal estrogen stimulation, subsides after several days.

Hormonal stimulation of the vulva and vagina, such as precocious development of pubic hair (adrenarche), clitorimegaly, estrogenization of the labia minora, or menstruation, should be investigated for signs of a systemic process. Exogenous sources of estrogen, such as ingestion of birth control pills, estrogen creams, autonomous ovarian or adrenal sources, or central nervous system lesions, must be excluded.

Imperforate hymen is generally not identified until menarche, when the patient may present with amenorrhea, abdominal pain, and lower abdominal swelling (hematocolpos) with or without a bulging introitus. Occasionally it may be identified in the newborn period by a bulging of the introitus due to the accumulation of vaginal secretions from the estrogenized vagina. When a large amount of secretions collects (hydrocolpos), lower abdominal swelling appears. Excision of the membrane is necessary for drainage. Vaginal or other defects are rarely associated.

With a transverse vaginal septum, symptoms similar to those seen with imperforate hymen may occur at any level above the hymen. The septum is usually resected.

Adhesions of the labia (labial agglutination) are extremely common. They usually occur in young girls 6 months to 6 years of age. The exact etiology of these lesions is unknown, but they are generally associated with mild vulvitis. Occasionally the vaginal orifice is completely covered, causing poor drainage of vaginal secretions. Urinary drainage may also be impaired. In mild cases, no treatment is necessary because the labia will separate completely with estrogenization at puberty.

When vaginal or urinary drainage is not impaired, an estrogen-containing cream (Premarin) should be applied twice a day for 2 weeks and then at bedtime for another 1 to 2 weeks, until the labia are separated. The cream must be rubbed into the area of the adhesion while the labia are gently separated. Treatment should be continued with a bland ointment at bedtime after the labia have separated. Forceful separation is discouraged because it is traumatic for the child and may cause the adhesions to form again.

CONGENITAL ABSENCE OF THE VAGINA

Vaginal Agenesis. Ultrasonography and laparoscopy should be done early to determine whether the uterus may be a source of pain. When the uterus is absent, a functional coital canal is created. When it is present, symptoms of primary amenorrhea and cyclic, recurrent abdominal pain are relieved by drainage of the retained blood; normal flow is maintained thereafter by the reconstructed vagina. Normal menstrual function, fertility, and vaginal delivery have resulted when the condition is promptly diagnosed and surgically corrected.

Testicular Feminization Syndrome. Testicular feminization syndrome (total androgen insensitivity) may be mistaken for vaginal agenesis. Patients have a male karyotype (46,XY), with testes that may be palpated in the labia or groin, a normal-looking vulva, and a blind vaginal pouch so short that it may be difficult to distinguish from vaginal agenesis. The cervix and uterus are absent. Pubic hair may be scanty or absent, and breast development is poor. Plasma testosterone is normal.

Testes are prophylactically removed after puberty (to retain the female habitus) because of the high rate of malignant degeneration. The patient's ability to have normal sexual relations, without menses and childbearing, should be discussed. After surgery, cyclic conjugated estrogen therapy (Premarin, 0.625 mg/day on days 1 to 21 of each month) is given.

TUMORS OF THE VULVA AND VAGINA

Fortunately, genital tumors in the child are rare.

Benign Cysts. *Mesonephric duct cysts* (Gartner's duct cysts) are common, representing wolffian duct remnants arising from the anterolateral vaginal wall. They present as a translucent, unilocular swelling that may protrude through the vaginal introitus. *Paraurethral duct cysts* are found in the urethrovaginal wall and may compress the hymenal opening or urethra. If they are symptomatic, simple surgical unroofing and marsupialization are preferred to total excision. *Inclusion cysts* on the vulva and vagina are secondary to trauma. They are simple cysts, lined by squamous epithelium, that contain cheesy material. They are treated by simple excision. *Cysts of the canal of Nuck* represent proximal obliteration of the processus vaginalis. If they are large or disfiguring they should be excised. *Bartholin's gland cysts* are treated by marsupialization. *Labial papillomas* (skin tags) are small, benign polyps. Excisional biopsy is mandatory if the diagnosis is in doubt. *Hymenal cysts* seen in the newborn period usually shrink and disappear.

Hemangiomas are the most common tumors of the vulva. They are of either the capillary or the cavernous type and generally tend to regress in time. Their treatment depends on size, distortion of adjacent structures, rapidity of growth, and susceptibility to injury (trauma). Recently, excision or cryotherapy of these vascular masses has been replaced by treatment with the argon laser. This technique effectively destroys large vascular tumors and has gained acceptance because bleeding is readily controlled and minimal scarring results. Lipomas, papillomas, and leiomyomas may be kept under observation and excised when symptomatic.

A *hydradenoma*, a cystic tumor of the sweat glands, presents as an umbilicated subcutaneous tumor. It should be removed only if the diagnosis is uncertain.

Tumors arising from mesodermal tissues are the fibroma, lipoma, leiomyoma, lymphangioma, and he-mangioma. Solid tumors are treated by local excision, while lymphangiomas and hemangiomas can be followed carefully.

Bleeding, ulceration, or distortion due to a large tumor mass is an indication for excision. Dysplastic epithelial changes of the vulvar skin, in the form of hypertrophic, atrophic, or mixed lesions, should be biopsied if the diagnosis is in doubt. Malignant precursors should be treated by local excision or laser techniques. Vulvectomy with lymph node dissection is reserved for the rare malignancies in the adolescent.

Urethral prolapse is often confused with neoplasm. It is treated by simple excision and suturing of the mucosal edges to the vestibular mucosa. Digital reduction should not be attempted because it is painful and recurrences are common.

Sarcoma Botryoides. This is the most common malignant tumor arising in the vagina during childhood and early adolescence. Complete vaginectomy and hysterectomy are indicated. When the tumor extends beyond the confines of the subepithelial tissue, exenterative procedures, possibly with excision of the vulva and rectum, may be required.

Adjunctive chemotherapy (combinations of actinomycin D, doxorubicin, vincristine, and cyclophosphamide) is effective in controlling these tumors. Radiation is often employed in the therapeutic regimen.

The preservation of ovarian function is determined by the extent of pelvic involvement of the malignant process. Vaginal reconstruction should be contemplated.

Diethylstilbestrol. In utero exposure to maternally administered diethylstilbestrol and related synthetic compounds (dienestrol and hexestrol), given to women from the 1940s to 1960s in an attempt to prevent fetal wastage, is associated with the development of vaginal adenosis and clear-cell adenocarcinoma in the vagina and cervix in young women.

Vaginal adenosis is the presence of glandular epithelium resembling that of the endocervix and associated with transverse cervical and vaginal ridges. It is almost always present if there is a vaginal clear-cell carcinoma. Treatment of clear-cell adenocarcinoma is aggressive, as the lesion is invasive. Early staging to determine the extent of spread will help in selecting the appropriate procedures. Vaginectomy, hysterectomy, extensive lymph node dissection, adjunctive chemotherapy, and radiation therapy may all be indicated.

INFECTIONS AND SKIN DISORDERS OF THE GENITALIA

Vulvovaginitis is a common gynecologic problem in childhood; it is strikingly different in the prepubertal child and in the adolescent. Usually there is a primary vulvitis with a secondary distal vaginitis; less often, there is a primary vaginitis, requiring more careful investigation, that might be due to a foreign body, trapped pinworms, gonorrhea, a specific bacterial infection, ectopic ureter, or a neoplasm. Management involves ruling out a specific cause of the vulvovaginitis other than poor hygiene; treating the specific cause, if there is one; reducing the inflammatory reaction and symptoms; and improving local hygiene.

Nonspecific Vulvovaginitis

For acute weeping pruritic dermatitis, give sitz baths in tepid water with colloidal oatmeal (Aveeno) or baking soda. Alternatively, wet compresses with Burow's solution (1:40) or saline may be applied at intervals of 3 to 4 hours. The skin is blotted dry, and a bland medication (e.g., Desitin or calamine shake lotion) is applied. Skin infections are treated systemically. Preventive care includes washing with nonmedicated, nonperfumed soap. The vulva is gently dried or exposed to dry air and dusted with cornstarch. After each bowel movement, the patient must wipe from back to front with soft, white, unperfumed toilet tissue. Loosely fitting white cotton undergarments are worn. Bubble baths and detergent washing of underpants should be avoided. Topical hydrocortisone or hydroxyzine hydrochloride (Atarax) may be given for itching. Bacterial infections of the vulva transmitted from extragenital primary sites (e.g., nasopharynx, intestine, skin) are treated according to the sensitivity of the offending organism. Topical estrogen cream or Premarin cream may be employed for 3 to 4 weeks for persistent or recurrent nonspecific vaginitis after negative vaginoscopy. Creation of a thickened vaginal wall and an acid vaginal pH usually result in a cure.

Nonspecific Vulvovaginitis Secondary to Foreign Bodies. This condition presents as a profuse purulent discharge, sometimes with blood, that lasts for weeks. The most common cause is toilet paper or stool and there is a high rate of recurrence. In adolescents, the cause is usually a retained tampon. Pelvic radiography is useful for diagnosis if the material is radiopaque. The extraneous object is removed using a cystoscope with a fiberoptic light source, and the vagina is irrigated with warm water.

Specific Vulvovaginitis

Diagnosis of specific vulvovaginitis requires close inspection, vaginoscopy, and a culture. Pathogens derived from other sites (e.g., pharynx, ear, skin) are treated with systemic antibiotics. The high or microperforate hymen may trap urine and mucus in the vagina, where it may become infected by stool bacteria and be a source of recurrent infection. Excision of some tissue is preferred to a simple incision.

Trichomonas **Vulvovaginitis.** This presents clinically as a frothy green yellow discharge with "strawberry cervix." Wet mounts contain trichomonads. Metronidazole (Flagyl) is the only effective therapy. The prepubertal child is given 125 mg three times daily for 5 days. In the adolescent female, 1.5 to 2 gm, given in a single dose, is effective in 90 per cent of cases. This drug is contraindicated in the first trimester of pregnancy, since its teratogenic potential is unknown. Treatment of sexual partner is recommended. Warn patients of side effects (e.g., minor gastrointestinal disturbances, neurologic signs, and depression). Patient should not ingest ethanol for 1 to 2 days after therapy because of disulfiram (Antabuse) effects.

Treatment failures may result from noncompliance, drug resistance, intolerance, or reinfection. Retreatment with metronidazole 500 mg twice a day for 7 days is recommended.

Vulvovaginal Candidiasis. This presents clinically as erythematous, itching external genitalia, cottage cheese–like whitish secretions, and budding hyphae in KOH preparations. Effective antifungal agents include miconazole nitrate (Monistat) cream, (one applicatorful intravaginally nightly for 7 days), or clotrimazole (Gyne-Lotrimin, Mycelex-G) (for 7 to 14 days or one tablet intravaginally for 7 days). Butaconazole nitrate (2 per cent vaginal cream one applicatorful [5 gm] intravaginally at bedtime for 3 days) has fungicidal activity against candida and several other fungal species, as does terconazole (80 mg suppository or 0.4 per cent cream intravaginally at bedtime for 3 days). Boric acid in size 0 gelatin capsules intravaginally for 7 days is effective in recurrent cases. Ketoconazole (Nizoral), an oral broad-spectrum antifungal agent (400 mg for 10 to 14 days), is treatment of choice in the management of frequently relapsing cases, followed by prophylactic ketoconazole. Liver function tests and informed consent should be obtained before starting prophylaxis.

Bacterial Vaginosis. This infection presents as a homogeneous, usually gray creamy or milky discharge. It is the most common form of bacterial vaginitis, formerly termed nonspecific vaginitis, *Gardnerella vaginalis* vaginitis, and *Hemophilus* vaginitis. G. vaginalis, considered a prime pathogen, may play a subsidiary role to anaerobes, which are usually isolated in high concentration in vaginal secretions with production of organic acids. The addition of KOH produces a fishy odor ("whiff test"). pH of the secretion is elevated above 4.7. The presence of "clue" cells formed by the adherence of organisms on epithelial cells in large numbers is diagnostic.

Metronidazole (Flagyl) 500 mg twice daily for 7 days is the treatment of choice, with a 90 per cent cure rate. A single oral dose of 2 gm is 65 to 70 per cent effective. This treatment is reasonably safe after the first trimester of pregnancy. Two per cent clindamycin cream (given in a dosage of 7 cc nightly for 7 days) is effective for patients unresponsive to metronidazole and has a 90 per cent reported cure rate.

Pinworm Vulvovaginitis. Pinworm infestations are common in preschool and school-aged children. Treatment with mebendazole (Vermox)—one chewable 100-mg tablet taken once only, regardless of weight—will clear the condition. Treat all other members of the family.

Gonorrheal Vulvovaginitis. Treatment is influenced by the spread of infections due to antibiotic-resistant N. gonorrhoeae, including penicillinase-producing N. gonorrhoeae (PPNG) and tetracycline-resistant N. gonorrhoeae (TRNG), by the high frequency of chlamydial infections in persons with gonorrhea, and by the absence of a fast inexpensive and highly accurate test for chlamydial infection. Children who weigh less than 45 kg are treated with ceftriaxone (Rocephin) 125 mg IM in a single dose. When this medication is mixed with a lidocaine diluent, local pain or discomfort is reduced. A dosage of 250 mg is given to patients who weigh more than 45 kg. Patients intolerant of ceftriaxone may be treated with spectinomycin (Trobicin) 40 mg/kg IM in a single dose to a maximum dose of 2 gm. Children above 8 years of age should also be given doxycycline (Vibramycin) 100 mg twice a day for 7 days to eradicate possible concomitant chlamydial infection. All children with gonorrhea should be evaluated for the possibility of sexual abuse.

Children with complicated infections such as peritonitis or arthritis should be hospitalized. Recommended regimens include ceftriaxone 0.5 to 1 gm IM or IV every 24 hours or ceftizoxime or cefotaxime 0.5 to 1 gm IV every 8 hours. Reliable patients with uncomplicated disease may be discharged 24 to 48 hours after all symptoms resolve and may complete the therapy for a total of one week with an oral regimen of cefuroxime 500 mg twice a day or amoxicillin 500 mg three times a day. Patients should be treated empirically for coexisting chlamydial infection.

***Chlamydia trachomatis* Infection.** This presents as scanty mucoid secretions with occasional dysuria and suprapubic pressure 7 to 10 days after coital exposure. Infection is asymptomatic in 50 per cent of cases. Cervicitis with mucopurulent exudate is common. Non-culture methods for diagnosis are rapid, reliable, and inexpensive and employ detection of fluorescein-conjugated monoclonal antibodies (Microtrak) or enzyme-linked immunoasay (ELISA) (Chlamydiazyme) for direct examination of cervical secretions.

Treatment of choice is doxycycline, 100 mg orally twice daily for 7 days, or tetracycline, 500 mg orally four times a day for 7 days. Erythromycin, 500 mg orally four times a day for 7 days, may be used, and if this is not tolerated because of side effects, sulfisoxazole, 500 mg four times a day for 10 days, may be effective.

Genital Herpes. Single or multiple vesicles occurring anywhere on the genitalia may rupture spontaneously to form shallow painful ulcers. The incubation period is about 4 days, with viral shedding lasting 12 days and another seven days elapsing until disappearance of crusting and healing. The entire process, however, may be asymptomatic. Recurrent infections are usually milder, with a duration of 4 to 5 days. Viral shedding occurs intermittently during the latency period. The diagnosis is usually confirmed by obtaining Pap smears or Tzanck preparations (by the presence of multinucleated giant cells) or recovering viral particles by culture. Microtrak monoclonal antibody test is 90 to 95 per cent positive.

Patients are advised to avoid transmission by abstinence from intercourse until crusts disappear and skin has healed. Patients late in the disease course and those who have mild episodes respond to treatment with analgesics, sitz baths, local hygiene, and treatment of secondary infection.

In primary genital herpes, oral acyclovir (200 mg 5 times daily for 10 to 14 days) decreases viral shedding, healing time, and number of new lesions. Treatment of recurrent episodes is less effective with this therapy but may be of marginal benefit if commenced at the beginning of the prodrome or within 2 days after onset of lesions. For severe disease, acyclovir is recommended in dosage of 5 mg/kg body weight IV every 8 hours for 5 to 7 days until clinical resolution occurs. Most episodes of recurrent herpes do not benefit from therapy with acyclovir. Acyclovir ointment applied topically is ineffective.

Continuous daily suppressive therapy with acyclovir (200 mg 2 to 5 times a day) reduces the frequency of recurrences by at least 75 per cent. Safety and efficacy have been clearly documented with treatment up to 3 years.

Condyloma Acuminatum. This is the most common sexually transmitted disease of viral origin, with increasing incidence among adolescents. The human papilloma virus (HPV), types 16, 18, and 31, is strongly associated with genital dysplasias and carcinoma. Atypical pigmented or persistent warts should therefore be biopsied.

The disease is highly infectious, presenting clinically as single or multiple soft fleshy papillary or sessile painless (unless confluent or secondarily infected) growths around the anus, vulvovaginal area, penis, urethra, or perineum. Subclinical infections are detectable by Pap smear or colposcopy, or blanching following the application of 3 per cent acetic acid. Incubation period is 6 weeks to 8 months.

Lesions respond to treatment with cryotherapy with liquid nitrogen or cryoprobe. Podophyllum (10 to 25 per cent) in compound tincture of benzoin is applied weekly to small areas and thoroughly washed off in 1 to 4 hours. Normal skin should be protected with petroleum jelly. Trichloroacetic acid (80 to 90 per cent) may be applied to the warts with repeat application at weekly intervals. Extensive lesions may require electrodesiccation, cryotherapy, laser therapy, or surgical excision under anesthesia. Excisional biopsy to exclude neoplasm is warranted when the diagnosis is in doubt.

COMMON SKIN DISORDERS AFFECTING THE GENITALIA

Vulvovaginitis may be secondary to staphylococcal skin infections, seborrhea, psoriasis, or atopic dermatitis; in such cases, it is usually associated with lesions in other parts of the body. Treatment includes hydrocortisone cream or Burow's solution soaks if the lesions are exudative. Secondary infection is treated.

Diaper Rash. Acute diaper rash may be treated with wet compresses of water, saline, or Burow's solution. The dermatitis usually responds to a 1 per cent hydrocortisone cream or lotion. Nystatin powder is applied to the skin when dry to treat monilial infection.

Lichen Sclerosus. In addition to the treatment outlined for nonspecific vulvovaginitis, a short course of topical corticosteroids, e.g., 0.025 per cent fluocinolone acetonide (Synalar), followed by a course of 1 per cent hydrocortisone ointment for a few more months, is useful in bringing the condition under control. Testosterone (2 per cent) in petrolatum gel may be effective; then testosterone propionate can be given once weekly as maintenance therapy.

TRAUMA

Vulvar and perineal ecchymoses, with significant vaginal lacerations and bleeding, are common with blunt trauma and straddle injuries. There can be significant vaginal laceration and bleeding or a transvaginal injury to the bladder, rectum, or peritoneal cavity even in the absence of external damage. Cold compresses will stop the bleeding. Lacerations may need sutures. Examination under general anesthesia may be necessary, with measures then taken as needed to prevent distortion of anatomy and secondary sepsis and to restore subsequent sexual and reproductive function. When child abuse or sexual molestation is suspected, attention is focused on evidence of vaginal penetration, abrasions, lacerations, contusions with hematomas, and spasm of the pubococcygeal muscle; laboratory work to check for seminal products should be performed.

With healing, multiple hymenal scars, rounded hymenal remnants with a large vaginal opening, and laceration extending to the perineum will be evident, in addition to an odorous vaginal discharge. The extent of anal injury may vary from acute spasm to swelling of the anal verge with abrasions, bruises, and localized hematomas. With chronic abuse, complete or partial loss of sphincter control may be found along with thickening of the skin mucous membranes and skin tags.

UTERUS, TUBES, AND OVARIES

VICTOR C. STRASBURGER, M.D.

COMMON MENSTRUAL DISORDERS

The average age of menarche (first menses) in American girls is 12.6 years, with a range from 10 to 15 years. Usually, menarche occurs an average of 2.3 years after breast budding, the first sign of puberty. "Normal" adolescent cycles may last 21 to 40 days, with 2 to 8 days of flow and an average blood loss of 20 to 80 ml each cycle. Four well-soaked tampons or pads per day is normal, and greater than six may suggest unusually heavy bleeding. Although many adolescents are initially anovulatory and take up to 20 months to establish normal cycles, as many as 45 per cent will be ovulatory from menarche. Up to half of all adolescent females may experience some menstrual dysfunction, including dysmenorrhea, dysfunctional uterine bleeding, or amenorrhea. Many of these disorders can be evaluated and treated competently by the pediatrician. The practitioner should realize that some problems may not require a full speculum examination, especially in virginal females, and that a thorough assessment can often be accomplished through visual inspection of the external genitalia and vaginal mucosa and a good bimanual or rectoabdominal examination.

Dysmenorrhea. The most common menstrual disorder in adolescents is dysmenorrhea, secondary to ovulatory periods, with increased progesterone and prostaglandin synthesis. Although 95 per cent of cases of dysmenorrhea are primary, a careful bimanual pelvic or rectoabdominal examination should be done to exclude the 5 per cent of cases that are secondary to other disease processes (e.g., pelvic inflammatory disease

[PID], endometriosis, cysts, congenital anomalies, and so on).

Mild dysmenorrhea may respond to simple analgesics, application of a heating pad, and rest. Moderate dysmenorrhea will usually respond to prostaglandin inhibitors:

1. Ibuprofen (Motrin), 400 mg orally four times a day for 3 to 5 days
2. Naproxen sodium (Anaprox), 550 mg orally as a loading dose, and then 275 mg three or four times daily for 3 to 5 days
3. Naproxen (Naprosyn), 500 mg orally as a loading dose, and then 250 mg two or four times daily for 3 to 5 days
4. Mefenamic acid (Ponstel), 500 mg orally as a loading dose, and then 250 mg three or four times daily for 3 to 5 days

Often, if one antiprostaglandin is ineffective, trying a different one may be useful. Side effects are minimal, usually limited to gastrointestinal symptoms. Although aspirin is a weak prostaglandin inhibitor and can be tried, patients do not place much faith in it.

Dysmenorrhea that is severe and unresponsive to prostaglandin inhibitors will usually respond to oral contraceptives (OCs), which substantially reduce menstrual flow. Any of the common OCs can be used (e.g., Ortho-Novum 1/35, Demulen 1/35, Norinyl 1/35, and Lo/Ovral). In patients who are already sexually active, using OCs is an ideal way to treat dysmenorrhea and provide contraception. Patients who have not had sexual intercourse but require further treatment should be told that they will be treated with "hormones," not "birth control pills."

Patients with dysmenorrhea that is unresponsive to all of the preceding measures should be referred to a gynecologist specializing in adolescents for consultation and further evaluation, which may include a pelvic ultrasonogram, luteinizing hormone (LH) and follicle-stimulating hormone (FSH) levels, or laparoscopy.

Premenstrual Syndrome (PMS). At present, much controversy surrounds the diagnosis and treatment of PMS. Typically, symptoms such as weight gain, headache, cramps, bloating, or mood swings occur 7 to 14 days before the onset of menses and resolve within a day or two of flow. No consistent hormonal patterns have been found, and a firm etiology has not been established. Therefore, no single treatment modality can be scientifically proposed. However, a number of different approaches have had some success.

Low-risk approaches include a well-balanced diet (limiting salt, refined sugar, red meat, fat, and caffeine), education of the patient, aerobic exercise, and relaxation techniques. Trials of medications that have few side effects include multivitamin and mineral supplements, prostaglandin inhibitors from day 14 of the cycle through the onset of menses, a progestin-dominant OC (e.g., Lo/Ovral) if associated with dysmenorrhea, or spironolactone, 50 mg daily from day 14 to the onset of menses for fluid retention. The use of progesterone, 200 to 400 mg rectally or vaginally, from day 14 to the onset of menses is controversial: In some studies, it is effective, but the long-term side effects are unknown. Treatments for which the risk may outweigh the potential gains are pyridoxine, 100 mg daily or from day 14 of the cycle through menses; danazol, 200 mg daily for severe breast pain; or bromocriptine, 5 mg nightly from days 10 to 26.

Dysfunctional Uterine Bleeding. Although early adolescent cycles are often irregular for the first 2 years, they should not be associated with excessive flow, duration, or frequency. Dysfunctional bleeding is usually anovulatory, secondary to an imperfect hypothalamic-pituitary-ovarian interaction, which causes the build-up of an overestrogenized endometrium without sufficient progesterone to cause normal sloughing. Bleeding is usually painless and occurs irregularly and unpredictably and at times can be life threatening. When dysfunctional bleeding begins at menarche, the likelihood of a concomitant bleeding disorder (e.g., von Willebrand's disease or idiopathic thrombocytopenic purpura) is increased.

Dysfunctional bleeding that is the result of physiologic immaturity is a diagnosis of exclusion and must be distinguished from bleeding secondary to an ectopic pregnancy, trauma, sexually transmitted disease, thyroid disease, cysts, or tumors. *A careful sexual history must be obtained and a pregnancy test performed if indicated.*

Treatment of "physiologic" dysfunctional bleeding is conveniently determined by the patient's blood pressure, hematocrit, and hemoglobin. Patients with mild cases have normal parameters, those with moderate cases have hemoglobins greater than 10 gm/dl, and those with severe cases have hemoglobins less than 10 gm/dl and may have orthostatic hypotension or shock. Patients with mild dysfunctional bleeding should be carefully followed, reassured, and placed on prophylactic ferrous sulfate. Patients with moderate bleeding will respond to immediate cessation of the bleeding, followed by treatment for 3 to 6 months with OCs. Bleeding will usually stop with the initial use of a 50-µg OC pill (e.g., Ovral), a 21-day package, one or two tablets orally at once, followed by one pill every 4 to 12 hours for the first 48 hours. Then the package is completed, and the patient either is allowed to have a withdrawal flow (which will be heavy) or is immediately switched to 28-day OCs for 3 to 6 months, along with ferrous sulfate supplements. An antiemetic agent (e.g., trimethobenzamide hydrochloride [Tigan] or promethazine hydrochloride [Phenergan] suppositories) may be required for the first 48 hours of treatment. The rationale is that after 3 to 6 months of imposing exogenous cycles, the hypothalamic-pituitary-ovarian axis may have matured enough to function appropriately, but retreatment may be required. The virginal patient should be told that she is being treated with "hormones," not "birth control pills." A less effective alternative is the use of medroxyprogesterone acetate (Provera), 10 mg daily for 5 days every 2 months, to induce a controlled slough of the endometrium.

Severe bleeding may respond to the preceding regimen but is best treated in the hospital. Patients unable to tolerate OCs up to every 4 hours may require treatment with conjugated estrogens (Premarin), 20 mg to 40 mg intravenously (IV) every 4 to 6 hours, followed by the use of OCs. Transfusion should be considered only in patients with unstable cardiovascular status, since cessation of the bleeding and long-term treatment with ferrous sulfate will restore normal hemoglobin levels, usually within a month. A dilatation and curettage (D & C)—a standard procedure for adult women with dysfunctional bleeding because of the incidence of endometrial pathology—is rarely indicated in adolescent patients, except as a last resort.

Primary Amenorrhea. The absence of menarche by age 16, the lack of pubic hair or breast development by age 14, or the failure of menarche to appear within 3 years of pubic hair or breast development constitute primary amenorrhea. Treatment depends upon establishing the correct diagnosis, which requires a careful history and physical examination, pelvic examination, and auxiliary laboratory tests, which may include an ultrasonogram of the pelvis; FSH, LH, prolactin, and testosterone levels; bone age films; and a karyotype. Reproductive prognosis depends on etiology.

Normal Tanner development and pelvic anatomy indicate probable immaturity of the hypothalamic-pituitary-ovarian axis. Menstrual cycles can be induced by administration of medroxyprogesterone acetate (Provera), 10 mg orally twice daily for 5 to 10 days, or progesterone-in-oil, 100 mg intramuscularly (IM). Indeed, this treatment can be used as a diagnostic aid, since withdrawal flow indicates that the endometrium is appropriately primed with estrogen. Spontaneous periods will sometimes commence following induction. Such patients may be overweight, underweight (e.g., may have anorexia nervosa), depressed or overly stressed, extremely athletic, or constitutionally delayed on the basis of family history or may suffer from a systemic disease (e.g., pituitary tumor, hypothyroidism, congenital adrenal hyperplasia, and inflammatory bowel disease).

Patients with normal pelvic examinations but no breast development and with elevated FSH or LH levels usually have hypergonadotropic hypogonadism, most typically seen in gonadal dysgenesis. However, the classic features of Turner's syndrome—especially short stature—may not be present if the patient has mosaicism. Treatment using conjugated estrogens (Premarin), medroxyprogesterone (Provera), and occasionally weak androgens like oxandrolone is best undertaken in conjunction with an experienced gynecologist specializing in adolescents or with an endocrinologist. Such treatment aims to maximize normal height and breast development.

Careful pelvic examination will reveal such causes as Rokitansky's syndrome (congenital absence of the vagina), transverse vaginal septum or imperforate hymen, hematocolpos, or Asherman's syndrome (uterine synechiae). Treatment is usually surgical. Normal breast development, sparse axillary and pubic hair, absence of a uterus, and normal male levels of testosterone indicate testicular feminization syndrome resulting from androgen insensitivity. Patients have XY chromosomes but are normal phenotypic females, often with blind vaginal pouches and with inguinal or abdominal testes that must be removed once full height and breast development have been reached because of the high incidence of malignant degeneration. Postoperatively, these young women need to be sensitively counseled about their femininity and their ability to have normal sexual relations, but childbearing is not possible. Counseling that discusses the fact that their "internal anatomy was never completely finished" is more productive than trying to inform them that they are genetic males (XY) but phenotypic females. Treatment also includes conjugated estrogen replacement (Premarin), 0.625 mg to 1.25 mg daily, to prevent osteoporosis and preserve breast development and normal vaginal estrogenization.

Secondary Amenorrhea. The pediatrician is far more likely to encounter a teenager who underwent a normal menarche but now has failed to have menses for 4 to 6 months or more. Since 50 per cent of 17-year-old girls have experienced sexual intercourse, *such patients must be considered pregnant until proved otherwise*. The second most common cause is transient hypothalamic disturbance, induced by illness, stress, weight changes, athletics, or ballet. During periods of enforced rest or injury, normal menses may return. A progesterone challenge test (Provera, 10 mg twice daily for 5 to 10 days, or progesterone-in-oil, 100 mg IM) may be both diagnostic and therapeutic. Normal withdrawal bleeding indicates that the patient is anatomically and physiologically normal.

Secondary amenorrhea may be the first sign of anorexia nervosa, even before weight loss becomes prominent. Normal adolescents will commonly cease menses with a 15 per cent weight loss. Although the prevalence of secondary amenorrhea is estimated at 5 per cent in the general population, it may reach 20 per cent in athletic women and 50 per cent in those involved in competitive athletes. Athletes should be encouraged to increase their caloric intake to compensate for their activity and to increase their calcium intake to 1500 mg per day (four to five glasses of milk). Ideally, the intensity of training should be cut back to a level at which regular menses can occur. If this is not possible, then cyclic estrogen and progesterone should be considered to try to prevent osteopenia and endometrial hyperplasia. The ideal regimen has yet to be determined, but OCs with 35 μg of estrogen or a combination of conjugated estrogens (Premarin), 0.625 mg to 1.25 mg daily for days 1 to 25, and medroxyprogesterone acetate (Provera), 10 mg daily for days 13 to 25, can be used. If the adolescent has a normal withdrawal flow with the progesterone challenge test, then she can also be cycled with medroxyprogesterone acetate (Provera), 10 mg daily for 5 to 13 days every 2 months.

Absence of withdrawal bleeding after progesterone indicates disorders such as polycystic ovary syndrome or other ovarian dysfunction secondary to infection, hemorrhage, or tumor; chronic illness; thyroid dysfunction; diabetes; or central nervous system tumors. Treatment depends on accurate diagnosis; and such tests as FSH, LH, and prolactin levels, 24-hour urine collections for 17-OH and 17-ketosteroids, thyroid functions, and skull radiographs may be indicated. Consultation with a gynecologist specializing in adolescents or an endocrinologist is recommended.

CERVICITIS AND CERVICAL DYSPLASIA

Gonorrhea. Whereas a man has only a 25 per cent chance of acquiring gonorrhea from an infected woman, a woman has a nearly 100 per cent risk of acquiring the organism from an infected man. The majority of young women with gonococcal infection of the cervix may be asymptomatic; but a purulent vaginal discharge, dysuria or frequency, and irregular menstrual bleeding are also common in symptomatic patients. Cervical cultures are plated on Thayer-Martin medium. Doing rectal cultures will increase the positive yield by 5 per cent, and pharyngeal swabs should be taken when there is a history of orogenital contact. Partners should be cultured *and* treated in the same visit, and the disease is reportable to the state or local health department. Patients should have a serologic test for syphilis, and repeat cultures should be taken as a test of cure within 10 to 14 days.

Because *Chlamydia trachomatis* can be found in up to 45 per cent of women and 25 per cent of men who have *Neisseria gonorrhoeae*, the Centers for Disease Control now recommend concomitant treatment for both organisms, even when only *N. gonorrhoeae* is isolated. Single-dose regimens for gonorrhea should be used before administering a doxycycline (or tetracycline) regimen to cover possible chlamydial infection. The following are treatment options:

1. Ampicillin, 3.5 gm orally, or amoxicillin, 3 gm orally, with probenecid, 1 gm orally given simultaneously. This is followed by doxycycline, 100 mg orally twice a day (or tetracycline hydrochloride, 500 mg orally four times daily) for 7 days.
2. Ceftriaxone, 250 mg IM. This is followed by doxycycline, 100 mg orally twice a day (or tetracycline hydrochloride, 500 mg orally four times daily) for 7 days. According to the 1989 CDC Guidelines, this is now the treatment of choice (Morbidity and Mortality Weekly Report, September 1, 1989, vol. 38/No. 5–8).
3. Aqueous procaine penicillin G, 4.8 million units IM, with probenecid, 1 gm orally. This is followed by doxycycline, 100 mg orally twice a day (or tetracycline hydrochloride, 500 mg orally four times daily) for 7 days. This is a less desirable alternative because of associated pain and toxicity.

For patients who cannot tolerate tetracyclines or who are pregnant, the single-dose regimen can be followed by erythromycin base or stearate, 500 mg orally four times daily for 7 days, or erythromycin ethylsuccinate, 800 mg orally four times daily for 7 days. Patients allergic to penicillin can be treated with spectinomycin, 2 gm IM, followed by doxycycline or tetracycline hydrochloride. For penicillin-resistant strains, ceftriaxone is highly effective and can be given in a single small-volume injection in the deltoid muscle. Spectinomycin is also effective.

Chlamydia. *Chlamydia trachomatis* has now become the most common sexually transmitted organism in the United States. It is a major cause of cervicitis, acute urethral syndrome, perihepatitis (Fitz-Hugh–Curtis syndrome), and pelvic inflammatory disease (PID).

Symptoms of chlamydial cervicitis may include a purulent or mucopurulent cervical discharge, a friable cervix, and a Papanicolaou (Pap) smear that displays inflammatory changes. Among adolescent girls, the prevalence of chlamydial infection ranges from 8 to 23 per cent. Rapid screening tests—employing either direct immunofluorescence or an enzyme immunoassay technique—are now widely available and are easier and cheaper alternatives to tissue cultures. In contrast to the treatment protocols for gonorrhea, patients with chlamydial infections are treated only for that organism:

1. Doxcyline, 100 mg orally twice daily for 7 days.
2. Tetracycline hydrochloride, 500 mg orally four times daily for 7 days.
3. Alternative for allergic or pregnant patients: erythromycin base or stearate, 500 mg orally four times daily for 7 days, or erythromycin ethylsuccinate, 800 mg orally four times daily for 7 days.
4. Sulfonamides are also active against *C. trachomatis.* Optimal dosages have not yet been determined, but sulfamethoxazole, 500 mg orally four times daily for 10 days, is probably effective.

Cervical Dysplasia. Surveys of Pap smears in 15- to 19-year-olds show cytologic abnormalities in as many as 11 per cent of sexually active young women. Abnormal Pap smears are associated with condyloma acuminata, early age of first sexual intercourse, multiple partners, and herpes simplex II infections. All sexually active adolescent girls should have Pap smears at least annually, and those at increased risk should have Pap smears every 6 months, or more frequently if abnormalities are present. If inflammation is present, a vigorous work-up should be pursued to find treatable causes (e.g., *Chlamydia* and *Trichomonas*). When dysplastic changes are present, the patient should be referred to an experienced gynecologist specializing in adolescents for colposcopy-directed biopsies and further treatment, which may include excisional biopsy, cryosurgery, or laser treatments. Early detection and treatment have resulted in a very high cure rate for cervical disease, as high as 90 per cent.

PELVIC INFLAMMATORY DISEASE

The risk of PID in sexually active young women aged 15 to 19 has been estimated to be as high as 1 in 8. In contrast, the lifetime risk of acute appendicitis is 7 per cent. *No evaluation of a sexually active woman with lower abdominal pain is complete without a pelvic examination.* Distinguishing between PID and acute appendicitis can sometimes be difficult, but PID typically occurs during or immediately following menses and usually involves bilateral lower abdominal pain, although one side may be more affected than the other. The classic criteria for making a diagnosis of PID are as follows:

1. History of lower abdominal pain
2. Lower abdominal tenderness
3. Cervical motion tenderness
4. Adnexal tenderness
5. One or more of the following: fever, leukocytosis, elevated erthyrocyte sedimentation rate (ESR), or adnexal mass on ultrasonography.

PID may have a single or polymicrobial etiology, but *N. gonorrhoeae, C. trachomatis,* anaerobes, and gram-negative bacteria are known to be the chief culprits. The risk of dissemination of cervicitis to PID is estimated to be 10 to 17 per cent, and approximately 1 to 3 per cent of cases then become systemic (e.g., gonococcal arthritis dermatitis syndrome, with tenosynovitis or arthritis, rash, fever, and leukocytosis). Adolescents with suspected PID should always be admitted to the hospital for observation and treatment. There are several reasons for this: Compliance with outpatient treatment regimens may be limited in adolescents; immediate, high-dose antibiotic treatment may help to preserve fertility; and the diagnosis may be in error. Even experienced gynecologists are accurate in diagnosing PID only 62 per cent of the time.

Inpatient therapy involves intravenous administration of antibiotics for at least 48 to 96 hours, or until the patient improves. A number of different regimens are available:

1. Cefoxitin, 2 gm IV every 6 hours or Cefotetan, 2 gm IV every 12 hours), and doxycycline, 100 mg IV every 12 hours. This is followed by doxycycline, 100 mg twice a day for 10 to 14 days after discharge from the hospital, or until the ESR is normal. This regimen covers gonorrheal and chlamydial PID but may not be adequate against certain anaerobes. Other cephalosporins such as ceftriaxone and cefotaxime can be used in appropriate doses and provide adequate coverage against gonococcal, gram-negative, and anaerobic organisms.
2. Clindamycin, 600 mg IV every 6 hours, and gentamicin or tobramycin, 2 mg/kg IV initially and 1.5 mg/kg every 8 hours, in patients with normal renal function. This is followed by clindamycin, 450 mg four times a day orally for 10 to 14 days. This regimen provides better coverage against anaerobes and gram-negative rods.
3. Metronidazole, 1 gm IV every 12 hours, and doxycycline, 100 mg IV every 12 hours. This is followed by doxycycline, 100 mg bid for 10 to 14 days. This regimen is ideal coverage for anaerobes and chlamydial infections but may be inadequate for some strains of *N. gonorrhoeae,* including pencillinase producers, and some gram-negative rods.

Consultation with a gynecologist or surgeon is advisable if the diagnosis is uncertain, the patient does not promptly respond to antibiotics, or a mass is present on pelvic or ultrasonographic examination. The risk of infertility approximately doubles with each succeeding episode of PID: 13 per cent after one episode, 35 per cent after two episodes, and 55 to 75 per cent after three or more episodes. Since the rate of infertility may be related to the interval between the onset of symptoms and treatment, prompt administration of intravenous antibiotics is desirable once the diagnosis has been made.

CHRONIC PELVIC PAIN

Chronic pelvic pain is often misdiagnosed in adolescent girls. It may occur with menses (cyclic pain) or not (acyclic). Cyclic pain associated with pelvic pathology could also be considered secondary dysmenorrhea. Adolescents with chronic pelvic pain most often have cyclic symptoms and abnormal findings on the pelvic examination (e.g., tenderness, cul-de-sac nodularity, or adnexal mass or thickening). Diagnostic laproscopy may be useful. Endometriosis is the most frequent cause of chronic pelvic pain, followed by adhesions, uterine abnormalities, PID, and functional ovarian cysts. Adhesions can sometimes be lysed through the laparoscope, and cysts may be punctured or biopsied. Treatment of endometriosis can be more problematic, usually involving the use of OCs or danazol for suppression of the aberrant tissue, sometimes in combination with surgery, and should be undertaken by an experienced gynecologist. The most benign cause of chronic pelvic pain is mittelschmerz, or pain on ovulation, often easily recognized by its mid-cycle occurrence but also visible on pelvic ultrasonography. Mittelschmerz is self-limited and responds to oral analgesics.

PELVIC MASSES

The most common pelvic mass in adolescent girls is *an enlarged uterus due to pregnancy*, even if sexual activity is denied. Ectopic pregnancy can also produce a pelvic mass but more typically manifests with abdominal pain and vaginal bleeding. Therapy for ectopic pregnancy involves immediate referral to a gynecologist for surgery, since it can be life threatening. With new microsurgical techniques, the fallopian tube can sometimes be preserved.

The ovary is the next most common source of pelvic masses in adolescents. By far, the most frequent ovarian mass is a follicular cyst, which develops from the unruptured follicle or corpus luteum. These cysts may or may not be hormonally responsive. A small cyst that is found incidentally on the pelvic examination should be followed routinely and does not require surgical intervention. Such cysts are frequently considered normal, "physiologic" findings. Cysts smaller than 5 cm that

cause pain or menstrual irregularities can be suppressed with OCs and usually resolve within 3 months. If they do not resolve, symptoms persist, or they are larger than 5 cm, laparoscopy can be utilized for aspiration. Pelvic ultrasonography is frequently useful to confirm the presence of a fluid-filled cyst versus a solid tumor.

Ovarian tumors are relatively rare, constituting only 1 to 2 per cent of all childhood tumors. Younger children may present with chronic abdominal pain or increasing abdominal girth. Occasionally, torsion or infarction of an ovary or an ovarian tumor can produce acute abdominal pain that mimicks appendicitis. The simplest method of detection is the bimanual pelvic or rectoabdominal examination. Thirty per cent of ovarian tumors are cystic teratomas or dermoid cysts, which often demonstrate calcification on radiography or ultrasonography and require surgical excision. They are bilateral in 10 to 25 per cent of patients and rarely undergo malignant degeneration (teratocarcinoma). Ten to twenty per cent of all ovarian tumors are cystadenomas, which are epithelial in origin and fluid filled. Other, rarer tumors include dysgerminomas, embryonal cell carcinomas, endodermal sinus tumors, granulosa-theca cell tumors, and gonadoblastomas. All require surgical consultation and excision. Radiation therapy and chemotherapy may be required for the rarer malignant tumors. When possible, a fragment of normal ovarian tissue should be preserved to allow normal menarche and development to occur. Otherwise, replacement hormonal therapy with conjugated estrogens (Premarin), 0.625 mg daily, should begin at 8 to 9 years of age.

Tumors of the fallopian tubes or uterus are exceedingly rare in childhood and adolescence. Uterine myomas may require excision, and uterine sarcomas or adenocarcinomas require radical surgery and radiation therapy. Cervical and vaginal lesions, such as polyps and papillomas, more typically manifest with vaginal bleeding and discharge; and prompt referral to a gynecologist for biopsy and treatment is indicated.

13

Bones and Joints

CRANIOFACIAL MALFORMATIONS

IAN T. JACKSON, M.D.

The treatment of craniofacial deformities is becoming better established in terms of what operation to perform and when to carry out corrective surgery. However, there are still areas of conflicting opinion, and it is not always possible to make hard and fast rules. The approach is multidisciplinary at the time of the initial assessment; the surgery is performed by the plastic surgeon and the neurosurgeon; occasionally an oral surgeon will be involved.

In some cases, total correction of the deformity can be achieved by initial repositioning of the skeletal component, followed by rearrangement of the soft tissue. In other conditions, however, a multistaged approach is necessary.

Bony defects, both those resulting from the deformity and those created by osteotomy, are reconstructed with bone. Usually this is accomplished using a free bone graft, but occasionally vascularized bone is employed. There are basically two methods of doing this. One is free vascularized bone transfer from a distant site using microvascular anastomosis or bone on its own vascular pedicle from the temporal area of the skull.

Microvascular techniques are now being used more frequently for reconstruction of soft tissue deficiencies. When indicated, soft tissue and bone can be replaced in this manner as a composite free tissue transfer.

Even in treating fairly standard, straightforward deformities (e.g., those of Crouzon's disease), it is usual that one major procedure is followed by one or two fairly minor ones in order to obtain the best possible end result. Recent advances in treatment include early correction of craniosynostosis, the use of skull as the primary bone graft site, the use of "mini" bone plates for stabilization in some situations, and—perhaps most important of all—a very considerable decrease in operating time.

CRANIOSYNOSTOSIS

All degrees of craniosynostosis, even the most minor, cause a rise in intracranial pressure. This may or may not be significant in terms of mental retardation, but high pressure levels may result in progressive papilledema, optic atrophy, and blindness. The advised timing of suture release is age 3 months. This allows the normal rapid brain growth during the first year to help improve the result of the osteotomy. There is good correction of the frontosupraorbital deformities associated with craniosynostosis, and it is hoped that in the long term the facial deformities resulting from coronal and basal craniosynostosis can be minimized. This, however, remains to be proved.

Scaphocephaly

A wide strip of cranium is removed in the region of the fused sagittal suture. In the past, silicone sheeting was used to line the edges of the craniotomy; however, this procedure has become less popular, since it seems ineffectual in preventing refusion of the cranium. In extreme cases of scaphocephaly, parallel vertical osteotomies anteriorly and posteriorly, running in a coronal direction, can be carried out; the lateral bone plates are then outfractured, the line of fracture being in the basal temporoparietal area. In some cases there is posterolateral rotation of the supraorbital rims, and in this situation the sagittal osteotomy is continued down to the glabellar area. A coronal craniotomy is performed behind the coronal sutures. The supraorbital rims and lateral orbital walls are mobilized as described for the correction of bicoronal craniosynostosis. This segment is split vertically in the midline. The two large frontal bone plates and supraorbital rims are derotated to improve the appearance of the forehead and the orbits. This frontal segment is wired to the glabellar area and to the lateral orbital walls but has no posterolateral fixation.

Trigonocephaly

Correction is similar to that described for the anterior portion of severe scaphocephaly. The frontal bone flap is removed, as are the supraorbital rims, both split in the midline. If the anterior cranial fossa is of adequate width (which is rather unusual in this condition), the frontal bone plates and the supraorbital rims can be rotated anteriorly by removing a wedge of bone based anteriorly along the central osteotomies; this flattens the forehead and supraorbital regions. In severe trigonocephalies, the two frontal bone plates and the supraorbital rims are left unsecured in the midline and are spread apart to widen the anterior cranial fossa. Fixation is to the lateral orbital rims and to the glabellar area. The two frontal bone flaps are wired to the supraorbital rims. This loose arrangement allows the expanding brain to remold the frontosupraorbital region. The bony gaps in the cranium are spontaneously filled with bone formed by the dura.

An alternative to the method described for reconstruction of the frontal bone is to harvest a suitably curved portion of bone from elsewhere in the skull using a metal template of the frontal area. This bone forms the new forehead, and the deformed frontal bone is morcellized and used to fill the donor defect.

Plagiocephaly

A frontal bone flap is removed, and the involved supraorbital rim is removed. The latter is shaped with bone-contouring forceps until it matches the contralateral side; it is then advanced by a lateral rotation to achieve symmetry and is fixed with wires at the lateral orbital rim and in the midline. If the zygomatic area is flattened, this is included in the osteotomy. The craniotomy is continued down along the sphenozygomatic suture to the inferior orbital fissure. The frontal bone flap is now rotated 180 degrees, and the former posterior border is wired to the supraorbital rim. The flattened front area is transferred to the opposite side but now lies within the hairline. In this way, symmetry is restored to the fronto-orbital region. An alternative technique is to cut through the bone at the edges toward the center—the "barrel stave" method—this weakens the bone and it can be molded. There is no posterior fixation, again allowing the pressure of the developing brain to hold the fronto-orbital region in the correction position.

In some cases, the orbit is narrowed transversely by as much as 10 to 15 mm. In these cases, a vertical cut is made in the supraorbital rim, and a bone graft of the required amount is inserted into this area. This enlarges the orbit and increases the fronto-orbital symmetry.

Bicoronal Craniosynostosis

This may or may not be associated with retrusion of the midface. To correct the condition, a frontal craniotomy is performed and the supraorbital area is freed by osteotomies laterally, across the orbital roof, anterior to the cribriform plate, and in the root of the nose. The supraorbital rims are advanced as a single unit and fixed to the nasal bones and to the lateral orbital walls. The oxycephalic skull anteriorly is reconstructed either by rotating it 180 degrees or by recontouring as seems appropriate. The bone flap is wired to the supraorbital rim; again, no posterior fixation is used in order to allow expansion of the brain to carry the frontosupraorbital area forward—the "floating forehead" technique. The amount of advancement required is that which will position the ridges 1 to 1.5 cm anterior to the cornea.

Warning

It is essential to establish the presence or absence of hydrocephalus prior to craniosynostosis correction. If in the opinion of the neurosurgeon this is significant and requires treatment, then a shunting procedure should be carried out *before* embarking on correction of the carniosynostosis.

CRANIOFACIAL DYSOSTOSIS (CROUZON'S SYNDROME) AND ACROCEPHALOSYNDACTYLY (APERT'S SYNDROME)

The frontosupraorbital deformities in these conditions are corrected at an early stage by the method described. Gross exorbitism is improved by the early surgery. The retrusion of the midface should be left until there is a strong reason for correcting it (e.g., peer or parental pressure or the danger of corneal exposure). When there is gross midface retrusion and airway compromise in babies, serious consideration should be given to advancement of the maxilla as a Le Fort III procedure at the same time as the fronto-orbital advancement ("monobloc technique"). The advanced maxilla is held in position with miniplates. This can lead to a connection between the nose and extradural space, and this must be closed carefully to avoid ascending infection. Galeal flaps can be used to effect this closure. The longer midface surgery can be postponed the better, as the dentition is increasingly able to cope with the fixation appliances required in the postoperative phase.

For the correction of the midface deformity, a Le Fort III osteotomy is performed, often with nasal bone grafting. In this procedure the approach is subcranial, but a coronal flap is used. Osteotomies are carried out at the root of the nose, the nasal septum, the medial orbital walls, the floor of the orbit, the lateral orbital walls, and then behind the maxillary tuberosites to separate them from the pterygoid plates. In this way, the maxilla can be separated from the skull base and moved forward and, if indicated, downward as required.

In some cases, because of the lateral rotational deformity of the maxilla caused by a slight hypertelorism (telorbitism), a central wedge based upward is taken out of the nasal bone area and a midline split of the palate is performed. This allows the maxilla to be rotated medially in order to level off the occlusion. In patients with a vertical shortness of the maxilla in the midline, a Le Fort I operation is selected, and the horizontal maxillary osteotomies are performed through a buccal sulcus incision. The dentoalveolar segment of the maxilla is placed in correct occlusion with the mandible. This may be done at the same time as the Le Fort III procedure or at a later date. In older patients, exactly the same procedures are carried out; however, in some cases these may have to be varied, since often some kind of limited cranial release has been performed in the past. Therefore, combinations of intracranial and extracranial procedures may be necessary when larger amounts of the orbit are to be moved forward. In selected cases, the frontosupraorbital advancement is performed with the Le Fort III osteotomy. Again, with this procedure, there is a danger of infection. This is particularly so in these patients, since the brain does not expand and fill the extradural dead space. Therefore, any connection into the nasal space or oropharynx is a considerable danger for extradural contamination.

Maxillary fixation is established by bone grafting the defects created by the osteotomies. Frequently "mini" bone plates are used in the lateral orbital wall and temporal region to establish rigid fixation. This can also be done on the zygomatic arch. The correct position of the maxilla is obtained using an acrylic wafer containing impressions of the ideal occlusion; this has been determined in the laboratory from dental models. Intermaxillary fixation is maintained for 6 to 8 weeks. However, with secure miniplate fixation and satisfactory bone grafts, the intermaxillary fixation is frequently removed a few days after surgery. This makes for airway safety and patient comfort.

HYPERTELORISM

This term is bandied about with little thought. Hypertelorism (telorbitism) indicates that the orbits are displaced laterally. Telecanthus, which may be of either bony or soft tissue origin, indicates that the medial canthi are displaced laterally. These two conditions tend to be lumped together into the category of hypertelorism, and therefore the wrong operation may be carried out. For example, frontonasoencephaloceles, extensive mucoceles, and some minor midface clefting syndromes produce bony telecanthus but rarely hypertelorism. Careful examination in these cases shows the lateral orbital walls to be in the correct position; for these a relatively minor procedure is indicated. This is frequently referred to as "mild to moderate hypertelorism."

Telecanthus

The position of the lateral orbital walls determines whether an extensive orbital shift is necessary. In patients with bony telecanthus or small degrees of hypertelorism, the correction can usually be subcranial, using a coronal flap approach, although frequently the cranium is entered because of the low position of the dura in the cribriform plate area. This is not an operation for practitioners inexperienced in this kind of surgery. The central segment of bone is removed, judging the size so as to leave a small segment of nasal bone laterally without disrupting the nasolacrimal apparatus. As this segment of bone is removed, the nasal mucosa is dissected very carefully in order not to damage it. The contents of the ethmoid sinuses are removed. The nasal septum may be resected from this extramucosal approach. Osteotomies are then made vertically far back on the medial wall of the orbit; horizontal osteotomies run out to the supraorbital rim and to the inferior orbital rim. If the anterior cranial fossa is entered, small dural tears can occur; if this happens, they should be carefully repaired. In the older patient, if there is a large frontal sinus, its lateral wall is actually freed and moved toward the medial wall, making the whole procedure much safer.

The orbital segments are mobilized, brought to-

gether, and wired in the midline; the medial canthal ligaments are identified and wired into position (transnasal canthopexy). A skull bone graft is used to build up the nasal bridge line. Bone grafts are not required in the orbit. In some cases with a low-lying cribriform plate, particularly those associated with frontonasal encephalocele, an intracranial approach may be used to remove the encephalocele and to make the operation much safer. In these cases, a trephine craniotomy is made in the frontal area just above the glabellar region. This allows very adequate exposure for performing the correction technique. The advantage of a limited approach like this is that any infection means only a loss of a small amount of bone rather than the large amount raised in a frontal craniotomy.

Hypertelorism

When the total orbital bulk has to be moved, a combined intracranial and extracranial approach is used. Again, the central segment is removed with careful preservation of the nasal mucosa. The septum is removed by an extramucosal approach, and the ethmoid sinuses are totally resected. An osteotomy is made above the supraorbital rim, down the lateral wall of the orbit, and across the front of the maxilla under the infraorbital nerve. The intraorbital osteotomy is made circumferentially, far back in the orbit. The orbital blocks are mobilized, brought together in the midline, and wired in position. Laterally, the orbits are held in position with miniplates wired from the temporal skull to the lateral orbital walls. Bone grafts are held in position using these miniplates and screws. Skull bone grafts are used to build up the dorsum of the nose and to fill in any lateral defects in the temporal area. Transnasal medial canthopexy and lateral canthopexies are performed.

Usually only a coronal approach is necessary; however, there may occasionally be some difficulty in gaining access to the floor of the orbit and the front of the maxilla. If this is the case, a conjunctival incision is used. This is made deep in the inferior fornix and allows good exposure to the floor of the orbit and to the anterior aspect of the maxilla. If the nasal mucosa is broached it should be very carefully repaired, since there is always the danger of infection ascending into the extradural space. If this risk exists in any craniofacial correcton, a galeal frontalis flap is used. This can be a long flap and is very vascular. It is based inferiorly on the supraorbital and supratrochlear vessels, then swung down to close off any openings into the nasopharynx, thus protecting the extradural space. Dural tears can be repaired with pericranium, fascia lata, or freeze-dried dura.

The timing of hypertelorism correction is dependent on the position of developing tooth buds; one must wait until there is enough room between the infraorbital rim and the tooth buds to perform the transverse osteotomy. Therefore, the correction is frequently delayed until around age 5, and many patients are much older.

HEMIFACIAL MICROSOMIA (LATERAL FACIAL DYSPLASIA)

The severity and extent of this condition are variable; frequently the cranium, orbit, maxilla, and mandible are involved. In addition to the skeletal anomalies, there is a shortage of skin and subcutaneous tissue and, in many cases, absence of masseter, temporalis, and pterygoid muscles. This latter situation is particularly significant in bilateral cases.

If there is cranio-orbital involvement, this can be corrected at any time either by onlay bone grafts or by osteotomies; a coronal flap approach is used. Often the zygomatic arch is missing, and in order to widen the involved side of the face, the zygomatic arch is reconstructed or augmented using vascularized cranial bone. This is taken from the temporal area. The blood supply is from the temporalis muscle and its overlying fascia or from the galea and the superficial temporal vessels. The bone is pedicled on these structures. The bone flap is swung down and fixed in position with wire or lag screws. Any onlay bone grafting of the orbit or the maxilla is performed with skull bone grafts. Correction of the enophthalmos involves advancement of the orbital contents and bone grafting deep in the orbit. If there is an associated macrostomia, this is corrected; any auricular tags are removed.

Should there be significant absence of the ascending ramus of the mandible, this can be re-established at the age of 5 or 6 years with a costochondral graft. However, vascularized iliac crest is being used more and more, with microvascular anastomosis of the deep circumflex iliac vessels to the facial vessels. If soft tissue bulk is required, it is supplied by the muscles surrounding the graft. If skin is necessary, an ellipse of skin overlying the iliac crest is added to the reconstruction. When soft tissue alone is required, the choice is between omentum, which frequently prolapses inferiorly, in spite of measures to prevent this, and de-epithelialized skin flaps, such as the scapular flap or groin flap. The use of free vascularized muscle flaps such as the rectus and latissimus has been abandoned because of atrophy of muscle bulk.

In the older child with a mild to moderate deformity, a functional orthodontic appliance is used to guide growth and development of the mandible and maxilla and to realign the teeth. At a later date a mandibular reconstruction, which usually involves a bilateral sagittal split and bone grafting to the deficient side, is carried out together with a Le Fort I osteotomy. In this way, tilt of the occlusal plane is corrected.

In adolescents and adults with severe deformities, the microvascular approach and the osteotomies described are used. Ear reconstruction is performed after the bony correction has been carried out. Costal cartilage is used to establish an ear skeleton; this is then elevated from the side of the head at a second stage, some 6 months later. No attempt is made to establish hearing in the unilateral case.

Bilateral cases of lateral facial dysplasia occasionally occur and are treated as outlined. In these cases, there may be airway problems due to bilateral absence of the ascending ramus of the mandible with posterior positioning of the tongue. This may necessitate early tracheostomy and occasionally gastrostomy for feeding. This severe involvement of the mandible presents a considerable challenge in treatment, since there are no

muscles present to power the mandible, and even after reconstruction, trismus and airway and feeding problems frequently persist.

TREACHER COLLINS' SYNDROME (MANDIBULOFACIAL DYSOSTOSIS)

This should be differentiated from Nager's syndrome, which has all the features of Treacher Collins' syndrome, but in addition has deformities of the radial side of the upper limb and a high incidence of mental subnormality. In addition, the familial incidence is much less frequent.

If there is a cleft palate, it is closed between 6 and 12 months of age. The recent tendency has been to do this earlier and earlier; thus, 6 months is the usual time. Correction of the skeletal deformity is being performed earlier than in the past, often within the first year of life and certainly before age 5.

The first procedure, using a coronal flap approach, consists of:

1. Osteotomy of the supraorbital rims—an ellipse of rim is removed laterally and is shifted up and wired to the frontal area to form a new, more prominent supralateral rim.
2. Skull bone grafting to the inferolateral portion of the internal aspect of the orbit. (Steps 1 and 2 change the orbital axis and thus alter the position of the eye.)
3. Reconstruction of the zygomatic arch and lateral orbital wall with a full-thickness vascularized skull graft based on temporalis muscle and temporalis fascia or galea and superficial temporal vessels.
4. Skull bone grafts to the anterior aspect of the maxilla.
5. Reconstruction of the coloboma of the lower lid with a full-thickness island flap of upper lid with a lateral skin pedicle.
6. Repositioning of the lateral canthus.

Additional bone grafts may be required at a later date, and extensive and prolonged orthodontic treatment is usually necessary. Correction of the mandibular and maxillary deformities is deferred until closer to adolescence. The osteotomies used are Le Fort II rotational advancement osteotomy of the maxilla and a sagittal split or C-osteotomy to advance and reposition the mandible with an advancement genioplasty to give better protrusion of the chin point. The final operation is usually a rhinoplasty to deal with the typical nasal deformity seen in this condition. The ear deformities are managed as for hemifacial microsomia, and a similar approach is adopted for the hearing problems.

DISORDERS OF THE SPINE AND SHOULDER GIRDLE

MICHAEL D. SUSSMAN, M.D.

Disorders of shoulder girdle and spine can be separated into those problems that are congenital, infectious or inflammatory, traumatic, and acquired or developmental. In this age group, one does not see degenerative changes, but some of these disorders may predispose to degenerative problems in later life. Disorders of the spine may affect neurologic function by applying pathologic mechanical stresses on the spinal cord, and this may have greater impact on function than the primary deformity.

SHOULDER GIRDLE

Congenital

Congenital Pseudarthrosis of the Clavicle. In this entity, there is a discontinuity, which is present at birth, in the midportion of the clavicle. The congenital pseudarthrosis can be easily distinguished from a birth fracture in that it is painless. The abnormality is usually found on the right side and is probably related to impairment of the development of the clavicle due to the juxtaposition of the subclavian artery to the underside of the midportion of the developing clavicle. Congenital pseudarthrosis of the clavicle may also occur in a bilateral form in association with cleidocranial dysostosis.

No treatment is required in infancy, and elective surgical repair of the pseudarthrosis to correct the cosmetic deformity is almost always successful (in contrast to congenital pseudarthrosis of the tibia, which is quite resistant to treatment) and can be accomplished when the child reaches a sufficient age that the structures are large enough for the fixation devices used at the time of surgery. No special treatment or handling is required prior to this time.

Sprengel's Deformity. The scapula lies in the cervical region during early fetal development and subsequently descends to its normal position on the posterior thorax. Failure of complete descent of the scapula results in a Sprengel's deformity. The scapula is in an elevated position, is small, malformed, and rotated so that the glenoid faces downward, and has a superomedial portion that hooks over the upper portion of the thorax. This results in a cosmetic deformity and also may limit the mobility of the shoulder due to the fixation and downward inclination of the glenoid. The deformity may be unilateral or bilateral. There is a female preponderance in most series, but this may be due to an ascertainment bias because of the cosmetic nature of this problem. Twenty to 30 per cent of patients may have a supernumerary bone known as the omovertebral bone which provides an osseous connection between the elevated, malformed scapula and the axial skeleton.

One third of these patients have a mild grade I deformity in which the shoulder joints are almost level, and the deformity cannot be seen with the patients dressed. These patients with mild deformities should be followed up throughout growth, as there may be progression in the severity of the deformity. Screening procedures for associated anomalies of the spine as well as renal anomalies should be done. One third of the patients have a grade II deformity, in which the asymmetry is mild to moderate but can be appreciated with the patients dressed owing to the asymmetry at the base of the neck. Another one third of patients have more severe deformities that are easily visible and can cause functional impairment.

Patients with grade II or III deformities may have surgery performed prior to the age of 5 or 6 years to correct the cosmetic appearance. In moderate cases, excision of the superomedial portion of the scapula in an extraperiosteal fashion, leaving the levator scapulae detached and excising the omovertebral bone, if present, may suffice. For more severe deformities the Woodward procedure is recommended, wherein the origin of the trapezius is detached and moved caudally in addition to excision of the superomedial angle of the scapula and omovertebral bone. If one waits to perform surgery until an older age (older than 7 years), the risk of brachial plexus palsy from compression of the plexus between the scapula and the first rib is increased, so that surgery at a younger age is preferred. The major goal of surgery is to reduce the cosmetic deformity; however, increased range of motion can also be expected. Scoliosis is common in these patients and may be due to congenital anomalies or may develop during the adolescent growth spurt in a pattern similar to that of idiopathic scoliosis. Other associated anomalies include the Klippel-Feil syndrome or may be found in the ribs and urogenital system.

Snapping Scapula. In this syndrome there is a palpable, audible, and sometimes painful click with elevation and declination of the scapula. This can be due to one or more osteochondromata on the costal surface of the scapula or may be a forme fruste of Sprengel's deformity with a prominent and curved superomedial portion of the scapula. These lesions can be excised surgically when identified.

Acquired

Birth-Related Brachial Plexus Palsy. The most common type of brachial plexus palsy affects the upper or C5-C6 distribution. This is usually found in large infants and is due to traction on the brachial plexus during delivery. These infants have limited active abduction, external rotation, and elbow flexion; therefore, the arm is held in an adducted, internally rotated, and extended posture. In the acute phase, no treatment is indicated, but the arm should be handled with care to avoid further traction on the injured nerves. At 2 to 3 weeks of age, gentle range of motion can be begun, concentrating on external rotation and abduction. Range of motion should not be forced, and long-term passive splintage should not be used. If elbow flexion is absent when sitting age is reached, an elbow splint should be used to maintain the elbow at 90 degrees to allow for development of active use of the hand. If the lower plexus is involved, then a hand and wrist splint may also be used. Since there are areas that are insensate, close observation should be made to avoid injury to these insensate areas. Improvement is seen until the age of 2, but subsequent to this, further improvement is unlikely. The percentage of children who achieve full recovery varies from 10 to 75 per cent, depending upon the series. If deficits persist, muscle releases and/or transfers may be done to improve range of motion. In some cases, a rotational osteotomy of the upper humerus may be done to improve function. Patients with severe defects persisting past 6 months of age may benefit from surgical exploration of the plexus and grafting to replace destroyed nerves.

Shoulder Dislocation. Traumatic shoulder dislocations are rare in the pediatric age group but may occur in older teenagers. More frequently fractures occur with traumatic episodes. Voluntary dislocation of the shoulder, however, may be seen in this age group, and the dislocation may be multidirectional, i.e., posterior as well as anterior. In general, surgery should be avoided on these patients, and physical therapy should be used to strengthen muscles that maintain shoulder alignment. In addition, patients should be counseled not to voluntarily dislocate their shoulders.

Fractures

Fractured Clavicle. Fractured clavicle is the most common fracture seen in the pediatric age group. Neonatal clavicle fractures occur with birth trauma and usually require no treatment other than gentle handling of the affected extremity. These fractures heal exceedingly rapidly, and infants are usually asymptomatic within a week to 10 days.

In children other than neonates, when clavicle fractures occur, these can be treated with a figure-of-8 dressing to reduce the symptoms. Healing is almost universal and no reduction is usually necessary, as bone remodeling is usually complete. A large amount of fracture callus may occur at the healing site, which may be cosmetically unpleasant, since the clavicle is directly subcutaneous. However, parents can be counseled that this will resolve in 6 to 12 months.

Fractured Scapula. Fractures of the scapula are very rare in this age group and are usually associated with major trauma. In most cases, they can be treated by immobilization of the extremity until healing occurs.

Fractures of the Upper Humerus. Fractures of the upper humerus usually occur in the proximal metaphysis, 1 to 2 cm distal to the growth plate and not through the growth plate. Although these fractures may be completely displaced, no reduction of the fracture fragments is necessary, and treatment with a collar and a cuff and swathe for 3 to 4 weeks is sufficient. Even in the severely displaced fractures, healing and subsequent remodeling can be anticipated and full recovery of function is likely.

SPINE

Congenital Muscular Torticollis. Congenital muscular torticollis results from a contracture of the sternomastoid muscle, which causes a tilting of the head to the side of the abnormal sternomastoid, associated with turning of the face to the opposite side. This condition is noted within the first few days of life and is believed to be secondary to ischemia of the sternomastoid muscle with subsequent fibrosis and contracture. The area of ischemia produces the so-called sternomastoid tumor, which appears during the first week of life and disappears by 6 to 8 weeks. The limitation of motion, however, persists. The asymmetric muscle pull results in plagiocephaly and facial asymmetry.

Most cases respond to gentle passive range of motion, rotating and tilting the head with each diaper change. If the deformity persists past 18 months, then surgical release of the tight sternomastoid should be done followed by maintenance of the head for 4 to 6 weeks in the overcorrected position using either an orthosis, cast, or halo vest. Radiographs of the cervical spine should be obtained to rule out the presence of congenital bony anomalies that may be the cause of torticollis. This should be done before attempts at vigorous manipulation.

Congenital Anomalies

Congenital anomalies can occur anywhere in the spine and may include only a single level or multiple levels or affect the entire spine. Most spine anomalies can be classified as either failure of segmentation of vertebrae, failure of formation of portions of vertebrae, or combinations of both of these. Failures of segmentation result in fusion of all or a part of one vertebral body to an adjacent vertebral body. If this fusion is partial, then the growth plate is absent in the area of fusion but may be present in the unfused area, leading to the development of a progressive deformity. Similarly, if a partially formed vertebra extends over only a portion of adjacent vertebral bodies, the deformity may increase with growth. Asymmetric growth and increasing deformity may occur, resulting in progressive scoliosis, kyphosis, or both. Lordosis may occur in those rare cases in which there are multiple congenital fusions of the posterior elements with intact bodies anteriorly.

As with other congenital anomalies, when congenital scoliosis is discovered, careful examination of the patient should be done to detect the presence of other anomalies. These may include hypothyroidism or hearing impairment with upper spinal anomalies and cardiovascular, gastrointestinal, or urogenital anomalies associated with anomalies lower in the spine. Spinal anomalies may also be associated with diastematomyelia or tight filum terminale, which may tether the spinal cord and result in progressive spinal cord dysfunction with growth. Patients with spinal anomalies who show evidence of neurologic dysfunction should have magnetic resonance imaging (MRI) or myelography to detect the presence of these problems.

In most cases of congenital spine deformity, careful serial follow-up is indicated until growth is finished, and if significant progression is documented, then posterior spinal fusion, usually without instrumentation, should be performed to prevent further progression of the deformity. Bracing may be indicated to control flexible curves adjacent to anomalous areas. Failure of segmentation may not be apparent radiologically in the first few years of life because of lack of ossification of the involved elements. If posterior fusion alone is insufficient to prevent progression of the deformity, then anterior fusion may also be required.

Congenital fusions of the cervical and upper thoracic spine tend to be less aggressive in terms of producing deformity than those in the lower thoracic and lumbar spine.

Klippel-Feil Syndrome. Congenital fusions in the

cervical spine are known as the Klippel-Feil syndrome. In most cases, this does not produce scoliosis or kyphosis but limits the linear growth of the cervical vertebrae, resulting in a short neck, low hairline, and limitation of motion of the cervical spine. A high percentage of these patients have hearing problems. No treatment is necessary for most of these cases. In exceedingly severe cases in which the cosmetic appearance is unacceptable, resection of the upper two or three ribs, with skin grafting to alter the contours in the shoulder area, may improve the cosmetic appearance.

Occipitocervical Instability. This form of instability, which may present with headache or pain with neck motion, is exceedingly rare and may be seen in combination with fusions in the cervical spine. When detected and documented radiologically, it should be treated by fusion of the occiput to the upper cervical spine.

Atlantoaxial Hypermobility. Excessive motion between C1 and C2 may occur in otherwise normal children with an os odontoideum (a hypoplastic odontoid with an ossicle superior to it), in children with skeletal dysplasia due to a hypoplastic odontoid (particularly Morquio's syndrome and spondyloepiphyseal dysplasia congenita), or in children with Down's syndrome (owing to alteration and laxity of the restraining ligaments). Diagnosis is made by interpretation of *voluntary* flexion-extension radiographs of the cervical spine with measurement of the distance between the posterior border of the anterior arch of C1 and the anterior border of the odontoid (atlanto-dens interval). It is important not to obtain these radiographs by passively forcing flexion of the neck, since this maneuver could result in injury or even death of patients with hypermobility. An absolute distance of greater than 4 mm of the atlanto-dens interval is abnormal. In the absence of neurologic findings, patients with instability of less than 6 to 7 mm should be followed up closely, and those with instability of greater amounts should have atlantoaxial fusion to prevent progressive myelopathy and/or acute spinal cord damage.

Atlantoaxial instability is prevalent in patients with Down's syndrome. Even if pathologic laxity is not documented in this group of patients, they should avoid activities that may place undue stress on the neck, such as tumbling and trampoline. They may participate in most recreational sports, recognizing that their risk of cervical injury is slightly increased. Patients with Down's syndrome should be radiographed initially at age 3 or 4; if the findings are within normal limits, radiography should be repeated every 2 to 4 years, or sooner if evidence of spinal cord compression such as hyperreflexia, weakness, or incontinence is detected. For instability with a dens interval of 7 mm or more or associated with evidence of cord compression, surgical fusion of C1-C2 may be indicated.

Pseudosubluxation of C2 to C4 in Children. After experiencing spinal trauma and receiving flexion-extension radiography of the cervical spine, some children exhibit what appears to be a subluxation of C2 on C3 and/or C3 on C4 on the lateral flexion view of the cervical spine. If this reduces fully in extension, is not greater than 5 mm, and is not associated with other evidence of fracture such as an increase in the prevertebral soft tissue space, then this can be considered normal. Patients should not be overtreated when they exhibit this normal pseudosubluxation.

Developmental

Idiopathic Scoliosis. Idiopathic scoliosis may present in infancy, although this occurs rarely in the United States and infrequently in the juvenile years. The most frequent onset of idiopathic scoliosis is during the pubertal growth spurt. Small spinal curvatures may occur in 5 to 10 per cent of the preadolescent population, but only 1 out of 20 of these requires treatment.

Curves of small magnitude in immature individuals have the potential to progress to severe deformities, so that patients with clinical evidence of spinal asymmetry should be evaluated and treated if progression occurs. Serial radiographs of all patients with spinal asymmetry document the degree of deformity and identify progressive curves, but this approach is costly and results in unnecessary radiation to adolescent children. Therefore, radiography should be reserved for those patients with significant deformities, whereas those with milder deformities can be followed up clinically. The degree of deformity may be assessed by measurement of the rib hump or lumbar hump in the forward bend position by using the "scoliometer," as described by Bunnell. This device, adapted from a nautical pitch gauge, is placed in the posterior midline at the point of maximum deformity with the patient in the forward bend position, and the angle with which the trunk deviates from the horizontal is read directly on the scoliometer. This angle of deformity is referred to as the angle of trunk rotation (ATR). Patients with curves of greater than 20 degrees had an ATR of less than 5 degrees in 99 per cent of the cases examined by Bunnell, giving a very low false-negative rate. There is, however, a significant false-positive rate, so some patients with mild curves have an ATR of 5 degrees or more. Therefore, patients with 5 degrees or less ATR do not require radiography. However, if these patients have growth remaining, they should be followed up at 6- to 12-month intervals by scoliometer in order to detect progression. If significant progression is detected (greater than 2 degrees ATR) or if the ATR is greater than 5 degrees, then a single standing AP radiograph in boys or PA radiograph in girls should be taken using high-speed screens and shields for breast and thyroid. Girls are seven times more likely to progress than boys, and the more immature the patient at the time of initial curve detection, the more likely the patient is to progress. In addition, there is a strong familial predisposition to scoliosis, and those patients with a positive family history should be followed up closely.

For curvatures having a Cobb angle of less than 25 to 30 degrees on radiograph, no treatment is necessary, but follow-up until 1 to 2 years after menarche in girls and after voice change in boys is indicated to ensure lack of progression. Curves that progress to the range of 25 to 45 degrees in skeletally immature individuals should be treated with an orthosis, usually of the underarm type, until skeletal maturity is achieved. The goal of bracing is to prevent progression of the curvature. In general, most physicians treating scoliosis require 23 hours a day of brace wear; however, there is some information that part-time brace wearing (16 hours per day) may be as effective as the 23-hour-a-day program that has been traditional. Electrical stimulation has been advocated by several groups to prevent progression of scoliosis. This is done at night only by use of transcutaneous electrodes attached to a stimulating device. However, there are several studies that show this approach to be ineffective, and at present this approach is not recommended.

Curvatures greater than 45 degrees will, in most cases, continue to progress following adolescence and require surgical treatment. Surgery consists of insertion of a metallic device onto the posterior (or in some cases, the anterior) spine, which partially corrects the deformity and holds the curvature in the corrected position, while the spine that has been prepared for fusion by removal of facet joints, decortication, and addition of bone graft heals solidly. Currently used devices, which include the Harrington rod along with the Drummond interspinous segmental spinal instrumentation or the Cotrel-Dubousset system, are more stable than the Harrington rod alone, and patients can be mobilized rapidly following surgery and may not require an external orthosis.

Neuromuscular Scoliosis. Scoliosis is found in a high incidence in quadriparetic cerebral palsy patients as well as in patients with degenerative neuromuscular diseases such as Duchenne muscular dystrophy and spinal muscular atrophy. Bracing may be indicated in younger patients with cerebral palsy and spinal muscular atrophy and may retard curve progression, but many of these children ultimately require surgery with sublaminar wiring by the Luque technique, which produces excellent curve correction and exceedingly stable fixation, allowing rapid mobilization following surgery. Bracing is not effective in scoliosis associated with Duchenne muscular dystrophy and may only delay surgery in these boys, thereby subjecting them to surgery at a time when their pulmonary function has deteriorated. Therefore, spinal bracing is contraindicated in Duchenne muscular dystrophy, and these patients should have early surgical stabilization as soon as it is apparent that they are developing a curvature.

Postural Roundback. Postural roundback is an increase in the normal thoracic kyphosis found in children and adolescents. As long as the kyphosis is flexible, no orthotic treatment is necessary, and these patients may respond to physical therapy in the form of thoracic hyperextension and pelvic tilt exercises. Occasionally, if the deformity is severe and progressive, an orthosis may be indicated. Patients should be followed up for progression or development of structural changes.

Scheuermann's Disease. Scheuermann's disease is increased thoracic or thoracolumbar kyphosis associated with changes in the vertebral body consisting of anterior wedging, endplate irregularity, and Schmorl's nodes. This usually presents in mid to late adolescence and may be associated with back pain and hamstring tightness. Boys are affected more frequently than girls. If the thoracic kyphosis is greater than 45 degrees and

there is significant growth remaining, the patient should be treated with an orthosis and physical therapy. Unlike scoliosis, in which the goal is to prevent progression, actual correction can be achieved and maintained in patients with Scheuermann's disease.

Spondylolisthesis. Spondylolisthesis is slippage forward of a vertebral body relative to the adjacent distal vertebral body. This usually occurs when L5 slips forward on S1, and in children this is usually due to a defect in the pars interarticularis, which appears in a predisposed individual during the first decade. Spondylolisthesis may also occur because of congenital deformity and elongation of the pars.

Patients with spondylolisthesis may present with back pain, posterior thigh pain, and evidence of tight hamstrings or may be asymptomatic but show evidence of deformity. Clinical examination demonstrates flattening of the buttocks, decreased range of flexion of the spine, and hamstring tightness. Radiographs document the presence of the pars defect and the presence and severity of the forward slippage. The upper border of the sacrum is divided into four quadrants, and grading ranges from grade I for slippage less than 25 per cent to grade V for complete slippage of L5 on S1 (spondyloptosis). Patients having grade I and II spondylolisthesis without significant symptoms should be followed up throughout growth for possible progression of the slippage by lateral standing radiographs of the lumbosacral spine on a yearly basis, or more frequently if symptoms indicate. If there is no evidence of increased slippage, no treatment other than avoidance of high-risk activities such as football and gymnastics is required. If the patient is symptomatic, then immobilization in an antilordotic lumbosacral orthosis or cast may decrease symptoms, and the patient may be weaned from the orthosis when asymptomatic. For patients with persistent symptoms or progressive slips of grade III or greater, spinal posterolateral fusion using a massive amount of autogenous graft, usually between L4, L5, and the sacrum, is performed. Only in very severe cases is decompression of the anterior sacrum, anterior fusion, or reduction indicated. Removal of the L5 lamina (Gill procedure) is not indicated and may actually aggravate the instability. When solid fusion is achieved, the symptoms, including the hamstring spasm, will resolve.

Traumatic Injury

Traumatic injuries to the spine may occur at any time during childhood and may be associated with injury to the underlying spinal cord. Injuries that occur at birth may be confused with anterior horn cell disease, since both of these conditions give signs of lower motor neuron damage. However, the spinal cord injury is nonprogressive. In infancy and childhood, spinal cord injury may occur in the absence of associated detectable bony injury.

The most common cause of vertebral and spinal cord trauma in children is motor vehicle accidents, and appropriate seat restraints are effective in prevention of these disastrous injuries. In the case of complete loss of spinal cord function, no recovery can be expected, whereas with incomplete injuries, recovery may occur. In either case, the bony injury and instability, if it exists, should be treated, and a rehabilitation program at a center accomplished in treatment of these patients should be instituted. Surgical decompression of the spinal cord is not of any benefit to patients with complete injuries but may, in selected patients with incomplete injuries, enhance the resolution of the deficits by removal of pressure on the spinal cord. Surgery may be necessary to stabilize the associated bony injury. In preadolescents with spinal cord injuries of the upper thoracic and cervical spine, the incidence of scoliosis is exceedingly high, and treatment of progressive deformity below the level of injury with an orthosis or surgery may be necessary.

Fractures of the Ring Apophysis. With hyperflexion or hyperextension injury of the spine, fragments of the ring apophysis may be separated from the main body of the vertebra and may impinge on the spinal cord, cauda equina, or nerve roots. When this occurs, the fragments must be surgically removed.

Causes of Back Pain in Children

There are a variety of entities that may cause back pain in children, and it is important to separate these from one another by careful history, physical examination, and follow-up of the clinical course. The major causes of back pain are as follows:

Spondylolisthesis. (See above discussion.) Patients with spondylolisthesis usually present with pain that may begin in the back and radiate into the posterior thighs, rarely prior to the age of 10.

Spinal Cord Tumor. The most common presentation of spinal cord tumor is back pain. However, careful physical examination may demonstrate the presence of neurologic dysfunction, and AP spinal radiographs may show evidence of increased interpedicular distance. Diagnosis is by MRI or myelography, and treatment is neurosurgical excision of the tumor.

Disc Disease. Disc disease may occur in young adolescents and is frequently due to a bulging annulus rather than a herniation of the nucleus. A trial of conservative therapy is indicated in most cases, but a high percentage of patients ultimately require surgical decompression. Since the bulging disc may be central rather than peripheral, patients may present with diffuse, nonradicular pain. Diagnosis can be made by MRI or myelography.

Osteoid Osteoma. Osteoid osteoma is an unusual condition that is thought to be neoplastic. Although these lesions generally appear in the second or third decade, they can occur in young children. They present with nonradiating back pain, which is usually increased at night and classically relieved by salicylates. Diagnosis can be made by plain radiography, tomography, and technetium-99 scan and confirmed by computed tomography. Treatment of these lesions is by surgical resection.

Discitis. Discitis may present as back pain with or without leg pain or as pseudoparalysis of the lower extremities. Radiographs may demonstrate a decreased disc space height and endplate irregularity. Although bacterial cultures of the disc are usually negative, many, if not all, of these cases may be secondary to focal osteomyelitis of the vertebral endplate. The usual organism is *Staphylococcus,* but occasionally other organisms, including gram-negative organisms, may be responsible. In the past, many children with discitis were successfully treated with cast immobilization alone. However, 3 to 6 weeks of antibiotic coverage along with cast or brace immobilization of the spine is probably indicated in most cases. An effort should be made to obtain a bacteriologic diagnosis by serial blood cultures and, on occasion, needle biopsy of the vertebral body prior to the institution of antibiotic therapy.

Cord Tether. Tethered cord may present with back pain, although it frequently presents with painless neurologic dysfunction in the lower extremities or secondary incontinence. Patients with a tethered cord secondary to a tight filum terminale also frequently have skin abnormalities such as a café-au-lait spot, hairy patch, or a dimple at the base of the spine. This entity may be diagnosed by MRI and is treated by surgical release of the tether.

Low Back Strain. Low back strain may be seen in teenagers with acute onset of low back pain without neurologic symptoms or radiographic evidence of bony abnormalities. This is not associated with any radicular pain or neurologic changes. Usual treatment is with salicylates or nonsteroidal anti-inflammatory drugs plus an active stretching program.

CONGENITAL DEFORMITIES OF THE ANTERIOR CHEST WALL

JOHN C. McQUITTY, M.D.

CONGENITAL ABSENCE OF THE RIBS

The most common ribs to be absent are the first and twelfth ribs; however, any ribs may be absent at birth. This may be associated with absence of the chest wall muscles and hemivertebrae. These defects are generally not associated with clinical or physiologic abnormalities. However, when clinical symptoms occur blood oxygen and carbon dioxide levels should be measured. Surgical repair is needed in some patients with clinical symptoms.

STERNAL DEFECTS

There can be partial or total midline vertical defects in the sternum. Defects can be isolated or associated with congenital heart disease, ectopia cordis, and the most severe associated defects in pentalogy of Cantrell, with defects in the abdominal wall, diaphragm, and pericardium. Prognosis in the uncomplicated cases is good, and surgery is performed for cosmetic reasons and to protect the underlying organs. Ectopia cordis and pentalogy of Cantrell are very difficult to correct surgically, with high surgical morbidity and often less than ideal surgical results.

ADDITIONAL ABNORMALITIES OF THE STERNUM

Pectus carinatum occurs predominantly in boys. Indications for surgery are cosmetic. Pectus excavatum (sternal chest) occurs structurally at birth and may increase or regress as the child gets older. In those cases in which the defect progresses, a careful history should rule out underlying increased resistance of the airways or decreased compliance of the lung and upper airway obstruction awake or asleep. Etiology of these defects is still debated in the literature. Some studies of pulmonary and cardiac function report minor abnormalities, particularly with exercise, and the indication for surgery is therefore generally cosmetic. Timing of surgery is debated, but it should be performed before adulthood.

ASPHYXIATING THORACIC DYSTROPHIES

In children born with small, abnormally formed chest walls, as accurate a diagnosis as possible should be made, allowing for prognosis, genetic counseling, and screening of associated organ abnormalities. Many of these infants die at birth. For those who survive with and without neonatal intensive care, we recommend quantitation of arterial blood oxygen and carbon dioxide levels and serial measurement of pulmonary and cardiac function with particular concern for pulmonary hypertension. There is as yet no satisfactory surgical correction for these infants. Medical treatment is bronchodilators, diuretics, and oxygen during the first several years of life, and throughout life with respiratory tract illnesses.

ORTHOPEDIC DISORDERS OF THE UPPER EXTREMITY

E. DENNIS LYNE, M.D.

In a recent survey of the American Academy of Pediatrics, it was found that 20 million school children take part in organized sports each year, and roughly 1 million are injured. Given these facts, plus the country's present preoccupation with both organized and recreational exercise, increasing attention should be given by pediatricians to sports medicine and its relationship to our children.

Although the focus of this article is on overuse syndromes in the upper extremities, a few basic principles should be established concerning children and their involvement in sports. In a recent survey, again from the American Academy of Pediatrics, 40 per cent of the children aged 5 to 8 had at least one risk factor for heart disease, with the three factors being increased blood pressure, increased cholesterol, and physical inactivity. What constitutes physical inactivity is not easy to define. Through the President's Physical Fitness Program it has been shown that about 40 per cent of boys between the ages of 6 and 12 can do one or no push-ups, and 60 per cent of girls between 6 and 17 can do one or no push-ups. Is that because they are not getting enough physical education in school and indeed are in poor physical shape? Eight states, including Michigan, have no physical education requirements at all; in contrast, Illinois requires daily physical education in all grades. Also, how important are sports, both recreational and organized, for the growing child?

In organized sports for the young child, several principles can be set forth which will be of help to the pediatrician.

1. Foremost is that between ages 6 and 12 sports should be fun, as sports are played by children in this age group for socialization rather than individual competition or achievement. The concept of winning and losing seldom plays a part in the child's involvement unless superimposed by adults. Only in the adolescent years should structured competitive sports assume a prominent role with individual and team achievement emphasized.

2. Boys and girls can, in general, play together until about age 10 or 11, after which it becomes advisable, in contact sports at least, to separate the sexes.

3. Weight training has no place in sports until the closure of growth plates, which in boys usually averages around 16 and in girls 12 or 13, and should be condemned in the immature athlete, in whom abuse of medications such as steroids also plays a part. It is estimated that approximately 500,000 schoolchildren are on anabolic steroids at the present time, mostly through nonphysician sources.

4. Collision sports, in general, are probably not appropriate until about age 14, and conversely, sports that stress agility, team organization, and collective winning should be emphasized. Sports such as racquet sports, swimming, track, and soccer should be emphasized to the young, reserving football, wrestling, and some of the high-injury sports for high school.

In teaching sports to the younger child, it is important to select teachers who are tuned in not only to the skill levels of the sport but also to the psychological needs of the child. In that respect, coaches should be mature people formally educated in both the psychology and the art of the sport and also very concerned about safety. Given these requirements, it is very often helpful to have as a coach a parent who has already raised his or her children and specifically whose own child(ren) is not directly involved with the team he or she is coaching. In the younger child, especially in the 6 through 10 age group, women coaches may actually be preferable, in that they are often better attuned to the young child's psychological needs. Verbal or physical abuse, of course, has no place in sports and is extremely detrimental to the child. Studies have clearly shown that the confident child athlete whose ego has been nurtured obtains superior levels of athletic achievement.

When dealing with injuries to the upper extremity, most of which are caused by overuse, one has to deal with subjective and objective signs, but pain and its relationship to athletic performance become paramount. Evaluation of the degree of pain has to take into consideration the typical teenager's response of hiding injury so that he or she will not miss out on a specific sports activity as well as the typical response of the child who is tired, frustrated, or otherwise looking for an out in a sport and is willing to exaggerate subjective complaints out of proportion to objective signs. Therefore, it should be emphasized that the treatment of most childhood injuries, which are usually due to overuse, is rest with occasional potions, but seldom is highly technical support necessary. Also, seldom does the adult model and treatment of the injury apply to the child. Two statements which I have found most useful in the treatment of overuse syndromes are: (1) "If it hurts, don't do it for a while" and (2) "If you still do it while it hurts, stop complaining to your parents."

OVERUSE SYNDROME OF THE UPPER EXTREMITY

Swimmer's Shoulder

Swimmer's shoulder is seen in approximately 47 per cent of competitive swimmers, some of whom are disabled by the condition and forced to stop their participation in the sport. Others seem to be able to handle the problem without treatment and continue their sport at a high level. This, of course, gets back to the age-old question of pain and a child's ability to handle it, and for what reasons. Swimmer's shoulder is particularly prevalent with free style, butterfly, and backstroke and is most painful during the pull-through and recovery phases. The etiology is irritation between the humeral head and the superior structures, such as the coracoacromial ligament and the acromium.

On examination, pain and tenderness are seen anteriorly over the coracoacromial ligament, and pain on flexion and internal rotation to 90 degrees is the most common clinical finding. One has to differentiate this from other problems, such as bicipital tendinitis and cuff tears. Radiographs in the child are usually normal. Treatment is decreased activity and anti-inflammatories such as ibuprofen (Motrin) for a 2- to 4-week period; seldom is surgery indicated in the growth plate–open child. When surgery is indicated in the older child, sometimes excision of coracoacromial ligament is adequate; I have yet to see acromioplasty necessary in this age group.

Little League Elbow

In a United States government study in 1981, elbow pain was noted in 20 per cent of pitchers under age 12, 40 per cent between age 13 and 14, and 58 per cent between 15 and 17. Pitchers and catchers are particularly susceptible to this problem. Painless asymptomatic loss of motion is frequently seen before pain becomes a paramount symptom and is most frequently seen at ages 12 to 14. It is most important to be able to differentiate the various types of Little League elbow, as they can be divided into three major categories: (1) the medial epicondyle, (2) the capitellum, and (3) the triceps insertion.

Medial Epicondyle. The medial epicondyle, which many people call the "funny bone," is usually inflamed owing to overuse from a rotary motion, although I recently saw a 15-year-old boy who threw his fast ball hard for an hour and ripped the entire flexor mass off after one particularly forceful pitch. In the younger child, with the apophysis open, it can occasionally lead to complete avulsion of the medial epicondyle, which of course will show on radiographs. Clinical symptoms are pain and tenderness over the funny bone area and pain on stressing the flexor muscles of the wrist and fingers. Radiographs may or may not be positive depending on whether there is some separation of the medial epicondyle; occasionally there may be some calcification 2 to 3 weeks after onset of symptoms just distal to the medial epicondyle.

Treatment for acute muscle avulsion is rest for 2 to 3 weeks and then gradual return to range of motion for a further 2 to 3 weeks. If there is an acute avulsion of the medial epicondyle, sometimes surgical replacement or excision and replacement of the flexor mass can be undertaken. It should be emphasized, however, that with complete avulsion of the flexor mass, full extension may never be achieved, even though there is complete healing of the lesion.

Capitellar Capitellum. A second type of Little League elbow is capitellar fragmentation, which may present with the symptoms of locking or loss of motion, especially extension, or may even present as pain over a palpable enlarged radial head area. Diagnosis can be made on examination with the loss of extension and tenderness over the radial capitellar joint and decrease in rotation and pain at extremes of supination and pronation. Radiography may often show, in a firmly established problem, fragmentation of the capitellum, enlargement of the radial head, and/or loose bodies. For the radiographically negative cases of relatively brief duration, rest and careful counseling about pitching habits usually suffice. When this does not promptly return range of motion to a reasonable level and/or a loose body is found, surgery may be indicated; although the results may be many months in coming, surgery can actually lead to a fairly decent return of motion, especially extension. Surgery can require anything from removal of loose bodies to an actual reconstruction of the articular surface of the capitellum.

Triceps Insertion. The final cause of Little League elbow is triceps insertion irritation. This is a very rare form of Little League elbow. On examination there is tenderness at the tip of the olecranon in the area of the insertion and tenderness on stress of the triceps. The radiographs may or may not show calcification in this area, and treatment is purely a decrease in activities. I have never seen a case in which surgical intervention was necessary.

de Quervain's Disease

Especially in the gymnastic, volleyball, and bowling sports, we see tenderness over the radial styloid characteristic of de Quervain's disease. At the radial styloid, the abductor pollicis longus tendon, accompanied by the extensor pollicis brevis, runs through a ligamentous synovium-lined sheath and is subject to considerable motion stress, especially ulnar deviation. Diagnosis may be made by simple palpation of the sheath. Also the Finkelstein test of flexion of the first metacarpal joint and increased pain over the radial styloid area caused by further ulnar flexion of the wrist joint are of use diagnostically. Treatment is usually conservative in nature, with immobilization of the wrist in a wrist splint and treatment with anti-inflammatories for 2 to 4 weeks.

If both wrists are involved, such as in gymnastic or volleyball type sports, the recovery period may be prolonged owing to an inability to rest both wrists completely. In the older child it is occasionally necessary to perform a surgical release of the sheath, with relatively careful follow-up thereafter.

THE HIP

LYNN T. STAHELI, M.D.

Hip problems in childhood are unusually serious for several reasons. First, the hip is normally only marginally competent; degenerative arthritis frequently occurs without known cause. Second, hip problems are often more difficult to diagnose than other joint disorders because of the hip's deep location under layers of muscle. Third, the blood supply to the proximal femoral epiphysis is tenuous. Trauma, inflammation, or compression can obstruct flow, cause necrosis, and permanently damage the hip in as short a time as 6 to 8 hours. Thus, early diagnosis of hip problems is critical. With early diagnosis and skillful management, deformity and disability can usually be prevented.

CONGENITAL DYSPLASIA OF THE HIP (CDH)

CDH includes a variety of deformities, from shallow acetabulum to frank dislocation. Effective management requires early diagnosis, which is not easy. The hip is primarily cartilaginous in the newborn, making radiography unreliable. Physical findings are subtle, and CDH can be missed by even the most skillful examiner. Thus, it is essential that the search for the problem continue throughout infancy.

Newborn Screening. The infant should be quiet and relaxed for the screening examination. The examiner employs Ortolani's or Barlow's maneuver to detect instability. "Clicks" are insignificant. "Clunks" or "jerks" are signs of instability felt by the examiner as the femoral head slides in and out of the socket. If screening is negative, the hip should be re-examined when the infant is next seen. If a "click" is heard, the infant should be examined at the next two or three visits to be certain that it is insignificant. If a "clunk" is felt, treatment is indicated. If the hip is stable in abduction, a simple, soft abduction splint is applied. If the hip is unstable, a "Pavlik harness" should be used. This harness is the most effective splint available.

If one is uncertain whether it is a "click" or a "clunk," the infant is either treated or referred. It is prudent to overtreat when in doubt. Triple diapers are not helpful and are often harmful. They become compressed between the thighs and provide little or no abduction. More importantly, they create the illusion that treatment is in progress when in fact valuable time is being wasted.

Early Infancy (1 to 3 Months). The physical findings change during the first weeks after birth. Hip instability signs, which are most reliable in the neonatal period, tend to disappear and are replaced by signs of limited abduction and limb shortening, which become more pronounced with increasing age.

HIGH-RISK INFANTS. The incidence of classic CDH is about 0.1 per cent. The chances increase 30 times when a positive family history is present. It is about 10 times more likely to occur in infants with metatarsus adductus. CDH is found in about 20 per cent of infants with torticollis. Infants at risk should have a single AP radiograph of the pelvis taken at 3 months of age. Some infants with a negative examination will have definite radiographic findings of CDH. Without treatment these children face early degenerative arthritis, perhaps as early as their teen years.

Radiography. Radiography in the newborn period is reliable in only about half of the cases. Reliability rapidly improves over the next 3 months, when it becomes the most definitive diagnostic method. A single AP radiograph of the pelvis is adequate for routine screening and follow-up evaluations. The slope of the acetabulum (acetabular index) is measured as an indicator of acetabular dysplasia. The relationship of the upper femur and acetabulum is assessed for evidence of dislocation. Ossification of the proximal femoral epiphysis, which normally occurs during the first 6 months, is often delayed in CDH. In its absence, the position of the upper femoral metaphysis is compared with the acetabulum. If the hip is reduced, the metaphysis will fall medial to a line (Perkin's) drawn vertically from the lateral margin of the acetabulum and at right angles to a line that passes through both triradiate cartilage clear spaces (Hilgenreiner's). If the epiphyseal ossification center is seen, it should fall in the inner lower quadrant created by the intersection of Perkin's and Hilgenreiner's lines.

The end point of treatment is a normal radiograph. After the hip is reduced, the physical examination becomes normal. Acetabular dysplasia may persist and must be corrected to ensure a lasting satisfactory result. This can only be assessed radiographically.

Older Infants and Children. Limited abduction, shortening of the limb, and limp are classic findings. Whenever the diagnosis is seriously considered, a radiograph should be taken.

Referral

The role of the primary care physician is diagnostic. Treatment should be provided by an orthopedic specialist. Objectives include achieving a concentric reduction, correcting acetabular dysplasia, and avoiding avascular necrosis. At present, Pavlik harness treatment is appropriate in infants under 6 months of age. Traditional traction, closed reduction under anesthesia, and cast immobilization are indicated if dislocation persists after a trial with the Pavlik harness, and for children first seen after 6 months of age. Open reduction is indicated if closed reduction fails or if the child is seen after about 2 years of age.

SEPTIC ARTHRITIS

Bacterial infection of the hip joint is one of the most urgent problems in orthopedics. It not only can damage the articular cartilage but also can obstruct the circulation to the epiphysis, causing avascular necrosis. The sequelae of necrosis include a severely shortened leg and a fused hip.

Early Infancy. Most sequelae of septic arthritis result from hip infections that occur during the neonatal period or early infancy. At that age diagnosis is difficult; systemic and localizing signs are few. The only reliable sign is "pseudoparalysis" of the involved limb. Spontaneous hip movement is absent. The cause should be determined. Trauma and true paralysis must also be considered.

Joint fluid examination is the only reliable method of establishing the diagnosis. Other studies are unreliable. When there is doubt, the joint is aspirated under image intensifier guidance. A negative study should be confirmed by arthrography. After aspiration, dye is instilled into the joint and a permanent radiograph is made. This confirms that the joint was entered.

In later infancy and childhood, diagnosing septic arthritis is less difficult. The patient is often ill, has guarding of the hip, resists rotational movement, and shows an elevated sedimentation rate. Again, these findings mandate the need for a diagnostic arthrocentesis. Studies such as bone scanning delay diagnosis and usually are of little help.

Radiography is of limited value. Fat pad signs are not reliable. It is a common mistake to rely on negative radiographs. Only a negative arthrocentesis documented with an arthrogram can rule out the presence of septic arthritis.

If purulent fluid is obtained from the arthrocentesis, the joint should be surgically drained. An open procedure makes certain the joint is completely evacuated and will remain free of fluid. Incomplete drainage by needle aspiration is too risky to be justified. The potential for disability is too great. About 20 per cent of purulent drainage will be culture and Gram stain negative. This is to be expected. Open drainage and antibiotic treatment should be provided. The antibiotic is selected empirically, using the age of the patient as a guide.

TOXIC SYNOVITIS

Toxic synovitis or "observation hip syndrome" is a benign inflammatory problem of the hip of unknown etiology. It commonly occurs in late infancy and childhood, and in 1 to 3 per cent of cases leads to Perthes' disease.

The major diagnostic problem is clearly separating this benign condition from septic arthritis. Differentiation is made by considering several factors: (1) The patient with synovitis is usually not as ill as the child with arthritis. The child's fever, malaise, and activity level are helpful guides. (2) In septic arthritis, joint guarding is more pronounced and the patient will usually refuse to walk. (3) The ESR is usually slightly elevated in synovitis and moderately or severely elevated

in septic arthritis. Leukocytosis is variable in both. (4) If the diagnosis remains uncertain, an arthrocentesis is indicated. It should be re-emphasized that radiographs and bone scans are seldom helpful in making this differentiation.

Synovitis is managed by rest. Traction on the limb is unnecessary and theoretically harmful. The hip joint capsule is most relaxed and, thus, the joint capacity the greatest, when the hip is flexed, slightly abducted, and laterally rotated. The patient will assume this position while resting. Traction is likely to alter this position, increasing the intra-articular pressure and possibly impairing circulation to the epiphysis.

Bed rest is continued until hip rotation is free and unguarded. A check-up should be made in a month or so to ensure that motion has completely returned. Persisting stiffness is an indication for a radiograph to rule out Perthes' disease.

PERTHES' DISEASE

Perthes' disease is commonly referred to as LCP disease, a name derived from the initials of those first describing the disease (Legg-Calvé-Perthes). LCP is an idiopathic avascular necrosis of the femoral capital epiphysis that occurs spontaneously during midchildhood. Healing occurs consistently but slowly over 2 to 3 years. Residual deformity may lead to degenerative arthritis in adult life. LCP tends to occur in some families, in children of delayed skeletal age, and occasionally following toxic synovitis. It affects boys most frequently, and in most cases the cause is unknown. During midchildhood, circulation to the femoral epiphysis is even more tenuous than at other ages, being almost totally provided by the lateral retinacular vessels. These may be obstructed by trauma, inflammation, coagulation defects, or other causes.

LCP disease results from one or more ischemic episodes occurring at different sites in the vascular network. In mild cases only the anterior portion of the head is involved; in severe cases the whole head is involved. The disease is also more serious in the older child.

Clinical Features. Onset is usually insidious. It commonly occurs in one hip of a boy between 4 and 8 years of age but may occur in either sex between ages 3 and 14 years. The child presents with a limp and mild discomfort. Often the symptoms are present for months before the family seeks medical attention. The physical findings include limitation of abduction and medial rotation of the affected hip. Radiographic features vary according to the stage of the disease. *Synovitic stage:* This stage has usually passed by the time the child is first seen. If the child is seen very early in the disease process, the radiographs may show slight joint space widening. *Necrotic or collapse stage:* The earliest definitive sign is a crescentic radiolucency just under the subchondral bone of the epiphysis on the lateral projection. More commonly there is a flattening, irregularity, and increased density of the epiphysis. *Fragmentation stage:* Replacement of necrotic bone with preossified fibrous tissue produces a "moth-eaten" appearance characteristic of this stage. *Consolidation stage:* Reossification progresses with increasing homogeniety of the epiphysis. Widening of the neck and head (coxa magna) and flattening of the epiphysis (coxa plana) are frequently seen.

These stages take several years to run their course. Treatment is usually started during the necrotic stage and continues through the fragmentation stage. This requires about 12 to 18 months.

Management. Treatment is controversial, but current management trends are conservative. Individualized management, fewer operative procedures, and shorter treatment periods with less cumbersome braces are currently favored. The first step is restoration of motion by rest. Activity causes microfractures of the soft, ischemic epiphysis. These fractures induce synovitis, which causes stiffness and adductor contracture. Rest reduces this inflammation and allows return of motion. Active motion is encouraged. Traction to immobilize the child and gently stretch the tight adductor muscles is appropriate in some cases. This can be done at home or in the hospital. The objective is to maintain the sphericity of the femoral head during the healing process by providing "containment." The uninvolved firm acetabulum is utilized as a mold to maintain the shape of the head. This requires that the hip be maintained in abduction, usually with an abduction brace. Currently, the smaller, lighter braces are most favored because they allow the child to maintain a nearly normal activity level.

No treatment is required for mild LCP disease. For severe cases, treatment is much less effective. In some cases, maintaining containment by operation is appropriate. The procedures alter the shape of the upper femur or acetabulum so that containment is provided with the child standing in the normal weight-bearing attitude.

SLIPPED CAPITAL FEMORAL EPIPHYSIS (SCFE)

SCFE is a fracture of the capital femoral epiphysis that usually occurs in the pubescent male and gradually produces progressive displacement (chronic slip). Occasionally, acute injury produces varying degrees of slip. Often these are superimposed on the chronic form.

SCFE is a serious condition. The slipping not only produces deformity but also stretches the vessels to the epiphysis. Prognosis depends upon the severity of displacement, which in turn is dependent upon the duration of the problem. Early diagnosis is critical.

SCFE is suspected when the pubertal patient complains of hip or knee pain. As the obturator nerve innervates both the hip and knee, referred pain to the knee is common. The physical examination demonstrates limited medial rotation of the hip. This is best evaluated with the patient prone and the knees flexed to a right angle. Both thighs are then rotated in (feet going out), while the pelvis is held in a level position. Asymmetry of rotation is consistent with the diagnosis. Diagnosis is established by a lateral radiograph. A so-called frog lateral of the pelvis is ordered. This view demonstrates the characteristic posterior displacement of the femoral epiphysis relative to the neck. In addition, diffuse rarefaction of the metaphysis and widening of the physis are seen.

After the diagnosis is established, the patient should be hospitalized without delay, since further slipping can occur at any time and fixation of the epiphysis by operation is essential. Fixation is achieved by passing two or three threaded pins across the physis. This promotes fusion, preventing further displacement.

INFANTILE CORTICAL HYPEROSTOSIS

DONALD B. DARLING, M.D.

Infantile cortical hyperostosis (ICH) is a disorder of unknown etiology characterized by the sudden development of soft tissue swelling, periosteal thickening of the underlying bone, and constitutional symptoms of variable severity. It can develop in utero and be present at birth; onset of the usual postnatal form is rare after 6 months of age. A sporadic type (now rare) and a familial form inherited as an autosomal dominant with variable expression and incomplete penetrance have been described. ICH occurs equally in boys and girls, is global in distribution, and is found in all ethnic, economic, and social groups.

The usual clinical presentation is the sudden appearance of deep soft tissue swelling over an affected bone (e.g., mandible, clavicle, ulna, tibia) in a previously well infant 7 to 10 weeks of age. The swelling is tender, wooden-hard, and firmly fixed to the bone; local warmth of the part, edema or discoloration of the overlying skin, and local lymphadenopathy are conspicuously absent. The infant is hyperirritable, usually febrile, and, when an extremity is involved, may refuse to move the part (pseudoparalysis). The erythrocyte sedimentation rate and serum alkaline phosphatase are elevated; leukocytosis and anemia may be present, but other laboratory tests are negative. A bone scan will be positive before radiographic changes are seen. Marked thickening of the entire shaft of the underlying bone will be found on radiography within 15 to 20 days of clinical onset.

In mild cases involving a single bone (usually the mandible), the soft tissue swelling and acute symptoms resolve in a few weeks; in infants with multiple sites of involvement, new areas of acute swelling may develop as the initial sites resolve, and local recurrences in previously involved areas may occur. As acuity of symptoms corresponds to the phase (developing or resolving) of the local lesions, clinical evolution in infants with multiple sites may last several weeks to months; in some cases, local swelling may persist for 18 to 20 months.

Twelve months after disappearance of the soft tissue swelling, the periosteal thickening evident by radiography has usually resolved; however, bony synostoses (ribs, radius/ulna, tibia/fibula), radial head dislocation, and anterior tibial bowing deformities are permanent residuals.

Osteomyelitis and the parent-trauma syndrome are differentiated from ICH by positive blood and bone cultures and by metaphyseal avulsion fractures and other evidence of trauma, respectively. Less frequent conditions to consider are healing scurvy, healing rickets, congenital syphilis, hypervitaminosis A, isolated trauma, and prostaglandin effect.

Treatment is generally supportive; infants with severe symptoms respond to steroids given for several weeks with slow withdrawal. Investigation of siblings and cousins should be considered in view of the familial pattern of the disorder as currently seen.

BONE AND JOINT INFECTIONS

NEIL E. GREEN, M.D.

The diagnosis of bone and joint infections is made on the basis of well-established clinical findings. Confirmation of the diagnosis may be sought with laboratory data, e.g., CBC and ESR, but normal laboratory findings do not rule out infection. Bacterial diagnosis of the infection is established through aspiration, which also yields information about the presence or absence of an abscess in acute osteomyelitis and about the status of joint fluid in patients with acute septic arthritis.

ACUTE SEPTIC ARTHRITIS

The most common infecting organisms are *Haemophilus influenzae* in children 6 months to 5 years of age, and *Staphylococcus aureus* in all age groups, although group B *Streptococcus* and gram-negative organisms are seen in neonates and gonococcus in teenagers.

The septic joint must be drained as part of the management of acute septic arthritis. This drainage may be performed either with needle aspiration or by open surgical drainage. The decision as to whether needle aspiration-irrigation or open drainage is necessary depends upon the duration and extent of the infection and the joint involved.

Needle aspiration-irrigation may be utilized for joint drainage in easily accessible joints, e.g., knee and ankle, and in early infections before precipitated fibrin has formed. Therefore, on initial aspiration, if the fluid is thin and contains no particulate matter, needle drainage may suffice. It is performed through a large-bore (18-gauge) needle. The involved joint is aspirated until dry and then irrigated until clear with normal saline through the aspirating needle.

Needle aspiration-irrigation is not appropriate treatment for the hip joint, which requires emergent open surgical drainage to preserve the blood supply to the femoral head. Other joints that are difficult to aspirate and irrigate, e.g., elbow, wrist, and tarsal joints, may also require open surgical drainage. Open drainage is also required if there is reaccumulation of pus with persistent sepsis 24 to 36 hours after initial aspiration-irrigation.

Open surgical debridement is necessary to remove debris within the joint and should be performed through a small incision. After thorough irrigation and debridement, the wound is closed over a drain. Some authors have recommended arthroscopic debridement; however, one may not be able to adequately debride all

of the precipitated fibrin through the arthroscope. Initially, the joint should be immobilized in the position of function, but early motion is started to prevent joint contracture.

Antibiotics are begun once cultures have been obtained using Gram's stain or best guess to assist in the choice of antibiotics while awaiting the culture results. *S. aureus* is the most common pathogen overall, and oxacillin is commonly used with this bacterium. In neonates, penicillin is added for coverage of group B *Streptococcus* and an aminoglycoside for gram-negative bacteria coverage. Since children between the ages of 6 months and 5 years are likely to have an infected joint secondary to *H. influenzae,* both this organism and *Staphylococcus* must be covered. Ampicillin should not be used initially, because of the high resistance rate of *H. influenzae* to this drug. Cefamandole also must not be used, because it does not cross the blood-brain barrier, and meningitis may occur along with septic arthritis. One may choose a semisynthetic penicillin such as oxacillin plus chloramphenicol, or a single antibiotic such as cefuroxime, which will cover both bacteria, is appropriate. Initially, antibiotics should be administered intravenously, but one may switch to oral antibiotics after 4 to 7 days if there has been a prompt response to intravenous therapy. Total treatment of 2 to 3 weeks is usually sufficient for the uncomplicated case. Gonococcal arthritis is usually treated with 3 days of intravenous penicillin followed by 4 days of ampicillin or amoxicillin therapy.

ACUTE HEMATOGENOUS OSTEOMYELITIS

The diagnosis of acute bone and joint infection is made on clinical grounds. Any child with a fever and bone and joint pain is considered to have an acute bone or joint infection until proven otherwise. Thus, the other studies that one may order are for confirmation or for bacterial identification. Bone aspiration is imperative for the identification of the infecting organism and also for the determination of the presence or absence of an abscess. The bone is aspirated both extraperiosteally and intraosseously. If no abscess is encountered, the marrow contents are cultured. The culture is positive 90 per cent of the time. Blood cultures should also be obtained even though the positive yield is only 50 per cent. Antibiotics are begun intravenously as soon as all cultures have been obtained. The most common organism by far is *S. aureus,* and a semisynthetic penicillin or a cephalosporin is begun while awaiting culture results (Table 1). In neonates, group B streptococci and gram-negative organisms are also seen, and therefore coverage for these organisms should be added until the cultures have been returned, at which time the antibiotics are adjusted to reflect the sensitivities of the infecting organism.

Intravenous antibiotic treatment should continue for 5 to 7 days, at which time oral antibiotics may be used if the patient has responded immediately, the organism is able to be treated with an oral agent, the patient is compliant, and the laboratory is able to perform serum bactericidal titers. The peak serum bactericidal titer should be at least 1:8 against *Staphylococcus.* The oral

TABLE 1. Antibiotic Dosage of Commonly Used Antibiotics

Antibiotic	Intravenous Dosage	Oral Dosage
Ampicillin	150 mg/kg/day q6h	
Amoxicillin		150 mg/kg/day q6h
Cefuroxime	100 mg/kg/day q8h	
Cephalexin		100 mg/kg/day q6h
Chloramphenicol	75 mg/kg/day q6h	50–75 mg/kg/day q6h
Clindamycin	30 mg/kg/day q8h	30 mg/kg/day q6h
Cloxacillin		100 mg/kg/day q6h
Dicloxacillin		50–75 mg/kg/day q6h
Gentamicin	6–7.5 mg/kg/day q8h	
Oxacillin	150–200 mg/kg/day q6h	

dosage of the antibiotic is much higher than is usually prescribed for routine infections (Table 1). The oral suspension of dicloxacillin and cloxacillin is not palatable, and therefore oral cephalexin may be preferred in patients unable to swallow capsules. The total duration of antibiotic therapy varies according to the type and location of the infection, the clinical response, and the amount of bone destruction seen. In general, 3 to 6 weeks of total antibiotic therapy are used.

If pus is encountered on initial aspiration or if there is lack of response with decrease in fever and pain in 24 to 36 hours, one must suspect the presence of an abscess, which requires drainage. Acute hematogenous osteomyelitis is neither a surgical nor a medical disease; rather, it is an infectious disease. Antibiotic treatment is always necessary, and surgical drainage is necessary if an abscess has formed. On the other hand, if the patient is seen early in the course of the disease and an abscess has not yet formed, antibiotic therapy alone will eradicate the infection as long as an abscess does not form during therapy.

SUBACUTE HEMATOGENOUS OSTEOMYELITIS

Children with a subacute bone infection do not have the severity of symptoms seen in an acute infection. There is usually radiographic evidence of bone involvement, which can occur anywhere in the bone. The treatment of these infections is usually surgical drainage and debridement in addition to anti-*Staphylococcus* antibiotics. The cultures are frequently sterile; nevertheless, the infecting organism is invariably *Staphylococcus*. Intravenous antibiotics may be switched to oral therapy within 5 days. Therapy is usually continued for at least 3 to 6 weeks or until there has been significant resolution of the bone changes seen radiographically.

CHRONIC OSTEOMYELITIS

Chronic osteomyelitis is rarely seen after appropriately treated acute hematogenous osteomyelitis, although it may occur after an open fracture. Regardless of the etiology of the chronic infection, the treatment of this infection requires surgical debridement of the sequestered bone in addition to appropriate antibiotic coverage for a prolonged period of time. We have generally used intravenous antibiotics for up to 3 weeks, followed by oral antibiotics until significant healing of the bone lesion has occurred. This may require months of antibiotic therapy.

DISC SPACE INFECTION

This is a distinct disease entity that can affect children of all ages but is most frequently seen in young children. The term "discitis" is sometimes used, but it should be remembered that this is a subacute osteomyelitis of the vertebral endplates which secondarily infects the disc. Needle aspiration of the infected disc is not recommended in young children because the organism is invariably *Staphylococcus*. However, aspiration or open biopsy is necessary if the lesion occurs in adolescents or teens, in whom the organism may be other than *Staphylococcus*, especially if drug abuse is suspected. Treatment with anti-staphylococcal antibiotics given intravenously initially and then switched to oral medication relieves symptoms in 24 to 36 hours. Cast immobilization is not required unless there has been bone destruction and stability of the spine is in question.

PSEUDOMONAS INFECTIONS OF THE FOOT AFTER PUNCTURE WOUNDS

Nail puncture wounds are relatively common, and fortunately most do not result in a bone or joint infection; however, if the nail has penetrated a bone or a joint, an infection is common. The organism is invariably *Pseudomonas*. This infection requires surgical debridement of the involved bone or joint along with appropriate coverage for *Pseudomonas* with an aminoglycoside. Antibiotic therapy is continued for 2 to 6 weeks depending upon the involvement. For joint infections, 2 weeks of medication is sufficient, whereas for a bone infection with significant bone involvement, 6 weeks of antibiotics may be required. One may use the sedimentation rate to guide therapy, and the drugs may be stopped after the erythrocyte sedimentation rate has stabilized in the normal range.

MALIGNANT BONE TUMORS

MARK C. LEESOM, M.D.

The incidence of primary malignant neoplasms arising in bone has been relatively unchanged over the past 30 years; however, as the population has increased in size, the absolute number of patients with primary malignancies of bone has steadily increased. An increase in the awareness of the problem and improvements in diagnostic technologies have led to earlier and more accurate diagnoses. This has allowed the orthopedic oncologist to successfully treat many of these patients in a more aggressive surgical fashion. Limb salvage procedures, not very long ago thought of as experimental in nature, are now not only acceptable but in many instances are the surgical treatment of choice. Changes in and combinations of chemotherapy have also led to improvements in survival rates. The remainder of this article details the current management strategies in the treatment of primary malignant tumors of bone in the pediatric population.

OSTEOSARCOMA

Osteosarcoma represents approximately 60 per cent of the primary malignant bone tumors in the pediatric population. The etiology remains unknown; however, a number of cases per year are secondary to therapeutic radiation (increased incidence in patients with retinoblastoma).

Careful evaluation of patients for pulmonary metastases is an integral part of preoperative staging and long-term follow-up. In the past, conventional tomography and plain films were the standard; however, recent studies clearly demonstrate that computed axial tomography detects pulmonary metastases with greater sensitivity than any other current test.

Surgery remains a mainstay in patient management. The goal of surgery is to remove the entire primary tumor with a wide margin of normal tissue. In the past, this has almost routinely meant an amputation. Currently, however, limb salvage procedures can be employed in up to 50 per cent of patients with osteosarcoma of the extremity.

Chemotherapy was initially used in patients with osteosarcoma that was metastatic or recurrent following initial surgery. Because the results of management with surgery alone are so poor, investigative trials of adjuvant chemotherapy following surgical resection were begun. This led to the decision to use chemotherapy "up front" or after biopsy and prior to definitive surgical procedure. The current treatment of choice is to use chemotherapy following biopsy and prior to definitive surgical intervention. Chemotherapy is also used following surgery for 12 to 18 months. A few centers are trying intra-arterial chemotherapy with and without preoperative radiation prior to surgical extirpation. The use of combination chemotherapy prior to and after surgery has increased the 5-year disease-free survival in osteosarcoma to 50 to 75 per cent. The main chemotherapeutic agent used in this regard is high-dose methotrexate. Other drugs used in combination include bleomycin, cyclophosphamide, and actinomycin-D. Following surgical resection, the pathologist studies the resected specimen and grades it with regard to tumor kill. Depending on the amount of tumor cell necrosis, the postoperative chemotherapy is either similar to the preoperative course, or if the tumor kill percentage is low, the postoperative chemotherapy is changed. *Cis*-platinum is often used in those cases with poor response to preoperative high-dose methotrexate.

Metastatic Disease

Approximately 15 to 25 per cent of the patients with osteosarcomas present with detectable metastatic disease at the time of primary presentation. The aggressive management of these metastatic lesions (surgery and chemotherapy) has produced an increased rate of survival and should be strongly considered in appropriate cases. A number of studies report disease-free survival as high as 40 per cent following the aggressive management of these metastatic lesions.

Pulmonary Metastases

Patients who develop pulmonary metastases may still have the opportunity for cure with surgical intervention. Depending on the number and location, either unilateral or bilateral thoracotomies may be performed. Up to 50 per cent of the patients who develop pulmonary metastases during treatment may still be rendered free of disease with the use of adjuvant chemotherapy, thoracotomy, and tumor resection.

Limb-Sparing Surgery

Since the large majority of osteosarcomas occur in the extremities of adolescents and young adults, the possibility of preserving limb function for this young and productive population is an appealing one. It should be continually stressed, however, that the primary objective in the management of osteosarcoma is disease-free survival. Limb preservation is a worthwhile but secondary objective. Limb salvage procedures are more complex than amputation. Wound healing, local recurrence, and overall limb function all must be considered in the individual case prior to initiating this type of surgery. Over the past few years, it has become clear that the use of limb salvage procedures in appropriate instances has little or no increased risk of local recurrence or distant metastases. Limb reconstruction may be accomplished in a variety of ways: large bone allografts, vascularized autografts, customized prostheses, or a combination of these.

PAROSTEAL OSTEOSARCOMA

Parosteal osteosarcoma is a less common, low-grade malignancy most often involving the long bones. In contrast to the classic high-grade osteogenic sarcoma, parosteal osteosarcoma has little or no response to chemotherapy or radiation. Surgical excision is the mainstay of management. Local resection (limb salvage) is the treatment of choice instead of amputation if a wide margin can be obtained. These are slow-growing neoplasms, and long-term follow-up is necessary to observe for local recurrence or distant metastases.

EWING'S SARCOMA

Ewing's sarcoma is the second most common primary malignancy of bone in the pediatric population. The management of patients with this neoplasm continues to evolve. Treated initially with surgery alone, the 5-year survival rate was less than 10 per cent. With the advent of radiation therapy and then chemotherapy, the role of surgery as part of the treatment protocol decreased. Although radiation and chemotherapy provide increased ability to "control" the tumor locally, local recurrence and/or metastatic disease are still very common, and the 5-year disease-free survival remains under 20 per cent. Patients with large central or axial lesions (pelvis, shoulder girdle, spine, ribs) tend to have a worse overall prognosis.

Management

The progress in the management of Ewing's sarcoma came following the introduction of systemic chemotherapy. The medications that have proved effective include vincristine, actinomycin-D, cyclophosphamide, and doxorubicin. Most chemotherapy protocols employ a combination of these medications along with the occasional use of prednisone. The major significant randomized trials have been performed by a multicenter study group and clearly demonstrate increased survival with the use of adjuvant chemotherapy along with surgery and radiation therapy. In another surgical study from the Mayo Clinic, patients who had surgical removal of confirmed Ewing's sarcoma along with chemotherapy and radiation had statistically significant improved survival, independent of primary site. Most patients have (wide surgical) local excisions. In this series, the overall 5-year disease-free survival rate in patients with complete surgical excision, chemotherapy, and radiation was 74 per cent, which is a dramatic improvement over the previous rates of 25 to 35 per cent.

Metastatic Disease

Patients who develop metastatic disease tend to have a dismal prognosis. Long-term disease-free survival in this group is less than 10 per cent. These patients are usually managed with systemic chemotherapy and radiation alone.

CHONDROSARCOMA

Chondrosarcomas are rare neoplasms and represent approximately 10 per cent of all malignant primary bone tumors. They appear more frequently in the adult or middle-aged patient, although the occurrence of chondrosarcoma in patients under 21 years of age represents approximately 10 to 16 per cent of all patients with chondrosarcoma. One of the most important parts of management may be the recognition of the lesion as a primary malignancy.

The treatment of new patients with chondrosarcoma remains predominantly surgical. An adequate margin of resection is essential and critical to the best chance for long-term survival. Limb salvage procedures may certainly be considered on an individual, case-by-case basis. In the past, chemotherapy such as doxorubicin and radiation therapy have been used, but neither has demonstrated any statistical success in the treatment of either primary or metastatic chondrosarcoma.

FIBROSARCOMA

Congenital or infantile fibrosarcoma is a rare but well-recognized malignancy, almost always involving soft tissue. It has rarely been reported in bone. It usually behaves as an aggressive, high-grade lesion most often requiring amputation.

Malignant Fibrous Histiocytoma

Malignant fibrous histiocytoma (MFH) is one of the most common primary malignancies in adults (bony and soft tissue) but is extremely uncommon in the pediatric population. It usually manifests itself in adolescents who already have closed growth plates. The mainstay of management is obtaining a wide or radical surgical excision (amputation versus limb salvage). Adjuvant chemotherapy is also being used, although there has been no good statistical evidence that it increases the disease-free survival or improves the overall prognosis.

14

Muscles

CONGENITAL MUSCULAR DEFECTS

BRUCE O. BERG, M.D.

These abnormalities of muscle include the congenital myopathies and those circumstances in which part or all of the entire muscle is absent. A myopathy is any abnormality of muscle—structural, biochemical, or electrophysiologic in which there is no related neurologic abnormality. A muscular dystrophy, on the other hand, is a genetically determined primary disease of muscle characterized by muscle fiber degeneration.

Congenital myopathies (Table 1) are apparent at birth or shortly thereafter and are characterized by weakness and usually hypotonia. Weakness is found primarily in proximal muscles. There is usually decreased muscle bulk, and the stretch reflexes are normal to decreased. Serum creatine phosphokinase is normal to mildly elevated; electromyographic studies may be normal but commonly demonstrate short-duration, low-amplitude polyphasic motor unit potentials. The congenital myopathies are named in accordance with the structural changes demonstrated on muscle biopsy.

Associated skeletal abnormalities, including elongation of facial features, narrow high arched palate, hip dislocation, lordosis, kyphoscoliosis, and pes cavus, are often present. A variety of orthotic and surgical procedures may be required for improvement or correction of skeletal deformities, particularly those affecting the hips, ankles, and feet.

The congenital absence of muscle may be partial or complete and, although primarily unilateral and involving one muscle, may be bilateral and symmetrical, affecting related muscle groups. The resulting disability is relatively stable. Muscles of the shoulder girdle, upper limbs, and neck are most commonly affected, particularly the sternocostal heads of the pectorals, the trapezius, and the sternocleidomastoids. Occasionally, the congenital absence of pectoral muscles may be accompanied by scoliosis and webbed fingers. No specific treatment is useful, and only a frank discussion of the matter with parents and child is required.

The absence or marked hypoplasia of abdominal muscles may affect respiration, coughing, and defecation. Impairment of normal thoracic excursion may be severe, resulting in pulmonary infection and further pulmonary insufficiency. Anomalies of the genitourinary and gastrointestinal systems are frequently associated with congenital absence of the abdominal muscles. Treatment consists of providing a functional abdominal support, a complete evaluation, and treatment of any concomitant anomaly.

Other skeletal muscles, including the levator palpebrae and external ocular muscles, have been reported as congenitally absent. A variety of ophthalmologic surgical procedures are available to effect not only visual but cosmetic improvement.

TORTICOLLIS

THOMAS S. RENSHAW, M.D.

Although torticollis, or "wry neck," is usually a benign cosmetic problem secondary to muscle tightness and responds successfully to stretching exercises during infancy, one must realize that there are causes of torticollis for which an exercise program could bring about catastrophic results. These include traumatic or congenital spinal lesions producing instability between the occiput and C1, or C1 and C2, such as congenital hypoplasia or aplasia of the odontoid, nonunion of an odontoid fracture, rupture of the transverse alar ligament of C1, and subluxation of C1 and C2. Torticollis can also result from a tumor in the bony vertebral column or brain or spinal cord. Infections in the neck involving the retropharyngeal space, a disc space, or upper respiratory tract have also caused torticollis. It is, therefore, essential in the evaluation to have good radiographs of the entire cervical spine in both frontal and sagittal planes, as well as dynamic flexion and extension lateral views to assess the stability from the occiput to C2. There is a 10 to 20 per cent incidence of congenital hip dysplasia associated with infantile idiopathic torticollis. In addition, approximately 15 per cent of all torticollis has an

TABLE 1. Congenital Myopathies*

Disease	Clinical Features	Muscle Biopsy
Central core disease	Hypotonia noted at birth or shortly thereafter; motor development delayed. Diffuse weakness, primarily proximal; stretch reflexes normal to reduced. Skeletal abnormalities may occur (hip dislocation, kyphoscoliosis, lordosis, pes cavus). Inherited as autosomal dominant trait, but sporadic cases occur. Serum CPK usually normal; EMG findings nonspecific. Malignant hyperthermia known to occur.	Variability of fiber diameter; often with predominance of type I fibers. Within the fiber, centrally or peripherally, are cores devoid of oxidative enzyme activity. Myofibrillary ATPase activity of cores normal to decreased.
Myotubular myopathy (centronuclear)	Hypotonic at birth with ptosis, external ophthalmoplegia, and occasionally facial weakness. Decreased muscle power throughout, greater distally than proximally. Neonatal type described with profound weakness at birth (may die in infancy). Inheritance reported as usually X-linked recessive, but autosomal dominant and recessive traits reported. Serum CPK normal to moderately increased. EMG nonspecific.	Predominance of type I fibers with central nuclei surrounded by clear area. Type I atrophy has been recorded. Increased central staining with oxidative enzymes and pale central area with ATPase reactions.
Congenital fiber type disproportion	Hypotonia and generalized weakness present at birth. Muscle contractures are often present with skeletal abnormalities (high arched palate, congenital hip dislocation, kyphoscoliosis, varus or valgus foot deformities). Rarely, external ophthalmoplegia occurs. Commonly, clinical status remains static or improves.	Type I fibers are more numerous and smaller than type II fibers.
Mitochondrial myopathies	Heterogeneous group of diseases with normal as well as abnormally shaped and enlarged mitochondria within muscle fibers. Symptoms usually begin in childhood but may appear at any time. External ocular muscle weakness a frequent finding. Excessive muscular fatigue following exercise is common. Inheritance is variable. Structural changes of muscle are nonspecific and have been reported in a variety of disorders (hypothyroidism, polymyositis, thyrotoxic myopathy, and spinal muscular atrophy).	Mitochondrial abnormalities suspected on light microscopy by accumulation of subsarcolemmal or intramyofibrillary granules, which are irregular and stain red with modified trichrome stain— "ragged red fibers."
Multicore disease	Several patients described with nonprogressive generalized hypotonia and weakness of trunk and limb muscles, proximal greater than distal. Stretch reflexes are decreased. Serum CPK is normal; EMG demonstrates short duration motor unit potentials or normal findings.	Predominance of type I fibers and numerous small randomly distributed areas of types I and II, with focal decreased oxidative enzyme activity and focal myofibrillary degeneration.
Nemaline myopathy	Hypotonia at birth; some mothers indicate decreased fetal movement. Poor suck, swallow, and respiratory embarrassment; delay in achieving milestones. Elongated face with narrow high arched palate, prognathism, dental malocclusion, and pigeon chest. Stretch reflexes reduced to absent. Inherited as autosomal recessive or dominant traits; sporadic cases known to occur. Serum CPK normal to mildly increased. EMG demonstrates brief, low amplitude, abundant, polyphasic motor potentials.	Usually a predominance of type I fibers; about half of type I fibers are small. Subsarcolemmal collection of ("nemaline") rods seen with vesicular nuclei and prominent nucleoli.
Trilaminar neuromuscular disease	Very rare congenital neuromuscular disease with muscular rigidity at birth. Muscles are hard on palpation. Stretch reflexes are normal. CPK in early infancy reported as markedly increased, but decreases near end of first year. EMG has been normal.	About 15% of fibers demonstrate three concentric zones of differential (trilaminar fibers). At EM, a sharp delineation is demonstrated between the outer and middle zones, but junction is not defined by membrane.
Reducing body myopathy	Profound hypotonia with decreased muscle bulk, generalized weakness, and stretch reflexes depressed to absent. Milestones delayed. Serum CPK normal to mildly elevated. EMG demonstrated myopathic potentials.	Variability of fiber size with predominance of type I fibers. Large numbers of fibers contain "reducing bodies" rich in sulfhydryl groups and RNA.
Fingerprint body myopathy	Hypotonia and generalized weakness, usually with sparing of external and bulbar muscles. Stretch reflexes reduced to absent. Muscle bulk reduced. Serum CPK normal to mildly elevated and EMG studies have varied from normal to "consistent with myopathy."	Small type I fibers and hypertrophied type II fibers. EM demonstrates inclusions composed of concentric lamellae resembling fingerprints. Similar structures also found in dermatomyositis, myotonic dystrophy, and oculopharyngeal muscular dystrophy.
Sarcotubular myopathy	One case report of two brothers whose parents were third cousins. Patients were clumsy and had mild weakness of proximal limb muscles and neck flexors. Stretch reflexes were normal to mildly decreased. Serum CPK normal to mildly decreased.	Vacuolar changes seen selectively affecting type II fibers. A "myriad" of small spaces were seen on cross-section in affected muscles and in longitudinal section; vacuolization was segmental.

*From Berg BO: Child Neurology. Jones Medical Publications, 1984, pp 116–117.

ophthalmologic basis, the most common cause being amblyopia.

Idiopathic muscular torticollis is a condition that usually presents in early infancy but can develop at any time during childhood. It may be caused by injury to the nerve or vascular supply to the sternocleidomastoid muscle. In children under age 1 year who have little or no facial asymmetry, an exercise program is almost always successful. The specific exercise is designed to place maximum distance between the ipsilateral sternoclavicular joint and mastoid process and is done by bending the neck laterally *away* from the torticollis and then slowly providing maximal rotation of the head and face to the side of the torticollis. This position should be held for about 5 seconds and then released and repeated ten times, at least four times a day, or better yet, with each diaper change. Another conservative therapeutic method involves positioning the infant prone in the crib with the normal side toward the wall, which may cause some rotation toward the affected side and help with the stretching exercise program. The exercises are worth trying in children beyond age 1 year, but often by that time surgical treatment will be necessary. There is a high failure rate with the exercise program at any age when the torticollis is accompanied by significant facial asymmetry and/or the restriction of neck rotation exceeds 30 degrees when compared with the normal side.

When surgical treatment is indicated, the treatment of choice is a distal release of both the sternal and clavicular attachments of the sternocleidomastoid muscle. As long as the incision is placed 1.5 to 2 cm above the clavicle, the cosmetic result is quite acceptable. It is rarely necessary to do bipolar tenotomy or a single release at the mastoid area. Surgical results are not age-dependent, and a good result may be expected up to and beyond age 10 years. Postoperative management usually consists of a brace for a period of approximately 4 weeks used in conjunction with an appropriate exercise program.

CONGENITAL HYPOTONIA

HERBERT E. GILMORE, M.D.

Normal body tone is maintained by the activity of the gamma-motor system. Central control is mediated through the basal ganglia, cerebellum, and brain stem (mainly vestibular) nuclei. Rubrospinal, reticulospinal, and other motor pathways carry impulses from these centers to the cells of the intermediate and anterior horns of the spinal cord. From there they are relayed through the nerve roots, peripheral nerves, and myoneural junction to the muscle spindle and somatic muscle cells. When the activity of any of these areas is disrupted, hypotonia can develop. Infantile hypotonia is caused by many disorders, which affect various levels of the nervous system. Table 1 lists the major diseases affecting each site. Appropriate evaluation of the hypotonic infant is dependent on a clinical and laboratory

TABLE 1. Causes of Congenital Hypotonia

Central Nervous System Diseases
  Perinatal hypoxia-ischemia
  Congenital infections (TORCH)
  Encephalitis, meningitis
  Trauma
  Hydrocephalus
  Syringobulbia
  Brain tumors: medulloblastoma, pontine glioma
  Chromosomal disorders: trisomy 13, 21
  Amino and organic acidopathies
  Progressive leukoencephalopathies (Pelizaeus-Merzbacher, Canavan's)
  Lysosomal storage diseases (Tay-Sachs, Gaucher's, etc.)
Spinal Cord Diseases
  Infantile spinal muscular atrophy (Werdnig-Hoffmann)
  Poliomyelitis
  Trauma: C1–C2 subluxation, C5–C6 distraction
  Severe perinatal hypoxia-ischemia
Nerve Root and Peripheral Nerve Diseases
  Postinfectious polyradiculoneuropathy (Guillain-Barré)
  Infantile neuropathies
Myoneural Diseases
  Myasthenia gravis: transient and persistent forms
  Infantile botulism
Muscle Diseases
  Congenital myopathies (myotubular, mitochondrial, nemaline rod, etc.)
  Infantile myotonic dystrophy
  Polymyositis
  Carnitine deficiency
  Pompe's disease
Combined Central and Peripheral Diseases
  Leigh's disease
  Prader-Willi syndrome
Non-Neurological Diseases
  Ehlers-Danlos disease
  Syndromes with congenital malformations
  Sepsis
  Dehydration
  Hypothyroidism
  Hypothermia

analysis based on these anatomic considerations. A careful history and thorough physical, neurologic, and developmental examinations are crucial to determine the direction of further laboratory investigations. After a specific diagnosis is established, the appropriate therapy can be instituted.

HISTORY

The family history can determine if other family members were hypotonic as infants; the age of onset, duration, and degree of impairment and the areas of involvement in those individuals are useful in determining the underlying disease and the patient's clinical course. The birth history should include a review of any infectious, toxic, or traumatic exposures during pregnancy. The absence of vigorous fetal movements is a symptom of some chromosomal disorders, congenital metabolic diseases, congenital infections, early fetal distress, fetal-onset Werdnig-Hoffmann disease, and arthrogryposis multiplex congenita. Particular note should be made of any difficulties at delivery or evidence for perinatal hypoxia-ischemia. The developmental history is critical in establishing a central nervous system disorder as the cause of infantile hypotonia. The age of onset of smiling; sitting without assistance; reaching for objects; crawling; standing; walking; speaking repetitive syllables, words, phrases, and short sentences; and the age of bowel and bladder control are the major milestones to be noted. Delay in the appropriate onset of these activities suggests central nervous system disease. The history of present illness should include the age at which the symptoms were first noted, the areas of the body most involved, the severity of hypotonia, the presence of deterioration, and progressive involvement of other body parts. Does the infant choke frequently during feeding? Is the hypotonia noted at any particular time of day? Does the older infant have frequent falling that is out of proportion to the level of gait development? Is tremor or dysmetria of the hands noted? Are the parents concerned about the infant's overall development?

EXAMINATION

Congenital hypotonia is occasionally noted at birth but is most often recognized by the parents or pediatrician sometime later in infancy. In its dramatic form it is seldom missed: the infant is "floppy," makes few spontaneous movements, and often has sucking and swallowing difficulties; when the infant is lifted up, the head, arms, and legs hang loosely from the trunk; the infant is described as feeling like a "dead weight" or "limp rag." Most often the hypotonia is subtle and first detected when the infant begins to sit, stand, or walk: The infant flops forward when sitting or has "rubbery legs" when standing or walking. Rarely, the hypotonia is so subtle as to be noted only during the physical examination: There is less resistance to passive movements of the limbs; it is easier for the examiner to passively "wave" the infant's hands and feet; often the infant will slip through the examiner's hands when held suspended under the axillae.

During the general physical examination particular note should be taken of the following: the ash-leaf or café-au-lait spots of phakomatosis; malformations associated with particular birth defect syndromes; the ligamentous laxity and double jointedness often seen in connective tissue disorders; the fixed contractures and joint deformity seen in arthrogryposis; the hepatosplenomegaly that is often seen in progressive metabolic disorders; the choreoretinitis or retinal scarring seen in fetal infections (TORCH infections); and the cherry red spot of some lysosomal storage diseases. Male infants with small hands and feet, failure to thrive, and undescended testicles are suspect for Prader-Willi syndrome.

The neurologic examination is critical for determining the anatomic locations of disease and directing further diagnostic investigations. The presence of cranial nerve abnormalities can be particularly helpful in this regard. Fasciculations and atrophy of the tongue are difficult to identify and are best seen in the resting infant with lighting over the surface of the tongue. They can be seen in Werdnig-Hoffmann disease, severe perinatal hypoxia-ischemia, and rarely syringobulbia and brain stem tumors. Strabismus, nystagmus, accentuated or depressed gag and jaw jerk reflexes, and sucking and swallowing difficulties are seen in many central diseases. Facial weakness (facial diplegia), trian-

gle-shaped mouth, or fish mouth suggest a congenital myopathy, myotonic dystrophy, or Prader-Willi syndrome. Extraocular muscle weakness is seen in myasthenia gravis, infantile myotonic dystrophy, and several congenital myopathies.

Muscle bulk, form, and strength should be examined carefully. Infants with hypotonia of central origin do not exhibit early weakness and atrophy; those with anterior horn cell, peripheral nerve, or muscle disease exhibit early, marked weakness and atrophy. These can progress rapidly, resulting in chest wall and extremity deformities (pectus carinatum, pes valgus, claw hand, and so on). The weakness of peripheral nerve disease is proportional to the atrophy and hypotonia; that of muscle disease is in excess. The deep tendon reflexes are normal or only slightly depressed early on in patients with muscle disease; in those with anterior horn cell or peripheral nerve disease they are markedly hypoactive or absent; and in those with central disease they are normal early and accentuated later in infancy. The presence of persistent ankle clonus and Babinski sign suggests central or spinal cord disease. The sensory examination of infants is very difficult and often requires repetitive testing for positive results. It is best performed with the infant resting after feeding, using a pin. It should proceed from the extremities toward the trunk and from the lower extremities upward. An appropriate or startle response should be noted. If performed carefully, the sensory examination can suggest spinal cord, nerve root, or peripheral nerve disease. If spinal cord disease is suspect, a digital rectal examination using the small finger will often demonstrate depressed anal sphincter tone.

The developmental examination should include techniques for determining fine motor adaptive and gross motor delay, as well as the stage of infantile reflex development (automatisms). The presence of the appropriate automatisms at a given age can greatly assist in ruling out central causes of hypotonia. Infants with peripheral nerve or muscle disease do not demonstrate a lag in infantile automatisms.

Some diseases can affect several levels of the nervous system at the same time, resulting in hypotonia with a mixture of central and peripheral symptoms and neurologic findings. Krabbe's disease, infantile metachromatic leukodystrophy, neuraxonal dystrophy, and Leigh's disease can produce progressive encephalopathy affecting the central and peripheral nervous system. Patients with these diseases often have hypotonia and hyperreflexia initially, and several months to years later the reflexes become markedly diminished or are totally absent. Perinatal hypoxia-ischemia can affect the basal ganglia, brain stem nuclei, and spinal cord concurrently, producing a variable clinical picture in addition to hypotonia.

LABORATORY INVESTIGATIONS

Despite a careful history and a thorough physical, neurologic, and developmental examination, the clinician often cannot determine the anatomic localization or a specific diagnosis. Laboratory investigations are therefore a necessary and important part of the work-up of patients with congenital hypotonia. The investigator should, however, have at least differentiated peripheral from central disease before laboratory tests are ordered, to avoid inappropriate, costly, and oftentimes painful laboratory procedures. If central disease is suspect, ultrasonography and CT scan of the head are invaluable in identifying intraventricular hemorrhage, periventricular leukomalacia, brain tumors, leukoencephalopathies, and other central diseases. If spinal cord disease is suspected, cervical or lumbosacral spine films are appropriate, and a myelogram should be considered. Nerve conduction velocity testing and electromyography (EMG) will identify and differentiate peripheral nerve from muscle disease. Muscle enzyme tests (CPK, SGOT, SGPT) should be performed before the EMG, since needle damage can cause a spurious elevation of these enzymes. Muscle (and often nerve) biopsies are required to differentiate peripheral nerve and muscle disease, since the infant EMG can be difficult to perform and correctly interpret.

Electromyography, nerve conduction velocity, and muscle biopsies are essential for diagnosing Werdnig-Hoffmann disease, congenital myopathies, and hereditary peripheral neuropathies. If progressive metabolic disease is suspected, serum amino acid and lysosomal enzyme and urinary organic acid tests should be performed. Chromosome analysis should be performed in patients with other congenital anomalies. Spinal fluid analysis is required if meningitis, encephalitis, or postinfectious polyradiculoneuropathy is suspected. In the latter disease, the spinal fluid should contain fewer than 10 WBC/ml and more than 60 mg protein/dl. The ability to diagnose this disease accurately in patients younger than 6 months on the basis of spinal fluid protein elevation alone is difficult, since the spinal fluid can normally contain 60 mg/dl or more of protein up to that age. Nerve conduction velocity studies, particularly F-wave determinations, can assist in making this diagnosis. Spinal fluid protein is also markedly elevated in Krabbe's disease, Leigh's disease, and metachromatic leukodystrophy.

If botulism is suspected, serum and stool should be sent for botulin determination; characteristic EMG and nerve conduction abnormalities are often present to assist in making this diagnosis.

Infants suspected of having myasthenia gravis should be given pyridostigmine (Mestinon) 0.05 to 0.15 mg/kg IM or IV. The onset of action is within 10 minutes and its duration of action is up to several hours. It is therefore more useful than the short-acting edrophonium (Tensilon) test, whose onset of action is within 30 seconds and duration of action only 5 minutes. This does not allow enough time for examination of the uncooperative infant. Tensilon (0.5 mg IV in an infant; 2 mg IV in children under 30 kg) can be used, however, in older children who are cooperative; then particular note should be made of improvement of eye closure, smile, and distal strength. Either test should be performed with equipment for endotracheal intubation and controlled ventilation available.

CLINICAL COURSE AND PROGNOSIS

The vigor with which one undertakes a diagnostic work-up of the hypotonic infant will depend on the clinical setting, severity, and course of the disease. Infants who present in the newborn period with severe hypotonia often require the full array of diagnostic tests available to arrive at a diagnosis. Infants in whom the hypotonia is mild and who present after 1 month of age with normal physical and developmental examinations can be followed periodically to determine the course of the hypotonia without any initial laboratory investigation. If other family members have had similar clinical presentations, the diagnosis of benign congenital hypotonia is likely. Infants with mild to moderate hypotonia and additional neurologic findings suggesting a specific anatomic localization or diagnosis should be investigated promptly with the appropriate laboratory tests. Male infants with small hands and feet, failure to thrive, and undescended testicles who later become obese most likely have Prader-Willi syndrome; the hypotonia in these infants resolves in early childhood and there is no need for further laboratory investigation. Hypotonic infants with fixed joint contractures (arthrogryposis) either had fixed posturing in utero (usually with breech presentation), fetal-onset Werdnig-Hoffmann disease, or a static fetal viral anterior horn cell infection. It is important to differentiate between these, since it is only patients with Werdnig-Hoffmann disease who will progress and often die within 1 year. Electromyography and muscle biopsy can often differentiate these diseases. Patients with group II Werdnig-Hoffmann disease (age of onset 2 to 12 months) may develop the ability to sit and stand but usually never walk and often die in the first decade; those with group III (age of onset 1 to 2 years) can sometimes walk but are often confined to a wheelchair. Neonatal myasthenia gravis is either transient or persistent. The former is due to passive transfer of antiacetylcholine receptor antibody from the myasthenic mother to the child. The time of onset is usually within hours or several days after birth, the patients develop a weak suck and few spontaneous movements, and they have dysphagia and ptosis. The symptoms last for several weeks. The persistent type usually has its onset after many days, and patients require prolonged treatment. Most of the congenital myopathies are benign and transient, but myotubular, mitochondrial, reducing-body, and carnitine-deficiency myopathy and congenital muscular dystrophy are progressive. Most patients with postinfectious polyradiculoneuropathy (Guillain-Barré syndrome) do well, with full recovery of function; a minority require prolonged ventilatory assistance. Most patients with amino and organic acidopathies and Leigh's disease improve or stabilize with appropriate dietary changes or restrictions. Patients with progressive metabolic encephalopathy due to lysosomal enzyme disease are usually severely involved and often progress to a spastic quadriparetic, bedridden state, with all of its attendant complications. Infants with hypotonia due to hypoxia-ischemia, neonatal meningitis, and birth trauma have a variable course dependent on other associated difficulties such as hydrocephalus and seizures.

THERAPY

Therapy for congenital hypotonia is directed at eliminating its cause and alleviating or preventing its effects. Metabolic insults such as hypoxia, hypoglycemia, and acidosis should be corrected promptly. Meningitis and sepsis should be treated with the appropriate antibiotics. Infants with myasthenia gravis should receive 4 to 10 mg pyridostigmine (Mestinon) syrup orally every 4 hours. Its onset of action is 15 to 30 minutes and its duration of action is 3 to 4 hours. If administered parenterally, 1/30 of the oral dose should be given. Patients with transient myasthenia gravis usually do not require treatment longer than 4 to 6 weeks. Patients with the persistent type require treatment indefinitely. Prednisone (2 mg/kg/day) and/or a thymectomy may be required in cases resistant to pyridostigmine treatment. Patients with polymyositis and postinfectious polyradiculoneuropathy (Guillain-Barré syndrome) can be treated with prednisone starting at 3 mg/kg/day, given daily and tapered over 10 days to 2 mg/kg/day; this dose is then given every other day until improvement is noted, at which time slow tapering can begin. Patients receiving prolonged steroid therapy should have long-bone roentgenography performed for osteoporosis and femoral head radiographs to determine necrosis; consideration should be given to supplemental calcium and vitamin D treatment in these patients. Other forms of congenital hypotonia have no specific cure, and treatment is directed at appropriate physical and occupational therapy programs, orthopedic procedures (bracing, tendon lengthening, and so on), and fitting of appropriate adaptive equipment (wheelchairs, Bliss Word Board). The parents of infants with progressive Werdnig-Hoffmann disease and muscular dystrophy should be informed that these infants will invariably develop life-threatening swallowing and respiratory difficulties often necessitating nasogastric or gastrostomy tube feedings and ventilatory support. A decision should be made early regarding the appropriateness of such heroic measures. The decision to withhold therapy from these patients often requires the involvement of other family members, hospital ethics committees, lawyers, and occasionally the courts. Intensive psychological and social support should be offered early. The approach to these difficult cases will vary according to physician and parental attitudes and medical and social standards.

MUSCULAR DYSTROPHY AND RELATED MYOPATHIES

IRWIN M. SIEGEL, M.D.

Muscular dystrophy is the general term for a group of chronic diseases that have in common abiotrophy with progressive degeneration of skeletal musculature, leading to atrophy and weakness, often contracture and deformity, and motor disability.

GENERAL THERAPY

Management of the patient with a muscle disease should be aggressive and multidisciplinary. Treatment is best administered by a team including pediatric, neurologic, genetic, physiatric, and orthopedic consultants. Additionally, occupational therapists, physical therapists, and medical social workers or psychologists can assist the patient and the family. Speech and dietary therapy, as well as subspecialty consultation (for instance, gastrointestinal and cardiopulmonary care), provide a thorough approach to the problems of comprehensive management.

Medications. Except in those myopathies due to the absence of a specific metabolite, for which replacement therapy will sometimes help (e.g., muscle carnitine deficiency), or in muscle disease secondary to endocrinopathy (e.g., hypothyroidism), in which appropriate therapy of the primary condition can alleviate the secondary myopathy, there is no effective drug treatment for muscular dystrophy. Although the myotonia of dystrophia myotonica can be relieved by a variety of agents, the dystrophia (weakness) remains. Agents used are phenytoin (Dilantin), 100 mg two or three times a day, or quinine,* 200 mg three times daily. Both procainamide and prednisolone, although mentioned in the literature, have undesirable side effects and are not suggested.

Cardiac. Cardiomyopathy is said to be present in over 80 per cent of patients with Duchenne muscular dystrophy (DMD), but the child may not show clinical evidence of heart disease because his restricted activity maintains a precarious status quo. Treatment is along conventional lines, with the administration of cardiac glycosides and diuretics when indicated.

Respiratory. Pneumonitis, secondary to decreased pulmonary function and poor respiratory toilet with aspiration, is frequently encountered in those in advanced stages of the muscular dystrophies, and periodic evaluation to monitor restrictive pulmonary disease is an integral part of any treatment regimen. Reduction in chest compliance, secondary to progressive weakness of respiratory musculature, requires an ongoing program of pulmonary rehabilitation. This may include diaphragmatic breathing exercises, postural drainage, chest percussion, proper humidification, and training in the use of various respiratory aids. Vigorous treatment of upper respiratory infections requires pharyngeal suction and intermittent positive pressure breathing as well as appropriate antibiotic therapy. Mechanical ventilation of patients in the terminal stages of DMD often can be managed at home without a tracheostomy, utilizing apparatus such as the rocking bed, plastic wrap ventilator, chest-abdomen cuirass respirator, and pneumobelt.

Dietary. Because obesity accelerates functional disability, nutrition should be carefully monitored throughout the course of muscular dystrophy but particularly after wheelchair confinement. A well-balanced vitamin-supplemented diet of no less than 1200 calories

---

*This use of quinine is not listed by the manufacturer.

is suggested. Patients are encouraged to choose fruits and vegetables as alternatives to high-calorie snacks, and high-fiber foods and fruit juices to aid in maintaining normal elimination. Only small amounts of dairy products are included because of their mucus-producing tendency.

When deglutition is difficult because of posterior pharyngeal and upper esophageal weakness, swallowing can be assisted by instruction in proper positioning, eating slowly, sitting upright for a time after meals, and introducing soft foods into the diet. Myotonic patients should avoid cold foods or fluids, which may cause pharyngeal myotonia.

Psychosocial. In addition to coping with the psychological problems imposed by a progressively disabling disease, children with muscular dystrophy face the same problems of peer interaction, body image, family adjustment, and sexuality that all normal youngsters must resolve in the process of maturing. Supportive psychiatric intervention made available at times of psychosocial crises can avert critical emotional damage, and empathic counseling of both the patient and family throughout the course of the illness is an important part of total management.

A higher incidence of mental retardation and decreased intellectual function has been noted in patients with DMD than in normal or other control groups. However, whenever possible, it is desirable to keep the child in the mainstream in the regular neighborhood school. Finally, in the treatment of muscular dystrophy the family is the patient. Group therapy has proved valuable in assisting parents and normal siblings by helping them develop insight and increasing communication through experience-sharing.

MOTOR DISABILITY

Physical Therapy/Occupational Therapy. Because muscular activity enhances protein synthesis (the danger of rapid loss of strength because of inactivity in DMD is well documented), it is imperative that the patient with muscular dystrophy be kept as mobile as possible for as long as feasible. The physical therapist systematically assesses weakness, imbalance, and contracture and provides submaximal exercise, gait training, and contracture stretching. As the child grows, surface area increases by the square of each linear increment and volume by its cube. This "scale effect" explains why a child with a condition limiting the ultimate muscle mass may eventually lose the ability to ambulate, even though the disease is arrested or only slowly progressive. Gradient measurement of strength and functional ability by the physical therapist aids in indicating appropriate times for contracture release and bracing.

The occupational therapist determines the patient's ability to attend to the tasks of daily living, assisting him or her through a variety of techniques and devices, such as lift and transfer equipment, clothing adaptations, special mattresses, and so on.

Wheelchair Care. Wheelchair confinement is a critical incident, both physiologically and psychologically, in the life of a patient with muscular dystrophy. Special wheelchair adaptations—for example, balanced forearm or-

thoses facilitating the use of the hands for feeding, writing, as well as other utilitarian tasks—can be prescribed to increase both comfort and function. Electric wheelchairs are available for those patients with insufficient strength to manage the standard model.

ORTHOPEDIC MANAGEMENT

Orthopedic complications are found in most of the muscular dystrophies. Central core disease (one of the congenital myopathies) can present at birth with congenital dislocation of the hips. Neonatal dystrophia myotonica is frequently complicated by severe clubfeet. In addition to weakness and contracture, particularly of the heel cords, children with dermatomyositis often develop subcutaneous or intramuscular calcification or both. In DMD, lower extremity contracture progresses until equinovarus and weakned pelvic balance, produced by hip flexion contracture, prohibit ambulation. Patients develop a stance and gait typified by hip flexion and abduction, increasing lumbar lordosis, and equinocavovarus. Eventually, they no longer can maintain a line projected from their center of gravity behind the center of rotation of their hips, in front of that of their knees and within their base of support. Ambulation stops at this point.

Properly timed surgery and bracing have helped selected patients to continue standing and walking anywhere from 2 to 5 years, thus significantly delaying confinement to a wheelchair with its inevitable downhill course.

Surgical management should permit early post-operative mobilization, as even brief restraint can lead to rapid loss of strength. Anesthesia must be closely monitored with particular attention to preventing gastric dilatation or potassium overload, to ensuring adequate ventilation, and to the singular danger of malignant hyperthermia in this class of disease.

For the patient experiencing increased difficulty with walking because of lower extremity contracture, percutaneous hip flexor, bipolar tensor fascia lata, and heel cord tenotomies, followed by extremity bracing, have proved effective in maintaining ambulation. Percutaneous tarsal medullostomy or osteoclasis with soft tissue release has been successful in treating late equinocavovarus with rigid bony deformity. Isolated forefoot adduction is corrected by percutaneous metatarsal osteotomy. Postsurgical orthotic management employs molded plastic appliances that are considerably lighter than steel or aluminum braces, yet equally sturdy. In those cases of facioscapulohumeral dystrophy in which shoulder weakness significantly interferes with upper extremity function, scapular stabilization has been performed.

Scoliosis. Because paraspinal weakness is symmetric, spinal curvature is unusual in the walking Duchenne dystrophic or the child with limb girdle dystrophy. Asymmetric muscle weakness, leading to scoliosis in the ambulatory patient, can occur in the Becker form of muscular dystrophy, sometimes in childhood dystrophia myotonica, and often with childhood facioscapulohumeral dystrophy. These spinal curves, when severe and progressive, can be surgically stabilized.

Most patients with DMD develop paralytic scoliosis as a complication of wheelchair confinement. A variety of external spinal containment systems, such as thoracic jackets or special wheelchair seating, designed to keep the pelvis level and to shape and hold the spine in the upright extended position, can retard such deformity.

Spinal fusion has been successfully used to correct and stabilize scoliosis in heritable neurologic conditions such as spinal muscular atrophy, familial dysautonomia, Charcot-Marie-Tooth disease, and Friedreich's ataxia. Such surgery is being increasingly performed in properly selected wheelchair-confined Duchenne dystrophics with rapidly decompensating scoliosis.

Fractures. Fractures in muscular dystrophy are most frequently seen in the long bones and are more common in patients falling from wheelchairs than in braced patients still ambulating. Such fractures are usually only slightly displaced, and there is not much pain as there is little muscle spasm. They heal without complication in the expected time and should be treated with minimal splintage (mold and sling for humeral fractures, light walking casts for fractures of the femur), encouraging continued independent function as long as possible.

MYASTHENIA GRAVIS

SUSAN T. IANNACCONE, M.D.

Myasthenia gravis is an acquired autoimmune disorder of the neuromuscular junction, although there are certain genetic predisposing factors that play a role in its incidence. The overall prevalence rate has been estimated to be between 13 and 64 per 1 million people, which translates to about 18,000 affected patients in the United States. About 1500 new cases occur each year. The relative proportion of these who are less than 20 years of age is quite small. Less than 10 per cent of new myasthenic patients are children.

The disease is characterized by fatiguability—weakness that increases with exertion. It is caused by the presence of an abnormal antibody—the acetylcholine receptor antibody—which attacks the acetylcholine receptor on the postsynaptic membrane of the muscle fiber. Myasthenia is frequently idiopathic but may be associated with other autoimmune disorders such as rheumatoid arthritis, systemic lupus erythematosus, diabetes mellitus, and thyroiditis. One form of the disease which accounts for 10 per cent of patients is paraneoplastic and may predate the identification of the carcinoma. The most commonly found tumor is thymoma, and thymic dysfunction without tumor plays a definite, but as yet undefined, role in the pathogenesis of the disease.

The weakness generally affects extraocular muscles and eyelids first, causing ptosis and diplopia. The young child with complete ptosis is at risk for amblyopia. Therefore, ophthalmologic consultation is indicated, and eyeglasses with lid crutches may be useful. Without treatment, the patient experiences spread of involvement to all voluntary muscles, including the bulbar musculature, causing dysphagia and aspiration. Death may occur from respiratory failure.

Myasthenia gravis has been classified in several ways. The most clinically useful system is that based on age of onset. The *transient neonatal form* occurs in babies born to mothers with the disease. It occurs in 10 per cent of such births and is caused by the circulating maternal acetycholine antibody. The antibody usually disappears from the infant's circulation by the age of 6 weeks, but the infant may require treatment until then if there are feeding or respiratory complications.

Congenital myasthenia is generally a different disease process than myasthenia gravis. It is a genetically determined abnormality of the presynaptic membrane that presents before the age of 2 years. Although the pathogenesis is not well understood, these extremely rare patients seem to respond to treatment with steroids.

Juvenile myasthenia gravis is associated with elevated acetylcholine receptor antibody levels, as is adult myasthenia. The spontaneous remission rate in juvenile myasthenia is higher than in adults, suggesting that conservative medical management is indicated for the first year following diagnosis. *Adult myasthenia* is more often associated with thymoma. The peak age of onset is 20 years, and women are affected two to three times more frequently than men. Past the age of 50 years, men are more likely to be affected and are more likely to have an associated carcinoma.

First, treatment should be symptomatic and supportive. This is most important for patients with severe weakness, as may be seen in myasthenic crisis when respiratory failure occurs. Once the crisis is recognized, the patient should be placed on ventilatory support and maintained in an intensive care unit. Treating underlying infection and maintaining adequate nutrition are crucial for the patient's recovery. Cholinergic crisis or overdose of anticholinesterase drugs may also cause respiratory failure and must be distinguished from myasthenic crisis before specific therapy can be given.

Secondly, diagnosis and treatment of an associated or underlying disorder such as thyroiditis or carcinoma may be crucial. Although such entities are rare in children, they should be ruled out in the initial evaluation. If the child suffers from an autoimmune disease, then pharmacologic management may begin with steroid therapy.

Thirdly, drug therapy is aimed at (a) increasing the availability of acetylcholine at the neuromuscular junction and (b) removing the abnormal acetylcholine receptor antibody and allowing the receptor membrane to repair itself.

Anticholinesterase drugs decrease the breakdown of acetylcholine and therefore increase the amount of neurotransmitter at the neuromuscular junction. These drugs are available in a number of forms for different routes of administration and different durations of action. Edrophonium chloride (Tensilon) is the most short acting (30 to 60 seconds duration) and is usually given as a test dose, 0.2 mg/kg intravenously, the "Tensilon test." Response to Tensilon may be difficult to interpret. Therefore, this test should be performed under controlled conditions in the presence of an experienced physician, usually a neurologist.

For a child who is combative in the presence of needles, intramuscular injection of an anticholinesterase drug is preferable to the intravenous Tensilon test. Neostigmine methylsulfate (Prostigmin), 0.04 mg/kg/dose, may be given intramuscularly and the effect observed 30 minutes later. Both oral Prostigmin (neostigmine bromide), 0.25 to 0.5 mg/kg up to every 4 hours, and Mestinon (pyridostigmine bromide), 15 to 60 mg every 4 to 8 hours, are commonly used for chronic management of myasthenia. The range of dosage is extremely wide because there is such variability in patients' responses. The dose must be titrated carefully so that the patient receives the maximum benefit with a minimum of side effects. For example, smaller, more frequent doses may be more beneficial than large doses 6 to 8 hours apart. Many patients do not require medication during rest, as during overnight sleep. Patients should be examined for muscle strength before their dose of anticholinesterase drug and at intervals afterward in order to determine their appropriate regimen. Inadequate therapy may provoke a myasthenic crisis, whereas overdose may result in respiratory failure from cholinergic crisis. The side effects of these drugs include increased oral secretions, cramping diarrhea, and flushing.

The following therapeutic options are thought to remove or inhibit the acetylcholine receptor antibody that causes myasthenia gravis.

Thymectomy is absolutely indicated if a thymoma is detected by radiologic imaging of the chest and anterior mediastinum. However, as many as 80 per cent of adult myasthenics without thymoma experience improvement or complete remission following thymectomy. Little more than anecdotal data is available regarding young children, but the juvenile myasthenic who is over 12 years old can be expected to have the same prognosis as an adult myasthenic. We do not yet know the possible immunologic risks of thymectomy in young children.

The thymus gland may be the source of abnormal lymphocytes, which either are directly responsible for producing the acetylcholine receptor antibody or fail to suppress its production by other lymphocytes. Cultures of thymic tissue from myasthenic patients have produced cells that attack the neuromuscular junction in vitro. Moreover, thymic tissue may share an antigen with the acetylcholine receptor, which stimulates production of abnormal lymphocytes. These mechanisms are consistent with the sometimes delayed and frequently permanent effect of thymectomy. Since all thymus tissue, including any ectopic material, must be removed in order to attain remission, a sternal splitting procedure should be done by an experienced thoracic surgeon. Postoperatively, the patient may require much less medication and thus careful monitoring.

Prednisone produces remission or cure in many myasthenics. It is occasionally given as the first line drug but more often is used when the patient has not done well on anticholinesterases and may not be ready for thymectomy. This drug should be given initially in high doses, 2 mg/kg/day, until there is a satisfactory clinical response. Some patients experience an increase in weakness during the first week of therapy. Such patients should be watched carefully but maintained on the drug, since they will most likely improve with continued treatment. After improvement is apparent, the dose of prednisone should be changed to every other day in order to avoid the long-term complications of its use. ACTH has also been used to treat juvenile myasthenia, but it is associated with more side effects than prednisone.

Immunosuppressant therapy, using cyclophosphamide or azathioprine, has been effective for some adults who did not respond to thymectomy. Fortunately, most children with myasthenia are not severely ill enough to warrant the use of these drugs, making an assessment of their effectiveness impossible at this time.

Gamma globulin given intravenously or intramuscularly is another adjunctive immunologic therapy that has been used too infrequently to judge its effectiveness. Anecdotal reports suggest that its use may be warranted in children who are not candidates for thymectomy and who have not responded or have become refractory to steroids.

Plasmapheresis or plasma exchange has become the most widely used adjunctive therapy for myasthenia gravis in both adults and children. The procedure is thought to work by removal of the acetylcholine receptor antibody from the circulation, but this has not been proven. It offers temporary albeit dramatic improvement in muscle strength. Antibody levels drop rapidly following exchange, and clinical improvement may be apparent within 24 hours. Although methods vary among centers, my recommendation is for a 1 volume exchange with Plasmanate every 3 to 5 days until the patient has improved to a satisfactory functional level and has remained stable for at least 5 days. Because of small blood volume, the risks of plasmapheresis are greater for children than for adults. They include hypotension, volume overload, sepsis, and cardiac arrest. Therefore, the procedure should be done on an inpatient basis with appropriate monitoring.

Some drugs may worsen myasthenia. Most medications that act at the neuromuscular junction to block acetylcholine transmission are contraindicated for use in myasthenia gravis. These include the aminoglycoside antibiotics, curare and curare-like drugs, lactate, lidocaine, phenytoin, procainamide, propanolol, quinidine, and quinine. Moreover, sedatives and narcotics that suppress normal respiration should be used with caution.

The prognosis for most children with myasthenia gravis is good. A thorough diagnostic evaluation is essential for choosing the appropriate management for an individual patient. Anticholinesterase drugs offer essentially symptomatic treatment, whereas thymectomy, prednisone, and immunosuppressants may produce remission or cure. Plasmapheresis and gamma globulin may be helpful adjunctive therapies.

PERIODIC PARALYSIS
ROBERT C. GRIGGS, M.D.

Recognition and accurate diagnosis are often the major challenges in the treatment of periodic paralysis.

Most patients present in childhood—usually in the first weeks of life for paramyotonia and hyperkalemic periodic paralysis and by adolescence in hypokalemic periodic paralysis. When diagnosis is first considered, careful exclusion of other disorders associated with weakness and abnormality of potassium (K) is necessary. Initial attacks require careful documentation before treatment is initiated. Provocative testing is necessary in most patients to establish diagnosis.

HYPOKALEMIC PERIODIC PARALYSIS

Acute Attacks. During paralytic episodes, potassium is invariably low, and, unless the patient is unable to swallow or is vomiting, potassium should be administered orally. A preparation of KCl that is free of sucrose and other carbohydrate should be chosen. A dosage of 0.5 mEq/kg as 25 per cent KCl is usually indicated and may have to be repeated. During severe attacks, serum electrolytes and electrocardiogram (ECG) should be monitored at half-hourly intervals until the attack resolves. The exact dosage of potassium depends on the severity and duration of the attack and on the response to the initial dose of potassium.

If patients are unable to take oral potassium, intravenous KCl may be necessary. The diluent for such treatment is of concern, since both 5 per cent glucose and physiologic saline cause a transient lowering of serum potassium. A concentration of at least 60 mEq/l of KCl must be used if either of these diluents is employed. Intravenous treatment is reserved for severely affected patients and requires careful monitoring of electrolytes, ECG, respiratory function, strength, and urinary output. Intravenous KCl-containing solutions should be administered slowly.

Prevention of Attacks. The prophylactic administration of potassium salts is seldom successful in preventing attacks, even when given in large doses on a daily basis. Patients subject to frequent attacks merit a trial of agents to prevent them. I have found that most patients respond to the carbonic anhydrase inhibitor acetazolamide with complete cessation of attacks. Treatment is usually effective within 24 to 48 hours, and attacks recur promptly after treatment is discontinued. The dosage is quite variable (2 to 20 mg/kg in divided doses) but is usually that required to produce metabolic acidosis, as indicated by serum chloride elevation and bicarbonate depression. In severe cases, an every-6-hours schedule is necessary.

In occasional patients acetazolamide may produce sufficient hypokalemia to worsen the disorder. In these patients, potassium-sparing agents such as triamterene may be effective. Dietary management, including the avoidance of carbohydrate and sodium loads, may be effective—occasionally as the sole, and often as adjunctive, treatment.

Chronic acetazolamide treatment presents certain hazards, most notably the occurrence of renal calculi. Patients on acetazolamide should have periodic abdominal radiographs and should maintain a high urine output. Sulfonamides should not be prescribed concurrently, since a sulfonamide nephropathy may be produced. Frequent but less troublesome side effects include dysgeusia for carbonated beverages, paresthesias, mild anorexia, and osteomalacia.

Treatment and Prevention of Progressive Weakness. Patients with frequent attacks of all types of periodic paralysis may develop persistent interattack weakness after repeated attacks. Acetazolamide prevents and improves such weakness in many patients. Patients unresponsive to acetazolamide may respond to the chloruretic carbonic anhydrase inhibitor dichlorphenamide.

Thyrotoxic hypokalemic periodic paralysis rarely occurs in childhood, and its treatment is markedly different from that of other hypokalemic periodic paralysis. Potassium administration is indicated for acute attacks, but acetazolamide markedly worsens patients. Treatment consists of management of underlying thyrotoxicosis. Propranolol is strikingly effective in preventing attacks, even while patients remain thyrotoxic.

POTASSIUM-SENSITIVE (HYPERKALEMIC) PERIODIC PARALYSIS

Acute Attacks. Hyperkalemic periodic paralysis is often a misnomer, since the serum potassium may remain within the normal range during attacks. The disorder is, therefore, defined by the development of weakness with potassium-loading. Acute attacks are often so mild that treatment is unnecessary. Oral carbohydrate administration in the form of sugar solutions is preferable to potassium-containing fruit juices and soft drinks. Attacks are seldom severe enough to require intravenous therapy. If a severe attack does occur, it will respond to standard measures used to treat hyperkalemia—intravenous glucose, insulin, or sodium bicarbonate.

Prevention of Attacks. Many patients do not require chronic treatment, particularly those with slight, infrequent attacks. Acetazolamide in dosage sufficient to produce a mild kaliopenia (usually 3 mg/kg two or three times a day) will prevent attacks and has the added benefit of ameliorating myotonia. Side effects (particularly paresthesias) often limit patient acceptability, and for this reason I have found thiazide diuretics the agent of choice. Chlorothiazide in a dosage of 10 mg/kg in two divided doses prevents attacks; *hypo*kalemia and weakness can develop in these patients as in normal people. Dosage should be kept low enough to prevent this occurrence. The use of inhaled beta-adrenergic agents such as albuterol (one or two puffs) has been found useful in alleviating attacks. Occasional patients with potassium-sensitive periodic paralysis have associated ventricular ectopy. Beta-adrenergic agents should not be used in such patients.

Normokalemic Periodic Paralysis. There are only rare, well-documented cases of patients with so-called normokalemic periodic paralysis who have not been found to have features identical to those of hyperkalemic periodic paralysis, and treatment is similar.

PARAMYOTONIA CONGENITA

Myotonia is the more disabling feature of paramyotonia, and episodic weakness is usually mild and infrequent. If the disorder requires treatment, it is important to distinguish the two types: (1) true paramyotonia, and

(2) paralysis periodica paramyotonica. Patients with the latter disorder are worsened by potassium administration and respond to agents such as acetazolamide and thiazides, which are kaliopenic. True paramyotonia is worsened by such treatment, and patients may develop quadriplegia with acetazolamide. Mexilitine, a drug recently used for treatment of cardiac arrhythmias, is useful for the myotonia and weakness of paramyotonia congenita. Simple maneuvers to avoid cold exposure are usually adequate treatment for mild cases of paramyotonia.

MYOSITIS OSSIFICANS

MARVIN L. WEIL, M.D.

Current therapeutic measures for the three types of myositis ossificans common to children involve symptomatic relief and treatment of complications. Disodium (1-hydroxyethylidene) diphosphonic acid (etidronate disodium), dichloromethylene diphosphonate (clodronate), and aminohexane diphosphonate (AHDP) used in adults to inhibit the formation, growth, and dissolution of hydroxyapatite crystals to regulate bone metabolism, are not approved for use in children, since they can modulate bone growth, lead to rickets, and cause proximal muscle weakness.

The progressive fibrodysplastic form of myositis ossificans has characteristic skeltal formations, with malformation of the big toes, reduction defects of the digits, and baldness. Deafness associated with this condition should be treated in order to minimize the symptoms of mental retardation, which may also occur. Exacerbating factors to be avoided as much as possible include trauma to muscle, intramuscular injections, careless venipunctures, biopsy of lungs, and operations to excise ectopic bone. Dental therapy may result in ossification of the masseter muscles. Surgical removal of the calcified tumor becomes necessary in cases with continued pain or significant functional limitation.

Postparalytic myositis ossificans, which can also occur after long-term coma, may be confused with deep venous thrombosis. Technetium 99m diphosphonate imaging can be used to recognize early heterotopic bone formation.

Post-traumatic myositis ossificans, which resembles the calcinosis seen in patients with dermatomyositis, is usually treated by nonoperative management. This circumscribed form must be distinguished from osteomyelitis and soft tissue abscesses.

Physical therapy to minimize limitation of movement and appropriate psychotherapy may be indicated in all forms of the disease.

15

Skin

TOPICAL THERAPY: A DERMATOLOGIC FORMULARY FOR PEDIATRIC PRACTICE

JO-DAVID FINE, M.D.,
and KENNETH A. ARNDT, M.D.

Many of the more common childhood dermatoses can be effectively managed by the pediatrician once a correct diagnosis has been established. However, more unusual diagnostic or therapeutic problems should be referred to a consultant dermatologist for further evaluation and intervention.

GENERAL PRINCIPLES

Acute Versus Chronic Inflammation. The ability to distinguish between acute and chronic inflammatory states will simplify diagnosis and initial skin care. Acute processes are often exudative, vesicular, and crusted and respond best to topical treatment with wet dressings, powders, lotions, and/or creams. In contrast, chronic eruptions often are dry, scaling, and lichenified and require more occlusive preparations, such as ointments, to lubricate and assist in the rehydration of the skin, thereby enhancing the percutaneous absorption of the active ingredients.

Role of Infection. The possibility of primary or secondary infection should be considered when initially evaluating a skin eruption. Information obtained from gross examination of the lesions may be sufficient to make a clinical diagnosis of an infectious process. For example, the presence of honey-colored or yellow crusting or exudate, frequently accompanied by a history of recent dermatosis, suggests secondary bacterial impetiginization. The use of appropriate systemic antibiotics to treat streptococcal and staphylococcal infections will result in marked improvement of such a patient. At other times, smears, microscopic examination, and cultures of the lesion (exudate; contents of pustules, vesicles, and bullae) or mass (skin biopsy with half the specimen submitted for cultures and half for histology) are required. Depending on the gross appearance of the lesion, bacterial, fungal, viral, and/or occasionally mycobacterial cultures of such biopsy-derived samples may be indicated.

Surface Area–to–Volume Ratio. Compared with adults, children have an increased surface area–to–volume ratio. Therefore, percutaneous absorption following application of topical agents over large body areas may result in clinically significant serum drug levels and subsequent acute toxicity or other unwanted systemic effects. For example, the former is seen with boric acid soaks (gastrointestinal symptoms, renal or hepatic failure, cardiovascular collapse, and central nervous system stimulation or depression), while the latter is found with the adrenal suppression that may occur as a result of widespread topical applications of potent corticosteroids. In addition, marked temperature lability may occur in small children when large surface areas are treated with wet compresses. To avoid such significant chilling and hypothermia resulting from the surface evaporation of water, only small areas should be treated simultaneously (i.e., a limb or part of the trunk).

Barrier Function and Penetration. In normal skin, an intact stratum corneum serves as a barrier to the absorption of external agents as well as to the excessive loss of internal fluids. Barrier function may be altered, however, when inflammation is present or when fissures or denuded areas develop. Skin hydration also significantly affects barrier function—that is, substances are absorbed far more readily through hydrated than through dry epidermis.

Ointments are more effective vehicles than creams for promoting percutaneous absorption, presumably by increasing surface hydration via occlusion. Similarly, the use of plastic gloves, vinyl exercise suits, or plastic wraps as occlusive dressings with topical corticosteroids will be advantageous in selected nonexudative dermatoses, such as psoriasis, chronic eczema, and lichen planus. Occlusion will also increase skin maceration, particularly in acute vesiculobullous and secondarily impetiginized disorders, and therefore is contraindicated in these situations.

When excessive scale is present (as in psoriasis), the efficacy of corticosteroids may be enhanced by prior or concomitant use of keratolytic agents under occlusion (see "Corticosteroids" later in this discussion).

421

Frequency of Application. Little is known about the optimal number of applications needed per day for most types of topical medications for effective treatment of a given skin disease. For example, some studies suggest that single daily applications of topical corticosteroids, with or without occlusion, may be as effective as multiple daily applications. The most usual practice is to apply medications two or three times daily. Potent and superpotent topical corticosteroids must be used only for limited periods.

Tachyphylaxis. The continued and uninterrupted use of topical corticosteroids may result in diminution in their effectiveness. This diminution may occur as early as 2 weeks into the course of treatment, but responsiveness returns after corticosteroids have been discontinued for 1 or more weeks. Intermittent use is best both to ensure optimal results and to decrease the risk of any adverse effects.

Adverse Systemic Effects. The prolonged use of even low-concentration topical corticosteroids over large surface areas may result in suppression of the pituitary-adrenal axis. Growth retardation in children has been reported from percutaneous absorption of topical steroids. Application of potent fluorinated corticosteroids can result in atrophy, telangiectasia, and striae formation within 1 month of use. The face, genitalia, and intertriginous areas are particularly at risk; therefore, corticosteroids must be used judiciously in these sites.

Boric acid compresses may result in significant systemic toxicity and should no longer be used.

Elevated phenol levels in blood and urine may result from the application of carbol-fuchsin solution (Castellani's paint) in children. Although an excellent astringent for macerated or fissured intertriginous skin folds or web spaces or for intertriginous candidiasis, it should be used only in very select situations.

Absorption of silver sulfadiazine (Silvadene) from extensively burned skin may result rarely in hyperosmolality from the propylene glycol in its vehicle and may thereby add to the metabolic instability of patients with burns.

Selection of Quantity and Generic Versus Brand Name Topicals. Careful thought must be given to the amount of topical medication needed by each patient to ensure that enough is dispensed to last for days or weeks and also to decrease the cost of the prescription. In an adult, 30 to 60 gm of an ointment or cream is required to cover the entire body in a single application. Most preparations are less expensive when purchased in larger prepackaged containers than in multiple small tubes or jars. If appropriate amounts are dispensed, the overall cost of care is reduced and the patient's compliance will be improved. Generic topical medications are often less expensive than brand-name products, but there is little information concerning their biologic equivalency. Generic topical corticosteroids have been shown generally to have less biologic effectiveness than their brand-name counterparts.

Fixed-Combination Preparations. One can usually provide more versatile and at least as effective therapy by using several single-component preparations in concert rather than fixed-combination medications. Fur-

thermore, use of many of the latter may result in unwanted side effects. As an example, an impetiginized inflammatory lesion may be better treated with oral antibiotics and topical corticosteroids than with a fixed combination of neomycin with steroid. Use of neomycin may actually exacerbate some skin disorders as a result of the development of allergic contact dermatitis. Positive patch test reactions have been reported in up to 20 per cent of patients subsequent to the use of neomycin on inflamed skin.

TYPES OF TOPICAL PREPARATIONS

"Wetness" provides benefit by cooling and drying through surface evaporation of water. *Wet dressings* also clean the skin of surface exudates and crusts and help drain infected sites. They are the principal form of therapy for acute exudative inflammation. *Powders* increase skin surface area, thereby enhancing drying and reducing maceration and friction. They are especially useful in body fold areas. *Lotions* are suspensions of powder in water. After the aqueous phase evaporates, a layer of protective or therapeutic powder is left on the skin.

Creams are emulsions of oil in water; they are less occlusive and more drying than corresponding ointments. *Ointments* either are suspensions of water droplets in oil or are inert bases such as petrolatum. They may not be miscible with water.

Gels are transparent, colorless, semisolid emulsions that liquefy when applied to skin.

Pastes are combinations of powder and ointment and are of stiffer consistency than ointments. Cornstarch is frequently the powder used, as in zinc oxide paste. Since application of cornstarch to intertriginous sites may enhance the overgrowth of yeast, pediatricians should be careful to use zinc oxide ointment rather than paste as a perianal barrier; otherwise, secondary *Candida albicans* infection might result.

FORMULARY

This formulary contains a representative list of commonly available topical agents that are beneficial in dermatologic therapy. Although more inclusive lists are available, we believe that this formulary is adequate for general pediatric use.

Acne Preparations

Benzoyl Peroxides. These preparations contain 2.5 to 10.0 per cent benzoyl peroxide. They are bacteriostatic for *Propionibacterium acnes* as well as mildly comedolytic. They are usually applied thinly once or twice daily to all acne areas but should be used less frequently or discontinued if excessive redness or dryness develops. The lower concentrations should be used initially to avoid unnecessary irritation. Higher concentrations of benzoyl peroxide should be used with caution, especially in darker complexioned individuals, because excessive irritation may lead to postinflammatory hyperpigmentation.

Numerous benzoyl peroxide solutions exist; some are now available over the counter. They differ from one another in the concentration of benzoyl peroxide and in the nature (i.e., lotion, cream, or gel) and specific composition of their vehicles. One oil-based lotion is Benoxyl (Stiefel), which is available in 5 per cent and 10 per cent concentrations. Benzagel (Dermik), 5 per cent and 10 per cent, and PanOxyl (Stiefel), 5 per cent and 10 per cent, have an alcohol gel base. A lotion with acetone gel base is Persa-Gel (Ortho Pharmaceutical, 5 per cent and 10 per cent), while an aqueous gel base can be found in Desquam-X (Westwood), 2.5 per cent, 5 per cent and 10 per cent gel and 10 per cent wash, and PanOxyl AQ (Stiefel), 2.5 per cent.

Retinoic Acid (Vitamin A Acid; Tretinoin). This agent is useful in comedonal acne because of its loosening effect on cellular debris impacted within sebaceous gland and follicular ostia. In children, this drug may also be useful in rarer disorders of keratinization or selected other conditions. Used nightly or every other night on acne sites (except eye and lip areas), retinoic acid induces comedones to be expelled. A transient flare in activity may be seen approximately 3 to 6 weeks into treatment. Because of the risk of exaggerated sunburn, retinoic acid preparations should be used with caution during summer months, and effective sunscreens with a sun protection factor (SPF) of 15 or higher should be used during any sun exposure. Lower concentrations and creams are initially used; in oilier skin, the gel may be more efficacious. Commonly used forms are Retin-A (Ortho Pharmaceutical) cream (0.025 per cent, 0.05 per cent, and 0.1 per cent) and gel (0.01 per cent and 0.25 per cent).

Topical Antibiotics. These agents may be quite effective in mild-to-moderate acne and are used often in conjunction with benzoyl peroxides or retinoic acid. Clindamycin, erythromycin, and tetracycline are all effective against *P. acnes,* generally in the order cited. Of the three, topical tetracycline is the least used currently in clinical practice. This latter drug may cause a temporary yellowish hue in the skin and also fluoresces when viewed under ultraviolet light; this may make it less cosmetically desirable for adolescent patients. Although pseudomembranous colitis has been seen in only a very few patients treated with topical clindamycin, its use is contraindicated in patients with ulcerative colitis, Crohn's disease, or pseudomembranous colitis; and it should be discontinued in otherwise healthy patients who develop persistent diarrhea.

Some of the liquid and gel preparations commercially available include clindamycin (Cleocin T solution or gel, Upjohn, 30-ml package, and other preparations), erythromycin solution or gel (T-Stat, Westwood; A/T/S, Hoechst-Roussel; EryDerm, Abbott; Erymax, Herbert; Erycette, Ortho Pharmaceutical; most of these are available in 60-ml packages), and tetracycline (Topicycline, Norwich Eaton, 70-ml package). A gel formulation of erythromycin compounded with 5 per cent benzoyl peroxide (Benzamycin, Dermik) is also available. Alternatively, one can extemporaneously formulate an approximately 1 per cent clindamycin solution in the following ways: one 600-mg Cleocin hydrochloride capsule in 50 ml of Neutrogena Vehicle/N or one 600-mg capsule of Cleocin hydrochloride in 54 ml of 70 per cent isopropyl alcohol and 6 ml of propylene glycol.

Acne Cleaners. Many products contain combinations of sulfur, salicylic acid, resorcinol, alcohol, and insoluble or slowly dissolving particles. These have, at best, only a minor role in acne therapy, providing mild drying and peeling of the skin. It must be emphasized that dryness and superficial peeling are not the desired endpoints of topical acne therapy. They are side effects of most of the effective topical agents and are not necessary for successful treatment. Therefore, we do not suggest these agents routinely, but they may be used at the patient's discretion, with care being taken to avoid excessive dryness and irritation.

Anesthetics (Topical)

Although usually ineffective in alleviating the pain or itching of inflamed skin, topical anesthetics may be beneficial in some inflammatory mucocutaneous conditions (aphthous stomatitis, herpes simplex infection of the oral cavity or anogenital area, and oral erosive lichen planus). However, benzocaine-containing preparations should be avoided because of their tendency for allergic contact sensitization.

Topical anesthetics include dyclonine hydrochloride (Dyclone, Astra, 0.5 per cent or 1.0 per cent solution, 30 ml); diphenhydramine hydrochloride (Benadryl elixir, Parke-Davis, 4 oz); lidocaine (Xylocaine, Astra, as a 2 per cent viscous solution, 100 ml, and as 2.5 per cent and 5.0 per cent ointment, 35 gm). These agents may be applied locally to the lesions or, in the case of elixirs, may be used as mouth rinses, four to six times daily as needed for symptomatic relief.

Anthralin

Anthralin, a chemical derivative of anthracene, is an effective topical agent used either alone or in conjunction with ultraviolet B (UVB) irradiation for the treatment of psoriasis. Like other tar by-products, anthralin probably is beneficial in psoriasis because of its antimitotic activity. Although used extensively in England and Europe, until recently anthralin was infrequently used in the United States because of its tendency to produce skin irritation and temporary staining. Anthralin is used in concentrations ranging from 0.1 per cent to 2.0 per cent, with usually the lowest concentration initially employed. Although in the past the drug was routinely left on the lesions for 4 to 12 hours prior to bathing, more recently it has been shown that anthralin may be just as effective but less irritating if one of the higher concentrations is applied for only 15 to 30 minutes ("short-contact therapy").

Antibacterial and Antiseptic Agents

Several preparations that contain bacteriostatic or bactericidal agents are available in both liquid and ointment form. Although most pyodermas are better treated with systemic antibiotics (e.g., penicillin for ecthyma and streptococcal impetigo, erythromycin or dicloxacillin for staphylococcal impetigo), localized superficial wounds often may be adequately treated with topical preparations. Such conditions include surgical sites, burns, areas of localized folliculitis, and abrasions. Combination formulations often broaden the effective antibacterial spectrum. Although a very effective antistaphylococcal agent, neomycin often causes an allergic contact sensitization, with subsequent worsening of the dermatosis. Systemic absorption and toxicity are highly improbable for these agents, owing to their poor percutaneous permeability.

Liquids and Surgical Cleansers. Chlorhexidine is antibacterial for both gram-positive and gram-negative organisms; it has immediate as well as continuing antibacterial effects and is not inhibited by the presence of blood. It is available as Hibiclens (Stuart) in a 4-oz package. Povidone-iodine has antibacterial coverage similar to that of Hibiclens. However, bacterial killing with povidone-iodine requires several minutes of direct contact with the skin and may be inhibited by blood. Furthermore, it may impart a slight yellow tint to the skin if it is not thoroughly removed by rinsing. It is available as Betadine (Purdue Frederick), as well as other brands, in the following liquid forms: solution, surgical scrub, shampoo, and douche.

Ointments. Bacitracin is bactericidal, especially for gram-positive organisms like streptococci and staphylococci. It may be dispensed simply in 15-gm tubes or in combination, as in Neosporin Ointment (Burroughs Wellcome) (containing 5000 units of polymyxin B sulfate, 400 units of zinc bacitracin, and 3.5 mg of neomycin sulfate per gram), 15 gm; Neo-Polycin Ointment (Dow Pharmaceuticals) (containing 8000 units of polymyxin B sulfate, 400 units of zinc bacitracin, and 3 mg of neomycin sulfate per gram), 15 gm; and Polysporin Ointment (Burroughs Wellcome) (containing 500 units of zinc bacitracin and 10,000 units of polymyxin B per gram), 30 gm.

Neomycin sulfate is effective against most gram-negative and some gram-positive organisms, but it has a significant potential as a contact allergen. It is available either alone in generic forms (15 gm) or in combination, as noted.

Polymyxin B is effective against most gram-negative organisms, but not *Proteus* and *Serratia*. It is available in combinations, as noted.

Povidone-iodine is also available in ointment form (30 gm) as Betadine or a generic brand.

Gramicidin is bactericidal against gram-positive organisms. It is available in combination with neomycin (Spectrocin Ointment, Squibb) and polymyxin B (Neosporin-G Cream, Burroughs Wellcome).

Mupiricin (pseudomonic acid; Bactroban, Beecham Laboratories), in the form of a 2 per cent ointment (15 gm), is a highly effective agent for the topical treatment of primary and secondary impetigo.

Any of these agents can be applied (or used as cleansers if liquid) four to six times daily to the affected sites, as needed.

Antifungal Medications

Dermatophyte Infections. Any agent listed in the following paragraph may be used twice daily for localized dermatophyte infections. Treatment is continued until approximately 2 weeks after all clinical signs of infection are gone—the average duration is about 1 month. However, systemic griseofulvin or ketoconazole is necessary for adequate treatment of dermatophyte involvement of hair and nails, when large surface areas of skin are involved, or for recalcitrant, persistently recurrent infection.

Clotrimazole is available as either Lotrimin (Schering) or Mycelex (Miles Pharmaceuticals); cream (30 gm) is usually used, but solution (30 ml) may be preferred for moist, macerated sites, such as interdigital web spaces of toes. Miconazole is similar in structure and mode of action. It is available as Monistat-Derm (Ortho Pharmaceutical), 30 gm of cream or 30 ml of solution. Other, newer imidazole agents include econazole (Spectazole, Ortho Pharmaceutical; 15, 30, and 85 gm) and ketoconazole (Nizoral, Janssen; 15 and 30 gm). An equally effective nonimidazole drug is ciclopirox olamine (Loprox, Hoechst-Roussel; 15, 30, and 90 gm). Others include haloprogin, available as Halotex (Westwood; 15- and 30-gm cream or 30-ml solution), tolnaftate (Tinactin, Schering; as 15- and 30-gm cream, 10-ml solution, 45-gm powder, and 100-gm aerosol), and naftine (Naftin, Herbert). Generic brands are also available.

Candida Infections. Clotrimazole, miconazole, econazole, ketoconazole, ciclopirox olamine, or haloprogin can be used as described.

Nystatin is found in many brands of medications, including Mycostatin (Squibb). The most commonly used forms are ointment, cream, and powder. All are available in 15-gm sizes. The use of topical nystatin in our experience seems to result in a slower clinical resolution of active lesions, and we therefore prefer the initial use of the broader spectrum antifungal agents previously described.

For *Candida* paronychial infections, any of the previously named preparations may be tried; occlusion under a fingercot may increase their effectiveness. If this treatment is unsuccessful, 2 to 4 per cent thymol in absolute alcohol (prescribed in 30 ml) may be compounded; this is applied two or three times daily to the nail fold areas until healing is complete. The area must be kept dry at all times during the latter nonaqueous therapy.

For oral *Candida* infection (thrush), 10-mg clotrimazole buccal troches taken five times a day for 2 weeks are highly effective; alternatively, nystatin oral suspension (100,000 units/ml; 2 ml for infants, 4 to 6 ml for older children and adults) may be swished in the mouth four times daily and swallowed. Another alternative therapy is 1 to 2 per cent gentian violet solution painted in the oral cavity one or two times a day.

Iodochlorhydroxyquin (Vioform, CIBA), 3 per cent cream or ointment (30 gm), may be used alone or combined with 1 per cent hydrocortisone (Vioform-Hydrocortisone, CIBA, 20 gm); generic preparations are also available. This agent has mild antifungal and antibacterial properties and is frequently used in diaper dermatitis, especially when the skin is mildly eczematous, impetiginized, or secondarily infected with yeast. Clothing and skin may be stained yellow by its use.

Topical amphotericin B (available as Fungizone Cream, Ointment, and Lotion; Squibb) is effective against *Candida* but not dermatophytes. Its use has no advantage over other anti-*Candida* therapies, and its yellow-orange color may stain.

Tinea Versicolor. This superficial infection, caused by *Pityrosporon orbiculare*, may be treated in many ways. Some effective approaches are as follows: (1) 2.5 per cent selenium sulfide suspension (available as Selsun, Abbott, and as Exsel, Herbert); this lotion is applied daily to all skin areas from the neck to the knees and is showered off after 5 to 10 minutes; this routine is repeated daily for 10 to 14 days; the scalp should also be shampooed with this solution on the first night of treatment; (2) shampoos containing zinc pyrithione (e.g., Head & Shoulders), applied 5 to 10 minutes nightly for 10 to 14 days; (3) 25 per cent sodium thiosulfite (available as Tinver Lotion, Barnes-Hind), applied twice daily for about 2 weeks to the affected areas; and (4) clotrimazole, miconazole, econazole, haloprogin, ketoconazole, or tolnaftate preparations.

Antipruritic Agents

If significant itching is present, the use of oral antihistamines as well as topical agents may be helpful. Baths containing Aveeno colloidal oatmeal are helpful for generalized eczematous or vesicular processes. For localized pruritic processes, however, drying and cooling preparations can be beneficial when applied four to six times a day. Examples of the latter include the following: (1) calamine or phenolated calamine lotion (drying); Caladryl (Parke-Davis) Cream or Lotion, frequently self-prescribed, should be avoided, since diphenhydramine, when applied topically, is both ineffective and a contact allergen; (2) Sarna Lotion (Stiefel), 0.5 per cent each of camphor, phenol, and menthol in an emollient lotion vehicle; (3) PrameGel (Gen Derm), 1 per cent pramoxine hydrochloride and 0.5 per cent menthol; (4) Schamberg's Lotion (somewhat oily), which contains menthol, 0.5 per cent gm; phenol, 1 gm; zinc oxide, 20 gm; calcium hydroxide solution, 40 ml; and peanut oil, to make 100 ml; (5) menthol, 0.25 gm, and phenol, 1 gm, in Eucerin Cream (Beiersdorf), to make 100 gm (lubricating).

Antiviral Agents

Acyclovir (ACV). ACV is an antiviral compound shown to be effective against herpes simplex. The drug is an acyclic nucleoside of guanine. Following phosphorylation by thymidine kinase, it becomes antiviral, causing inhibition of herpes simplex DNA polymerase. ACV is also somewhat effective against varicella-zoster virus.

This drug may be beneficial topically in the first episode of genital herpes but is ineffective in recurrent disease. It is also effective systemically in primary genital or generalized herpes simplex infections and may be useful in bone marrow recipients to prevent or attenuate the course of cutaneous herpes infections.

ACV is available as 5 per cent ointment (Zovirax, Burroughs Wellcome, 15 gm) as well as forms for oral or intravenous use.

Burn Preparations

One of the most frequently used agents for first-, second-, and third-degree burns is silver sulfadiazine (available as Silvadene, Marion, in 50- and 400-gm packages). It is bactericidal against a wide spectrum of organisms, allowing wound healing to occur under rather sterile conditions. However, it should be avoided in patients allergic to sulfa because of its potential for systemic absorption and subsequent allergic response.

Corticosteroids

Topical corticosteroids are often the most effective single therapy for a variety of inflammatory and hyperplastic cutaneous disorders. The pediatrician will have the most frequent need of them in eczematous dermatitis (including allergic contact dermatitis and atopic dermatitis) and psoriasis. Sensible and effective use of these agents necessitates not only a correct diagnosis but also an understanding of tachyphylaxis, the use of occlusion, and the potential for systemic and cutaneous side effects, all of which have been discussed. Although many preparations exist, it is necessary to become familiar with only a few of these to treat most steroid-responsive dermatoses effectively.

Table 1 lists representative topical corticosteroids of varying strength. Each of these creams and ointments may be applied thinly two to four times daily to affected skin areas. They are most effective if applied to well-hydrated skin. Corticosteroid solutions are applied one or two times daily after shampooing and drying of the scalp; they are used for 7 to 14 days as needed and for psoriasis should be occluded overnight by use of a plastic shower cap. After a few days of treatment with

TABLE 1. Representative Topical Corticosteroids for Dermatologic Disorders

Super potency	Clobetasol propionate, 0.05%; Temovate Cream and Ointment (Glaxo), 15, 30, and 45 gm; *Note:* May be too potent for routine use in children
High potency	Fluocinonide, 0.05%; Lidex Cream, Ointment, and Gel and Lidex-E Cream (Syntex), available in 15-, 30-, and 60-gm sizes Halcinonide, 0.1%; Halog Cream and Ointment (Squibb), available in 15-, 30-, and 60-gm sizes; Halog also comes as 0.1% solution (2 oz), as well as 240 gm in both cream and ointment
Middle potency	Betamethasone valerate, 0.1%; Valisone (Schering), 15- and 45-gm ointment and creams, 60-ml solution Betamethasone dipropionate, 0.05%; Diprosone Cream and Ointment (Schering), both available in 15- and 45-gm sizes; lotion (0.05%) and topical aerosol (0.2%), available in 20- and 60- ml and 85-gm sizes, respectively; Diprolene Ointment (Schering) is available in 15- and 45-gm sizes Fluocinolone acetonide, 0.025%; Synalar (Syntex), available in 30, 60, and 425 gm in both 0.025% cream and ointment; 2 oz as 0.01% solution Hydrocortisone valerate, 0.2%; Westcort Cream and Ointment (Westwood) in 15, 45, and 60 gm
Low potency	Hydrocortisone, 1%; Nutracort (Owen), 120-gm cream and ointment; Hytone (Dermik), Synacort (Syntex) in 30- and 120-gm cream and ointment; others

potent topical corticosteroids, facial, genital, and intertriginous areas are more safely treated with 1 per cent hydrocortisone to avoid the side effects of steroids.

Moist or vesicular lesions (acute inflammatory lesions) are better treated with creams, while corticosteroid ointments are better suited for dry, lichenified areas (chronic inflammatory or hyperplastic lesions). If excessive scale is present (e.g., psoriasis, hypertrophic lichen planus), pretreatment or concomitant treatment with Keralyt Gel (Westwood, 30 gm) under occlusion (e.g., plastic gloves, bags, or wraps) for 2 to 4 hours will enhance the effect of subsequent corticosteroid applications.

Emollients

Many emollients are readily available and inexpensive. If hydrophobic (greasy) substances are applied to skin surfaces after adequate hydration (immersion in water for at least 10 minutes), they will add to the surface barrier and impede water loss. In pediatric practice, they are most frequently used for children with atopic dermatitis. By decreasing dryness, they help prevent further fissuring, itching, and subsequent inflammation and possibly impetiginization. Some emollients are greasier than others; choice of emollient will depend on expense and cosmetic acceptance. Commonly used emollients include lotions, such as Alpha Keri (Westwood), Lubriderm (Ortho Pharmaceutical), U-Lactin (T/I Pharmaceutical), Cetaphil (Parke-Davis), Lubrex (T/I Pharmaceutical), Moisturel (Westwood), and Wibi (Owen); creams, such as Nivea (Beiersdorf), Eucerin (Beiersdorf), Carmol (Syntex), and Keri (Westwood); and ointments, such as Aquaphor (Beiersdorf) and hydrated petrolatum USP.

Keratolytics

Propylene glycol solutions, with or without added salicylic acid, are excellent agents for loosening and removing scales; they are especially effective when applied to affected skin for 2 to 4 hours under plastic wrap occlusion after adequate prior hydration by soaks or bathing. Patients with conditions such as ichthyosis (vulgaris and X-linked), psoriasis, hypertrophic lichen planus, and tinea manuum and pedis will benefit from this treatment. Commonly used keratolytic agents include Keralyt Gel (Westwood, 30 gm), Lac-Hydrin (Westwood, 6 and 12 oz), and 40 per cent propylene glycol solution, the last prepared by a pharmacist. Whitfield's ointment (as half-strength concentration, 3 per cent salicylic acid and 6 per cent benzoic acid, in 30-gm tube) is mainly used either alone or in conjunction with other antifungal creams for the treatment of hyperkeratotic dermatophyte infections of the palms and soles. In isolated cases of dense scalp psoriasis, nightly treatment under a plastic shower cap with either Keralyt Gel or P & S liquid (Baker) helps in the debridement of scale.

Minoxidil

A topical preparation of minoxidil (Rogaine, Upjohn), a potent vasodilator antihypertensive agent, has recently been released for use in male pattern hair loss.

Although the latter is not of clinical importance in pediatric dermatology, it is of interest that this drug has been reported to be of benefit in some adult patients with alopecia areata. Although minoxidil is not yet formally approved by the Food and Drug Administration (FDA) for use in the latter disorder, and little information is currently available regarding its safety in children, use of this drug may be of possible benefit in those rare children with widespread alopecia areata or totalis.

Scabicides and Pediculocides

Gamma benzene hexachloride (Kwell Lotion or Shampoo, Reed & Carnrick, 60 ml, and other generic brands) is effective for both mites (scabies) and lice (pediculosis). When treating scabies, all skin below the angle of the jaw is covered; medication should be applied to dry skin (i.e., the patient should not shower first) and washed off 8 hours later. The treatment may be repeated in 7 days to protect against possible reinfection by hatched larvae. Because of its potential for percutaneous absorption, lindane must be used with great caution, if at all, in pregnant women, in neonates and very young children, and in those with widespread cutaneous disease and an abnormally permeable skin barrier; isolated cases of central nervous system side effects in children have been reported when the agent has not been used properly.

Permethrin (Nix, Burroughs Wellcome; as 2-oz cream rinse) is a synthetic pyrethroid active against lice, ticks, mites, and fleas. It has 70 to 80 per cent ovicidal activity and no reported adverse effects. The cream rinse is applied for 10 minutes and is rinsed off with water. This agent, as well as the pyrethrins and lindane, is highly effective for the treatment of pediculosis capitis. Nits must be combed out of the hair after all of these treatments.

Pediculosis pubis is treated by the application of lindane to the groin and other affected areas, with rinsing after 8 hours. Pediculosis capitis may be treated with a single lindane shampooing, although some advocate repeat treatment in 4 to 7 days.

Crotamiton (Eurax Cream and Lotion, Westwood, 60-gm and 2-oz packages) is an alternative to lindane for the treatment of scabies. This is applied twice daily for 2 days.

Six to 10 per cent precipitated sulfur in petrolatum (30 or 60 gm), the initial antiscabetic therapy to be used in pregnancy and infancy, is applied daily for 3 days. It is messy and malodorous but has no risk of systemic side effects.

Effective over-the-counter alternate treatments for pediculosis are pyrethrin-containing agents, such as A-200 Pyrinate Liquid (Norcliff Thayer) and Rid (Pfipharmecs).

Involved eyelashes may be treated by the careful application of petrolatum twice daily for 8 days, 0.025 per cent physostigmine ophthalmic ointment (5 gm), or yellow oxide of mercury.

Shampoos

Although nonmedicated shampoos are certainly useful in routine scalp hygiene, shampoos containing selenium sulfide, zinc pyrithione, tar, or salicylic acid–sulfur are more beneficial for seborrheic dermatitis and psoriasis. These are initially used daily, with a second application after the first rinsing; after the scalp improves in appearance, shampooing may be done every other or every third night as necessary. Useful agents include selenium sulfide, available as Selsun (Abbott) and Exsel (Herbert); zinc pyrithione, available as Zincon (Lederle), Head & Shoulders (Proctor & Gamble), and others; tar (particularly useful in psoriasis), available as Sebutone (Westwood), Pentrax (Cooper Care), T-Gel (Neutrogena), and others; and salicylic acid–sulfur, available as Sebulex (Westwood), Vanseb (Herbert), TiSeb (T/I Pharmaceutical), and others.

Soaps

In children with eczema or atopic dermatitis, skin irritation from harsh soaps may develop. The least irritating soaps have been found to be Dove, followed by a group include Aveenobar, Purpose, Basis, Dial, Alpha Keri, Neutrogena, Ivory, and Oilatum. In children more severely affected by atopic dermatitis, a reasonable alternative to soap is Cetaphil Lotion (Owen Laboratories, 8 oz).

Sunscreens

Sunscreens are agents containing chemicals that absorb ultraviolet light from the sunburn spectrum. The use of sunscreens permits increased exposure time to sunlight without development of sunburn. Their use is especially important in light-aggravated diseases, such as lupus erythematosus and polymorphous light eruption, as well as in chronic protection against the known aging and carcinogenic effects of ultraviolet light. The individual usefulness of a sunscreen to prevent sunburn depends on its relative efficacy in blocking or absorbing UVB radiation (280 to 320 nm), as well as its SPF rating. In general, the higher the SPF rating, the more effective the protection provided by a sunscreen. Within the past few years, many sunscreens have been produced with SPF ratings of at least 15 and extending to at least SPF 50. Four of the more effective and popular sunscreens are PreSun 15, 29, and 39 (Westwood) and Total Eclipse (Herbert). Several para-aminobenzoic acid (PABA)–free sunscreens are available for patients with known sensitivity to PABA. Most sunscreens should be reapplied after sweating or swimming, although some are well retained on the skin despite either of these situations. For more complete sunlight exclusion, sunshades containing opaque substances can be used; these include Clinique Continuous Coverage, zinc oxide paste, A-Fix (Texas Pharmacals), and RVPaque. Lipstick sunscreens are also available.

Synthetic Dressings

A variety of synthetic semipermeable sterile dressings are now available, differing primarily in extent, if any, of adhesiveness to the skin. Representative products include Op-Site (Acme United Company), an adhesive dressing, and Vigilon (Bard Home Health Division), a nonadhesive dressing. Although reported to be beneficial in several conditions, they are primarily useful in promoting the healing of erosions and superficial abrasions of the skin. Only nonadhesive dressings should be employed in patients having mechanically fragile skin (e.g., epidermolysis bullosa and pemphigus vulgaris).

Tar Compounds

Coal tar preparations have long been known to be effective in psoriasis and eczematous dermatitis, although their exact modes of action are still not understood. Tars are anti-inflammatory, inhibit DNA synthesis, and photosensitize to long-wave ultraviolet light (UVA). Among commonly used preparations are the following.

Liquids. For chronic eczema of the hand or foot, soaks or compresses for 30 minutes twice daily with Balnetar (Westwood, 8 oz) or Zetar Emulsion (Dermik, 6 oz) are useful, especially if areas are fissured. When more widespread areas are involved, as in generalized atopic dermatitis or psoriasis, tar baths taken twice daily, followed by application of other medication or emollients, are beneficial.

Another useful liquid tar preparation for the treatment of scalp psoriasis is T/Gel (Neutrogena). This solution contains 2 per cent coal tar extract and a keratolytic agent (2 per cent salicylic acid); it is applied to the scalp following shampooing in the evening, occluded overnight with a plastic shower cap, and rinsed off the following morning.

Oils. Tar body oils (such as T/Derm, Neutrogena) may be useful in the treatment of psoriasis and other inflammatory skin conditions associated with dry skin. They may be applied to the skin following routine bathing.

Ointments and Pastes. In some patients, a better response occurs when tar ointments or pastes are used. Two frequently prescribed forms are 5 per cent crude coal tar or Zetar Ointment (Dermik). These preparations are quite messy and malodorous and will stain clothing and sheets if not adequately removed; mineral oil may be useful in cleansing them from the skin.

Tar Shampoos. These have been previously discussed. Descriptions of other multicompound formulations containing tar can be found in any of the current dermatology textbooks or monographs.

Wart Remedies

Many modes of therapy are available for warts, depending on type, location, number of lesions, and previous responses to treatment. These include chemicals, liquid nitrogen application, and electrodesiccation curettage.

Condylomata acuminata usually respond to the application of podophyllin, but there is a high potential for cutaneous burns and possible systemic toxicity secondary to overaggressive treatment.

Isolated common warts can be self-treated with daily applications of combined salicylic and lactic acids in collodion (Duofilm, Stiefel, 15 ml); Occlusal (17 per cent salicylic acid) or Occlusal HP (26 per cent salicylic acid) in a polyacrylic vehicle (Gen Derm, 15 ml); or other agents. Two to four drops daily are applied to the wart after hydration (5 to 10 minutes of soaking in warm water). The lesion is then covered with adhesive or plastic tape for 12 to 24 hours. If the area becomes red and tender, treatment is withheld for a few days. The resultant whitened surface of the wart is gently filed down daily with a callus file or pumice stone, and the medication is reapplied. Using this approach, the majority of warts can be cured, but at least 6 to 12 weeks of daily applications may be required. Plantar warts can be treated similarly or by the daily application of 40 per cent salicylic acid plaster carefully cut just to cover the area of the wart. This plaster is then covered with tape. The wart should be frequently debrided.

Wet Dressings and Compresses

Weeping, exudative, crusted, and vesicular eruptions require the use of wet dressing to aid in drying and surface debridement. As mentioned, boric acid solutions are no longer used because of the risk of absorption and toxicity. We no longer use potassium permanganate solutions because of the difficulty in mixing, the potential for chemical burn from undissolved crystals, and the rather dramatic and persistent staining of skin and nails.

Wet dressings of comfortable temperature are applied using several layers of sterile gauze, Kerlix, or clean old linens. The dressings are removed, remoistened, and reapplied every 5 to 10 minutes, for a total of 15 to 30 minutes three or four times a day as needed. As mentioned, in children, only small surface areas are treated simultaneously to avoid chilling from evaporative heat loss. Solutions include (1) aluminum acetate (Burow's solution), available as Domeboro Powder or Tablets (Dome Laboratories, box of 12); one tablet or packet is added to a pint of water (makes a 1:40 solution); a fresh solution should be made daily, but it can be refrigerated for storage; however, it should be allowed to warm to room temperature prior to application; (2) acetic acid solution, 0.25 per cent to 1.00 per cent; the higher concentration has been suggested as having the added benefit of killing *Pseudomonas aeruginosa;* (3) normal saline; (4) povidone-iodine (Betadine), which is less advantageous than the others because of its color, which may make subsequent wound observation somewhat more difficult unless the wound is first irrigated.

Cosmetic Masking Agents

Some vascular or pigmentary congenital lesions are cosmetically unsightly and deforming. An excellent approach to therapy is the use of Covermark Makeup (Lydia O'Leary, 22.5- and 85.5-gm cream) or Dermablend. Many of these lesions can be completely masked in this manner.

SKIN DISEASES OF THE NEONATE

SHARON S. RAIMER, M.D.

INITIAL SKIN CARE

The skin of a normal term infant requires no special care other than gentle cleansing to remove excess ver-

nix, blood, and meconium, both for aesthetic reasons and to discourage the colonization of pathogenic organisms. Cleansing should be postponed until the body temperature has become stable. Warm, sterile water applied with cotton balls generally will cleanse the infant adequately. Vernix, which frequently remains in body folds, will gradually disappear during subsequent days. The use of 3 per cent hexachlorophene detergent cleanser (pHisoHex), once routinely employed in the newborn nursery, is recommended only during an outbreak of staphylococcal infection because of the potential neurotoxicity of the compound if absorbed.

Care of the umbilical cord area is important to limit colonization by pathogenic organisms. The application of triple dye to the umbilicus is frequently recommended, but alcohol or antibacterial ointments have also been used.

Desquamation of the skin in some neonates may be prominent during the latter part of the first week of life. Lubrication is unnecessary, as the desquamation will resolve spontaneously.

As in any age group, the skin of the newborn serves as an effective barrier against organisms and harmful or toxic substances. The outermost layer of the skin, the stratum corneum, is most critical for providing barrier function. Mechanical removal of the stratum corneum occurs from removing adhesive tapes or bandages; thus, these should be avoided on the skin of newborns whenever possible. Maceration of the stratum corneum from excessive humidity will also reduce barrier function and may provide a portal of entry for pathogenic organisms. The permeability of the skin of the term newborn does not differ from that of older persons, but greater care should be exercised in applying topical medications because the body surface–to–body volume ratio is greater in infants; therefore, higher serum levels of topically applied medications may be obtained. Inflamed or disrupted skin will also permit a greater penetration of topically applied compounds.

The general principles of skin care applicable to the term infant are also acceptable for the preterm infant; however, the earlier in gestation, the thinner the integument of the infant. These infants, therefore, are more vulnerable to the effects of trauma, maceration, and occlusion, and their skin may be more permeable to topically applied substances than that of term infants.

BIRTH TRAUMA

Ecchymoses. Ecchymoses and petechiae, which are regularly found over the presenting part of the newborn infant, resolve spontaneously over the first few days of life. After difficult deliveries, hemorrhage and erosions may also be present. These generally require no special therapy but should be kept clean and dry. The use of vacuum extractors during delivery may cause large ecchymoses and resultant jaundice in the newborn.

Caput Succedaneum. Caput succedaneum is an edematous swelling resulting from pressure changes over the presenting part of the infant. Even when alarming, the edema generally decreases markedly in the first 24 hours following birth, and treatment is unnecessary.

Cephalhematomas. Cephalhematomas result from rupture of blood vessels that traverse the cranial periosteum. The swelling that results is limited to the surface of one cranial bone because of adherence of the periosteum at the suture lines. Regression is slow, and the edges may calcify during healing. Aspiration is contraindicated, as infection may be introduced by the needle. Subgaleal hemorrhage has been erroneously referred to as giant cephalhematoma. Without the constraint of the periosteum, hemorrhage in this area may be serious enough to induce cardiac failure from hypovolemia and may require urgent transfusion.

Pressure Necrosis. Pressure necrosis may occur following prolonged labor and delivery, particularly in large infants. The lesions may be mistaken for aplasia cutis congenita. Treatment is aimed at preventing secondary infection and minimizing scarring. Exudate from the lesion should be stained for organisms and cultured for pathogens. A Tzanck smear should be done on cells scraped from the base of the lesion to rule out herpetic infection. Saline compresses are useful for moist or exudative lesions. If pathogens are demonstrated, appropriate antibiotic therapy should be instituted but is otherwise unnecessary. Gas-permeable dressings, such as Vigilon, may be of benefit in speeding re-epithelialization, particularly for large, superficial erosions. After re-epithelialization, scarring is generally minimal, and infants may be discharged from the nursery during the healing process.

Iatrogenic Lesions. Diagnostic testing and monitoring in the prenatal period, during delivery, and in the immediate postnatal period may result in skin lesions of minimal consequence. Midtrimester amniocentesis may cause dimple-like or linear scars on the skin. The lesions are of minor cosmetic importance, but infants should be examined for the rare occurrence of injury beneath the scar. Fetal skin biopsy may leave depressed scars at the site of biopsy. Internal fetal monitoring during delivery may result in pressure necrosis at the site of the monitor placement. Oxygen monitors on the skin, which are employed in many intensive care nurseries, may occasionally cause small burnlike lesions, which may heal with slight scarring. Small cutaneous calcifications resulting from heel sticks generally will resolve spontaneously with time but rarely may require excision if they persist and cause pain with ambulation.

TRANSIENT LESIONS OF THE NEWBORN'S SKIN

Milia. Milia are superficial epidermal inclusion cysts that are 1 to 2 mm in diameter and white. They are found most commonly on the face but occasionally occur on the foreskin or elsewhere on the body. Milia will resolve spontaneously in the first weeks of life and require no special treatment.

Sebaceous Gland Hyperplasia. These lesions are pinpoint-sized, closely grouped, yellow or white spots, generally most prominent on the nose, which occur as a result of the stimulation of the sebaceous glands by maternal androgens. The lesions disappear spontaneously during the first several days of life.

Miliaria Crystallina. Miliaria occurs with increased frequency in infants subjected to high ambient temperature or phototherapy. The condition is harmless and requires no therapy except for alteration of the environmental temperature and humidity.

Erythema Toxicum. This is an extremely common benign, self-limited condition of healthy term newborns. The lesions generally occur during the first 4 days of life but, rarely, may be present at birth. Erythema toxicum rarely develops in preterm infants. Lesions may range from blotchy erythematous macules to frank pustules, but the most typical lesion is a small papulopustule set on a wide erythematous base. A smear of the lesional contents demonstrates numerous eosinophils and differentiates erythema toxicum from an infectious process or other eruptions of the newborn. The lesions are evanescent and asymptomatic, and treatment is unnecessary.

Transient Neonatal Pustular Melanosis. This benign, self-limited eruption is present at birth and is seen most commonly in dark-skinned infants. Any or all of three characteristic types of lesions may be present: vesicopustules on a nonerythematous base or with a narrow rim or erythema; ruptured vesicopustules, identifiable by their characteristic collarette of scale; and hyperpigmented macules, which may persist for several months. Smears of the subcorneal pustules show variable numbers of polymorphonuclear leukocytes and cellular debris. Cultures are sterile. No treatment is necessary.

Sucking Blisters. Sucking blisters are generally solitary and are located on the radial surface of the forearm or the dorsum of the hand and fingers. They are caused by vigorous sucking, and the diagnosis can generally be confirmed by observing the sucking activity of the infant. They are harmless and require no treatment if infections and congenital blistering disorders can be excluded as possibilities. Sucking pads or calluses are found frequently on the lips of newborn infants. The lesions resolve spontaneously with peeling of the lips.

Aplasia Cutis. The congenital absence of skin occurs most commonly in the occipital region of the scalp. If the condition is not recognized, the lesions may be attributed falsely to obstetrical trauma and may lead to malpractice litigation. If the diagnosis is in question, a biopsy from the margin of the defect may be helpful by demonstrating the absence of normal skin architecture and appendages. The lesions should be cultured, but only true infections should be treated with antibiotics. Open lesions should be kept clean with compresses, using saline or Burow's solution. The lesions may be superficial, with the absence of only epidermis and dermis, or may occasionally be characterized by the absence of subcutaneous tissue and periosteum as well. When the defect is small, the course is usually benign, and epithelialization results in scar tissue devoid of appendages. Deep lesions may require excision with primary closure, and lesions large in area may require grafting. A skull film is advised, as an underlying bony defect may be present.

Acne Neonatorum. True neonatal acne with inflammatory papules and open and closed comedones may develop when the infant is 2 to 4 weeks of age. The process, which has been blamed on maternal androgens, is self-limited and rarely produces scars in this age group. Gentle washing of the face generally is sufficient, but 2.5 per cent benzoyl peroxide or 2 per cent erythromycin solution or gel may be used safely for severe or protracted cases.

NEVI

Vascular Lesions. The nevus simplex or salmon patch caused by ectatic dermal capillaries occurs in approximately 40 per cent of infants and almost always regresses spontaneously. Lesions on the nape of the neck may remain in approximately 5 to 10 per cent of individuals but are of little cosmetic significance.

Capillary or strawberry hemangiomas and cavernous hemangiomas either are present at birth or develop in the first few weeks of life. Ninety per cent of capillary hemangiomas and 70 per cent of cavernous hemangiomas resolve spontaneously, with excellent cosmetic results, during the first 5 to 7 years of life and therefore require no treatment. Lesions in critical locations, such as those on the face or near vital structures, should be observed carefully for rapid initial growth. Large hemangiomas in any location may threaten the welfare of the infant by trapping platelets (Kasabach-Merritt syndrome) or by sequestering bacteria and serving as a source of sepsis. For hemangiomas impinging on vital structures or causing systemic complications, oral prednisone, in an initial dosage of 2 to 3 mg/kg/24 hr for 4 weeks, may be effective in invoking involution of lesions. The prednisone dosage should then be tapered over the next 2 to 3 weeks. Repeat courses of prednisone are occasionally needed but should be postponed as long as possible to allow recovery of the adrenal glands and to allow growth of the infant. Intralesional triamcinolone in a concentration of 10 to 20 mg/ml may be effective in shrinking relatively small but rapidly growing hemangiomas in critical locations on the face. Radiation therapy and surgery are reserved for those lesions that threaten the life of the child but that are unresponsive to corticosteroids.

Port-wine stains do not resolve and actually become more prominent with time. When in the area of the trigeminal nerve, they may be associated with the Sturge-Weber syndrome. A careful ophthalmologic examination should also be done when lesions are present in the trigeminal nerve area to detect possible associated glaucoma. Pulsed-dye laser therapy in early studies shows promise of good cosmetic improvement of treated lesions, with a low incidence of hypopigmentation and scarring. Pulsed-dye laser therapy may be used in infants and young children, whereas argon laser therapy is not recommended during childhood because of the high incidence of scarring that occurs in children under the age of 16 years who are treated with argon lasers. Covering the lesions with cosmetics matched to the skin tone, such as Covermark, is recommended early in the child's life.

Pigmented Nevi. Congenital melanocytic nevi are estimated to occur in 1 to 2 per cent of the population. They appear to have a greater potential for developing melanomas within the lesions than do nevi appearing after 2 years of age, but the exact incidence of malignant transformation is not known. The presence and size of congenital pigmented lesions should be well documented in the neonatal record. Giant pigmented nevi should be removed early in life, when feasible, because they appear to have the greatest risk of malignant transformation. Tissue expanders now available have made primary excision and closure of many large pigmented lesions possible. For very large "bathing trunk" lesions requiring multiple procedures, the morbidity of the multiple procedures must be weighed against the possible benefits for the child. There is debate over whether small congenital nevi should be removed. Until more data are available, it seems prudent at least to remove the very darkly pigmented lesions, in which early development of melanoma would be difficult to detect.

Sebaceous Nevi. Sebaceous nevi are slightly yellowish, hairless plaques on the head and neck of newborn infants. They can be ignored safely during childhood but should be excised with close margins near puberty, as basal cell carcinomas and, rarely, sebaceous carcinomas may develop within the lesions after puberty.

Epidermal Nevi. Epidermal nevi require no treatment during infancy, but infants should be evaluated for the possible association of skeletal abnormalities or neurologic or ocular defects.

INFECTIONS

Herpes Simplex. A Tzanck smear to detect multinucleated giant cells should be taken from the base of any vesicular or bullous eruption or from any erosive lesions in a newborn infant. Viral cultures should be obtained for confirmation of the diagnosis. Because of the devastating effects of herpes simplex infections in the neonatal period, the infant should be treated with intravenous acyclovir if a positive Tzanck smear is obtained.

Staphylococcal Infections. Pustular or purulent lesions in the newborn should be Gram stained and cultured for organisms, and appropriate antibiotic therapy should be instituted if pathogenic organisms are found. Staphylococcal scalded skin syndrome develops occasionally in newborns, particularly in an intensive care nursery setting. A condition of bright red erythema and peeling of the skin caused by circulating staphylococcal toxin generally begins periorificially, around the neck, and in the groin and axillae. Frozen sections of the peeling skin, which show a midepidermal split in the epidermis, may be helpful for rapid diagnosis. Antistaphylococcal antibiotic therapy should be instituted; corticosteroids are contraindicated. Semipermeable dressings, such as Vigilon, may speed the reepithelialization of eroded areas.

Congenital Candidiasis. Congenital candidiasis manifests as multiple pustules that are sometimes as large as 3 to 4 mm in diameter on an erythematous base. Diagnosis is made by a Gram stain or potassium hydroxide examination, which demonstrates candidal spores and pseudohyphae, or by culture. The infection of term infants will generally clear rapidly with topical imidazole or nystatin cream. Premature infants must be observed carefully for the development of candidal sepsis.

Dermatophyte Infections. Dermatophyte infections, most commonly caused by the organism *Trichophyton tonsurans,* are increasing in frequency in infants and may develop as early as 3 days of age. Infections are generally acquired from the infant's mother. The diagnosis can be made by potassium hydroxide examination of skin scrapings or by fungal culture. Lesions generally respond well to topical antifungal therapy.

ERUPTIONS IN THE DIAPER REGION
GARY M. GORLICK, M.D., M.P.H.

GENERAL MEASURES

These measures are aimed at the prevention of the most common diaper rashes as well as their early treatment by simple, effective, and safe measures.

Most importantly, parents must be educated in correct cleaning, bathing, and diaper care of the infant; they in turn must transmit this to the infant's babysitters and/or day-care and nursery school personnel, especially when a rash is present. After birth, the umbilicus should be cleaned with isopropyl alcohol tid–qid and continued for approximately 1 week after it has detached and become dry at the stump, to prevent a focus from which bacterial dermatitis might develop. Signs of infection at the umbilicus or circumcision must be brought to the physician's attention and treated. Tub-bathing is not begun until the umbilicus is dry and fully healed. Either type of diaper, permanent (cloth) or disposable, is currently acceptable inasmuch as there is inadequate evidence at this time that one type predisposes to increased incidence of rash. If a disposable type is used, the plasticized outer covering should be folded away from the baby's skin at the back, front, and thigh regions if not pleated. Cloth diapers are best washed in Ivory Snow and rinsed thoroughly. Fabric softeners should not be used if a rash develops. The diaper is to be removed and changed as soon as stooling is noted; with the onset of a rash, quickly changing the diaper after urination also becomes important, as does a change late in the evening hours. The infant's room should not be overheated and should be kept at normal humidity. Skin cleansing is best done with cool or tepid water on a soft and nontraumatic (not heavy and rough-surfaced) washcloth or cotton pledgets. Particular care is necessary to clean and dry all creases well. If soap is used, a mild one is recommended, such as Dove or Neutrogena Baby Soap. Oils should not be used, particularly in the diaper region. Avoid overdressing the infant; consequent heat and sweat retention may lead to miliaria and/or intertrigo. When early chafing or eruption is noted, allow open air exposure as often as feasible, decrease the use of outer plastic pants, and apply a protective ointment such as Desitin, A and D, or zinc oxide to the involved areas.

There appears to be a role for dietary management in some diaper eruptions. The infant should have adequate fluid intake. Some rashes respond to water supplements alone. At times, empiric stopping of juices will clear the eruption. The prevention and treatment of diarrheal stools by diet manipulation (e.g., adding banana or rice foods for a binding effect, decreasing or stopping juices or other known diarrhea-producing agents) often help. Although there is strong evidence against "ammoniacal dermatitis," at least as a primary entity, oral cranberry juice bid–tid may be tried. Any new food introduced and soon followed by a rash should be discontinued and reintroduced carefully when the rash has abated. Cow's milk should not be introduced until an infant is at least 6 to 12 months of age (the American Academy of Pediatrics recommends 12 months), and dermatitis should be carefully watched for on any area of the body, including the diaper region. Obesity should be prevented; the friction of opposing skin creates a greater than normal propensity for intertrigo to develop.

Many contactants must be avoided. Oils applied directly to the skin or placed in the bath water should be avoided, as should "bubble-baths" for the young child. The infant's skin should be kept free of cosmetics and other skin and hair preparations. Creams, ointments, oils, talcs, and emollients being used at the time of an eruption may be etiologic and should be empirically stopped. Careful review of all aspects of bathing, cleansing, and diaper care may be necessary to identify contactants that are causing a dermatitis.

SPECIFIC MEASURES

These measures are aimed at the treatment of the conditions listed below. Reference to *Topical Therapy: A Dermatologic Formulary for Pediatric Practice* is herein made for dosage schedules not repeated in this section.

Chafing, Irritant Dermatitis, Intertrigo, and Perianal Dermatitis. Ointments such as Desitin, A and D, Diaparene, and zinc oxide may be applied as often as each diaper change. Talcum powder is useful, especially in the creases, but must not be used if the skin is denuded, and care must be taken that it is not inhaled by the infant, as it is easily airborne. Corn starch is less likely to be inhaled but may enhance the growth of *Candida albicans* (monilial dermatitis).

Monilial Dermatitis. Therapy consists of applying Mycostatin cream or ointment bid–qid to the rash. Another technique is to alternate the application of hydrocortisone cream 1 per cent with either Mycostatin cream or Mycostatin dusting powder at each diaper change. The dusting powder can also be applied bid–tid when the skin is clear in the infant who is prone to repetitions of this condition. Oral Mycostatin is added to the local treatment in the following situations: when thrush is present; when the baby is breast-fed and the mother has monilial mastitis; when the diaper eruption is extensive; when there is nonresponse to local therapy alone; or when the eruption recurs soon after local treatment. One to 2 ml of oral Mycostatin is given tid–qid until finished (60-ml bottle), with particular attention to its contact with all areas of thrush before being swallowed. A mother with active monilial vaginitis may be a source of reinfection and should be treated. The treatment of oral lesions with topical gentian violet is messy and is rarely used today. Oral ketoconazole is *not* to be used for simple monilial dermatitis. In addition to Mycostatin, there are many topical antifungals that are applied bid and are active against *C. albicans,* e.g., clotrimazole (Lotrimin, Mycelex), miconazole (Monistat-Derm), haloprogin (Halotex, Tinactin). Use of topical ketoconazole is not advised unless the eruption has not responded to other treatments in the immunologically deficient patient.

Seborrheic, Atopic, and "Psoriasiform" Dermatitis. Apply hydrocortisone cream 1 per cent on a "least-often" as necessary basis, that is, once to qid prn. Stronger topical corticosteroids are rarely necessary, but if they are, use one from the next higher potency group and stop it as soon as response is noted and return to the very safe hydrocortisone 1 per cent cream. Never use fluorinated corticosteroids or oral/parenteral steroids, or occlusive technique, in the diaper region. The therapeutic role of biotin for generalized seborrhea (not Leiner's) is uncertain at the present time.

Bacterial Dermatitis. Controversy exists over the therapeutic effectiveness of topical antibiotics for skin infections. In addition, the potential for allergic contact sensitization is of concern. However, if the diaper dermatitis area is small, topical Neosporin-G *cream* (not ointment) qid alone may suffice. Since *Staphylococcus aureus* is by far the most common cause of diaper area bacterial infection, cloxacillin sodium (Tegopen) is given orally at 25 to 50 mg/kg/day in four divided doses for 7 to 10 days when more than local treatment is necessary.

"Ammoniacal Dermatitis." As mentioned before, controversy exists as to whether ammonia causes dermatitis, or if it exacerbates an existing dermatitis. Some clinicians, however, believe the following measures may be efficacious: oral cranberry juice or oral methionine (Pedameth), and/or Caldesene Medicated Powder or Ointment. Pedameth liquid contains 75 mg of racemethionine per 5 ml, and the recommended dosage for infants 2 to 6 months old is 5 ml tid (in formula, milk, or juice) for 3 to 5 days. For infants 6 to 14 months of age the same dosage is given but at a qid frequency and also for 3 to 5 days.

Psoriasis. The ideal therapy for the infant and very young child with psoriasis in the diaper region has not yet been established. Corticosteroids probably should be avoided as much as possible. Treatment with tars such as 2 per cent crude coal tar in a zinc oxide ointment (removed with warm mineral oil) once or twice a day has been effective. Estar, a 5 per cent coal tar, may also be used once or twice a day. Should corticosteroids be used because of nonresponse to the above, it is best to attempt control with mild 1 per cent hydrocortisone ointment. Since this dermatitis is often chronic, it might be best to treat only flare-ups with these specific agents. Preventing Koebner reaction by the most atraumatic hygienic methods is important.

Granuloma Gluteale Infantum. In this uncommon condition symmetric nodular lesions occur in the diaper region following diaper dermatitis with or without candidiasis, previously often treated with fluorinated ste-

roids. It resolves without therapy, and therefore all agents should be stopped. In some cases it is best to taper corticosteroid agents gradually from those of strongest to those of mildest potency to avoid a "flare-up" when they are abruptly stopped.

Recalcitrant Diaper Eruptions. Rule out pinworms and/or urinary tract infection when appropriate. Rule out *Tinea corporis* infection on rare occasion. Consider dermatitis medicamentosa—especially when Mycolog *cream* has been used, for this contains a potent corticosteroid as well as potential allergic sensitizers. Mycolog II is a safe re-formulation of Mycolog and can be used in the cream form without risk of these problems. Look for signs of telangiectasis or bleeding within the rash, and for anemia, fever, hepatosplenomegaly, and intractable diarrhea in the child who shows signs of failure to thrive, for these may herald serious systemic conditions such as congenital syphilis, acrodermatitis enteropathica, Wiskott-Aldrich syndrome, or Letterer-Siwe disease.

Agents Not to Be Used. Boric acid, baking soda, mercurials, hexachlorophene, fluorinated corticosteroids, and oral ketoconazole should not be used to treat diaper eruptions. The *cream* form of Mycolog should be avoided; if the physician wishes to use Mycolog, the *ointment* form is strongly advised, as is the precaution to stop as soon as the rash improves and to continue therapy with hydrocortisone cream 1 per cent with or without anticandidal therapy as necessary.

CONTACT DERMATITIS

WILLIAM L. WESTON, M.D.

The two prevailing strategies for the management of contact dermatitis in children are the administration of glucocorticosteroids and the avoidance of allergens. Clinicians should appreciate that once a contact allergy is established, the redness, itching, and other skin changes persist for at least 3 weeks and frequently longer. This observation is particularly true when a child has developed an allergic contact dermatitis to a strong allergen such as poison ivy or poison oak. Thus, any treatment protocol should be designed to treat the child for at least 3 weeks.

Glucocorticosteroids are anti-inflammatory agents that produce cutaneous vasoconstriction and prevent the egress of leukocytes from cutaneous vessels, thus reducing the signs and symptoms of contact dermatitis. As a general guideline, most authorities select a topical glucocorticosteroid ointment or cream if less than 10 per cent of the skin surface is involved with the dermatitis and choose oral steroids if greater than 10 per cent of the body surface is involved.

For topical steroids, an ointment or cream of moderate potency is selected, and the patient is treated two or three times daily for at least 3 weeks. I recommend one of the following preparations: mometisone furoate, 0.1 per cent (Elocon), ointment or cream; hydrocortisone valerate, 0.2 per cent (Westcort), ointment or cream; or fluocinolone acetonide, 0.025 per cent (Synalar), ointment or cream. Each is supplied in 15- or 45-gm tubes. As a guideline, 1.8 gm/m² of area treated per dose will be used.

For systemic steroids, oral prednisone is preferred at doses of 1 mg/kg/24 hr. Treatment for at least 2 weeks at the starting dose is recommended, with reduction of the dose to 0.5 mg/kg/24 hr for the last week. Intramuscular steroids are irregularly and unreliably absorbed and are not recommended. The popular dose packs of oral steroids in decreasing doses often result in a recurrence of the contact dermatitis, since the steroid effect is of short duration.

Some authorities also use oral antihistamines to help reduce the itching. I have not observed any additional benefit from adding antihistamines to steroids in the treatment of contact dermatitis.

For most children with allergic contact dermatitis, avoidance of allergens simply involves awareness of the location of poison ivy or poison oak plants within their area, and the reaction itself is sufficient to motivate the child toward avoidance. In children whose allergic contact dermatitis is not due to plants and is persistent or recurrent, further attempts to identify an allergen are warranted. This is accomplished with patch testing, which should be performed by one experienced in epicutaneous (patch) testing and usually requires referral to a dermatologist. Patch testing involves placing suspected substances upon the skin of the back of the child for 48 hours and then removing the patches and reading the test at 72 hours. Usually, 20 patches are applied, and interpretation of the test requires an experienced observer. A positive test result reproduces the dermatitis in a small (1.0 cm) area of the skin of the back.

The most frequently observed contact allergens in children are neomycin, nickel, and potassium dichromate. Neomycin is a popular topical antibiotic, and neomycin-free antibiotic ointments can be recommended if the child requires them in the future. Nickel is found in jewelry, and dermatitis of the ear lobes caused by earrings is commonly seen. Metal belt buckles, watches, and necklaces are other common sources. Contact with nickel can be avoided by wearing no jewelry or by substituting nonmetal jewelry. Covering the metal with nail polish occasionally is effective and allows the child to continue wearing the jewelry. Hypoallergenic posts for ear piercing are widely available. Potassium dichromate is used to tan leather and is usually the cause of shoe-induced dermatitis in children. Wearing canvas or vinyl shoes will prevent the problem, or special shoes made of leather tanned without potassium dichromate can be specially ordered from several manufacturers but are expensive.

For children with recurrent or persistent allergic contact dermatitis, patch testing for allergen identification and subsequent strategies for allergen avoidance are most useful. Most physicians who perform patch testing have written lists of allergen sources and allergen-free products to provide the patients.

ATOPIC DERMATITIS

ALVIN H. JACOBS, M.D.

Atopic dermatitis is a genetically determined abnormality of the skin that often occurs in association with allergic diseases, probably as a linked inheritance. It is manifested as dry, itchy skin, which is subjected to many internal and external factors that tend to increase the pruritus, thereby stimulating the "itch-scratch" cycle. These factors include environmental temperature changes, stimulation of sweating, external irritants such as rough clothing, bacterial infection, emotional stress, antigen-antibody reactions, bathing with soap and water, and many others.

In managing patients with atopic dermatitis, the physician must recognize that the only primary skin manifestations are pruritus, dryness, and a generalized "goose-pimple" appearance. All other skin findings, such as oozing, weeping, crusting, or cracking, are secondary to scratching, rubbing, and secondary infection.

GENERAL MANAGEMENT

Psychological Factors. Successful management is time consuming for both parents and physician. At the outset, the parents must understand that this is a chronic disorder for which there is no complete and quick cure; rather, the therapy is aimed at controlling factors that contribute to the eruption and its attendant discomforts.

During the introductory discussions, the physician must be alert to the mother's emotional reactions to her child's disorder, since in many mothers guilt feelings arise from the fear that they are in some way responsible for the skin problem, as well as from their frequent feelings of rejection of the child and his or her ugly skin. The mother's emotional involvement is further complicated by the consumption of time in taking care of this crying, fussing, irritable, scratching infant or child. The physician must try to relieve the mother of her guilt feelings and express understanding of the rejection phenomenon. The treatment program must take into account the time the mother will have to devote to the care of her child's skin problem and must allow her periods of relief when she may be away from the child and without anxiety. I feel quite strongly that maternal anxiety transmitted to the infant or child may make the itching worse and aggravate the disease.

Infection. When first seen, most patients with atopic dermatitis have secondary infection, usually due to *Staphylococcus aureus*. This infection manifests as oozing, crusting, and fissuring of the skin. This infection must be adequately treated before other steps will be effective. Locally applied antibiotics are of little use in this situation, although 2 per cent mupirocin (Bactroban), a recently introduced topical agent, seems to be effective in clearing small areas of infection. Systemic antibiotic therapy should be given for at least 2 weeks to eliminate the secondary infection. Recurrent infection is common, requiring prolonged antibiotic therapy with eventual reduction to a maintenance dose. The most useful antibiotic in most cases of atopic dermatitis is erythromycin in a dosage of 50 mg/kg/day. Occasionally, it is necessary to use cloxacillin or cephalexin in the same dosage.

Clothing. The individual with eczema has a tremendous tendency to itch, and anything that irritates the skin will cause him or her to scratch. The child should, therefore, avoid irritating materials, especially woolens. Cotton and some of the softer synthetics are preferable for the patient with atopic dermatitis. Wool-upholstered chairs and wool carpets are also a source of irritation.

Sweating. Another important factor in the stimulation of pruritus is perspiration. Atopic dermatitis is always associated with a degree of sweat retention that will produce itching. Therefore, excessive clothing, high environmental temperatures, and overactivity will increase perspiration and promote itchiness.

Antipruritic Medication. The antipruritic action of antihistamines is beneficial in the treatment of atopic dermatitis, and long-term use may be necessary. Hydroxyzine (Atarax) appears to be the most effective, starting with 10 mg every 4 to 6 hours, and increasing the dose by 5-mg increments every 3 to 5 days until itching is minimized or intolerable sleepiness occurs. Since patients with atopic dermatitis itch more at night, it is advisable to double or even triple the bedtime dose. In fact, in some patients, it is possible to minimize side effects with acceptable therapeutic effects, with a single moderate-to-large dose at bedtime. If increased doses of hydroxyzine do not give sufficient night-time relief, diphenhydramine (Benadryl), in doses of 25 to 50 mg, can be added at bedtime because of its greater sedative effect. It is important to emphasize that antihistamines must be prescribed on a regular basis to help or control pruritus, thus interrupting the itch-scratch cycle.

Diet. Dietary management may be useful in only a small percentage of patients with atopic dermatitis. Diets that arbitrarily eliminate certain foods or types of foods rarely are helpful, and most often lead to malnutrition. A complete dietary history and the use of a food diary will occasionally bring out revealing information, but whether a suspected food is indeed responsible must be confirmed by a challenge test. If a food is related to exacerbation of the disease, administering the suspected food will cause marked redness and severe pruritus within 2 hours.

Hyposensitization. Skin tests, RAST tests, and hyposensitization therapy are of very little use in the management of the patient with atopic dermatitis. However, such testing may be used as a guide in conjunction with dietary history in selecting foods for challenge tests.

Systemic Corticosteroids. Oral or intramuscular corticosteroids should be avoided in the treatment of atopic dermatitis. On rare occasions, a burst of systemic steroids may be necessary for the initial control of a very severe dermatitis while instituting proper general and topical therapy. However, it should be kept in mind that the dermatitis often flares when the steroid is stopped.

Topical Therapy. When eczema is first seen in the acute phase, with inflammation, oozing, and crusting, it is important to recognize that secondary infection is present, and systemic antibiotic therapy must be promptly instituted (see previously). Reduction of inflammation and removal of crusts and exudate are best done with intermittent cool, wet dressings applied by the open method. Two or three layers of gauze, Kerlix, or linen are thoroughly moistened with Burow's solution and loosely applied to the involved areas without occlusion. One-half to 1 hour of application four times daily is usually sufficient, with remoistening by complete removal of the dressing every 10 minutes to prevent drying and sticking. Burow's solution, 1:40, is prepared by dissolving one tablet or packet (Domeboro tablets and powder packets) in 1 quart of cool tap water. Wet compresses should not be used for longer than 3 days.

At this point, or if the patient is first seen while in the dry, itchy phase, one may proceed with the modified Scholtz regimen, the prime feature of which is the complete avoidance of bathing with water. The dry skin of atopic dermatitis is due to a lack of sufficient water in the stratum corneum. The drier the skin, the greater is the pruritus. Washing with water removes the water-soluble substances that retain the water in the horny layer, thus resulting in increased dryness and itchiness after bathing.

The modified Scholtz regimen is instituted as follows:

1. No bathing with either soap or water is allowed. The only exception to this rule is the use of a moist washcloth to cleanse the groin and axillary areas if necessary.

2. The entire skin surface is cleansed at least twice daily with a nonlipid cleansing lotion consisting primarily of cetyl alcohol, sodium lauryl sulfate, propylene glycol, and water (Cetaphil Lotion or Aquanil Lotion.) The lotion is applied liberally and rubbed in until it foams. It is then gently wiped off, leaving a film of the lotion on the skin. This film aids in the retention of water in the horny layer of the skin.

3. No oily or greasy lubricants are allowed, since these will further occlude sweat pore openings and contribute to sweat retention.

4. Inflamed or pruritic areas of the dermatitis are treated by topical corticosteroids in a solution or cream formulation, not an ointment base. In relatively mild or moderate cases, 1 per cent hydrocortisone cream is effective. However, some generic preparations of hydrocortisone do not have a satisfactory base and may even be irritating. Several hydrocortisone preparations have been found to have smooth, nonirritating vehicles (1 per cent Nutracort, 1 per cent Hytone, and 1 per cent Synacort). In more severe cases, a medium-strength steroid, such as 0.1 per cent triamcinolone cream, may be used. However, as soon as improvement is evident, one should shift down to hydrocortisone. In any case, only 1 per cent hydrocortisone should be used on the face, groin, and genitalia.

All acutely inflamed areas can be cleared with the topical steroid preparation. If the entire program is followed, clearing usually occurs in 2 to 3 weeks. After the acutely inflamed areas have responded, it is possible to maintain the improvement by adhering to the no-bath policy and cleansing with the nonlipid lotion. The topical steroid is then needed only occasionally when there is a brief flare of the dermatitis.

5. When the skin has remained clear of eruption for several months, a brief cool bath is allowed once or twice monthly, always followed immediately by the liberal application of Cetaphil Lotion. Most patients are eventually able to tolerate a brief, not hot, bath as often as once weekly after they have remained clear for several months. It is essential that they learn never to bathe more often than once weekly and that they continue indefinitely to use Cetaphil or Aquanil Lotion for daily cleansing and lubrication.

URTICARIA

BERNICE R. KRAFCHIK, M.B., Ch.B., F.R.C.P.(C)

Urticaria is a pruritic dermatitis; it manifests as a series of red, raised dermal wheals. Angioedema occurs in the subcutaneous tissues and is usually asymptomatic. Both conditions are produced by fluid accumulation. The individual lesions appear and then disappear within a few hours. Urticarial reactions are arbitrarily divided into acute and chronic, depending on whether individual attacks last for less than 6 weeks or longer. The acute cases are usually self-limited, persisting for 10 to 14 days, whereas in chronic urticaria, clearing occurs spontaneously in 1 to 5 years without treatment.

Instrumental in causing urticaria is histamine, which is the main documented chemical substance released by the degranulation of mast cells. This process may be on an immunologic or nonimmunologic basis. Other substances released by mast cell degranulation include slow-reacting substance of anaphylaxis (SRS-A) and kinins; both of these are also potent causes of tissue edema and of wheal-flare reactions.

More than 20 per cent of individuals have at least one episode of urticaria during their lifetime. In only 10 to 20 per cent of cases does the etiology become apparent in spite of thorough history taking, complete physical examination, and laboratory work-up.

Treatment is often initiated without an apparent cause.

TREATMENT OF URTICARIA

With regard to treatment, it is useful to divide urticaria into three distinct groups, depending on its severity and duration: (1) life-threatening, (2) acute urticaria, and (3) chronic urticaria.

Treatment of the Life-Threatening Condition

Although rare, life-threatening angioedema results in airway obstruction, which requires emergency treatment. This is usually given in the hospital and consists of intramuscular or subcutaneous epinephrine (Adrenalin), 1 mg (concentration 1:1000), repeated in 2 to 5 minutes if necessary. A tracheostomy may be required. If obstruction is not life threatening but worsening, epinephrine, 0.5 mg subcutaneously, may be adminis-

tered. A mini-jet epinephrine and a pressurized aerosol epinephrine, one to three puffs per minute, are available for home use in cases in which patients are highly sensitive, such as reactions to the ingestion of nuts or to bee stings. Both subcutaneous injection and inhalation rapidly relieve obstructive symptoms.

While epinephrine is being administered, an intravenous steroid infusion should be started and continued over a period of 24 to 48 hours while the patient remains in the hospital. Hydrocortisone (Solu-cortef), either as 100 mg every 8 hours or as 4 mg/kg/day, is given initially and then changed to oral prednisone. In children, the dosage is 2 mg/kg/day, whereas in adults the dosage varies between 60 and 120 mg/day according to weight. The steroid dosage should be slowly decreased over a period of weeks.

In acute urticaria in which airway obstruction is not imminent, intramuscular or intravenous diphenhydramine (Benadryl), 25 to 50 mg, or other histamine$_1$ (H$_1$) blockers constitute the treatment. This agent may be combined with intravenous cimetidine, 300 to 600 mg injected slowly to avoid asystole, as studies have shown that H$_1$ and histamine$_2$ (H$_2$) blockers given simultaneously preserve vascular integrity and sustain blood pressure more effectively than an H$_1$ agonist used alone.

General Measures for Treating Acute Urticaria

In the minority of cases in which the etiology is apparent, it is imperative to address the precipitating factors by stopping drugs (e.g., penicillins and sulfas), treating a systemic illness (e.g., systemic lupus), or avoiding any of the causes of physical urticarias (e.g., sunlight, cold, exertion, and so on).

Heat, aspirin, and morphine may aggravate urticaria of any cause and should be avoided during acute episodes if possible.

Soaking in a cool bath once or twice a day with colloidal oatmeal is soothing, and a steroid cream mixed with 0.25 per cent camphor or 0.25 per cent menthol helps relieve the pruritus.

Specific Treatment of Acute and Chronic Urticaria

The mainstay of treatment for non–life-threatening urticaria is the H$_1$ antihistamines. There are now seven groups of these agents, which act on receptor sites around blood vessels to prevent the action of histamine (Table 1). Antihistamines do not prevent the production of histamine; therefore, treatment should be continued until symptoms do not recur when therapy is terminated. These measures are palliative without being curative.

Differences in the clinical efficacy of available H$_1$ classes are minor, although some studies have shown hydroxyzine hydrochloride to be the most effective, particularly in controlling cholinergic urticaria. Cyproheptadine is the drug of choice in the treatment of cold urticaria (it also has a hypothalamic effect and may stimulate appetite).

H$_1$ blockers are generally sedating, but drowsiness may be prevented by early evening administration and once-a-day dosage, as their effect is much longer lasting than previously thought. The newer antihistamines,

TABLE 1. Major Group of H₁ Antihistamines

General Class	Generic Name	Trade Name
Ethanolamines	Diphenhydramine	Benadryl
	Carbinoxamine	Clistin
	Clemastine	Tavist
Ethylenediamines	Pyrilamine	Triaminic
	Tripelennamine	PBZ
Alkylamines	Chlorpheniramine	Chlor-Trimeton
	Brompheniramine	Dimetapp
	Triprolidine	Actidil
Piperazines	Hydroxyzine	Atarax
	Cyclizine	—
Phenothiazines	Promethazine	Phenergan
	Trimeprazine	Temaril
	Methdilazine	Tacaryl
Piperidines	Cyproheptadine	Periactin
		Loratadine
	Azatadine	Optimine
Miscellaneous	Terfenadine	Seldane
	Astemizole	
	Ketotifen	

such as astemizole, 10 mg daily, and terfenadine, 60 mg twice a day, do not penetrate the blood-brain barrier and are, therefore, nonsedating and, in addition, have no anticholinergic effect, such as dryness of the mucosa. The latter product is equal but not superior to the classic H₁ antihistamines. When using astemizole, a therapeutic dosage takes some days to establish, so that initially double amounts may be required. The bioavailability of astemizole is reduced 60 per cent when taken with meals.

When single agents are ineffective, combinations of two H₁ antihistamines of different classes may be indicated. The addition of an agent acting on beta-adrenergic receptors, such as ketotifen, 1 to 2 mg twice daily, or an H₂ antihistamine (cimetidine, 300 to 600 mg twice a day) may also increase the therapeutic response.

Danazol (an attenuated androgen), 400 to 600 mg daily, has been shown to be effective for prophylactic and preoperative treatment of patients with hereditary angioedema.

Newer Agents in the Treatment of Urticaria

Loratadine, 10 mg, is a cyproheptadine derivative newly marketed, which is suitable for once-a-day dosage. It appears to be as efficacious as the conventional and newer antihistamines and does not exhibit sedating effects.

Ketotifen has a potent H₁ blocking effect and antianaphylactic activity. It acts by inhibiting mediator release and action and optimizing the expression of beta-adrenergic receptors. It is promising in the treatment of chronic urticaria, cold urticaria, and cholinergic urticaria.

Doxepin hydrochloride, 10 to 25 mg three times a day, a tricyclic antidepressant, has also been used in urticaria and is more effective than diphenhydramine.

ERYTHEMA NODOSUM

LAWRENCE SCHACHNER, M.D.

Erythema nodosum is not a simple clinical diagnosis, nor is it an entity whose pathogenesis is well understood.

It is believed to be a Type 3 hypersensitivity reaction to a myriad of agents, including infectious diseases, inflammatory diseases, drug reactions, and disorders that may frequently be of undiagnosed or unknown origin. The clinical appearance of erythema nodosum may be mimicked by various focal infections and inflammations of the subcutaneous fat and soft tissues with a predilection for the lower extremities.

On clinical examination in the acute stage, one will note multiple tender red nodular lesions. Although the lesions are most frequent and obtain their greatest size on the lower extremities, more generalized lesions, including facial erythema nodosum, have been seen. A characteristic color change from red to blue to yellow-green before resolution is probably commensurate with the degree of focal subcutaneous hemorrhage. Fever and malaise may precede the cutaneous lesions and/or accompany the acute stage of these lesions. Patients often complain of arthralgias, usually in the lower extremities, during the acute course of this disorder. While all ages and races, and both sexes, may be involved, there is an increased incidence in females versus males and in young people versus old people.

The etiology of erythema nodosum cases seen by a pediatrician may be determined by the ages and even the socioeconomic class of the patients he or she sees. For example, a practitioner who sees many school-age children may see many cases of *Streptococcus*-evoked erythema nodosum. A practitioner who services indigent populations or an area with a recent influx of immigrants from South America or Asia may see a fair amount of tuberculosis-associated erythema nodosum. Similarly, a pediatrician with a large adolescent practice may find many cases of oral contraceptive-associated erythema nodosum.

THERAPY

The initial therapeutic approach should be conservative but strict. At least 2 to 3 weeks of bed rest is usually optimal when patients are seen at the onset of disease. Every 3 hours throughout the day, cool water soaks should be placed wet over the lesions and allowed to dry for 20 minutes. If fever, malaise, or joint pain is significant, nonsteroidal acute inflammatory drugs (NSAIDs) or salicylates in dosages appropriate for age should be administered. It should be stated here that the most effective therapy for the specific case of erythema nodosum requires discovery of the etiology of the underlying infection.

Of the many etiologies of erythema nodosum, perhaps those most appropriately diagnosed are the infectious diseases. The most common causes, such as group A beta-hemolytic streptococcal infection, may be diagnosed by throat culture or streptozyme titer. A purified protein derivative (PPD) test is worth applying to any previously PPD-negative erythema nodosum patient. *Yersinia* species have been associated with gastrointestinal complaints and erythema nodosum.

Lymphogranuloma venereum, cat-scratch fever, and deeper fungal infection including coccidioidomycosis, blastomycosis, histoplasmosis, and deep *Trichophyton* infections may also be associated with erythema nodosum.

Frequently associated inflammatory disorders include sarcoidosis, regional enteritis, ulcerative colitis, and Behçet's syndrome. Various medications have been associated with eruptions of erythema nodosum, and many contemporary cases have accompanied the use of oral contraceptives, phenytoin, sulfa-related drugs, and halogens.

A minimal diagnostic work-up would include a streptozyme test, a PPD, a chest radiograph, skin tests for fungi, and a skin biopsy to rule out the various infections and inflammatory conditions that mimic erythema nodosum clinically but can be distinguished histologically.

Bed rest, wet soaks, and salicylates will usually alleviate pain and tenderness. Rarely, one finds persistent erythema nodosum in a patient whose clinical diagnosis has been confirmed by biopsy and in whom both infectious and noninfectious etiologies have been ruled out. In these rare instances, the use of intralesional corticosteroids may hasten involution of the lesions and relieve discomfort. Although the use of oral corticosteroids has been advocated in the literature, I have not found them to be necessary.

DRUG REACTIONS AND THE SKIN

LAWRENCE SCHACHNER, M.D.

Cutaneous drug reactions include both immunologic reactions of all classes of hypersensitivity and nonimmunologic reactions. The class of hypersensitivity reaction in the immunologic type often determines the appropriate therapy. In Type 1 hypersensitivity reactions, IgE antibodies are produced and reactions ranging from urticaria to angioedema and anaphylaxis may occur. In Type 2 reactions, drugs may form an antigenic complex with the surface of red blood cells or platelets. Thrombocytopenic purpura may be observed. Type 3 hypersensitivity reactions with drugs inducing an antigen-antibody and complement immune complex may result in cutaneous signs such as urticarial vasculitis. Indeed, a Type 3 reaction may be manifested by the persistence of urticarial-wheal type lesions that may progress to purpura. Severe cutaneous reactions of erythema multiforme, Stevens-Johnson syndrome, and toxic epidermal necrolysis might also be examples of Type 3 reactions. Further immune complex–mediated cutaneous reactions to medications include specific reactions, such as fixed drug reaction and erythema nodosum. Type 4 cell-mediated hypersensitivity may occur as an eczematous dermatitis with eruptive distribution in areas where topically applied medications have been used. Photoallergic reactions may be induced by either internal or external use of various medications.

In the pediatric population, the drugs most often associated with immediate or Type 1 hypersensitivity drug reaction are the penicillins, which may also be associated with Type 3 hypersensitivity drug reaction. In addition, numerous other drugs can produce a serum sickness syndrome with urticarial vasculitis and/or angioedematous components. These drugs include the commonly used childhood medications phenytoin and the sulfonamides. In Type 2 hypersensitivity reactions, again penicillin and the more rarely used quinidine class drugs may be associated with characteristic reactions. Topical medications, including antibiotics such as neomycin as well as numerous ointments with parabens and ethylenediamine as components, may induce a Type 4 or cell-mediated drug reaction.

Nonimmunologic drug reactions may take several forms. Long-term use of gold- or mercury-based drugs may lead to cutaneous or mucous membrane changes. Drugs may also be capable of a nonimmunologic activation of mast cell– and complement-mediated pathways inducing cutaneous reactions such as acute and chronic urticaria and angioedematous changes.

One may see among the common drug eruptions not only urticarial and vasculitic lesions but also acne type lesions, erythema multiforme, erythema nodosum, exanthem type lesions, eczematous dermatitis, fixed-drug eruptions, lichen planus–like eruptions, lupus-like eruptions, photosensitive eruptions, pigmentary changes, and blistering reactions.

THERAPY

Whenever the diagnosis of a drug eruption is made, if possible, the offending agent should be replaced by a non—cross-reacting medication. Many drug reactions are mild and require little more than discontinuation of the offending medication, followed by simple supportive measures. When pruritus is intense, oral antihistamines as well as mentholated topical preparations can offer considerable relief. The combination of hydroxyzine (Atarax) and pseudoephedrine (Sudafed) has been particularly successful in our more pruritic patients with drug reactions. Mentholated petrolatum or calamine with 0.25 per cent menthol is also quite soothing.

In drug reactions of more emergent nature such as the various severe hypersensitivity reactions, therapy must be individualized. A patient with a Type 1 hypersensitivity reaction of the anaphylaxis class will require emergency preservation of airway supplemental oxygen and intravenous use of epinephrine, Benadryl, and systemic steroids as the clinical manifestations mandate. Patients in whom the drug reaction may provoke considerable loss of cutaneous surfaces, such as drug-induced toxic epidermal necrolysis or Stevens-Johnson type erythema multiforme, may require fluid and electrolyte monitoring identical to that of patients with extensive burns. Indeed, the epidermal barrier function may be as disturbed as in a severe burn. In such patients I have used wet to dry soaks and Silvadene as topical therapy. In severe drug reactions, antibiotic treatment for secondary infection is often necessary. Although controversial, toxic epidermal necrolysis associated with several medications, including Dilantin, and Stevens-Johnson syndrome invoked by a number of medications, may necessitate the use of systemic steroids as a life-saving step when steroids are begun in the first days of the eruption.

Lastly, cutaneous reactions to topical medication may

be approached as any eczematous dermatitis. In the acute stage, it is important to apply wet to dry soaks to induce drying of the lesions. This may be followed with topical steroid cream preparations to induce added drying and decrease inflammation. Concomitant utilization of oral antihistamines may hasten the patient's relief.

ERYTHEMA MULTIFORME

JAMES E. RASMUSSEN, M.D.

The treatment of erythema multiforme depends upon the severity of the disease. Varieties with only a few papular or bullous lesions, primarily on the extremities, are usually referred to as erythema multiforme minor. Erythema multiforme major encompasses a spectrum of disease ranging from widespread blisters to severe involvement of the ocular and oral mucous membranes (Stevens-Johnson syndrome) to widespread sheet-like necrosis of the epidermis (toxic epidermal necrolysis). Minor varieties usually require no specific therapy, since the disease is short term and self-limited and has no common complications. Patients with erythema multiforme major usually require admission to hospital because of the severity of the disease as well as to maintain adequate fluid intake. The care of patients with erythema multiforme major can be divided into general (supportive) care, specific therapy, and management of complications.

GENERAL CARE

Patients with erythema multiforme major usually have substantial involvement of ocular, oral, and urethral mucosa. These patients usually have decreased fluid intake coupled with widespread loss of the protective epidermal barrier. Therefore, it is necessary to maintain adequate oral or intravenous intake of fluids, electrolytes, calories, and proteins. An occasional patient may also have moderate-to-severe kidney disease such as glomerulonephritis or acute tubular necrosis. Consequently, urine output, specific gravity, hemoglobin, hematocrit, serum electrolyte levels, and total body weight should be monitored diligently. Although most patients do not require intravenous therapy for more than 5 to 6 days, an occasional patient will have an extended recovery that necessitates parenteral feedings for several weeks.

Local wound care depends upon the extent of the cutaneous erosions. A few small lesions on the extremities can be treated with topical antiseptics such as silver sulfadiazine cream and dressings. In my experience, petrolatum gauze dressings are frequently all that is necessary. More widespread loss of the epidermis will probably require therapy similar to that for an extensive burn. Admission to a burn unit may be useful, but the problem of cross-infection should always be considered in an endemically colonized unit.

SPECIFIC THERAPY

There is a substantial controversy over whether patients with severe erythema multiforme should be treated with systemic doses of corticosteroids. While clinicians believe that these preparations are definitely helpful, six analyses have not shown any benefit. In fact, one showed that patients treated with corticosteroids had a greater incidence of bleeding and infection. If corticosteroids are to be used, the dose should be high enough to produce a response (1 mg/kg/day) and the duration short enough not to impede healing—no more than 4 to 7 days. Topical application of steroids has little or no place in the treatment of erythema multiforme.

Every patient with involvement of the ocular mucosa should be seen by an ophthalmologist. Topical application of corticosteroids and antibiotics is frequently recommended, but whether their use prevents complications and speeds healing is not known.

COMPLICATIONS

Patients with erythema multiforme may suffer a variety of complications, including infection, gastrointestinal bleeding, renal failure, and eye disease. Blood and wound cultures should be done at the first sign of a deterioration in the patient's condition and may be useful on admission as well, since some patients initially have erythema multiforme—associated infection. Prophylactic doses of antibiotics are not generally recommended, since they may be associated with overgrowth of antibiotic-resistant organisms. Gastrointestinal bleeding is surprisingly common in this group of patients and can often be massive and life-threatening. Whether cimetidine and antacids should be given is not known at this time, but it seems a reasonable precaution. Renal failure can be due to hypovolemia, acute tubular necrosis, or glomerulonephritis. Eye complications, including synechia and xerosis, are common.

GIANOTTI DISEASE

SILVIA IOSUB, M.D.

Gianotti disease, or papular acrodermatitis of childhood (PAC), is a distinctive erythematopapular rash with a peculiar distribution on the limbs and face. It is preceded by an upper respiratory tract infection and accompanied by generalized lymphadenopathy, mild constitutional symptoms, and anicteric hepatitis. In the cases described by Gianotti, hepatitis B surface antigen was invariably present and the virus was of the subtype ayw. The skin lesions are monomorphic, flat papules, 2 to 3 mm in diameter, that are nonpruritic and last 15 to 20 days.

In the past 10 years cases of PAC-like eruptions have been reported in association with other viruses: Epstein-Barr virus, cytomegalovirus, Coxsackie virus A-16, and parainfluenza virus. These eruptions are called "PAC with [the respective viral condition]." The term "Gianotti-Crosti syndrome" is used when the etiology is unknown.

Since Gianotti disease is self-limited, only symptomatic treatment is indicated.

PAPULOSQUAMOUS DISORDERS

DEBRA A. HORNEY, M.D.

SEBORRHEIC DERMATITIS

Seborrheic dermatitis of the scalp is best managed by frequent shampooing, preferably with antidandruff or antiseborrheic shampoos. Active agents and shampoos containing these include selenium sulfide (Exsel [prescription], Selsun [prescription], Selsun Blue), zinc pyrithione (Danex, DHS-Zn, Head & Shoulders), and tar derivatives (DHS Tar, Polytar, Zetar).* Combination products including sulfur, salicylic acid, and coal tar are also very effective (Ionil T, Sebulex, Sebutone, Vanseb T, and X Seb T).

Several factors influence the effectiveness of therapy. One is frequency of shampooing. Most patients require daily shampooing. However, this is determined on an individual basis, and some children do well with every-other-day or twice-weekly shampooing. Particularly with black patients, daily shampooing is not well tolerated. The hair of blacks is generally drier and more brittle than the hair of nonblacks. Conditioners, oil sprays, and glycerin-containing preparations are useful to keep the hair better hydrated and less susceptible to breakage.

For best results, the shampoo should be lathered and in contact with the scalp for 5 to 10 minutes before rinsing. In addition, to prevent the development of tolerance to a given shampoo, three different effective shampoos should be rotated on a weekly basis. Heavy scales and thick crusting of the scalp, as seen in "cradle cap," often require softening with mineral oil or petrolatum for 15 to 20 minutes prior to shampooing. For persistent cases, topical application of a steroid lotion or spray may be added to the regimen.

Eyelid dermatitis (blepharitis) may be managed with gentle warm water compresses and cleansing with an amphoteric "no sting" baby shampoo.

Seborrheic dermatitis of the face and intertriginous areas may be treated with 1.0 to 2.5 per cent hydrocortisone, e.g., Westcort or Tridesilon cream. Because of their cutaneous side effects (atrophy and telangiectasias), fluorinated topical steroid preparations should not be used on the face. Seborrheic dermatitis of the diaper area is often complicated by a candidal infection, which requires appropriate therapy.

PSORIASIS

Psoriasis is a common inherited disorder affecting 1 to 3 per cent of the population. The nails are affected in 25 to 50 per cent of patients. Psoriatic involvement of the nail matrix causes small pits in the nail plate, the most characteristic nail change in psoriasis. Other psoriatic nail changes include discoloration, subungual hyperkeratosis, crumbling of the nail plate, and onycholysis (separation of the nail plate from the nail bed). Psoriatic nails are difficult to treat. They should be kept closely trimmed, and subungual debris should be gently removed.

Psoriasis of the Scalp. The scalp is often the initial site of psoriatic involvement. The well-demarcated erythematous plaques with thick, adherent silvery scales may be diffuse or localized. Frequent shampooing is the key to effective management. Tar shampoos (Zetar, Polytar, Neutrogena T-Gel) are generally best but may be rotated with other keratolytic shampoos (see Seborrheic Dermatitis). When shampooing alone is ineffective, Baker's P & S (phenol, paraffin oil, and saline) solution, mineral oil, or baby oil should be massaged into the scalp at bedtime and the head covered with a shower cap. This will soften the scales, allowing their easy removal in the morning with a tar shampoo. Immediately after shampooing, while the scalp is still wet, apply a steroid lotion (Synalar or Valisone) or aerosol spray (Valisone).

Guttate Psoriasis. The sudden appearance of small guttate (droplike) psoriatic lesions over the trunk and extremities is a common and, sometimes, first presentation of psoriasis in a young child. The eruption is often preceded 1 to 3 weeks by an upper respiratory infection, such as a streptococcal pharyngitis. A 2- to 3-week course of erythromycin is warranted even in the absence of etiologic documentation. Additional topical therapy is discussed later.

Generalized Pustular Psoriasis. This rare, sometimes fatal, form of psoriasis is characterized by an explosive generalized eruption of superficial pustules associated with high fever and toxicity. The cause is unknown, but precipitating factors include acute infection and abrupt discontinuation of systemic or topical steroids. When possible, it is best to admit these very sick patients to a burn unit for total-body whirlpool therapy. Bland emollients and hydrocortisone cream are applied after whirlpool treatments. Short-term use of 13-cis-retinoic acid (Accutane)* (1.0 to 1.5 mg/kg) early in the course of the disease has shown great promise.

Death, when it occurs, is often associated with electrolyte imbalance or secondary infections.

Psoriatic Arthritis. Psoriatic arthritis occurs in about 5 to 10 per cent of patients with psoriasis and is seen only rarely in the pediatric patient. This painful arthropathy most commonly affects the distal interphalangeal joints of the hands and feet. There appears to be no relationship between the severity of the cutaneous disease and the development of joint disease. Therapy of psoriatic arthritis consists primarily of aspirin and other nonsteroidal antiinflamatory drugs, as well as physical therapy to minimize or prevent the flexural deformities that are known to occur.

Topical Therapy

The key to successful therapy of psoriasis is for patients to understand that although there is no cure

---

*All shampoos listed are available over the counter unless otherwise indicated.

*This use is not listed by the manufacturer.

for the disease, its satisfactory control is largely in their hands. That is, with daily attention to topical therapy, the average psoriatic patient will do well. Various topical agents are used. These include topical steroids, tar derivatives, anthralin, and keratolytic agents, such as salicylic acid.

For infants and young children, and for the face and genital areas in adolescents, 1 to 2.5 per cent hydrocortisone cream, applied twice daily, is recommended. Otherwise, mid-potency topical steroids (triamcinolone, Cyclocort, Synalar) in an ointment base are good for long-term use. High-potency topical steroids (Lidex, Diprosone, Topicort) should be reserved for recalcitrant disease and short-term use. A steroid ointment under occlusion (e.g., Saran Wrap) at bedtime is helpful for thickened, scaly plaques. Topical steroids should not be used more than twice daily. Other topical preparations, or even bland emollients, may be applied other times during the day.

To enhance penetration of the steroid, a keratolytic agent may be added. Salicylic acid (3 to 5 per cent) with 25 per cent Lidex cream in Aquaphor or Eucerin base is very effective.

Tar preparations, which decrease epidermal proliferation, remain a highly effective therapeutic modality. LCD (liquor carbonis detergens), 3 to 10 per cent, in Nivea oil or Eucerin cream, may be applied once or twice daily. Over-the-counter, cosmetically acceptable tar preparations are now available for baths and direct application. Three or four capfuls of Balnetar bath oil (2.5 per cent coal tar) or Zetar emulsion (30 per cent coal tar) is added to the bath water, in which the patient sits for 20 minutes. PsoriGel and Estar gel are applied directly to the lesions but are most effective when mixed with Aquaphor or Eucerin cream to prevent the drying effect of gel preparations. T-Derm body oil (5 per cent coal tar) may be applied directly to psoriatic plaques.

Tar preparations should not be used for inflammatory lesions or acute erythroderma. To avoid a tar folliculitis, the product should be applied down the extremity rather than up. Some tar products may stain hair and fabric.

Phototherapy

Most psoriatic patients are benefited by exposure to sunlight and, accordingly, have less cutaneous disease during the summer months. There is an occasional patient, however, who does worse with sun exposure. In all patients, appropriate sunburn precautions must be taken, since severe sunburn is likely to cause an exacerbation of the disease due to the Koebner phenomenon. Although natural sunlight is superior to artificial ultraviolet therapy, it is frequently helpful for the patient to have access to ultraviolet therapy (UVB) either at home or in the office. To optimize ultraviolet therapy, a tar preparation should be applied at least 2 hours prior to exposure and removed with mineral oil just before the treatment.

Recently, psoralen and long-wavelength ultraviolet light (UVA) have been used successfully in psoriatic patients.* However, the long-term toxicity of such ther-

---
*This therapy is still considered investigational.

apy has yet to be fully ascertained, and its use in children is not endorsed by the American Academy of Pediatrics.

Systemic Therapy

Only under rare circumstances should systemic therapy for psoriasis be required in children. Systemic steroids result in a dramatic clearing of psoriasis, but once discontinued, or even tapered significantly, there is often a serious rebound in disease activity. Prednisone does, however, have a role in the management of severe exfoliative erythroderma that is unresponsive to intensive topical therapy.

Methotrexate, a folic-acid antagonist, is highly effective in the management of recalcitrant, wide-spread psoriasis and psoriatic arthritis. Side effects include gastrointestinal disturbances and bone marrow, renal, and hepatic toxicity. It is used by dermatologists only under extreme conditions in children in a dose of 10 to 25 mg orally or intramuscularly once weekly.

The use of 13-*cis*-retinoic acid (Accutane) in pustular psoriasis has been described.

LICHEN PLANUS

The etiology of lichen planus is unknown. Thus there is no specific therapy, but the eruption generally resolves within 6 months to 3 years. Treatment is mainly symptomatic, aimed at reducing the pruritus that is the primary complaint in this disease. Orally administered antihistamines and mid- to high-potency topical steroids (Valisone, Lidex cream) are helpful. Hypertrophic plaques, which are recalcitrant to standard therapy, must be treated with Cordran tape or 0.1 per cent triamcinolone ointment covered with Saran Wrap overnight. The rare patient will require a short course of systemic steroids.

A variety of medications have been reported to cause a lichen planus–like drug rash. Thus, suspicious medications should be discontinued or substituted for whenever possible.

Since even minor surface injury is known to aggravate lichen planus, care must be taken to avoid unnecessary trauma. This is especially important in the mouth, where ill-fitting or rough-edged dental appliances and foods such as popcorn or peanuts may cause minor tears in the buccal mucosa along the bite line, where many lichen planus lesions are found. Intraoral lesions may be treated with topical anesthetics (Benadryl elixir mixed in equal parts with Maalox), topical steroids (Kenalog in Orabase), or topical 0.025 per cent Retin-A gel, applied three or four times daily.

PITYRIASIS RUBRA PILARIS

The treatment of pityriasis rubra pilaris (PRP) depends upon suppression of hyperkeratinization. For severe cases, this involves oral vitamin A therapy, 25,000 to 100,000 units twice daily. An adequate trial requires treatment for at least 3 to 6 weeks. If the therapy is effective and vitamin A is continued, it is important to watch for signs of vitamin A toxicity (anorexia, pruritus, hair loss, dry skin). To help prevent this, a 1-week drug-free holiday every 4 to 6 weeks should be considered.

13-*cis*-Retinoic acid (Accutane)* may also be effective, but side effects, including hypertriglyceridemia and skeletal hyperostoses, limit its usefulness in PRP. Methotrexate† is used in adults, but because of its potential toxicity this drug should be used with great caution in children.

Topical therapy includes mid- to high-potency topical steroid (Synalar, 0.1 per cent triamcinolone, Lidex) in an ointment or emollient base twice daily. Less potent topical steroids should be substituted once a response is seen. For the hyperkeratosis of the palms and soles, keratolytic agents—such as 3 to 5 per cent salicylic acid or 10 to 20 per cent urea in Aquaphor or petrolatum—applied two to four times a day are helpful.

Patients and parents should be counseled that PRP tends to be persistent and is characterized by spontaneous remissions and exacerbations.

PITYRIASIS ROSEA

If the rash of pityriasis rosea does not itch, no treatment is required. It is important, however, to advise patients and their parents that the rash may last for 6 to 12 weeks. Simple lubrication with bland emollients (Lubriderm, Keri lotion, Nivea) or an antipruritic lotion containing menthol and phenol (Sarna lotion) provides relief when pruritus is minimal. For more severe itching, a medium-strength steroid (Synalar, Aristocort, Cordran), applied alone or mixed in equal parts with a bland emollient, may be used twice daily. Antihistamines (hydroxyzine or diphenhydramine) and acetaminophen or aspirin also help relieve pruritus. Early in the course of the disease, exposure to ultraviolet light or sunshine may reduce the pruritus as well as hasten resolution of the eruption.

MUCHA-HABERMANN DISEASE

Mucha-Habermann disease, also known as pityriasis lichenoides et varioliformis acuta, or PLEVA, is characterized by crops of scaly papules or papulovesicles that tend to develop central hemorrhagic necrosis and crusts soon after they arise. Lesions may involve the entire body but are most pronounced on the trunk and the flexor aspects of the extremities. The etiology is unknown. Most acute cases resolve spontaneously within a few months and require no therapy other than antihistamines and emollients. Topical corticosteroids and natural or artificial ultraviolet light exposure are sometimes helpful. Likewise, oral administration of erythromycin, 40 mg/kg, or tetracycline, 1 or 2 gm/day, seems to shorten the course or minimize flares in some patients. Tetracycline, however, should not be used in children under 8 years of age because of the possibility of damage to teeth. These antibiotics are used on an empirical basis. The pathogenesis of this disease is not clear.

---

*This use of Accutane is not listed by the manufacturer.
†This use of methotrexate is not listed by the manufacturer.

CHRONIC NONHEREDITARY VESICULOBULLOUS DISORDERS OF CHILDHOOD

MARY K. SPRAKER, M.D.

The child with a blistering disease, especially when the problem is extensive, is a diagnostic and management challenge for the physician. Therefore, it is important to have a logical approach. The first step is to make sure that the child does not have an acute blistering disease such as bullous impetigo, the staphylococcal scalded skin syndrome, or toxic epidermal necrolysis; these diseases are discussed at length elsewhere in this text. Genetic blistering diseases are also seen in childhood; they are discussed later in this section under the heading Genodermatoses.

DERMATITIS HERPETIFORMIS

Dermatitis herpetiformis (DH) is an intensely pruritic, chronic recurrent eruption characterized classically by the presence of grouped erythematous papules and vesicles distributed symmetrically over the body, usually on extensor surfaces such as the elbows, knees, sacrum, buttocks, and shoulders. Patients with DH seem to have a gluten sensitivity, since therapy with a gluten-free diet is highly effective. Also, many patients are positive for the HLA-B8 antigen. Therefore it is hypothesized that, in genetically susceptible individuals, gluten causes the formation of IgA antibodies that initiate the alternate complement cascade, the end result of which is the inflammatory response we see in the skin. Unlike patients with celiac disease, another gluten-sensitive condition, patients with DH do not have diarrhea or malabsorption.

Treatment consists of medication or dietary restriction. It is said that 75 per cent of patients can be controlled with a strict gluten-free diet that removes the antigen. I encourage all my patients to become familiar with this diet, which requires referral to an experienced dietician, since a strict gluten-free diet is complicated. Because the diet usually takes 4 to 12 months to control the disease, and because it is extremely difficult for adults—let alone children—to follow, I find that therapy with medication is more practical. DH can be treated with either sulfapyridine or dapsone, a sulfone derivative. Either drug can cause a severe hemolytic anemia, which can be idiopathic or related to a glucose-6-phosphate dehydrogenase (G-6-PD) deficiency. Therefore, a G-6-PD level should be established prior to therapy with either drug.

The initial dose of sulfapyridine in children is usually 100 to 200 mg/kg/day in four divided doses, to a maximum of 2 to 4 gm daily. When existing lesions have been suppressed, the dosage may be tapered at weekly intervals. Frequently a maintenance dose of 0.5 gm or less may control the disease. Pretreatment and follow-up blood counts must be done at monthly intervals.

The sulfone derivative dapsone is better tolerated, more economical, and probably more effective than sulfapyridine, although some feel that its side effects may be more severe. A G-6-PD level, complete blood count (CBC), renal and liver function studies, and urinalysis must be obtained prior to therapy. The usual starting dose is 2 mg/kg/day, to a maximum of 400 mg daily, although some patients respond to lower doses. Patients respond rapidly within 4 to 48 hours. Then the dose can be decreased gradually to a minimum maintenance level, often as little as 25 to 50 mg daily. A CBC should be obtained two times per month for the first 3 months and then every 6 to 8 weeks. Liver function tests should also be given periodically.

BULLOUS PEMPHIGOID

Bullous pemphigoid is usually a disease of older adults, but occasionally it is seen in children. The etiology of this rare disease is unknown. The response to therapy is variable, but systemic and often high-dose corticosteroids on a chronic basis are usually required to suppress the eruption. In severe or resistant cases, a combination of sulfones or sulfapyridine in conjunction with systemic corticosteroids may be helpful.

CHRONIC BULLOUS DERMATOSIS OF CHILDHOOD

There is a great deal of controversy regarding this blistering disease. Some argue that it is the most common of the chronic bullous diseases of childhood, and others insist that there is no such disease, that the lesions are merely a form of either dermatitis herpetiformis or bullous pemphigoid. Most pediatric dermatologists believe that chronic bullous dermatosis of childhood is a separate entity because the direct immunofluorescent findings are distinctive: linear deposits of IgA are seen along the basement membrane.

The cause of the disorder is unknown. Like DH, chronic bullous dermatosis of childhood responds to either sulfapyridine or dapsone.

PEMPHIGUS VULGARIS

Fortunately, pemphigus is extremely uncommon in childhood, for it can be severe and sometimes fatal. The disease tends to be chronic, although spontaneous remissions occur rarely. It is usually fatal if not treated aggressively. The treatment of choice is systemic steroids. Once the disease is controlled, the dose should be slowly reduced and preferably administered on an alternate-day schedule. Immunosuppressive drugs such as methotrexate, azathioprine, or cyclophosphamide may be used in addition for patients with severe disease that is not controlled with steroids alone or to help reduce the need for high-dose steroids.

HERPES GESTATIONIS

Herpes gestationis is a rare blistering disease that occurs during pregnancy. The mother is primarily affected, but there seems to be an increased risk of fetal morbidity and mortality, and occasionally the infant has a similar dermatitis during the newborn period. The dermatitis clears spontaneously in most mothers within a few days after delivery, but in some it can persist for many months. There may be recurrences during subsequent pregnancies, after oral contraceptive treatment, and sometimes at the time of menstruation.

The mainstay of treatment for the mother is the systemic administration of steroids. These should be withheld during the first trimester of pregnancy, if possible, to avoid potential abnormalities in fetal development. Also, the dose should be reduced to a minimum during the final weeks of pregnancy to avoid adrenal suppression in the fetus. There have been some reports of therapy with pyridoxine, estrogen and progesterone, and plasma exchange. In the infant the disease is self-limited and requires no treatment.

DISCOID LUPUS ERYTHEMATOSUS
RONALD C. HANSEN, M.D.

The skin lesions of discoid lupus erythematosus characteristically appear in the chronic cutaneous form of the disease but may also be found in systemic and neonatal lupus erythematosus. The lesions should be approached as a separate problem when associated with the systemic disease.

Although the degree of induction or aggravation of the cutaneous lesions by sunlight varies from patient to patient, it is prudent to assume that photosensitivity is a feature in each case. Hence, a sunscreen lotion with a sun protection factor (SPF) of 15 should be applied to all lesional and exposed skin on a daily basis. Caution in sun exposure must be advised as well.

Topical corticosteroid creams are the mainstay of therapy. Here one is forced to use potent fluorinated steroid creams, even on the face, since the disease is difficult to control. It is advisable to review the possibly poor outcome of the lesions, noting that atrophy and telangiectasia are usually the results of the disease rather than of the therapy. Cordran tape is a convenient method by which to occlude a topical steroid.

In refractory cases, intralesional corticosteroid injections can be very beneficial. Intralesional steroids produce temporary atrophy, and this must be discussed in the context of an atrophy and scarring-prone disease such as discoid lupus erythematosus. Antimalarial agents such as hydroxychloroquine (Plaquenil) can be very helpful when the above measures have failed. However, there are finite risks, chiefly retinal toxicity requiring close ophthalmologic follow-up. Hence, antimalarials should be prescribed only by physicians who are knowledgeable about these agents and experienced in the management of childhood lupus erythematosus.

A brief course of systemic steroids is of occasional value in bringing an acute flare of discoid lesions under control, but systemic steroids have no place in chronic therapy of discoid lupus erythematosus in childhood. When systemic steroids are used for other organ system involvement, there is likely to be concurrent improvement in the discoid lesions.

KAWASAKI SYNDROME
(Mucocutaneous Lymph Node Syndrome)

MARIAN E. MELISH, M.D.

Although prevention and truly effective therapy for Kawasaki syndrome await the discovery of its etiology and pathogenesis, remarkable strides have been made within the last 5 years. For cases diagnosed within the first 10 days of illness, the early provision of intravenous gamma globulin and aspirin will result in a prompt defervescence in two-thirds of the patients and will reduce the likelihood of the development of coronary aneurysms from over 20 per cent to under 5 per cent.

DIAGNOSIS

Management of Kawasaki syndrome starts with diagnosis. Kawasaki syndrome should be considered in the differential diagnosis of patients with fever and any of the following: generalized polymorphous erythematous rash, conjunctival injection, characteristic changes in the mouth, characteristic changes in the hands and feet, and unilateral cervical lymph node swelling measuring greater than 1.5 cm. A secure diagnosis of Kawasaki syndrome is made in patients who fulfill five of the six criteria and in whom other illnesses that may mimic Kawasaki syndrome are excluded. Diseases to be excluded include (1) nonspecific exanthems, presumably viral; (2) measles; (3) streptococcal and staphylococcal scarlatiniform eruptions; (4) infectious mononucleosis; and (5) hypersensitivity reactions. There are "incomplete" cases of Kawasaki syndrome in which patients are at risk for the development of coronary artery aneurysms. Therefore, this illness should be considered even if diagnostic criteria are not fulfilled and, in some cases, patients with incomplete forms of Kawasaki syndrome should receive the same care as patients who fulfill all the clinical criteria. The laboratory tests provide modest diagnostic support. An elevated C-reactive protein or elevated sedimentation rate is almost universal in Kawasaki syndrome and not commonly found in viral exanthems, hypersensitivity reactions, or measles. Platelet count elevation greater than 450,000 is usually seen in patients presenting after the seventh day of illness, but platelet count is usually normal for the first week.

MANAGEMENT

Intravenous Gamma Globulin

As soon as the disease can be diagnosed, patients should have a baseline echocardiogram and receive intravenous gamma globulin, 2 gm/kg, given in a 10 to 12 hour infusion. This dosage schedule has recently been demonstrated to be equally efficacious in reducing the risk of coronary disease as a schedule of 400 mg/kg/day given for 4 consecutive days. The single-dose schedule is superior to the four-dose schedule in rapidity of return of fever and acute phase reactant to normal. Single-dose infusion is safe, having been given to approximately 300 children in a controlled trial with no significant adverse effects. Pulse, heart rate, and blood pressure should be monitored at the beginning of infusion, 30 minutes, one hour, and then q 2 hours during infusion. Although this dose does provide a substantial fluid and protein load, it has not been found to increase the risk of congestive heart failure, even in patients with decreased myocardial function.

There are no data available to guide therapy of patients encountered later than 10 days from onset. If patients are still febrile or have other signs of active disease including progressive coronary dilation, gamma globulin therapy should be instituted, as it may result in prompt clinical improvement. Patients who have become afebrile and have normal coronary arteries by day 21 of illness are unlikely to benefit from gamma globulin but should be placed on aspirin, 3 to 5 mg/kg once daily. There is currently no evidence suggesting any beneficial effect of gamma globulin in patients who have already developed coronary aneurysms once active inflammation has subsided.

Aspirin

On the same day that gamma globulin is administered, the patient should receive aspirin. The dose of aspirin best studied in the United States is 100 mg/kg/day until the fever is controlled or until day 14 of illness, followed by a dose of 5 to 10 mg/kg/day (40 to 80 mg p.o. given once daily) until sedimentation rate and platelet count are normal, which is approximately 3 months from onset of illness. The appropriate dose of aspirin in Kawasaki syndrome has been controversial. As gamma globulin appears to have potent anti-inflammatory effects, a lower dose of aspirin throughout the illness may be more appropriate. A study to answer this important question is currently under way. Salicylate level should be obtained if symptoms of vomiting, hyperapnea, lethargy, or liver function abnormalities develop while the patient is on high-dose aspirin. To decrease the risk of Reye's syndrome, aspirin can be interrupted if patients develop varicella or influenza during the follow-up phase.

Monitoring

All patients should be admitted to the hospital to receive their gamma globulin infusion and to be observed until fever is controlled. Cardiovascular function should be carefully monitored. Once a child's fever has decreased, it is unlikely that significant congestive heart failure or myocardial dysfunction will occur. The patient should be evaluated within a week after discharge and should have an echocardiogram between 21 and 28 days after onset of fever. If baseline and 3 to 4 week echocardiogram are normal with no evidence of coronary abnormality, further echocardiograms are unnecessary. The peak period to demonstrate coronary abnormalities detectable by echocardiogram is at 3 to 4 weeks after onset. In a recent study of >800 patients, we found no new abnormalities at 8 weeks if the 3 to 4 week echocardiogram was normal. Patients with no evidence of coronary abnormalities should receive 80 mg of aspirin per day for approximately 3 months, the period required for both platelet count and sedimentation rate to return to normal.

MYOCARDIAL INFARCTION

Myocardial infarction occurs most commonly in patients with giant coronary aneurysms > 8 mm in the first year after onset. Patients with a history of giant aneurysms are also at higher risk for later coronary thrombosis than are those with smaller lesions. Parents of all children with coronary abnormalities should be instructed to contact a physician and alert the emergency medical system if chest pain, dyspnea, extreme lethargy, or syncope develop. Prompt fibrinolytic therapy with streptokinase, urokinase, or tissue plasminogen activator should be attempted at a tertiary care center if acute coronary thrombosis is diagnosed.

NONCARDIAC COMPLICATIONS

Kawasaki syndrome is a multi-system disease but, except for cardiac complications, other systemic involvement is generally self-limited. In most cases, arthritis occurs in the acute stage and is intense and painful but self-limited, usually lasting less than 2 weeks. Although we have treated patients with both high-dose aspirin (100 mg/kg/day) and with other nonsteroidal anti-inflammatory drugs, particularly Tolmetin sodium (20 mg/kg/day in three divided doses), we have not been impressed with prompt temporal response to anti-inflammatory therapy. Many patients with large effusions appear to benefit most from arthrocentesis, which usually has to be done only once. Abdominal pain/diarrhea complex, also a feature of the early acute stage, usually responds to intravenous hydration and supportive care. Gallbladder hydrops, presenting clinically as a right upper quadrant mass, sometimes in association with obstructive jaundice, can be confirmed by diagnostic ultrasonography and monitored until resolution occurs. Surgical removal of the dilated gallbladder is not necessary as this complication is self-limited. A rare complication seen in the acute febrile stage is peripheral vasoconstriction threatening distal extremities. This is usually seen only in severe systemic illness with widespread vascular involvement. This complication has been managed with either prostaglandin E_1 infusion, 0.007 to 0.03 mg/kg/min maintained over several days in an intensive care unit with constant hemodynamic monitoring, or with systemic heparinization and corticosteroid pulse therapy (methyl-prednisolone 25 mg/kg IV push). There are anecdotal reports of success with both approaches but no controlled experience. Telephone consultation with a center treating large numbers of these patients should be sought by the physician whose patient has rare or serious complications.

LONG-TERM MANAGEMENT

Patients with No History of Coronary Artery Abnormalities. There is no need for aspirin or other antiplatelet medications beyond 3 months or for restriction of physical activities. Cardiac evaluation and EKG every 2 to 3 years may be warranted.

Patients with Transient or Small Coronary Aneurysms. These patients should be on long-term antiplatelet therapy with aspirin 3 to 5 mg/kg/day at least until resolution of abnormalities, preferably indefinitely.

There is no need for restriction of physical activities unless cardiac stress test abnormalities occur. Patients older than age 5 should be followed with yearly cardiac evaluations and periodic stress testing. Angiography is indicated if EKG or stress test abnormalities develop.

Patients with Giant Aneurysms. For patients with aneurysms 8 mm or larger, indefinite therapy with aspirin 3 to 5 mg/kg once daily with or without dipyridamole 3 to 4 mg/kg/day in 3 doses is given. Anticoagulant therapy with coumadin and/or subcutaneous heparin may be added, especially during the first 2 years after onset. Cardiac evaluation should be performed every 6 months with periodic stress testing. Angiography should be performed to define the extent of disease and whenever symptoms or stress tests indicated myocardial ischemia. Physical activity should be regulated on the basis of stress test results and level of anticoagulation. Patients with obstructive lesions or signs of ischemia may need to be evaluated for possible surgical intervention. These patients require consultation by a pediatric cardiologist with extensive experience managing Kawasaki syndrome patients.

FUNGAL INFECTIONS
LAWRENCE SCHACHNER, M.D.

The use of creams and lotions with combined antifungal and anti-yeast action, such as miconazole (Micatin), clotrimazole (Lotrimin), and haloprogin (Halotex) have made the treatment of superficial mycosis somewhat simpler. However, their appropriate use, as well as that of griseofulvin in tinea capitis and tinea unguium, can maximize their effectiveness and enhance the rate at which the patient is helped. Adjuncts that enhance the therapeutic action of these medications in specific mycosis and the substitution of often less expensive preparations such as selenium sulfide (Selsun) or sodium thiosulfate (Tinver) in tinea versicolor have also been very effective.

Specific diagnostic tests for cutaneous fungal infections should not be allowed to become a lost art. Correct performance of potassium hydroxide (KOH) preparations and Wood's lamp examination can lead to immediate and inexpensive confirmation of the diagnosis of cutaneous fungal infections. Fungal cultures, particularly in tinea capitis, can lead to confirmation that a clinical finding such as alopecia is appropriately attributed to a dermatophyte and is not a clinical sign of mild or severe underlying disease.

It is worth reiterating briefly the technique of KOH preparation. Hair specimens, scale from the border of the cutaneous eruption, nail scrapings, or blister roofs are placed on a microscope slide with a cover slip. Ten to 20 per cent KOH may be added to the side of the cover slip and will disperse itself equally over the covered material by flowing under the edge of the cover slip. KOH solutions free of dimethylsulfoxide (DMSO) should be heated until they begin to boil. If the KOH solution contains DMSO, the preparation should not be heated. Scanning the field under low power, with the condenser lowered to a position that allows for reduced amounts of illumination, will often aid in finding characteristic hyphae in dermatophytes, or pseudohyphae and budding spores in candidiasis.

The Wood's lamp is a valuable diagnostic tool in a number of cutaneous and systemic diseases, not the least of which are tinea capitis and tinea versicolor. In a totally darkened room, the patient's scalp or skin is illuminated with the Wood's lamp. The microsporum species causing tinea capitis reveals a characteristic green fluorescence that is most notable in the areas of inflammation and loss of the acral hair shafts. The Wood's lamp produces an orange or yellow fluorescence over areas of involvement of the skin with tinea versicolor.

There are several media to choose among when preparing fungal cultures. Dermatophyte test medium (DTM) is a reliable diagnostic adjunct. The presence of a dermatophyte is confirmed not only by colony growth but also by the change in color of the media from gold to red in the presence of a dermatophyte. Mycosel agar is another good diagnostic culture medium for identifying dermatophytes and *Candida albicans*.

THERAPY

Two dermatophytoses that always require griseofulvin therapy are tinea capitis and tinea unguium. Tinea capitis, caused by species of *Trichophyton* and *Microsporum*, presents as an inflammatory or noninflammatory scalp disorder featuring scaling and alopecia. Inflammation, when present, can vary from mild to a suppurative boggy mass, replete with pustules and swelling, called a kerion. Griseofulvin should be started in doses of 10 to 20 mg/kg in the microcrystalline forms and half that dose in the ultra-microcrystalline griseofulvins, such as Gris-PEG. Since griseofulvin absorption seems to be enhanced by fatty food, I recommend that it be given after meals including milk or ice cream products. Griseofulvin should be given for a minimum of 4 weeks and preferably for at least 2 weeks after all clinical signs of disease have abated. Additional benefit may be gained by the use of keratolytic shampoos, such as Sebulex, which have been reported to decrease dissemination of spores and infected particles to the patient and to others who may physically contact the patient. Topical antifungal solutions including clotrimazole, haloprogins, and miconazole preparations may enhance the rate of clinical improvement.

When tinea capitis has evolved to the point of kerion formation, the choice of therapies to clear the infection and minimize permanent hair loss and scalp scarring takes on added importance. In addition to griseofulvin, a course of prednisone at 1 mg/kg/day for 1 to 2 weeks will greatly decrease the inflammation and help attenuate the course of the kerion. Although the subject is certainly controversial, I among others feel that a 10-day course of oral antibiotics such as cloxacillin or erythromycin also may be helpful when kerions are

present. If griseofulvin is not tolerated or is ineffective, oral ketoconazole (Nizoral) may be tried.

Tinea unguium is a chronic infection of finger- and toenails that is fortunately rare in childhood. Culture and KOH can help distinguish onychomycosis caused by *Trichophyton* or *Epidermophyton* from that caused by *Candida albicans*. The latter often is limited to the nails of the upper extremities, and concurrent paronychial inflammation is characteristic. Topical medications are effective in candidal nail infections, and any of the medications mentioned above, such as clotrimazole or nystatin preparations, would be useful. The onychomycoses due to *Trichophyton* and *Epidermophyton* species require long-term griseofulvin therapy. Similar dosages as for tinea capitis are appropriate; however, therapies must extend for at least 4 to 6 months for potential cure.

Tinea corporis, tinea cruris, tinea faciei, and tinea pedis, when acute, merit wet to dry soaks to decrease the inflammation and the oozing associated with the eczematous state. Tap water soaks are both effective and most inexpensive; if soaks are applied for 20 minutes every 4 hours for 2 days, most patients with these forms of tinea are ready for topical therapy. Most will respond nicely and completely to 2 to 3 weeks of twice-daily therapy with clotrimazole, haloprogin, miconazole, or tolnaftate (Tinactin), although the latter is effective only against dermatophytes and is not active against *Candida albicans*. Recurrences of tinea may be decreased by the prophylactic administration of topical antifungal creams or powders. Only the most chronic severe and unresponsive forms of the above-mentioned tineas will require the addition of griseofulvin.

Tinea versicolor is a common chronic cutaneous infection that may be entirely asymptomatic. Although any of the above-mentioned topical antifungal preparations can be effective, the widespread distribution of the lesions makes selenium sulfide (Selsun) or sodium thiosulfate (Tinver) an effective and less expensive therapeutic approach. Overnight applications of either of these preparations to the entire affected area for a period of 2 weeks often leads to resolution. Pigment changes will take longer to resolve. Prophylactic therapy with these two preparations or with the above-mentioned antifungals can prevent recurrence, especially in more temperate months and climates.

Candidiasis, whether of the oral mucous membrane, the perineum, the flexural surfaces of the body, or the nails or interdigital spaces of the upper extremities, is responsive to nystatin preparations. Oral administration of nystatin suspension is useful not only in thrush but also in decreasing the bowel contamination that can seed candidal diaper dermatitis. The candidal dermatitis of the newborn infant is also nystatin responsive as is candidal vulvovaginitis, which can be treated with vaginal preparations. Much previous enthusiasm for Mycolog cream and similar polyformulary preparations has waned because of the presence of topical corticosteroids and sensitizing compounds in their formulation.

WARTS AND MOLLUSCUM CONTAGIOSUM

LAYNE HERSH, M.D.

WARTS

Warts are benign growths caused by the human papilloma virus. Originally warts were thought to be caused by a single DNA virus type; however, there has recently been evidence to suggest at least seven antigenically distinct viruses. Warts often last 1 to 2 years but may regress spontaneously. The choice of treatment depends on the age of the child and the location of the warts.

Lesions of the hands and extremities respond best to liquid nitrogen applied with a cotton-tipped applicator. Freezing time varies with the size of the wart but is usually around 15 to 30 seconds. Parents should be told that a blister may occur and will fall off by itself. In very young children cantharone can be applied sparingly. This works best if the area is then covered with tape for 4 to 6 hours. Treatments are given once or twice a month, and the wart may take weeks or months to resolve.

Flat warts on the face, arms, and knees are usually treated with retinoic acid (Retin-A cream or gel) daily until erythema and scaling are produced. If this treatment is too irritating, a light freeze with liquid nitrogen, 5 to 10 seconds, can be tried instead. Shaving can spread warts and should be avoided.

Plantar warts are notoriously difficult to treat. The least painful way to begin therapy is with 40 per cent salacid plaster, applied daily and secured with tape. As the wart softens it is pared, with a No. 15 blade, once a month. An alternative to the plaster is topical salicylic acid and lactic acid liquid (Duofilm) applied daily. This also works better if occluded with tape.

Condylomata acuminata and penile warts in uncircumcised boys can be treated with 25 per cent podophyllin in tincture of benzoin. Care should be taken to apply the chemical only to the wart. It should be washed off in 2 to 4 hours to avoid a severe reaction. As the treatment is repeated weekly, the time it is left on can be increased gradually to 6 to 8 hours. These lesions are rarely encountered in very young children and raise the possibility of sexual abuse.

Treatments still considered experimental include wart vaccine, intralesional bleomycin, topical acyclovir (Zovirax), and topical 5 per cent 5-fluorouracil cream. For recalcitrant warts a laser may be helpful.

Susceptibility to warts and the rate of their resolution depend on the child's immune system. The incidence of warts is higher in immunosuppressed transplant patients and in children with Hodgkin's disease, lymphomas, and leukemias. It has been hypothesized that both cell-mediated immunity (T cells) and complement-fixing antibodies (B cells) may play an important role in the immune response.

MOLLUSCUM CONTAGIOSUM

Molluscum contagiosum is a viral infection of the skin characterized by a pearly-white papule with central umbilication. The treatment usually includes cantharone, with or without occlusive tape, for 4 to 6 hours or a light liquid nitrogen freeze of 5 to 10 seconds. Occasionally it may be preferable to use a local anesthetic and open each papule with a No. 11 blade, then curette out the contents of the sac. Treatment can be repeated once or twice a month, depending on the number of lesions and the rate of appearance of new papules.

SCABIES AND PEDICULOSIS

SIDNEY HURWITZ, M.D.

SCABIES

The treatment of scabies consists of topical application of 1.0 per cent gamma benzene hexachloride (lindane; available as Kwell, Scabene), 10 per cent crotamiton (Eurax), 6 to 10 per cent precipitate of sulfur in petrolatum, 5 per cent permethrin cream (available as Elimite cream 5 per cent) or a suspension of benzyl benzoate in a 12.5 to 25 per cent concentration. Application of lindane from the neck down in older children and adults and to the entire body, including the head and neck, in infants and young children is curative in 96 per cent of patients. The medication is applied to dry skin for a period of 6 to 12 hours and is then removed by a thorough washing (shower or bath). One application is usually curative, but when necessary, lindane may be reapplied in 1 week for another 6 to 12 hours. The vulnerability of small infants to percutaneous absorption of this potentially neurotoxic substance warrants caution in prescribing lindane for infants and small children. Although most cases of adverse reaction have been caused by misuse of the preparation, the problem of possible toxic effects is more acute in infants and small children, owing to a relatively greater skin surface and possibly higher blood level accumulations in this age group.

For infants and small children (those 1 year of age or younger), alternative therapy includes 5 per cent permethrin cream (Elimite cream 5 per cent) applied from the scalp to the feet, including the soles, for 8 to 14 hours (overnight), and 10 per cent crotamiton cream or lotion (Eurax) applied twice a day for 5 days or 6 per cent sulfur in petrolatum applied nightly for 3 nights. Again, the therapy may be repeated in 1 week if necessary.

Pruritus due to hypersensitivity to the mite antigens may persist for days or weeks despite adequate therapy. It may be treated by oral doses of antihistamines or hydroxyzine, by topical application of antipruritic lotions containing menthol or phenol (Cetaphil or Keri lotion with 0.25 per cent menthol), or by topical application of pramoxine, available as Prax or Pramosone (1 per cent hydrocortisone in combination with pramoxine), in cream or lotion. Postscabietic nodules, which represent a hypersensitivity to the mite, frequently persist for many weeks to months. Although therapy is not necessary, they can be treated with variable degrees of success by application of topical corticosteroids alone or in combination with tar formulations (Estar gel, PsoriGel, or Fototar cream), intralesional steroids, or corticosteroids under occlusion.

When treating an individual patient, the entire family and close personal contacts should be examined and, if affected, treated appropriately. Since the hypersensitivity state and associated pruritus and nodular lesions frequently do not cease immediately after eradication of the infestation, the patient and his family should be alerted to this possibility so that they will not be tempted to continue excessive, unnecessary, and potentially hazardous therapy.

PEDICULOSIS

Head Lice. Pediculosis capitis, except under crowded and unsanitary conditions, is the most common form of louse infestation. Lindane (Kwell, Scabene) is a highly effective treatment. One tablespoon, approximately 15 ml of 1 per cent shampoo is massaged into the scalp for 4 minutes and followed by a thorough rinsing. If the lotion is used, it may be applied to the scalp, left on overnight, and then washed out carefully. A second treatment may be repeated after 1 week if viable eggs persist. Other members of the family should be examined, and those with evidence of infestation should be treated. Pyrethrins (RID, A-200) are also effective and are available as over-the-counter formulations. It should be noted, however, that corneal damage, namely ulceration and scarring, has been reported with the use of A-200, which contains 5 per cent denatured kerosene.

An alternative treatment for pediculosis capitis is malathion 0.5 per cent (Ovide Lotion, Gen Derm) or a 1 per cent permethrin formulation (available as Nix Creme Rinse). Since nits are firmly attached to the hair shaft, their removal may be facilitated by the use of a fine-toothed comb or tweezers. When nits are resistant to removal, a formic acid formulation available as Step 2 Creme Rinse will help facilitate their removal.

Pediculosis Pubis. Pediculosis pubis normally involves the hairs of the pubic region but may also involve the eyelashes, beard, mustache, and axillary and other body hairs. Infestation of the pubic region is most frequently seen in adolescents and young adults as a result of transmission by sexual intercourse, but the lice may also be transmitted by clothing, bedding, or towels. The treatment of pediculosis pubis is similar to that of pediculosis capitis. Sexual contacts should be treated simultaneously, but other household members need not be treated. At the conclusion of therapy, treated individuals should change their underclothing, pajamas, sheets, and pillowcases. These articles should be washed and dried by machine, ironed, or boiled to destroy remaining ova and parasites.

Pediculosis Palpebrarum. Pediculosis of the eyelashes may be treated by petrolatum applied thickly to the eyelashes twice daily for 8 days, followed by mechanical removal of remaining nits. Although this appears to be the treatment of choice, physostigmine ophthalmic preparations (Eserine) are also effective when applied topically to the eyelid margin twice daily for 24 to 48 hours. Because of the parasympathetic effect of physostigmine, miosis is a possible side effect.

Fluorescein eyedrops may also be utilized to treat pediculosis of the eyelids.

Pediculosis Corporis. The body louse generally lives in clothing or bedding, lays eggs along the seams of the clothing, and visits the human host only long enough to feed. This disorder is rarely seen in children, except under conditions of poor hygiene. The treatment of pediculosis corporis mainly consists of proper hygiene, with frequent showers or baths and frequent changes of underclothes and bedding. Underclothing and bedding should be laundered with hot water or boiled; dry-cleaning destroys lice in articles that cannot be laundered. Pressing woolens with a hot iron, with special attention given to the seams of the clothing, is also satisfactory. All likely contacts (members of the household and close contacts in an institution) should be examined and treated if there is evidence of infestation.

DISORDERS OF PIGMENTATION

ROBERT A. SILVERMAN, M.D.

Cutaneous chromophores are compounds within the skin that absorb specific wavelengths of light to produce skin color. Hemoglobin (red) and melanin (brown, blue-gray, or black) are examples of intrinsic chromophores, while carotene (yellow) is an example of an external agent that may affect skin color. Disorders of pigmentation are due to increases or decreases in the amount of chromophores or to the manner in which they are dispersed in the skin (superficial, deep, clumped, or diffuse). This discussion will be limited to melanin pigment disorders.

Superficially, generalized or localized pigment anomalies are only of cosmetic significance; however, some may portend serious underlying illness. In addition, the location and extent of pigmentation may adversely affect a child's psychosocial development and self-image. These factors should be considered when a diagnostic work-up is considered or a therapeutic intervention is contemplated. Treatment of pigment disorders is directed at lessening the contrast between dark and light areas of skin.

HYPERPIGMENTATION

Freckles. Freckles (ephelides) are small (less than 6 mm in diameter), light brown macules with ill-defined borders, which may darken significantly in response to sun exposure. They occur on individuals who burn easily and tan poorly. Freckles are not present at birth and usually develop during later infancy or early childhood.

Common freckles should not be confused with the axillary freckles of neurofibromatosis. In addition, freckling during early infancy may be a sign of xeroderma pigmentosum or other photosensitivity diseases.

Since melanin pigment in freckles is located in the epidermis, it is amenable to therapy with hydroquinone bleaching agents or light freezing with liquid nitrogen. However, such treatments may be irritating, sensitizing, or painful and are inappropriate for use in children. Strong consideration should be given to the routine application of a sunscreen agent (sun protection factor of 15 or above) or an opaque sun block (that contains zinc oxide) to all children who freckle easily. This practice minimizes the appearance of these macules and protects the fair-skinned child from other acute and chronic ultraviolet light effects, which include sunburn and potential skin cancer.

Lentigines. Lentigines are medium to dark brown macules that are similar in size to freckles. However, these proliferations of melanocytes have distinct borders and remain heavily pigmented even when located on skin not exposed to sun. They may be found on the lips and mucosal surfaces. The LEOPARD syndrome, Peutz-Jeghers syndrome, and LAMB syndrome are characterized by a myriad of these macules.

Treatment of lentigines is not indicated, but cryotherapy or hydroquinone bleaches (e.g., Solaquin, Melanex, and Eldoquin) will lighten the lesions. Lentigines may also be removed by shave biopsy or laser photocoagulation.

Postinflammatory Hyperpigmentation. Postinflammatory hyperpigmentation is common in children with dark skin color or in those who tan easily. It occurs most commonly in response to insect bites, trauma, pityriasis rosea, or various exanthems. The neonatal "freckles" of pustular melanosis are also a form of this condition.

Postinflammatory hyperpigmentation lasts for months, since there is retention of melanin in dermal macrophages. Therefore, topically applied depigmenting agents are generally not useful. Topical hydroquinone bleaches may produce partial hypopigmentation. Cosmetic cover-ups (e.g., Covermark and Dermablend) and the "tincture of time" are the most judicious approaches to the problem. The prompt treatment of preexisting inflammatory conditions with topical corticosteroids may minimize the complication of postinflammatory hyperpigmentation in susceptible patients.

Melasma (Chloasma). Melasma is a patchy, often symmetric light to dark brown skin condition located on the face of women who are pregnant or are receiving estrogens. The condition becomes more obvious after sun exposure. Cases in children or men are distinctly unusual and should prompt careful diagnostic consideration. Melasma is easily distinguished from the more uniform blue-gray nevus of Ota. Sunscreens, cosmetic cover-ups, and bleaches containing 2 per cent hydroquinone combined with tretinoin may be helpful in some patients.

Incontinentia Pigmenti (Bloch-Sulzberger Syndrome). Incontinentia pigmenti is an X-linked dominant condition characterized by vesicular, eczematoid, hyperpigmented, and hypopigmented stages that occur sequentially from birth. The macular pigmentation has a peculiar whorled or "marble-cake" pattern, which usually fades over a period of years. The pigmentary stage is rarely present at birth and should be distinguished from a zosteriform lentiginous nevus. No treatment is required, but the physician should be aware of associated abnormalities of the auditory, ophthalmic, musculoskeletal, and central nervous systems.

Dysplastic Nevus Syndrome (BK Mole Syndrome). It is now recognized that at least some melanomas in adults (5 to 35 per cent) arise in association with a peculiar type of nevocellular nevus, the dysplastic nevus (or the Clark nevus). Dysplastic nevi are first manifest during puberty and have been recognized in 2 to 5 per cent of white adults.

Dysplastic nevi share certain clinical and pathologic features with melanoma, including large size (greater than 6 mm in diameter), irregular or ill-defined ("smudged") borders, asymmetric shape, and several shades of color (brown, red, white, blue, or black). Dysplastic nevi may be located on the head, neck, trunk, or non–sun-exposed areas of the scalp, interdigital web spaces, or buttocks.

Although dysplastic nevi are benign, a change in the appearance of these lesions should prompt immediate excision. The presence of dysplastic nevi increases one's risk for melanoma, especially in a familial setting with melanoma in two or more relatives. Routine complete cutaneous examination and regular use of sunscreens should be stressed. Pigmented lesion clinics have been organized in many academic centers as one approach to the management of these patients.

Congenital Nevocellular Nevus. Congenital nevi are tan to black pigmented lesions found in approximately 1 per cent of newborn infants. These benign proliferations of nevus cells and melanocytes are usually larger than 1.5 cm in diameter and are always raised above the skin surface when observed in tangential light (as opposed to café au lait spots). In a minority of cases, small and medium-sized congenital nevi have been associated with contiguous malignant melanoma that develops during adulthood. Malignant degeneration of giant or garment nevi may occur during early childhood.

The management of congenital nevi is controversial. Prophylactic surgery to remove the nevus is currently advocated by many investigators. Small lesions may be electively removed when a child is old enough to tolerate local anesthesia, while staged surgical procedures should be planned during infancy for "bathing trunk" lesions. Alternatively, the physician may wish to observe, measure, and photograph congenital nevi and teach families self-examination techniques if surgery is not desired. Currently, there are no nonsurgical methods that produce satisfactory removal of congenital nevi. Bleaching agents, dermabrasion, and chemical peels should be avoided.

Café au Lait Spots. Café au lait spots are uniform, light brown macules found in 10 to 20 per cent of normal children. Five or more café au lait spots greater than 0.5 mm in diameter on an infant or six or more café au lait spots greater than 1.5 cm in diameter on an older child or adolescent are presumptive evidence for type I (peripheral) neurofibromatosis. Other disorders with increased numbers of café au lait spots include Watson's syndrome, tuberous sclerosis, Turner's syndrome, and Russell-Silver syndrome. Unilateral or segmental large café au lait spots are suggestive of McCune-Albright syndrome (precocious puberty, polyostotic fibrous dysplasia, and endocrine dysfunction). A single large macule that develops on the shoulder just before puberty is characteristic of a Becker nevus. Treatment of café au lait spots is not advised or necessary.

HYPOPIGMENTATION

Vitiligo. Vitiligo is a common acquired condition characterized by somewhat symmetric, irregular macular patches of depigmentation in which melanocytes are absent. Spontaneous resolution is unusual. Treatment for 3 to 6 months may be attempted with daily applications of midpotency corticosteroid creams. The ivory-white patches located around the eyes and mouth and over the knees, elbows, and digits may repigment if melanocytes remain in the hair bulbs of the affected areas. Ultraviolet light by itself is not useful; however, topical or systemic photosensitizers (psoralen), in combination with ultraviolet A radiation, administered in a carefully supervised setting is useful in older, motivated patients. This modality (PUVA) may require months of administration and may entail acute and chronic risks, such as phototoxicity, cataracts, and potential skin cancer induction. Routine sun protection is mandatory and will minimize differences in pigmentation between affected and nonaffected areas. Vegetable dyes (e.g., Vytadye, Dye-O-Derm) as well as cosmetics (Dermablend or Covermark) are useful camouflage agents. Proper application of these products is very important for optimal results. Punch grafts and in vitro melanocyte cultures with autotransplantation are new techniques that may restore pigment to small patches of vitiligo. The widespread application of these techniques is not currently expected. Since vitiligo has been associated with other autoimmune disorders, a careful history, a physical examination, and laboratory studies (e.g., thyroid antibodies) may be obtained.

Piebaldism. Piebaldism is a congenital absence of pigment that at first glance may be confused with vitiligo but is distributed in a widespread truncal or midline pattern. A white forelock is a forme fruste of this disorder. Piebaldism may be associated with Hirschsprung's disease. Repigmentation is currently not possible. Cosmetic cover-ups are helpful, and sunscreens are necessary to diminish contrast.

Waardenburg Syndrome. This congenital depigmentation resembles piebaldism except that it is associated with sensorineural deafness, laterally displaced medial canthi, and heterochromic irides. A white forelock is also present. Protection from sunburn should be stressed.

Tuberous Sclerosis. Tuberous sclerosis is an autosomal dominant condition characterized by lance-ovate–shaped, hypopigmented macules that may resemble an ash leaf. Larger hypopigmented patches and small confetti-like macules may also be observed, especially when a Wood light is employed to accentuate the lesions. White spots are also found on a significant number of normal, unaffected individuals. Therefore, other stigmata, such as angiofibromas, a shagreen patch, periungual fibromas, intracranial calcification, seizures, mental retardation, renal cysts, or cardiac rhabdomyomas, should be present in the patient or a family member to suspect a probable diagnosis of tuberous sclerosis. There is no treatment for the hypomelanotic macules.

Hypomelanosis of Ito (Incontinentia Pigmenti Achromians). Hypomelanosis of Ito is a sporadic condition recognized at or soon after birth that is characterized by whorled, marble-cake hypopigmentation. Unlike incontinentia pigmenti, there are no preceding inflammatory stages. However, abnormalities in other organ systems similar to those in incontinentia pigmenti may be found in hypomelanosis of Ito. There is no treatment.

Disorders of Generalized Pigment Dilution. Genetic abnormalities of melanin production, packaging, or transfer result in generalized pigment dilution. For instance, there are at least 17 forms of albinism that affect the skin or eyes or both. Functional or structural abnormalities or an absolute decrease in the enzyme tyrosinase (necessary for melanin synthesis) has been documented in many of these cases. The cofactor for tyrosinase, copper, is known to be diminished in the serum of patients with Menkes' kinky hair syndrome, in which the complexion is very sallow. Chédiak-Higashi syndrome is characterized by pale skin color from abnormal melanosomes that are not transferred to other skin cells and characteristic giant lysosomes in peripheral blood leukocytes that are dysfunctional and predispose affected individuals to pyogenic infections. No satisfactory treatment for pigment dilution in these disorders is currently available. For patients with defects compatible with relatively normal lifespans, sun protection is necessary to reduce the risk of basal cell and squamous cell carcinomas during adulthood.

Pityriasis Alba. Pityriasis alba is an inflammatory skin condition frequently observed in atopic children that is characterized by hypopigmented, slightly scaly patches of skin located primarily on the cheeks. A more generalized form comparable to folliculopapular eczema due to external irritants may be observed on the trunk and extremities. The "ashy" appearance is most distressing to parents of darkly pigmented individuals. Moisturizers, 1 per cent hydrocortisone preparations, and avoidance of irritants will improve the appearance of children affected by this transient, self-resolving, benign condition.

Postinflammatory Hypopigmentation. Postinflammatory hypopigmentation may be observed after severe eczema, burns, erythema multiforme, psoriasis, or a host of other conditions. Tinea versicolor, found commonly on the neck, shoulders, and back of adolescents, should not be confused with this condition. Localized areas of postinflammatory hypopigmentation may be camouflaged with agents used to treat vitiligo. Small areas may resolve spontaneously over a period of years.

PHOTODERMATOSES

MOISE L. LEVY, M.D.

Dermatoses caused by exposure to sunlight are generally easy to appreciate from the distribution of the cutaneous findings in affected individuals. The challenge to physicians is dealing with the wide variety of potential causes for the photosensitivity disorder seen in a particular patient. Such problems can be purely environmental in origin, based in genetic or metabolic diseases, the result of systemic illnesses, drug related, or idiopathic.

POLYMORPHOUS LIGHT ERUPTION

This group of diseases is characterized by a predisposition to a photodistributed skin eruption marked by eczematous patches, erythematous papules or plaques, or sometimes vesicles, which may resolve with superficial scarring. This group of diseases is felt to result primarily from short-wavelength ultraviolet light (UVB), although some cases are demonstrated to result from long-wavelength ultraviolet (UVA) exposure. It must be emphasized that the diagnosis of this disease is one of exclusion.

Treatment is necessarily based on sun avoidance and protection from excessive sun exposure. The routine use of sunscreens is essential. In selected individuals, the use of antimalarial agents, such as hydroxychloroquine, or beta-carotene has proved useful in controlling these eruptions.

DRUG-INDUCED PHOTOSENSITIVITY

The finding of a photodermatitis in a child receiving medications such as tetracycline derivatives, sulfonamides, phenothiazines, and thiazides should raise concern for the role of such medications in the appearance of the skin disease. Additional medications such as amiodarone and certain nonsteroidal anti-inflammatory agents have been implicated in this setting as well. Obviously, discontinuation of the suspected drugs should be attempted if at all possible. Diligent application of sunscreens should also be employed.

COLLAGEN VASCULAR DISEASES

Lupus erythematosus (LE) is a well-known systemic illness that can be marked by acute or chronic photosensitivity. The diagnosis can, at times, be difficult to confirm. An "acquired" form of LE, neonatal lupus erythematous (NLE), is essential to recognize. This condition is often marked by a photodistributed dermatitis and, in some infants, by congenital heart block. Dermatomyositis, like LE, will frequently show varying degrees of photosensitivity.

Treatment of each of these diseases should include sun control measures, including liberal and frequent sunscreen use, as part of their overall management. Topical corticosteroids can be used to modify the local inflammatory response, as needed for limited times. The lowest potency steroid to obtain the desired result should be utilized. In selected individuals with LE or dermatomyositis, antimalarial agents have proved to be useful adjuncts in the control of the photodermatitis.

GENETIC AND METABOLIC DISEASES

A myriad of such diseases can be included in this section and can usually be distinguished on the basis of clinical or laboratory data. Examples would include Rothmund-Thomson syndrome, ataxia-telangiectasia, Bloom and Cockayne syndromes, xeroderma pigmentosum, and the group of porphyrias.

Of the last-named diseases, erythropoietic protoporphyria (EPP) is dominantly inherited and is seen in children aged 2 to 5 years. This condition is marked by itching or burning, followed by vesiculation and ultimately scarring over exposed surfaces after exposure to UVA. Other porphyrias may be seen in children but are much rarer.

Management again involves sun protection. Betacarotene has proved quite useful in EPP. Many of the other diseases carry an increased risk of developing cutaneous or internal malignancies, which necessitates cautious, long-term evaluation of affected patients.

ENVIRONMENTAL PHOTODERMATITIS

Photodermatitis can result from a variety of agents found in deodorant soaps, perfumes, and plants, such as limes and figs. Many of these photoreactions are due to furocoumarins, which, when exposed to light, result in erythema, vesiculation, and oozing. The often bizarre-shaped hyperpigmentation that results is sometimes confused with bruising from physical abuse. Management, of course, involves avoidance of sun exposure and treatment of the acute reaction with mild topical corticosteroids. The postinflammatory hyperpigmentation will generally resolve spontaneously over weeks to months.

NEVI AND NEVOID TUMORS

ANDREA M. DOMINEY, M.D.,
and MOISE L. LEVY, M.D.

The term nevus is derived from the Latin word *naevus*, meaning mark. Nevus can be used clinically to describe a congenital or acquired lesion, or it can be used histopathologically to describe a cell that is presumably related to the melanocyte. Nevi may be divided into several categories, including nevocellular, melanocytic, vascular, and epidermal.

NEVOCELLULAR NEVI

Congenital Nevocellular Nevus

Congenital nevocellular nevi occur in approximately 1 per cent of neonates. By definition, they are lesions that appear at birth or shortly thereafter. Some studies show that female infants are affected twice as often as male infants; the most common locations of involvement include the face, chest, and buttocks.

Large congenital nevi have a 5 to 15 per cent risk of malignant degeneration. Malignant melanoma generally develops during the first 15 years of life. Therefore, patients with large congenital nevi should be referred to a pediatric or plastic surgeon for excision as soon as possible. Disseminated nevi or large nevi affecting the head and neck area may be associated with central nervous system abnormalities.

The management of small congenital nevi should be individualized. Some studies have shown that small nevi have a 3 to 10 times increased risk of developing malignant melanoma. Parents should be counseled regarding the potential risk of malignant melanoma and the need for close observation. Onset of bleeding or changes in size, color, and thickness may signal the development of a mitotic process. Excision prior to puberty may be advisable.

Acquired Nevocellular Nevus

Acquired nevocellular nevi generally appear several years after birth. The peak age of incidence is the second decade. Treatment is cosmetic except in the case in which malignant degeneration is suspected. Lesions may be shaven, saucerized, or excised.

Halo Nevus

Nevi that are surrounded by a rim of depigmentation are called halo or Sutton's nevi. This phenomenon usually occurs in acquired nevi, although congenital nevocellular nevi, blue nevi, and malignant melanoma may be similarly affected. Vitiligo may be an associated finding. The appearance of halo nevi should trigger a careful examination of the integument, looking for signs of atypical nevi or malignant melanoma. If no abnormalities are found, treatment should consist of expectant observation. A large proportion of halo nevi will spontaneously resolve.

Nevus Spilus

Nevus spilus represents a special subset of nevocellular nevi characterized by brown macular pigmentation studded with dark brown to black macules or papules. These lesions may be present at birth or may develop at any age. Because there is no increased risk of malignant melanoma, treatment is cosmetic.

Spitz Nevus

Spitz nevi, also called spindle cell nevi or benign juvenile melanoma, are benign lesions that usually appear on the face during the first decade of life. Generally solitary, they appear as red to red-brown, smooth, dome-shaped papules or nodules. They are usually less than 1.5 cm in diameter. Surgical excision may be desired and is frequently performed owing to the potential histologic confusion with malignant melanoma.

Dysplastic Nevus

Another subset of acquired nevocellular nevi is the dysplastic nevus. These occur in fewer than 10 per cent of the population older than 14 years of age, and onset is during the first two decades of life. Certain familial forms with at least two family members affected by malignant melanoma have up to a 100 per cent lifetime risk of developing malignant melanoma. Sporadic forms and familial forms with fewer than one family member affected by melanoma have a sevenfold increased risk of malignant melanoma.

The management of these patients should include inquiry about a family history of melanoma or atypical nevi, confirmation of the diagnosis of dysplastic nevus by biopsy, self-examination every 1 to 2 months, and annual examination by a dermatologist to document changes in pre-existing nevi or the development of new dysplastic nevi. Prophylactic removal of all dysplastic nevi is usually neither feasible nor desirable. All blood relatives of patients with dysplastic nevi and a family history of melanoma or atypical nevi should also be evaluated. Sun exposure should be avoided.

MELANOCYTIC NEVI

Becker's Nevus

Becker's nevi are light brown macules with splotchy pigmentation that appear during the second decade of life, around the time of puberty. They are usually found in boys, although female patients have been reported. The lesion is usually solitary and located on the upper trunk, especially the scapular area. Coarse hair develops with advancing age. Treatment is cosmetic.

Mongolian Spots

Mongolian spots are benign, single or multiple, ill-defined, blue to blue-gray macules of varying size and shape. They are present at birth and occur in approximately 25 per cent of all newborns. They tend to fade with time and are of no significance except that they are sometimes mistaken for bruises.

Nevus of Ota and Nevus of Ito

Nevus of Ota, also called nevus fuscoceruleus ophthalmomaxillaris, is a unilateral slate gray to blue macule seen in the periorbital, temporal, malar, or frontal area of the face. Bluish pigmentation may be noted in the ipsilateral sclera. The lips, palate, and nasal mucosa may also be affected. Approximately 50 per cent are congenital, with the remainder developing by the second decade of life. Nevus of Ito, or nevus fuscoceruleus acromiodeltoideus, has the same clinical features as nevus of Ota, except that it is located on the scapula and deltoid area. Malignant degeneration is very rare, and treatment is cosmetic. Excision, dermabrasion, or laser surgery should be considered on an individual basis.

Blue Nevus

Blue nevi are sharply demarcated, oval to round, blue-gray to blue-black, dome-shaped lesions that are generally less than 1 cm in diameter. A variant of the blue nevus is the cellular blue nevus, which is greater than 1 cm in diameter and usually located on the buttocks. The risk of malignant melanoma is small, and treatment is elective surgical excision.

VASCULAR NEVI

Nevus Simplex

One of the most common congenital skin lesions is the nevus simplex, also called salmon patch, angel's kiss, stork bite, or Unna nevus. The vast majority, with the exception of nuchal lesions, fade with time, and no treatment is necessary.

Nevus Flammeus

Clinically, these nevi manifest as flat to minimally elevated, red to purple lesions that may darken and develop papules or nodules with time. The most common location is the face.

The Sturge-Weber syndrome consists of a nevus flammeus involving the first branch of the trigeminal nerve with ipsilateral vascular malformations of the meninges and cerebral cortex. If the second branch of the trigeminal nerve is also involved, congenital glaucoma may be associated. Since the characteristic cerebral calcifications do not develop until the child is 1 to 2 years of age, evaluation of the newborn should include computed tomography with contrast used in visualizing the head, electroencephalograms, and ophthalmologic examination when indicated. Treatment of nevus flammeus includes cosmetic camouflage or argon laser therapy (in older children and adolescents); the tunable dye laser can be used in younger children.

Capillary Hemangioma

Capillary or strawberry hemangiomas may appear at birth, but they usually are first seen at 1 to 2 months of age. The period of rapid growth is during the first 7 months of life, and over the next few years, the vast majority spontaneously involute. Generally, no therapy is needed; however, if the lesion encroaches on vital structures, such as the eye, intervention is necessary. These lesions may respond to systemic steroids. Surgical excision and cryotherapy are other options.

Cavernous Hemangioma

Cavernous hemangiomas appear at birth as bluish-red, subcutaneous nodules that tend to be soft and compressible. Unlike strawberry hemangiomas, cavernous hemangiomas grow in proportion with the child. They may spontaneously involute with time. Up to 90 per cent have some degree of resolution by age 9, and treatment is generally not warranted.

Syndromes Associated with Vascular Lesions

Blue rubber bleb nevus syndrome is the association of cavernous hemangiomas with gastrointestinal hemangiomas. Gastrointestinal bleeding and anemia are common problems with this syndrome. *Maffucci's syndrome* manifests after the time of birth as cavernous hemangiomas, phlebectasias, lymphangiomas, and dyschondroplasia. The vascular lesions do not necessarily overlie the bone lesions. This syndrome occurs more frequently in male babies and has a 30 per cent incidence of malignancy. *Klippel-Trenaunay-Parkes-Weber syndrome* consists of vascular malformations such as port-wine stains, capillary hemangiomas, cavernous hemangiomas, phlebectasias, or lymphangiomas associated with hypertrophy of the soft, hypertrophic area. *Kasabach-Merritt* syndrome is the development of a consumptive thrombocytopenia because of a capillary or cavernous hemangioma. The hemangioma may be as small as 5 to 6 cm in diameter.

ORGANOID NEVI

Epidermal Nevus

Clinically, these nevi appear as single or multiple, well-demarcated, linear, flesh-colored to hyperpigmented, verrucous plaques. These nevi may appear at birth or in childhood or even early adulthood. The epidermal nevus syndrome consists of large or generalized epidermal nevi, as well as bone, central nervous system, cardiovascular, and ophthalmologic abnormalities. Malignant degeneration of epidermal nevi is unusual. Therapy should be individualized and includes surgical excision, cryotherapy, and dermabrasion.

Nevus Sebaceous

Nevus sebaceous occurs in fewer than 1 per cent of births and appears as a flat to slightly elevated, yellow to orange, linear to oval plaque. The risk of malignant degeneration is 10 to 20 per cent; and treatment consists of surgical excision around the time of puberty or earlier. Like epidermal nevi, large midline or extensive nevi may be associated with central nervous system, cardiovascular, or ophthalmologic abnormalities.

OTHER SKIN TUMORS

MARY K. SPRAKER, M.D.

Most skin tumors are uncommon in children, but when a lesion does occur it is important that it be diagnosed accurately, since some of these tumors indicate underlying systemic disease, some require surgical intervention, and an occasional lesion is malignant.

FACIAL LESIONS

The following lesions are most frequently found on the face and therefore may be confused with acne if they are not carefully examined.

Angiofibromas, inaccurately called *adenoma sebaceum* in the older literature, are the small (1 to 4 mm) pink or flesh-colored papules seen in association with tuberous sclerosis. They generally begin during early childhood but occasionally are not present until puberty. As the patient ages, the lesions become somewhat larger. They can be effectively treated with cryosurgery, electrodesiccation and curettage, or dermabrasion if removal is necessary for cosmetic reasons. Occasionally a lesion may be solitary; in that case it is not associated with tuberous sclerosis.

Although *trichoepitheliomas* may occur as solitary lesions in early adult life, the other form of the disorder, which is dominantly inherited, begins during childhood or at puberty and is associated with multiple lesions. Small (2 to 5 mm) flesh-colored papules and nodules are seen on the central area of the face. Solitary lesions should be excised, but with multiple lesions excision is unnecessary. Instead, they are treated with electrodesiccation, cryotherapy, or dermabrasion. While most trichoepitheliomas are benign, there is disagreement in the literature about whether some of these lesions eventually evolve into basal cell carcinomas.

Trichofolliculomas also occur on the face. These flesh-colored papules or dome-shaped nodules classically have a central pore with a protruding tuft of fine hair. The lesion is best treated by surgical excision.

Syringomas frequently first appear during adolescence.

Small (1 to 3 mm) skin-toned or yellowish papules or nodules are seen. They occur on the lower eyelids in more than half of affected patients. Other common locations include the sides of the neck, trunk, extremities, and genital area. It is estimated that one-fifth to one-third of children with Down's syndrome have syringomas. Treatment is necessary only for cosmetic reasons and consists of destruction by electrodesiccation, cryotherapy, or surgical excision.

Basal cell carcinomas are slow-growing, locally invasive but rarely metastasizing malignant skin tumors that are all too common in older adults but are also seen occasionally in children. They occur most commonly in individuals with fair skin who have been exposed to the sun. Over the past decade we have been seeing more adolescents with basal cell carcinomas on the face, which are frequently mistaken for acne. The lesions begin as small (2 mm) erythematous papules that have a clear or translucent quality and often contain telangiectasias. They enlarge slowly and may undergo some central necrosis and crusting. Occasionally basal cell carcinomas are pigmented and resemble nevi, or they may be sclerosing and resemble scars.

In the *basal cell nevus syndrome*, multiple basal cell carcinomas are associated with other abnormalities including temporal bossing, dental cysts, bifid ribs, intracranial calcifications, ovarian fibromas, and, rarely, medulloblastoma. The disorder is inherited in an autosomal dominant fashion. Skin lesions usually first appear at puberty, although they may occur much earlier.

It is important that basal cell carcinomas be completely removed, since the carcinoma may recur locally if the excision is not complete. The lesions can be surgically excised or removed by curettage and electrodesiccation.

RED-BROWN LESIONS

Pyogenic Granulomas. These solitary, red-to-brown, vascular pedunculated nodules, 5 mm to 1 cm in diameter, may develop rapidly on any cutaneous surface. The lesions are round and well circumscribed and clinically may resemble small capillary hemangiomas. The etiology is unclear, but it is thought that trauma to the skin in the presence of pyogenic bacteria causes a reactive proliferative vascular process. These lesions are usually easy to treat. They can be shaved or snipped off parallel to the skin and the base electrodesiccated. The specimen is usually sent for a pathologic examination to confirm the diagnosis and to differentiate this benign lesion from other conditions, including a Spitz nevus or amelanotic melanoma.

Urticaria Pigmentosa. It is not uncommon for the pediatric dermatologist to see children with one or two localized lesions of urticaria pigmentosa known as *mastocytomas*. These red-brown or yellow-brown papules or nodules urticate when rubbed (Darier's sign). They are composed of collections of mast cells in the dermis that release histamine when the skin is traumatized, resulting in the characteristic urtication. Children with just a few of these lesions rarely have systemic symptoms.

Other children, however, have myriads of smaller yellow to red-brown macules or papules that are also composed of mast cells and therefore urticate with stroking. When the disease is this extensive it is known as *urticaria pigmentosa*. Many children have only cutaneous symptoms of the disease, consisting of itching and, sometimes, blister formation. Approximately 10 per cent of patients, however, have systemic involvement, since mast cells can also accumulate in almost any body organ or tissue, including the bones, liver, spleen, and lymph nodes. Patients with systemic symptoms may have flushing attacks, hypotension, headaches, tachycardia, pruritus, diarrhea, and, rarely, blood clotting abnormalities. These symptoms can be severe and life threatening.

Patients with cutaneous disease alone generally require no therapy unless the lesions are symptomatic; then antihistamines usually help to control pruritus or blistering. The prognosis in most patients is excellent, since the lesions resolve spontaneously in time. Children with numerous lesions should avoid aspirin, codeine, morphine, procaine, and polymyxin B because these nonspecific releasers of histamine may cause systemic symptoms. Patients with systemic symptoms may be treated with oral cromolyn, cimetidine combined with an H_1 antihistamine, or UVA light therapy with psoralen. Children with many cutaneous lesions should have a complete blood count periodically to check for the presence of mast cell leukemia, which has been reported in a small number of patients.

Juvenile Xanthogranulomas. These yellow to red-brown papules and nodules can be solitary or multiple. They may occur anywhere on the body but are common on the head and neck. They resolve spontaneously after several years. In most patients this is a benign and self-limited problem. However, the disease can also occur in other body organs, including the lung, pericardium, meninges, liver, spleen, and testes. Systemic involvement usually is asymptomatic and requires no treatment or evaluation. However, if lesions are present in the eye, glaucoma or hemorrhage may occur in the absence of treatment. Therefore, any child with this disease should be examined by an ophthalmologist.

Eccrine Poromas. This benign cutaneous tumor, which arises from the sweat duct unit, usually occurs in older adults but has been reported in adolescents. Firm, reddish nodules, 2 to 12 mm in diameter, are usually seen on the dorsal surface of the foot. The treatment of choice is surgical excision.

FLESH-COLORED LESIONS

Follicular Cysts. This lesion, which is also known as an *epidermal* or *sebaceous cyst*, is a discrete, slowly growing, elevated, firm nodule that may occur anywhere on the body but is commonly seen on the face, scalp, and back. The cyst contains a cheesy white material that has a sour odor. The treatment is surgical excision. The entire cyst, with its epidermal lining, must be removed to prevent recurrence.

Pilomatrixomas. These uncommon solitary deep nodules occur only in children and adolescents. A 0.5 to 2 cm flesh-colored or reddish-blue nodule is seen on the face, neck, or upper extremities. Treatment is surgical excision.

Neurofibromas. These soft polypoid lesions, which "buttonhole" or invaginate into the underlying dermis when pressure is applied to their surface, may first appear in childhood. Solitary lesions may occur in otherwise normal individuals. However, when multiple lesions are present they are a cutaneous marker for the dominantly inherited disease *neurofibromatosis.*

Connective Tissue Nevi. These single or multiple, slightly raised, skin-colored oval lesions may occur anywhere on the body and may be a sign of an inherited condition. Biopsy shows them to be composed of collagen or elastic fibers. The *shagreen patch* seen in tuberous sclerosis is actually a large connective tissue nevus. In the *Buschke-Ollendorff syndrome*, multiple widespread connective tissue nevi are present in association with osteopoikilosis.

Lipomas. These benign nodules, which are soft and rubbery in consistency, may occur on any part of the body. They are composed of mature fat cells. Treatment is not required unless the lesions are large enough to cause a cosmetic problem.

Recurring Digital Fibromas of Childhood. These smooth, shiny, erythematous nodules occur on the distal phalanges of infants and young children. The management of these lesions is controversial. There are several case reports of spontaneous involution. Of lesions surgically excised, 70 per cent recur. Dissection down to the periosteum is necessary.

Dermatofibromas. Dermatofibromas are small (1 mm to 3 cm) dermal nodules that are fixed to the skin but move freely over the subcutaneous fat. They may occur anywhere on the body. They range from flesh colored to brown. Treatment is unnecessary unless there is a cosmetic problem. Treatment options include cryotherapy and surgical excision.

SCARS AND KELOIDS

Damaged dermis heals with a *scar* that is initially pink. The color gradually fades to a permanent white, and the scar appears shiny. New scars may be elevated or *hypertrophic* before they finally flatten and contract, within 6 months to 1 year after the original injury. They must be differentiated from *keloids*, which are an exaggerated connective tissue response to skin injury. Keloids appear long after the original injury and slowly increase in size beyond the area of the original wound. While hypertrophic scars usually require no therapy, as they will flatten in time, keloids do not resolve spontaneously and may continue to enlarge slowly. They can be treated with intralesional injections of corticosteroids; if this fails, surgery can be attempted if it is needed for cosmetic reasons. Surgical excision must be done with care, and intralesional steroids are usually injected both at the time of excision and periodically during the postoperative period to prevent recurrence of the keloid.

THE GENODERMATOSES
SIDNEY HURWITZ, M.D.

The genodermatoses are a group of cutaneous disorders with genetic rather than environmental causes.

These include the ichthyoses, ectodermal dysplasias, disorders of collagen and elastic tissue, and diseases of metabolism. Appropriate management requires knowledge of the conditions and their clinical features and of the genetic risks for patients and their families. An important aspect of therapy for the genodermatoses is genetic counseling, so that families of affected individuals can evaluate the risk of future pregnancies for themselves and their offspring.

ICHTHYOSIS

Icthyosis refers to a group of hereditary cutaneous conditions characterized by dryness and scaling. The management of all forms of ichthyosis consists of retardation of water loss, rehydration and softening of the stratum corneum, and alleviation of scaliness and associated pruritus. Ichthyosis vulgaris and X-linked ichthyosis can be managed quite well by the topical application of emollients and the use of keratolytic agents to facilitate the removal of scales from the skin surface. Limited baths with a mild soap, prolonged baths followed by the application of petrolatum, and hydration of skin by frequent use of lubricating creams or lotions are helpful. Urea, in concentrations of 10 to 20 per cent in a cream, lotion, or ointment base, has a softening and moisturizing effect on the stratum corneum and is helpful in the control of dry skin and pruritus. Propylene glycol (40 to 60 per cent in water), applied overnight under plastic occlusion, helps hydrate the skin and assists in the desquamation of scales.

Salicylic acid is an effective keratolytic agent, and concentrations between 3 and 10 per cent promote shedding of scales and softening of the stratum corneum. When these agents are used to cover large surface areas for prolonged periods, however, care should be taken to ensure that salicylate toxicity does not occur. Keralyt Gel (Westwood Pharmaceuticals), a proprietary preparation containing 6 per cent salicylic acid in propylene glycol, is frequently helpful after hydration of the involved area. Alpha-hydroxy preparations, such as lactic, glycolic, or pyruvic acid, are also beneficial for the treatment of ichthyosiform dermatoses. Lactic acid is available as Epilyt Lotion (Stiefel Laboratories), Lac-Hydrin Lotion (Westwood Pharmaceuticals), and LactiCare or LactiCare HC Lotion (Stiefel). Although 5 to 12 per cent concentrations of lactic acid are frequently utilized, lower concentrations of 2 to 5 per cent and LactiCare HC lotion are less irritating and usually better tolerated by young children and individuals with atopic dermatitis or open, raw, or irritated cutaneous eruptions. Glycolic acid is available in a 5 per cent concentration as Aquaglycolic Lotion (Herald Pharmacal).

Lamellar ichthyosis can be treated with lubricating lotions containing urea, salicylic acid, or lactic acid. Although this approach is somewhat beneficial, it is not as effective as in the treatment of ichthyosis vulgaris and X-linked ichthyosis. The treatment of epidermolytic hyperkeratosis (bullous ichthyosiform erythroderma) is similar to that of lamellar ichthyosis, with the exception that antibiotics are frequently required for the control of secondary infection (particularly in young individuals). Oral vitamin A has also been used for the treatment of lamellar ichthyosis. Since, however, it is ineffective except in large dosages, the hazards of toxicity preclude its use in infants and small children with this disorder.

Topically applied vitamin A acid (tretinoin [Retin-A]) is also beneficial for the treatment of lamellar ichthyosis and epidermolytic hyperkeratosis. This preparation, however, because of potential irritation, should be used cautiously on a daily or alternate-day regimen. The recently introduced oral retinoids (Accutane or Tegison, Roche Laboratories) have also been utilized for patients with severe, recalcitrant ichthyosis. Since long-term management is generally necessary, complications associated with long-term oral retinoids preclude their routine use for patients with chronic ichthyoses.

PALMOPLANTAR KERATODERMAS

Palmoplantar keratodermas are a large, heterogeneous group of disorders with punctate or diffuse thickening of the stratum corneum of the palms, soles, or both. The mechanical removal of thickened stratum corneum can be accomplished by soaking the hands or feet in water for 15 to 20 minutes, followed by the application of an effective keratolytic agent, such as Keralyt Gel. This agent is best utilized under occlusion, and its effect can be enhanced by gentle rubbing with a pumice stone while the skin is wet. Salicylic acid in a 10 per cent concentration in Aquaphor (under occlusion) is also helpful. Oral retinoids, although beneficial, are not curative and give only temporary relief. Accordingly, although they can be utilized for temporary relief of severe, disabling forms of this disorder, they should not be used for long-term therapy.

ECTODERMAL DYSPLASIA

Hidrotic ectodermal dysplasia is an autosomal dominant disorder of keratinization characterized by dystrophy of the nails, hyperkeratosis of the palms and soles, and defects of the hair. *Anhidrotic ectodermal dysplasia* is an X-linked recessive disorder in which more than 90 per cent of affected patients have been male. It is characterized by partial to complete absence of eccrine sweat glands, hair and dental abnormalities, and associated congenital defects. Therapy for anhidrotic ectodermal dysplasia is directed toward temperature regulation, restriction of excessive physical exertion, choice of a suitable occupation, and avoidance of warm climates. Cool baths, air conditioning, light clothing, and reduction of the causes of normal perspiration are beneficial. Dental supervision may help to preserve teeth and reduce cosmetic disfigurement. Artificial tears are helpful for individuals with defective lacrimation, and saline sprays and topical application of petrolatum can help individuals with dry nasal mucosa. Plastic surgery and psychiatric assistance can help severely affected individuals adjust to their appearance and limitations in lifestyle.

APLASIA CUTIS CONGENITA

Aplasia cutis congenita is a localized congenital absence of the epidermis, the dermis, and, at times, the subcutaneous tissue. Whether this disorder is inherited is uncertain, but a number of familial cases suggest an autosomal mode of inheritance. The disorder is present at birth, and although it generally occurs on the scalp, it may also involve the skin of the face, trunk, and extremities. Treatment during the newborn period consists of controlling secondary infection. As the child matures, most scars become inconspicuous and require no correction. Obvious scars may be treated by multiple punch-graft hair transplants or surgical excision with plastic repair when the child becomes older.

PACHYONYCHIA CONGENITA

Pachyonychia congenita is an unusual congenital and sometimes familial disorder inherited in an autosomal dominant fashion and characterized by dyskeratosis of the fingernails and toenails, hyperkeratosis of the palms and soles, follicular keratosis (especially about the knees and elbows), hyperhidrosis of the palms and soles, oral leukokeratosis, and, in some instances, epidermal inclusion cysts and steatocystoma multiplex. The lesions persist for life, and treatment is directed toward relief of the hyperkeratosis by the use of oral vitamin A in large doses, 20 per cent urea in an emollient cream, 60 per cent propylene glycol in water under occlusion, or 6 per cent salicylic acid in a gel containing propylene glycol (Keralyt Gel), which aids in the debridement of the excessive keratin. The nails may be treated by surgical avulsion, with scraping of the matrix to prevent regrowth.

ACRODERMATITIS ENTEROPATHICA

Acrodermatitis enteropathica is a hereditary disorder that appears in early infancy and is characterized by acral and periorificial vesicobullous, pustular, and eczematoid skin lesions, alopecia, nail dystrophy, diarrhea, glossitis, stomatitis, and frequent secondary infection due to bacterial or candidal organisms. Diiodohydroxyquin is no longer considered the treatment of choice for this disorder. Zinc gluconate or zinc sulfate is highly effective in dosages of 5 mg/kg/day given two or three times a day. With adequate therapy (100 to 200 mg/day), most patients improve in temperament, showing a decrease in irritability (usually within 1 or 2 days). The appetite improves in a few days, and diarrhea and skin lesions begin to respond within 2 to 3 days after the initiation of therapy. Hair growth begins after 2 or 3 weeks of therapy, and an increase in the growth rate of the infant generally occurs in approximately 2 months. Once the patient is stabilized on a given dosage of zinc, the physician should check serum zinc levels at periodic (6- to 12-month) intervals, followed by the adjustment of supplemental zinc to the lowest effective dosage schedule.

FAMILIAL BENIGN PEMPHIGUS

Familial benign pemphigus (Hailey-Hailey disease) is an autosomal dominant genodermatosis characterized by recurrent vesicles and bullae that most often appear on the sides and back of the neck, the axillae, the groin, and the perianal region. Exacerbations commonly occur during the hot summer months, in the form of small vesicles or, more usually, superficially crusted erosions in intertriginous areas. Therapy should be directed at relief of the precipitating factors: heat, humidity, and friction. Although topical antibiotics may be helpful in some cases, systemic antibiotics chosen on the basis of bacterial culture and sensitivity studies seem to be most effective in the treatment of this disorder. Topical and systemic corticosteroids may also be useful in some cases. Systemic corticosteroids, however, are not generally recommended, since the disorder frequently recurs when the dosage levels are reduced. In persistent cases, when patients have been disabled by painfully eroded plaques unresponsive to other therapeutic measures, excision of the involved regions, followed by split-thickness skin grafts, has been helpful.

EPIDERMOLYSIS BULLOSA

Epidermolysis bullosa (EB) is a term applied to a group of inherited disorders characterized by bullous lesions that develop spontaneously or as a result of varying degrees of trauma.

Mild cases of the dystrophic and nondystrophic types of EB may be compatible with a nearly normal existence. Severe disease, however, remains a challenge and requires cooperation by the patient, parents, and physician. Nursing care and adequate dental attention for patients with severe EB are time consuming and difficult. Since lesions result from mechanical injury, measures should be taken to relieve pressure and to prevent unnecessary trauma. A cool environment, avoidance of overheating, and lubrication of the skin to decrease friction help control blister formation. Extension of blisters may be prevented and pain may be reduced by aseptic aspiration of blister fluid.

A water mattress with a soft fleece covering limits friction. Daily baths, nonadherent dressings such as petrolatum-impregnated gauze, and topical antibiotics control infection and promote spontaneous healing. Of these, topical mupirocin (Bactroban) appears to be safe and particularly beneficial. Large denuded areas may be treated by the open method (as in the treatment of burns) with intravenous fluids and systemic antibiotics.

Dysphagia is a major symptom of esophageal involvement in recessive dystrophic EB. Softening of the diet may improve symptoms, but if conservative management fails, bougienage or surgery, or both, may be considered. Restoration of function in severe fusion and flexion deformities of the hands and feet will be helped by physiotherapy and plastic surgery. Although early studies suggested that oral phenytoin (Dilantin) was helpful in patients with recessive dystrophic EB, subsequent double-blind studies failed to confirm this. Accordingly, use of phenytoin is no longer recommended.

It is the responsibility of the physician to inform parents of the risks associated with transmitting genetic abnormalities. Support and information groups are beneficial to many families who have children with epidermolysis bullosa. The Dystrophic Epidermolysis Bullosa Research Association is an international group dedicated to research and support for patients with all forms of EB and their families. For information regarding this organization, one should contact D.E.B.R.A. of America, Inc., 141 Fifth Avenue, Suite 7S, New York, NY 10010, USA.

DISORDERS OF THE HAIR AND SCALP
ANNE W. LUCKY, M.D.

INFECTIOUS DISEASES

Bacterial Folliculitis and Impetigo of the Scalp. Scalp folliculitis is most commonly caused by *Staphylococcus aureus* and less commonly by Group A *beta-hemolytic streptococci*. Clinically, the primary lesions are pustules surrounding hair follicles, but secondary erythema, oozing, crusting, edema, tenderness, pruritus, and, ultimately, abscess formation with cervical lymphadenopathy are common. Predisposing factors include occlusion by greasy hair preparations, impetigo, and trauma. Bacterial folliculitis must be distinguished from a kerion, a hypersensitivity reaction to fungal infection. A diagnosis of folliculitis is confirmed by culturing the pustules. Fungal and bacterial disease may coexist. Treatment should be tailored to the particular bacterial organism found on culture using systemic antibiotics such as erythromycin in doses of 30 to 50 mg/kg/day, dicloxacillin in doses of 25 to 100 mg/kg/day, or cephalexin, 25 to 40 mg/kg/day orally. A 10- to 14-day course is usually sufficient but may be prolonged if infection lingers. Adjunctive local care should consist of a keratolytic shampoo (see discussion on seborrheic dermatitis) when scale is present and warm soaks with an antiseptic such as Burow's solution to remove accumulated crusts. The family should be instructed in careful hygiene, separating the infected patient's personal items (e.g., towels, combs, and hats) from those of other family members until infection has cleared. Resistant or recurrent cases may result if pathogenic organisms are harbored in the nasopharynx or on the skin of the patient or close contacts. Nasopharyngeal colonization requires topical therapy with an antibiotic ointment such as bacitracin or polymyxin (Polysporin).

Seborrheic Dermatitis, Eczema, and Psoriasis. In infancy, seborrheic dermatitis (cradle cap) and atopic dermatitis (eczema) involving the scalp are similar clinically and pathogenetically and will be considered together. "Cradle cap" of infancy is responsive to therapy. If scaling and pruritus persist or appear in later childhood, we often consider that the entire picture had been a manifestation of atopic dermatitis. The typical lesions are adherent, greasy, white to yellow scales, which appear first in patches on the scalp and eventually may cover the entire scalp surface. The scalp is pruritic, and secondary excoriations with infection are frequent. There is erythema, scale, fissuring, and weeping behind the ears. Greasy yellow scales and erythema can be found in the eyebrows, along the nasolabial folds, and in the neck folds, axillae, and groin. Tinea capitis due to *Trichophyton tonsurans* must always be considered in the differential diagnosis of seborrheic dermatitis, especially in older children.

Treatment consists of antiseborrheic shampoos that

may contain any of a number of products to reduce itching, scaling, and erythema. Such products include sulfur and salicylic acid, pyrithione zinc, coal tar, or selenium sulfide. The shampoo should be applied at least three times weekly to the scalp and left on for at least 5 minutes before washing off. This should be continued until all scale is removed. Shampooing can be reduced in frequency as clinical improvement occurs. In persistent cases, overnight applications of a phenol and saline solution (Baker's P&S) is helpful in removing excessive scale. If antiseborrheic shampoos irritate the scalp, a mild, bland shampoo plus topical steroid lotions such as 1 per cent hydrocortisone lotion or, in more severe cases, 0.1 per cent triamcinolone lotion will hasten resolution and rapidly bring relief of pruritus.

Psoriasis may appear in childhood as single or multiple stubborn plaques of scale in the scalp or as generalized scaling. Erythematous plaques with silvery scale may be present on elbows, knees, genitalia, and intergluteal clefts and diaper area in infants. Nails are often studded with 1-mm pits. Psoriasis is usually not as pruritic as atopic dermatitis. Scalp lesions may be the only sign of psoriasis in childhood. Treatment of scalp psoriasis is similar to that outlined for seborrheic dermatitis, with tar shampoos and topical steroids being especially useful.

Tinea Capitis (Scalp Ringworm). Tinea capitis is fungal infection of the scalp and hair shaft. *Trichophyton tonsurans* is now the infective agent in over 90 per cent of cases in many areas of the United States, whereas *Microsporum audouinii* once was the primary dermatophyte. A few cases acquired from kittens and puppies are caused by *Microsporum canis* or *Trichophyton mentagraphytes*. The most common presentation is diffuse scaling mimicking seborrheic dermatitis with patchy and diffuse hair loss. Since *T. tonsurans* invades the hair shafts (endothrix infection), hairs become fragile and break at the level of the scalp, leaving characteristic "black dots." *T. tonsurans* differs from *Microsporum* infection in that it does *not* fluoresce with a Wood light examination and is *not* limited to prepubertal children. *T. tonsurans* is a chronic disorder, carried asymptomatically by many children. It can produce lesions on the skin (tinea corporis), which serve as reservoirs of infection. In some cases, an inflammatory reaction, a kerion, may occur. A kerion is a boggy, erythematous, tender mass studded with perifollicular pustules. These pustules may be sterile or may contain *S. aureus*. A kerion is the host's cellular immune response to the fungal infection. Systemic symptoms such as fever, diffuse maculopapular rash (or "id"), leukocytosis, and lymphadenopathy may accompany a kerion.

The only effective treatment is systemic griseofulvin. Topical antifungal agents are ineffective. Griseofulvin (microsize) is given in a single dose of 15 mg/kg/day. It is available as a suspension (Grifulvin V, 125 mg/tsp), or appropriately sized capsules may be opened and fed to young children who cannot swallow tablets. Absorption is enhanced by a fatty meal (e.g., milk, ice cream, yogurt). Adjunctive therapy includes 2.5 per cent selenium sulfide lotion (Selsun Brown, Excel) used as a shampoo twice weekly. This acts as a sporicidal agent

and reduces shedding of spores significantly. Topical antifungal agents are not sporicidal and do not penetrate the hair follicle. They have no role in the treatment of tinea capitis. Systemic griseofulvin treatment usually requires 6 to 8 weeks for fungal cultures to become negative, unless a sporicidal shampoo is used. In refractory cases, the dose of griseofulvin should be raised to 20 mg/kg/day and the length of treatment increased. Complete blood counts and liver function tests may or may not be measured when treatment is initiated but should certainly be followed with prolonged therapy or therapy at increased dosage. Treatment of a kerion requires griseofulvin and systemic antibiotics if secondary infection with *S. aureus* is documented. Systemic or intralesional glucocorticoids have been advocated by some physicians to hasten resolution of kerions, but there are no data to support the contention that kerions resolve faster or that scarring is reduced. Systemic ketoconazole may be a useful alternative for tinea capitis.

SCARRING ALOPECIAS

Aplasia Cutis Congenita. Congenital absence of the skin in single or multiple patches on the scalp leaves a thin, shiny, parchment-like, hairless scar that is prone to breakdown, secondary infection, and crust formation. Such lesions are often mistaken for trauma secondary to a fetal monitor. Underlying bone defects may be present and skull radiographs should be taken. In later life, excision of small lesions that do not have underlying skeletal defects may be warranted for cosmetic purposes. Nonhealing lesions may require excision and primary closure or grafting in infancy.

Nevus Sebaceus of Jadassohn. Nevus sebaceus is a benign skin hamartoma. There is overgrowth of sebaceous and apocrine elements and underdevelopment of hair follicles. Such lesions are present at birth and are usually found on the scalp and face. Nevus sebaceus is one of the main causes of localized congenital alopecia. The lesions are yellow to orange, pebbly plaques that become more prominent at puberty. In the fourth and fifth decades of life, tumors such as basal cell epitheliomas or squamous cell carcinomas may develop. Because of the cosmetic appearance and the malignant potential, excision in the prepubertal years is recommended. Excision prior to that time may not fully remove the lesion, since the borders may be difficult to define.

Other Scarring Alopecias. Scarring alopecias may occur as a result of a number of infections and inflammatory disorders affecting the scalp, such as bacterial folliculitis and tinea capitis. Systemic disorders such as lupus erythematosus, morphea, and lichen planus can result in permanent hair loss. Scarring alopecia of unknown etiology, leaving a "footprint in the snow" pattern, has been termed pseudopelade of Brocq. Traction from tight braids or pony tails may at first cause transient hair loss but eventually will permanently destroy hair follicles. No therapy short of localized hair transplantation is effective.

NONSCARRING ALOPECIAS

Alopecia Areata. Alopecia areata is one of the most common causes of alopecia in childhood. It is probably autoimmune in origin. There is a spectrum from single to multiple coin-sized areas of spontaneous complete hair loss (alopecia areata) to total loss of all scalp hair (alopecia totalis) to universal loss of scalp and body hair (alopecia universalis). Occasionally, diffuse hair loss precedes the patchy lesions. Histopathologically, alopecia areata is characterized by swarms of lymphocytes surrounding the hair bulb. Other autoimmune disorders such as vitiligo, Hashimoto's thyroiditis, diabetes, and hypoparathyroidism may be associated with alopecia areata. Many patients will have characteristic linear pitting of the nails. Alopecia areata has spontaneous remissions and exacerbations. Theories that alopecia areata is a psychosomatic disorder have not been well substantiated. As a rule, the younger the child and the more extensive the hair loss, the less likely it is that regrowth will occur. Loss in the ophiasis pattern, around the margins of the scalp, also indicates a poor prognosis.

Treatment must be individualized and is often not successful. Therapy with intralesional steroids (triamcinolone acetonide, 1 ml of 5 to 10 mg/ml suspension) can be successful in limited cases but may require multiple and repeated courses of therapy. No more than 10 mg of triamcinolone should be given every 4 to 6 weeks to avoid systemic effects from the intralesional steroids. High-potency topical steroids may be useful in a child too young or too afraid to cooperate with intralesional injections. Systemic steroids are *not* recommended in growing children. There are serious side effects, not the least of which is growth retardation. Even if systemic steroid therapy is successful in allowing regrowth of hair, when the steroids are tapered, hair loss usually recurs. Newer forms of therapy promoted in the recent literature include sensitization to dinitrochlorobenzene (DNCB) or to squaric acid ester, with subsequent application of the antigen to the affected areas of the scalp to produce a contact dermatitis and hypersensitivity reaction. (This form of therapy has raised questions about potentially stimulating the immune system and causing malignancy.) Simple irritation of the scalp with substances such as anthralin cream (0.25 to 1.0 per cent) has met with moderate success. Topical minoxidil, 2 to 5 per cent, has had limited success in approximately one third of patients. Although some groups have advocated the use of systemic psoralens and ultraviolet A light (PUVA), the efficacy and safety of this procedure in childhood has not yet been established. Psychological adjustment of the child to alopecia areata is best reflected by the attitude of the parents and the physician. Support and encouragement without specific therapy is often the best treatment.

Traumatic Hair Loss. Traumatic hair loss is usually either self-induced by compulsive hair pulling (trichotillomania) or inappropriate use of hair cosmetics or hair styling. Hair loss secondary to trauma is usually nonscarring and is a combination of traction from the bulb and breakage of the shaft. Repeated trauma to the hair bulb may eventually cause permanent scarring alopecia. Trichotillomania appears as isolated or multiple areas of alopecia. It is identified by the presence of fractured, unevenly broken off, short hairs. Histologically, twisted medullary shafts with pigment casts are

diagnostic. It is a sign of underlying emotional or psychological conflict, and if persistent and severe, the family should be referred for appropriate counseling. It is often impossible to obtain a positive history of compulsive hair pulling from parent or child. Traction alopecia occurs primarily in small children whose hair is kept in tight braids or pony tails. Rubber bands can sever the hair shafts, but the traction itself will cause disruption of the hair bulb and a permanent hair loss pattern, especially around the scalp margins. The only treatment is advice on hair styling. Overzealous cosmetic treatments can produce broken hairs, secondary to increased fragility. Home permanent waves, chemical hair straighteners, blow dryers, and hot combs are major causes of traumatic hair loss. In this condition, the number and density of hairs in the scalp are normal but the hairs are broken. Discontinuation of all treatment to the hair except a mild shampoo and conditioner is warranted. Conditioners render the hair easier to comb with fewer tangles. Hair is more fragile when wet and thus combing should be done after drying.

Diffuse Hair Loss. Diffuse hair loss may result from a wide variety of causes. Normal hair loss occurs at the rate of 100 hairs per day. Thinning of the scalp hair may not be noticeable until a large percentage of scalp hair is gone, and thus increased shedding of hair may be the initial complaint. Telogen effluvium is the term used for the phenomenon of a large number of hairs going into the resting (telogen) stage of growth at the same time and then falling out. Telogen effluvium may follow 2 to 3 months after a severe illness with high fever (e.g., typhoid fever, scarlet fever, or Kawasaki disease) or surgery with general anesthesia. It is physiologic in infants and their mothers approximately 3 months post partum. Occasionally, alopecia areata may begin with diffuse hair loss. Endocrine disorders such as hypothyroidism or hyperthyroidism and excessive masculinizing levels of androgens from ovarian or adrenal origin may manifest with diffuse hair loss. Female pattern baldness, or so-called "androgenetic" alopecia, consists of thinning of the hair predominantly over the crown of the scalp. It may be a familial trait or result from elevated circulating plasma androgens in teenage girls. Deficiencies of trace elements such as zinc or iron, essential fatty acids, or proteins or multiple nutritional losses such as seen in marasmus or anorexia nervosa can produce diffuse hair loss. Finally, a careful history of drug exposure, including thallium, mercury, propranolol, and chemotherapy or radiation therapy, must be considered in the differential diagnosis. Treatment is decided depending on the underlying cause.

DISORDERS OF SEBACEOUS GLANDS AND SWEAT GLANDS

ANNE W. LUCKY, M.D.

DISORDERS OF SEBACEOUS GLANDS

Acne. Acne vulgaris affects nearly all adolescents at some time during puberty, starting as early as 8 years of age. The basic lesion is a *comedo,* which is a plugged sebaceous follicle. Comedones may be closed (whiteheads) or open (blackheads) to the surface of the skin. Comedones form under the stimulatory influence of androgens on the sebaceous glands at puberty. Increased growth of bacterial flora of the face *(Propionibacterium acnes)* and an acceleration of the immune response on the part of the host to this infection result in inflammation and pustule formation, producing *papules* and *pustules.* When papules or pustules from single follicles coalesce into groups with multiple follicular openings and invade deep into the dermis, *nodules* and *cysts* are formed. The acne-prone areas of the body are the face, anterior chest, and back. The earliest acne lesions are comedones in the external ears and on the nose. Girls will often note flares of their acne 1 or 2 weeks prior to onset of menstrual periods. Acne usually improves dramatically in summer. Stress precipitates acne flares. Although acne is characteristically transient, there is a broad spectrum of severity.

There is no best treatment, just as there is no single cause of acne. The causes are multiple and include endocrine, infectious, and immunologic factors. Occlusion with oily makeup or hair grease may exacerbate acne. There is little evidence that diet and dirt are factors. Therapy for the individual patient depends on the severity of the disease and the predominant type of lesion. The number of acne preparations available, both over the counter and by prescription, is overwhelming. It is advisable to become familiar with one or two products of each type. Therapy will be discussed on the basis of mild, moderate, and severe acne.

Mild acne is primarily comedonal with occasional papules and pustules. Benzoyl peroxide gels (2.5, 5, and 10 per cent) are the first choice for treatment. Gels are more effective than lotions or washes but may cause more irritation. Water-based and emollient gels are less irritating. Benzoyl peroxide acts like a topical antibiotic to reduce local skin flora and seems to have anticomedonal action. Most often, patients are started on a preparation of 5 per cent benzoyl peroxide gel twice daily, with increase or decrease in strength and/or frequency of applications, depending on tolerance. Major side effects are redness and dryness of the skin. A small percentage of patients develop true contact allergy to benzoyl peroxide. Fair-skinned individuals are more sensitive to benzoyl peroxide. Benzoyl peroxide can act like a bleach and may discolor clothing.

For more persistent or more numerous comedonal lesions, the use of topical retinoic acid (tretinoin [Retin-A]) has made a marked difference in acne therapy in the past decade. Topical retinoic acid acts to prevent comedo formation by altering the faulty keratinization process that plugs the follicular orifice. Without comedones, there is no chance for secondary papules, pustules, or cysts to develop. Topical retinoic acid comes in a cream (0.025 per cent, 0.05 per cent, and 0.10 per cent), a gel (0.01 per cent and 0.025 per cent), and a liquid (0.05 per cent) form, which is the strongest. The cream is tolerated with the least amount of irritation. Therapy is begun with 0.025 per cent Retin-A cream or 0.01 per cent Retin-A gel once every second or third

night. Application is advanced in strength and frequency to a nightly application as tolerated. Patients must be forewarned that they will look worse for the first few weeks of treatment because of erythema, peeling, and appearance of more acne lesions. Some patients can develop an inflammatory papulopustular flare with initiation of treatment. The skin develops tolerance to the drug in the first month, and the strength of the preparation can be increased. The back and chest are less sensitive than the face. It takes 3 months to judge whether the therapy is successful in preventing formation of new comedones. The combination of topical benzoyl peroxide and retinoic acid, each used once daily, appears to be very effective. Because of increased sensitivity to sun and a theoretical tumorigenic potential in animals when retinoic acid is used with ultraviolet light, some dermatologists discontinue topical retinoic acid during the summer months or at other times of intense exposure to sunlight. Sunscreen should be applied, using at least SPF 15.

Many topical antibiotics have become available in the past few years. Tetracycline, erythromycin, and clindamycin are now commercially available. Their primary action appears to be to reduce bacterial colonization of the skin. Topical antibiotics can be applied as alcohol-based liquids, gels, or saturated pads, once or twice daily alone or in combination with benzoyl peroxide or retinoic acid, or they may be reserved for cases in which the former combination is not tolerated. Topical tetracycline may fluoresce with "Disco" black lights.

For *moderate acne,* which includes more persistent and numerous papules and pustules in addition to comedones, systemic antibiotics are essential. They should be used in conjunction with the topical medications described previously. The mainstay of systemic treatment for acne is tetracycline. It is used starting at 1 to 2 gm daily divided into three or four doses. Tetracycline is poorly absorbed with food and must be taken 30 minutes before or 2 hours after a meal. Dairy products are especially inhibitory to absorption. Minocycline, a close cogener of tetracycline, does not need to be taken on an empty stomach but is many times more expensive. It can be used in a dosage of 50 mg to 100 mg once or twice daily.* Limitations of the use of the tetracyclines are gastrointestinal intolerance and vaginal candidiasis in some women. The latter may be treated with local antifungal preparations (nystatin, clotrimazole, or miconidazole) and the tetracycline may be continued. Tetracycline induces hepatic enzymes that also metabolize estrogens, and warnings that oral contraceptives may become less effective and that breakthrough bleeding may occur must be given to patients. Although tetracycline has been used safely in an enormous number of patients continuously for many years without ill effect, there are occasional severe reactions, such as photosensitivity and liver and renal abnormalities. In

---

*The use of all tetracyclines, including minocycline during tooth development (last half of pregnancy to the age of 8 years), may cause permanent tooth discoloration. Similar discoloration has been seen with high-dose, long-term Minocycline in adult patients. Minocycline has also caused reversible blue/black pigmentation of the skin, especially in scars.

patients who do not tolerate tetracycline, erythromycin, 1 to 2 gm divided into three or four doses, may be equally effective. As acne improves, the dose of medication is slowly reduced to a maintenance of 250 mg once daily of tetracycline or erythromycin or 50 mg once daily of minocycline (Minocin). A course of oral antibiotics usually requires 9 to 12 months, and premature withdrawal may result in exacerbation or recurrence of acne. In a rare few patients treated with long-term antibiotics, the facial flora may change to gram-negative organisms such as *Escherichia coli, Pseudomonas,* or *Klebsiella*. Antibiotics such as trimethoprim and sulfamethoxazole (Bactrim) may be useful.

Severe acne, which is most often cystic in nature, is the most devastating and most difficult form to treat. It can be psychologically and socially crippling. It is most severe in boys and is often familial. Cystic acne may take a chronic severe form called *acne conglobata* or an acute explosive form termed *acne fulminans*. In addition to high doses of systemic antibiotics, such as tetracycline or erythromycin, and topical treatment with benzoyl peroxide, retinoic acid, and topical antibiotics, systemic treatment with glucocorticosteroids or dapsone may be necessary to reduce acute inflammation in extreme cases of acne fulminans. Individual cystic lesions respond well to cautious intralesional injections of steroids (triamcinolone acetonide, 2.5 to 5.0 mg/ml), reducing the inflammatory response and, it is hoped, preventing severe scarring.

The drug 13-*cis*-retinoic acid (Accutane) has been available since 1983 for severe, disfiguring cystic acne. A limited course of this potent drug lasting 16 to 20 weeks has produced excellent, prolonged remissions of severe cystic acne in clinical trials. However, there may be troublesome side effects, such as cheilitis, dry skin, radiographic skeletal changes, hepatic dysfunction, pancytopenia, hypercholesterolemia, and hypertriglyceridemia. It is extremely expensive. Accutane is a well-known teratogen, and its use in reproductive-aged female patients should include contraception counseling and written informed consent. There are no known mutagenic effects, and long-term problems with future birth defects in boys and girls are *not* a concern. The use of Accutane should be limited to severe, disfiguring cystic acne treated by practitioners who use the drug enough to become familiar with the dosages and side effects.

There are many adjunctive measures for acne that may help but are not essential to successful treatment. These include comedo extraction for cosmetic purposes, abrasive scrubs (which may be useful in some patients but often irritate and worsen lesions), sulfur preparations either in liquid form or as a mask, and various alcohol-containing astringents. Oil-containing makeup and hair grease should be eliminated from use. Although there are many so-called "acne" soaps on the market, patients should be advised simply to wash their faces two or three times daily with any mild soap. For scarring that remains after acne has become quiescent, new techniques such as dermabrasion, plastic repair, collagen implants, and autotransplants of plugs of skin

may be useful. In some women, excessive production of androgenic hormones from the ovary (polycystic ovarian disease) or adrenal gland may contribute to acne flares or persistence of acne. Careful specific hormonal treatment such as with estrogens (oral contraceptives) or low-dose glucocorticoids may be of use in well-documented selected cases of this type. Antiandrogens such as spironolactone, in doses of 50 to 200 mg/day, may also have a role in well-documented cases of endocrine imbalance.

Sebaceous Hyperplasia of Infancy, or Neonatal Acne. Infants in the first 6 months of life may have prominent sebaceous follicles and/or frank acneiform lesions, both of which spontaneously resolve. Maternal and endogenous androgen stimulation of sebaceous glands in the young infant is the presumed cause of these disorders. When hormone levels become normal in the first year of life, the skin lesions disappear. No treatment is necessary, but 2.5 or 5 per cent benzoyl peroxide may be appreciated in severe cases.

DISORDERS OF SWEAT GLANDS

Miliaria. Miliaria is caused by obstruction of the sweat ducts. *Miliaria crystallina* is seen often in the newborn as tiny (1 mm) crystal-clear vesicles that can be ruptured by gentle pressure on the skin surface, leaving a fine collarette of scale. It is caused by sweat duct obstruction high in the stratum corneum of the skin. Obstruction of the sweat ducts at a slightly lower level produces *miliaria rubra*, known as "prickly heat" or "heat rash." Miliaria rubra presents as 1- to 2-mm punctate red papules in occluded sweaty areas, such as underarms, neck, chest, or back. It may be quite pruritic. Treatment of both types of miliaria includes keeping the skin dry and cool. *Miliaria profunda* is deep obstruction in the eccrine ducts, producing white papules on the skin and inhibition of normal sweating. It is seen in adolescents and young adults after extensive exercise and may lead to profound heat retention and collapse. Fortunately, it is rare. Susceptible persons should avoid heat and strenuous exercise.

Hypohidrotic Ectodermal Dysplasia. The most common form of hypohidrotic ectodermal dysplasia is an X-linked recessive trait affecting only men. Patients are unable to sweat and have associated defects in hair, nails, and teeth. Such children may present in infancy with hyperpyrexia. It is important to recognize this disorder to prevent central nervous system damage. Patients should be counseled to avoid heat and strenuous exercise and to have immediate cooling during febrile illnesses by physical methods such as cold water and alcohol baths, as well as antipyretics.

Hyperhidrosis. Hyperhidrosis is exaggerated sweating of the palms, soles, and underarms. It is triggered by emotional as well as thermal stress. Aluminum chloride 20 per cent (Drysol), applied once or twice weekly to palms and soles, may be very useful. In milder cases, Zeasorb Powder inside socks and shoes will help to absorb sweat.

MISCELLANEOUS DERMATOSES

STEPHEN E. GELLIS, M.D.

Juvenile plantar dermatosis is a condition seen in children ages 3 to 10 that appears symmetrically in the weight-bearing areas of the feet as shiny and fissured skin. It is thought to result from the chronic exposure of the feet to a humid environment produced by occlusive footwear. The condition may also have an association with atopic dermatitis. Treatment consists of the avoidance of occlusive footwear, such as running shoes and rubber boots. The purchase of well-aired shoes and the placement of insoles may be helpful. In acute flare-ups, topical steroids and soaks in an oil and tar preparation (Polytar, Balnetar) are somewhat useful.

Perioral dermatitis is an eruption of unknown etiology that appears as small, asymptomatic papules and scaling surrounding the skin of the nose and mouth. It is usually seen in young girls and younger children and may be a variant of acne. A brief course of tetracycline, 250 mg twice a day for 3 weeks, will clear most cases. For children under age 12, tetracycline should not be prescribed because of its potential for producing dental staining. In this age group, topical keratolytics, such as benzoyl peroxide, and topical antibiotics may be tried. Topical steroids may aggravate the condition and should be avoided.

Keratosis pilaris is a common condition in children who have either a personal or a family history of atopy. It consists of keratotic papules 1 to 2 mm in size over the extensor aspect of the arms, the thighs, and occasionally the cheeks. At times, entrapped hairs may be seen within the papules. The eruption is more prominent in dry environments. Treatment consists of the use of emollients, particularly those containing urea or lactic acid (U-Lactin, Nutraplus, Lacticare, Aquacare). Increasing the humidity in the bedroom at night with a vaporizer or humidifier is also effective. In extensive cases, a keratolytic gel (Keralyt or Epilyt), applied daily, will remove the keratotic papules temporarily. Manual removal by rubbing with a pumice stone while the skin is wet may also be tried.

Perianal cellulitis occurs in young children with an average age of 4 and is due to group A streptococcus. Patients present with a persistent perianal rash often accompanied by painful defecation leading to stool retention. The symptoms may persist for weeks to months. On examination, there is intense erythema and oozing in the perianal area. The treatment consists of a systemic antibiotic, either penicillin VK, 25 to 50 mg/kg/day in four divided doses, or erythromycin ethylsuccinate, 40 mg/kg in four divided doses for 10 to 14 days. A more prolonged treatment is sometimes required.

16

The Eye

THE EYE

LEONARD APT, M.D.,
and PAUL T. UREA, M.D., M.P.H.

GENERAL CONSIDERATIONS OF EYE DISORDERS

Eye disorders that may be recognized and treated by the pediatric practitioner are stressed in this section. For the most part these disorders are the simple inflammations of the eye and its adnexa. Most other ocular diseases should be referred to an ophthalmologist. It is our recommendation that instrumentation other than that required to remove a superficial foreign body be avoided by the nonophthalmologic physician.

As in other areas of medicine, the key to successful therapy of eye disorders is precise diagnosis. An accurate diagnosis is derived from a careful history, a systematic inspection of the visible eye structures, ophthalmoscopy, and appropriate laboratory studies. The history should include details about the symptoms and their duration, preceding illnesses or trauma, and contact with others with similar symptoms. Thorough inspection of the eye with good illumination is imperative. One must gain the child's confidence and cooperation to accomplish this. Forceful closure of the eyelids by the patient causes the eyeball to roll up and thus conceal the cornea. Forceful separation of the eyelids by the physician with the placement of inadvertent pressure on the globe may rupture a thin or perforated cornea or globe in patients having a history of trauma. In some instances a sedative or general anesthetic may be necessary in order to satisfactorily relax a child for an ocular examination.

Since a child's primary care physician is often consulted first when an eye problem arises, it is necessary that he or she be aware of the manifestations of a serious eye disease. Knowledge of certain danger signs is of particular importance in dealing with "red eye," a common presenting complaint that varies in significance from a benign conjunctivitis to a blinding or life-threatening intraocular disease. A serious or potentially serious eye disease should be considered if any of the following signs or symptoms is present:

Visual disturbance—reduced acuity, diplopia, "spots" before the eyes, reduction in part of the field of vision.

Severe *pain* or *photophobia* suggests corneal, intraocular, or orbital disease. A corneal abrasion or foreign body may be the cause.

Opacities in the cornea, lens, or vitreous. A corneal opacity may be overlooked if a bright focal light aimed obliquely is not used. Opacities in the lens or vitreous can be seen as dark areas outlined in the red ophthalmoscopic reflex.

Pupils—irregularities in size or shape are seen after trauma or with intraocular inflammation.

Persistent *discharge* or *red eye* after several days of supposedly adequate treatment.

General Remarks About Local Therapy

In young children medication in ointment form has certain advantages over liquid preparations. There is less tendency for the ointment preparation to undergo dilution from crying, with subsequent loss of the medication. As a consequence, less frequent instillations of ointments are required. On the other hand, drops may be easier to instill, are less messy, and do not temporarily blur the vision. In some children it is often more convenient to use drops during the day and ointment at bedtime.

The pediatric practitioner should not prescribe local eye anesthetics for a painful eye for use at home. Local anesthetics tend to retard corneal healing. Furthermore, injury to an anesthetized eye by the parent or child may occur unintentionally.

A plea is made for the nonophthalmologic physician to avoid the indiscriminate use of local corticosteroids or combination drug products that include corticosteroids for the treatment of nonspecific inflamed or irritated eyes. Corticosteroids are effective antiallergic and anti-inflammatory agents, but they may retard healing, allow the progression of serious viral (e.g., herpes simplex) and/or fungal infections of the eye, or lead to glaucoma and cataract with prolonged use. The pediatric practitioner should make it a general rule that when an antibiotic or corticosteroid eye preparation is given without a definitive diagnosis, the patient is to be referred to an ophthalmologist if no distinct improvement occurs in 1 or 2 days.

Useful Local Eye Preparations

Diagnostic Stain. Stains are used to delineate abrasions, ulcerations, and foreign bodies of the cornea and conjunctiva.

FLUORESCEIN STRIPS. Strips of filter paper impregnated with fluorescein are commercially available in sterile packages. Fluorescein strips are desirable because the sterility of a fluorescein solution is difficult to maintain, particularly against contamination with *Pseudomonas* organisms. The dry or slightly moistened strip is merely touched to the conjunctival fornix. No flushing of the eye is needed.

ROSE BENGAL SOLUTION. This dye stains devitalized epithelium. It is useful in demonstrating changes in the conjunctiva and cornea in Sjögren's syndrome and in exhibiting the dendrites in herpes epithelial keratitis.

Local Anesthetics. Local anesthetics are used to alleviate pain in order to examine the eye with convenience or to anesthetize the cornea and conjunctiva prior to the removal of a foreign body (Table 1).

The most widely used local anesthetics are tetracaine and proparacaine. Tetracaine aqueous solution has the advantages of high anesthetic potency, great stability, resistance to bacterial and fungal contamination, and low cost. The disadvantages are the moderate burning sensation with initial instillation of the drug and the mild congestion of the conjunctival vessels that it evokes. Proparacaine causes little or no discomfort on instillation, is not toxic, and has a rapid onset, but it has a much shorter duration of action than tetracaine. The minimal stinging and burning of proparacaine is a practical advantage of its use in infants and children.

Mydriatics and Cycloplegics. Weak mydriatics merely dilate the pupil. Strong mydriatics, in addition to dilating the pupil, temporarily relax or paralyze accommodation (the act of focusing at near) by acting on the ciliary muscle. For ophthalmoscopy alone, a weak mydriatic is all that is needed, since relaxation of accommodation often is unnecessary. Mydriasis lasts only a few hours. Cycloplegic drugs are used principally to measure refractive errors, to immobilize the ciliary muscle in inflammatory conditions of the uveal tract, and to dilate the pupil to avoid posterior synechiae formation in cases of iridocyclitis.

The useful drugs for this purpose are as follows:

Mydriatics (minimal or virtually no cycloplegic effect)
Tropicamide (Mydriacyl) 0.5%

TABLE 1. Local Anesthetics for Ocular Use

Generic Name	Trade Name	Concentration
Tetracaine solution	Pontocaine	0.5%
Tetracaine ointment	Pontocaine	0.5%
Proparacaine solution	AK-Taine	0.5%
	Alcaine	0.5%
	I-Paracaine	0.5%
	Kainair	0.5%
	Ophthaine	0.5%
	Ophthetic	0.5%

Cyclopentolate 0.2% with phenylephrine 1% (Cyclomydril)
Phenylephrine (Neo-Synephrine) 2.5, 10%
Cycloplegics
Atropine 0.5, 1, 2%
Tropicamide (Mydriacyl) 1%
Cyclopentolate (Cyclogyl) 0.5, 1, 2%
Homatropine 2, 5%
Scopolamine 0.25%

Atropine is the most potent cycloplegic drug and is the longest acting: 7 to 14 days. Mydriasis begins within 30 to 40 minutes after instillation of the drug, and maximum cycloplegia occurs in about 32 hours. The lower concentrations of the drug should be used in infants and young children because toxic amounts of the drug may be absorbed systemically. It is important to realize that toxic quantities of atropine can be absorbed. For example, a 1 per cent solution provides 0.5 mg of atropine with each drop, or 1 mg when a drop is instilled into each eye. Assuming that only 50 per cent of the administered drug is absorbed systemically, a 5-kg infant receives 10 times the usual systemic therapeutic dose (0.05 mg) and a 20-kg child receives 2.5 times the usual therapeutic dose (0.2 mg). Similar comparisons can be made for other topically applied drugs. Pressure over the lacrimal sac when the solution is instilled will help to prevent absorption of the drug through the nasopharyngeal mucosa. Use of atropine in ointment form allows less chance of absorption of the drug through the lacrimal drainage system.

Scopolamine is also a potent cycloplegic. It produces the same toxic symptoms as atropine. Mydriasis begins within 40 minutes; cycloplegia is maximal in 60 to 90 minutes, and gradually subsides in 3 to 6 days.

Homatropine is a less potent cycloplegic drug than atropine or scopolamine. The higher concentrations produce full mydriasis within 30 minutes, and maximum cycloplegia is reached in 1 to 2 hours. Recovery from cycloplegia occurs in 36 to 48 hours. Toxicity from homatropine eye drops is infrequent. Instillation causes a burning sensation.

Cyclopentolate (Cyclogyl) produces rapid mydriasis and cycloplegia. Mydriasis appears in 15 minutes, and maximum cycloplegia is reached in 30 to 75 minutes after instillation of the drug. Recovery of accommodation takes place in 6 to 24 hours; mydriasis can persist for 24 hours. The cycloplegia, when maximal, is as profound as that obtained with atropine. Systemic toxicity is similar to that produced by atropine except that visual and tactile hallucinations are a more striking feature. Avoid the 2 per cent concentration in infants.

Tropicamide (Mydriacyl) in the 1 per cent concentration is an ultrashort-acting cycloplegic. The 0.5 per cent preparation is principally a mydriatic. Mydriasis and cycloplegia occur simultaneously in 15 to 30 minutes. The duration of maximal cycloplegia is only 10 to 20 minutes. Recovery from cycloplegia likewise is rapid: 30 minutes to 4 hours. Tropicamide is used primarily as a mydriatic in pediatric patients because of its transient effect on accommodation. Local or systemic toxic effects are rare.

EYELID DISORDERS

Blepharitis ("Granulated Eyelids")

Blepharitis is a common, chronic, recurrent inflammation of the lid margins characterized by redness, crusting, burning, irritation, itching, loss of eyelashes, and conjunctival irritation.

Two types are recognized by inspection. Clinical differentiation is of practical importance because knowledge of the cause aids in determining the specific treatment.

Staphylococcal Blepharitis. The most common cause of inflammation, crusting, and irritation along the lid margins in children is staphylococcal blepharitis. Although the findings of accumulated secretions with inflammation of the eyelid margins are quite characteristic, smears, cultures, and sensitivity tests can readily be obtained to confirm the diagnosis. The scales at the base of the lashes often are hard and tenacious. In more severe cases ulcers and pustules may appear on the eyelid margins. Toxic products of the bacteria may cause an accompanying conjunctivitis. A hypersensitivity reaction to staphylococcal antigens may produce an inflammatory keratitis.

TREATMENT. Lid hygiene, whereby scales are removed from the eyelid margins, is the mainstay of treatment of staphylococcal blepharitis. Moist compresses for 5 to 10 minutes may be needed to first loosen the scales before they are removed by mechanical scrubbing with a clean washcloth or cotton-tipped applicator moistened with diluted baby shampoo or I-Scrub (a detergent made by Spectra Pharmaceutical Services, Hanover, MA). The topical antistaphylococcal preparations most useful for treatment are erythromycin, bacitracin, and sulfacetamide ophthalmic ointments or drops (Table 2). After removal of the scales the medication is placed between the eyelid and globe at bedtime. In severe cases a combined antimicrobial-steroid agent (Table 3) is sometimes helpful to reduce the inflammation in the eye and on the eyelid caused by the *Staphylococcus* itself or by the hypersentivity reaction that may accompany the infection. The use of drops during the day and ointment at bedtime often is more convenient. Prolonged use of neomycin should be avoided because of the risk of an allergic reaction. Tonometry is indicated if corticosteroid therapy is long-term. General measures, such as the daily use of antibacterial soap to control skin staphylococci, also are worthwhile.

Seborrheic Blepharitis. In seborrheic blepharitis greasy scales and flakes are found along the eyelashes; seborrhea of the scalp usually coexists. A helpful sign in differentiating staphylococcal from seborrheic blepharitis is that conjunctivitis or keratitis usually is absent in the latter.

TREATMENT. Lid hygiene, as described above, is similarly effective in the treatment of seborrheic blepharitis. Sulfacetamide has antiseborrheic activity, but the commonly used antibiotics do not. For the successful therapy of seborrheic blepharitis, it is imperative to treat the seborrhea that usually exists in other areas, e.g. scalp, eyebrows, or ears. Diluted baby shampoo or I-

TABLE 2. Topical Antibiotic and Sulfonamide Eye Preparations

Generic Name	Trade Name	Concentration
Drops		
Chloramphenicol solution	Chloromycetin	0.16–0.5%
	Chlorofair	0.5%
	Chloroptic	0.5%
	Ophthochlor	0.5%
Gentamicin solution	Garamycin	0.3%
	Genoptic	0.3%
	Gentacidin	0.3%
	Gentafair	0.3%
	Gent-AK	0.3%
Polymixin-B solution		10,000–25,000 U/ml
Sulfacetamide solution	AK-Sulf	10% & 15%
	AK-Sulf Forte	30%
	Bleph-10	10%
	Isopto Cetamide	15%
	Ophthacet	10%
	Sodium Sulamyd	10% & 30%
	Sulf-10	10%
	Sulfair-15	15%
	Sulten-10	10%
Sulfisoxazole solution	Gantrisin	4%
Tetracycline suspension	Achromycin	1%
Tobramycin solution	Tobrex	0.3%
Ointments		
Bacitracin	AK-Tracin	500 U/gm
Chloramphenicol	Chlorofair	10 mg/gm
	Chloromycetin	10 mg/gm
	Chloroptic	10 mg/gm
Chlorotetracycline	Aureomycin	10 mg/gm
Erythromycin	AK-Mycin	5 mg/gm
	Ilotycin	5 mg/gm
Gentamicin	Garamycin	3 mg/gm
	Genoptic S.O.P.	3 mg/gm
	Gentacidin	3 mg/gm
	Gentafair	3 mg/gm
	Gent-AK	3 mg/gm
Sulfacetamide	AK-Sulf	10%
	Bleph-10 S.O.P.	10%
	Cetamide	10%
	Sodium Sulamyd	10%
Sulfisoxazole	Gantrisin	4%
Tetracycline	Achromycin	10 mg/gm
Tobramycin	Tobrex	3 mg/gm

Scrub may similarly be used to facilitate hygiene of the lid margins and lashes.

Hordeolum (Stye)

External Hordeolum. This is an acute localized pyogenic infection (usually staphylococcal) of the sebaceous glands (Zeis or Moll) along the lid margin. The localized area of redness, swelling, and tenderness appears on the lid margin at the base of the eyelash. A small yellow area of suppuration appears in a day or so. With rupture of the abscess, pain diminishes. Recurrences are common.

TREATMENT. In the early stages warm, moist compresses applied for 20 minutes three or four times daily hasten localization of the infection. Pressure should not be applied to speed up this process. When the hordeolum is entirely localized, pointing through the epidermis, it is then incised to allow the pus to drain. An antistaphylococcal ointment (bacitracin, erythromycin, or sulfacetamide) applied locally four to six times daily is helpful in aborting the suppuration and preventing

TABLE 3. Topical Antimicrobial-Corticosteroid Eye Preparations

Generic Name	Trade Name
Drops	
Chloramphenicol + hydrocortisone (suspension)	Chloromycetin-hydrocortisone
Gentamicin + prednisolone (suspension)	Pred-G
Neomycin + hydrocortisone (suspension)	AK-Neo-Cort
	Cort-Oticin
	Neo-Cortef
	Ortho
Neomycin + prednisolone (suspension)	Neo-Delta-Cortef
Neomycin + dexamethasone (solution)	Neo-Decadron
Neomycin + polymyxin + hydrocortisone (suspension)	Cortisporin
	Triple-Gen
Neomycin + polymyxin B + prednisolone (suspension)	Poly-Pred
Neomycin + polymyxin B + dexamethasone (suspension)	AK-Trol
	Dexacidin
	Maxitrol
Sulfacetamide + prednisolone (suspension)	AK-Cide
	Blephamide
	Isopto Cetapred
	Metimyd
	Ophtha P/S
	Or-Toptic M
	Predamide
	Predsulfair
	Sulfamide
	Sulphrin
Sulfacetamide + prednisolone (solution)	Optimyd
	Vasocidin
Tobramycin + dexamethasone (suspension)	Tobradex
Ointments	
Chloramphenicol + polymyxin + hydrocortisone	Ophthocort
Neomycin + prednisolone	Neo-Delta Cortef
Neomycin + dexamethasone	Neo-Decadron
Neomycin + polymyxin B + bacitracin + hydrocortisone	Coracin
Sulfacetamide + prednisolone	AK-Cide
	Blephamide
	S.O.P.
	Cetapred
	Metimyd
	Predsulfair
	Vasocidin

spread of the infection. Treatment should be continued for about 1 week after the sty has healed to prevent further infection in other hair follicles.

Internal Hordeolum. This acute purulent infection involves one of the meibomian glands (meibomian sty). The area of localized redness, pain, swelling, or abscess appears on the conjunctival rather than the skin side corresponding to the location of the gland. Spontaneous rupture is less frequent than with the external sty. Recurrences are common.

Treatment is the same as for external hordeolum.

Chalazion

Chalazion is a common, chronic granulomatous meibomian gland infection of unknown cause. In contrast to the acute purulent infection of this gland (internal hordeolum), there is little or no pain or tenderness unless there is a superimposed secondary pyogenic infection. Symptoms are slight. A slow-growing, hard, round mass localized in the tarsus points more commonly to the conjunctival than to the skin side. If large

enough, the mass will distort vision. The tumor may remain the same size, ulcerate through the surface and leave some remains, or be absorbed gradually over a few weeks or months.

TREATMENT. If warm moist compresses and topical antibiotic-corticosteroid therapy do not appreciably reduce the size of the mass in a few weeks, an intralesional injection of a corticosteroid or incision and evacuation of the chalazion should be performed. For recurrent chalazia the use of an antibacterial ointment at bedtime and several times a day and weekly massage of the meibomian glands to express secretions may be helpful.

CONJUNCTIVAL DISORDERS

Conjunctivitis

Conjunctivitis ranks with blepharitis as one of the most common external ocular inflammations. Inflammation of the conjunctiva may be microbial, allergic, or traumatic in origin. It may be acute, subacute, or chronic. In the differential diagnosis of the acutely inflamed eye, conjunctivitis can be differentiated from iritis and glaucoma by the presence of a discharge (often bilateral), normal or unaffected vision, normal pupil size and reaction to light, and normal intraocular pressure.

Bacterial Conjunctivitis. Because certain bacteria cause distinct clinical features of bacterial conjunctivitis, the following classification is possible:

ACUTE BACTERIAL (MUCOPURULENT) CONJUNCTIVITIS ("PINK EYE"). The most common causative microorganisms are *Staphylococcus aureus*, pneumococcus, *Haemophilus influenzae,* and beta-hemolytic *Streptococcus*. Intense bulbar but minimal tarsal inflammation is seen. Epithelial keratitis is rare except in the staphylococcal form. Petechial hemorrhages are most common with pneumococcal and *H. influenzae* infections. The disease is highly contagious. It may last several weeks if untreated. The eyelids seal overnight from drying of the products of inflammation.

HYPERACUTE (PURULENT) CONJUNCTIVITIS. Purulent discharge occurs with intense bulbar and tarsal conjunctivitis and chemosis. The gonococcus and, much less commonly, the meningococcus are the main etiologic agents. Meningococcal conjunctivitis may accompany meningitis.

CHRONIC BACTERIAL CONJUNCTIVITIS. *S. aureus* is not only a frequent cause of acute conjunctivitis but is the most common microorganism causing chronic bacterial conjunctivitis. Aerobic, gram-negative bacilli may also cause acute, subacute, and chronic conjunctivitis. *Proteus mirabilis, Klebsiella pneumoniae, Serratia marcescens,* and *Escherichia coli* are common organisms implicated in such cases. Any of the bacteria that cause the more acute forms of conjunctivitis may be found here. Typically the eye feels worse (itching, irritation, foreign body sensation) at night or in the morning. Blepharitis is common. The palpebral conjunctiva is chronically inflamed, but the bulbar conjunctiva is little affected, if at all. In the staphylococcal type, marginal infiltrates, ulcers, and epithelial erosions of the cornea are frequently seen. Loss of cilia may result. *Moraxella lacunata* characteristically produces redness, most intense near the inner and outer canthi (angular conjunctivitis). *Staphylococcus* can also cause an angular conjunctivitis.

TREATMENT. The best guide for specific therapy is established by showing etiologic bacteria in smears and cultures and then testing the sensitivity to various antimicrobial agents. From a practical standpoint this seldom is done. Often the conjunctivitis is treated empirically with a topical broad-spectrum antibiotic or sulfacetamide (Tables 2 and 4). The drug prescribed should produce few or no local sensitivities and should be one that is used infrequently in the treatment of systemic disease. Bacitracin, neomycin, polymyxin B, and sulfacetamide are such drugs. If no improvement occurs in several days, cultures and antibiotic sensitivity studies are done and the appropriate antibiotic is used.

Corticosteroids have been combined with antimicrobial agents in ophthalmic preparations (Table 4) to reduce the inflammatory and possibly the allergic reactions to the bacterial infection. It is best to avoid corticosteroids because of their adverse effect on latent or potential herpes simplex infections and because of a false impression of control of the inflammatory response by the anti-inflammatory action of corticosteroids. Prolonged corticosteroid use also can cause increased intraocular pressure and cataract.

In severe forms of bacterial conjunctivitis, systemic therapy may be needed. Patients with uncomplicated conjunctivitis should not have the eyes patched. To avoid infections of other sites or other people, clean and separate cloths should be used for cleansing the eye area.

Viral Conjunctivitis. There is no specific therapy for viral conjunctivitis. The adenovirus is one of the most common agents. Therapy consists in combating secondary bacterial infections by the local use of broad-spectrum antibiotics or a sulfonamide and in relieving symptoms by the use of hot or cold compresses and local astringents or vasoconstrictors (Table 5).

ADENOVIRAL CONJUNCTIVITIS. The adenoviruses produce two well-organized infections: pharyngeal-conjunctival fever and epidemic keratoconjunctivitis.

Phayrngeal-conjunctival fever is seen mostly in children and is characterized by fever, malaise, sore throat, preauricular and cervical lymphadenopathy, and a fol-

TABLE 4. Topical Antimicrobial Combination Eye Preparations

Generic Name	Trade Name
Drops	
Polymixin B + neomycin	Statrol
Polymyxin B + neomycin + gramicidin	AK-Spore
	Neocidin
	Neosporin
Ointments	
Polymyxin B + bacitracin	AK-Poly-Bac
	Polysporin
Polymyxin B + neomycin	Statrol
Polymyxin B + bacitracin + neomycin	AK-Spore
	Neosporin
	Neotal
	Mycitracin
Polymyxin B + chloramphenicol	Chloromyxin
Polymyxin B + oxytetracycline	Terramycin

TABLE 5. Topical Vasoconstrictor, Astringent, and Antihistaminic Preparations

Generic Name	Trade Name
Vasoconstrictors	
Naphazoline (0.1%)	AK-Con
	Albalon
	Muro's Opcon
	Nafazair
	Naphcon Forte
	Vasocon Regular
Naphazoline (0.05%)	(various mfg.)
Naphazoline (0.03%)	Comfort Eye Drops
Naphazoline (0.02%)	Vasoclear
Naphazoline (0.012%)	Allerest
	Clear Eyes
	Degest 2
	Naphcon
Phenylephrine (0.12%)	AK-Nefrin
	Isopto Frin
	Prefrin
Tetrahydrozoline (0.05%)	Murine Plus
	Optigene
	Soothe
	Visine
Vasoconstrictors with Astringent or Antihistamine	
Naphazoline (0.02%) + zinc sulfate (0.25%)	Vasoclear A
Naphazoline (0.05%) + antazoline (0.5%)	Albalon-A
	Vasocon-A
Naphazoline (0.025%) + pheniramine (0.3%)	AK-Con-A
	Muro's Opcon-A
	Naphcon-A
Phenylephrine (0.125%) + pheniramine maleate (0.5%)	AK-Vernacon
Phenylephrine (0.12%) + pyrilamine (0.1%)	Prefin-A
Phenylephrine (0.12%) + zinc sulfate (0.25%)	Phenylzin
	Zincfrin
Tetrahydrozoline (0.05%) + zinc sulfate (0.25%)	Collyrium-2
	Visine A.C.

licular conjunctivitis. The palpebral conjunctiva is red, and there is a copious watery discharge. The disease usually is caused by adenovirus type 3 and less frequently by types 4 and 7 or other serotypes. It is self-limited, lasting about 10 days. Contaminated swimming pools, even chlorinated, are frequent sources of infection. There is no specific therapy. Isolation precautions should be taken. Symptomatic relief can be given with cold compresses, topical decongestants (Table 5), and sunglasses. Sulfacetamide ophthalmic ointment has been used to prevent secondary bacterial infection.

Epidemic keratoconjunctivitis is highly contagious and actually may occur in epidemics. Types 8 and 19 adenovirus are the most frequent causes, but other serotypes may be etiologic. There is a sudden onset of conjunctival congestion, chemosis, profuse tearing, and epithelial keratitis but little secretion. The infection may also be manifested as a pseudomembranous conjunctivitis. Physicians and hospital clinics may spread the disease. The exudate contains predominantly mononuclear cells, sometimes many polymorphonuclear cells if there is a pseudomembranous reaction, but no inclusions. A few days after onset, preauricular lymphadenopathy appears on the affected side. After about 15 days subepithelial infiltrates may develop in the cornea. The corneal opacities usually clear in several months but on occasion may never clear completely. Because of its communicability, great care should be exercised in the handling of objects used around the eye. Patients admitted to the hospital should be isolated. Topical broad-spectrum antibiotics have been used to prevent secondary infection. In severe cases topical corticosteroids in low concentrations may be used to treat the severe conjunctivitis or keratitis if herpes simplex infection is excluded.

Chlamydial Conjunctivitis. INCLUSION CONJUNCTIVITIS. The disease takes different forms in newborns (see Conjunctivitis Neonatorum for treatment details) and in older children and adults (usually referred to as adult inclusion conjunctivitis). The causative organism is *Chlamydia trachomatis* serotypes D, E, F, G, H, I, J, and K.

In newborns a mucopurulent or purulent papillary conjunctivitis appears 5 to 14 days after vaginal delivery. Sequelae usually do not occur, but occasionally a mild superior micropanus and flat conjunctival scarring are seen, especially if treatment is delayed. Diagnosis can be made easily by microscopic examination of a Giemsa-stained conjunctival smear because the typical basophilic granular intracytoplasmic inclusions in epithelial cells are prevalent. (Additional diagnostic tests are given in the discussion of ophthalmia neonatorum.)

In adolescents and adults chlamydial conjunctivitis most often results from exposure to infected genital secretions. Occasionally transmission of inclusion conjunctivitis occurs in poorly chlorinated swimming pools. An acute mucopurulent follicular conjunctivitis appears, usually in one eye and often with preauricular adenopathy. Corneal involvement with superficial epithelial keratitis and marginal subepithelial infiltrates can occur. Because few inclusions are seen in Giemsa-stained conjunctival smears in adult inclusion conjunctivitis, diagnosis usually is made by isolation of the agent in cell culture or by immunofluorescent assay. Treatment consists of full doses of oral tetracycline (in children over 8 years) or erythromycin for 2 or preferably 3 weeks. Sexual consorts should also receive systemic antibiotic therapy. Pregnant women are treated with oral erythromycin. Topical 1 per cent tetracycline or 0.5 per cent erythromycin is not necessary for patients on full oral therapeutic doses of antibiotics, but local therapy often is prescribed for additional relief and prevention of bilateral infection. Topical therapy alone is not advisable because the effect is slow or partial and the infection usually is not limited to the eye.

Trachoma. This disease is one of the leading causes of blindness in some parts of the world. Contrary to general belief, it exists also in the United States. Trachoma is endemic among the native American Indians, in a few localities in the South and Southwest, and in immigrant populations from endemic areas. The causative organism is *Chlamydia trachomatis* serotypes A, B, and C. It is of low infectivity but occurs under conditions of poor sanitation and hygiene. The clinical picture is that of chronic bilateral conjunctival redness, mild itching, and watery discharge with scant exudate. In the early stages trachoma is indistinguishable from a mild bacterial conjunctivitis. Cytoplasmic inclusion bodies, morphologically identical to those found in inclusion blennorrhea, although fewer in number, are found in conjunctival scrapings. In untreated cases inflammation of the conjunctiva continues over a period of months or years, producing papillary and then follicular hypertrophy followed by scarring. With progression of the disease the cornea becomes opacified, vascularized, and scarred, and vision is severely impaired. Some of the ocular complications are due to secondary bacterial infection.

TREATMENT. Trachoma is effectively treated with a 3-week course of oral tetracycline or erythromycin (30 mg/kg/day in four divided doses). Erythromycin is used instead of tetracycline in pregnant women and children under 8 years old. Topical tetracycline or erythromycin therapy alone can cure trachoma, but the response time is longer. Topical antibiotic therapy usually is given along with systemic therapy because it decreases the intensity of the conjunctival inflammation and counteracts secondary bacterial infection—a factor contributing to scar formation. Concurrent topical corticosteroids should be avoided because (1) signs and symptoms of the primary eye disease could be masked, (2) rebound of the disease may occur when the corticosteroid is discontinued, and (3) reactivation of a concomitant herpes virus infection is liable to occur. Eyelid deformities are treated surgically.

Exanthematous Conjunctivitis. The exanthems such as measles, chickenpox, and smallpox may be accompanied by an acute conjunctivitis. No specific treatment is given unless secondary bacterial infection occurs. If the cornea becomes involved, an ophthalmologist should be consulted for further treatment.

Vaccinial Conjunctivitis. Ocular vaccinia is rarely seen now since smallpox vaccination no longer is routinely recommended. Autoinoculation or inoculation from a contact may lead to a conjunctivitis or serious corneal involvement. Treatment of the conjunctival lesions with a topical antiviral agent may help prevent development of keratitis. Vidarabine (Vira-A) and trifluridine (Viroptic) are probably more effective than idoxuridine (Stoxil, Herplex). Vidarabine is given as a 3 per cent ointment five times daily. Trifluridine 1 per cent drops are given every 2 hours while the patient is awake (maximum 9 drops/day). Idoxuridine is given as a 0.1 per cent solution every hour during the day and every 2 hours at night or as a 0.5 per cent ointment every 6 hours. Hyperimmune vaccinial gamma globulin (VIG) may be used topically (100 mg/ml) every 2 hours. If there is considerable eyelid and conjunctival involvement but no keratitis, VIG may be given intramuscularly (0.6 ml/kg body weight) and repeated in 48 hours if no improvement occurs. VIG is not given or is used with caution if the cornea is involved because of experimental evidence that antigen-antibody complexes within the cornea from administration of VIG may aggravate the keratitis and cause persistent stromal edema. Topical antibiotics may be used to prevent superinfection.

Conjunctivitis Neonatorum (Ophthalmia Neonatorum). Any inflammation of the conjunctiva of the newborn is considered in this category. The inflammation may be due to the chemical irritant silver nitrate or to an infection acquired from an infected birth canal during parturition. The infection may be (1) bacterial (*Staphylococcus; Streptococcus;* pneumococcus; *Neisseria* species, e.g., gonorrhoeae, meningitidis; *Haemophilus* species; coliform organisms; or other bacteria), (2) chlamydial (see Inclusion Conjunctivitis), or (3) viral (herpes simplex).

The incidence of blindness from gonococcal conjunctivitis has been dramatically reduced by prenatal treatment of the mother and by routine topical use of 1 per cent silver nitrate solution or an appropriate antibiotic in each eye of the infant within 1 hour after birth. Erythromycin, and less commonly tetracycline, in recent years have replaced silver nitrate as the prophylactic agents of choice in most newborn nurseries. The reason for the change is that these antibiotics are effective against *Chlamydia trachomatis* as well as *Neisseria gonorrhoeae.* Silver nitrate, however, is not effective against *C. trachomatis*—currently the most common cause of infectious ophthalmia neonatorum. In addition, the antibiotics do not cause a chemical conjunctivitis. Although most strains of *N. gonorrhoeae* at present are sensitive to erythromycin and tetracycline, there is the distinct danger of encountering an increasing number of resistant strains. Resistance to silver nitrate over the years has not been a factor. Since gonococcal ophthalmia neonatorum is a rapidly blinding disease when not treated promptly, whereas chlamydial ophthalmia neonatorum is not, some pediatricians still prefer the use of silver nitrate. They fear that they may encounter an antibiotic-resistant strain of *N. gonorrhoeae.* Thus, until we find a more desirable antimicrobial drug for ophthalmia neonatorum prophylaxis, it is not unreasonable to use topically both silver nitrate and erythromycin (or tetracycline) for prophylaxis in situations or areas where gonococcal and chlamydial ophthalmia are more likely to occur. Infants born to mothers with untreated gonorrhea should be treated prophylactically with a single injection of aqueous crystalline penicillin G 15,000 units intravenously or intramuscularly if full-term and 20,000 units if birth weight is under 2000 gm.

The time of onset of conjunctivitis after exposure to the etiologic agent is helpful in the diagnosis. In general, the times in days are silver nitrate, 1 to 2; *N. gonorrhoeae,* 2 to 4; other bacteria, 4 to 7; herpes simplex, 2 to 4; and *C. trachomatis,* 5 to 14. The definite diagnosis, however, is made from studies that include (1) examination of Gram- and Giemsa-stained scrapings from the tarsal conjunctiva, (2) bacterial cultures of scrapings and exudates, (3) additional chlamydial identification tests such as cell culture of conjunctival scrapings, immunoglobulin antibody titers, monoclonal antibody test on conjunctival smears, and enzyme-linked immunoassay, and (4) other herpes simplex identification tests such as viral culture, recognition of specific herpes simplex virus antigen by immunofluorescence in conjunctival scrapings, and detection of herpes simplex virus particles by electron microscopic examination.

TREATMENT. Active treatment of neonatal gonococcal ophthalmia consists of (1) hospitalization with isolation for 24 hours after initiation of treatment, and (2) aqueous crystalline penicillin G 50,000 units/kg/day intravenously in two doses or 100,000 units/kg/day intramuscularly in four doses. For penicillinase-producing and chromosome-mediated resistant *N. gonorrhoeae* infections either cefotaxime 100 mg/kg/day is given intravenously in three doses for 7 days or ceftriaxone 125 mg is given intramuscularly as a single dose. Topical erythromycin ointment commonly is instilled four to six times daily even though local therapy is not required when systemic therapy is used. Frequent irrigation of the eye with saline to eliminate discharge is helpful. Both parents should be treated with tetracycline or an appropriate penicillin taken orally.

Other bacteria cause neonatal conjunctivitis but have less propensity to corneal involvement. Microscopic examination of Gram-stained conjunctival scrapings and discharge is useful for selection of initial antibiotic therapy. Bacterial cultures of conjunctival scrapings and discharge along with antibiotic sensitivity tests should be obtained at the outset to properly guide further therapy. Most gram-positive pathogens respond to 0.5 per cent erythromycin ointment; gram-negative organisms are treated with 0.3 per cent gentamicin or tobramycin drops or ointment. If initially the etiologic agent is in doubt, a broad-spectrum antimicrobial drug or drug combination (see Tables 2 and 4) may be given until results of the culture and sensitivity studies are returned. *Pseudomonas* conjunctivitis can be particularly serious, especially in premature infants. Prompt topical therapy with gentamicin or tobramycin for several weeks is indicated. If response is poor, subconjunctival injections are given twice daily until cultures are negative. Systemic gentamicin or tobramycin is given if there are other foci of infection or if the conjunctivitis continues to progress.

Chlamydial conjunctivitis is treated with systemic therapy because many infants also have nasopharyngeal infection and may develop chlamydial pneumonia. Oral erythromycin 30 to 50 mg/kg/day is given in four divided doses for 2 weeks along with topical tetracycline or erythromycin ointment instilled four times daily. Both parents should be treated with erythromycin 30 mg/kg/day for 3 weeks to avoid reinfecting the infant.

Herpes simplex conjunctivitis should be treated in association with an ophthalmologist because serious ocular sequelae may occur, namely, keratitis, cataracts, chorioretinitis, and optic neuritis. Infected infants must be isolated. Topical antiviral therapy consists of 1 drop of 1 per cent trifluridine instilled every 2 to 3 hours while the infant is awake, with 0.5 per cent idoxuridine ointment used at bedtime until 3 days after healing appears complete (usually within 2 weeks). If no response occurs within 1 week, therapy with systemic acyclovir may be considered. Topical and systemic corticosteroids should be avoided because they exacerbate herpes simplex infections.

Mucocutaneous Ocular Diseases. Treatment of the conjunctivitis associated with the mucocutaneous diseases, such as erythema multiforme, Stevens-Johnson syndrome, and Reiter's syndrome, is mostly nonspecific, since the etiologic agent is unknown. Precipitating factors may be drugs, food allergy, or infections. Mild soothing eye drops with or without astringent and vasoconstricting properties (Table 5) may be used. Steroids used locally (Table 6) or systemically may be helpful in controlling the allergic and inflammatory phases of the disease, but they must be used judiciously. Drugs such as the sulfonamides and antibiotics should be avoided, for they have been known to precipitate erythema multiforme and Stevens-Johnson disease. A local antibiotic should be used only when a secondary bacterial infection occurs. Choose a suitable one that the patient has not previously used or one that unquestionably was not associated with the present episode. In severe cases visual function can be seriously impaired because of lack of tears, symblepharon formation, corneal ulcer, perforation, and panophthalmitis in Stevens-Johnson disease and scleritis, interstitial keratitis, and hypopyon uveitis in Reiter's disease. Because of the seriousness of the eye complications it is advisable to have an ophthalmologist treat the ocular aspects of these diseases.

Allergic Forms of Conjunctivitis. SIMPLE ALLERGIC CONJUNCTIVITIS. The clinical manifestations of these nonspecific conjunctival inflammations are acute edema of the lids and conjunctiva, itching, photophobia, lacrimation, mild injection of the palpebral and bulbar conjunctiva, and a scanty, stringy discharge. Conjunctival papillae and follicles are not present. An occasional eosinophil is present in the smear of the conjunctival scraping. There may or may not be a direct relation to an allergen such as a pollen (hay fever), cosmetic, or drug.

Treatment consists in (1) removal of the offending agent if possible, (2) desensitization to the allergen, and (3) symptomatic relief with the use of local vasoconstric-

tors with or without antihistamines, astringents, cromolyn sodium 4 per cent solution (Opticrom), and only during the acute phase of severe cases, corticosteroids (Tables 5 and 6). Steroids should be avoided if possible and used only under special circumstances supervised by an ophthalmologist. The disadvantages of the steroids, i.e., activation of herpes simplex keratoconjunctivitis and of bacterial and fungal infections, must be kept in mind. Cataracts and glaucoma have been seen in children as well as in adults who have used topical corticosteroids for long periods. If vasoconstrictors with or without antihistamines (local and systemic) or cromolyn sodium drops control the allergic reaction, steroids should not be used.

VERNAL CONJUNCTIVITIS. This is a bilateral chronic conjunctivitis with symptoms that usually become worse in the spring and last throughout the warm months. The cause is thought to be allergic. The onset is between 5 and 15 years. The severity of the symptoms tends to become milder with the passing years. This condition is characterized by intense itching, lacrimation, photophobia, conjunctival injection, a stringy conjunctival discharge, and, at times, a milky pseudomembrane. Giant papillary hypertrophy develops in the tarsal conjunctiva, especially the upper, to give the typical "cobblestone" appearance. The lesions may cause a corneal "shield ulcer" (called such because of the shape of the epithelial defect). Papillary hypertrophy in the limbal region appears as gray elevated lesions. Many eosinophils are seen in the smear of the conjunctival exudate.

In mild cases symptoms may be relieved by topical vasoconstrictors, topical and oral antihistamines, and cold compresses. More serious disease warrants topical cromolyn 4 per cent (Opticrom) eye drops instilled four times daily. Cromolyn inhibits the degranulation of conjunctival mast cells, thereby preventing the release of histamine. The action of cromolyn is prophylactic in that it prevents the release of this mediator of inflammation. If further control of the disease is required, topical corticosteroids (Table 6) are used. To suppress symptoms in severe disabling disease it may be necessary to use the corticosteroid every 2 hours, perhaps supplemented by small oral doses. As improvement occurs corticosteroid therapy is reduced as soon as possible to the minimum therapeutic dosage. Fluorometholone (FML) is the topical corticosteroid often preferred over the more potent preparations such as dexamethasone and prednisolone because it is effective locally yet has less tendency to increase intraocular pressure with continued use. The prolonged use of any corticosteroid, however, carries the risk of glaucoma, herpes simplex infection activation, and cataract. Topical cromolyn sodium in many cases has eliminated the need for topical corticosteroids or has reduced its use to once or twice a day. Beta-radiation, cryoablation, and surgical excision of giant papillae have been used, but the papillae usually recur. Desensitization of the patient to allergens has had little effect on the disease. Symptoms usually subside or disappear with cool or cold weather.

PHLYCTENULAR KERATOCONJUNCTIVITIS. The phlyctenule is a small, hard, red elevated nodule surrounded by hyperemic vessels. It appears most commonly at the

TABLE 6. Topical Corticosteroid Eye Preparations

Generic Name	Trade Name	Concentration
Drops		
Dexamethasone alcohol (suspension)	Maxidex	0.1%
Dexamethasone sodium phosphate (solution)	AK-Dex	0.1%
	Decadron	0.1%
Fluorometholone (suspension)	FML	0.1%
	Fluor-op	0.1%
	FML Forte	0.25%
Medrysone (suspension)	HMS	1%
Prednisolone acetate (suspension)	AK-Tate	1%
	Econo-pred	0.125%
	Econopred Plus	1%
	Pred Mild	0.12%
	Pred Forte	1%
Prednisolone sodium phosphate (solution)	AK-Pred	0.125% & 1%
	Inflammase Mild	0.125%
	Inflammase Forte	1%
	Metreton	0.5%
Ointments		
Dexamethasone sodium phosphate	AK-Dex	0.05%
	Decadron	0.05%
	Maxidex	0.05%
Fluorometholone	FML S.O.P.	0.1%

limbus to involve both the bulbar conjunctiva and the cornea. The lesion is a subepithelial collection of neutrophils and mononuclear cells including lymphocytes, macrophages, and plasma cells that ulcerate but usually heal. Recurrences, especially with secondary infection, may result in corneal opacification. The outstanding clinical manifestations are intense photophobia and lacrimation. The disease has been regarded as a hypersensitivity reaction of the conjunctiva and cornea to a product of the tubercle bacillus, to other bacteria such as the *Staphylococcus*, or to fungi.

Since malnutrition is frequently a part of the disease, general measures such as improving the diet and hygiene are important. A topical corticosteroid or antimicrobial-corticosteroid combination (see Tables 3 and 6) is effective in treating the disease and the secondary infection that may be present. For patients who do not respond to corticosteroids or develop corticosteroid complications, oral erythromycin or tetracycline (for patients older than 8 years) has proven effective. Investigation for a systemic disease such as tuberculosis should be made.

Nonspecific Conjunctival Hyperemia. External irritants such as smoke, smog, fumes, or swimming pool or ocean water or factors such as inadequate rest or asthenopia (eyestrain) may produce conjunctival hyperemia. Astringent eye drops with or without a vasoconstrictor (Table 5) relieve this nonspecific inflammation. A complete eye examination should be performed if the symptoms are associated with eyestrain.

The pediatrician must consider specific diseases, such as ataxia-telangiectasia and familial dysautonomia (Riley-Day syndrome), before settling on a diagnosis of nonspecific conjunctival hyperemia.

CORNEAL DISORDERS

In general, diseases of the cornea require early attention by an ophthalmologist. Even so-called minor infections of this portion of the eye can lead to serious ocular complications, including blindness, if they are not promptly and correctly handled by the skilled specialist. A safe rule for the nonophthalmologic physician to follow is that all diseases and injuries of the cornea (including foreign bodies) should be seen promptly by an ophthalmologist. It is important, therefore, for the pediatrician to learn the symptoms and signs of corneal disease to enable him to recognize this diagnostic possibility.

Patients with corneal disease may have photophobia, lacrimation, blepharospasm, pain, decreased vision, ocular discharge, hyperemia of the superficial and deep conjunctival vessels (circumlimbal flush), corneal opacity, small pupil if secondary iritis exists, and often a history of trauma. Inspection of the cornea with intense oblique focal illumination is often necessary to see a foreign body or a lesion.

The treatment of corneal diseases will not be reviewed in detail because therapy should be carried out by the ophthalmologist.

Corneal Ulcers and Infections

Careful examination of the ocular adnexa is important because inflammation of the cornea may be secondary to other diseases, e.g., blepharitis, trichiasis, trachoma, the "cobblestone" papillae of vernal conjunctivitis, conjunctivitis, scleritis, iritis, or dacryocystitis. Systemic disease and poor general physical condition must be evaluated, for they may contribute to the development of a corneal infection.

Ulcers of the cornea can be easily seen by placing a drop or two of sterile fluorescein solution or a moistened fluorescein paper strip (Fluor-I-Strip) into the conjunctival sac and then washing out the excess with isotonic saline solution. Studies to determine the cause of corneal ulcer include Gram and Giemsa stains of smears and scrapings, cultures (bacterial, viral, and fungal), and antimicrobial sensitivity tests when cultures are positive.

Simple Corneal Ulcer. This lesion may result from direct infection after a break of the epithelial barrier by trauma or by disturbances in the metabolism of the epithelium from causes such as vitamin A deficiency, corneal exposure, and neurotrophic disease.

Central Corneal Ulcer. Central ulcers have an intense purulent reaction in and around the ulcer, with occasional extension into the deeper layers of the cornea or an exudative reaction in the anterior chamber (hypopyon); most are bacterial. The gram-positive cocci most likely to produce central corneal ulcers are *Staphylococcus aureus, Staphylococcus epidermidis, Streptococcus pneumoniae,* and *Streptococcus pyogenes.* The most common gram-negative causative bacteria are *Pseudomonas aeruginosa, Moraxella lacunata,* and Enterobacteriaceae *Proteus, Serratia, E. coli,* and *Klebsiella).* The ulcers may develop after trauma or appear in association with a dacryocystitis.

TREATMENT. Before antimicrobial treatment is started, smears and cultures of the ulcer material should be prepared and sensitivity studies to various antimicrobial agents should be pursued. A young child may require a general anesthetic to accomplish these studies. Until these studies indicate the antimicrobial drug of choice, fortified topical antibiotics, such as cefazolin (50 mg/ml) and gentamicin or tobramycin (15 mg/ml), effective against a wide range of gram-positive and gram-negative bacteria, should be used at hourly intervals. Mixtures that contain bacitracin or gramicidin, neomycin, and polymyxin B are available (see Table 4). Gentamicin plus bacitracin may also be used. Local therapy alone may be all that is required in the superficial ulcers. In the more severe corneal ulcers, systemic and subconjunctival antibiotic therapy may be necessary. Cycloplegic medication is usually given because of the accompanying iridocyclitis. Local corticosteroid therapy is avoided because it interferes with tissue reparative processes and immune responses. Ulcers that progress in spite of vigorous medical therapy may benefit from covering the ulcer with a conjunctival flap, closure of the eyelids with adhesions (tarsorrhaphy), or replacement of the ulcer site by a keratoplasty.

Marginal Corneal Ulcer. Marginal ulcers are usually sterile and probably represent a toxic or hypersensitivity reaction to bacterial infection of the conjunctiva or eyelid. The acute type is seen with staphylococcal or *H. influenzae* conjunctivitis. The chronic type is secondary to staphylococcal, diplobacillus or *Moraxella lacunata,* and streptococcal conjunctivitis.

TREATMENT. Topical corticosteroids usually cure the sterile toxic or hypersensitivity type of ulcer in 3 to 4 days. The infectious blepharitis and conjunctivitis should be treated with bacitracin if the primary infection is due to *Staphylococcus, Streptococcus,* or *H. influenzae.* A tetracycline or sulfonamide is also effective against these bacteria as well as the diplobacillus or *Moraxella lacunata.*

Phlyctenular Keratoconjunctivitis. This is discussed on pages 469 to 470.

Herpes Simplex Virus Keratitis (Dendritic Keratitis). This form of keratitis is a common corneal disease in childhood. The widespread and indiscriminate use of local steroids increases the severity of the infection and the ocular complications such as corneal perforation and loss of the eye. Dendritic keratitis is the most important corneal disease leading to loss of vision in the United States. Herpes simplex infections of the cornea tend to be chronic, leaving opaque scars that impair vision. Recurrent infections are frequent.

The patient complains of mild irritation and has photophobia, lacrimation, and blurred vision. A recent history of an infection of the respiratory tract with "cold sores" on the face is often elicited. Fever, trauma, menstruation, and psychic stress may be other precipitating factors. The dendrite-shaped ulcer (seen best with fluorescein or rose bengal staining) and decreased corneal sensitivity characterize this type of keratitis.

TREATMENT. The principal treatment previously had been the removal of the virus-containing epithelium by mechanical debridement. Chemotherapy with the topical antiviral drugs idoxuridine (Herplex, Stoxil), vidarabine (Vira-A), and trifluridine (Viroptic) is known to be effective against herpes simplex keratitis. They interfere with DNA synthesis. The response to topical antiviral therapy is best when the infection is limited to the epithelium. With stromal involvement these drugs are less effective or ineffective. Of the three antiviral agents trifluridine has been the most effective, probably because of its greater solubility than either idoxuridine or vidarabine. One drop of the 1 per cent solution is instilled every 2 hours while the patient is awake for a maximal daily dose of 9 drops. Healing of uncomplicated ulcers occurs in 1 to 2 weeks. As the epithelial defect heals the antiviral therapy can be tapered to 5 drops daily, but it should be continued for about 1 week after healing to prevent immediate recurrences. Although corticosteroids are generally contraindicated in herpes simplex keratitis, in the less acute inflammatory form with stromal involvement known as *disciform herpetic keratitis,* restricted use of a topical corticosteroid such as prednisolone acetate 1 per cent can be helpful if used concurrently with trifluridine if the epithelium is healed. Disciform herpetic keratitis is believed to be a hypersensitivity reaction to the viral antigens. If the keratitis is progressive in spite of medical treatment, a conjunctival flap, tarsorrhaphy, or lamellar keratoplasty may be required. A topical cycloplegic agent such as 1 per cent atropine or 0.25 per cent scopolamine is helpful to keep the eye comfortable.

Herpes Zoster Keratitis. The diagnosis is usually made from the characteristic skin lesions and their distribution along the ophthalmic division of the trigeminal nerve. The skin of the tip of the nose and the eye are often simultaneously involved, since the nasociliary nerve innervates both sites (positive Hutchinson's sign). An iridocyclitis usually accompanies the corneal involvement.

TREATMENT. Topical antiviral agents are ineffective. Although corticosteroids (without antiviral agents) are contraindicated in herpes simplex keratitis, they frequently relieve the keratitis and iridocyclitis of herpes zoster. Severe involvement and alleviation of postherpetic neuralgia may be benefitted by systemic administration of corticosteroids. The incidence of neuralgia, however, is not high in young patients. The steroids act primarily as an anti-inflammatory agent. Corticosteroids should be avoided or used with extreme caution in immunosuppressed patients for fear of dissemination of the disease. Correspondingly, fulminating herpes zoster has developed in patients who were receiving systemic corticosteroids for other diseases. Thus it is wise to delay start of corticosteroid therapy in the otherwise healthy patient for 3 to 5 days after appearance of the eruption to enable the host's immune system to be mobilized. Intravenous or oral acyclovir given within the first 72 hours of the onset of herpes zoster ophthalmicus has been particularly beneficial. Its use, especially in immunosuppressed patients, is indicated for severe corneal or uveal involvement and visually threatening complications such as proptosis, chorioretinitis, or optic neuritis. Cycloplegic eye drops are used along with topical corticosteroids for the iridocyclitis. Antibiotics to reduce secondary bacterial infection may reduce severe scarring of the cornea.

Vaccinia Keratitis. Topical antiviral drugs are used for vaccinia infection of the cornea (see Vaccinial Conjunctivitis). Trifluridine is the agent of choice because of better corneal permeability. Cycloplegics are used to relieve the iritis. Vaccinia immune globulin (VIG) is not used because experimental studies indicate that delayed immune reactions occur in the cornea from its use, and these reactions lead to prolonged stromal edema. Topical antibiotics may be given twice daily to prevent superinfection.

Exanthematous Keratitis. Measles (rubeola) and its complications are less often seen now because of routine immunization of young children with live attenuated measles virus. A keratitis with multiple epithelial erosions causes photophobia. The keratoconjunctivitis usually is mild and self-limited. The available topical antiviral agents are not effective. Microbial superinfection is prevented or treated with topical antibiotics.

Chickenpox (varicella) rarely causes serious ocular disease. In addition to a mild conjunctivitis varicella may produce a punctate or dendritic keratitis that is similar to but not caused by herpes simplex infection. Although there is no conclusive evidence that topical antiviral drugs are efficacious, claims of their value in the acute phase of epithelial keratitis have been made. Trifluridine 1 per cent (Viroptic) 1 drop five times daily may be helpful. Cycloplegics are used for the uveitis that may accompany the keratitis. Topical antibiotics are given to prevent or treat microbial superinfection.

Smallpox (variola) has been essentially eliminated by vaccination measures. Direct corneal involvement can occur, but most lesions heal spontaneously and leave minimal scars. Severe infections, however, may lead to corneal ulcers that become secondarily infected with bacteria and result in dense scars. Adequate antiviral therapy is not available. Cycloplegics are used for any accompanying iridocyclitis. Topical antibiotics prevent secondary bacterial infections.

Superficial Punctate Keratitis. Thygeson's superficial punctate keratitis is characterized by scattered, fine punctate infiltrations in the superficial corneal layers, usually of both eyes. The lesions favor the pupillary area and require magnification to be seen. Vision may be appreciably reduced. The lesions are nonulcerative, but most stain with fluorescein. Healing may take several years in the untreated case, but no scarring or vascularization occurs. The disease is thought to be caused by a virus. Drugs, exposure, and staphylococcal infections, however, may produce the same signs and symptoms. The symptoms are photophobia, lacrimation, pain, conjunctival infection, and decreased vision. Preauricular lymphadenopathy may be present.

TREATMENT. Topical use of a corticosteroid such as fluorometholone (FML) usually is beneficial. Steroid dosage is tapered rapidly. Since recurrence of keratitis is common, periodic use of the steroid (e.g., 1 drop once or twice weekly) may be sufficient to keep the patient asymptomatic. Antiviral drugs are not recommended because they can cause scarring beneath the lesions. Cycloplegics usually are not needed. Local antibiotics are used if there is a bacterial infection. The use of soft contact lenses has also been helpful.

Fungal Corneal Ulcers. The incidence of keratomycosis has increased in recent years. Local antibiotic and steroid therapy seems to be an important factor in this increase. Fungi infect the cornea after a break in the epithelium from trauma or damage by inflammation. Numerous fungi, including those previously regarded as nonpathogenic, have been cultured from these indolent, slowly progressive corneal ulcers. Consider a fungal etiology if an ulcer does not respond to antibiotic therapy. Identification of the fungus is made by examination of scrapings obtained with Gram, Giemsa, and potassium hydroxide stains and by culture on Sabouraud's agar or blood agar at room temperature.

TREATMENT. Natamycin (Natacyn) is the initial drug of choice for both yeast and filamentary forms; a 5 per cent suspension is given every 1 to 2 hours for 3 to 4 days, then reduced to 1 drop six to eight times daily for 2 to 3 weeks. If no response occurs and filamentous organisms are isolated, miconazole (Monistat) 1 per cent prepared from the injectable solution is given every hour initially. If yeast forms (Candida) do not respond to topical natamycin, then nystatin (Mycostatin, Nilstat) is used—1 drop of 25,000 units/ml hourly—or the powder may be dusted onto the lesion. Flucytosine 1 per cent prepared from oral capsules has been used hourly for Candida infections. Amphotericin B (Fungizone) 0.15 per cent solution applied hourly is effective against a group of pathogenic and saprophytic fungi including Candida, Coccidioides, Cryptococcus, Histoplasma, Blastomyces, and Sporotrichum. For corneal perforations or intraocular extension of Candida and filamentous fungi (except Fusarium), miconazole may be given subconjunctivally and intravenously. Oral flucytosine may also be effective. Oral ketaconazole has been reported to be helpful for severe keratomycoses. Nonhealing ulcers may require a conjunctival flap. A penetrating keratoplasty may provide a cure if the entire area of infection can be encompassed. Cycloplegics are used for an accompanying iridocyclitis. Broad-spectrum antibiotics are applied to combat bacterial superinfection.

Interstitial Keratitis. Most cases in children occur as complications of congenital syphilis. Tuberculosis and leprosy are rare causes. Symptoms of intense photophobia, lacrimation, pain, and gradual loss of vision, ultimately in both eyes, occur between 5 and 15 years of age. Inflammation and vascularization involve the deep layers of the cornea. The cornea assumes a ground-glass appearance with orange-red areas ("salmon patches") due to vascularization. The reaction normally begins to subside in 1 to 2 months, sooner when topical or systemic corticosteroids are given. Ghost vessels, seen with magnification, remain in the corneal stroma after the inflammation has subsided. An associated uveitis or choroiditis is common. These serious ocular manifestations are less often seen today because of intensive systemic antiluetic and topical corticosteroid therapy. Other signs of congenital syphilis may be seen, such as saddle nose, deafness, and notched teeth. The serologic tests for syphilis give positive results. Interstitial keratitis may represent an allergic response, since Treponema pallidum is not found in the cornea during the acute stage.

TREATMENT. There is no specific treatment for syphilitic interstitial keratitis. Systemic acute syphilis should be treated with penicillin, but the treatment does not affect the corneal disease. Topical steroids relieve the symptoms. Systemic steroids are valuable if the local steroids do not adequately control the symptoms. Some physicians believe steroid therapy may prolong the disease. The accompanying iridocyclitis is helped by the local steroids, but in addition a strong cycloplegic such as atropine 1 per cent should be instilled daily. For severe corneal scarring a corneal transplant is indicated, but only if damage to other parts of the eye does not preclude a good visual outcome. In the rare case when tuberculosis is the cause of the interstitial keratitis (usually unilateral), the systemic infection is treated.

Corneal Drying and Exposure. The following diseases are associated with the complications of corneal drying and exposure: (1) keratitis sicca, the result of a lacrimal gland insufficiency; (2) exposure keratitis, developing after facial nerve palsies, exophthalmos, and prolonged periods of unconsciousness; (3) neuroparalytic keratitis, seen after interruption of function of the trigeminal nerve; (4) familial dysautonomia (Riley-Day syndrome), corneal complications occurring from the congenital absence or deficiency of tears and corneal hypesthesia. Corneal infection may lead to intraocular infection and loss of the eye.

TREATMENT. The cornea should be protected with artificial tears used hourly or less often as needed. The many different products available commercially attest to the variability in patient relief. The principal bases in the liquid preparations include (1) methylcellulose, (2) ethylcellulose, (3) polyvinyl alcohol, and (4) polyvinylpyrrolidone polymer. The lubricant ointments contain petrolatum, lanolin, and mineral oil. For patients who need frequent tear replacement a soluble insert of hydroxypropylcellulose (Lacrisert) is available. Sodium hyaluronate (Healon) 0.1 per cent solution has been helpful in some patients. The use of a soft contact lens in association with frequent artificial tear instillation helps maintain a satisfactory precorneal tear film. To conserve tears, temporary closure of the lacrimal punta can be accomplished with silicone or Teflon plugs or with cyanoacrylate glue; permanent closure is achieved with electrocautery or argon laser. Temporary closure of the puncta may be used to predict whether the patient will have epiphora following permanent closure. In severe cases a moist chamber can be made by applying an occlusive plastic shield across the eyes or by wearing flush-fitting goggles. Lastly, a temporary or permanent tarsorrhaphy may be required to protect the cornea.

SCLERAL AND EPISCLERAL DISORDERS

Episcleritis

A localized inflammation of the tissue between the conjunctiva and sclera is characteristic of episcleritis. The patient has slight pain, photophobia, and tenderness in the area. The localized patch of hyperemia and the absence of a discharge distinguish episcleritis from conjunctivitis. Episcleritis can occur as an isolated disease or in association with a systemic disorder, most commonly a collagen disease such as rheumatoid arthritis. The condition often is self-limited. About one third of the patients have uveitis as well.

TREATMENT. Local vasoconstrictor drops (Table 5) are helpful, but topical steroid medication (Table 6) may give better relief of symptoms. A cycloplegic such as scopolamine 0.25 per cent, 1 drop two times daily, is instilled into the eye if there is an anterior uveitis. A systemic disorder should be sought and treated. Oral oxyphenbutazone (Tandearil) or indomethacin (Indocin) has been reported to be effective in the treatment of persistent episcleritis. Oxyphenbutazone is not available at present in the United States.

Scleritis

Inflammation of the deeper scleral tissue is more severe and appears more purplish than in episcleritis. It may be localized, diffuse, or nodular. Pain, photophobia, and tenderness may be intense. An associated anterior uveitis is frequently present. Scleritis may be seen with systemic diseases such as the collagen diseases (particularly rheumatoid arthritis), tuberculosis, syphilis, brucellosis, and gout. The severity of the scleritis is often directly related to the severity of the systemic disease.

TREATMENT. In the acute phase an occasional patient may respond to topical corticosteroid therapy, but topical anti-inflammatory agents usually are ineffective. Systemic nonsteroidal anti-inflammatory drugs or a corticosteroid generally is necessary. The nonsteroidal drugs are tried first. If long-term corticosteroid therapy is needed for recurrent or persistent episcleritis or scleritis, periodic examination for increased intraocular pressure and cataract should be performed. In the severe necrotizing form of scleritis, topical steroids may hasten corneal and scleral melting. Systemic steroids may be needed for severe posterior scleritis. Scopolamine 0.25 per cent is instilled into the eye two times daily if an anterior uveitis is present. The systemic disease is actively treated.

It is of interest that scleritis may develop in patients receiving salicylates or systemic corticosteroids for a disease such as rheumatoid arthritis. The addition of topical steroid therapy is rarely of value in such a situation. Subconjunctival corticosteroid injections must be avoided because the sclera often is thin and may perforate after injection of the drug. Cases of severe scleritis may require immunosuppressive drugs. If scleral ectasia and impending perforation of the globe occur, scleral grafting may be necessary.

UVEITIS

Inflammation of the uveal tract is a serious disease because it often leads to severe visual impairment or blindness. Early diagnosis and treatment are important to prevent the ocular complications. The damaging effect of the disease often is subtle in children. There may be few or no subjective complaints or obvious signs of the disease during episodes of recurrent or chronic inflammation.

Uveitis has been popularly classified as nongranulomatous and granulomatous. *Nongranulomatous uveitis* more often involves the anterior uvea, producing the following symptoms and signs: acute onset with pain, redness, photophobia, blurred vision, circumcorneal flush, miotic or irregular pupil, and on slit-lamp examination the presence of fibrin and cells in the anterior chamber and fine white keratic precipitates on the posterior surface of the cornea. *Granulomatous uveitis* appears more frequently as a posterior uveitis with a slow onset, minimal redness, pain or photophobia, normal or slightly miotic pupil, and vision less than one would expect from the mild external manifestations of the disease. Large, yellow-gray "mutton-fat" keratitic precipitates are seen on the posterior surface of the cornea with the slit lamp. Iris nodules are often visible. On ophthalmoscopy single or multiple yellow or white exudative lesions are seen in the choroid with or without vitreous haze.

Uveitis presents a difficult therapeutic problem because, although numerous causes are suspected, in only relatively few cases is a specific etiologic agent detected. Studies indicate that there is a higher incidence of nongranulomatous uveitis in patients with autoimmune disorders such as juvenile rheumatoid arthritis, sarcoidosis, systemic lupus erythematosus, and the like. Granulomatous uveitis may result from the actual invasion of the uveal tract by an organism, but organisms are rarely isolated or demonstrated. Granulomatous uveitis may be caused by toxoplasmosis (the infection most frequently incriminated), syphilis, tuberculosis, brucellosis, leptospirosis, viruses, fungi, nematodes, and sarcoidosis.

TREATMENT. The management of uveitis consists of (1) thorough medical evaluation of the patient in search for a specific cause (the primary care physician should work closely with the ophthalmologist), (2) specific treatment if the cause is found or if one is highly suspected, and (3) nonspecific ocular treatment to minimize the complications from the inflammatory process (often this is all that is or can be done).

Nonspecific treatment should include the following:

Cycloplegics to dilate the pupil to prevent posterior synechiae and to put the iris and ciliary body at rest. This reduces pain from the ciliary and pupillary spasm and decreases the inflammatory protein response in the aqueous humor. Scopolamine 0.25 per cent or atropine 1 per cent solution or ointment, instilled once or twice daily, is the favored cycloplegic agent.

Mydriatics further help the cycloplegic in obtaining wide pupillary dilatation and thus prevent or break up posterior synechiae. A drug such as phenylephrine 2.5 per cent (Neo-Synephrine) is an effective mydriatic and also decreases hyperemia by its vasoconstricting properties.

Corticosteroids, applied locally or given by subconjunctival injection, may be used to treat anterior uveitis. The subconjunctival route is usually reserved for the more severe forms of anterior uveitis in which a higher and prolonged concentration of the drug is desired. Topical steroid drops or ointment (see Table 6) can be used initially every 1 to 4 hours, depending on the severity of the disease, then less often as improvement occurs.

Steroids should be given systemically in the more severe forms of anterior uveitis if local or subconjunctival medications are not beneficial. Posterior uveitis also usually requires systemic therapy. The daily dosage in children is 1 to 2 mg/kg body weight of prednisone up to a maximum of 80 mg. The equivalent dose of another corticosteroid may be used. One should use the minimum dose necessary to achieve a reasonable effect and for the shortest time needed to control the inflammation. The toxic effects and contraindications to the corticosteroids for short- and long-term therapy must be kept in mind.

Treatment for active *ocular toxoplasmosis* deserves special mention. It consists in the combined use of pyrimethamine (Daraprim) and sulfadiazine. The concomitant use of systemic corticosteroids is controversial and generally is reserved for acute, progressive lesions in the macular area or optic nerve. Pyrimethamine is given orally twice daily in the total daily dosage of 2 mg/kg body weight up to 150 mg for 1 to 3 days, then 1 mg/kg up to 25 mg daily for 4 weeks. The sulfadiazine* dosage is 120 to 150 mg/kg/day orally in four divided doses up to 4 gm/day for 4 weeks. In the acute fulminating cases clinical improvement is seen in 2 to 3

weeks. Pyrimethamine should be avoided in pregnant patients because it can cause congenital malformations. Clindamycin and (in Europe) spiramycin have been used instead of pyrimethamine.

Weekly urinalysis for sulfadiazine crystaluria or evidence of kidney irritation should be done. Since pyrimethamine is a folic acid antagonist, folinic acid, 3 mg intramuscularly or orally twice weekly, should be given to prevent hematologic toxicity, e.g., bone marrow suppression, especially thrombocytopenia.

LACRIMAL APPARATUS DISORDERS

Infantile Dacryostenosis

Normally the nasolacrimal drainage system is patent throughout its length at birth. Failure of the nasolacrimal duct to canalize completely leads to persistent tearing *(epiphora)* of one eye or both eyes in the first weeks of life. Contrary to a common belief, most newborn infants tear in the first week of life. Persistent tearing from dacryostenosis without dacryocystitis can be differentiated from conjunctivitis and corneal disease by the lack of conjunctival inflammation. The diagnosis of infantile glaucoma must also be excluded. Usually, significant dacryostenosis is followed promptly by dacryocystitis.

TREATMENT. Most cases of infantile dacryostenosis clear spontaneously with further canalization of the nasolacrimal duct in the first 6 to 8 months of life. Massaging the contents of the lacrimal sac properly down through the nasolacrimal duct four to six times daily may be helpful. Topical antibiotics usually are not prescribed if there is no secondary infection. Persistent obstruction generally leads to dacryocystitis (see Infantile Dacryocystitis treatment).

Infantile Dacryocystitis

Obstruction of the nasolacrimal duct usually leads to infection of the lacrimal sac (dacryocystitis) by the common pyogenic bacteria. Excess tearing is then replaced by mucopurulent discharge and some conjunctival redness. There may be an acute distention of the lacrimal sac with overlying redness, pain, and tenderness. Occasionally a lacrimal sac abscess ruptures and forms a draining fistula. In the differential diagnosis of infantile dacryocystitis one must exclude infantile glaucoma as well as conjunctival or corneal disease.

TREATMENT. Since most cases of obstructed nasolacrimal ducts clear spontaneously in the first 6 to 8 months of life, medical treatment consisting of massage and topical antibiotic medication is advisable in this age period. Massaging the nasolacrimal sac area properly empties the sac of purulent material, and the downward pressure tends to increase hydrostatic pressure to rupture the obstructing membrane located usually at the lower end of the duct. The authors' preferred treatment program consists of massage of the nasolacrimal sac area four to six times daily followed by the instillation into the inner canthus of a broad-spectrum drop (not ointment) such as gramicidin-neomycin-polymyxin B (see Table 4) for 4 to 7 days. Sulfacetamide drops may be used if the discharge is not predominantly purulent.

---

*Manufacturer's precaution: Sulfadiazine is not for use in children under 2 months of age.

If signs of obstruction reappear, a second course of massage and topical antimicrobial therapy is given. If the two separate courses of treatment are not curative, we then irrigate the lacrimal sac and probe the nasolacrimal duct under light general anesthesia. By this time the infant usually is over 6 months of age, but age is no contraindication to this procedure if skillful anesthesiologists are available. The success rate of simple irrigation and probing begins to diminish after 12 months of age and even more so after 18 months of age. Severe infections of the lacrimal sac are treated with systemic antibiotics. An abscess of the lacrimal sac should be probed. If unsuccessfully decompressed it requires incision and drainage.

To properly guide antimicrobial therapy in cases of chronic, recurrent, or severe infection, it is advisable to obtain smears for Gram-stain examination, cultures, and antibiotic sensitivity studies.

A single probing with irrigation usually eliminates the obstruction and infection. Occasionally the procedure must be repeated. If the nasolacrimal duct cannot be opened by probing, intubation of the nasolacrimal system with silicone tubing for a short period or an external dacryocystorhinostomy may be required to restore drainage of tears into the nose. The operation usually is not done before the age of 3 years.

One exception to delaying the probing of obstructed ducts until after 6 to 8 months of age or after several trials of medical treatment is in the management of congenital nasolacrimal duct obstruction associated with congenital mucocele (dacryocystocele). This condition usually is apparent in the newborn nursery and is manifested by a bluish swelling over the lacrimal sac, occasionally mistaken for a hemangioma. Diagnosis is aided by ultrasonography. Treatment is immediate probing of the lacrimal system.

OCULAR TRAUMA

Prompt and appropriate care after eye injury often saves useful vision; poor management may lead to blindness. Improper initial eye care by the nonophthalmologic physician usually results from unfamiliarity with a few fundamental rules in the correct handling of the patient with ocular trauma.

To determine the ocular structures involved and the extent of the injury, it is imperative to examine closely the external and visible structures of the eyes with good illumination and magnification, and to perform ophthalmoscopy. An accurate history is essential. Testing the patient's visual acuity before treatment is important for diagnostic, prognostic, and medicolegal reasons. If an adequate examination cannot be performed by the nonophthalmologic physician, the patient should be referred to an eye physician for further care. The nonophthalmologic physician should not be the one to decide whether or not an eye injury is minor except in obvious situations such as occur with a superficial conjunctival foreign body.

Foreign Bodies

Conjunctival foreign bodies can usually be safely flushed out with a stream of isotonic saline solution or removed with a sterile moistened cotton applicator. If the history suggests that a foreign body is the likely cause of the eye symptoms and none is found on the bulbar or lower palpebral conjunctiva of the cornea, then the upper eyelid should be everted for inspection. The use of a local anesthetic such as 0.5 per cent proparacaine (see Table 1) facilitates the examination.

Corneal foreign bodies may be difficult to see unless adequate local anesthesia, oblique lighting, and magnification (loupe or slit-lamp biomicroscopy) are used. Fluorescein stain helps to delineate the foreign body. One drop of sterile 2 per cent fluorescein solution or a fluorescein strip is placed in the conjunctival sac and the excess washed out with isotonic saline solution. Corneal foreign bodies that are not easily removed by irrigation or with the wipe of a moistened sterile cotton applicator should be referred to an ophthalmologist for further treatment. If the foreign body is dislodged, fluorescein is again added to the eye to determine the extent of the corneal abrasion. Unless the abrasion is minute (less than 1 mm), a broad-spectrum antimicrobial agent such as sulfacetamide or a combination of bacitracin or gramicidin, neomycin, and polymyxin B is instilled into the eye and the eye is covered with a patch for 24 hours. If the abrasion is not superficial or is large (more than a few millimeters), an antibiotic is instilled and a patch is applied. The patient should then be seen by an ophthalmologist. The cornea should be re-examined in 24 hours in all cases after the removal of a foreign body for the presence of a secondary infection in the abraded area. Metallic foreign bodies frequently leave a localized rust stain (rust ring). This is best removed by an ophthalmologist under slit lamp magnification. An untreated corneal infection may lead to corneal ulceration, intraocular infection, and loss of the eye.

Intraocular foreign bodies (suspected or known) must be referred immediately to an eye physician. If there will be a delay of a few hours before the child is seen by an ophthalmologist, the physician should test the visual acuity, instill a cycloplegic drug and a broad-spectrum antibiotic into the eye, and start systemic antimicrobial therapy. Ampicillin, gentamicin, or chloramphenicol in full dose has been widely used for potential or active intraocular infections because of the broad spectrum of antibacterial activity and the ability to penetrate the ocular tissues. It is important to know that small, missile-like foreign bodies may penetrate the globe and cause transient pain or no pain at all. When a history suggests the possibility of penetration of the eye by a high-velocity foreign body, the patient should be referred to an ophthalmologist for thorough evaluation. Radiographs and computed tomography may help confirm the suspicion of an intraocular foreign body.

Corneal Abrasions

Corneal abrasions are handled in the same way as described for the abrasion that remains after removal of a corneal foreign body.

Lacerations

Lacerations that involve the eyelid margin or the lacrimal apparatus should be treated by the ophthalmologist. Permanent notching may result from improper lid margin repair. Superficial minor lacerations of the eyelid and brow, however, may be closed with fine sutures by the experienced nonophthalmologic physician after careful evaluation of the levator palpebrae for normal function, determination of good visual acuity, and examination to rule out trauma to the globe. Lacerations or perforating injuries to the globe are an ocular emergency. Examination by the nonophthalmologist should be limited because lid squeezing may cause expulsion of intraocular tissues. The eye should be covered and the patient sent immediately to an ophthalmologist.

Contusions

Contusion injuries of the globe and the surrounding tissues are usually produced by blunt objects. The effects may be minor or serious, obvious or inapparent, immediate or delayed. Therefore careful study by an ophthalmologist and sufficient follow-up are necessary. A blunt injury to the eye may result in ecchymosis of the eyelid ("black eye"), subconjunctival hemorrhage, abrasion or rupture of the cornea, anterior chamber hemorrhage (hyphema), laceration of the iris, cataract, dislocated lens, vitreous hemorrhage, retinal edema or hemorrhage, retinal detachment, rupture of the choroid, optic nerve injury, or rupture of the globe. All these complications, except for the eyelid ecchymosis, require expert eye care.

Traumatic hyphema is defined as the presence of blood in the anterior chamber of the eye. It commonly results from a contusion injury to the eye or may stem from a perforating eye injury. Child abuse may be suspected. It may appear as a blood/fluid level in the anterior chamber between the cornea and the iris, or as a diffuse hemorrhage in the aqueous humor. It is imperative that a patient with a hyphema be referred for ophthalmologic evaluation promptly, as more extensive injury to the internal and more posterior structures of the eye may be present.

An important goal of treatment is to prevent vision-threatening complications. A particularly serious complication is recurrent or secondary hemorrhage. The occurrence ranges from 3 to 38 per cent. It is difficult to predict which patients will rebleed. Rebleeding may occur within the first 6 days of injury, most often between 3 and 5 days. Secondary hemorrhage predisposes to (1) elevated intraocular pressure with subsequent optic nerve damage and atrophy, (2) corneal blood staining, a particular concern in children younger than 6 years because amblyopia may result from visual deprivation, and (3) peripheral anterior synechiae formation, which may lead to chronic glaucoma. Glaucoma may also ensue from traumatic recession of the iris angle where aqueous fluid normally leaves the eye.

Controversy exists over the ideal treatment plan for hyphema patients. Disagreement prevails regarding the value of absolute bed rest, binocular patching, need for hospitalization, use of various drug regimens, and surgical procedures. Lack of agreement probably is due in part to the types of cases encountered. In general we prefer to hospitalize infants and children to permit close observation. In the uncomplicated case wherein most hyphemas clear in 5 to 6 days, ordinarily the management plan consists of bed rest with bathroom privileges and monocular eye patch for 5 days, cautious ambulation on the sixth day, and discharge from the hospital on the seventh day. Aspirin is avoided because of its possible effect on bleeding time. Miotics and cycloplegics usually are not used. A topical corticosteroid and atropine are prescribed if iritis develops.

To reduce the incidence of secondary hemorrhage, some physicians recommend the prophylactic use of an antifibrinolytic agent such as aminocaproic acid (Amikar) in the dosage of 50 to 100 mg/kg body weight up to 30 gm/day orally for 5 days. Another antifibrinolytic drug, tranexamic acid (Cyklokapron), was recently marketed in the United States in tablet and intravenous injection forms for use in hemophiliacs who are to undergo dental extraction; the drug has been used abroad to prevent rebleeding in traumatic hyphema. These drugs reduce lysis of the initial clot until the primary ruptured blood vessels heal. Systemic corticosteroids (equivalent to adult dosage of 40 mg prednisone/day for 5 days) also have been advocated by some ophthalmologists to prevent secondary hemorrhage. Although some ophthalmologists recommend the systemic use of either aminocaproic acid or corticosteroids in all cases of traumatic hyphema (because the rebleeding rate may not depend on the size of the hyphema), the low incidence of rebleeding, especially in the less severe hyphemas, coupled with the high cost (principally aminocaproic acid) and possible side effects of these drugs has deterred their routine use. The fibrinolytic agent tissue plasminogen activator (tPA) may prove of clinical value in the future when used at the proper time. It has been reported to be effective in accelerating the clearance of hyphema in the experimental animal.

If glaucoma occurs, a topical beta-blocker such as timolol maleate is given. If it is ineffective, ocular hypotensives such as oral acetazolamide (Diamox) or intravenous mannitol may be needed. If medical therapy fails to control elevated intraocular pressure, surgical removal of the aqueous humor or clot material may be necessary.

Sickle cell hyphema merits special attention. Patients with either the trait or the disease are at increased risk for complications of hyphema because their circulating erythrocytes tend to sickle in the acidic, hypoxic environment of the aqueous humor. Sickle cells have difficulty passing through the outflow drainage system of the eye and thus can lead to an acute secondary glaucoma with blindness from retinal or optic nerve infarction. Initial laboratory screening for sickle cell trait or disease therefore is important for patients who are black, Hispanic, or of Mediterranean origin. These patients must be observed closely for a rise in intraocular pressure so that medical or surgical treatment can be initiated promptly.

Burns

Thermal burns of the eyelids are treated as burns of the skin elsewhere. Burns of the cornea are treated by irrigation with water or saline solution and an antibiotic ointment before sending the patient to an ophthalmologist.

Chemical burns of the conjunctiva and cornea are treated immediately by irrigation with water or isotonic saline solution. Time should not be lost in trying to neutralize the chemical. Serious damage may occur in a matter of minutes. Moreover, the heat generated by such a reaction may lead to further damage. Alkali burns of the cornea are more serious than those caused by acids because alkalis are not precipitated by the tissue proteins as are the acids.

Immediate irrigation should be carried out for at least 30 minutes in the case of alkalis. The eye can be held under the water faucet stream. Local anesthetics may be used to relieve the pain. A local antibiotic ointment can be inserted into the conjunctival sac and the patient sent as soon as possible to an ophthalmologist for further care.

RETINOBLASTOMA

Retinoblastoma, although a relatively rare malignant tumor, is the most common primary intraocular malignancy in infants and children. The incidence of retinoblastoma is about one case in every 20,000 live births. The tumor may be present at birth (detected often by routine examination in families known to have retinoblastoma) but most often is discovered before 3 years of age. The average age of detection is about 17 months. Extraocular extension with histologically proved orbital retinoblastoma has an overall 3-year mortality rate of 91 per cent. Mortality from retinoblastoma results from central nervous system involvement by extension along the optic nerve or by hematogenous metastases from the choroid to other organs, most commonly bone, liver, kidney, and adrenal glands. In the United States advanced disease at presentation is rare. In cases of early diagnosis, in which the tumor remains confined within the eye and early treatment is provided in modern centers, the mortality rate is much decreased. In the past 100 years, the overall mortality rate of retinoblastoma has decreased from 95 per cent to 9 per cent in the United States.

The occurrence of retinoblastoma is largely sporadic (i.e., there is no previous history of the tumor), but a significant proportion are familial. Nonhereditary retinoblastoma, comprising 60 per cent of all cases, represents a sporadic somatic mutation and tends to be unilateral and unifocal. It is estimated that 10 to 15 per cent of patients with sporadic, unilateral retinoblastoma transmit the disease to their offspring. In contrast, hereditary retinoblastoma, comprising approximately 40 per cent of all patients, can arise after inheritance of a predisposing germ-line mutation from an affected parent (approximately 10 per cent of cases) or through acquisition of a new germinal mutation (approximately 30 per cent of cases). Hereditary retinoblastoma cases have a high degree of penetrance, are usually bilateral and multifocal, and have an earlier age of onset. The hereditary, bilateral cases often do not have a previous family history of the tumor. A patient with bilateral retinoblastoma or a family history of retinoblastoma has

a 50 per cent probability of transmitting the disease to his or her offspring. The risk estimate of the offspring of healthy siblings or healthy children of a patient with familial retinoblastoma is about 1 in 15. An affected child born to such a person, however, identifies that individual as an unaffected carrier and the risk factor becomes 1 in 2. Patients with hereditary retinoblastoma are also at increased risk of developing not only "radiation-induced" neoplasms in the field of ocular irradiation but also second cancers different from retinoblastoma. Most are osteogenic sarcomas in and out of the field of radiation.

The risk to children of patients with unilateral sporadic cases of retinoblastoma (usually the nonhereditary type) is about 5 per cent. The risk of disease in siblings of the sporadic cases is about 1 per cent.

Genetic predisposition to the inheritence of retinoblastoma has been demonstrated in those born with a partial deletion of the long arm of chromosome 13. Partial loss of band 14 (region 13q14) has been hypothesized to result in faulty retinal development, which may predispose to the development of retinoblastoma. Patients with small 13q14 deletions usually have no phenotypic abnormalities other than retinoblastoma. Patients with larger deletions often have other congenital abnormalities, including mental retardation. Studies have demonstrated that the locus for autosomal dominant retinoblastoma is closely linked to the locus for the enzyme esterase D. Quantitation of esterase D levels has been shown to be a quick and objective means of identifying 13q14 deletion carriers in cases in which conventional chromosomal analysis has proved inadequate. Other studies have demonstrated the location of the gene responsible for the nondeletion form of hereditary cases to be also in region 13q14. In order to provide accurate counseling to the parents of a child with retinoblastoma, genetic evaluation of all retinoblastoma patients should include chromosome analysis using high-resolution prophase banding, determination of esterase D activity, and family studies.

The gene for retinoblastoma recently has been partially cloned. There is little doubt that the process will be completed. Genetic evaluation in the future with all the new developments at hand will then enable the physician or counselor to specify which patients with retinoblastoma are at risk for developing second nonocular malignancies and for producing future children with the tumor.

Awareness of a positive family history results in earlier diagnosis of the tumor in both unilateral and bilateral cases. The most common presenting sign of retinoblastoma is leukokoria, or "white pupil." Other presenting signs may include strabismus resulting from impairment of vision, ocular inflammation, anisocoria, heterochromia iridis, red painful eye, glaucoma, hyphema, and hypopyon.

Before initiating treatment, a number of diagnostic studies may be performed to help establish an accurate diagnosis and the degree of tumor involvement. They include (1) the basic diagnostic evaluation (history, physical, and ocular examination); (2) ocular ultrasonography (A and B scans); (3) computed tomography (also detects an associated pinealoblastoma or "trilateral retinoblastoma"); (4) aqueous enzyme levels of lactic dehydrogenase (LDH) and phosphoglucose isomerase (PGI), including plasma concentrations of these enzymes for ratio comparisons; (5) anterior chamber tap for cytologic studies of possible tumor cells; and (6) bone marrow and cerebrospinal fluid samples for cytologic studies if tumor spread is suspected.

TREATMENT. Of greatest significance in determining the treatment modality for retinoblastoma is the stage of the disease at the time of diagnosis. For this reason it is imperative that the patient with leukokoria be referred to an ophthalmologist immediately. Extraocular extension of the tumor invariably is associated with a poor prognosis. The classification of eyes with retinoblastoma is based on tumor size, number of tumors, and location. The smaller, the fewer, and the more posteriorly located in the retina the tumors are, the better is the overall prognosis. If the disease is unilateral, examination of the fellow eye reveals no disease, and the search for metastasis is negative, enucleation of the involved eye is usually advised. In rare instances, unilateral cases with a favorable classification may be treated in lieu of enucleation.

Generally in bilateral cases one eye has far-advanced changes requiring enucleation, whereas the remaining eye has a more favorable classification allowing nonsurgical therapy. In rare instances, in cases with far advanced bilateral disease which would result in complete blindness despite treatment, bilateral enucleation is indicated to ensure the best chance for survival. It should be noted that some parents may refuse permission to remove both eyes.

In cases requiring enucleation, the surgeon should attempt to remove at least 10 mm of optic nerve to determine whether invasion has occurred. If the tumor has spread to the optic nerve and there is no evidence of extraocular spread, external beam radiation and chemotherapy have been used. The remaining eye must be examined thoroughly at 3- to 6-month intervals for several years.

Supravoltage external beam irradiation may be recommended as a primary mode of therapy if useful vision is salvageable and tumor growth is not advanced enough to require enucleation. The total tumor dose is about 400 rads. Episcleral plaque radiotherapy (Cobalt-60, Iridium-192, Iodine-125) has been used to treat solitary tumors less than 12 mm in diameter and 8 mm thick; a target dose of 3500 to 4000 rads is given to the apex of the tumor.

The indications for chemotherapy in retinoblastoma are controversial. The merit of using chemotherapy as a prophylactic measure following enucleation for unilateral sporadic retinoblastoma and for patients having local treatment of tumors confined to the eye is unsettled. A combination of antitumor drugs such as cyclophosphamide (Cytoxan) and vincristine (Oncovin) has been used when there is metastatic disease or extraocular orbital involvement. Nonetheless, extraorbital spread invariably is fatal.

Photocoagulation and cryotherapy have been used as primary modes of therapy when a tumor is small, solitary, unilateral, and extrafoveal. These modalities have been used most often for recurrent or residual tumors following incomplete destruction by radiation therapy.

The prognosis for survival has been dramatically improved in recent years because of earlier diagnosis, better visualization of the entire retina by the use of indirect ophthalmoscopy, and improved radiotherapeutic and chemotherapeutic techniques. No longer is retinoblastoma a hopeless disease. A survival rate up to 90 per cent has been reported in patients whose prognosis was favorable at the time that treatment was begun.

Preseptal and Orbital (Postseptal) Cellulitis

Preseptal cellulitis refers to an inflammation located anterior to the orbital septum. Thus signs of orbital involvement (i.e., proptosis, ophthalmoplegia, decreased vision) are absent. The clinical findings are limited to the eyelids and periorbital tissues and are characterized by erythema and edema of these tissues; conjunctivitis, chemosis, and fever may also be present. Preseptal cellulitis may result from eyelid trauma with subsequent infection; skin infections; spread of infection in the eyelid or periorbital region (e.g., hordeolum, conjunctivitis, dacryocystitis); upper respiratory infection; sinusitis; and bacteremia. Causative organisms include staphylococci, streptococci, *H. influenzae,* and anaerobes. The *H. influenzae* organism is more likely to be encountered in children, especially those younger than 5 years; a magenta discoloration of the skin of the eyelids is distinctive.

Preseptal cellulitis should not be considered a benign disease. Infections caused by virulent organisms may enter the vascular system and progress to orbital and intracranial involvement. Therefore, most patients are hospitalized for treatment.

Bacteriologic studies involving the conjunctiva, nasopharynx, and blood (Gram-stained smears, cultures, antibiotic sensitivity tests) should be obtained. Radiography and computed tomography of the orbital and sinus areas are ordered if there is any indication of orbital inflammation, sinusitis, fracture, or foreign body. If a fluctuant mass is present, surgical drainage of the mass is performed, and smears and cultures of the drained material are carried out. If no area of fluctuation is present, percutaneous aspiration of the swollen area with smear and culture of the aspirated material should be considered for possible detection of the causative organism. If a causative organism cannot be found, broad-spectrum antibiotic therapy is recommended until results of the bacteriologic studies are returned. At present our preference is full parenteral doses of a penicillinase-resistant penicillin such as oxacillin or nafcillin and chloramphenicol. The latter drug is effective against *H. influenzae,* including ampicillin-resistant strains, streptococcal species, and anaerobes, and it has good tissue penetration ability. For patients allergic to penicillin, vancomycin is given. An alternative regimen is the use of cefuroxime. Antibiotic therapy usually is given for 1 to 2 weeks. Appropriate antibiotics may be given orally when there is clear clinical improvement.

Orbital (postseptal) cellulitis designates an inflammation behind the orbital septum. Most often the cause is direct extension of a bacterial infection from the paranasal sinuses. Other causes include extension of infection from facial cellulitis, orbital trauma, dental abscess, and bacteremia. The organisms most frequently responsible are *Streptococcus pneumoniae,* group A beta-hemolytic streptococci, *Staphylococcus aureus, H. influenzae* (especially in young children), and non–spore-forming anaerobes. The characteristic clinical findings are erythema and edema of the eyelids and periorbital tissues, proptosis, painful limitation of eye movement (ophthalmoplegia), decreased vision, and often symptoms of toxicity with fever and leukocytosis.

It is imperative that orbital cellulitis be recognized promptly and treated aggressively. Progressive inflammation within the orbit may lead to decreased vision and blindness. Extension of the process may result in meningitis, central nervous system abscess, and death from cavernous sinus thrombosis.

Treatment is carried out in the hospital. Consultation with an otolaryngologist is advisable. Bacteriologic studies, orbit and sinus radiographs, and orbital computed tomography scans as described for prespetal cellulitis should be obtained. If on admission Gram-stain smears of material obtained from the nose and throat, infected sinus, or surgical drainage of an acutely compromised orbit are not informative for selection of appropriate initial antibiotic therapy, then broad-spectrum antibiotic therapy is given as for preseptal cellulitis. Results of culture and antibiotic sensitivity studies may dictate a change in the choice of antibiotics. Treatment usually is given for 2 to 3 weeks or at least 7 to 10 days after the patient is afebrile and decided clinical improvement has been seen.

A subperiosteal or orbital abscess may result from progression of an acute ethmoiditis and could lead to compression of the optic nerve and blindness. Intensive antibiotic therapy early in the formation of the periosteal abscess, that is, when limitation of globe movement is minimal and vision is unaffected, may make surgical intervention unnecessary. The diagnosis of early subperiosteal abscess by CT scan is not always accurate.

STRABISMUS

Strabismus is a misalignment of the eyes which occurs in about 3 per cent of children. Depending on the nature of the eye misalignment, strabismus is categorized as esotropia (eyes turned in), exotropia (turned out), hypertropia (up), or hypotropia (down). Strabismus can occur in the newborn (most commonly congenital esotropia), but it is most likely to occur in infancy or early childhood (most commonly accommodative esotropia). Many young infants appear to have strabismus but actually have normal ocular alignment. This false strabismus, or pseudostrabismus, is usually caused by a wide nasal bridge and prominent epicanthal folds, which obscure the medial conjunctiva and give the appearance of esotropia (pseudoesotropia). The apparent resolution of a pseudostrabismus as the child grows older is the basis for the mistaken notion that some infants outgrow their strabismus. This can lead to a false sense of security, which delays referral of an infant or child to an ophthalmologist for evaluation and treatment of a true strabismus.

Monocular strabimus is a common cause of amblyopia, that is, decreased vision or "lazy eye." At least 3 per cent of children have amblyopia. Approximately half of the cases are secondary to strabismus, and most of the others are due to an uncorrected refractive error in one eye. The unfortunate aspect of the problem is that in most instances this form of visual impairment could have been prevented if the patient had been seen early in childhood by an ophthalmologist.

When strabismus is present in an infant or child, the brain actively suppresses the image from the strabismic eye to avoid double vision and confusion. As a consequence, vision fails to develop properly in the deviating eye, and it becomes amblyopic ("lazy"). Normal vision and binocular function are not present at birth. These functions mature rapidly during the first years of life and become relatively fixed by the age of about 6 years. To reach the goal of 20/20 vision with normal binocular fusion, clear images must be presented to both foveae simultaneously throughout the early years of life. With proper ocular alignment, similar images from each eye are relayed along the visual pathway in the brain, where the two images are ultimately perceived as one. This binocular visual fusion permits the appreciation of depth perception, or stereopsis. In the presence of monocular strabismus, vision does not fully develop. If normal binocular vision does not develop by about age 4 years because of amblyopia and strabismus, correction of the strabismus after this age is unlikely to provide fully normal fusion. If amblyopia is not treated by appropriate occlusion of the normal eye, or by other means, before the age of about 6 years, it is unlikely that one can effect substantial improvement of vision in the amblyopic eye thereafter.

It is important for the pediatrician to keep in mind that diseases such as retinoblastoma, intraocular infection, congenital cataract, or other eye abnormalities may be manifested early in life as a transient or constant strabismus. The pediatrician should not take the responsibility of delaying the referral of the patient unless he can absolutely rule out serious ocular disease or the presence of a true strabismus rather than pseudostrabismus.

The earlier strabismus therapy is initiated, the better is the prognosis for a functional as well as a cosmetic cure. No infant or child is too young to have an eye examination and to have treatment initiated. Although fusion is not necessary for good vision, its presence is a powerful force for maintaining ocular alignment after treatment of strabismus.

The first goal in the treatment of strabismus is obtaining good vision in each eye. The best way to stimulate vision in an amblyopic eye is to correct an underlying refractive error (if present) and to patch the good eye. Occlusion therapy generally is full time if vision is poor and is tapered to part time as the vision improves. Occlusion therapy is continued until the best visual acuity is reached.

The second goal is correction of the strabismus. This

commonly is accomplished by one or more of the following measures: corrective glasses, miotic therapy, orthoptics, and surgery. Corrective glasses generally are effective for the accommodative forms of esotropia. In children with moderate or high degrees of hyperopia, greater accommodation is required to see clearly. Because of the synkinetic reflex of accommodation and convergence, the eyes may overconverge and become esotropic. Proper correction of the refractive error with glasses decreases the need for accommodation and thus lessens convergence.

Another type of accommodative strabismus is seen in children who are not highly hyperopic but who have an exaggerated accommodative-convergence ratio at near fixation. These patients usually respond to bifocals to reduce the need for increased accommodation with near targets. Also effective in selected cases are the cholinesterase inhibitor miotics isoflurophate (Floropryl, DFP) and echothiophate iodide (Phospholine iodide). These drugs induce "peripheral" rather than "central" accommodation by their action on the ciliary body and thus lessen convergence. Potential toxic effects (usually from excessive dosage or use) must be kept in mind. They include headache, conjunctival hyperemia, rhinorrhea, abdominal pain, nausea, vomiting, diarrhea, salivation, hypotension, and potential ocular (iris cysts) and systemic side effects (such as prolonged apnea if a general anesthesia should need to be administered).

Orthoptics (eye exercises) conducted by a trained technician (orthoptist) or doctor in certain circumstances may help to treat amblyopia and suppression, increase fusion ability, and stereopsis. Orthoptics are more commonly effective in cases of intermittent strabismus and may be useful before or after surgery or during both periods.

When nonsurgical methods of treatment do not or cannot satisfactorily correct the strabismus, surgery is performed on the extraocular muscles. Although surgery at times may be performed for "cosmetic reasons," it is often performed with the goal of promoting binocular fusion by aligning the eyes in those patients in whom there is a reasonable expectation of obtaining some fusion. Fusion is more likely to be achieved if the strabismus is corrected early in life. The most common strabismus procedures performed are recession and/or resection operations. In a recession procedure a rectus muscle is cut from its insertion onto the sclera and recessed, or moved back, from its insertion to weaken the pull of the muscle. In a resection operation, a segment of the rectus muscle is removed and the shortened muscle is then reattached to its site of original insertion in order to strengthen the action of the muscle. Surgery may be performed on one or both eyes in spite of the appearance of a monocular strabismus. More than one operation may be needed to correct the strabismus. In older children and adults an "adjustable suture" technique may be used to "fine tune" the eye position later on the day of surgery or on the first postoperative day.

A recent alternative to surgery in special circumstances is the injection of botulinum toxin (Oculinum) into an overacting rectus muscle to temporarily weaken its action. This drug was released in early 1990 for the treatment of strabismus and blepharospasm associated with dystonia, including benign essential blepharospasm, in patients 12 years of age and older. It has been found successful, for example, in patients with transient sixth nerve palsies to prevent contracture of the opposing overactive medial rectus muscle. The younger patient may require a general anesthetic for the procedure. Treatment with Oculinum in patients younger than 12 years remains investigational.

17

The Ear

FOREIGN BODIES IN THE EAR

VICTOR E. CALCATERRA, M.D.

Removal of foreign bodies from the external ear canal is made difficult by the extreme sensitivity of the medial portion of the canal. In addition, it is often in children too young to cooperate who accidentally insert a foreign body into the ear. The situation may be complicated by the development of a secondary external otitis.

The method of removal is dictated by the location of the foreign body and the ability of the patient to cooperate. As in cerumen removal, irrigation with water by a syringe is often a useful method of foreign body removal but should be avoided if it consists of a material that swells with water. Purulent material from an accompanying external otitis or other debris may obscure visualization of the foreign body, and cleaning of the canal with an angled tube-suction device becomes necessary. Extraction can be done using either an otoscope with an operating head or a handheld aural speculum with appropriate lighting, such as a headlight or head mirror. Various instruments for extraction are available. A small alligator-jaw ear forceps is most useful for removing foreign bodies. Larger or friable foreign bodies are best removed with a currette. Often a large-caliber, angled suction tube may be sufficient to pull out the foreign body. Complete cooperation of the patient is essential, and it may be necessary to use general anesthesia in children.

Secondary lacerations of the ear canal usually heal without difficulty. Secondary infections respond well to otic drops.

OTITIS MEDIA

JEROME O. KLEIN, M.D.

Antimicrobial treatment of otitis media is based on knowledge of the bacterial pathogens. *Streptococcus pneu-moniae* is the most important bacterial cause of otitis media in all age groups (35 percent of cases of acute otitis media). Until recently, *Haemophilus influenzae* was considered a pathogen only in preschool children; new information indicates that this organism is also a significant cause of otitis media in older children, adolescents, and adults (20 percent of cases of acute otitis media). *Moraxella catarrhalis* was found to be an important cause of otitis media in recent studies from Pittsburgh and Cleveland but of lesser incidence in reports from other cities (approximately 10 percent). Of limited importance as causes of otitis media are group A beta-hemolytic streptococci, *Staphylococcus aureus*, and anaerobic bacteria.

Choice of Initial Therapy

Some children with acute otitis media improve without the use of antimicrobial agents. Studies employing a placebo control suggest that the number of cases of bacterial otitis media that resolve spontaneously may be as large as one third of enrolled children, presumably healing takes place by drainage of the abscess through the eustachian tube or a perforation of the tympanic membrane. Without antimicrobial treatment, however, many children will have persistent acute signs and some may develop suppurative complications. The limited incidence of suppurative complications of otitis media in areas in which antimicrobial agents are used extensively in comparison with the period of time when these drugs were unavailable, or with areas of the world in which drugs are not available today, speaks for their beneficial effects.

The preferred antimicrobial agent for the patient with otitis media must be active against *S. pneumoniae* or *H. influenzae*. Amoxicillin is the drug of choice for initial treatment of otitis media, since it is active in vitro and in vivo against these organisms and is less expensive than alternative drugs. About 20 to 30 percent of recently isolated strains of *H. influenzae* and 60 to 70 percent of strains of *M. catarrhalis* produce beta-lactamase and are resistant to amoxicillin. Therefore, about 10 to 14 percent of cases of acute otitis media are caused by beta-lactamase producing strains of bacteria and

TABLE 1. Daily Dosage Schedule for Oral Antimicrobial Agents Useful in Otitis Media

Drug	Dosage/kg/24 hr
Amoxicillin	40 mg in 3 doses
Amoxicillin and clavulanic acid	40 mg in 3 doses
Cefaclor	40 mg in 3 doses
Cefixime	8 mg in 1 dose
Cefuroxime axetil*	30 mg in 2 doses
Erythromycin	40 mg in 4 doses
Sulfisoxazole*	120 mg in 4 doses
TMP-SMZ†	8 mg TMP and 40 mg SMZ in 2 doses

*Available only in tablets.

†Manufacturer's warning: Not recommended for infants less than 2 months of age.

require therapy with an antibacterial drug resistant to this enzyme. Since about one third of cases of acute otitis media resolve without antimicrobial agents, we may expect that about 10 percent of children who receive amoxicillin for acute otitis media will not respond because of bacterial resistance. Other drugs that are satisfactory include trimethoprim-sulfamethoxazole (TMP-SMZ), the fixed combination preparation of erythromycin and sulfisoxazole (Pediazole), amoxicillin-clavulanate (Augmentin) and the cephalosporins cefaclor (Ceclor), cefuroxime axetil (Ceptin), and cefixime (Suprax). TMP-SMZ and the combination of erythromycin or cephalosporin are acceptable combinations for the child with allergy to penicillin. If the child has had a major reaction to a penicillin (an immediate or accelerated reaction), crossreactivity of penicillins and cephalosporins should be considered and use of the cephalosporin avoided.

With appropriate antimicrobial therapy, most children with acute otitis media are significantly improved within 48 to 72 hours. If there is no improvement the patient should be re-examined. Tympanocentesis to identify the microbiology of the middle ear infection may be considered for children who are toxic; the appropriate antimicrobial agent may be chosen on the basis of review of Gram's stain and subsequent results of culture of the fluid. A change in initial antimicrobial regimen should be considered if signs persist but the child is not toxic and tympanocentesis is not performed. The new regimen should include drugs that are effective for all strains of *H. influenzae*, including those that produce beta-lactamase, and the pneumococcus. If ampicillin or amoxicillin was given initially, then amoxicillin plus clavulanic acid, TMP-SMZ, erythromycin-sulfisoxazole, cefaclor, cefuroxime axetil, or cefixime should be administered.

Management of the Child with Recurrent Episodes of Acute Otitis Media

The bacteriology of middle ear infection in children who have recurrent episodes of acute otitis media is qualitatively similar to that for the first episode; the predominant pathogens are *S. pneumoniae* (though of different serotypes) and *H. influenzae*. Two methods of prevention should be considered: immunoprophylaxis (use of pneumococcal vaccine) and chemoprophylaxis (use of a modified course of an antimicrobial agent).

Chemoprophylaxis. The data about use of chemoprophylaxis are persuasive that children who are prone to recurrent episodes of acute infection of the middle ear are benefited. I believe it is reasonable to consider the following program:

1. Criteria for usage: children who have had three documented episodes of acute otitis media in 6 months or four episodes in 12 months.

2. Antimicrobial agents: sulfisoxazole or ampicillin (amoxicillin has advantages of ease of administration) were the drugs used in published studies and provide advantages of demonstrated efficacy, safety, and low cost.

3. Dosage: half the therapeutic dose—amoxicillin 20 mg/kg or sulfisoxazole* 50 mg/kg—administered once a day at bedtime offers maximal compliance. Administration at any single time during the day would probably be satisfactory.

4. Duration: during the winter and spring when respiratory tract infections are most frequent, for a period up to 6 months.

5. Observations during prophylaxis: children should be examined at 1-month intervals to determine if middle ear effusion is present. Management of the middle ear effusion should be considered separately from prevention of recurrences of the acute infection.

6. Management of acute infections during prophylaxis: acute infections should be treated with an alternative regimen. Amoxicillin plus clavulanic acid would be an appropriate drug to use as an alternative without regard to initial therapy. If a sulfonamide is used for prophylaxis, ampicillin or a cephalosporin would also be appropriate. If ampicillin is used for prophylaxis, erythromycin-sulfisoxazole, TMP-SMZ, or a cephalosporin would be adequate to treat the acute infection.

Immunoprophylaxis. The currently licensed pneumococcal vaccines contain purified polysaccharide antigens of the types of pneumococci most frequently associated with otitis media. Available data suggest that the older children who still have problems with recurrent acute otitis media have received some benefit from the use of the vaccine. I recommend its usage in children over 2 years of age, although I recognize that it will prevent only a fraction of cases of acute otitis media. Nontypable strains are responsible for most acute otitis media caused by *H. influenzae;* therefore, it is unlikely that the available polysaccharide vaccine will alter the incidence of this disease.

Management of the Child with Persistent Middle Ear Effusion

Many children have fluid that persists in the middle ear for weeks to months. Most children with middle ear effusion have some impairment of hearing; the audiogram reveals a conductive loss in the range of 15 to 40 dB. With such deficits, the softer speech sounds and voiceless consonants may be missed. The results of more than a dozen studies suggest that children with histories of recurrent episodes of acute otitis media score lower on tests of speech and language than do disease-free

*Manufacturer's warning: Not recommended for infants less than 2 months of age.

peers. These data are controversial, but the physician must consider the consequences of prolonged periods of impairment of hearing due to middle ear fluid in the young child.

Medical Therapy. No medical therapy has been found to be uniformly effective in ridding the middle ear of fluid. Nasal and oral decongestants, administered either alone or in combination with an antihistamine, are very popular for this purpose. The results of clinical trials, however, indicate no significant evidence of efficacy for any of these preparations used alone or in combination for relief of signs of disease or decrease in time spent with middle ear effusion.

Surgical Management. The value of myringotomy for persistent middle ear effusion alone is of benefit in some children, but in many the fluid reaccumulates once the incision heals.

Adenoidectomy alone or in combination with tonsillectomy may benefit some children with recurrent and persistent otitis media.

Tympanostomy or ventilating tubes allow for egress of secretions produced by the middle ear mucosa and maintain ambient pressure in the middle ear and mastoid. The insertion of tubes in children who have had persistent middle ear effusion appears to be beneficial in most children; hearing is restored and permanent structural changes that might occur due to persistent fluid are prevented.

LABYRINTHITIS

STEVEN D. HANDLER, M.D.

Purulent Labyrinthitis. Purulent labyrinthitis occurs when bacterial agents invade the inner ear from adjacent sources, such as the middle ear or meninges, or through hematogenous spread. Proper management requires treatment of the bacterial source of the inner ear infection. If a purulent acute otitis media is the cause of the infection, wide-field myringotomy for drainage and intravenous antibiotics are required. Chronic otitis media requires intravenous doses of antibiotics and surgical drainage in the form of a middle ear exploration and mastoidectomy. Meningitis as a cause of purulent labyrinthitis is treated aggressively with intravenous antibiotics. If the purulent labyrinthitis persists, with symptoms of incapacitating vertigo and permanent sensorineural hearing loss, a labyrinthectomy may be indicated.

After the acute process has been treated, full audiometric testing is mandatory to determine the presence and nature of any hearing loss. Children who are too young or not cooperative enough to undergo conventional audiometric testing should be evaluated with brain stem evoked audiometry. Persistent serous otitis media is managed with myringotomy and ventilation tube placement. Persistent tympanic membrane perforation requires surgical closure with tympanoplasty and possible ossicular reconstruction. Sensorineural hearing loss must be detected and followed closely. Hearing aid

amplification is required in some cases of unilateral and in almost all cases of bilateral sensorineural hearing loss in children. If any vestibular imbalance is present, the child must be monitored carefully when he engages in activities in which any vestibular dysfunction might be dangerous, e.g., swimming.

Viral Labyrinthitis. Viral labyrinthitis occurs when viral agents invade the inner ear. In cases of prenatal viral labyrinthitis there is no active treatment for the infection, which has usually subsided by the time the diagnosis is made.

Complete audiometric and, if indicated, vestibular evaluation should be performed. Appropriate habilitative measures (e.g., special education, amplification with hearing aids) must be started as soon as possible to maximize speech and language development.

Postnatal viral labyrinthitis is usually associated with viral upper respiratory infections. The treatment of this condition is supportive. Vertiginous symptoms are treated with bed rest, fluids, and antivertigo or sedative drugs, if necessary. Once again, hearing and vestibular evaluations are required after the resolution of the acute infection. Appropriate intervention can then be planned, with special schooling, close observation in swimming activities, amplification with hearing aids, and so forth.

Serous Labyrinthitis. Serous labyrinthitis is a sterile inflammatory process that is usually secondary to an adjacent infection such as otitis media or meningitis. The treatment requires proper diagnosis and treatment of the adjacent infection, i.e., otitis media or meningitis. Recovery is usually complete, with normal hearing and absence of vertigo.

Syphilitic Labyrinthitis. Treponemal infection of the labyrinth occurs in syphilitic labyrinthitis. Treatment requires high doses of penicillin and a long course of corticosteroids. While the vertigo and hearing loss often stabilize on this regimen, the latter may progress once the steroid doses are tapered or stopped.

Perilymph Fistulas. Perilymph fistulas are an infrequent cause of labyrinthitis. In addition to treatment for bacterial or viral labyrinthitis, middle ear exploration and closure of the fistula are required for control of the vertigo and stabilization of the hearing loss.

INJURIES OF THE MIDDLE EAR

VICTOR E. CALCATERRA, M.D.

Perforations of the Tympanic Membrane

A sudden increase of pressure in the ear canal can produce a blowout or rupture of the tympanic membrane. This typically occurs either from a sharp blow over the pinna, such as from a slap, or from a nearby explosion, such as a land mine. Direct tympanic membrane injuries occur from sharp, penetrating objects. No treatment is necessary because the perforation usually heals. Unless there is an infection with otorrhea, otic drops are unnecessary and should be avoided, since they will cause severe pain when instilled in an uninfected middle ear. If, however, there is purulent discharge indicating an infection, a culture is advised, and antibiotics are prescribed based on the sensitivities. If the perforation is extremely large and especially if fragments of the tympanic membrane are displaced deeply into the middle ear, an attempt should be made to realign the torn fragments into normal position and to maintain their position with a patch of Gelfoam. If the tympanic membrane has not healed after several months, a tympanoplasty will usually be successful and will restore hearing to normal.

Fractures

Fractures involving the middle ear are commonly part of a larger fracture of the temporal bone and base of skull. Injuries to the facial nerve, tympanic membrane, and ossicles must be considered. A hemotympanum is very common and will usually disappear in a few weeks, presumably by clearance through the eustachian tube. Tears and perforations of the tympanic membrane usually require no treatment, and otic drops should be avoided. Infections should be treated with systemic antibiotics. Facial nerve function should be assessed as early as possible in a fracture involving the temporal bone and middle ear. Immediate and complete facial paralysis suggests transection of the nerve, which usually requires surgical exploration and repair of the nerve.

Ossicular Discontinuity

Discontinuity of the ossicles from trauma is recognized by a persistent conductive hearing loss after the tympanic membrane has healed. The stapes and incus are most commonly affected and may be either displaced or fractured. Treatment is surgical realignment of the ossicles.

Occasionally the stapes, including the footplate, is dislocated from the oval window, allowing leakage of perilymph from the inner ear into the middle ear, resulting in a sensorineural hearing loss and dizziness. Treatment involves surgically plugging the oval window with fat and replacing the stapes by interposing a prosthesis from the incus. If there is only a crack or minor defect in the stapedial footplate, the leak may be corrected by a soft tissue patch without a stapedectomy.

HEARING LOSS

ARNOLD E. KATZ, M.D.,
and HUBERT L. GERSTMAN, D.Ed.

MEDICAL AND SURGICAL MANAGEMENT OF CONDUCTIVE HEARING LOSS

The external and middle ears constitute a system that gathers and transmits sound to the inner ear. This system is connected and suspended in an optimal manner so that its mass and tension characteristics efficiently transmit sound. Addition of mass (e.g., wax, fluid, tumors) or alterations in tension (e.g., otosclerosis, adhesions) impair the efficiency of the system and result in

hearing loss. Conductive hearing impairments are usually treatable medically or surgically or both. They are also frequently effectively treated with amplification (hearing aids).

Congenital Conductive Hearing Loss

Congenital conductive hearing losses may be unilateral or bilateral. Although the maximum conductive loss can be no greater than 60 decibels or so, bilateral losses in this range can impair greatly the child's ability to develop speech. The severity of congenital impairment must be considered in outlining therapy. Surgical correction of total aplasia of the external auditory canal or middle ear is fraught with the real possibility of facial nerve injury. Surgical correction of anomalies of the ossicles is accompanied by a much smaller risk of facial paralysis. These risks must be fully discussed with the patient's family. In unilateral conductive losses, surgery should probably be delayed until the child is able to participate in the selection of therapy. Amplification is frequently a good choice.

Inflammatory Conductive Hearing Loss

External Otitis. This infection may cause a conductive hearing loss, depending on how much inflammation and debris are in the canal. When the canal is filled with debris, pain is usually a major symptom and must be controlled with salicylates or codeine. Removal of debris is accomplished with a gentle suction and small wisps of cotton wound on metal cotton carriers. A wick must also be inserted so that the otic drops used will reach the site of infection. The otic drops usually employed and quite effective contain hydrocortisone, polymyxin B, and neomycin: 4 drops four times a day. After the swelling of the canal has decreased, the wick may be eliminated; however, the drops should be continued at least 3 days after the relief of pain. Recurrences may be prevented by routine use of acid-alcohol drops (mix white vinegar and rubbing alcohol 50/50) after swimming or bathing. Any signs of systemic involvement necessitate the culturing of the exudate and the immediate institution of systemic antibiotics. *Staphylococcus aureus*, group A beta-hemolytic streptococcus, micrococci, diphtheroids, and *Pseudomonas aeruginosa* are the organisms most usually encountered.

Secretory Otitis Media. The therapy of this most common cause of hearing loss must be based on the knowledge of the natural history of this disease. By far most of these patients will experience spontaneous remission without any treatment. Medical or surgical therapy should not be instituted until the patient has been followed up for at least 1 month without improvement in symptoms.

If the fluid persists for over a month, one must then ask how this fluid is affecting the patient. If speech has developed normally and the child is doing very well in school, one can feel comfortable about following up the child. It would be wise to advise the school that the child may suffer from an intermittent increase in the severity of the hearing problem. He or she should be seated in the front row with the better ear toward the teacher, and any deterioration of the child's work should be brought to the attention of parents and physician.

If speech or school work is suffering (even if the hearing loss is 25 decibels or less) aggressive therapy should be instituted in the following order:

1. The child should be instructed to perform the Valsalva maneuver several times a day.

2. The chewing of sugarless gum should be recommended.

3. If the child is atopic, antihistamines or decongestants or both may be of value. If there is no response to these for 1 month, they should be discontinued. If the fluid clears while the child is taking this type of medication, parents should be instructed to reinstitute this therapy at the first sign of a runny nose or other clinical symptoms of increased antigenic exposure. No group of drugs has enjoyed such widespread advocacy without demonstration of efficiency in these cases as have antihistamines and decongestants. It is highly likely that if these drugs are effective, they are only of value in a minority of patients with this disease. It has been estimated that less than 30 per cent of patients with chronic secretory otitis media have an underlying allergic etiology.

4. Although advocated by some, the efficency of prophylactic antibiotics in this disease has not been established. If the fluid is associated with recurrent attacks of acute suppurative otitis media, trimethoprim/sulfamethoxazole or sulfisoxazole,* 100 mg/kg/24 hr, may be of value.

5. Myringotomy with aspiration of fluid and placement of a ventilating tube is remarkably effective in immediately relieving the hearing loss caused by this disease. Unfortunately, the ventilating tubes remain effective for only about 6 months to a year. Occasionally, after the tubes are obstructed or expelled, the fluid recollects. In these patients, replacement of the tubes is sometimes necessary. It must be remembered, however, that amplification (hearing aids) remains a viable option in the treatment of these very difficult management problems. Adenoidectomy, with or without tonsillectomy, probably does not affect the natural history of this disease.

Acute Suppurative Otitis Media. Treatment of this entity is discussed beginning on page 481.

Chronic Suppurative Otitis Media. Intermittent foul-smelling drainage from one or both ears usually heralds a perforation of the tympanic membrane or a cholesteatoma. Both of these conditions are usually accompanied by a conductive hearing loss and the patient should be referred to an otolaryngologist. Surgery is indicated to remove the infected bone of the middle ear and mastoid, which frequently are affected by this disease.

Traumatic Causes of Conductive Hearing Loss

Foreign Bodies. These may cause a conductive hearing loss in various ways. Their presence may prevent sound from reaching the tympanic membrane. They

---

*Sulfisoxazole is contraindicated in infants less than 2 months of age.

may also cause a conductive hearing loss by perforating the tympanic membrane or fracturing or dislocating the ossicles. If there is no damage to the tympanic membrane or ossicles, removal of the foreign body will restore hearing. If there is middle ear damage, further surgery may be necessary to restore hearing. Foreign bodies in the ear of an uncooperative child should be removed by an otolaryngologist, frequently with general anesthesia.

Trauma to the Tympanic Membrane or Ossicles. Blast injuries or penetrating wounds to the external ear can result in conductive hearing loss. Immediate treatment should include examination under an otoscope, if possible, and assessment of the amount of hearing loss. Most traumatic perforations heal spontaneously. Parents should be advised to keep water out of the ear during bathing or washing the child's hair. This is best accomplished by placing a cotton ball to which has been applied a small amount of petroleum jelly in the external canal to seal it. Do not fill the canal with petroleum jelly. Dry cotton will act as a wick and allow water to contaminate the middle ear. Antibiotic drops are also helpful in preventing or treating an ear infection while the tympanic membrane is healing.

If a conductive hearing loss persists after the eardrum is healed, one must suspect ossicle damage. Exploratory tympanotomy with an ossiculoplasty may be necessary to restore the hearing.

Fractures of the External Auditory Canal. Fractures of the external auditory canal may accompany other types of facial and temporal bone trauma. Trauma to the mandible may result in a posterior displacement of the anterior wall of the canal with obstruction. Sound is prevented from vibrating the tympanic membrane, and a conductive hearing loss will result.

If this fracture is diagnosed early (within 7 to 10 days) it can be reduced easily with a nasal speculum. The speculum is inserted into the canal and opened. If weeks elapse between the time of the fracture and the time of the diagnosis, much more extensive surgery is necessary to enlarge the canal.

Neoplastic Causes of Conductive Hearing Loss

Benign and malignant tumors of the external and middle ears may reach sufficient size to cause a conductive hearing loss. If the tumor is benign (e.g., osteoma), local surgical excision is indicated. If it is malignant, treatment of the malignancy must assume prime importance. Treatment of the malignancy will probably necessitate sacrifice of hearing in the affected ear. Malignancy must be suspected in a chronic external otitis with pain and blood-tinged purulence, and a biopsy must be performed on the canal. Even in the absence of the hallmarks of malignancy, a firm, granular-appearing external canal should have a biopsy to rule out an early squamous cell carcinoma or rhabdomyosarcoma.

Conductive Hearing Loss—General Considerations

In general, pure conductive hearing loss is defined by the fact that the patient has normal "cochlear reserve." When the sound is loud enough, the hearing loss is compensated for by amplification. Thus, when medical or surgical treatment fails to fully restore hearing, a mild amount of gain in a hearing aid may be safely used. In chronic otitis, as in other conditions characterized by intermittent reductions in hearing acuity, a hearing aid is sometimes utilized on an "as needed" basis.

Except in rare cases, "pure" conductive pathologies seldom require significant other supportive treatment. However, if the illness is a concomitant, subsequent, or consequent condition to etiologies affecting motor speech, language, or cognitive development, the matter requires prompt treatment and frequent follow-up visits and supportive training. For instance, a cleft palate problem invariably is accompanied by some otitis media. Such a child already is impaired to a degree by a communication deficit. The added illness hinders perceptual skill to the extent that loss of acuity affects perception. Therefore, particular attention must be paid to the status of the middle ear.

When conductive pathology is overlaid on a significant sensorineural hearing loss, the conductive components must be remedied so as to allow other habilitation training and amplification to be optimal. The fitting of hearing aids requires attention to the amount of gain, the intensity of sound to be allowed into the auditory system, the frequency range or spectrum to be admitted, and the varied patterns in the different portions of the frequency bands amplified. These specific differences in amplification properties are fitted to the patients' perceptions of clarity, intelligibility, pitch, quality, and sound comfort in search of a perfect union of person to machine. The compensation for conductive loss may be markedly different from that for sensorineural loss; thus additional or intermittent conductive impairment may be doubly disturbing to the basic sensorineural patient.

SENSORINEURAL HEARING LOSS

Medicine's best contribution to the area of sensorineural hearing loss is probably in its prevention. Immediate treatment of toxic conditions, conservative use of ototoxic medications, genetic counseling for parents who have already produced hearing-impaired off-spring, and efficient treatment of upper respiratory infections or other diseases apt to produce damage to the cochlea or the auditory nervous system are the most productive for management of those at high risk.

Except for that caused by certain specific disease states (e.g., viral labyrinthitis) and certain medications (aspirin may produce ototoxic reactions that are reversible when use is discontinued), sensorineural hearing loss is permanent, irreversible, and frustrating.

Audiologic and Other Management

Audiologic evaluation, coupled with variously required other evaluations, such as those performed by psychologists and speech/language pathologists, contributes to the diagnosis regarding site of lesion and, more importantly, regarding degree of impairment. An understanding of specific effects of patterns of hearing loss contributes more to habilitation and rehabilitation than any other single factor.

Once the basic diagnostic activity is under way, management plans may begin for infant stimulation, specifically of language. Later, stimulation for speech and consideration of cognitive development may be included in the management plan. Before the child is at the preschool level, treatment proceeds on several fronts, including any medical and surgical intervention that is necessary, fitting of hearing aids when appropriate, counseling of parents, plans for preschool educational programs, and general long-term plans.

In addition to hearing aids, specific activities may also take place in the area of auditory training, which teaches the child to differentiate specific warning sounds in the environment and later other alerting sounds and the various meanings of sounds that the child may be capable of heeding on both an uncompensated and a compensated basis. Other training forms take advantage of the visual modality for the benefit of communication and the other sensory modalities in training for speech production.

Training in sign language contributes to children's ability to develop symbolic behaviors, to increase their use of language, and to maintain other such linguistic shortcuts in categorizing their experience to the benefit of cognitive skills.

18

Infectious Diseases

NEONATAL SEPTICEMIA, MENINGITIS, AND PNEUMONIA

JOSEPH W. ST. GEME, III, M.D.,
and RICHARD A. POLIN, M.D.

Despite the rarity of proven bacterial sepsis (1 to 5 cases per 1000 live births), systemic bacterial infections during the first month of life remain a major cause of morbidity and mortality. Although the mortality rate for most noninfectious diseases in the neonate has plummeted during the past 5 to 10 years, the incidence of fatality for documented sepsis has not substantially decreased. Approximately one third of neonates with "early onset" bacterial infections develop central nervous system involvement, and of these, 20 to 50 per cent ultimately display neurologic handicaps.

Most neonatal bacterial infections occur during the first week of life (early onset sepsis) and result from the spread of microorganisms colonizing the maternal genital tract into the amniotic cavity. Susceptible infants either inhale or swallow contaminated amniotic fluid and develop generalized sepsis. Common pathogens responsible for early onset disease in neonates include group B streptococci (*Streptococcus agalactiae*), *Escherichia coli*, *Listeria monocytogenes*, group D streptococci, *Klebsiella-Enterobacter* species, and nontypable *Haemophilus influenzae*. During the past decade, however, improvements in neonatal intensive care have permitted the survival of a population of very low birth weight infants, who are hospitalized for many months and who are at increased risk for nosocomial infection. Nosocomial infections developing after the first week of life (late onset sepsis) are caused by a different spectrum of microorganisms (*Staphylococcus aureus*, coagulase-negative staphylococci, *Pseudomonas aeruginosa*, and so on); however, any of the bacteria causing early onset infections can be responsible for late onset disease.

The primary objective of the clinician caring for infants at risk for neonatal infection is to identify all potential cases of bacterial disease quickly and begin antibiotic therapy promptly. The secondary goal should be to determine which of these cases initially identified represent true infection, and therefore require a full course of antibiotics, and which do not. We make decisions regarding initiation and maintenance of antimicrobial therapy based upon the infant's gestational age and the presence of clinical signs or risk factors for neonatal infection, as is summarized in Figures 1 to 3. We consider these decision trees to be guidelines and use them to supplement, rather than replace, clinical judgment.

SEPTICEMIA

Septicemia is a clinical syndrome resulting from invasion of the bloodstream by microorganisms. Treatment for this disease should begin immediately after appropriate cultures have been obtained. Infants who present with infection during the first week of life should receive combined therapy with a penicillin and an aminoglycoside. Ampicillin and gentamicin are generally used for the following reasons: (1) Ampicillin is effective against group B streptococci, *Listeria monocytogenes*, enterococci, and some gram-negative rods, including most nontypable *Haemophilus influenzae*; and (2) gentamicin provides broader coverage of the Enterobacteriaceae. Empiric therapy for infants with suspected nosocomial infections must include coverage for hospital-acquired organisms in addition to the pathogens listed previously. In our nursery, coagulase-negative staphylococci are the most common cause of nosocomial infections, and there is a high incidence of gentamicin resistance among hospital-acquired coliforms. Therefore, we use vancomycin and netilmicin as initial therapy for infants with nosocomial infections.

After an organism has been isolated from culture, antibiotic therapy should be tailored according to the results of in vitro susceptibility testing. *Listeria monocytogenes* and enterococci can usually be treated with ampicillin alone, while group B streptococci can be satisfactorily treated with either penicillin or ampicillin. If a gram-negative enteric isolate is susceptible to both ampicillin and aminoglycoside antibiotics, treatment with either drug alone may be adequate; however, we generally continue treatment with both drugs for their synergistic effect. *Staphylococcus aureus* should be tested

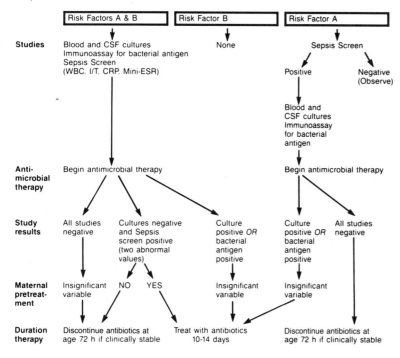

Figure 18–1. Evaluation of the high-risk asymptomatic term infant.

Sepsis screen tests, with criteria for abnormal results: WBC (white blood count), total white blood count <5000/mm³ or absolute neutrophil count <1750/mm³; I/T (immature to total neutrophil ratio) >0.2; CRP (C-reactive protein), positive latex agglutination test with undiluted serum; Mini-ESR (capillary tube erythrocyte sedimentation rate) ≥10 mm/hr, age 0 to 3 days, ≥15 mm/hr thereafter.

*PROM >18 h. maternal fever. uterine tenderness. cloudy or foul smelling amniotic fluid. fetal tachycardia

for resistance to methicillin or nafcillin. If the organism is resistant, vancomycin is the antibiotic of choice. Coagulase-negative staphylococci are almost universally sensitive to vancomycin and on occasion will be susceptible to nafcillin as well. *Pseudomonas* infections should be treated with ticarcillin or carbenicillin and an aminoglycoside. For gram-negative bacteria that are resistant to aminoglycosides, cefotaxime is a suitable alternative drug. This third-generation cephalosporin has a wide therapeutic index and lacks the ototoxicity or nephro-

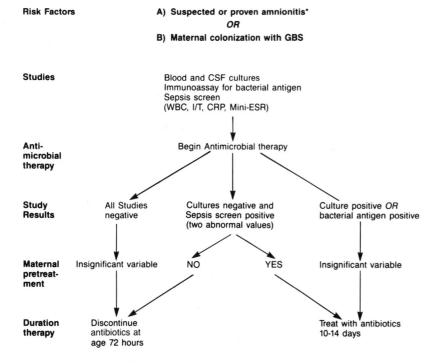

Figure 18–2. Evaluation of the high-risk asymptomatic preterm infant.

Sepsis screen tests, with criteria for abnormal results: WBC (white blood count), total white blood count <5000/mm³ or absolute neutrophil count <1750/mm³; I/T (immature to total neutrophil ratio) >0.2; CRP (C-reactive protein), positive latex agglutination test with undiluted serum; Mini-ESR (capillary tube erythrocyte sedimentation rate) ≥10 mm/hr, age 0 to 3 days, ≥15 mm/hr thereafter.

*(PROM >18 h, maternal fever, uterine tenderness, cloudy or foul smelling amniotic fluid, fetal tachycardia)

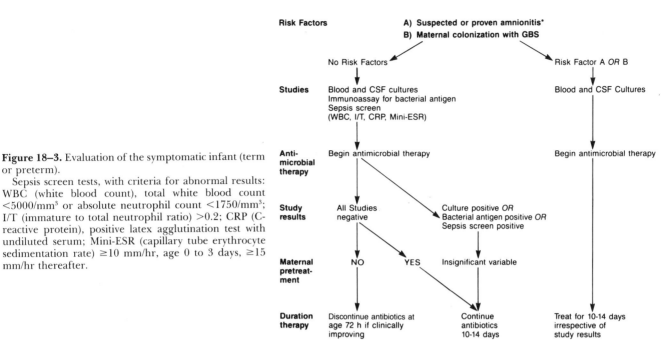

Figure 18–3. Evaluation of the symptomatic infant (term or preterm).

Sepsis screen tests, with criteria for abnormal results: WBC (white blood count), total white blood count <5000/mm³ or absolute neutrophil count <1750/mm³; I/T (immature to total neutrophil ratio) >0.2; CRP (C-reactive protein), positive latex agglutination test with undiluted serum; Mini-ESR (capillary tube erythrocyte sedimentation rate) ≥10 mm/hr, age 0 to 3 days, ≥15 mm/hr thereafter.

toxicity of the aminoglycosides. Unfortunately, emergence of resistance to cefotaxime can develop rapidly, so it should not be used routinely.

Blood cultures should be repeated 24 to 48 hours following the institution of antibiotic therapy to document clearing of bacteremia. Persistently positive cultures suggest errors in antimicrobial dosage, infection with a resistant or tolerant organism, or an occult focus of infection, such as an abscess or infected catheter. The duration of parenteral therapy for confirmed septicemia without focal infection should be 10 to 14 days. Dosage recommendations for antibiotics commonly used in premature and full-term infants are shown in Table 1. During the course of treatment with aminoglycoside antibiotics or vancomycin, one should carefully monitor serum levels because of the low therapeutic index of these drugs. Recommended peak serum levels are 4 to 8 µg/ml for gentamicin and tobramycin, 5 to 10 µg/ml for netilmicin, 15 to 25 µg/ml for kanamycin and amikacin, and 20 to 30 µg/ml for vancomycin. Trough serum levels should be less than 2 µg/ml for gentamicin, tobramycin, and netilmicin, less than 10 µg/ml for kanamycin and amikacin, and less than 12 µg/ml for vancomycin.

In addition to appropriate antimicrobial therapy, supportive therapy is vital to optimize recovery from septicemia. Common problems encountered during the course of sepsis include circulatory failure and acidemia, requiring fluids, alkali therapy, and occasionally vasopressors; respiratory failure, treated with supplemental oxygen and mechanical ventilation; coagulopathy, requiring transfusion of platelets or plasma or both; and hypoglycemia, managed with additional intravenous dextrose. Because caloric needs are increased during infection, intravenous nutritional support is also vital.

Although there have been several recent studies recommending adjunct immunologic therapies for infected infants (e.g., granulocyte transfusion, intravenous gamma globulin, and exchange transfusion), a role for these agents has not been substantiated.

MENINGITIS

Meningitis in the neonate is usually a sequela of bacteremia and shares a common etiology and pathogenesis with neonatal septicemia. Since the pathogens responsible for meningitis are identical with those that cause sepsis, the initial empiric antimicrobial selection for neonatal meningitis is the same as for neonatal sepsis. Therefore, infants who present with meningitis during the first week of life are usually begun on ampicillin and gentamicin. The final antibiotic selection for treatment of meningitis is again based on susceptibility testing of the pathogen causing disease.

For group B streptococci, ampicillin or penicillin alone is generally adequate. It should be noted, however, that some group B streptococci demonstrate in vitro tolerance to penicillin, which may be clinically important in cases of meningitis. Tolerant group B streptococci can be identified by a minimal bactericidal concentration (MBC)/minimal inhibitory concentration (MIC) ratio greater than 32:1. For meningitis due to tolerant group B streptococci, we recommend treatment with a combination of penicillin or ampicillin and gentamicin. Ampicillin is the preferred agent for meningitis due to *Listeria monocytogenes*, though some physicians advise combination therapy with gentamicin for part or all of the course.

Treatment of gram-negative meningitis is somewhat controversial. The combination of ampicillin and an aminoglycoside has been the traditional therapy for

TABLE 1. Dosage of Antibiotics for Neonates

Antibiotic	Age	Weight Group	mg/kg/Dose	Dosage Interval
Amikacin		Any weight	7.5	q 12 hr
			Loading dose 10	
Ampicillin	<1 wk	>2000 gm	50	q 12 hr
	<1 wk	<2000 gm	25	q 12 hr
	>1 wk	Any weight	75	q 6 hr
Carbenicillin		>2000 gm	75	q 6 hr
		<2000 gm	75	q 8 hr
Cefazolin		Any weight	25	q 12 hr
Cefotaxime	<1 wk	Any weight	50	q 12 hr
	>1 wk	Any weight	50	q 8 hr
Chloramphenicol	<1 wk	Any weight	25	q 24 hr
	>1 wk	Any weight	25	q 12 hr
Clindamycin		>2000 gm	5	q 6 hr
		<2000 gm	5	q 8 hr
Gentamicin	<1 wk	>2000 gm	2.5	q 12 hr
netilmicin	<1 wk	1500–2000 gm	2.5	q 18 hr
tobramycin	<1 wk	<1500 gm	2.5	q 24 hr
	>1 wk	>1500 gm	2.5	q 8 hr
	>1 wk	<1500 gm	2.5	q 12 hr
Kanamycin		>2000 gm	10	q 12 hr
		<2000 gm	7.5	q 12 hr
Oxacillin		>2000 gm	50	q 12 hr
		<2000 gm	25	q 12 hr
Penicillin G		Any weight	25,000–50,000 units	q 12 hr
Piperacillin		>2000 gm	50	q 6 hr
		<2000 gm	50	q 8 hr
Polymyxin B		Any weight	2	q 12 hr
Ticarcillin		>2000 gm	75	q 6 hr
		<2000 gm	75	q 8 hr
Vancomycin	<1 wk	>2000 gm	10	q 12 hr
	<1 wk	1000–2000 gm	10	q 18 hr
	<1 wk	<1000 gm	10	q 24 hr
	7–30 d	>2000 gm	10	q 8 hr
	7–30 d	1000–2000 gm	10	q 12 hr
	7–30 d	<1000 gm	10	q 18 hr
	31–60 d	Any weight	10	q 8 hr
	>60 d	Any weight	10	q 6 hr

meningitis caused by coliform bacteria. However, the spinal fluid concentrations of these antibiotics are often at or below the MBCs necessary to eradicate these organisms. As a consequence, sterilization of cerebrospinal fluid (CSF) is often delayed, which may contribute to the high incidence of neurologic sequelae seen in these infants. The instillation of gentamicin directly into the lumbar subarachnoid space or cerebral ventricles (in addition to systemic antimicrobial therapy) has not been shown to lessen the mortality or improve outcome. Third-generation cephalosporins achieve higher concentrations in the spinal fluid but are not associated with either more rapid sterilization of the CSF or decreased morbidity or mortality. Therefore, we still recommend ampicillin and an aminoglycoside for gram-negative meningitis and reserve cefotaxime as an alternative treatment for pathogens resistant to the aminoglycosides.

Citrobacter deserves special mention as a cause of gram-negative meningitis because of its unique virulence and propensity to produce brain abscess. One of three infants with *Citrobacter* meningitis dies, and at least three of every four survivors suffer severe neurologic sequelae. More than 70 per cent of newborn infants with this infection develop brain abscess. In patients who have abscesses that are accessible and are not multiple, surgical drainage is indicated. *Citrobacter* men-

ingitis should probably be treated with a combination of cefotaxime and an aminoglycoside antibiotic.

All neonates with meningitis should have a repeat lumbar puncture performed 24 to 48 hours into therapy and then every 2 days until spinal fluid cultures are negative. In infants with infections due to group B streptococci or *Listeria monocytogenes*, the CSF is generally sterilized by 24 to 48 hours. In contrast, infants with meningitis due to coliform organisms may have CSF cultures that remain positive for 3 or 4 days. Persistently positive CSF cultures beyond these norms should suggest one of the following possibilities: a resistant or tolerant organism, an error in antibiotic dosage or administration, or the presence of ventriculitis, subdural empyema, or brain abscess. Therefore, we recommend computed tomography scans for all neonates with persistently positive spinal fluid cultures as well as those with focal neurologic deficits, persistently elevated CSF protein, seizures beyond 3 days of therapy, *Citrobacter* meningitis, or increasing head circumference, as determined by daily measurements. The duration of therapy for uncomplicated meningitis caused by group B streptococci or *Listeria monocytogenes* should be 14 days following sterilization of the CSF. For gram-negative meningitis, we recommend a minimum of 21 days of antibiotics from the time of the first negative spinal fluid culture.

As with septicemia, supportive therapy is critical in the treatment of neonatal meningitis. Fluid therapy should be adequate to maintain perfusion and ideally no more than the normal daily maintenance requirements. If frequent monitoring of electrolytes demonstrates evidence of inappropriate antidiuretic hormone (ADH) secretion, fluids should be restricted to two thirds of maintenance. Seizures should be managed with phenobarbital and, if necessary, phenytoin or other anticonvulsants. If hydrocephalus develops, surgical intervention with a ventricular shunt is generally necessary. At the conclusion of therapy, we evaluate hearing in all neonates, using brain stem auditory evoked responses.

PNEUMONIA

Most neonates with early onset bacterial infections present with signs of respiratory distress, and the vast majority of these infants have pneumonia. As noted previously, newborn infants become infected when they come in contact with infected amniotic fluid. Pneumonia results from direct inhalation of contaminated amniotic fluid or bacteremic spread from a colonized nasopharynx. Therefore, initial empiric antimicrobial therapy is the same as for early onset septicemia or meningitis and consists of ampicillin and gentamicin. For pneumonia caused by group B streptococci, either ampicillin or penicillin is satisfactory therapy. Infants with pneumonia caused by *Listeria monocytogenes* are best treated with ampicillin. Enterobacteriaceae are generally treated with either ampicillin or an aminoglycoside, depending upon antibiotic susceptibility testing.

The organisms most commonly responsible for nosocomial pneumonia in the neonate are *Staphylococcus aureus*, coagulase-negative staphylococci, *Pseudomonas aeruginosa*, and other gram-negative rods. If *Staphylococcus aureus* is suspected, oxacillin or nafcillin should be included in the initial antibiotic regimen. For coagulase-negative staphylococci, vancomycin should be employed while awaiting the results of susceptibility testing to oxacillin and nafcillin; either of these latter drugs is preferred if the isolate is sensitive. Infants with pneumonia caused by *Pseudomonas* spp. require combination therapy with ticarcillin or carbenicillin and an aminoglycoside.

Another important etiology of pneumonia in the neonate is *Chlamydia trachomatis*. Infants acquire this pathogen during passage through a birth canal colonized with *Chlamydia*. Signs generally appear sometime after 3 to 4 weeks of age and include mild-to-moderate respiratory distress and a dry, harsh, repetitive cough described as staccato. Fever is often absent, chest roentgenography reveals bilateral diffuse interstitial infiltrates, and peripheral eosinophilia with greater than 400 cells per cubic millimeter is common. Erythromycin (40 mg/kg/day) is considered the drug of choice, though sulfisoxazole (150 mg/kg/day) is a suitable alternative. *Pneumocystis carinii* and *Ureaplasma urealyticum* may also be responsible for pneumonia in infants 3 to 4 weeks of age. *Pneumocystis* infections are treated with trimethoprim-sulfamethoxazole, and *Ureaplasma* infections may be treated with erythromycin.

The other group of pathogens responsible for pneumonia include those transmitted transplacentally, such as *Toxoplasma gondii*, *Treponema pallidum*, rubella virus, cytomegalovirus, and mycobacteria. Though less common as causes of neonatal pneumonia than the pathogens discussed previously, these organisms deserve consideration when there is evidence of congenital infection or when diagnostic testing is unrevealing and there is no response to antibiotic therapy.

The duration of antibiotic therapy for pneumonia depends upon the etiologic agent. In general, pneumonias caused by *Staphylococcus aureus*, *Pseudomonas*, or coliforms are treated for 3 weeks, while those caused by group B streptococci, *Listeria monocytogenes*, coagulase-negative staphylococci, or *Chlamydia* are treated for 10 to 14 days.

Supportive therapy is often as important as specific antimicrobial treatment in the management of neonatal pneumonia and frequently includes supplemental oxygen and mechanical ventilation, along with chest physiotherapy and nutritional support. In addition, closed-chest tube placement is required for drainage of pleural empyema, a complication that occurs most frequently with staphylococcal pneumonia.

BACTERIAL MENINGITIS AND SEPTICEMIA BEYOND THE NEONATAL PERIOD

JAMES K. TODD, M.D.

Severe infection (including meningitis) in children is often accompanied by bacteremia (i.e., septicemia). In the absence of focal infection, the precise bacteriologic diagnosis and definitive treatment must await the results of blood cultures and antimicrobial susceptibility testing. Because of the inherent diagnostic delays necessitated by culture techniques, an empiric approach to diagnosis and initial therapy has evolved. The causative organisms of septicemia in children beyond the newborn period differ with the focus of infection as well as with the age and underlying host defense status of the patient. Therefore, the general approach to diagnosis and treatment requires a progression of considerations that include the age and underlying host defense status of the patient, the diagnosis (e.g., focal infection, meningitis), the severity of illness, and the probable organisms involved and their common antimicrobial susceptibility patterns. Appropriate cultures of blood and any possible focus of infection (e.g., spinal fluid, abscess, septic arthritis) are essential to clarify ultimately the true nature of the infection. In children with suspected sepsis, these cultures should be obtained expeditiously and empiric treatment begun that will cover the likely organisms, with modification of therapy dependent upon the result of cultures. This general approach to the diagnosis and treatment of suspected sepsis in children is of critical importance to be sure that the initial treatment broadly covers the possible infecting organisms and also to allow modification to more specific therapy (including, in some cases, appropriate oral antibiotics), as indicated.

SEPTICEMIA IN CHILDREN WITH HOST DEFENSE DEFICIENCY

There are many causes of fever in children with host defense deficiency states (e.g., asplenia, immunodeficiency, leukemia, neutropenia, and so on), some of which may be benign (e.g., some viruses) or may be life threatening with accompanying septicemia. Many patients may have an indwelling central venous catheter that serves as an extra focus of bacterial infection. All patients who have a host defense deficiency, which puts them at increased risk of bacterial infection, should have a thorough evaluation of any illness that causes fever with a high suspicion of septicemia. Appropriate cultures of blood and any possible focus of infection should be obtained prior to initiating antimicrobial therapy. Such therapy should include antibiotics that cover a broad range of organisms, including *Staphylococcus aureus*, coagulase-negative *Staphylococcus* (if an indwelling central venous catheter is present), *Pseudomonas aeruginosa*, the Enterobacteriaceae (e.g., *Escherichia coli*), as well as other pathogens more commonly seen in normal children (e.g., *Streptococcus pneumoniae*, *Haemophilus influenzae*, and *Neisseria meningitidis*). Vancomycin is administered intravenously at a dose of 40 to 50 mg/kg/24 hr, given four times a day (each dose slowly over at least 1 hour), along with ceftazidime at a dose of 150 mg/kg/24 hr given three times a day. Because excessively high levels of vancomycin may be achieved with intravenous usage in patients with renal failure, some assessment of renal function (e.g., blood urea nitrogen [BUN] or creatinine) should be obtained at the time of initiation, and vancomycin levels should be measured to ensure safe but therapeutically adequate levels if the drug is continued on the basis of culture results. Other broad-spectrum combinations of antibiotics may be selected for initial therapy, depending on the type of population and common infecting organisms.

Of course, because septicemia in patients with host defense deficiency may occasionally occur with uncommon organisms having unusual antimicrobial susceptibilities, it is very important to tailor the specific antimicrobial therapy to in vitro susceptibility results of the isolated organism, based on a good understanding of the pharmacology of the selected antimicrobial agents. Any focus of infection should be treated until all evidence of active infection is resolved. Treatment should continue for a documented septicemia for 7 to 14 days and, in neutropenic patients, until the neutrophil count is greater than 1000 per cubic millimeter.

BACTEREMIA ASSOCIATED WITH FOCAL INFECTION

Many focal infections caused by bacteria may occasionally or even frequently be associated with bacteremia. The actual organism may vary somewhat, depending on age (see further on). Pneumonia associated with bacteremia may be caused by *S. pneumoniae*, *H. influenzae* Type b, *S. aureus*, or group A streptococci.

Skin and soft tissue infections (e.g., cellulitis or abscess) are commonly caused by group A streptococci or *S. aureus* and may be associated with lymphangitis or bacteremia. Other organisms causing cellulitis after trauma or a bite wound may less likely be associated with bacteremia, which nonetheless should be suspected in the patient who has systemic signs and symptoms that go beyond those usually associated with an isolated focal infection.

Osteomyelitis and septic arthritis are often (but not always) accompanied by bacteremia. Although *S. aureus* is a common cause in all age groups, in children under 5 years of age, arthritis is ordinarily caused by *H. influenzae* Type b; in older, sexually active children, it may be associated with *Neisseria gonorrhoeae*. Osteomyelitis is more commonly caused by *S. aureus* and occasionally other gram-positive organisms, although children with sickle cell disease and other hemoglobinopathies may also have *Salmonella* strains isolated. Children with underlying heart lesions may have endocarditis associated with many different organisms frequently isolated from the mouth—most commonly *Streptococcus viridans*. In all cases in which a focus of infection is present and systemic signs suggest bacteremia, a culture of both the focus and the blood is indicated prior to initiating empiric therapy based on the patient's age, severity of illness, and site of infection. If purulent material is obtained from the focus, a Gram stain may help direct antimicrobial selection.

When *S. aureus* is suspected, an intravenous beta-lactamase–resistant penicillin, such as nafcillin, 150 mg/kg/24 hr given four times a day, should be initiated. A first- or second-generation cephalosporin, such as cefazolin (100 mg/kg/24 hr) or cefuroxime (150 mg/kg/24 hr) given four times per day, is also effective. These antibiotics should be adequate initial treatment for other gram-positive organisms, including *S. pneumoniae* and group A streptococci, although therapy should be modified based upon the final culture results and antimicrobial susceptibility tests. For penicillin-allergic patients, clindamycin (40 mg/kg/24 hr given every 6 hr) or vancomycin is an adequate substitute; vancomycin (see previously) should be considered for patients with life-threatening symptoms if methicillin-resistant organisms are possible.

When *H. influenzae* is suspected, appropriate therapy includes intravenous treatment with a second- or third-generation cephalosporin (cefotaxime, 150 to 200 mg/kg/24 hr given every 6 hours, or ceftriaxone, 100 mg/kg/24 hr given every 12 hours). Other related antibiotics are currently being tested in children and may prove to have similar efficacy, although their routine use should await sufficient clinical data published in the peer-reviewed literature. It should be emphasized that these third-generation cephalosporins are not particularly effective antistaphylococcal therapy, and when *S. aureus* is thought to be a likely possibility, additional coverage should be achieved, as indicated previously.

When multiple organisms are potentially present (e.g., as in septic arthritis in an infant), it always is appropriate to cover more broadly and then to narrow therapy based upon the culture results. Cultures become imperative when the potential for multiple organisms requires the initial selection of multiple antibiotics at the outset, since the isolation of the causative organism is the only way to narrow appropriately what appears to be effective empiric therapy.

For focal infections not mentioned here, it is appropriate to remember that many other organisms can occasionally be associated with bacteremia (e.g., the Enterobacteriaceae with urinary tract infection), and appropriate selection of empirical therapy includes consideration of the focus involved, the common organisms etiologically associated with that focus, and their usual antimicrobial susceptibility pattern.

Treatment of the focal infection should continue until adequate healing has occurred as well as for a period sufficient to eradicate the bacteremia fully. This period may range from 7 to 10 days for many organisms to a few days of intravenous treatment for some gram-positive infections, followed by a longer period with appropriate oral therapy. Articles describing the treatment of these infections in greater detail should be consulted. For serious infections or those that are difficult to treat, especially with antimicrobials to which the organism is not highly susceptible, measurement of serum killing powers (serum bactericidal levels) may be important, especially to document adequate absorption of oral therapy or to monitor optimal parenteral therapy. Peak serum killing powers should be obtained one-half hour after completion of an intravenous dose or one and one-half hours after an oral dose, and a trough specimen can be obtained just prior to any dose. Appropriate therapy may range from a peak of greater than 1:8 for osteomyelitis and septic arthritis to a peak of greater than 1:32 for bacterial endocarditis. It should also be remembered that the healing of many foci of infection (abscesses or osteomyelitis) may be hastened by appropriate drainage procedures.

BACTEREMIA ASSOCIATED WITH SEVERE ILLNESS

Some patients may present with fever and signs of severe illness, including shock, purpura, meningeal signs, or altered state of consciousness, which require immediate evaluation and treatment at any age. A thorough history and physical examination may point the way to a more specific diagnosis; however, in children in whom such a diagnosis cannot be definitively established, bacteremia must always be ruled out. Appropriate cultures should be taken, and the patient should be thoroughly evaluated for focal infection that might give a clue to the causative organism and point the way to appropriate selection of therapy. Patients appearing with severe symptoms with a scarlatiniform rash may have toxic shock syndrome associated with a focal *S. aureus* infection or bacteremia or severe group A streptococcal septicemia, both of which require appropriate supportive care and antimicrobial therapy. If no focal signs exist, the encapsulated bacteria should be strongly considered as a possible cause, including *S. pneumoniae*, *N. meningitidis*, and *H. influenzae* Type b. Other organisms (e.g., group A streptococci, Enterobacteriaceae, and anaerobes) may occur in occasional cases. The therapy for fever associated with these signs

and symptoms should proceed quickly to maintain adequate blood pressure and tissue perfusion as well as to initiate broad-spectrum antibiotics, which should include an antistaphylococcal penicillin or first- or second-generation cephalosporin and appropriate therapy for *H. influenzae* and *N. meningitidis* (cefotaxime or ceftriaxone), as indicated previously. Appropriate cultures, including blood cultures and spinal fluid cultures as well as the focal cultures mentioned previously, should be obtained quickly, and the emphasis should be on supporting system failure (see under the specific disease) and providing appropriate antimicrobial coverage until culture results are obtained.

SEPSIS WITH MENINGITIS

Older children presenting with classic symptoms of meningitis may have fever, stiff neck, and headache; however, the younger the child, the less specific the signs and symptoms, so that in a child under 2 years of age only fever, lethargy, malaise, and/or poor feeding may be present. Therefore, the younger the febrile child, the higher the suspicion that bacteremia and meningitis might be present. In any child presenting with severe illness or in children presenting with any possible signs of meningitis, it is appropriate to obtain blood cultures as well as cerebrospinal fluid (CSF) cultures if deemed safe by the apparent lack of cerebral edema and focal neurologic signs). Often, the CSF Gram stain will help determine appropriate therapy. Antigen detection for *H. influenzae* will always yield a few false-negative results, and those tests for *S. pneumoniae* and *N. meningitidis* are currently undependable and should not be relied upon. Again, it is appropriate to obtain a complete range of cultures (i.e., blood, CSF, urine, any focus of infection) in the patient suspected of having meningitis and to initiate antimicrobial therapy pending culture results. This therapy should include ampicillin, 300 mg/kg/24 hr given every 4 hours, and cefotaxime, 200 mg/kg/24 hr given every 6 hours, in children under 2 to 3 months of age in whom other organisms, such as group B streptococci and *Listeria monocytogenes*, may occasionally occur. In children older than 3 months, the common organisms (*S. pneumoniae*, *H. influenzae*, and *N. meningitidis*) can be adequately covered with a single third-generation cephalosporin, such as cefatoxime, 200 mg/kg/24 hr given every 6 hours or ceftriaxone, 100 mg/kg/24 hr given twice a day. Although the combination of ampicillin and chloramphenicol may still be appropriate therapy in some areas, ampicillin- and chloramphenicol-resistant *H. influenzae* strains do occur, suggesting the greater initial coverage of the third-generation cephalosporins.

Of course, antimicrobial therapy should be modified once susceptibility tests are available. For the most part, *S. pneumoniae* and *N. meningitidis* will be susceptible to penicillin G, 300,000 units/kg/24 hr in six divided doses, or ampicillin, 300 mg/kg/24 hr given every 6 hours. Patients with documented penicillin allergy should be treated with chloramphenicol (100 mg/kg/24 hr in four divided doses). It should be remembered that chloramphenicol metabolism is affected by liver function and perfusion. All patients should have liver function studies monitored at the initiation of chloramphenicol therapy, and levels should be followed to ensure adequate therapeutic levels without exceeding toxic levels (a peak of >25 µg/ml). Some *S. pneumoniae* strains are now resistant to penicillin, so that all strains should have appropriate susceptibility testing by a laboratory experienced with the procedure. When resistance is identified, patients should be treated with vancomycin or chloramphenicol, depending upon susceptibility results. Many *H. influenzae* strains produce a beta-lactamase, which renders them ampicillin resistant. Most of these strains can be treated with either chloramphenicol or a third-generation cephalosporin, as indicated previously. It should be remembered that in some areas strains may also be chloramphenicol resistant, and the combination of ampicillin and chloramphenicol should not be used for initial therapy.

For the great majority of patients, if the organism is analyzed in an experienced microbiology laboratory using approved techniques, proper selection of antimicrobial therapy should result in eradication of the organism from the blood and spinal fluid. Routine repeat spinal fluid examination is therefore not required for these common organisms (i.e., *H. influenzae*, *N. meningitidis*, and *S. pneumoniae*). When an unusual organism is present, or one with unpredictable susceptibilities, or when less common antibiotics are being used, a repeat tap may be necessary to document bacteriologic cure.

Ordinarily, with the large experience that we now have with the common organisms, a repeat tap is not necessary to assure bacteriologic cure as long as the patient is showing signs of gradual improvement. The patient's response may be misleading in the first few days of illness, as fever and irritability may persist and meningeal signs may actually increase as the patient's developing inflammatory response plays an increasing role in meningeal irritation. Nonetheless, the child's level of consciousness in response to external stimuli should improve, and when there is any doubt, a repeat spinal tap should be considered. Fever may persist throughout the course of treatment. Most patients with *H. influenzae* meningitis become afebrile by the fifth day, but approximately 10 per cent may remain febrile throughout the treatment course, and an additional 10 to 20 per cent may have a secondary fever. For the most part, these persistent or secondary fevers are not due to persistent infection when treating the common causes of meningitis but rather are due to a secondary nosocomial infection acquired within the hospital, drug fever, or phlebitis. Subdural effusions occur commonly in children with meningitis but are rarely infected and are rarely a cause of persistent fever. The head circumference should be monitored on a daily basis; concern regarding symptomatic subdural effusions should occur only if the patient has an increasing head circumference or development of focal neurologic signs or deteriorating mental status. The total course of antimicrobial therapy is currently 14 days for *S. pneumoniae*, 10 days for *H. influenzae* Type b, and 7 days for *N. meningitidis*. Shorter periods have been reported to be successful for treating some of these organisms and may be possible when supported by additional confirmatory clinical data.

It should be remembered, however, that the treatment of meningitis only begins with the selection of antimicrobial therapy and that there are many other therapeutic issues that need to be addressed. Those patients most severely ill with shock associated with *H. influenzae* meningitis may have as a mechanism the presence of cerebral edema causing brain stem herniation, which is a medical emergency that should be treated with intubation and hyperventilation, with mannitol (0.25 to 1 gm/kg per dose given intravenously [IV] over 10 to 30 minutes). Serum glucose should be maintained, and the serum osmolality should be carefully monitored to avoid any decrease that could exacerbate the cerebral edema. In general, in patients who do not have evidence of cerebral edema, some element of dehydration may be present. Although many authors advise the routine restriction of fluids for fear of exacerbating the inappropriate antidiuretic hormone syndrome, other data suggest that it is appropriate to rehydrate the patient carefully, avoiding any drop in serum sodium level or osmolality and then restricting fluids once normal hydration and perfusion are reestablished.

Vital signs (blood pressure, pulse, respiratory rate, and temperature), as well as urine output, level of consciousness, and neurologic status, should be monitored frequently. Those patients with seizures should be treated with appropriate anticonvulsants. The use of systemic corticosteroid therapy has been recently reevaluated in patients with meningitis. Although the debate continues, there are now data suggesting that the early initiation of corticosteroid therapy (dexamethasone, 0.6 mg/kg/24 hr divided four times a day for 4 days) may be effective in reducing the incidence of deafness and may reduce the cerebral vasculitis that seems to be associated with cortical sequelae. Clinical data are not sufficient at present to establish fully the benefits of such therapy compared with the known risks (gastrointestinal bleeding and relapse); however, the risks and benefits should be weighed in individual patients on the basis of the best data available.

The sequelae of bacterial meningitis in children are related to three different pathophysiologic mechanisms. Death is most commonly associated with severe cerebral edema and brain stem herniation. Cortical sequelae are related to the development of a sterile cerebral vasculitis. Both sequelae are predicted by a clinical scoring system that can be applied at the time of admission. Patients receive the following scores: coma requiring intubation (3); seizures (2) or hypothermia (2); shock (1), age less than 12 months (1), a CSF white blood cell count less than 1000 (1), or a hemoglobin lower than 11 gm/100 ml (1); febrile symptoms that have persisted for more than 3 days prior to admission (1/2) and CSF glucose levels less than 20 mg/100 ml (1/2). Patients having a cumulative score of 4.5 points or more are at greater risk of death or severe cortical sequelae owing to the above mechanism and may respond more favorably to the administration to corticosteroids (see above dose) and mannitol if cerebral edema is present. This scoring system does not predict hearing loss outcome, which seems to be related to inner ear inflammation.

Children with *H. influenzae* or *N. meningitidis* infection may frequently carry the causative organism in their nasopharynx even after a course of systemic antibiotic therapy. There are two concerns regarding the further spread of these organisms. The first is that at the time of admission other family members may already be colonized with the organism and thus may be at risk of developing secondary infections. In addition, the patient may return home after hospitalization with the organism still in the nasopharynx and put subsequent contacts at some risk. Because of this, it is important to observe all exposed household or daycare contacts carefully and to evaluate any ill contacts with a full understanding of their prior exposure. To minimize the risk of secondary cases of *H. influenzae* infection, rifampin prophylaxis is recommended for all household contacts, including adults, in those households with at least one contact younger than 48 months old, regardless of the immunization status of the contacts. This therapy should be initiated as soon as possible after hospitalization. Prophylaxis is not recommended for pregnant women. All others should receive 20 mg/kg of rifampin once a day for 4 days, with a maximum of 600 mg per dose. The dose for chemoprophylaxis of *N. meningitidis* infections is 20 mg/kg/24 hr divided into two doses for 2 days, with a maximal unit dose of 600 mg. For daycare center and nursery school contacts, prophylaxis may be recommended by the local or state health department.

BACTEREMIA WITHOUT A FOCUS
Children Less Than 2 to 3 Months of Age

Fever without a focus of infection occurs commonly, especially in young children. Prospective studies suggest that occult bacteremia may occur in 5 to 10 per cent of these patients. This figure may be higher in those patients with host defense deficiency states or severe illness or both, as mentioned above. The risks and consequences of bacteremia in young infants (less than 2 to 3 months of age) may be greater than in older children. In addition, the signs of meningitis are the most difficult to detect in such young children, so that it is traditional in many training programs to suggest the admission of all febrile children under 3 months of age (in some programs, as old as 6 months of age) for a mandatory work-up and intravenous antibiotics until cultures are negative. Clinical evaluation will certainly detect some infants with severe illness who should always be admitted for empiric therapy, whereas there will be many infants with fever who otherwise look well. The work-up for this latter group may be especially difficult, as routine hospitalization of all such patients may lead to unnecessary complications. However, observation outside the hospital may lead to the occasional patient with bacteremia who is missed and progresses to more severe illness. There is no current laboratory test or clinical evaluation that permits one to resolve this diagnostic dilemma successfully. Some authors recommend the use of a white blood cell count and differential count to help detect those infants at risk of sepsis; however, there are always patients with normal studies who have bacteremia and many with abnormal studies who do not.

For those young children with fever who look clinically ill, hospital admission and thorough culturing (of blood, CSF, urine, and any other focus) are indicated, followed by initiation of antibiotics pending the culture results. Ampicillin, 300 mg/kg/24 hr in four doses, and cefotaxime, 200 mg/kg/24 hr given every 6 hours, should be used. If *S. aureus* infection is suspected, an antistaphylococcal penicillin (e.g., nafcillin) or cephalosporin (e.g., cefazolin) should also be prescribed.

For those young infants with fever who do not appear ill and are alert and responsive, a blood culture and urine culture are indicated, followed by close observation. A chest radiograph is indicated in any infant with tachypnea or respiratory distress. Broad-spectrum antimicrobial therapy (e.g., ceftriaxone, 50 mg/kg/24 hr as a single dose) may be prescribed but is of unproven efficiency, and frequent re-evaluation is still required. It is important to emphasize that in those patients who are started on empiric antibiotics, cultures of blood, urine, *and spinal fluid*, as well as of any focal infection sites, should be obtained prior to the initiation of therapy. In the final analysis, the management of the young infant with fever and no localizing signs requires careful evaluation and frequent re-evaluation until the fever is resolved or the diagnosis is clarified.

Children Older Than 2 to 3 Months of Age

Similar diagnostic considerations exist in older infants and young children with fever and no localizing signs. Occult bacteremia may occur at any age; beyond 3 months, *S. pneumoniae, H. influenzae, N. meningitidis*, and assorted other, less common organisms may be associated with an occult bacteremia that may ultimately progress to cause focal infection or meningitis but that in some cases may resolve spontaneously. At the outset, however, neither the diagnosis nor the outcome is clear, and as in the younger infant, the white blood cell count and differential, urine antigen testing, and even clinical evaluation are not always diagnostic. Patients with a severe febrile illness or suspected meningitis should have cultures done and should be admitted to the hospital and treated as indicated in the previous section, although ampicillin may not be required beyond 3 months of age. In those patients who have no underlying host defense deficiency and a normal physical examination (with special care being taken in evaluating the child's level of consciousness, neurologic condition, and laboratory tests), careful outpatient observation and re-evaluation may be appropriate. In cases in which there is some doubt about the severity or nature of the child's illness, a blood culture and urine culture may be indicated, followed by empiric antibiotic therapy with close observation. In those patients with suspected occult bacteremia, oral therapy (e.g., amoxicillin-clavulanate, 40 mg/kg/24 hr given three times a day) may be effective in more rapidly improving symptoms in some patients; however, others may subsequently develop meningitis in spite of this therapy. This finding has prompted some investigators to study (and many practitioners to advocate) the use of a long-acting third-generation cephalosporin (e.g., ceftriaxone, 50 mg/kg/day as a single dose) as appropriate "coverage" for all eventualities. It should be emphasized that even then such therapy may not be adequate for some organisms (e.g., *S. aureus*) and that breakthrough meningitis can still occur. Thus, again, careful follow-up of the potentially bacteremic patient is essential whether or not antimicrobial agents are prescribed. If there is any doubt about the patient's condition, reculturing is recommended prior to hospitalization and the initiation of appropriate intravenous therapy.

ENDOCARDITIS

T. G. CLEARY, M.D.

Although endocarditis is an infrequent pediatric problem, corrective surgery for congenital heart disease, use of intravascular catheters, rheumatic fever, drug abuse, and sepsis continue to put children at risk of this life-threatening disease. Since children often lack the textbook physical findings, the diagnosis must be considered in every febrile child, particularly if recognizable risk factors are present. Among the congenital defects, tetralogy of Fallot, ventricular septal defect (especially with aortic regurgitation), aortic stenosis (even after valvotomy), patent ductus arteriosus, mitral valve prolapse, and transposition of the great vessels are more commonly complicated by endocarditis than are isolated secundum atrial septal defects or pulmonic valve lesions. Palliative or corrective surgery does not always eliminate the risk of endocarditis. Prosthetic valves continue to be a risk long after insertion. Although normal heart valves may be infected during sepsis, there is a much higher risk of endocarditis in the setting of congenital heart disease (0.8 per cent versus 10.0 per cent in an autopsy series). The patient with a normal heart may also develop endocarditis when there is an infected intravascular catheter, a large burn, or intravenous drug abuse. In addicts, because tricuspid valve infection is particularly common, the easily heard murmurs, congestive heart failure, and peripheral embolic phenomena so prominent in left-sided infections may be replaced by symptoms of septic pulmonary emboli that can be misinterpreted as pneumonia.

Although the first blood culture is positive in the vast majority of cases, multiple positive blood cultures are required for a firm diagnosis. Multiple positive blood cultures, although necessary for diagnosis, are not sufficient. Generally, additional physical findings and laboratory data are required to make a diagnosis with confidence. Some organisms (e.g., *Escherichia coli* or *Klebsiella* spp.) so infrequently cause endocarditis that multiple positive blood cultures must be coupled with other very convincing data to make a diagnosis of endocarditis. Other organisms, such as viridans streptococci or *Staphylococcus aureus*, so commonly cause endocarditis that multiple positive blood cultures should be interpreted as indicating endocarditis unless strong data to the contrary exist. For *S. aureus*, the presence of teichoic acid antibodies strengthens the case for endocarditis, since these antibodies are almost always present in *S. aureus* endocarditis. About 10 per cent of patients with a clinical diagnosis of endocarditis have negative blood cultures. To optimize blood culture yield, cultures should be held in the laboratory for 4 weeks and blindly subcultured. Other sometimes helpful maneuvers include culturing for L-forms with hypertonic media, using media supplemented with vitamin B-6 for nutritionally deficient streptococci, using media containing penicillinase or the Antibiotic Removal Device when prior therapy has been used, venting blood cultures when *Pseudomonas* is a consideration, culturing blood in vented bottles containing biphasic media kept at 30°C when fungi are suspected, and obtaining serologies for Q fever, *Brucella* spp., and teichoic acid antibodies. Although these laboratory maneuvers may diagnose some difficult cases, usually negative blood cultures are due to previous, often inappropriate, antibiotic use.

PRINCIPLES OF ANTIBIOTIC THERAPY

Bactericidal rather than *bacteriostatic* agents should be used. Drugs such as chloramphenicol, tetracycline, clindamycin, and erythromycin, which slow the growth of bacteria but do not consistently kill, are generally inadequate as single agents because of the risk of relapse. Therapy is generally continued for 4 to 6 weeks, although 8 to 12 weeks may be required in selected cases. No compromise in treatment plan should be made once the diagnosis is certain. Rapid improvement of the sort often seen with viridans streptococci should not tempt the physician to utilize less than optimal therapy. Dosage should be monitored with the aid of the serum bactericidal titer (SBT). The SBT is determined by testing the ability of serial dilutions of the patient's serum to kill a standard inoculum (5×10^5 organisms per milliliter) of the bacteria isolated from the patient's blood. The standard microdilution method using Mueller-Hinton broth mixed 1:1 with pooled human serum should be used. An SBT of 1:64 or more at peak (30 minutes after an antibiotic dose) and 1:32 or more at trough (30 minutes before a dose) predicts bacteriologic cure. Lower levels do not always predict failure. However, antibiotic doses should be raised or alternate drugs selected, when possible, to achieve these high levels. The peak concentration of antibiotic is used to adjust the milligram per kilogram per dose; the trough concentration is used to adjust the interval between doses. Both peak and trough drug concentrations should be followed regularly during the course of endocarditis therapy because changes in hemodynamic status and renal function (sometimes associated with endocarditis-induced glomerulonephritis) alter drug distribution and excretion. In the occasional child who has fungal endocarditis, there currently is no satisfactory way of predicting adequacy of therapy.

Optimal drug selection is based on the sensitivity data obtained by inoculating the bacteria isolated from the patient's blood in serial dilutions of a potentially useful antibiotic to define the lowest antibiotic concentration that inhibits bacterial growth (minimal inhibitory concentration, or MIC) and the lowest concentration that kills the bacteria (minimal bactericidal concentration, or

MBC). Combinations of antibiotics are often used in endocarditis therapy. This is particularly appropriate when the organism isolated from the patient's blood is resistant to usual first-line antibiotic choices, when a very unusual organism with unpredictable antibiotic sensitivity is isolated, and when the organism has a marked disparity between the MIC and the MBC (tolerance). Tolerance (MBC/MIC >16) is a clinically significant problem, particularly with enterococcal and *S. aureus* endocarditis. The antibiotic choice in these settings is guided by determining the killing of the organism in the face of serial dilutions of each of the prospective drugs in a checkerboard fashion. Synergistic combinations are preferred over those that show antagonism or simple additive killing.

MICROBIOLOGY

Empiric antibiotic therapy is based on predicted bacteriology. Acute fulminant endocarditis is most often due to *S. aureus*, although *Streptococcus pyogenes, Streptococcus pneumoniae*, and *Neisseria gonorrhoeae* occasionally cause this syndrome. An indolent subacute illness with emboli, low-grade fever, and constitutional symptoms is most likely to be caused by an alpha-hemolytic (viridans) streptococcus. Infections with some organisms, such as enterococci and *S. aureus*, may manifest acutely or subacutely. In the drug-addicted adolescent, *S. aureus, Pseudomonas aeruginosa* and other gram-negative rods, *Candida* spp., viridans streptococci, and enterococci all occur. Endocarditis occurring in the first 2 months after cardiac surgery is typically due to *Staphylococcus epidermidis, S. aureus*, or Enterobacteriaceae, while later cases usually result from viridans streptococci or *S. epidermidis; S. aureus* and gram-negative enteric organisms occur less commonly in late onset prosthetic valve endocarditis. Endocarditis occurring with an intravascular catheter in place is typically due to *S. aureus* or *S. epidermidis*; other organisms sometimes occur.

The alpha-hemolytic streptococci, particularly *S. sanguis* I, *S. sanguis* II, *S. mutans*, and *S. milleri (M.G.-intermedius)*, are the most common organisms causing endocarditis. *S. mitior (mitis)* and pyridoxal-dependent *S. mitior* are of special concern because unlike most viridans streptococci they are relatively resistant to penicillin. For viridans streptococci, which have low MICs to penicillin (≤0.1 µg/ml), regimens of proven efficacy (>98 per cent cure) include intravenous aqueous crystalline penicillin G given at a dose of about 25,000 to 35,000 units/kg per dose (maximum of 20 million units/day) every 4 hours for 4 weeks or intravenous aqueous crystalline penicillin G for 4 weeks, combined with intramuscular streptomycin at a dose of 15 mg/kg per dose (maximum of 500 mg per dose) given every 12 hours during the first 2 weeks of penicillin therapy. Two-week courses of combined parenteral penicillin and streptomycin are also very effective, but there is little experience with this regimen in pediatric patients. Those whose course is complicated should not be considered candidates for short-course therapy. Patients with impaired renal function or ototoxicity ought to receive 4 weeks of penicillin without the aminoglycoside. In the penicillin-allergic patient, cephalothin, 100 to

150 mg/kg/day in six divided doses intravenously (maximum of 12 gm/day), and vancomycin, 40 mg/kg/day in four divided doses intravenously (maximum of 2 gm/day), are appropriate alternative agents. For viridans streptococci having relatively high MICs (>0.1 µg/ml) to penicillin, the regimen that includes both penicillin for 4 to 6 weeks and streptomycin for 2 weeks is favored.

Enterococcal *(Streptococcus faecium, Streptococcus faecalis*, and *Streptococcus durans)* infections are usually treated with combinations of antibiotics because of "tolerance" to penicillin. All enterococci are resistant to 0.2 µg/ml of penicillin G. *S. faecium* has a higher MIC to penicillin and is more resistant to kanamycin, tobramycin, and netilmicin than is *S. faecalis*. Although many enterococci show high-level in vitro resistance to streptomycin (MIC >2000 µg/ml) and do not respond in vitro to penicillin and streptomycin in a synergistic fashion, failures on penicillin-streptomycin regimens are uncommon. We prefer to treat enterococcal endocarditis with combinations of ampicillin or penicillin and gentamicin because gentamicin is synergistic with penicillin and serum concentrations of gentamicin can easily be measured. Generally, a dose of 1 to 2 mg/kg per dose (maximum of 100 mg per dose) of gentamicin is given intravenously every 6 to 8 hours to maintain peak concentrations of 3 to 5 µg/ml. Higher doses of gentamicin do not improve outcome. Vancomycin combined with an aminoglycoside is appropriate for the penicillin-allergic patient. Cephalosporins are *not* adequate because they appear to be ineffective in enterococcal endocarditis. Desensitization to penicillin is another option in the penicillin-allergic patient. Those who have been symptomatic for longer than 3 months prior to diagnosis and those with mitral disease ought to be treated for 6 weeks. Uncomplicated enterococcal endocarditis can be treated with 4 weeks of therapy.

S. aureus is generally treated with nafcillin at a dose of 25 to 35 mg/kg per dose (maximum of 2 grams per dose) given intravenously every 4 hours for a total of 4 to 6 weeks. We do not use methicillin in this setting because of the nephrotoxicity associated with prolonged courses of methicillin therapy. Although the data in humans suggest no advantage with combined therapy, many infectious disease specialists recommend adding an aminoglycoside to the regimen during the first 1 to 2 weeks of therapy. *S. aureus* strains that exhibit "tolerance" to penicillins should be treated more aggressively than those that do not. Infections with "tolerant" *S. aureus* are associated with prolonged fever and bacteremia. We use nafcillin for 6 weeks along with gentamicin in the first 2 weeks in this setting. Methicillin-resistant *S. aureus* (MRSA) are resistant to naficillin and oxacillin as well as methicillin. Vancomycin is the drug of choice for MRSA. Cephalosporins are not recommended despite occasional in vitro sensitivity because treatment failures appear to be common. For the rare *S. aureus* that is sensitive to penicillin G, doses of penicillin similar to those used with viridans streptococci may be given.

Infections caused by *S. epidermidis* and other coagulase-negative staphylococci, particularly when acquired

TABLE 1. Prophylaxis for Patients at Risk of Bacterial Endocarditis

Operation or Instrumentation Involving	Parenteral	Oral	Regimen (Penicillin Allergic)
Teeth or upper respiratory tract	Ampicillin *or* Penicillin G *plus* Gentamicin	Penicillin V	Vancomycin *or* Erythromycin
Gastrointestinal or genitourinary tract	Ampicillin *plus* Gentamicin	Amoxicillin	Vancomycin *plus* Gentamicin

Doses of antibiotics for prophylaxis:
Penicillin G: 50,000 units/kg (maximum, 2×10^6 units) IM or IV 30 to 60 minutes before and 25,000 units/kg 6 hours after procedure
Ampicillin: 50 mg/kg (maximum, 2 gm) IM or IV 30 to 60 minutes before and 6 to 8 hours after procedure
Gentamicin: 2 mg/kg IM or IV 30 to 60 minutes before and 8 hours after procedure
Vancomycin: 20 mg/kg (maximum, 1 gm) IV infused during the 1 hour before procedure
Penicillin V: 2 gm PO 60 minutes before and 1 gm PO 6 hours after procedure; if <27 kg, give half this dose
Amoxicillin: 50 mg/kg (maximum, 3 gm) PO 60 minutes before and 25 mg/kg (maximum, 1 gm) PO 6 hours after procedure
Erythromycin: 20 mg/kg (maximum, 1 gm) 120 minutes before and 10 mg/kg PO (maximum, 500 mg) 6 hours after procedure

in a hospital, are often resistant to multiple antibiotics. Because these infections may be very difficult to cure, two or three drug regimens should be routinely used. When the organism is sensitive to a semisynthetic penicillin, nafcillin, rifampin, and gentamicin can be used. Vancomycin is generally substituted for nafcillin when the organism is resistant to semisynthetic penicillins or when the patient is allergic to penicillins.

Gram-negative enteric rod endocarditis is usually treated with an aminoglycoside (gentamicin, tobramycin, or amikacin) plus a penicillin (carbenicillin, ticarcillin, piperacillin, or mezlocillin) or a cephalosporin (cephalothin, cefotaxime, ceftazidime, ceftriaxone, or cefoperazone). The prognosis in these patients is generally worse than in those with infections caused by the more common gram-positive cocci.

Fungal endocarditis (typically due to *Candida* spp.) has a very poor prognosis. Amphotericin B, at a maintenance dose of 0.5 to 0.6 mg/kg/day given intravenously over 6 hours (maximum dose of 30 mg/day), and 5-fluorocytosine, at a dose of 150 mg/kg/day orally in four divided doses, are given for *Candida* spp. Although the optimal duration is uncertain, we generally continue therapy for a very prolonged period (6 to 12 weeks). We discontinue 5-fluorocytosine if the organism is resistant or if the patient develops toxicity (particularly bone marrow depression). The dosage needs to be lowered when renal function is impaired. Levels of 5-fluorocytosine should always be kept below 100 µg/ml. Valve replacement is usually indicated in *Candida* endocarditis and should be done within a few days of starting antifungal therapy.

When the diagnosis of endocarditis seems clear-cut, but no cultures are positive, we give combined ampicillin-gentamicin therapy for a 4- to 6-week period, since many of the culture-negative cases are due to routine pathogens that the laboratory has failed to isolate.

SUPPORTIVE MEASURES

Nonantibiotic medical measures such as digitalization, maintenance of fluid and electrolyte status, diuretics, and anticoagulants may be required. A daily physical examination, close monitoring of hemodynamic data,

and frequent laboratory evaluation are essential. A team approach involving cardiologists, a cardiac surgeon, an infectious disease specialist, a medical microbiologist, and a general pediatrician is needed to give the patient the best chance for cure.

Aggressive surgical management is nearly always indicated in the face of uncontrolled infection, heart failure unresponsive to medical management, and an unstable, infected prosthetic valve. Relative indications include multiple large emboli, fungal endocarditis, relapse after presumed effective therapy, evidence of intracardiac extension of infection, and early prosthetic device infection. Some experts also recommend an aggressive surgical approach in the settings of gram-negative endocarditis, *S. aureus* infection of the aortic or mitral valve, left-sided vegetations large enough to be seen on M-mode echocardiography or right-sided vegetations larger than 1 cm, and aortic insufficiency with mild heart failure or with new conduction abnormalities that are persistent and unrelated to drugs or ischemia in a patient with aortic valve involvement. Late prosthetic valve endocarditis can sometimes be treated without removal of the prosthetic device. The major indication for cardiac surgery in regard to infection is continued bacteremia despite optimal antibiotic therapy. Repeat blood cultures during the course of therapy and after therapy is completed are essential, as most relapses occur within 2 months after the end of therapy. Fortunately, prosthetic devices inserted shortly after the institution of adequate antibiotic therapy generally do not get infected.

ANTIBIOTIC PROPHYLAXIS FOR PREVENTION OF ENDOCARDITIS

Antibiotic prophylaxis continues to be controversial both because no regimen has ever been shown in controlled studies to affect the incidence of endocarditis in humans and because failures with recommended prophylactic regimens are well documented. Prophylaxis has been advised for those who have valvular heart disease, prosthetic heart valves, idiopathic hypertrophic subaortic stenosis, mitral valve prolapse, and congenital heart disease (excluding isolated secundum atrial septal defect). In general, recent recommendations have favored parenteral rather than oral therapy in those patients who are at highest risk of endocarditis (Table 1).

STAPHYLOCOCCAL INFECTIONS

PAUL G. QUIE, M.D.

Staphylococci cause a wide variety of serious infectious diseases. *Staphylococcus aureus* is an opportunistic pathogen associated with both abscess-type lesions such as boils and osteomyelitis and toxin-related diseases such as toxic shock syndrome. *S. epidermidis* is primarily a nosocomial pathogen colonizing vascular catheters and other foreign bodies and producing systemic disease.

Superficial staphylococcal skin infections may not require antibiotic therapy, and *S. epidermidis* bacteremia may clear with removal of foreign bodies, but most staphylococcal infections require treatment with penicillinase-resistant antibiotic agents. Staphylococcal abscesses frequently require incision and drainage in addition to antimicrobial agents. Staphylococci may develop tolerance for antibiotics and persist in tissues so that long-term therapy is frequently necessary.

Selection of the antimicrobial agent and the route of administration for treating staphylococcal disease will be conditioned by the severity of infection, the patient's age, and the antibiotic sensitivity of the strain causing infection (Table 1).

SERIOUS INFECTIONS

In general, systemic administration of bactericidal antibiotics is necessary for treatment of serious staphy-

lococcal disease. Since most staphylococci are penicillin resistant, a semisynthetic beta-lactamase–resistant penicillin is the drug of choice. Nafcillin and oxacillin are highly effective beta-lactamase–resistant penicillins.

Hypersensitivity reactions such as skin rash, leukopenia, and nephropathy occur in 0.1 per cent of treated children. Renal reactions consisting of hematuria and dysuria usually do not appear until high-dose intravenous therapy is continued for 10 days or more. These toxic or irritative reactions disappear when dosage of the drug is reduced or therapy is changed to a nonpenicillin drug.

First-generation cephalosporins such as cephalothin and cephapirin, as well as clindamycin and vancomycin, are effective antistreptococcal agents useful for treating patients allergic to penicillin. Cephalosporins should not be used for central nervous system staphylococcal infections, since they diffuse poorly into cerebrospinal fluid.

The newer cephalosporins such as cefamandol, cefotaxime, and cefuroxime are not first-choice antibiotics for treating staphylococcal infections. In vitro sensitivity data show them to be less effective than less expensive first-generation cephalosporins.

The aminoglycosides, gentamicin and amikacin, are effective antistaphylococcal agents used in combination with beta-lactamase–resistant penicillins for initial therapy of serious staphylococcal infections. Aminoglycosides have bactericidal activity, and synergism can be demonstrated between other antistaphylococcal agents and aminoglycosides against most strains of *S. aureus* in vitro. It is reasonable, although controversial, to initiate therapy with a combination of aminoglycoside and nafcillin, clindamycin, or vancomycin when life-threatening *S. aureus* infection is suspected. The serious side effects

TABLE 1. Dosage Schedule of Drugs Useful in Treatment of Staphylococcal Infections *(Continued on p. 500)*

Antibiotic	Oral (for mild to moderate infection)	
	1 Month to 50 kg	*>50 kg or Maximum*
PENICILLINS		
Benzyl (Penicillin G)	50,000–150,000 units/kg/24 hr (4)	1.6–4.8 million units/24 hr (4)
Phenoxymethyl (Penicillin V, V-Cillin, Pen-Vee K, others)	50–100 mg/kg/24 hr (4)	1–4 gm/24 hr (4)
Methicillin (Staphcillin)	—	—
Oxacillin (Prostaphlin)	50–100 mg/kg/24 hr (4)	1–2 gm/24 hr (4)
Nafcillin (Unipen)	50–100 mg/kg/24 hr (4)	1–2 gm/24 hr (4)
Cloxacillin (Tegopen)	25–50 mg/kg/24 hr (4)	1–4 gm/24 hr (4)
Dicloxacillin (Dynapen, Pathocil, Veracillin)	12.5–25 mg/kg/24 hr (4)	0.5–2 gm/24 hr (4)
CEPHALOSPORINS		
Cephalothin (Keflin)	—	—
Cephapirin (Cefadyl)	—	—
Cefazolin (Ancef, Kefzol)	—	—
Cephalexin (Keflex)	25–50 mg/kg/24 hr (4)	1–4 gm/24 hr (4)
Cephradine (Anspor, Velosef)	25–50 mg/kg/24 hr (4)	1–4 gm/24 hr (4)
OTHERS		
Erythromycin lactobionate (Erythrocin-Lactobionate-IV) *AND* Erythromycin gluceptate (Ilotycin Gluceptate)	—	—
Erythromycin stearate and estolate (Erythrocin, E-mycin, Ilosone, others)	25–50 mg/kg/24 hr (4)	1–2 gm/24 hr (4)
Clindamycin (Cleocin)	10–20 mg/kg/24 hr (4)	600–1200 mg/24 hr (4)
Vancomycin (Vancocin)	—	—
Gentamicin (Garamycin)	—	—
Rifampin		10–20 mg/kg/day

Note: Numbers in parentheses: Number of doses into which the daily dose should be equally divided.

TABLE 1. Dosage Schedule of Drugs Useful in Treatment of Staphylococcal Infections *(Continued)*

Parenteral (for severe infection)			
<1 Week	*1 to 4 Weeks*	*1 Month to 50 kg*	*>50 kg or Maximum*
100,000 units/kg/24 hr IV every 12 hr	100,000–250,000 units/kg/24 hr IV every 6 hr	200,000–400,000 units/kg/24 hr IV every 4 hr	8–24 million units/24 hr IV every 4 hr
—	—	—	—
50–100 mg/kg/24 hr IV every 12 hr	100–200 mg/kg/24 hr IV every 6 hr	200–300 mg/kg/24 hr IV every 4 hr	6–12 gm/24 hr IV every 4 hr
50–100 mg/kg/24 hr IV every 12 hr	100 to 200 mg/kg/24 hr IM or IV every 6 hr	100–200 mg/kg/24 hr IV every 4 hr	4–8 gm/24 hr IV every 4 hr
40–60 mg/kg/24 hr IV every 12 hr	60 to 100 mg/kg/24 hr IM or IV every 6 hr	100–200 mg/kg/24 hr IV every 4 hr	4–8 gm/24 hr IV every 4 hr
—	—	—	—
40 mg/kg/24 hr IV every 12 hr	60 mg/kg/24 hr IV every 6 hr	100 mg/kg/24 hr IV every 4 hr	6–12 gm/24 hr IV every 4 hr
40 mg/kg/24 hr IV every 12 hr	60 mg/kg/24 hr IV every 6 hr	100 mg/kg/24 hr IV every 4 hr	6–12 gm/24 hr IV every 4 hr
40 mg/kg/24 hr IV every 12 hr	50 mg/kg/24 hr IV every 8 hr	50 mg/kg/24 hr IV every 6 hr	3–6 gm/24 hr IV every 6 hr
—	—	—	—
Not recommended	10–20 mg/kg/24 hr IV every 8 hr, infuse over 0.5–1 hr	10–20 mg/kg/24 hr IV every 6 hr, infuse over 0.5–1 hr	1.5–4 gm/24 hr IV every 6 hr, 1 gm diluted in 100 ml
—	—	—	—
Not recommended	20–40 mg/kg/24 hr IV every 6 hr, infuse over 30 min	20–40 mg/kg/24 hr IV every 6 hr, infuse over 30 min	1.2–2.4 gm/24 hr IV every 6 hr, 1 gm diluted in 100 ml
30 mg/kg/24 hr IV every 12 hr, infuse over 30 to 60 min	45 mg/kg/24 hr* IV every 8 hr, infuse over 1 hr	40–60 mg/kg/24 hr* IV every 6 hr, infuse over 1 hr	2 gm/24 hr IV every 6 hr, infuse over 1 hr
5 mg/kg/24 hr† IV every 12 hr	7.5 mg/kg/24 hr† IM every 8 hr	5 mg/kg/24 hr† IM every 8 hr	5 mg/kg/24 hr† IM every 8 hr

*These doses may exceed the manufacturer's recommended dosage.
†May be given IV slowly over 20 to 30 minutes.

glycosides to special circumstances once the in vitro antibiotic sensitivities of the infecting *Staphylococcus* are known. Aminoglycoside therapy can be stopped and the primary antistaphylococcal agent continued when patients improve clinically.

Vancomycin is an important antistaphylococcal agent. It is frequently used for treating systemic infections with *S. epidermidis* because of the frequent resistance of these organisms to penicillins, cephalosporins, and aminoglycosides. Vancomycin must be administered intravenously for treating staphylococcal infection, since it is not absorbed from the gastrointestinal tract. This property makes it useful for oral treatment of *Clostridium difficile* toxin–related pseudomembranous enterocolitis.

Vancomycin has been considered a highly toxic agent with serious side effects of ototoxicity and nephrotoxicity; however, these reactions were related to impurities in older preparations of the drug. Vancomycin is now highly purified and therapy is relatively free from serious side effects in patients with normal renal function.

Antibiotics may be administered by the intravenous route either continuously or intermittently. However, practical considerations usually make intermittent administration over a 10- to 20-minute period at 4- to 6-hour intervals the preferred schedule.

Rifampin is a valuable antibiotic for treating severe staphylococcal infections. *S. aureus* resistant to beta-lactamase antibiotics are usually exquisitely sensitive to rifampin, and synergistic or additive effects of rifampin can be demonstrated in vitro. Rifampin should always be used with another antibiotic, since staphylococci

rapidly develop resistance to rifampin. Rifampin is able to penetrate phagocytic cells, and since *S. aureus* may survive intracellularly, this property provides a clinical advantage.

Trimethoprim-sulfamethoxazole is another effective oral antistaphylococcal combination with an excellent spectrum of activity against beta-lactamase–producing *S. aureus*. The drug has been available in oral form for several years and has been licensed for intravenous administration to very sick patients.

Combination therapy with rifampin and trimethoprim-sulfamethoxazole has recently been shown to be effective for serious staphylococcal infections.

MILD TO MODERATE STAPHYLOCOCCAL INFECTIONS

Oral administration of antibiotics is acceptable when treating soft tissue infections that are considered mild or moderate. Cloxacillin and dicloxacillin are the beta-lactamase–resistant penicillins of choice, since absorption from the gastrointestinal tract is reliable and adequate serum levels are attained. Cephalexin or erythromycin may be used for patients allergic to penicillin.

Clindamycin is highly effective for treating staphylococcal infections in pediatric patients. The frequent occurrence of colitis limits its usefulness in adults, but this complication is much less frequent in pediatric age patients. Clindamycin is concentrated in phagocytes, which is a therapeutic advantage in certain clinical situations.

Duration of therapy is arbitrary, but the notorious difficulty in eradicating staphylococci from necrotic lesions and the frequency of recurrences dictate at least

2 weeks for most lesions. Nonspecific agents still being used for staphylococcal lesions include vaccines, toxoids, gamma globulins, and bacteriophages. None has survived the rigor of controlled trials and their use is not recommended.

SPECIFIC STAPHYLOCOCCAL INFECTIONS

Bullous Impetigo and Staphylococcal Scalded Skin Syndrome. *S. aureus* bullous impetigo can usually be treated with hygienic measures and topical antibiotic therapy. However, when extensive lesions are present, systemic antibiotics are necessary. Oral therapy with a beta-lactamase–resistant antibiotic such as dicloxacillin should be used. When large areas of the body are denuded, the disease is described as "scalded skin syndrome" and intravenous therapy with nafcillin should be used. Cephalothin or clindamycin may be used in patients allergic to penicillin. Once patients are stabilized, oral therapy is effective.

Abscesses. Furuncles and other skin lesions are the most common clinical infections caused by *S. aureus*. These lesions are often self-limited and heal spontaneously, but if there are systemic symptoms or cellulitis is present, antibiotic therapy and incision and drainage are indicated. Antibiotic choice is similar to that described for patients with *S. aureus* impetigo and scalded skin syndrome. Recurrent furunculosis is a difficult clinical problem and often requires prolonged antibiotic therapy; fortunately the oral route is satisfactory. Several family members may be involved and exquisite hygiene for all family members is necessary. Artificial colonization of the nasal mucosa with a strain of *S. aureus* of low virulence (502A, available from Henry Shinefield, M.D.) may interfere with autoinoculation by a patient's or family's more virulent resident strain. Care must be taken to assure that patients are immunologically normal before this form of therapy is employed.

Metastasis of *S. aureus* from skin lesions to bone or soft tissues such as liver, kidney, lung, and brain may occur. Deep abscesses require intravenous antibiotic therapy and drainage of accessible lesions after localization. If abscesses are present in the vicinity of foreign bodies, removal is necessary to prevent chronic suppuration. *S. epidermidis* may be the basis for suppurative lesions or bacteremia associated with vascular catheters and other foreign bodies and intensive prolonged antibiotic therapy is necessary for *S. epidermidis* as well as *S. aureus*. Appropriate antibiotics need to be administered for 6 to 12 weeks in order to eradicate staphylococci from deep-seated abscesses. Since many strains of *S. epidermidis* are insensitive to beta-lactamase–resistant penicillins, vancomycin therapy is necessary.

Septicemia, Osteomyelitis and Endocarditis. Staphylococcal bacteremia is a relatively frequent occurrence, and septicemia (symptomatic bacteremia) and endocarditis are constant threats. Secondary bacteremia, i.e., when a focus of infection is defined, can be treated by drainage, removal of vascular catheters or foreign bodies, and conventional antibiotic therapy for 1 to 2 weeks. Oral therapy with cloxacillin, clindamycin, or cephalexin is satisfactory. It must be remembered that patients with congenital or postoperative heart lesions and drug abusers are highly susceptible to endocarditis. *S. aureus* septicemia or endocarditis must be treated promptly and aggressively with intravenous antibiotics. The necrotizing properties of *S. aureus* lesions are especially dangerous when they involve the heart valves or brain, and combination therapy with nafcillin (vancomycin in penicillin sensitive individuals) and gentamicin should be given intravenously for maximum bactericidal action. Vancomycin should be the antibiotic of first choice when treating *S. epidermidis* endocarditis. Since many patients with staphylococcal endocarditis have artificial valves or other heart prostheses, removal of these foreign bodies may be necessary for cure.

Poor response to antibiotic agents that should be satisfactory by in vitro sensitivity testing may result from occult staphylococcal lesions or from "tolerance" of *S. aureus* to the agent. Tolerance, defined as dissociation between minimal inhibitory and minimal bactericidal concentrations of an antibiotic, is usually associated with beta-lactamase antibiotics that primarily act on staphylococcal cell walls. If tolerance is suspected, rifampin or an aminoglycoside should be added to the therapeutic regimen.

Infections of the Central Nervous System. Neurologic procedures using plastic tubes to relieve congenital or acquired obstructions to the flow of cerebrospinal fluid have resulted in susceptibility of the CNS to staphylococcal infections. Infections secondary to neurologic procedures are usually caused by *S. epidermidis*, and vancomycin is used for initial therapy. *S. aureus* infections of the CNS may be related to primary lesions at a distant site. High-dose intravenous nafcillin or vancomycin is necessary to treat *S. aureus* meningitis or brain abscess. Intrathecal medication should not be used. It is necessary to remove CNS shunts that have become infected with staphylococci. Antistaphylococcal therapy should be continued for at least 2 weeks after an infected shunt is removed, and if signs and symptoms of increased intracranial pressure dictate that a new shunt is needed, antibiotics should be continued for several days after the surgery.

Toxic Shock Syndrome. The toxic shock syndrome is secondary to infection with a toxin-producing strain of *S. aureus*. It occurs most frequently in young menstruating women presumably because tampon use favors *S. aureus* replication and production of toxin that is absorbed through mucous membranes and results in shock, rash, and severe diarrhea. Supportive therapy and replacement of fluid and electrolytes are critical in toxic shock syndrome. Antistaphylococcal therapy is aimed at preventing recurrences in toxic shock syndrome associated with menstruation. When the syndrome occurs in young children or males, identification of the site of infection, drainage, and therapy with beta-lactamase–resistant antibiotics are necessary. Shock may be associated with other serious staphylococcal infections as a consequence of massive fluid accumulation in local infections, a direct effect on cardiac function, or activation of complement and coagulation systems; therefore aggressive intravenous therapy with nafcillin or other beta-lactamase–resistant antibiotics is mandatory.

Pyomyositis. Pyomyositis is a staphylococcal disease associated with the tropics and primarily affects malnourished individuals. However, pyomyositis does occur in the United States. Staphylococci are present in the muscle or fasciae in this disease, and although there may be few objective signs of infection aside from muscle pain and swelling, a fatal outcome is frequent. When *S. aureus* organisms are identified, the infected site *must* be drained surgically and the patient treated aggressively with intravenous nafcillin or other beta-lactamase antibiotics.

GROUP A STREPTOCOCCAL INFECTIONS
BASCOM F. ANTHONY, M.D.

The group A beta-hemolytic streptococcus is the leading bacterial cause of acute pharyngitis. Streptococcal pharyngitis is a significant entity because of its continued high prevalence in children, the associated acute morbidity, and the potential complications. Correct diagnosis and appropriate treatment are desirable for several well-established reasons: (1) Antistreptococcal therapy is highly effective in the prevention of acute rheumatic fever; the resurgence of rheumatic fever in several regions of the United States since 1985 reinforces the importance of this rationale in the management of streptococcal pharyngitis; (2) therapy also reduces the frequency of the suppurative complications of streptococcal pharyngitis; (3) eradication of virulent group A streptococci from the pharynx prevents further spread to the patient's contacts; and (4) treatment significantly shortens the clinical illness associated with streptococcal pharyngitis, as confirmed in recent pediatric studies.

RECOGNITION OF STREPTOCOCCAL PHARYNGITIS

Most cases are not easily distinguished on clinical grounds alone from pharyngitis due to other causes. Clinical and epidemiologic clues are best used to determine patients who need laboratory evaluation for the presence of group A streptococci. Some selectivity in testing patients with symptoms of pharyngitis minimizes unnecessary procedures and reduces the number of carriers of streptococci (as opposed to patients with bona fide infection) who will be detected.

A throat culture that is properly processed and interpreted is considered the "gold standard" for identifying group A streptococci in the pharynx. However, this requires 1 or 2 days, and more rapid tests to detect specific streptococcal antigen in throat swabs are commonly used, primarily latex agglutination and enzyme-linked assays. With careful attention to quality control, the specificity of the better antigen tests is high enough that a positive test can be accepted as such, without the need for confirmation by culture. However, a negative antigen test should be followed by a standard throat culture, because of the decreased sensitivity of antigen detection when the swab contains only a few streptococci.

THERAPY AND FOLLOW-UP

Immediate antistreptococcal therapy is indicated when there is a positive test for group A streptococcal antigen, a high level of clinical suspicion, or severe symptoms compatible with streptococcal pharyngitis. Withholding antibiotics in other patients pending culture results is justified by the fact that many (the majority, in most studies) will not have a streptococcal etiology and will not require antimicrobial therapy and by the fact that rheumatic fever is prevented even when the treatment of streptococcal pharyngitis is delayed for several days.

Penicillin is the drug of choice, and both intramuscular and oral regimens are acceptable. A single injection of benzathine penicillin—600,000 units for patients weighing 60 pounds or less and 1.2 million units for larger patients—is considered optimal therapy by some experts. Alternatively, oral penicillin should be given as penicillin V, 125 or 250 mg three or four times a day. There is a tendency to discontinue treatment as symptoms resolve, but 10 days of oral penicillin is an absolute requirement for acceptable rates of success. Erythromycin is the drug of choice in penicillin-allergic patients and should be given as erythromycin estolate (20 to 40 mg/kg/day) or erythromycin ethylsuccinate (40 mg/kg/day) divided into three or four doses each day. Available evidence suggests that oral therapy may be simplified to two doses per day of penicillin or erythromycin, but one-a-day regimens are not recommended. Various other antibiotic agents are active against group A streptococci but are more expensive, provide excessively broad antimicrobial therapy, or have not been adequately evaluated for streptococcal pharyngitis. Drugs that are not recommended include the sulfonamides and tetracyclines.

After 24 hours of effective therapy, the patient is unlikely to infect others and can return to school or daycare and other normal activities if justified by clinical improvement. Follow-up throat cultures at the completion of therapy are not recommended in the absence of recurrent symptoms of pharyngitis, cases of rheumatic fever in the patient's immediate environment, or an outbreak of acute glomerulonephritis. Similarly, throat cultures of asymptomatic contacts are unnecessary except under unusual circumstances, such as those mentioned previously.

RHEUMATIC FEVER PROPHYLAXIS

Patients with a well-documented rheumatic fever history or rheumatic heart disease should be placed on an acceptable regimen of continuous prophylaxis against group A streptococcal infection. The best established of these is intramuscular benzathine penicillin, 1.2 million units every 4 weeks. Oral prophylaxis with sulfadiazine, 0.5 gm daily for patients under 60 pounds and 1.0 gm for others, or penicillin V, 125 to 250 mg twice a day, is also effective if patient and family are compliant.

It should be stressed that the preceding regimens are inadequate for the prevention of bacterial endocarditis in patients with valvular rheumatic heart disease and certain other cardiac lesions. Such patients undergoing dental or surgical procedures should receive prophylaxis as recommended in the article on Endocarditis and by the American Heart Association.

STREPTOCOCCAL IMPETIGO

Group A streptococci play a dominant role in common impetigo, which is to be distinguished from bullous impetigo caused by unique strains of *Staphylococcus aureus*. Systemic antibiotic therapy should be considered for all but the mildest cases to speed the healing of lesions, control such complications as cellulitis and lymphangitis, and limit the spread of infection. Effective therapy includes a single injection of Bicillin or 7 days of oral penicillin in the doses recommended for pharyngitis. Erythromycin is recommended for the penicillin-allergic patient. Good skin hygiene is recommended, and topical antimicrobials (e.g., bacitracin or mupirocin) may be useful for treating a single lesion or a few mild impetigo lesions. Although there is no evidence that antibiotic treatment prevents acute glomerulonephritis in the patient infected with a nephritogenic streptococcus, prophylaxis with benzathine penicillin may be useful in controlling outbreaks of acute poststreptococcal glomerulonephritis.

GROUP B STREPTOCOCCAL INFECTIONS

CAROL J. BAKER, M.D.

In the usual clinical setting, antimicrobial therapy for infection due to group B streptococci (GBS) must be initiated before culture results are known. Initial therapy generally consists of intravenous ampicillin and an aminoglycoside for the treatment of this as well as other neonatal pathogens. This combination has been shown to be more effective than ampicillin or penicillin G alone in the in vitro and in vivo killing of most GBS strains. However, synergy is not observed among isolates that are tolerant in vitro, an uncommon laboratory phenomenon that has no documented clinical relevance. Once GBS has been identified and its penicillin susceptibility verified, penicillin G or ampicillin alone is sufficient for the treatment of these infections.

Penicillin G remains the drug of choice for the treatment of infections caused by GBS, since susceptibility to this agent is uniform. However, the optimal dose and duration of therapy are dictated by the focus and severity of infection, since most reported relapses of infection can be attributed to inadequate dosage or length of therapy. Other facts important when considering appropriate dose are the following: (1) The minimal inhibitory concentration (MIC) of GBS to penicillin G is approximately 10-fold greater than that of group A streptococci; (2) the amount of penicillin G achievable in the cerebrospinal fluid (CSF) is at best 10 to 20 per cent of serum levels; (3) the inoculum of GBS in the CSF of infants with meningitis is often high (10^7 to 10^8); and (4) high doses of penicillin G and ampicillin are safe in the newborn. Therefore, to ensure rapid bacterial killing, especially in patients with meningitis, rela-

tively high doses of penicillin G or ampicillin are recommended for both early onset and late onset infections.

Irrespective of birth weight, infants with suspected or proven meningitis and those in whom the clinical condition will not permit lumbar puncture should receive ampicillin at a dose of 300 mg/kg/day in combination with an aminoglycoside, usually gentamicin. Once CSF sterility is documented in infants with meningitis (usually within 36 hours of therapy) *and* susceptibility to penicillin G is verified, penicillin G alone at a dose of 500,000 units/kg/day is given. Intravenous therapy should be continued for a minimum of 14 days, and longer if the course is particularly severe, if the infant has concomitant ventriculitis, or if there is delayed sterilization of the CSF. In the last circumstance, the presence of an unsuspected suppurative focus (subdural empyema, brain abscess, obstructive ventriculitis, or septic thrombophlebitis) should be suspected and excluded by appropriate studies. At the completion of therapy, a lumbar puncture should be repeated to determine whether the CSF findings are consistent with adequate therapy or suggest the need for additional treatment. Examples of the latter include polymorphonuclear cells in excess of 20 per cent of the total cells or a protein level in excess of 150 to 200 mg/dl. These findings may occur in infants with severe cerebritis, extensive parenchymal destruction with focal suppuration, severe vasculitis, or a combination of these.

Infants with bacteremia *without* meningitis should receive intravenous ampicillin (150 mg/kg/day) or penicillin G (200,000 units/kg/day) for 10 days. A shorter duration of therapy has no documented efficacy, and relapses, although rare, have been reported under these circumstances. Patients with septic arthritis, osteomyelitis, or endocarditis should be treated with intravenous penicillin G (200,000 to 300,000 units/kg/day) for 2 to 3 (arthritis), 3 to 4 (osteomyelitis), and 4 weeks (endocarditis). Oral therapy has no place in the management of infants with GBS infections. Alternative agents, such as the cephalosporins and vancomycin, are active against GBS in vitro, but their efficacy is unknown, and they are not recommended in the usual clinical situation.

When they occur, suppurative foci should be drained. For septic arthritis, involvement of the hip, and often the shoulder, dictates open surgical drainage. For other joints, needle aspiration on one or two occasions usually achieves adequate drainage. For osteomyelitis, open curettage of necrotic metaphyseal bone is required in most patients, and all should have diagnostic needle aspiration of the involved metaphyseal area to determine the etiologic agent *before* or within 24 hours of the initiation of antibiotic therapy. In the infant less than 2 months of age who presents with an indolent course, pseudoparalysis of an arm, and a metaphyseal lytic lesion, the propensity of GBS for the humerus, especially the proximal end, is an important clue that this agent is involved.

The importance of prompt, vigorous, and careful supportive therapy in the successful treatment of serious GBS infections in infants cannot be overstated. In infants with early onset infection accompanied by pneumonia, the need for ventilatory assistance should be anticipated before the onset of apnea or respiratory failure. The prompt treatment of shock in its early phases is critical. Persistent metabolic acidosis and delayed capillary refill are characteristic of this phase. All patients with signs of circulatory or respiratory failure or meningitis should be cared for in a neonatal or pediatric intensive care unit or transferred to one as promptly as possible. When present, hypoxemia or severe anemia should be corrected, seizures should be controlled with anticonvulsants, and acidosis should be treated. In addition, fluid and electrolyte status should be monitored meticulously. Adjunctive therapies for life-threatening GBS infections that are aimed at correction of "deficient" host defense mechanisms are under investigation. These include use of intravenous human immune globulins, nonsteroidal anti-inflammatory agents, and leukocyte transfusions in neutropenic patients. None has proven efficacy, and although they might be employed for individual patients, they should be considered experimental.

In infants with recurrent infection, suppurative foci should be excluded or treated if present, as should humoral immune deficiency. Quantitative immunoglobulins should be determined to exclude the latter. The GBS isolate should have tube dilution susceptibility testing to ensure in vitro susceptibility to penicillin G. If the reason for the recurrence remains unknown, it is likely that mucous membrane infection with GBS, which is not predictably eradicated by even parenteral therapy with penicillins, is the source. Although controlled studies supporting the use of oral rifampin at a dose of 10 mg/kg/day for 4 days at the *conclusion* of parenteral therapy have not been performed for such patients, such use of this agent may eradicate the source of infection.

The continuing magnitude and severity of GBS infections in infants has led to many investigations aimed at their prevention. Administration of penicillin G at birth is not effective in the prevention of early onset infection, since most have their onset in utero. However, selective intrapartum prophylaxis for women known to have genital or anorectal GBS infection during pregnancy is effective in the prevention of early onset GBS infections in infants. Maternal prophylaxis consists of intravenous ampicillin (an initial dose of 2 gm followed by 1 gm every 4 hours) until delivery. Selection criteria are based on the known increased risk of systemic infections in infants when predisposing conditions exist in maternal GBS carriers, including premature rupture of membranes, preterm delivery, prolonged rupture of membranes, chorioamnionitis, and/or intrapartum maternal fever. Therapy in the infant born to women given prophylaxis should be individualized. Term, healthy infants may require none, symptomatic infants obviously should be treated with broad-spectrum antibiotics pending laboratory results, and preterm infants may be given empiric therapy until laboratory results and clinical course clarify their need.

The second mode of prevention, immunoprophylaxis, remains investigational. This prevention method is based upon the observation that immunity to GBS depends on antibody to the capsular polysaccharides of these organisms. These antibodies, in combination with complement and polymorphonuclear leukocytes, allow for opsonization, phagocytosis, and bacterial killing of GBS. Since most pregnant women are "deficient" in these type-specific GBS antibodies, active immunization of women with polysaccharide or polysaccharide-protein vaccines has been advocated as a method for prevention. Similarly, use of human immune globulins has been suggested as a method to correct antibody "deficiencies." This method has the problem that existing intramuscular and intravenous preparations contain low concentrations of antibodies specific for GBS, suggesting that the volume required would be prohibitive. Further, if globulins were administered to the infant, these would be suitable only for prevention of late onset infections. Before recommendations concerning these methods of prophylaxis can be made, additional studies must be done.

LISTERIA MONOCYTOGENES INFECTION
ANNABEL J. TEBERG, M.D.

Listeria monocytogenes is a small, aerobic, motile, grampositive rod widely distributed in animal species and in the environment. Human infections occur both sporadically and in epidemics and arise primarily through consumption of contaminated food products. Since the *Listeria* organism continues to grow at temperatures as low as 4 to 6°C, refrigeration of contaminated food does not provide protection.

The organism is a relatively mild pathogen that affects primarily the immunocompromised host. Colonization is common; however, the attack rate in humans, although unknown, appears to be uncommon. Infection during pregnancy may be mild or even unrecognized in the mother but may result in abortion, preterm labor, infection of the fetus, or serious, often fatal, disease in the newborn. Mild or inapparent maternal infections during pregnancy are transmitted transplacentally or during delivery.

Neonatal listeriosis has been classified as "early onset" when intrauterine infection results in symptomatic illness at or soon after birth or as "late onset" when symptoms occur after the child is 5 days of age. In the infant, the disease may manifest as a generalized illness with septicemia or meningitis or both, as primarily a respiratory illness, or as a localized form, such as conjunctivitis. Although granulomatosis infantiseptica with disseminated abscesses and granulomas in multiple internal organs is considered characteristic of neonatal listeriosis, the more common presentation at birth is an acutely ill, normally grown infant, often premature, with severe respiratory distress but without evidence of prolonged intrauterine infection. The usual presenting picture of neonatal listeriosis is indistinguishable from that of other congenital infections. Although listerial meningitis is a serious neonatal problem, the primary pneumonic presentation may be the most difficult to manage and has the greatest degree of mortality. This infection must be considered in any normally grown preterm infant with evidence of fetal distress during labor and with meconium- or brown-stained amniotic fluid who has depression or respiratory distress at birth. Because of the severity of listerial disease, rapid institution of therapy is important; antimicrobials effective against *Listeria* should be administered after appropriate cultures are taken but before reports are available.

Ampicillin is considered the drug of choice for the treatment of listeriosis. Penicillin is also highly effective. Resistance to either of these two drugs is rare, and most clinical failures can be related to treatment begun too late or given for too short a time or characterized by inadequate drug dosage.

During the first week of life, therapy should be with ampicillin, 100 to 200 mg/kg/day given intravenously (IV) in two divided doses, and from the second to fourth week of life, 200 to 300 mg/kg/day in three divided doses. Thereafter, the dosage recommended should be 200 to 400 mg/kg/day in four to six divided doses, depending upon the severity of the infection. Although maintenance of therapy for 2 weeks is usually sufficient, 3 weeks of therapy or longer may be necessary in cases of *Listeria* meningitis.

Ampicillin and penicillin have been shown to act synergistically with an aminoglycoside against *Listeria*, so that combination therapy is recommended in newborns and in patients with systemic listeriosis. Gentamicin is currently the aminoglycoside of choice. Dosage in the first week of life is 5 mg/kg/day IV, divided into two doses. Consideration of the immaturity of the renal system of the premature infant requires that drug serum levels be monitored to ensure continued appropriate dosage levels. After 1 week of life (in the term infant), 7.5 mg/kg/day IV in three divided doses is recommended, again monitoring the drug serum levels as indicated. Usually, after 2 weeks of combined therapy, all cultures are negative, and gentimicin may be discontinued.

Listeria monocytogenes is also susceptible in vitro to tetracycline, erythromycin, sulfonamides, cephalosporins, chloramphenicol, trimethoprim-sulfamethoxazole, and rifampin, any of which may be used when an allergy to penicillin exists. Chloramphenicol is preferred for intracranial infections, and tetracyclines should not be used in children under 8 years of age.

Supportive measures are important, particularly in the premature infant, in whom infection with *Listeria* is an additional, often fatal, complication of the many problems so often found in the immature infant.

The woman who is pregnant or in the postpartum period and who has symptomatic listeriosis may be treated with ampicillin. However, the ability to prevent abortion, preterm labor, or an affected newborn by treating the asymptomatic pregnant woman with positive cultures remains unclear, especially since the majority of these pregnancies are uncomplicated and unrecognized for involvement with *Listeria* until the onset of labor.

DIPHTHERIA

C. GEORGE RAY, M.D.

The most important agent for the treatment of diphtheria is specific antitoxin, preferably given intravenously. A single dose should be promptly administered on the basis of a clinical diagnosis alone, even before culture results become available. This is because *Corynebacterium diphtheriae* exotoxin can rapidly attach to cells, and only free, unattached toxin can be neutralized by the antitoxin. It has been shown that such treatment begun on the first or second day of illness, compared with the fourth day or later, is associated with a reduction in the case fatality rate from 16.9 to 1.3 per cent; however, antitoxin should be administered even if the duration of symptoms prior to presentation may appear to be prolonged. Since diphtheria antitoxin is a horse serum, testing for sensitivity is required as a prelude to administration. This testing can be done with a 1:10 antitoxin dilution in saline for conjunctival testing or 1:100 dilution for intradermal testing. If the patient is sensitive, careful desensitization is necessary. An intravenous protocol is suggested as the safest approach.

Antitoxin dose ranges are as follows: pharyngeal or laryngeal disease of a duration of 48 hours or less, or cutaneous disease, 20,000 to 40,000 units; nasopharyngeal lesions, 40,000 to 60,000 units; and extensive disease of more than 2 days' duration or brawny swelling of the neck, 80,000 to 100,000 units.

Although antimicrobial therapy is required to eradicate the organism and prevent spread, it is not a substitute for antitoxin. The choice is 14 days of either erythromycin (given parenterally or orally) at 40 mg/kg/day (maximum, 2 gm/day) or intramuscular procaine penicillin G, 300,000 units/day for those weighing 10 kg or less and 600,000 units/day for others. Eradication of the organism should be documented by three consecutive nasopharyngeal and throat cultures after completion of treatment. If this has not been achieved, a second 5-day course of oral penicillin or erythromycin should be given and the cultures repeated.

COMPLICATIONS

Myocarditis, respiratory obstruction, oculomotor, palatal, and pharyngeal weakness or paralysis, peripheral neuritis, and thrombocytopenia represent the major complications that can occur. Of these, myocarditis and respiratory obstruction are the most life threatening. Evidence of myocarditis can be found in the first week of illness in 50 per cent of patients with respiratory tract involvement if electrocardiography is performed frequently. Any electrocardiographic abnormalities or cardiac symptoms that develop are indications for continuous cardiac monitoring. Atrioventricular block and left bundle branch block have been associated with a greater than 50 per cent mortality risk, and electric pacing with temporary transvenous electrodes or a myocardial demand pacemaker may be required. Otherwise, arrhythmias are treated with agents such as procainamide, lidocaine, and isoproterenol. For congestive heart failure, short-acting digitalis preparations are given, and fluid and sodium are restricted. One randomized (but not double-blinded) study of 132 patients has also suggested that early initiation of oral L-Carnitine, 50 mg/kg twice daily for 4 days, may result in decreased incidences of heart failure, the necessity for pacemaker implantation, and mortality. On the other hand, there is no proven benefit of corticosteroid therapy in preventing either diphtheritic myocardial or neurologic complications.

Laryngeal, tracheal, and bronchial obstruction by pseudomembranes may require treatment by intubation, aspiration, bronchoscopy, or tracheostomy. If swallowing difficulties are present, measures to prevent aspiration, such as frequent pharyngeal suction, are required. All patients with diphtheria should be kept in bed and should avoid exertion for at least 2 weeks, until it is certain that all danger of cardiac damage has passed. Peripheral neuritis involving the extremities may not appear for a month or more after the initial illness. This neuritis is usually mild and self-limited, requiring no specific treatment. In rare instances, respiratory muscles are affected, and the patient may need assisted ventilation.

In contrast to nasal or pharyngeal diphtheria, skin infections are much less likely to be accompanied by toxic symptoms. Thorough cleansing of the lesion and administration of antimicrobials for 10 days are recommended. The need for antitoxin in cutaneous infections is debatable but is recommended by some authorities.

Not all patients who recover from diphtheria will develop adequate antitoxic immunity. Therefore, active immunization should be undertaken, commencing during convalescence.

CONTACTS

Household and other close contacts of a diphtheria patient who show clinical evidence of diphtheria should be cultured and treated with antitoxin and penicillin or erythromycin at once. Close contacts who are asymptomatic and have been immunized previously should have cultures done (nasopharynx, throat, and any skin lesions) and should receive a booster dose of either pediatric- or adult-type diphtheria toxoid, depending upon their age. They should also be observed carefully for 7 days. If *C. diphtheriae* is isolated, the contact should be treated with penicillin or erythromycin.

Asymptomatic close contacts with a negative or doubtful history of previous immunization should have cultures done and should be given 40 mg/kg/day of erythromycin orally for 7 days or one dose of 600,000 to 1,200,000 units of benzathine penicillin G intramuscularly. Immunization with either diphtheria-pertussis-tetanus (DPT) vaccine or pediatric- or adult-type diphtheria and tetanus toxoids, depending upon age, should be started. They should also be observed daily for 7 days. We do not believe that the prophylactic use of antitoxin is warranted because of the risk of allergic reactions to horse serum.

Medical and nursing attendants of a diphtheria patient should also be considered close contacts and treated accordingly.

PERTUSSIS

MELVIN I. MARKS, M.D.

Pertussis continues to be a major problem in developing countries and in other poorly immunized populations. The term "pertussis" is reserved for respiratory infection due to the bacterium *Bordetella pertussis*; however, pertussis-like syndromes are occasionally noted in association with infection due to *B. parapertussis*, *B. bronchiseptica*, *Chlamydia trachomatis*, adenovirus, and combinations of these microorganisms. The age of the patient, immunization status, virulence of the bacteria, and stage of the disease are major determinants of the clinical expression.

Supportive Care. The younger the patient, the more important the supportive care in cases of pertussis due to *Bordetella pertussis*. In fact, respiratory compromise due to obstructive secretions, aspiration of secretions and/or vomitus, and central nervous system complications (apnea, seizures) are the major causes of severe morbidity and death in this infectious disease. These are most prevalent in infants in the first year of life, particularly those under 6 months of age. Hence, these patients with pertussis need to be assessed very carefully for two features. One is the severity of the clinical disease, and the other is the ability of the family to provide appropriate supportive care. There should be no hesitation about admitting such patients to the hospital. This should probably be done with all infants under 6 months of age and with many under 1 year of age. For example, a brief period of in-hospital training may be necessary to help parents learn how to observe the child and how to manage the secretions, vomiting, and paroxysmal episodes.

These patients most commonly come to medical attention during the early paroxysmal stage. During this stage, a variety of stimuli will precipitate a paroxysm in infants, which is often followed by vomiting and occasionally by apnea, cyanosis, and severe distress. It is important, therefore, to provide the most comforting, quiet environment. This is often achieved by the parent or nursing staff, provided these caretakers have appropriate expectations about the clinical expression of disease and its complications. Pollutant-free air and a solicitous, caring observer are most important. Infants are often most calm in the arms of their mother or other caretakers in such a situation. Invasive procedures, such as blood taking, suctioning, and measurement of vital signs, should be kept to a minimum and are probably best done immediately after a paroxysm, when there is some refractoriness to further coughing. Suctioning should be gentle and should be used in addition to the head-down position for handling excessive secretions and vomitus. Adequate hydration and nutrition are important, since excessive secretions and vomiting can disturb fluid and electrolyte balance and the nutritional status of the host in a dramatic fashion. Humidified oxygen should be administered to patients with cyanosis and apnea and when blood gas levels indicate true hypoxemia. The risks and benefits of masks, tents, and other methods for administering oxygen need to be weighed carefully in such cases. Humidified air in a mist tent is contraindicated.

Respiratory isolation is important, since pertussis is so highly contagious. Nonetheless, immune individuals (e.g., the child's mother) who are providing constant care for the patient should avoid wearing masks if possible. Similarly, isolation should be carefully done but should not be a deterrent to observation. Infants with paroxysmal pertussis under 6 months of age and those with apnea should never be left alone, because apnea, convulsions, and aspiration are frequent and life-threatening complications.

Antibiotic Therapy. Erythromycin estolate is the most active drug against *B. pertussis* in vitro and in vivo and should be administered in all cases. This is done primarily to reduce contagiousness, although administration of the drug may reduce the severity of the disease if given during the catarrhal phase. The appropriate dosage of erythromycin estolate is 50 mg/kg/day given orally in divided doses every 6 hours, for 14 days. Respiratory isolation can be relaxed after approximately 5 days of erythromycin therapy, since the bacteria will be eliminated from the nasopharynx during this period of time in almost all patients. Fourteen days of therapy are recommended, since bacteriologic relapses have been reported with shorter durations. Although chloramphenicol, trimethoprim-sulfamethoxazole, ampicillin, and some cephalosporins (cefoperazone and cefotaxime) are active in vitro against *B. pertussis*, there is limited clinical experience with these agents and additional side effects are expected with their use, particularly in infants.

Occasionally Useful Therapy. Adrenal corticosteroids have been used in infants with particularly severe paroxysmal disease in an effort to reduce the host's inflammatory response, which is thought to be mediated by toxins elaborated by these bacteria. Although preliminary studies indicate this, and some bronchodilators, such as albuterol* and salbutamol,* reduce the severity of paroxysms and other complications of the disease, there are insufficient controlled studies to justify their use on a routine basis. Currently, prescription of these pharmacologic agents should be limited to hospitalized infants with severe paroxysmal disease and with careful observation for the known toxicities of these agents. Corticosteroids (beta-methasone in oral doses of 0.075 mg/kg/day or hydrocortisone in intramuscular doses of 30 mg/kg/day) can be given for two days and then in gradually tapered dosages for one week. Albuterol* can be given at a dosage level of 0.5 mg/kg/day during the severe paroxysmal stage. Intubation and ventilation may be useful in selected cases.

Knowledge of the complications of pertussis is important in order to diagnose and manage bronchopneumonia, otitis media, apnea, and convulsions. Other manifestations of the disease, such as rectal prolapse and petechiae, may be referable to the extreme pressures developed during the paroxysmal stage and may occasionally be attributed to therapies as well.

*The safety and efficacy of these agents in children less than 12 years of age have not been established.

Prevention. Avoidance of exposure and appropriate immunization with pertussis vaccine are most effective. Exposed susceptible individuals under 6 years of age should receive a booster dose of vaccine if their primary series of immunizations (three doses, each separated by at least 4 weeks, plus a booster dose at 1 year and 18 months) is incomplete, or if more than 2 years have elapsed since immunization. Immunization can be initiated shortly after birth in epidemic situations and in highly endemic regions. Erythromycin can also be administered at the time of exposure or at the earliest onset of catarrhal symptoms in exposed susceptible individuals at any age. To avoid outbreaks in closed populations, erythromycin and strict respiratory isolation may be necessary for all subjects over 6 years of age. Immune globulin has no proven value in the prevention or treatment of pertussis.

PNEUMONIA

SHELDON L. KAPLAN, M.D.

Although the diagnosis of pneumonia in infants and children can be readily established by a chest roentgenogram once it is suspected after a history is obtained and the physical examination is performed, the etiology of the pneumonia is much more difficult to determine. Only a small percentage (5 per cent) of children with "outpatient" pneumonia will have positive blood cultures. Bacterial antigen can be detected in sera, urine, or pleural fluid in up to 25 per cent of such patients. According to most studies, in young children, the majority of cases in which an etiologic diagnosis of pneumonia is established have a viral cause. Many children appear to have both a viral and a bacterial component to their illness; presumably, the viral infection predisposes the child to the bacterial infection. Furthermore, from a clinical standpoint and from findings on a chest roentgenogram, viral and bacterial pneumonia cannot be easily distinguished. The white blood cell count offers no help in this regard either. Unfortunately, under ordinary circumstances, no etiology is established in most children with pneumonia. Therefore, antimicrobial therapy is initiated and continued on the basis of the most likely pathogens for age, immunologic competence of the host, clinical appearance of the patient, and the mode of acquisition, that is, community versus hospital acquired. As with any infection, the most specific antibiotic is administered when a bacterium is isolated and the antimicrobial susceptibility is determined.

SPECIAL CONSIDERATIONS IN TREATMENT

The decision to treat a child with either parenteral (Table 1) or oral antibiotics is dependent on several factors. Hospitalization for close observation and intravenous antibiotic therapy for pneumonia are indicated for infants, children with underlying deficiencies in host defense, and patients who are acutely ill and have respiratory distress, including tachypnea, accessory res-

TABLE 1. Parenteral Antibiotics and Doses for Children with Pneumonia

Agent	Spectrum of Activity	Dose (mg/kg/day)	Comments
Ampicillin	*Streptococcus pneumoniae* Other streptococci (Groups A and B) *Streptococcus faecalis* *Haemophilus influenzae* Type b (ampicillin susceptible)	150–200 q 6 hr	See text for discussion concerning neonates
Aminoglycosides Gentamicin Tobramycin Amikacin	Gram-negative enterics (*Escherichia coli,* *Klebsiella pneumoniae, Proteus* spp.) *Pseudomonas* spp.	Gentamicin, 4.5–7.5 q 8 hr Tobramycin, 6–9 q 8 hr Amikacin, 15–30 q 8 hr	Which aminoglycoside to use depends upon susceptibility pattern in the hospital; must monitor levels; dose reduced in renal dysfunction
Extended-spectrum Penicillins Ticarcillin Piperacillin Azlocillin Mezlocillin	Gram-negative enterics *Pseudomonas* Streptococci	200–300 q 6 hr	Used in combination with aminoglycosides
Nafcillin/oxacillin	*Staphylococcus aureus* *S. pneumoniae*	150–200 q 4–6 hr	
Vancomycin	Methicillin-resistant staphylococci	40–60 q 6 hr	Monitor levels; dose reduced in renal dysfunction
Cefazolin	*S. aureus* Streptococci *S. pneumoniae*	50–100 q 6–8 hr	For use in penicillin-allergic patient
Cefuroxime	*S. pneumoniae* *Branhamella catarrhalis* *S. aureus* Streptococci *H. influenzae* Type b	100–150 q 8 hr	Not approved for children <3 months of age
Cefotaxime	*H. influenzae* Type b Gram-negative enterics Streptococci, *B. catarrhalis* Moderate activity against *S. aureus*	100–150 q 6 hr	—
Ceftriaxone	Same as cefotaxime	50–75 q 12–24 hr	—
Ceftazidime	Gram-negative enterics *Pseudomonas*	150 q 6–8 hr	—
Chloramphenicol	*H. influenzae* *B. catarrhalis* Streptococci *S. pneumoniae* Anaerobes	50 q 6 hr	Must monitor levels
Erythromycin gluceptate or lactobionate	*M. pneumoniae* *Chlamydia trachomatis* *Legionella* spp.	15–20 q 6 hr	Thrombophlebitis may occur
Trimethoprim-sulfamethoxazole	Mainly for *Pneumocystis carinii*	100 of the sulfamethoxazole component q 6 hr	
Acyclovir	Herpes simplex Varicella zoster	250 mg/m² q 8 hr 500 mg/m² q 8 hr	Neonatal dose, 10 mg/kg q 8 hr; Dose requires adjustment in renal failure; Neurotoxicity with excessive levels
Amantadine (oral)	Influenza A	5 q 12 hr × 7 days	Do not exceed 150 mg/day for children <10 yr
Ribavirin	Respiratory syncytial virus (RSV)	Aerosol for 3 to 7 days	Expensive
Amphotericin B	*Candida* spp.	1.0 once daily	Must monitor renal function and serum potassium concentrations

piratory muscle use, or hypoxemia, if arterial blood gas measurements have been obtained. In addition, the physician must assess the ability of the patient to ingest and keep down medicine as well as the compliance of the family or caretaker in giving the antibiotic.

Neonates. The pathogens recovered from neonates with perinatally acquired pneumonia most commonly include group B streptococcus, other streptococci, and gram-negative enteric bacteria, especially *Escherichia coli*, and nontypable *Haemophilus influenzae*. Thus, empiric administration of ampicillin plus an aminoglycoside is reasonable. Since the incidence of ampicillin resistance is unclear for *H. influenzae* isolates recovered from

vaginal sources or from neonates, and since *Pseudomonas* spp. are unlikely pathogens for early onset pneumonia in the neonate, cefotaxime could be substituted for the aminoglycoside for initial therapy. Severe pneumonia that develops after the first few days of life can be due to herpes simplex. Acyclovir should be added to the antimicrobial coverage if herpes simplex pneumonia is suspected.

Infants 1 to 3 Months of Age. In this age group, viruses are the predominant cause of pneumonia. Nevertheless, bacteria, including *Staphylococcus aureus*, that are encountered in the neonate, as well as pathogens seen in older infants and children (namely, *Streptococcus* *pneumoniae* and *H. influenzae* Type b), can cause pneumonia in this age group. *Chlamydia trachomatis* classically causes an afebrile pneumonitis in infants of this age but can also cause the child to present with apneic episodes.

In the febrile, ill-appearing infant, empiric therapy with a penicillinase-resistant penicillin (nafcillin or oxacillin) plus cefotaxime will cover most of the common bacterial pathogens for this age group. If *S. aureus* is isolated, a sweat test should be performed, since staphylococcal pneumonia can be the initial presentation of cystic fibrosis. When *Chlamydia* pneumonia is suspected, erythromycin ethylsuccinate (40 mg/kg/day for 2 weeks) is the drug of choice. This infection can be rapidly confirmed by direct immunofluorescence microscopy or enzyme immunoassay of nasopharyngeal secretions.

Respiratory syncytial virus (RSV) is an important cause of pneumonia in infants in this age group and can cause apnea in addition to the respiratory infection. Again, this agent can be rapidly detected in nasopharyngeal secretions by commercially available enzyme immunoassays. In young infants with underlying immune or cardiopulmonary diseases or those with severe RSV infection (hypoxia and rising P_{CO_2}), ribavirin administration may be beneficial. Ribavirin is expensive to administer and should not be prescribed for infants who are mildly ill with RSV pneumonitis.

Children 3 Months to 5 Years. Again, in this group of children, the most common proven etiology of pneumonia is a virus. *S. pneumoniae* and *H. influenzae* Type b are clearly the most important bacterial causes. For children who require hospitalization because of either age or degree of illness, intravenous cefuroxime is a convenient single agent with in vitro activity against the most common bacterial pathogens causing pneumonia, including ampicillin-resistant *H. influenzae* Type b. Cefuroxime is also active against strains of *S. pneumoniae* that are relatively resistant to penicillin and currently account for 5 to 15 per cent of pneumococci isolated from normally sterile sites in children. Cefuroxime also covers *S. aureus* adequately, so that a specific penicillinase-resistant penicillin is not required initially to treat the patient. Ceftriaxone is an alternative for initial monotherapy of pneumonia in this age group. If no organism is isolated, pneumococcal polysaccharide antigen is not detected in serum or urine, or an ampicillin-resistant *H. influenzae* Type b is recovered, cefuroxime can be continued. If *S. pneumoniae* or an *H. influenzae* Type b susceptible to ampicillin is isolated, aqueous penicillin or ampicillin can be administered, respectively.

Once the child is afebrile, has improved symptomatically, and is able to take oral medication, an oral antibiotic can be substituted for the parenteral agent. If an organism has been isolated, it is not difficult to decide which oral agent to administer. On the other hand, since a bacterium is recovered or an antigen detected in the minority of children, the selection of an oral drug to complete parenteral therapy is more problematic. Amoxicillin, amoxicillin plus clavulanic acid, trimethoprim-sulfamethoxazole, erythromycin-sulfisoxazole, and cefaclor are all reasonable choices. Which antibiotic to administer is based on price, adverse effects, and personal preferences, unless ampicillin-resistant *H. influenzae* Type b is highly suspected, in which case amoxicillin is not appropriate therapy. These same oral antibiotics are employed for the initial therapy of outpatients with pneumonia. Amoxicillin is generally used as the initial oral antibiotic for pneumonia in a child who has not recently received this antibiotic for some other infection, such as otitis media. Influenza virus is an important cause of pneumonia during the influenza season. If the child has other clinical features consistent with influenza A, which is known to be circulating within the community, administration of amantadine should be considered.

Children Older Than 6 Years. In this age group, *S. pneumoniae* and *Mycoplasma pneumoniae* are the major bacterial agents causing pneumonia in outpatients. Cold agglutinins tested at bedside may help one determine if an *M. pneumoniae* infection is likely to be present. If the bedside cold agglutinin test is strongly positive, erythromycin therapy is appropriate and will also treat pneumonia due to *S. pneumoniae*. Otherwise, penicillin is adequate therapy.

Intravenous aqueous penicillin G or cefuroxime is sufficient initial therapy for the normal child over 6 years of age who is hospitalized with pneumonia. If pneumonia complicates a preceding viral infection, such as influenza or varicella, *S. aureus* is a likely pathogen, and thus nafcillin or oxacillin should be included in the initial antibiotic regimen.

Repeat Chest Roentgenogram. If a normal child with pneumonia responds promptly to antibiotic therapy, is clinically well, and has a normal physical examination at follow-up, a repeat chest roentgenogram is optional. However, a repeat chest roentgenogram at 6 weeks after initial treatment is indicated if the child has continuing symptoms and signs of pneumonia or if a foreign body aspiration or congenital malformation is suspected. The possibility of primary pulmonary tuberculosis should always be kept in mind, and an intermediate-strength purified protein derivative (PPD) should be placed if the child does not respond to therapy as expected or has any history suggestive of exposure to tuberculosis.

Duration of Therapy. Except in complicated cases, such as those involving pleural empyema, or disease due to *S. aureus*, a total of 10 to 14 days of parenteral or oral therapy, or both, is generally adequate to treat bacterial pneumonia in otherwise normal children.

Nosocomial Pneumonias and Pneumonias in Immunocompromised Children. Hospital-acquired pneumonias occur most commonly in children who are intubated and dependent upon mechanical ventilation. The bacteria causing the pneumonias usually are the organisms that colonize the orotracheal tree. Fever, a change in sputum characteristics, and new pulmonary infiltrates on a chest roentgenogram generally raise the possibility that pneumonia has developed in such patients. Initially, antibiotic therapy is directed against the organisms colonizing the patient or known nosocomial pathogens within the intensive care unit in accordance with their established antimicrobial susceptibility patterns. In general, an aminoglycoside is included in the initial antibiotic regimen, since gram-negative pneumonias are common in this setting. If methicillin-resistant staphylococci are endemic within a unit, vancomycin should also be considered in the initial therapy. A Gram stain of material obtained through the endotracheal tube may be useful if polymorphonuclear leukocytes are abundant and one organism is predominant. Unfortunately, unless the patient is bacteremic or other invasive procedures are undertaken, the exact etiology of these hospital-acquired pneumonias cannot be determined precisely. One should not forget that viral pneumonia can be nosocomial in origin, especially when RSV or influenza viruses are prevalent in the community.

Deciding which antimicrobial agent to administer empirically to children with pneumonia and deficiencies in host defense is particularly difficult. The likely pathogens differ to some degree with the nature of the underlying host immune compromise. Children with leukemia and neutropenia secondary to chemotherapy are very susceptible to gram-negative organisms. Usually, an aminoglycoside plus an extended-spectrum penicillin (ticarcillin, piperacillin, and so on) is administered. An antistaphylococcal penicillin or vancomycin is appropriate if the child has an indwelling central line that frequently is infected with gram-positive organisms.

Cefuroxime covers the common organisms isolated from children with sickle cell anemia and pneumonia. Since encapsulated bacteria are the predominant pathogens from children with acquired immunodeficiency syndrome (AIDS) or congenital hypogammaglobulinemia, cefuroxime again is a logical choice for initial monotherapy. *Pneumocystis carinii* is always a consideration when any of these patients present with fever, coughing, hypoxia, and diffuse alveolar infiltrates. In such cases, parenteral trimethoprim-sulfamethoxazole should be administered promptly. Other opportunistic organisms, such as fungi, *Legionella* spp., and cytomegalovirus, must also be considered in these patients.

MENINGOCOCCAL DISEASE

ELI GOLD, M.D.

The choice of antimicrobial agents for meningococcal infection in children is dependent upon the certainty of a specific diagnosis. In most situations, treatment is initiated when a child is acutely ill with fever, toxicity, and a petechial or maculopapular rash suggestive of meningococcal disease. There may or may not also be an abnormal spinal fluid. Treatment should be immediate before laboratory studies are complete and in the young child should include antimicrobial coverage appropriate for the major causes of bacteremia and meningitis in that age group. The choices are several. I still prefer ampicillin, 300 mg/kg/24 hr in six divided doses intravenously (IV), plus chloramphenicol sodium succinate, 100 mg/kg/24 hr IV in four divided doses. Cefotaxime, 200 mg/kg/24 hr or ceftriaxone, 100 to 150 mg/kg/24 hr, is an acceptable alternative. When the etiology is confirmed, which may require 24 to 48 hours,

one may switch to penicillin G, 400,000 units/kg/24 hr IV in six divided doses, or, for the child with allergy to penicillin, chloramphenicol or either of the cephalosporins. Whenever chloramphenicol is administered beyond 3 days, the serum concentration is measured and the dose modified to maintain a peak level below 25 µg/ml. The duration of therapy is usually 10 days but can be shortened to 7 with either meningococcemia or meningococcal meningitis if the response is rapid and the patient has been afebrile for at least 72 hours.

Children with meningococcal infection may develop a fulminant form of disease with disseminated intravascular coagulation, profound hypotension, and coma or may have involvement of joints, heart, or lungs. Careful monitoring of vital organs should be performed during the first hours of treatment, and appropriate additional therapy should be initiated as indicated. Intravenous hydrocortisone in doses of 10 mg/kg repeated at variable frequency has been used to treat shock, along with blood and fluids. (See "The Management of Septic Shock.")

Correlates of a poor prognosis are meningococcemia without meningitis, hypotension with a systolic blood pressure of less than 70 mm Hg in children up to 14 years of age, presence of petechiae for less than 12 hours prior to admission, hyperpyrexia (rectal temperature of greater than 40°C), peripheral leukocytosis of less than 15,000 per cubic millimeter of blood, or thrombocytopenia (<100,000 platelets per cubic millimeter of blood). Patients who have two or more of these signs are severely ill and require constant vigilance and intense care.

Patients with meningococcal infection should be maintained in "respiratory isolation" until treatment has been given for 24 hours. Rifampin is recommended for the prophylaxis of close contacts at a dosage of 600 mg orally every 12 hours for four doses in adults, 10 mg/kg every 12 hours for four doses in children 1 to 12 years of age, and 5 mg/kg every 12 hours for four doses in infants less than 1 year of age. Observation for onset of illness of exposed individuals even after prophylaxis is prudent.

Meningococcal vaccine is available for children at risk for meningococcal disease, especially those with complement deficiency, asplenism, or other forms of immune deficiency.

INFECTIONS DUE TO *ESCHERICHIA COLI, PROTEUS, KLEBSIELLA-ENTEROBACTER-SERRATIA, PSEUDOMONAS,* AND OTHER GRAM-NEGATIVE BACILLI

HARRIS D. RILEY, Jr., M.D., *and* MICHAEL J. MUSZYNSKI, M.D.

Although the management of infections due to these organisms must be individualized, certain generalizations can be made. Few infections that the physician is called upon to treat pose as difficult a problem as do those due to gram-negative coliform bacilli. Infections with these organisms are increasing in frequency, particularly as a hospital-associated phenomenon. Although new antibiotics have become available to which certain of these organisms are susceptible, the susceptibility of a given strain is unpredictable, and susceptible strains may develop resistance relatively rapidly. Furthermore, most of the antimicrobials that have activity against these organisms are accompanied by a significant risk of toxicity.

The fact that infections due to these organisms are particularly common in postoperative patients and in those debilitated by other disorders or therapies compounds the difficulties by limiting the choice of available therapeutic agents and makes evaluation of antibacterial treatment more perplexing. Because of the variability in response to therapy, careful bacteriologic study and in vitro susceptibility tests should precede initiation of therapy.

In general, comparatively large doses of the selected antimicrobial agent(s) should be utilized and should be continued for relatively long periods. Infection, especially bacteremia, due to these and other gram-negative bacteria, may be accompanied by clinical shock secondary to the elaboration of endotoxins. Appropriate supportive therapy for this complication is an important phase of the total management.

Antimicrobial agents of choice against the relatively common gram-negative bacilli are shown in Table 1. The most reliable guide to the choice of an antimicrobial agent is the result of in vitro antibiotic susceptibility tests. However, in many instances, particularly in infants and children, treatment must be initiated after appropriate cultures are obtained but before the results of these studies are known. Table 1 can be used as a general guide in such situations. The choice of a particular drug depends upon many different circumstances: epidemiologic information, particularly whether the infection is community or hospital acquired; the clinical picture, including the site of infection and presence of underlying disease; the frequency of resistance to various antimicrobials among various organisms in the local area; and others.

The dose, route of administration, and other details of therapeutic use of the various antimicrobial agents useful in the treatment of infections due to these organisms are listed in Table 2. Since these infections occur frequently in the neonatal and infancy periods, the difference in the pharmacology and metabolism of drugs in patients in these age groups, as well as in patients with impaired renal function, should be recalled. The dosage schedule for newborn and low birth weight infants is also included.

INFECTIONS

Escherichia coli Infections

Escherichia coli are gram-negative, motile rods normally found as part of the bacterial flora of the gastrointestinal tract. They have the capacity to produce a

powerful endotoxin, which enters the circulation and induces shock and the clinical pathologic picture of the Shwartzman phenomenon.

Infection in the Neonate. Gram-negative bacilli, particularly *E. coli*, are among the most common causes of septicemia and meningitis in the neonate. In most areas of the United States, *E. coli* and *Klebsiella-Enterobacter-Serratia* account for a large segment of the cases. *E. coli* bacilli are also a significant cause of pneumonia in this age group and have been shown, along with other gram-negative enteric organisms, to be a cause of otitis media in infants less than 6 weeks of age. *E. coli* also produces urinary infection often associated with jaundice in infants less than 2 months of age.

Supportive measures are critically important in the neonate with a systemic infection, irrespective of type or cause. In general, antimicrobials should be administered by the intravenous route because the depressed infant has decreased gastrointestinal absorption and microcirculatory changes in sepsis can lead to poor absorption of intramuscular drugs. Re-establishment and maintenance of body temperature in a heated environment are important, and urinary output should be monitored. Intravenous fluid and electrolyte therapy should be meticulously provided by standard methods. The complications of hyponatremia, hypoglycemia, or hypocalcemia may mimic or complicate septicemia. Thus, appropriate diagnostic biochemical determinations must be repetitively carried out and appropriate replacement therapy instituted. Lumbar punctures should be performed at frequent intervals in meningitis due to *E. coli* or other gram-negative enteric bacilli until sterilization of the cerebrospinal fluid (CSF) has occurred, which is usually by the fourth or fifth day of therapy. Treatment should be continued for 3 total weeks or 2 weeks after cerebrospinal fluid sterilization.

Antibiotic therapy is of cardinal importance in the management of infections due to *E. coli*. Because of changing patterns of resistance, in vitro susceptibility studies are essential. For example, kanamycin has been the drug of choice for *E. coli* infections in the neonate; however, in recent years kanamycin-resistant strains of *E. coli* have become more widespread. In many geographic areas, more than 40 per cent of strains are resistant. In hospitals in which the majority of *E. coli* strains remain susceptible to kanamycin, this drug may be used. The intramuscular or intravenous dosage is as follows: infants 1 to 7 days of age weighing less than 2000 gm, 7.5 mg/kg every 12 hours; infants 1 to 7 days of age weighing more than 2000 gm, 10 mg/kg every 12 hours;* infants 8 to 30 days of age weighing less than 2000 gm, 10 mg/kg every 12 hours;* infants 8 to 30 days of age weighing more than 2000 gm, 10 mg/kg every 8 hours.*

In most areas, gentamicin plus ampicillin is the preferred combination of drugs for *E. coli* septicemia of the neonate. For infants under 1 week of age, the dosage is 5 mg/kg/24 hr in equally divided doses every 12 hours. Beyond 1 week of age, the dosage is 5 to 7.5

---

*These doses exceed the manufacturer's maximum recommended daily dosage of 15 mg/kg/day.

Text continued on page 517

TABLE 1. Antimicrobial Agents for Infections Due to Gram-Negative Bacilli of Relatively Common Clinical Occurrence*

Organism	Drug	
Escherichia coli† Community acquired	Ampicillin Kanamycin Tobramycin Gentamicin	Cephalosporin[1] Chloramphenicol Tetracycline
Hospital acquired	Ampicillin Gentamicin Kanamycin Amikacin[3] Quinolones	Tobramycin[3] Cephalosporin[1] Ticarcillin Chloramphenicol
Enterotoxigenic and enteroinvasive‡	Polymyxin (oral) Neomycin (oral) Kanamycin (oral)	Ampicillin Gentamicin (oral)
Enterobacter spp.	Gentamicin Tobramycin[3] Cephalosporins Carbenicillin or ticarcillin Nalidixic acid Kanamycin	Polymyxin or colistin Chloramphenicol Ticarcillin Amikacin[3] Tetracycline
Klebsiella pneumoniae	Gentamicin with or without a cephalosporin Tobramycin[3] Kanamycin	Tetracycline Cephalosporin[1] Chloramphenicol Amikacin[3]
Proteus mirabilis	Ampicillin Penicillin G Cephalosporin[1] Gentamicin	Kanamycin Tobramycin[3] Nalidixic acid Chloramphenicol
Indole-positive *Proteus* (*P. vulgaris, P. morgani,* *P. rettgeri*)	Gentamicin Kanamycin Tobramycin Chloramphenicol Carbenicillin or ticarcillin	Nalidixic acid Tetracycline Amikacin[3] Sisomicin[2,3] Cephalosporin[4]
Pseudomonas aeruginosa†	Tobramycin[3,5,6] Polymyxin or colistin Ticarcillin Gentamicin[6]	Piperacillin Azlocillin Mezlocillin Aztronam[2] Tobramycin[3,5] Imipenem-cilastatin Amikacin[3,5,6] Carbenicillin
Serratia marcescens	Tobramycin Amikacin[3] Gentamicin Kanamycin Trimethoprim- sulfamethoxazole	Chloramphenicol Nalidixic acid Carbenicillin Ticarcillin Cephalosporin[1]

*In most instances, the drug of first choice is listed first. Susceptibility tests are important in determining therapy for infections due to any of these organisms. However, in many instances, the drug of choice depends on susceptibility results.

†For treatment of urinary tract infections, see text.

‡Indications tentative.

[1]Refers to one of the cephalosporins, administered parenterally or orally, depending upon drug and nature of infection. See text and Table 2 for further details and information on new cephalosporins.

[2]Investigational drug.

[3]See text for discussion of indications and use.

[4]Cefoxitin appears to be the most effective cephalosporin.

[5]Combination of gentamicin or other aminoglycoside and carbenicillin or ticarcillin is usually synergistic. Both can be used in serious life-threatening infections. Use of carbenicillin or ticarcillin alone is associated with emergence of resistant *Pseudomonas* and superinfection with resistant *Klebsiella*.

[6]Synergistic with carbenicillin and ticarcillin against many strains.

TABLE 2. Daily Dosage Schedule for Antimicrobial Agents*

Drug	Oral	Intramuscular (IM)	Intravenous (IV)	Intrathecal	Adult or Maximum Dose
Penicillin G[1]	500,000–2,000,000 units in 5 doses ½ hr	20,000–50,000 units/kg in 4–6 doses	20,000–100,000 units/kg in 4–6 doses		20–100 million units/24 hr
Neonate and premature[2]	50,000 units/kg in 4 doses	20,000–50,000 units/kg in 2–4 doses	20,000–50,000 units/kg in 4 doses		
Chloramphenicol[3]	50–100 mg/kg in 4 doses[4]		50–100 mg/kg in 3–4 doses (10% solution)		3–4 gm/24 hr; maximum in child, 2 gm/24 hr
Neonate and premature[2, 4]	25[a]–50[b] mg/kg in 4 doses		15[a]–25[b] mg/kg in 2–4 doses (0.5 mg/ml)		
Tetracycline[5, c]	20–40 mg/kg in 4 doses	12 mg/kg in 2 doses	12 mg/kg in 2 doses (1 mg/ml)		2 gm/24 hr
Neonate and premature[2]	10–20 mg/kg in 4 doses	6 mg/kg in 2 doses	6 mg/kg in 2 doses (1 mg/ml)		
Kanamycin[6]	100 mg/kg in 4 doses	30 mg/kg in 3 doses	30 mg/kg in 3 doses (2.5 mg/ml)		Oral, 3–4 gm/24 hr; IM, 1.0–1.5 gm/24 hr
Neonate and premature[2, 17]	50 mg/kg in 4 doses	15–20 mg/kg in 2–3 doses (see text)	(see text)		
Neomycin[d]	100–150 mg/kg in 4 doses[f]				Oral, 6 gm/24 hr; IM, 1 gm/24 hr
Neonate and premature[2]	50 mg/kg in 4 doses				
Streptomycin sulfate[7, d]		20–40 mg/kg in 2–3 doses		1 mg/kg or 20 mg/24 hr (5 mg/ml)	2 gm/24 hr
Neonate and premature[2]		10–20 mg/kg in 2 doses			
Sulfonamides[8]	120–150 mg/kg in 4 doses		120 mg/kg (24 mg/ml) in 2–4 doses		3–4 gm/24 hr
Neonate and premature[2, 4]	50 mg/kg/day[c] in 2–3 doses				
Polymyxin B[9]	15–20 mg/kg in 4–6 doses	2.5–5.0 mg/kg in 4–6 doses	2.5–5.0 mg/kg in 3 doses (0.4 mg/ml 5% dextrose in endocarditis)	<2 yr, 2 mg/24 hr or every other day	Oral, 500 mg/24 hr; parenteral, 200 mg/24 hr
Neonate and premature[2]	10–15 mg/kg in 4 doses	3[a]–4[b] mg/kg in 4 doses		>2 yr, 5 mg/24 hr (0.5–1.0 mg/ml)	Intrathecal, 10 mg/24 hr
Colistin[9]	15–30 mg/kg in 4 doses	5–8 mg/kg in 3 doses	1.5–5.0 mg/kg in 2–4 doses	<1 yr, 2 mg/24 hr[14] >1 yr, 5 mg/24 hr	5 mg/kg/24 hr IM
Neonate and premature[2]	10–20 mg/kg in 4 doses	1.0–2.0 mg/kg in 2–4 doses			
Novobiocin[10]	20–45 mg/kg in 4 doses				Oral, 2 gm/24 hr
Neonate and premature[2, 4]	10–15 mg/kg in 2–3 doses				
Gentamicin[11]	5–10 mg/kg in 1 dose[26]	3.0–7.5 mg/kg in 3 doses		1–2 mg/24 hr	IM, 5 mg/kg/24 hr[11]
Neonate and premature[2, 12]		5 (3.0–7.5) mg/kg in 2–3 doses[18]			
Cephalothin[13]		80–160 mg/kg in 4–6 doses	80–160 mg/kg in 4–6 doses or in continuous infusion		Parenteral, 2–6 gm/24 hr
Neonate and premature[2]		50–100 mg/kg in 2–3 doses	50–100 mg/kg in 4 doses or in continuous infusion		
Ampicillin[15]	100–200 mg/kg in 4 doses	150–400 mg/kg in 4 doses	150–400 mg/kg in 4 doses		Oral, 2–6 gm/24 hr; parenteral, 2–4 gm/24 hr
Neonate and premature[2]	25–200 mg/kg in 4 doses	50–200 mg/kg in 2–3 doses[19]			
Paromomycin[9]	50–100 mg/kg in 4 doses[f]				2 gm/24 hr
Neonate and premature[2]					
Cephaloridine		50–100 mg/kg in 3 doses	30–100 mg/kg in 2–3 doses		4 gm/24 hr
Neonate and premature[2]					
Nystatin	1,000,000–2,000,000 units in 3–4 doses				
Neonate and premature[2]	400,000 units in 4 doses				

Table continued on following page

TABLE 2. Daily Dosage Schedule for Antimicrobial Agents* *Continued*

Drug	Oral	Intramuscular (IM)	Intravenous (IV)	Intrathecal	Adult or Maximum Dose
Amphotericin B[16]			1 mg/kg given over 6- to 8-hr period		1 mg/kg
Neonate and premature[2]					
Methenamine mandelate	100 mg/kg first dose; then 50 mg/kg/24 hr in 3 doses				4 gm/24 hr
Nitrofurantoin	5–7 mg/kg/24 hr; reduce dosage after 10–14 days to 2.5–5.0 mg/kg/24 hr				400 mg/24 hr
Neonate and premature[2]	Contraindicated				
Carbenicillin	100 mg/kg/day in 4 doses		400–600 mg/kg in 4–6 doses		40 gm/24 hr
Neonate and premature[2]			300 mg/kg/24 hr		
Carbenicillin indanyl sodium	30–50 mg/kg in 4 doses				2–3 gm (max)
Cephalexin	50–100 mg/kg/24 hr in 4 doses				12 gm/24 hr
Nalidixic acid[g]	12 mg/kg/24 hr				4 gm/24 hr
Cefazolin		50–100 mg/kg in 3 doses	50–100 mg/kg in 3 doses		6 gm/24 hr
Neonate and premature[2]		Not recommended	Not recommended		
Tobramycin		8–10 mg/kg in 3 doses	8–10 mg/kg in 3 doses		5 mg/kg/24 hr
Neonate and premature[2]		5 mg/kg in 2–3 doses	5 mg/kg in 2–3 doses		
Clindamycin	10–25 mg/kg in 4 doses	10–40 mg/kg in 4 doses	10–40 mg/kg in 4 doses		4.8 gm/24 hr
Neonate and premature[2]	Unknown	Unknown	Unknown		
Cloxacillin	50–100 mg/kg in 4 doses				4 gm/24 hr
Neonate and premature[2]	Not recommended				
Dicloxacillin	25–100 mg/kg in 4 doses				4 gm/24 hr
Neonate and premature[2]	Not recommended				
Methicillin		100–300 mg/kg in 4–6 doses	100–300 mg/kg in 4–6 doses		12 gm/24 hr
Neonate and premature[2]		50–200 mg/kg[20] in 2–3 doses	50–100 mg/kg[20] in 2–3 doses		
Nafcillin	50–100 mg/kg in 4 doses	100–200 mg/kg in 4–6 doses	100–200 mg/kg in 4–6 doses		12 gm/24 hr
Neonate and premature[2]		75–100 mg/kg in 2–4 doses[20]	75–100 mg/kg in 2–4 doses[20]		
Oxacillin	50–100 mg/kg in 4 doses	100–200 mg/kg in 4–6 doses	100–200 mg/kg in 4–6 doses		12 gm/24 hr
Neonate and premature[2]		50–200 mg/kg in 2–4 doses[20]	50–200 mg/kg in 2–4 doses[20]		
Penicillin V	25,000–400,000 units/kg in 4 doses				6.4 million units/24 hr
Neonate and premature[2]	25,000–200,000 units/kg in 3 doses				
Amoxicillin	40–100 mg/kg in 3 doses				3 gm/24 hr
Neonate and premature[2]	40–100 mg/kg in 3–4 doses				
Amikacin		20 mg/kg in 2–3 doses	20 mg/kg in 2–3 doses		
Neonate and premature[2]		Initial dose, 10 mg/kg[21]	Initial dose, 10 mg/kg[21]		
Ticarcillin			300 mg/kg in 4–6 doses		
Neonate and premature[2]			Initial dose, 100 mg/kg[22]		
Lincomycin	30–60 mg/kg in 4 doses	20 mg/kg in 2 doses	20 mg/kg in 2 doses		Oral, 2 gm/24 hr IM, 8 gm/24 hr IV, 8 gm/24 hr
Cefaclor	40 mg/kg in 3 doses				2–3 gm/24 hr

TABLE 2. Daily Dosage Schedule for Antimicrobial Agents* *Continued*

Drug	Oral	Intramuscular (IM)	Intravenous (IV)	Intrathecal	Adult or Maximum Dose
Cefadroxil[h]	40 mg/kg in 2 doses				2 gm
Neonate and premature	Not recommended				
Cephradine	40–60 mg/kg in 4 doses	50–100 mg/kg in 4 doses	50–100 mg/kg in 4 doses		2–3 gm
Neonate and premature	Not recommended	Not recommended			
Cephapirin		40–80 mg/kg in 4 doses	40–80 mg/kg in 4 doses		
Cefamandole[23, 24]		50–150 mg/kg in 4–6 doses	50–150 mg/kg in 4–6 doses		4–6 gm
Cefoxitin		50–150 mg/kg in 3–4 doses	50–150 mg/kg in 3–4 doses		12 gm
Neonate and premature		Not recommended	Not recommended		
Hetacillin	50–100 mg/kg in 4 doses				
Cyclacillin	0.5–1.0 gm in 4 doses				2 gm
Neonate and premature	Not recommended				
Bacampicillin	25–50 mg/kg in 2 doses				3.2 gm
Cefotaxime		150–200 mg/kg in 4 doses	150–200 mg/kg in 4 doses		
Ceftriaxone		75 mg/kg in 2 doses	75 mg/kg in 2 doses		
Cefuroxime		75 mg/kg in 3 doses	75 mg/kg in 3 doses		
Cinoxacin for urinary tract infection only for those >12 yr old	1000 mg in 2–4 doses				
Doxycycline	4–5 mg/kg in 2 doses				
Erythromycin	30–50 mg/kg in 4 doses		40–70 mg/kg in 4 doses		
Neonate and premature[2] and <4 mo	20–40 mg/kg in 3 doses				
Flucytosine	150 mg/kg in 4 doses				
Ketoconazole	5–15 mg/kg in 1 dose				
Metronidazole	20–30 mg/kg in 3 doses		20–30 mg/kg in 3 doses		
Neonate and premature[2]	Not recommended		15 mg/kg loading dose, then 15 mg/kg in 2 doses		
Mezlocillin		300 mg/kg in 6 doses	300 mg/kg in 6 doses		24 gm
Neonate and premature[2]		≤2000 gm: <1 wk, 150 mg/kg in 2 doses; >1 wk, 225 mg/kg in 3 doses >2000 gm: <1 wk, 150 mg/kg in 2 doses; >1 wk, 300 mg/kg in 4 doses	<2000 gm: <1 wk, 150 mg/kg in 2 doses; >1 wk, 225 mg/kg in 3 doses >2000 gm: <1 wk, 150 mg/kg in 2 doses; >1 wk, 300 mg/kg in 4 doses		
Miconazole			30 mg/kg in 3 doses		
Minocycline	4–5 mg/kg in 2 doses				
Neonate and premature[2]	Not recommended				
Moxalactam[2, 24, 25]		100–200 mg/kg in 4 doses	100–200 mg/kg in 4 doses		
Neonate and premature[2, 10]		100 mg/kg in 2 doses, >1 wk, 150 mg/kg in 3 doses	100 mg/kg in 2 doses, >1 wk, 150 mg/kg in 3 doses		
Piperacillin *Not recommended in those <12 yr old		100–300 mg/kg in 4 doses			20 gm
Rifampin	15 mg/kg in 1 dose				120 mg/kg
Meningococcal prophylaxis × 2 days	1200 mg in 2 doses; 1–12 yr old, 20 mg/kg in 2 doses; <1 yr old, 10 mg/kg in 2 doses				
Haemophilus prophylaxis × 4 days	20 mg/kg/day in 1 dose				1200 mg/kg

Table continued on following page

TABLE 2. Daily Dosage Schedule for Antimicrobial Agents* *Continued*

Drug	Oral	Intramuscular (IM)	Intravenous (IV)	Intrathecal	Adult or Maximum Dose
Trimethoprim *Not recommended in those <12 yr old	200 mg/kg in 2 doses				
Trimethoprim (TMP)-sulfamethoxasole (SMX)	5–10 mg/kg TMP 25–50 mg/kg SMX } in 2 doses		5–10 mg/kg TMP 25–50 mg/kg SMX } in 3 doses		
Neonate and premature[2] and <2 mo			2 mg/kg TMP, 10 mg SMX loading dose, then 2 mg/kg TMP, 10 mg/kg SMX in 2 doses		
Pneumocystis prophylaxis	5 mg TMP/25 mg SMX/kg in 1 dose		5 mg TMP/25 mg SMX/kg in 1 dose		
Pneumocystis treatment	20 mg TMP/100 mg SMX/kg in 3 doses		20 mg TMP/100 mg SMX/kg in 3 doses		
Vancomycin	50 mg/kg in 4 doses		40 mg/kg in 2–3 doses		
Neonate and premature[2]			30 mg/kg in 2 doses		
Azlocillin Neonate and premature			300–600 mg/kg divided q 4 hr; <1 wk, 100–150 mg/kg in 2 doses; >1 wk, 200 mg/kg in 2 doses		
Cefoperazone[24, 25] Not yet approved for pediatric use					2–4 gm/day divided q 6–12 hr

*Some of these agents may be administered by other routes. For intrapleural, intra-articular, intraperitoneal, ocular, aerosol, and topical use, see Report of the Committee on the Control of Infectious Diseases, American Academy of Pediatrics, Evanston, Ill., 1964. Some, such as neomycin, are specifically contraindicated by the intrapleural and intraperitoneal routes.

[1] Phenoxymethyl penicillin or phenethicillin is preferred for oral therapy. Procaine penicillin should not be used in neonates. Sodium penicillin contains 1.5 mEq of sodium, and potassium penicillin G, 1.69 mEq of potassium per 1 million units. The latter should be avoided intravenously in neonates and in patients with impaired renal function.

[2] If renal output is reduced, decrease the dose still further.

[3] Should not be used for minor infections or when less hazardous agents are effective. Observe for bone marrow depression.

[4] Avoid during first week of life unless essential. Desirable to follow treatment with serial blood levels to avoid "gray" syndrome.

[5] Any of the tetracycline group of antibiotics may be used.

[6] With parenteral administration, auditory nerve and renal injury may occur; frequent audiometric and renal tests are essential. *Manufacturer's note:* The intravenous dose of kanamycin should not exceed 15 mg/kg/24 hr.

[7] Auditory nerve damage can occur.

[8] A soluble sulfonamide should be used. *Manufacturer's precaution:* Systemic sulfonamides are contraindicated in infants under 2 months of age.

[9] Observe for renal and neural toxic effects.

[10] Severe skin and liver toxicity occasionally occurs. *Manufacturer's warning:* Use should be avoided in premature and newborn infants because it affects bilirubin adversely.

[11] In general, the dose by the intramuscular route should not exceed 5 mg/kg/24 hr for no longer than 7 to 10 days except in serious or life-threatening situations. Observation for vestibular and renal toxicity should be carried out. Desirable to follow therapy with serial blood levels if renal function is impaired. The intrathecal use of gentamicin is not mentioned in the manufacturer's instructions.

[12] For neonates, see No. 18.

[13] Doses up to 200 mg/kg/24 hr in infants and children have been utilized without untoward effect.

[14] For intrathecal use, colistin without dibucaine should be used.

[15] In severe infections, may be necessary to increase oral and intramuscular dose as much as 3 times that listed.

[16] Fever, thrombophlebitis and renal, hepatic, and bone marrow damage may occur.

[17] Infants <7 days, <2000 gm, 15 mg/kg in 2 doses; >2000 gm, 20 mg/kg in 2 doses. Infants >7 days, <2000 gm, 20 mg/kg in 2 doses; >2000 gm, 20 mg/kg in 3 doses.

[18] Dose should be given in 2 divided doses in infants <7 days and in 3 divided doses in infants >7 days.

[19] In infants <7 days, 50–100 mg/kg in 2 doses; >7 days, 100–200 mg/kg in 3 doses.

[20] In infants <7 days, 50–100 mg/kg in 2 doses; >7 days, 100–200 mg/kg in 3–4 doses. Pediatric IV doses not known due to rarity.

[21] After initial loading dose of 10 mg/kg, follow with 7.5 mg/kg dose every 12 hr. (Can be given IM or IV.)

[22] After initial loading dose of 100 mg/kg, dose is as follows: <2000 gm = 225 mg/kg in 3 doses during first week of life; 600 mg/kg in 6 doses after 7 days of age; >2000 gm, 300–400 mg/kg in 4–6 doses; 600 mg/kg in 6 doses after 2 weeks of age. Can be given IM or as 15- to 20-minute IV infusion.

[23] CSF penetration not adequate. "Breakthrough" meningitis may occur during therapy.

[24] Bleeding due to hypoprothrombinemia is a possible complication. Administer prophylactic vitamin K.

[25] Displaces bilirubin from albumin. Use with caution with patients under 2 weeks of age.

[26] Oral preparation is an investigational drug.

[a] Premature.

[b] Full-term.

[c] *Manufacturer's warning:* The use of drugs of the tetracycline class during tooth development (last half of pregnancy, infancy, and childhood to the age of 8 years) may cause permanent discoloration of the teeth. This adverse reaction is more common during long-term usage of the drugs but has been observed following repeated short-term courses.

[d] In general, limit parenteral therapy to 10 days.

[e] First dose should be doubled. Do not use sulfonamides in premature infants or infants under 2 months of age.

[f] May exceed manufacturer's recommended dosage.

[g] *Manufacturer's warning:* Do not administer to children less than 3 months of age.

[h] Safety and dosage in children have not been established.

mg/kg/24 hr in divided doses every 8 hours for both full-term and low birth weight infants. For intravenous administration, the dose is diluted in sterile normal saline and infused over a 1- to 2-hour period. If necessary, the drugs can be given intramuscularly except to infants with poor circulation. If renal function is impaired, the dosage of aminoglycosides must be reduced and serum levels monitored to avoid potential toxicity.

Ampicillin administered parenterally may be effective in infections caused by susceptible strains, especially those that are community acquired. The daily dose administered intravenously for infants 1 to 7 days of age is 50 to 200 mg/kg in two doses, and for infants 8 to 30 days of age, 75 to 250 mg/kg divided into three doses. A combination of ampicillin and gentamicin or another aminoglycoside is preferred initially because of possible synergism in action and broad-spectrum coverage. Other drugs listed in Table 1 may be used if susceptibility studies show the organism to be sensitive. Amikacin and tobramycin are effective, but their use should be reserved for strains resistant to other antibiotics.

For the initial treatment of neonatal meningitis, many clinicians now prefer the combination of ampicillin and cefotaxime over the use of ampicillin and gentamicin. Cefotaxime is a third-generation cephalosporin with a wide spectrum of activity against gram-negative organisms and group B streptococci; in meningitis in the neonate and young infant, it should be used in combination with ampicillin because of its poor activity against *Listeria*. Advantages of cefotaxime over aminoglycosides include higher CSF concentrations, lower concentrations required for bacterial killing, and lower potential for toxicity, which obviates monitoring serum concentrations. Other third-generation cephalosporins have similar properties but are not recommended for use in neonates. Experience with these agents in neonates is limited, especially when compared with cefotaxime. For example, the pharmacokinetics of ceftriaxone are largely undefined, and the half-life may be quite prolonged in many of these patients, especially premature infants. Ceftriaxone, moxalactam, and other third-generation cephalosporins will displace bilirubin from albumin, whereas this is not a problem with cefotaxime. In addition, compared with cefotaxime, ceftriaxone results in much higher concentrations in bile, which can result in bile sludging, the elimination of gastrointestinal flora, and the potential for intestinal colonization with resistant, hospital-acquired organisms, such as *Pseudomonas*, *Candida*, and enterococcus. The incidence of antibiotic-associated diarrhea may also be higher.

Empiric use of the ampicillin-cefotaxime combination in the neonatal intensive care unit should be limited to treatment of patients with suspected meningitis or those in whom the offending pathogen is susceptible to it. Indiscriminate use of this combination in place of ampicillin and an aminoglycoside for empiric therapy of neonatal sepsis may ultimately lead to the emergence of resistant strains in the nursery environment.

The dosage for cefotaxime for serious infections such as meningitis is 50 mg/kg per dose given every 12 hours for patients aged 7 days and less, every 8 hours for patients older than 7 days but less than 1 month, and every 6 hours after 1 month of age.

Second-generation cephalosporins such as cefamandole and cefuroxime show increased activity against enteric organisms; however, CSF penetration is poor with cefamandole, and "breakthrough" meningitis during therapy is a possibility. Cefuroxime achieves reasonable CSF concentrations but has spotty activity against many Enterobacteriaceae, and thus its use in neonates is not recommended.

General supportive care depends on the underlying problem. Serious *E. coli* infections in older infants and children should be treated with parenteral gentamicin alone or in combination with ampicillin. Ampicillin given intravenously in a dose of 200 mg/kg/24 hr at 4- to 6-hour intervals, plus gentamicin, 3 to 7.5 mg/kg/24 hr in three divided doses, is the initial treatment of choice. Other drugs may be used, depending upon the results of susceptibility tests.

Urinary Tract Infection. *E. coli* remains the most common cause of primary uncomplicated urinary tract infection. The strains are usually quite susceptible to the sulfonamides or to ampicillin. Sulfisoxazole,* 150 mg/kg/24 hr in four divided doses for a period of 2 weeks, affords effective therapy in most patients. Ampicillin, 50 to 100 mg/kg/24 hr orally in four divided doses, is equally effective but not superior. Amoxicillin (20 to 40 mg/kg/24 hr in three divided doses) is often used instead of ampicillin, since gastrointestinal side effects (especially diarrhea) are less frequent and compliance may be improved with dosing three times a day. The sulfonamides are still preferred for urinary tract infection of this nature, since they are usually effective, the cost and incidence of associated untoward reactions are low, and dosing is twice a day.

Because these drugs are effectively concentrated in the renal parenchyma and urine, favorable treatment response may be observed even when in vitro susceptibility testing shows the organism to be resistant. For this reason, if a favorable clinical response has been achieved after 48 to 72 hours and pyuria has been diminished and the urine sterilized, treatment may be continued with the drug initiated. If this has not been accomplished by this time, it is likely that the organism is resistant.

In recurrent disease, the infecting *E. coli* is likely to be sulfonamide resistant, and antibiotic susceptibility data must be used as guidelines for selecting alternative drugs. However, the trimethoprim-sulfamethoxazole combination or cephalosporins administered orally are often useful in such situations.

It is most important to ensure that the patient demonstrates both a clinical and a bacteriologic cure and that an asymptomatic bacteriologic relapse does not occur. If the repeat urine cultures at 48 to 72 hours are sterile, treatment should be presumed effective. After the 2-week course of therapy, repeat urinalysis and quantitative urine cultures should be performed within several days and repeated at monthly intervals there-

---

*Contraindicated in infants younger than 2 months of age.

after for 3 months and again at 6 months and a year. Shorter courses of antimicrobial administration may be effective in uncomplicated lower urinary tract infections. However, differentiation between upper and lower urinary tract infection in children and infants is often difficult. Short courses of antimicrobial therapy in these patients with urinary tract infection may be associated with unacceptable rates of relapse of infection. Drugs for oral therapy of urinary tract infection in children over 12 years include trimethoprim alone, trimethoprim-sulfamethoxazole, or amoxicillin. If urinary tract infections recur, especially if polymicrobial in type, the presence of abnormalities of the urinary tract, especially those producing obstruction, should be suspected.

Diarrheal Disease. The association of *E. coli* with diarrheal disease has been known for years. Numerous outbreaks of diarrhea occurring in nurseries have been investigated, and certain antigenetically distinct strains of *E. coli* have been connected with these epidemics.

In recent years, the possible pathogenic mechanisms for the diarrhea associated with *E. coli* have been elucidated by the demonstration of the toxigenic and invasive properties of some of the strains. Stool isolates of *E. coli* can be characterized as being (1) enteropathogenic; (2) enterotoxigenic (ETEC), by their ability to produce toxins; or (3) enteroinvasive (EIEC), by their capacity to penetrate mucosal cells. It is now known that strains may have none, one, two, or all three of these characteristics. Recent evidence also suggests that the intestinal mucosal adherence of some *E. coli* strains may be related to their pathogenicity.

E. coli has been shown to cause diarrhea by two separate mechanisms: enterotoxin production and mucosal invasion. Strains with enteroinvasive capacity produce the characteristic findings of bacterial dysentery, namely, local inflammation with hyperemia, ulceration, and intraluminal exudate composed of polymorphonuclear leukocytes. Enterotoxigenic *E. coli* causes diarrhea by two means: (1) production of an antigenic heat-labile toxin that resembles cholera toxin, in that it activates cellular adenyl cyclase, thereby increasing intracellular cyclic adenosine monophosphate and promoting secretion of sodium and water; (2) production of a nonantigenic heat-stable toxin, the exact action of which is not completely understood. Heat-labile enterotoxin has been shown to cause diarrhea in humans; heat-stable enterotoxin, although known to be a major cause of diarrhea in animals, has also recently been shown to be associated with diarrheal disease in humans.

Supportive therapy for *E. coli*–mediated diarrhea, irrespective of pathogenesis, consists mainly of maintaining adequate fluid and electrolyte intake. Patients with evidence of dehydration should be hospitalized and managed with intravenous fluids and electrolyte therapy, details of which are described elsewhere. In these patients, it is important to determine serum electrolyte concentrations, since hyponatremia and hypernatremia occur fairly commonly.

Infants who are not significantly dehydrated can be managed as outpatients. The details of management are described in other sections, but two points must be mentioned. Homemade salt solutions should *not* be prescribed because of the risk of inducing hypertonic dehydration. Certain commercially available oral rehydration fluids can be used successfully in the outpatient treatment of mildly dehydrated children. Adsorptive agents that firm the stool or narcotic-containing agents that decrease bowel motility have *no* place in the treatment of diarrheal disease in infants and young children. None of these agents is specifically directed toward the primary cause of the diarrhea. None has been shown to decrease the fluid and electrolyte loss across the bowel mucosa in *E. coli* diarrhea, but by decreasing bowel motility they may mask the amount of fluid accumulated in the bowel lumen. They may also allow heavier colonization of the offending organism, with greater enterotoxin production in the jejunum. Deaths or severe central nervous system depression have occurred when atropine- or diphenyoxylate-containing antidiarrheals have been used in infants and children.

The effectiveness of antimicrobial therapy in *E. coli* diarrhea is open to some question. Specific antimicrobial therapy appears to shorten the severity and duration of diarrhea. Neomycin sulfate oral solution is the drug of choice in areas where neomycin resistance is not encountered frequently. It is administered in a dosage of 100 mg/kg/24 hr divided into doses every 6 to 8 hours for 5 days. This dose is higher than that recommended by the manufacturer but has been found safe and effective. Continuation of therapy for more than 5 days is not advised because the bacteriologic cure rate is not improved and because neomycin may cause a malabsorptive state. Colistin sulfate oral suspension is the alternative drug of choice and is given in dosages of 10 to 15 mg/kg/24 hr every 6 to 8 hours for 5 days. Antibiotic susceptibility testing should be performed because when resistant organisms are involved, treatment has resulted not only in failure but also in spread of the infection, presumably by suppression of competing normal bacterial intestinal flora.

To date, controlled studies evaluating the effectiveness of antibiotic therapy in the treatment of diarrhea due to enterotoxigenic and enteroinvasive strains have not been performed. Because the bacteria remain within the intestinal lumen in enterotoxigenic *E. coli* disease, it seems logical to speculate that nonabsorbable antibiotics might be useful in treatment. However, in an outbreak of diarrheal disease due to a strain of *E. coli* elaborating a heat-stable enterotoxin but that did not belong to an enteropathogenic serotype, oral colistin therapy was ineffective in eradicating the organisms from the stools of culture-positive infants and in preventing illness or shortening the carrier state. It is reasonable to presume that drugs effective against these strains in vitro might be beneficial in decreasing the severity and duration of diarrhea in those patients, as has been shown with *Shigella* dysentery. If strains susceptible to ampicillin are involved, this drug should be administered at a dosage of 100 mg/kg/24 hr in four to eight divided doses, preferably intravenously. In a double-blind, placebo-controlled study of 110 older patients with "traveler's diarrhea," a 5-day course of oral trimethoprim-sulfamethoxazole or trimethoprim alone significantly reduced the gastrointestinal distress and number of diarrheal stools in a majority of the patients. Oral bismuth preparations (e.g., Pepto-Bismol) may also be helpful. Ciprofloxacin, an oral quinolone, has been shown to be effective in traveler's diarrhea but is not recommended for use in prepubescent patients because of potential toxicity to growing cartilage.

It is not clear at this time whether older children with *E. coli* diarrhea should receive antimicrobial therapy.

Outbreaks of *E. coli* diarrhea in newborn nurseries can be catastrophic. Such outbreaks can be controlled by the use of rapid fluorescent antibody techniques to detect the presence of organisms in the stool and by segregation of infants found to be colonized and treatment with oral neomycin or colistin in the dosages mentioned.

Other Infections. A variety of other infections, including pneumonia, peritonitis, and abscesses, may be caused by *E. coli*. The information in Tables 1 and 2 can be used for selection of antimicrobial therapy pending susceptibility test results. Surgical intervention and supportive measures depend upon the disease. *E. coli*, including nonenteropathogenic strains, has been causally linked to necrotizing enterocolitis in neonates. Therapy for *E. coli* infections, other than uncomplicated urinary tract infections, should be provided by the parenteral route.

Proteus-Providencia-Morganella Infections

The variable, unpredictable response to antibacterial therapy for *Proteus* and *Morganella* infections is striking, and prolonged therapy is often necessary. In addition to in vitro susceptibility studies, *Proteus* isolates should also be classified with regard to species because of the variability in the susceptibility of various species and strains to different antibacterial agents. For example, *P. mirabilis* is usually susceptible to ampicillin (or occasionally to large doses of penicillin G), and it is the drug of choice in most infections due to this species. Many strains of *P. mirabilis* are also susceptible to gentamicin, cephalosporins, including many third-generation cephalosporins, ticarcillin, and kanamycin. Indole-positive species such as *P. vulgaris* and *Morganella morganii*, for practical purposes, are always resistant to ampicillin and penicillin G. The drug of choice must be governed by the results of in vitro susceptibility tests as well as the clinical condition of the patient. Many strains are susceptible to gentamicin, kanamycin, tobramycin, and nearly all to amikacin; these are usually the drugs of choice in infections due to these species. Some strains are susceptible to carbenicillin and ticarcillin and others to one of the cephalosporins, particularly the second- and third-generation agents.

Most strains of *P. vulgaris* are two- to fourfold more sensitive in vitro to tobramycin than to gentamicin. In vivo, however, strains resistant to gentamicin are likely to be resistant to tobramycin. Amikacin and sisomicin show increased activity against most strains of indole-positive *Proteus*. The use of these two agents should be reserved for infections due to organisms resistant to other available agents. Cefoxitin and cefotaxime also show activity against certain strains of indole-positive

Proteus. Cefuroxime, cefoperazone, and ceftazidime are much less active. Alternate drugs for infections due to susceptible strains are listed in Table 1. Some strains of *Proteus* are moderately susceptible to novobiocin, but this drug has a significant toxicity risk, and the response to therapy is often variable.

Organisms of the genus *Providencia* were formerly known as *P. inconstans* and included with "paracolon bacilli." They are easily differentiated from *Proteus* and *Morganella* by their lack of urease. Members of the group have been isolated from human feces during outbreaks of diarrhea but also in normal individuals. They are primarily associated with urinary tract infections but may also cause sepsis and localized infections. *Providencia* organisms are highly resistant to antibiotics, except for carbenicillin and ticarcillin and the aminoglycosides; some strains are inhibited by cefamandole or cefoxitin and some by trimethoprim-sulfamethoxazole.

Providencia stuartii has recently emerged as a hospital pathogen in burned patients, appearing first in burn wounds but subsequently as a cause of pulmonary and urinary infections.

Klebsiella-Enterobacter-Serratia Infections

Klebsiella-Enterobacter-Serratia organisms have variable susceptibility to antimicrobial agents and must be tested in vitro. Frequently, however, antimicrobial therapy must be instituted before results of antibiotic susceptibility tests are available. An aminoglycoside antibiotic, such as gentamicin, amikacin, or tobramycin (the choice depending upon the susceptibility patterns of organisms in the local area), is usually the drug of choice, with certain exceptions. For example, many strains of *K. pneumoniae* are susceptible to cephalothin, and some strains of *Enterobacter* are inhibited by carbenicillin and ticarcillin and by cefamandole, moxalactam, and cefotaxime and other third-generation cephalosporins. Trimethoprim-sulfamethoxazole and second- and third-generation cephalosporins inhibit some strains of *Serratia*. In contrast to *Klebsiella* and *Enterobacter*, almost all strains of *Serratia* are resistant to the polymyxins. For serious *Klebsiella* and *Enterobacter* infections, it is usually desirable to utilize a third-generation cephalosporin such as cefotaxime, especially for meningitis. Other drugs for treatment of infections due to members of the *Klebsiella-Enterobacter-Serratia* group, depending upon susceptibility results, are shown in Table 1.

Pseudomonas Infections

The *Pseudomonas* group is composed of gram-negative, motile rods, which are nonfermenters and occur widely in soil, water, sewage, and air. *P. aeruginosa* is the member of the genus most commonly pathogenic for human beings. *Pseudomonas* occurs in several antigenic types and several phage types that are equally pathogenic. Because of its ability to form a pigment that colors inflammatory exudate blue or green, the epidemic spread of *P. aeruginosa* in hospital wards has long been recognized. It is found in small numbers in the intestinal tract and on normal skin, particularly when other coliforms are suppressed.

P. aeruginosa is resistant to the more commonly used antimicrobial agents and therefore assumes prevalence and importance when more susceptible bacteria of the normal flora are suppressed. Although most strains of *P. aeruginosa* are susceptible to the polymyxins, these agents have been relatively ineffective in eradicating bacteremia and deep-seated tissue infections. Gentamicin and other aminoglycosides and carbenicillin or ticarcillin are usually more effective. In other instances, the organism may be eradicated, but the ultimate results are often unsatisfactory because of the poor host defenses in debilitated patients.

Carbenicillin is effective against susceptible strains, but some 30 per cent of strains are resistant to it. It must be given in relatively large doses intravenously. During prolonged therapy with carbenicillin alone, organisms initially susceptible may become resistant. Most strains of *Pseudomonas* are inhibited by gentamicin, but recently an increasing number of strains have been found to be resistant. Ticarcillin, a semisynthetic penicillin similar to carbenicillin, has excellent activity against *Pseudomonas*, with 90 per cent or more of isolates being susceptible. Presumptive therapy for systemic *Pseudomonas* infection is a combination of tobramycin and ticarcillin. The two drugs appear to act synergistically in vitro, and coadministration may delay emergence of *P. aeruginosa* resistant to ticarcillin.

Tobramycin has been found to be two to four times more active against *Pseudomonas* than is gentamicin. It is particularly valuable in treatment of infections due to gentamicin-resistant strains. When tobramycin is used in combination with ticarcillin, higher antibacterial serum titers are achieved than with either agent alone. See Table 2 for dosage.

Amikacin inhibits many strains of *P. aeruginosa*. It may be used alone or in combination with carbenicillin or ticarcillin. At the moment, its most valuable use is in the treatment of *Pseudomonas* infections due to strains resistant to gentamicin or to other agents.

The broad-spectrum ureidopenicillins, mezlocillin and azlocillin, have good activity against *P. aeruginosa*. In general, mezlocillin is equal to ticarcillin in activity, and azlocillin is approximately twice as active. The minimal inhibitory concentrations (MIC) of the new piperazine penicillin, piperacillin, for *P. aeruginosa* are fourfold lower than those of mezlocillin or ticarcillin. Advantages of these newer agents over carbenicillin and ticarcillin include greater CSF penetration, lower sodium load, and a broader antimicrobial spectrum. Piperacillin and azlocillin are generally reserved for use against isolates with high MICs to ticarcillin and, like ticarcillin, are used in combination with an aminoglycoside. Adverse reactions with piperacillin (fever, rash, lymphadenitis, and eosinophilia) have been reported to occur with greater frequency in patients with cystic fibrosis.

The recently marketed ticarcillin-clavulanate combination may be useful in the therapy of some *Pseudomonas* infections. It is especially helpful when empiric therapy for coverage of multiple pathogens such as *Pseudomonas*, other gram-negative organisms, *Staphylococcus aureus*, and anaerobes, is required. Examples might include infected animal bites, puncture wounds, and pulmonary exacerbations in patients with cystic fibrosis. Clavulanic acid is an effective inhibitor of beta-lactamase, and isolates highly resistant to ticarcillin may be inhibited by 64 mg/ml or less of ticarcillin in the presence of clavulanic acid. However, many beta-lactamases produced by *P. aeruginosa* are not affected by clavulanic acid.

Aztreonam is a monobactam antimicrobial with a spectrum of activity very similar to that of the aminoglycosides. It is highly active against most Enterobacteriaceae, *P. aeruginosa*, *Enterobacter* spp., and *Serratia marcescens*. Similar to some of the newer cephalosporins, aztreonam is not active against facultative aerobic gram-positive or anaerobic bacteria. As with the antipseudomonas beta-lactams, it is frequently synergistic with aminoglycosides against *P. aeruginosa*.

Imipenem (thienamycin) is a novel, broad-spectrum beta-lactam antibiotic with activity against many aerobic and anaerobic gram-positive and gram-negative bacteria, including *P. aeruginosa*. Of the pseudomonads, only *P. maltophilia* and *P. cepacia* are resistant. This agent may prove useful as an alternative to antibiotic combinations currently employed to provide initial broad-spectrum coverage (especially in situations in which infection with *P. aeruginosa* is a possibility).

Antibiotics in the quinolone class (e.g., ciprofloxacin, enoxacin, ofloxacin, and amifloxacin) are under investigation as orally effective agents against *P. aeruginosa* and other gram-negative as well as gram-positive bacteria. Unfortunately, the quinolones cannot be used before puberty in pediatric patients until the question of toxicity to growing cartilage is resolved.

Pseudomonas is a pre-eminent opportunist, and the vast majority of infections caused by it occur in hospitals, particularly those housing patients with serious diseases. Since 1961, the incidence of *P. aeruginosa* bacteremia has increased, and the respiratory tract has become an increasingly important source of infection. The use of gentamicin, carbenicillin, and colistin has not changed the outlook of *Pseudomonas* bacteremia. A polyvalent vaccine has limited usefulness in burned patients; further attention needs to be given to immunoprophylaxis. At the present time, control of the underlying disease condition contributes most toward survival of patients with bacteremia and other serious *Pseudomonas* infections.

The pseudomallei group of the genus *Pseudomonas* consists of *P. mallei*, *P. pseudomallei*, and *P. cepacia*. The first-named is the cause of glanders, a severe infectious disease of horses that can be transmitted to humans. Human infections can usually be treated with sulfonamides.

Melioidosis due to *P. pseudomallei* is a disease resembling glanders in humans and occurs chiefly in Southeast Asia but perhaps also in the Western hemisphere. *P. pseudomallei* is susceptible to many antibiotics in vitro. Tetracycline, chloramphenicol, or gentamicin, alone or in combination, may be the treatment of choice. Tetracycline-streptomycin and chloramphenicol-streptomycin combinations have also been used. Trimethoprim-sulfamethoxazole may be effective.

Outbreaks of nosocomial bacteremia due to *P. cepacia* secondary to contaminated antiseptics and disinfectants used in cleaning equipment or in skin asepsis for intravenous infusions have been described. Environmental isolates are frequently sensitive to chloramphenicol and trimethoprim-sulfamethoxazole and occasionally to kanamycin. *P. cepacia* has been isolated with increasing frequency from the sputum of cystic fibrosis patients. Such patients are usually adolescents and young adults with a history of long-term, intensive antipseudomonas therapy. Cystic fibrosis patients who acquire *P. cepacia* tend to have a poorer prognosis than those from whom *P. cepacia* has never been isolated. Cystic fibrosis isolates of *P. cepacia* are often resistant to standard antipseudomonas agents as well as to chloramphenicol and trimethoprim-sulfamethoxazole. The new third-generation cephalosporin, ceftazidime, demonstrates good in vitro activity against all *P. cepacia*, but early trials in cystic fibrosis patients with this difficult organism have been disappointing. It is interesting that *P. cepacia* is now recognized as an important cause of infection in patients with chronic granulomatous disease and other disorders of phagocytic cells. Certain other pseudomonads may cause infections in humans. These include *P. fluorescens*, *P. maltophilia*, and *P. putida*. Less frequent are *P. acidovorans*, *P. alcaligenes*, *P. putrefaciens*, *P. pseudoalcaligenes*, *P. testosteroni*, *P. diminata*, and *P. mendocina*. These organisms vary widely in their antimicrobial susceptibility, and treatment should be guided by in vitro susceptibility tests.

Aeromonas and *Plesiomonas* Infections

The *Aeromonas* and *Plesiomonas* genera have characteristics in common with both the Enterobacteriaceae and *Pseudomonas* in that they ferment carbohydrates and are oxidase positive. They may be easily mistaken in the laboratory for *E. coli* unless oxidase testing or selective media are used. The most important members are *A. hydrophila*, *A. sobria*, and *P. shigelloides*. These organisms are found in natural water sources and soil and are frequent pathogens for cold-blooded marine and freshwater animals. In humans, *A. hydrophila* has been associated with cellulitis and wound infections (especially those acquired in natural water environments), hepatobiliary infection, and septicemia, mainly in immunocompromised patients. Both *Aeromonas* and *Plesiomonas* have been implicated as etiologic agents in patients with gastroenteritis. Enteropathogenic strains of *Aeromonas* have been described. Diarrhea is usually mild and clinically indistinguishable from certain types of gastroenteritis, although a dysentery-like illness requiring hospitalization can occur. *Plesiomonas* is a rare cause of a devastating meningitis in the newborn. It has become increasingly recognized as a pathogen in compromised patients, especially those with acquired immunodeficiency syndrome (AIDS).

Resistance to cephalosporins and penicillins is common. The latter has led to the incorporation of ampicillin into isolation media to select for *Aeromonas*. Most strains of *Aeromonas* and *Plesiomonas* are susceptible to chloramphenicol and tetracycline, with variable sensitivity to the aminoglycosides. Of the newer cephalosporins, only moxalactam demonstrates reasonable activity. Most strains are susceptible to the monobactam aztreonam, and trimethoprim-sulfamethoxazole may be effective against selected isolates. Whether or not antimicrobial therapy will alter the clinical course of gastroenteritis related to these agents is not yet known.

Noncholera *Vibrio* Infections

Noncholera vibrios are commonly found in the coastal waters of the world. *Vibrio parahaemolyticus* is the most important species. Illnesses have been reported after ingestion of incompletely cooked or raw seafoods (especially oysters) contaminated with these organisms. Gastroenteritis is the most common presentation. Wound infection and bacteremic illness have been described with other halophilic vibrio species.

Noncholera vibrios are inhibited by a variety of antibiotics. Gentamicin is the drug of choice against infections due to *V. parahaemolyticus*, but ampicillin, tetracycline, chloramphenicol, cephalothin, and kanamycin are frequently effective. Most strains of *V. fetus* are inhibited by tetracycline, chloramphenicol, ampicillin, streptomycin, and kanamycin.

Campylobacter Infections

Campylobacter organisms are small, curved, gram-negative rods that were previously classified among the vibrios. *Campylobacter fetus* (formerly *C. fetus*, subspecies *fetus*) is best recognized as a cause of puerperal infection. Reports of bacterial endocarditis, thrombophlebitis, and meningitis can also be found in the literature. Most isolates were found to be sensitive to aminoglycosides and tetracycline. Chloramphenicol and clindamycin may be effective as well. Clinical experience and pharmacokinetic data with clindamycin in neonates are limited. *C. fetus* is generally resistant to cephalosporins, colistin, polymyxin B, rifampin, and vancomycin. Sensitivity to erythromycin is variable.

Campylobacter jejuni (formerly *C. fetus*, subspecies *jejuni*) is now known to be a common cause of infectious diarrhea. The illness typically presents in early childhood and is usually self-limited; however, cases of rather severe colitis have been described. The onset is acute with diarrhea, fever, vomiting, and abdominal pain. Septic complications, such as bacteremia, arthritis, and osteomyelitis, have been reported occasionally. Uncomplicated *Campylobacter* enteritis usually does not require antimicrobial therapy. Whether or not treatment early in the disease may affect the clinical course is still unclear. Erythromycin therapy (40 mg/kg/24 hr divided every 6 hours for 7 days) shortens the duration of excretion of organisms in the stool and is the drug of first choice. Chloramphenicol, gentamicin, and tetracycline may also be effective. A *Campylobacter*-like organism *(C. pylori)* has been implicated as an etiologic agent in gastroduodenal disease, including gastritis, duodenitis, and peptic ulcer disease. The organism is morphologically similar to other *Campylobacter* species but with biochemical differences. It is characterized by a strong production of urease, believed to be important in the pathogenesis of gastric and duodenal mucosal damage. The diagnosis can be made by histologic examination of mucosa with direct visualization of organisms, by culture, or by serologic methods. The last cannot differentiate between acute and past infection. Direct histologic examination with Giemsa and hematoxylin-eosin staining is the most satisfactory technique. Urease production serves as a rapid diagnostic test to confirm the histologic finding of this organism. Initial therapy emphasizes the use of histamine$_2$ (H$_2$) antagonists, and patients in whom this approach fails may be helped by oral ampicillin in combination with oral bismuth preparations. Eradication of the organism from the mucosal surface has been associated with resolution of symptoms and histologic findings, but, disappointingly, relapse rates on long-term follow-up are high.

Infections Due to Other Gram-Negative Bacilli

Other Enterobacteriaceae. Certain other members of the Enterobacteriaceae sometimes cause infection in humans. *Arizona* organisms are now considered among the salmonellae. However, nosocomial infections caused by members of this group, notably *Arizona hinshawii*, have been described. Poultry, contaminated eggs and dairy products, and reptiles (especially snakes) have been identified as vectors of infection. Ampicillin, chloramphenicol, or trimethoprim-sulfamethoxazole are the agents that are usually effective in treatment.

Edwardsiella. *Edwardsiella* includes a group of motile, lactose-negative organisms that resemble salmonellae in some biochemical features and sometimes in pathogenicity for humans. They ferment only glucose and maltose. *E. tarda* has been isolated from a variety of mammals and reptiles. It is occasionally found in the human intestinal tract, especially in acute gastroenteritis, and it can produce serious septic conditions, usually in debilitated or immunocompromised hosts. Patients appear to be infected or colonized through inoculation of a wound or ingestion of the organism. *Edwardsiella* are susceptible in vitro to many antibiotics, including tetracycline, chloramphenicol, trimethoprim-sulfamethoxazole, cefotaxime, gentamicin, quinolones, and occasionally ampicillin.

Citrobacter. The *Citrobacter* group is composed of Enterobacteriaceae previously designated as *Escherichia freundii* and the Bethesda-Ballerup of "paracolon" organisms. *Citrobacter* strains occur infrequently in normal feces. They have been recovered from urinary tract infections in various septic processes. *Citrobacter* is also an occasional cause of neonatal meningitis. A significant number of these infants will develop brain abscesses, often despite early and appropriate antimicrobial therapy. Nosocomial outbreaks have been reported. Drugs of choice are aminoglycosides or third-generation cephalosporins. Some strains are susceptible to chloramphenicol and tetracycline.

Other Gram-Negative Bacilli

ACINETOBACTER. *Acinetobacter lwoffi* (previously *Mimia polymorpha* and *Achromobacter lwoffi*) neither ferments nor oxidizes carbohydrates, whereas *Acinetobacter calcoaceticus* (previously *Herellea vaginicola* and *Achromobacter anitratus*) utilizes glucose oxidatively and produces acid from 10 per cent (but not from 1 per cent) lactose-containing medium. These organisms are frequently antibiotic resistant, and antibiotic susceptibility tests are required as a guide to therapy. Drugs likely to be effective are ticarcillin, gentamicin, tobramycin, polymyxins, and the new agents aztreonam and imipenem. Ceftazidime (a third-generation cephalosporin) has activity against *Acinetobacter* spp. and other nonfermenters. The ampicillin-sulbactam combination (sulbactam is a nonreversible or "suicide" inhibitor of beta-lactamase) has shown promise in treating serious *Acinetobacter* infections.

MORAXELLA. *Moraxella* are similar to *Acinetobacter* but are oxidase positive and highly susceptible to penicillin. They are primary animal parasites, most commonly present on the mucous membranes. Most of these organisms do not utilize carbohydrates.

ALCALIGENES.* *A. faecalis* fails to ferment or oxidize any of the usual carbohydrates; it is usually motile. It may occasionally be confused on initial isolation with other nonlactose fermenters, chiefly *Salmonella* or *Shigella*. These organisms are not uniformly sensitive to any antibiotic; tetracycline and chloramphenicol are usually the most effective.

FLAVOBACTERIUM. *Flavobacteria* are widely distributed in soil and water and are encountered as opportunistic pathogens in humans. *F. meningosepticum*, which has high virulence for the neonate, has an unusual antibiotic susceptibility pattern for a gram-negative bacillus. It is usually susceptible in vitro to erythromycin, novobiocin, and rifampin—and, to a lesser degree, to chloramphenicol and streptomycin—but is resistant to gentamicin and polymyxins. Trimethoprim-sulfamethoxazole and cefoxitin may also be effective.

STREPTOBACILLUS MONILIFORMIS. *Streptobacillus moniliformis*, the cause of one type of rat-bite fever, is carried by many rats presumably as a saprophyte. Penicillin G is the treatment of choice, but streptomycin and tetracycline are also therapeutically effective. The wound should be immediately cleansed with soap and water. Tetanus prophylaxis should be carried out by standard methods.

CALYMMATOBACTERIUM (DONOVANIA) GRANULOMATIS. Granuloma inguinale is an indolent, ulcerative disease, caused by a gram-negative bacillus that is antigenically similar to, but not identical with, *Klebsiella pneumoniae* and *K. rhinoscleromatis*. It can be treated successfully with tetracyclines, chloramphenicol, or streptomycin. Penicillin G is not effective.

BARTONELLA BACILLIFORMIS. *Bartonella bacilliformis* is a gram-negative, very pleomorphic, motile organism that in humans causes two different clinical manifestations of the same geographically restricted bacterial disease.† The collective designation of the two syndromes is Carrión disease.

Penicillin, streptomycin, and chloramphenicol are dramatically effective in Oroya fever and greatly reduce the fatality rate, particularly if blood transfusions are also given. Control of the disease depends upon the

---

*Also "nonfermenter."

†Recently, cases of anemia involving *Bartonella*-like bodies have been reported from Southeast Asia.

elimination of the sand fly vectors. Insecticides, chlorophenothane (DDT), insect repellents, and elimination of breeding areas are of value. Prevention with antibiotics may be useful. Chloramphenicol should be used when the patient is also suffering from secondary *Salmonella* infection.

Others. There are a few other gram-negative bacilli that very rarely cause human infection but have been reported to do so. Members of a group of slow-growing, fastidious, gram-negative bacilli or coccobacilli, often referred to as the HACEK group (*Haemophilus* spp., *Actinobacillus* spp., *Cardiobacterium* spp., *Eikenella* spp., and *Kingella [Moraxella]* spp.), have been shown to cause a variety of infections, most notably endocarditis and skeletal infections. Other types of infection they cause are variable but may be bacteremic or localized to various organ systems. These organisms can require days to weeks to grow in standard blood culture systems and might be missed if cultures are not observed for a sufficient time.

Selection of antimicrobial therapy is based on in vitro susceptibility test results. The agents that are usually effective are listed here, but some of the newer agents mentioned, especially the newer aminoglycosides and third-generation cephalosporins, may prove useful with further experience.

Actinobacillus actinomycetemcomitans	Cephalosporins Tetracycline Streptomycin Chloramphenicol
Actinobacillus lignieresii	Kanamycin
Bordetella bronchiseptica	Tetracycline Polymyxins Chloramphenicol
Chromobacterium violaceum	Kanamycin or gentamicin Tetracycline Chloramphenicol
Comamonas terrigenia	Chloramphenicol Tetracycline
Enterobacter agglomerans	Gentamicin Chloramphenicol Colistin Kanamycin

Haemophilus aphrophilus
  (HB group) and
  Paraphrophilus
	Penicillin G
	Gentamicin
	Cephalothin
	Chloramphenicol
	Tetracycline
	Cephalosporins

INFECTIONS DUE TO ANAEROBIC COCCI AND GRAM-NEGATIVE BACILLI

ITZHAK BROOK, M.D., M.Sc.

The recovery of a child from an anaerobic infection depends on prompt and proper management. The strategy for therapy of anaerobic infections consists of surgical drainage of pus, débridement of any necrotic tissue, and appropriate antibiotics. Certain types of adjunct therapy such as hyperbaric oxygen may also be useful. Antimicrobial therapy is in many patients the only form of therapy required, whereas in others it is an important adjunct to a surgical approach.

Surgical therapy may be the only therapy required in some cases, as for localized abscesses or decubitus ulcers without signs of systemic involvement. In the treatment of such lesions, antibiotics are indicated whenever systemic manifestations of infection are present or when suppuration has either extended or threatened to spread into surrounding tissue. Antibiotics are needed in the majority of cases, however. Selection of antimicrobial agents is simplified when a culture result of a reliable specimen is available. This may be particularly difficult in anaerobic infections because of the problems encountered in obtaining appropriate specimens. Because of this difficulty, many patients are treated empirically on the basis of suspected, rather than established, pathogens. Fortunately, the types of anaerobes involved in many anaerobic infections and their antimicrobial susceptibility patterns tend to be predictable. Some anaerobic bacteria have become resistant to antimicrobial agents, however, and many can become resistant while a patient is receiving therapy.

Aside from susceptibility patterns, other factors influencing the choice of antimicrobial therapy include the pharmacologic characteristics of the various drugs, their toxicity, their effect on the normal flora, and their bactericidal activity.

Since anaerobic bacteria generally are recovered mixed with aerobic organisms, selection of proper therapy becomes more complicated. In the treatment of mixed infection the choice of the appropriate antimicrobial agents should provide for adequate coverage of most of the pathogens. Some broad-spectrum antibacterial agents possess such qualities, while for some organisms, additional agents should be added to the therapeutic regimen.

Antimicrobial Drugs

Penicillins. Penicillin-G is the drug of choice when the infecting strains are susceptible to this drug. These include the majority of anaerobic strains other than those belonging to the *B. fragilis* group. Other strains that may show resistance to penicillins are growing numbers of *Bacteroides*, such as the *B. melaninogenicus* group and *B. oralis*, strains of *Clostridium*, *Fusobacterium* species, and microaerophilic streptococci. Some of these strains show minimal inhibitory concentration (MIC) in dosages of 8 to 32 units/ml of penicillin G. In these instances, administration of very high dosages of penicillin G may eradicate the infection. Ampicillin, amoxicillin, and penicillin generally are equally active, but the semisynthetic penicillins are less active than the parent compound. Methicillin, nafcillin, and the isoxazolyl penicillins have unpredictable activity and frequently are inferior to penicillin G against anaerobes. Carbenicillin and ticarcillin are active against *B. fragilis* because of the high serum level that can be achieved; however, penicillin G is also active against *B. fragilis* in this concentration. Resistance to these agents is present in up to 30 per cent of *B. fragilis* strains.

Clavulanic acid is combined with amoxicillin for an oral preparation or with ticarcillin for parenteral use. Sulbactam is combined with ampicillin for parenteral use. Over 98 per cent of *B. fragilis* group are susceptible to these agents; however, resistance due to other mechanisms of resistance to penicillins is present in aerobic and facultative anaerobic bacteria.

Imipenem-cilastatin (athienamycin) is effective against a wide variety of aerobic and anaerobic gram-positive and gram-negative organisms. It possesses excellent activity against beta-lactamase–producing *Bacteroides* species and is an effective single agent for the therapy of mixed aerobic-anaerobic infections. However, at present, data in children are limited, and it is not yet approved for use in this age group.

Chloramphenicol. Although it is a bacteriostatic drug, chloramphenicol is one of the antimicrobial drugs most active against anaerobes, and resistance to this drug is rare. Although several failures to eradicate anaerobic infections, including bacteremia, with chloramphenicol have been reported, this drug has been used for over 25 years for treatment of anaerobic infections. It is regarded as a good choice for treatment of serious anaerobic infections when the nature and susceptibility of the infecting organisms are unknown. Because of its good penetration through the blood-brain barrier it is used in infections of the central nervous system. The toxicity of chloramphenicol must be borne in mind, however. This includes the low risk of aplastic anemia, dose-dependent leukopenia, and "gray baby syndrome" in the newborn.

Cephalosporins. The antimicrobial spectrum of the first-generation cephalosporins against anaerobes is similar to that of penicillin G, although they are less active on a weight basis. Similar to what is seen with penicillin G, most strains of the *B. fragilis* group and many of the *B. melaninogenicus* group are resistant to cephalosporins as a result of cephalosporinase production. Cefoxitin, a second-generation cephalosporin, is relatively resistant to this enzyme and is therefore effective against the *B. fragilis* group. Cefoxitin is active in vitro against at least 95 per cent of strains of *B. fragilis* at a level of 32 µg/ml, but cefoxitin is relatively inactive against most species of *Clostridium* (including *C. difficile*) other than *Clostridium perfringens*. Clinical experiences with cefoxitin in anaerobic infections have shown it to be effective in eradication of these infections. It has often been used for surgical prophylaxis because of its activity against enteric gram-negative rods. Cefotetan is equally as effective as cefoxitin against *B. fragilis* but is less effective against all members of the *B. fragilis* group. These

members represent 35 to 50 per cent of *B. fragilis* group isolutes recovered from patients. Third-generation cephalosporins, with the exception of moxalactam, are effective only against about 50 per cent of *B. fragilis* groups.

Clindamycin. Clindamycin has a broad range of activity against anaerobic organisms and has proved its efficacy in clinical trials. Approximately 95 per cent of the anaerobic bacteria isolated in clinical practice are susceptible to easily achievable levels of clindamycin. *B. fragilis* is generally sensitive to levels below 3 µg/ml. There are, however, reports of resistant strains associated with clinical infections, although these are uncommon.

Several reports have described the successful use of this drug in the treatment of anaerobic infection. Clindamycin does not cross the blood-brain barrier efficiently and should not be administered in cases of central nervous system infections. Because of its effectiveness against anaerobes it is frequently used in combination with aminoglycosides for the treatment of mixed aerobic-anaerobic infections of the abdominal cavity and obstetric infection. The primary manifestation of toxicity with clindamycin is colitis. It should be kept in mind that colitis has been associated with a number of other antimicrobial agents, such as ampicillin and all the cephalosporins, and has been described in seriously ill patients in the absence of previous antimicrobial therapy. The occurrence of colitis in pediatric patients is very rare, however.

Metronidazole. This drug shows excellent bactericidal activity against most obligate anaerobic bacteria, such as *B. fragilis* group, other species of *Bacteroides*, fusobacteria, and clostridia. Occasional strains of anaerobic gram-positive cocci and nonsporulating bacilli are highly resistant. Microaerophilic streptococci, *Propionibacterium acnes*, and *Actinomyces* species are almost uniformly resistant. Aerobic and facultative anaerobes, such as coliforms, are usually highly resistant. Over 90 per cent of obligate anaerobes are susceptible to less than 2 µg/ml metronidazole.

Clinical experience in adults and limited experience in children indicate its efficacy in the treatment of infections caused by anaerobes, including intra-abdominal sepsis, infections of the female genital tract, and especially infections of the central nervous system. However, it does not seem to be as effective in therapy of anaerobic gram-positive pulmonary infection. Because of its lack of activity against aerobic bacteria, additional antimicrobial agents effective against these organisms should be administered whenever they are also present. The use of metronidazole seems advantageous in central nervous system infections because of its excellent penetration into the central nervous system.

Tetracyclines. Tetracycline has currently limited usefulness because of the development of resistance to it by virtually all types of anaerobes. Currently only about 45 per cent of all *B. fragilis* strains are susceptible to this drug. The new tetracycline analogues, doxycycline and minocycline, are more active than the parent compound. The use of tetracycline is not recommended before 8 years of age because of its adverse effect on teeth.

Other Drugs

Vancomycin is effective against all gram-positive anaerobes but is inactive against gram-negative ones. Little clinical experience has been gained in the treatment of anaerobic bacteria using this agent.

Clavulanic acid and sulbactam are beta-lactamase inhibitors that resemble the nucleus of penicillin but differ in several ways. They irreversibly inhibit beta-lactamase enzymes produced by some Enterobacteriaceae, staphylococci, and beta-lactamase–producing *Bacteroides* species (*B. fragilis* group and strains of *B. melaninogenicus* and *B. oralis*). When used in conjunction with a beta-lactamase antibiotic, they are effective in treating infections caused by beta-lactamase–producing bacteria. Its usefulness in the therapy of human infections is currently being evaluated. Clavulanic acid and other beta-lactamase inhibitors may prove to be effective adjuncts to penicillins in the treatment of resistant organisms.

HAEMOPHILUS INFLUENZAE INFECTIONS

JANET R. GILSDORF, M.D.

Haemophilus influenzae type b is the most common cause of serious systemic bacterial infections in children. Invasive diseases caused by this organism are limited almost exclusively to children between 2 months and 6 years of age; approximately 75 per cent of illnesses occur before age 18 months. Although the encapsulated type b *H. influenzae* is responsible for the majority of invasive bacteremic diseases caused by this organism, nonencapsulated, nontypable *H. influenzae* is an important cause of local, mucosa-associated infections, such as otitis media and sinusitis.

GENERAL ANTIBIOTIC THERAPY

A number of antibiotic regimens are now available for the treatment of infections caused by invasive *H. influenzae* type b. Newer drugs, including cephalosporins, appear to offer the same therapeutic efficacy as ampicillin or chloramphenicol but may offer certain advantages because of their different toxicities and pharmacokinetics. In addition, carefully monitored home antibiotic therapy, using either oral or parenteral drugs, may be considered in selected patients.

In many invasive *H. influenzae* infections, empiric antibiotic therapy is initiated before the etiologic agent is identified. This empiric therapy is broad spectrum, designed to treat the most likely infecting organisms until more definitive therapy, based on culture and sensitivity results, can be chosen.

Antibiotic Resistance

The prevalence of ampicillin-resistant *H. influenzae* strains may be as high as 30 per cent in some areas of the United States. The majority of these strains may be rapidly identified by their production of β-lactamase. However, rarely, ampicillin resistance is mediated by other mechanisms, including alteration of penicillin-binding proteins. These organisms produce no β-lactamase and can be identified only by standard sensitivity testing. Chloramphenicol-resistant strains remain rare and are often ampicillin resistant as well. However, because of the possible increased spread of chloramphenicol-resistant strains, sensitivity testing to chloramphenicol should be done on all invasive *H. influenzae* type b strains. No *H. influenzae* type b isolates resistant to the newer cephalosporins have been reported.

Ampicillin

Ampicillin was the major drug for treatment of *H. influenzae* infections prior to the emergence of resistant strains in the late 1970s. The drug continues to be effective treatment in patients infected with organisms that are known to be ampicillin susceptible.

Chloramphenicol

Serum chloramphenicol levels following oral administration may be identical with, or higher than, those following the same dose of intravenous chloramphenicol. Thus, oral chloramphenicol is adequate therapy in patients tolerating oral feedings. Because of bone marrow suppression associated with high serum chloramphenicol levels, the use of this drug requires the ready availability of reliable tests for monitoring serum levels after two or three doses. Peak serum levels (samples drawn 30 minutes after completion of an intravenous infusion or 90 minutes after an oral dose) should be maintained between 15 and 25 μg/ml to ensure an adequate therapeutic level and to avoid toxicity. Limited data are available on the clinical use of trough serum levels (samples drawn immediately prior to administration of a dose), but a trough level between 5 and 10 μg/ml ensures continuous levels of chloramphenicol above the minimal inhibitory concentration of the drug for most strains of *H. influenzae* b. Serum chloramphenicol levels may vary widely and may be affected by the concurrent administration of anticonvulsive drugs or rifampin.

Newer Cephalosporins

Cefotaxime, ceftriaxone, and cefuroxime all penetrate the blood-brain barrier, and thus are very useful in treating young children in whom bacteremic *H. influenzae* b infections may be associated with meningitis. Ceftriaxone offers the advantage of twice-daily dosing (intravenous or intramuscular) for meningitis and once-a-day dosing (intravenous or intramuscular) for non-meningitis infections. Cefuroxime has the possible disadvantage of slightly delayed sterilization of the cerebrospinal fluid (CSF) in some patients with meningitis.

MENINGITIS

Empiric therapy for bacterial meningitis in children should include an antibiotic effective against ampicillin-resistant *H. influenzae* (Table 1). Such drugs include chloramphenicol, 75 to 100 mg/kg/day divided into four doses, or one of the new cephalosporins, such as ceftriaxone, 100 mg/kg/day divided into two doses, cefotaxime, 200 mg/kg/day divided into four doses, or

TABLE 1. Therapy for *H. influenzae* Type b Systemic Infections

Infection	Empiric Drugs (Prior to Confirmation of *H. influenzae* b)	Comments	Subsequent Drugs (After Confirmation of *H. influenzae* b)	Duration of Therapy
Meningitis	1. Chloramphenicol, 75–100 mg/kg/day intravenously (IV) in 4 doses, *or*	Monitor serum levels to maintain peak at 15–25 μg/ml	1. Ampicillin, 200–300 mg/kg/day IV in 4 to 6 doses for ampicillin-sensitive strains, *or*	10–14 days
	2. Ceftriaxone, 100 mg/kg/day IV in 2 doses, *or*		2. Chloramphenicol, 75 mg/kg/day po in 4 doses, *or*	10–14 days
	3. Cefotaxime, 200 mg/kg/day IV in 4 doses, *or*		3. Ceftriaxone *or* 4. Cefotaxime *or* 5. Cefuroxime — Same as empiric therapy	10–14 days / –14 days / 10–14 days
	4. Cefuroxime, 250 mg/kg/day IV in 4 doses			
Bacteremic, nonmeningeal infections	1. Chloramphenicol, 75–100 mg/kg/day IV in 4 doses, *or*	Monitor serum levels to maintain peak at 15–25 μg/ml	1. Ampicillin, 100–200 mg/kg/day IV in 4–6 doses for ampicillin-sensitive strains, *or*	Varies with clinical entities
	2. Ceftriaxone, 50–75 mg/kg/day IV in 1 or 2 doses, *or*		2. Chloramphenicol, 75 mg/kg/day po in 4 doses, *or*	*Note:* Oral antibiotics may be used to complete therapy in some clinical entities (see text)
	3. Cefotaxime, 100–150 mg/kg/day IV in 4 doses, *or*		3. Ceftriaxone *or* 4. Cefotaxime *or* 5. Cefuroxime — Same as empiric therapy	
	4. Cefuroxime, 100–150 mg/kg/day IV in 3 doses			

cefuroxime, 250 mg/kg/day divided into four doses. If the infecting organism is known to be ampicillin sensitive, therapy with ampicillin, 200–300 mg/kg/day in four to six divided doses, may be used.

Recent studies have suggested that dexamethasone (0.15 mg/kg every 6 hours for 4 days) may reduce the incidence of deafness following *H. influenzae* b meningitis, particularly when cefuroxime is used for treatment. These recommendations for the use of steroids in acute bacterial meningitis are very controversial, and confirmation of their value in preventing deafness or other neurologic sequelae awaits results of ongoing, additional studies.

With appropriate antibiotic treatment, a clinical response (decreased temperature, normalized peripheral blood leukocyte count, and improved neurologic status) should be noted in 24 to 36 hours. Failure of a patient to respond clinically to initial antibiotic therapy within 48 hours is an indication for repeat lumbar puncture. If the CSF is not sterile, a resistant organism should be suspected and alternate antibiotic therapy instituted. If an organism resistant to multiple agents is suspected, trimethoprim-sulfamethoxazole, 20 mg of trimethoprim and 100 mg of sulfamethoxazole per kilogram per day in four divided doses, could be considered, although controlled trials documenting its efficacy in *H. influenzae* meningitis have not been conducted.

Initial fluid management needs to be approached with care. Many children with meningitis may be dehydrated and may require rehydration to ensure adequate cerebral perfusion. Children who are adequately hydrated should not receive fluids in excess of maintenance requirements, and the osmolality of serum and urine should be monitored for evidence of inappropriate antidiuretic hormone secretion. This entity is managed by decreasing fluid intake to about 75 per cent of maintenance. Rarely, endotoxemia and septic shock may occur and are treated with intensive care supportive measures.

Antibiotic therapy for uncomplicated *H. influenzae* meningitis should continue for at least 10 days, although some centers have reported good outcome with 7 days. Patients with prolonged fever, slow neurologic recovery, or otherwise complicated courses are usually treated for longer periods, 10 to 14 days or longer. If the patient's course is uncomplicated, repeat lumbar puncture is not necessary, either during therapy or when treatment is terminated. Relapse is rare and usually occurs 48 to 96 hours after stopping antibiotic therapy. If recurrent infection occurs more than 7 days following the end of therapy, reinfection rather than relapse is likely. Typical CSF findings from a lumbar puncture done at 10 to 12 days after the initiation of therapy include an elevated protein level and lymphocytosis, although about 30 per cent of patients may have persistent neutrophils. Decreased glucose levels in the CSF or the presence of polysaccharide antigen in the CSF may persist for weeks.

Acute Complications

In all children with bacterial meningitis, the possibility of increased intracranial pressure should be considered, and repeated physical examination, careful neurologic examination, and monitoring of vital signs should be performed frequently. Once increased intracranial pressure is recognized, therapy should be instituted immediately. Severe intracranial hypertension may require the insertion of an intracranial pressure monitoring device to assess the adequacy of therapy with mannitol or other osmotic agents. Airway maintenance and oxygen administration are important to ensure adequate oxygenation of the cerebral tissue. Anti-inflammatory agents, such as steroids, have been used to control acute intracranial pressure, but there are no data supporting their efficacy in meningitis. Seizures may occur early owing to small areas of infarction secondary to cerebral vasculitis and may be controlled with phenobarbital, phenytoin (Dilantin), or other anticonvulsant agents. Inappropriate antidiuretic hormone effect is managed with fluid restriction and careful monitoring of serum and urine osmolality. Ventriculitis, especially in infants younger than 6 months of age, may cause prolonged fever and hydrocephalus. Disseminated intravascular coagulation occurs uncommonly and is managed with fresh frozen plasma, platelet transfusions, and supportive measures as necessary.

Secondary and Persistent Fevers

Fever persists beyond 10 days after the initiation of therapy in about 10 per cent of patients. These prolonged (persistent) fevers may be due to drug fever, subdural effusions, nosocomial infections, unrecognized and undrained secondary foci (septic arthritis or pleural or pericardial empyema), or recurrent meningitis. Secondary fever occurs in 20 to 50 per cent of patients and may be associated with intercurrent viral illness, drug fever, phlebitis, or subdural effusion.

The occurrence of subdural effusions during the resolution of meningitis is common. If the effusions, as seen on computed tomographic scan, are large or are associated with increased irritability, neurologic deficit, persistent seizures, or persistent fever, the fluid should be evacuated and cultured. Rarely, subdural effusions will contain infected, loculated fluid. Such subdural empyemas should be surgically drained to shorten the duration of hospitalization and decrease morbidity. Increasing head size may indicate subdural effusion, communicating hydrocephalus, or inadequately treated ventriculitis. Brain abscess secondary to *H. influenzae* meningitis is rare but is more common than with other meningotrophic organisms and is usually apparent on computed tomographic scan (demonstrating enhancement of the vascular rim). Surgical drainage or prolonged antibiotic therapy, or both, may be required.

Outcome

The mortality of *H. influenzae* type b meningitis is 3 to 7 per cent, and the morbidity may be up to 50 per cent. About 10 per cent of children may suffer unilateral or bilateral deafness, and comprehensive hearing evaluation should be done during recovery from the infection. Other neurologic sequelae include seizure disorders, learning disability, mental retardation, blindness, and spastic diplegia or quadriplegia. Cranial nerve palsies are generally transient.

BACTEREMIC INFECTIONS WITHOUT MENINGITIS

Empiric therapy for patients with possible bacteremic *H. influenzae* infections without meningitis (Table 1) should include a parenteral antimicrobial agent that will be effective against ampicillin-resistant strains and that will achieve bactericidal levels in the CSF, as central nervous system seeding may accompany any bacteremic

H. influenzae type b infection. Such empiric therapy should include parenteral chloramphenicol, 75 to 100 mg/kg/day divided into four doses, or one of the third-generation cephalosporins, such as ceftriaxone, 50 to 75 mg/kg/day divided in one or two doses, cefotaxime, 100 to 150 mg/kg/day divided into four doses, or cefuroxime, 100 to 150 mg/kg/day divided into three doses. If the organism is known to be ampicillin sensitive (beta-lactamase negative), parenteral ampicillin, 100 to 200 mg/kg/day in four to six divided doses, may be used.

Epiglottitis

Acute epiglottitis, which is nearly always caused by *H. influenzae* Type b, is a true medical emergency requiring immediate measures to maintain an adequate airway. Nasotracheal intubation, orotracheal intubation, and tracheostomy have been used successfully with comparable rates of morbidity. The use of a technique for which there is readily available expertise and back-up is more important than the specific procedure. Most patients with epiglottitis have an associated *H. influenzae* bacteremia, so initial antibiotic therapy should follow the above guidelines for bacteremia without meningitis and should be continued for at least 7 days. In most instances, with adequate therapy, the signs and symptoms of the acute infection abate within 48 hours, and the tracheal cannula may be removed 2 to 3 days after the initiation of antibiotic therapy. Secondary foci of infection are uncommon but may include pneumonia and, very rarely, meningitis.

Septic Arthritis

Septic arthritis of the hip is a surgical emergency and should be externally drained immediately at the time of diagnosis. In contrast to *Staphylococcus aureus* septic arthritis, *H. influenzae* b infections of the shoulder, knee, and elbow joints rarely require surgical drainage when appropriate antibiotic therapy is used. Needle aspiration to confirm the etiologic agent and to provide some drainage is recommended.

Initial empiric antibiotic therapy for patients with septic arthritis should include antimicrobial agents that are effective against the most likely pathogens and that achieve adequate bactericidal levels within the joint spaces. Coverage for *H. influenzae* type b is accomplished by following the previously given guidelines for treatment of bacteremic *H. influenzae* type b infections without meningitis. If β-lactamase antibiotics (ampicillin or new cephalosporins) are used, they should be given by the intravenous route until the child is afebrile, the erythrocyte sedimentation rate is significantly decreased, and local inflammation has decreased (usually 5 to 7 days). Then oral antibiotics (amoxicillin or amoxicillin–clavulanic acid, 100 to 150 mg/kg/day in four divided doses; cefuroxime axetil, 30 mg/kg/day in two divided doses; cefixime, 8 mg/kg/day in one or two divided doses; or cefaclor, 100 to 150 mg/kg/day in four divided doses) may be used to complete a minimal antibiotic course of 2 to 3 weeks. Peak serum bactericidal levels of 1:8 or more ensure continued adequate therapy. Antibiotic therapy needs to be continued until the sedimentation rate returns to normal. If chloramphenicol is used as initial therapy, the oral form of the drug may be used to complete the entire 2- to 3-week course, with careful monitoring of serum drug levels and hematopoietic status. Decreased reticulocyte count is the first indication of marrow suppression; however, the drug may be safely continued until the peripheral leukocyte count decreases below 3000 cells per cubic millimeter.

Osteomyelitis

H. influenzae type b osteomyelitis tends to be a less destructive process than that caused by staphylococci, and thus surgical drainage may not be necessary. In most instances, the extremity is immobilized, often with casting. The initial antibiotic therapy is identical with that recommended for septic arthritis. Parenteral administration of ampicillin or new cephalosporins should be continued until the child is afebrile, all local signs of inflammation have abated, and the erythrocyte sedimentation rate has significantly decreased (1 to 3 weeks). For infections caused by ampicillin-sensitive strains, oral therapy with amoxicillin (100 to 150 mg/kg/day in four divided doses) may then be continued for an additional 2 to 4 weeks (6 weeks total for the course) and until the erythrocyte sedimentation rate is normal. As a guide to adequate therapy, the peak serum concentration of oral amoxicillin (sample drawn 2 hours after an oral dose) should be 8 to 20 μg/ml, with a bactericidal titer of 1:8 or more. For infections caused by ampicillin-resistant organisms, the remainder of the 6-week course may be completed with cefaclor, 100 to 150 mg/kg/day in four divided doses; cefuroxime axetil, 30 mg/kg/day in two divided doses; cefixime, 8 mg/kg/day in one or two divided doses; or amoxicillin–clavulanic acid, 100 to 150 mg/kg/day in four divided doses.

Pneumonia

H. influenzae pneumonia is commonly segmental or lobar and may be associated with pleural effusion. Initial antibiotic therapy should include antimicrobial agents that ensure adequate bactericidal levels in lung tissue and is accomplished using the previously given guidelines for bacteremic *H. influenzae* type b infections without meningitis.

After the child's condition has clinically stabilized, and the child is no longer tachypneic and tolerates oral feedings (3 to 5 days), oral amoxicillin may be used for infections caused by ampicillin-sensitive strains. For ampicillin-resistant strains, cefaclor or amoxicillin–clavulanic acid (both at 100 to 150 mg/kg/day in four divided doses), or cefuroxime axetil (30 mg/kg/day in two divided doses) or cefixime (8 mg/kg/day in one or two divided doses) may be used. Effective treatment of uncomplicated pneumonia is achieved with 10 to 14 days of total antibiotic therapy. However, in the presence of large pleural effusions, prolonged antibiotic therapy may be necessary. Needle aspiration of large pleural effusions should be performed early to evacuate the fluid as well as to recover the causative organism, and empyema is treated with a closed-chest tube until drainage substantially decreases (usually 2 to 3 days).

Cellulitis

The most serious aspects of this illness are the associated bacteremia, seen in 70 to 80 per cent of patients, and the possibility of a secondary focus of infection, such as meningitis, septic arthritis, or pericarditis. Most infants defervesce within 18 to 24 hours of appropriate antibiotic therapy; persistence of fever more than 48 hours after starting treatment suggests the possibility of a resistant organism or the occurrence of a secondary focus. The empiric antibiotic therapy for *H. influenzae* type b cellulitis is outlined in the previously given guidelines for treatment of bacteremic infections without meningitis. After the child is afebrile and inflammation has decreased (2 to 4 days), an antibiotic course totaling 7 to 10 days may be completed with an oral antibiotic, such as amoxicillin (100 to 150 mg/kg/day in four divided doses) for ampicillin-sensitive organisms or cefaclor or amoxicillin–clavulanic acid (both 100 to 150 mg/kg/day in four divided doses), or cefuroxime axetil (30 mg/kg/day in two divided doses) or cefixime (8 mg/kg/day in one or two divided doses) for ampicillin-resistant organisms.

Periorbital cellulitis may be associated with underlying sinusitis or orbital cellulitis; computed tomographic scans may be useful in defining the extent of the infection.

Bacteremia Without Apparent Focus

Occult *H. influenzae* type b bacteremia occurs among infants under 2 years of age; these infants present with high fever, leukocytosis with a marked shift to the left, and no apparent focus of infection on initial evaluation. If untreated, many of these children ultimately develop clinically apparent infection, such as pneumonia or meningitis. Since the child with *H. influenzae* bacteremia without focus is at increased risk of invasive disease, treatment should be identical with that of a systemic *H. influenzae* infection, with admission to the hospital and initiation of appropriate antibiotic therapy. If the CSF cultures are sterile, no secondary foci of infection are found, and the child is afebrile and clinically improved, the antibiotics may be discontinued after 7 days.

Uncommon Systemic Infections

The following may be complications of acute *H. influenzae* type b bacteremia:

Pericarditis. *H. influenzae* type b pericarditis is generally associated with another focus of infection, such as meningitis, septic arthritis, facial cellulitis, or pneumonia. In these patients, the duration of antibiotic therapy is dictated by the primary site of infection. Pericarditis may be a life-threatening infection, and the patients should be carefully monitored for evidence of cardiac tamponade. Early surgical drainage of the pericardial empyema will decrease morbidity.

Endocarditis. H. influenzae type b endocarditis may occur in children with cyanotic congenital heart disease; these children have persistent *Haemophilus* bacteremia and low-grade fever. Most case reports document successful therapy with 6 weeks of intravenous ampicillin or with intravenous or oral chloramphenicol if the organism is ampicillin resistant.

Central Nervous System Shunt Infections. Patients with indwelling ventricular drainage systems may be at increased risk for meningitis following *H. influenzae* bacteremia. These patients have been successfully treated with 2 to 3 weeks of antibiotics without replacement of the shunt apparatus. However, sterilization of the ventricular fluid obtained from the shunt reservoir during antibiotic therapy must be documented.

Neonatal Sepsis. *H. influenzae*, both type b and nontypable varieties, may produce a clinical picture similar to group B streptococcal sepsis in neonates. These premature or term infants present with apparent respiratory distress syndrome and may develop shock within the first 24 hours. Optimal antibiotic therapy for preterm infants includes newer cephalosporins, such as cefotaxime, 100 mg/kg/day in two daily doses for infants younger than 7 days of age and 150 mg/kg/day in three daily doses for babies 1 to 4 weeks of age. For term infants, the dose of cefotaxime is 100 mg/kg/day in two daily doses for neonates younger than 7 days and 150 mg/kg/day in three daily doses for babies 1 to 4 weeks of age. Ceftriaxone, 50 mg/kg once a day, may also be used in neonatal infections. If the organism is shown to be ampicillin sensitive, ampicillin, 100 mg/kg/day in two divided doses for babies up to 7 days of age or 150 to 200 mg/kg/day in three or four divided doses for neonates beyond 7 days of age, may be used. Therapy should continue for 14 days in infants showing a rapid clinical response; prolonged clinical illness requires longer therapy and a search for another focus of infection. Chloramphenicol is not used in the neonatal period.

MUCOSAL SURFACE INFECTIONS

The following respiratory mucosal infections are generally caused by nonencapsulated, nontypable *H. influenzae* but may occasionally be caused by encapsulated type b organisms.

Otitis Media

Approximately one third of all otitis media infections are due to *H. influenzae*, and approximately 30 per cent of these may be due to ampicillin-resistant organisms. In general, oral amoxicillin (40 mg/kg/day in three divided doses) remains the drug of choice for otitis media of unknown etiology. In patients who fail to respond to this therapy (e.g., continued fever, irritability, and poor feeding), several alternative antimicrobial agents may be used, all of which appear to have equal efficacy against *H. influenzae*. These include cefaclor (40 mg/kg/day orally in three divided doses), erythromycin-sulfisoxazole (40 mg/kg/day of erythromycin in three or four divided doses), trimethoprim-sulfamethoxazole (6 to 8 mg/kg/day of trimethoprim in two divided doses), cefuroxime axetil (30 mg/kg/day in two divided doses), cefixime (8 mg/kg/day in one or two divided doses), or amoxicillin–clavulanic acid (40 mg/kg/day of amoxicillin in three divided doses). Antihistamines, decongestants, and nasal drops have not been shown to be effective in preventing acute otitis media or in facilitating drainage of the middle ear effusion following acute infection. However, these agents may provide symptomatic relief for children with viral upper respiratory infections often associated with acute otitis media. In most instances, the antibiotic therapy is continued for 10 days,

with a follow-up evaluation 2 to 3 weeks following discontinuation of therapy. Asymptomatic sterile middle ear effusions may persist for at least 4 weeks after acute infection in half of the adequately treated patients.

Sinusitis

The antimicrobial therapy for *H. influenzae* sinusitis is identical with that for acute otitis media. However, adequate resolution may require continued antibiotic therapy for 2 to 3 weeks, along with the use of systemic or topical decongestants or both. If clinical improvement does not occur within 48 to 72 hours, surgical drainage may be indicated.

Bronchiectasis

Long-term (6 weeks) administration of amoxicillin or another of the drugs used to treat acute otitis media usually results in symptomatic improvement of children with chronic pulmonary disease and bronchiectasis. In controlled studies, long-term sulfonamide administration has decreased the frequency of recurrence in individuals with *Haemophilus* bronchiectasis.

Conjunctivitis

Systemic antibiotic therapy is generally not required for *H. influenzae* conjunctivitis unless it is associated with periorbital cellulitis. Administration of topical antibiotic ophthalmic drops (such as gentamicin or sulfacetamide) every 2 hours or ointment every 4 to 6 hours for 5 to 7 days generally controls this infection.

PREVENTION OF *H. INFLUENZAE* TYPE b INFECTION

Two approaches to the prevention of serious *H. influenzae* b infections in young children are available. Rifampin prophylaxis to all household or daycare contacts in some situations may prevent the spread of the bacteria from asymptomatic carriers of any age to young, susceptible children. Vaccination of young children who are old enough to mount a high and sustained immune response may also prevent *H. influenzae* infections.

Prophylaxis of Contacts

Clusters of systemic *H. influenzae* type b infections have recently been recognized among household and daycare contacts of children with invasive *H. influenzae* b disease, and the asymptomatic nasopharyngeal carriage rates of *H. influenzae* b may be much higher in contacts compared with the general population. Rifampin has been shown to eliminate the nasopharyngeal carrier state, at least in the short term, from household and daycare contacts, thus decreasing the spread of *H. influenzae* organisms to young, susceptible children.

Household Contacts. Among household contacts of a child with systemic *H. influenzae* b infection, the risk of the occurrence of secondary disease in children under age 4 years has been well documented and is significantly higher than in age-matched children in the general population. The risk is particularly great for children under age 1 year (6 per cent). Thus, the American Academy of Pediatrics Committee on Infectious Diseases has recommended that rifampin prophylaxis be used in all household contacts of children with invasive *H. influenzae* type b disease if any of the household members are under 4 years of age.

Daycare Contacts. The risk of occurrence of secondary invasive disease among daycare contacts is less well understood, and the efficacy of rifampin in preventing secondary disease in the daycare setting has not been established. Thus, the prophylaxis of daycare contacts needs to be considered on an individual basis for each daycare situation. Caregivers in the daycare facility and parents of the other children need to be notified of the potential risk to ensure prompt evaluation of febrile illnesses in the contacts. While secondary cases in day care contacts over age 2 are very rare, contacts under age one year may be at greater risk. An outbreak of multiple cases of invasive *H. influenzae* b infections in a daycare setting may indicate the presence of as yet unrecognized risk factors among these children. Thus, rifampin prophylaxis should be instituted when an outbreak is suspected (more than one case within 60 to 90 days), and all daycare children and adult caretakers should be treated simultaneously.

Administration of Rifampin. Rifampin is given at a dose of 20 mg/kg once a day for 4 days to children and 600 mg once a day for 4 days to adults. No pediatric suspension of rifampin is commercially available, so liquid preparations must be freshly prepared by a pharmacist, or the correct daily dose of the powder must be prepared to be administered in a suitable vehicle, such as applesauce or ice cream. Rifampin is available in 300-mg and 150-mg capsules. Contraindications to rifampin use include pregnancy and known allergy to rifampin. All household contacts are treated simultaneously and as soon as possible following diagnosis of the index case. If the patient's household or daycare facility has children younger than 4 years, the patient should receive 4 days of rifampin upon hospital discharge, as treatment of systemic disease may not eradicate the carriage state and he or she may continue to spread the organism to the young, susceptible contacts. No data are available to suggest that rifampin may protect the patient from reinfecting himself or herself. The risk of spread to contacts from patients with systemic nonmeningeal *H. influenzae* b infections (such as pneumonia, cellulitis, and so on) is identical with that from children with meningitis, and the prophylaxis recommendations apply to situations involving all forms of invasive *H. influenzae* b infections.

Vaccines

Several vaccines have been developed for the prevention of *H. influenzae* b infections, and the spectrum of available vaccines and the recommended age of immunization are constantly changing. The most recent vaccines consist of the capsular polysaccharide of *H. influenzae* b (PRP) conjugated to a protein carrier (such as diphtheria toxoid, CRM-197, or *Neisseria meningitidis* outer membrane protein). These vaccines are licensed for use in all children at age 18 months, with permissive use at age 15 months, based on studies of antibody responses; additional data in younger children may lead to licensure at younger ages. Efficacy trials of these vaccines (the ability to prevent natural disease) in various population groups have given disparate results, and ongoing trials are in progress.

All of these vaccines protect against invasive *H. influenzae* b infections and cannot prevent nontypable *H. influenzae* infections. Therefore, they are not effective in preventing recurrent otitis media or sinusitis.

TETANUS NEONATORUM
JAMES M. ADAMS, M.D.

Although neonatal tetanus is now rare in the United States, it is most prevalent among infants delivered at home and in segments of the population with inadequate maternal immunization. It must be differentiated primarily from neonatal seizures, but trauma, hypoxic injury, septicemia, and other diseases of the perinatal period are common in this group of patients and may coexist with neonatal tetanus.

General Supportive Care. Programs for outpatient management of tetanus have been implemented in developing nations, but the disease should be considered an indication for hospitalization of the newborn infant even if initial spasms are mild. The baby should be admitted to a neonatal intensive care unit or a unit able to provide electronic cardiac monitoring, a controlled thermal environment, skilled nursing care, and mechanical ventilatory support, if necessary.

The infant should be placed initially in a servocontrolled or manually controlled incubator, protected from light and noise. This environment reduces the spasm-provoking external stimuli that reach the baby. Swaddling and minimal handling and disturbance of the infant further reduce the tendency of environmental stimuli to provoke self-perpetuating spasms. Such minimal intrusion into the environment of the infant requires close observation by trained personnel as well as careful electronic monitoring. Swaddling may result in overheating if the temperature of both the infant and its environment is not properly monitored and controlled.

Serum electrolytes, blood urea nitrogen, albumin, and urine specific gravity determinations aid in guiding metabolic and nutritional management. All infants should receive 1 mg of vitamin K_1 initially, and a VDRL specimen should be obtained. Prophylactic eye care should be administered with erythromycin ointment.

Fluids should be administered intravenously initially as 10 per cent glucose in water with appropriate electrolytes at an infusion rate of 100 to 125 ml/kg/24 hr. Once spasms are controlled, or if mechanical ventilation has been instituted and the condition stabilized, enteral feedings can be initiated by nasogastric tube if bowel sounds are present. A formula of 24 calories per ounce should be given initially at 25 ml/kg/24 hr by continuous nasogastric infusion and advanced progressively until intravenous fluids can be discontinued. For long-term growth and nutrition, formula intakes of 140 to 150 ml/kg/24 hr will be necessary. When the infant's course is stabilized on full milk drip feedings, intermittent gavage may be attempted. This feeding program is designed to avoid gastric distention, impairment of mobility of the diaphragm, and regurgitation. In term infants, if the formula utilized meets the recommendations of the American Academy of Pediatrics Committee on Nutrition, vitamin and mineral supplementation will not be required unless specific deficiencies are identified.

Bacteriologic Management. Because septicemia or meningoencephalitis cannot be ruled out during the initial hours of hospitalization, ampicillin (150 mg/kg/24 hr in three divided doses) and kanamycin (15 mg/kg/24 hr in two divided doses) should be administered parenterally following blood and cerebrospinal fluid cultures. When a diagnosis of tetanus has been confirmed, these antibiotics may be discontinued and 100,000 units/kg/24 hr of aqueous penicillin G given alone to finish a 10-day course of therapy.

Human tetanus immune globulin, 500 units, should be given in divided doses intramuscularly. All babies should receive an initial dose of diphtheria-tetanus vaccine prior to discharge, as no permanent immunity results from *Clostridium tetani* infections treated with antitoxin. The initial immunization should be delayed, however, until 4 to 6 weeks after administration of antitoxin.

Positive cultures of *C. tetani* from the umbilicus are rarely obtained, even with anaerobic techniques. Antibody tests may confirm the diagnosis, but results are usually not available in the early days of the disease.

Control of Tetanic Spasms. Various tranquilizers and sedating drugs have been utilized to control the violent spasms of tetanus. At best, these agents can be expected to modify the frequency or severity of the spasms rather than abate them. In general, slightly better results can be expected from combination regimens and very high dosage ranges. The incidence of apnea, retention of pulmonary secretions, and other complications of central nervous system depression, however, is also increased. The potential for addiction with these drugs, particularly chloral hydrate, must be considered.

Phenobarbital 10 to 15 mg/kg/day may be given by nasogastric tube in two or three divided doses. Chloral hydrate, 40 to 60 mg/kg/day, may be added. Good results have been achieved abroad using a continuous infusion of diazepam, 20 to 40 mg/kg/day. This is combined with phenobarbital, 10 mg/kg/day. The safety of parenteral diazepam in the neonate has not been established, however, and respiratory depression requiring mechanical ventilation should be anticipated in some patients receiving this high-dose regimen.

During the recovery phase of the disease, intermittent spasms, usually less severe, may require continuation of phenobarbital or diazepam, 2 to 4 mg/kg/day per nasogastric tube, for muscle relaxation.

Pulmonary Care. Virtually all deaths in tetanus neonatorum are respiratory. Specific pulmonary complications include apnea, hypoventilation, hypoxemia, pneumothorax, infection, and airway obstruction from retained secretions. Constant observation of color, respiratory rate, heart rate, and work of breathing is necessary. Arterial blood gases should be obtained as a guide to respiratory management and warm, humidified oxygen given as necessary to maintain PaO_2 at 60 to 80 torr. Transcutaneous oxygen monitoring or pulse oximetry may be helpful in determining trends in oxygenation during spasms and at rest. Indications for mechanical ventilation are (1) apnea, (2) recurrent hypoxemia during spasms, and (3) continuous or rapidly recurring spasms.

Infants may initially require ventilation in conjunction with neuromuscular blockade. Pancuronium bromide is given intravenously in an initial dose of 0.05 mg/kg. This may be increased to 0.1 mg/kg, given as frequently as needed to keep the infant quiet and immobile. Complete muscular paralysis is not necessary. As lung function in these babies is essentially normal but chest compliance and airway resistance are subject to change throughout the course, we prefer a volume-controlled ventilator. As the infant receiving neuromuscular blockade is at the mercy of the environment, strict attention must be paid to suctioning, changes of position, chest percussion, and maintenance of sterile technique.

Infants should be maintained on mechanical ventilation until respiratory compromise is no longer produced by residual spasms. This may require 3 to 4 weeks. Tracheostomy should be the exception rather than the rule in neonatal tetanus. Modern neonatal intensive care has produced a low incidence of complications of prolonged endotracheal intubation, and tracheostomy itself is not without serious consequences in this age group.

Pulmonary infection is a constant threat, and the clinician should be alert to changes in temperature control, glucose metabolism, or pulmonary function as early warning signs. If changes in pulmonary function suggest pneumonia, complete blood count, blood culture, chest radiograph, and Gram's stain and culture of tracheal secretions should be performed. Gram's stain may aid in the initial choice of antibiotics, but in most instances appropriate therapy would include methicillin (200 mg/kg/24 hr in three divided doses) or vancomycin (20 to 30 mg/kg/24 hr in two divided doses) plus gentamicin (7.5 mg/kg/24 hr in three divided doses) or amikacin (20 to 30 mg/kg/24 hr in three divided doses). It is important to recognize that a significant proportion of staphylococcal infections in the newborn are resistant to methicillin.

INFANT BOTULISM

JOEL A. THOMPSON, M.D.

Infant botulism occurs when a susceptible infant (age 2 months to 1 year) ingests *Clostridium botulinum* spores. The organism colonizes the bowel and elaborates an extremely potent toxin, which, when absorbed, blocks release of acetylcholine from the terminal axon, causing bulbar weakness and, to a lesser extent, weakness of the appendicular and axial musculature. Infant botulism is differentiated from *botulism food poisoning*, in which toxin elaborated in improperly preserved foods is ingested and absorbed from the intestine, and from *wound botulism*, in which toxin is elaborated by organisms infecting a wound.

TREATMENT

Recognition. Therapeutic success depends on the rapid recognition of infant botulism, which may manifest in a spectrum ranging from feeding difficulties caused by bulbar weakness to acute respiratory arrest over a period of a few hours. If the correct diagnosis is established before respiratory arrest, the survival rate should be near 100 per cent, and the risk of hypoxic ischemic encephalopathy should be minimized.

Respiratory Management. Respiratory arrest is the primary cause of morbidity and mortality in infant botulism. It usually occurs secondary to bulbar, intercostal, and diaphragmatic weakness. Because respiratory failure may occur so quickly, the patient must be observed in an intensive care unit with constant cardiac, apnea, and oximetry monitoring. A ventilator needs to stand in readiness. Optimal positioning, frequent suctioning, and nasojejunal feedings may help the borderline patient avoid endotracheal intubation, which is necessary if more severe respiratory failure occurs. Tracheostomy has not been necessary in patients who have been ventilator dependent for as long as 106 days. Patients with "pneumonia" *and* an absent gag reflex probably have infant botulism and should not be given aminoglycoside antibiotics, which increase neuromuscular blockade and may accelerate respiratory failure.

Nutrition. Enteral feedings should be instituted within a few days of diagnosis. Nasojejunal feedings minimize the risk of aspiration in infants with an absent gag reflex, but gastric residuals should still be checked regularly. Hyperalimentation may be employed as an alternate method of feeding but is rarely needed. Oral feedings should not be resumed until the gag reflex and swallowing return to normal.

Bowel Care. Constipation is common on presentation and may persist for months after resolution of muscle weakness. Cathartics are not recommended, since they do not increase bowel motility and may simply remain in an atonic loop of bowel, perhaps osmotically breaking down organisms, with release of toxin. Digital evacuation of stool, judicious use of saline enemas, and use of stool softeners will generally be sufficient.

Antibiotic Therapy. Antibiotics effective against *C. botulinum* do not appear to shorten the course of the illness. Destruction of organisms may cause the release of substantial amounts of toxin and worsen the patient's condition. If secondary systemic infections with other organisms occur, it may be of theoretical advantage to avoid antibiotics effective against *C. botulinum*.

Antitoxin Therapy. *C. botulinum* antitoxin has not been widely used to treat infant botulism and has not been demonstrably successful when used. The antitoxin is made from horse serum and causes an unacceptable percentage of side effects, including serum sickness. Although a human antitoxin may prove to have fewer side effects, its efficacy will still need to be determined. Any use of a serum product needs to be done with the knowledge that supportive care alone should result in 100 per cent survival.

Hospital Precautions. There are no reported cases of transmission of infant botulism from infant to infant. It would appear prudent to use thorough hand washing when going from infant to infant. Diapers and bedding should be placed in closed containers. Although contact with the stool of an infected infant could represent a risk to children in the community, the organism is widely distributed in this environment as well.

Psychosocial Factors. Infants with infant botulism are usually hospitalized for an average of 30 days. This hospitalization results in prolonged separation from the family and often significant financial strain. Parents should be encouraged to visit their infant frequently. Mothers who breast feed can pump their breasts, and the milk can be fed to their infant. Most mothers abandon plans to breast feed if the hospitalization is prolonged.

Infant botulism is a disease that should be associated with a 100 per cent survival rate if the diagnosis is made early and meticulous respiratory support and supportive care are instituted. Children should not be discharged from the hospital until the gag reflex is normal and feeding has returned to normal.

SHIGELLOSIS

LARRY K. PICKERING, M.D.

Shigellosis is defined as infection of the gastrointestinal tract by *Shigella* organisms. Bacillary dysentery is a form of shigellosis characterized by passage of stools of small volume that contain blood, mucus, and inflammatory cells. *Shigella* are divided into four serogroups and at least 40 serotypes: (a) group A, *S. dysenteriae*, (b) group B, *S. flexneri*, (c) group C, *S. boydii*, and (d) group D, *S. sonnei*. Currently, *S. sonnei* accounts for between 60 and 80 per cent of cases of shigellosis reported in the United States, and *S. flexneri* serotypes account for most of the remaining cases. *S. boydii* and *S. dysenteriae* are rare causes of diarrhea in the United States. *Shigella* is a highly infectious organism; the infectious dose for healthy adults is 10 to 100 organisms.

Antimicrobial therapy is administered to patients with shigellosis to abbreviate the clinical course and/or decrease excretion of the causative organisms. A stool culture should be obtained and antibiotic susceptibility testing of the suspected pathogen performed to ensure optimal therapy. The organisms do not survive well in fecal specimens, so that freshly passed stool specimens should be plated directly onto culture media such as xylose-lysine-deoxycholate, salmonella-shigella, and MacConkey agars. Changing susceptibility patterns often make the initial selection of an antimicrobial agent difficult. Antimicrobial agents should not be used routinely or liberally for gastroenteritis of unknown etiology. In addition, antidiarrheal agents with antiperistaltic activity should not be used in patients with shigellosis, since they may prolong the fever, diarrhea, and excretion of the organism.

Several antibiotics have been used successfully in eradicating clinical symptoms and fecal shedding of *Shigella*. Approximately half of the *S. sonnei* strains are resistant to ampicillin, whereas *S. flexneri* strains have remained relatively susceptible to ampicillin. Table 1 outlines suggested antimicrobial therapy for children and adults who are presumed to have shigellosis or from whom *Shigella* organisms are isolated from stool. Trimethoprim plus sulfamethoxazole is the treatment of choice for shigellosis because of ampicillin resistance among *Shigella* isolates. In children with known ampicillin-susceptible strains, ampicillin is a treatment of choice and can be given either orally or intravenously. Single-dose tetracycline therapy is effective in the treatment of *Shigella* infection in adults, but it must be limited to adults because of the side effects, including discoloration of teeth, that occur in children under 8 years of age who receive tetracycline. Patients who are transient asymptomatic carriers may be managed without antimicrobial therapy if they understand and employ excellent standards of personal and public hygiene. Treatment of these patients, however, may reduce fecal shedding of the organism and prevent spread of infection.

Sulfonamides are as effective as ampicillin if the organism is susceptible, but most *Shigella* strains are resistant to sulfonamides. Nonabsorbable antibiotics such as neomycin, kanamycin, and gentamicin will not alter the course of the disease or the fecal excretion of *Shigella*. Amoxicillin is not as effective as ampicillin in the treatment of shigellosis and should not be used. In shigellosis caused by antibiotic-resistant strains, nalidixic acid (55 mg/kg/24 hours given four times daily for 5 days to children) may be effective but has not been approved for this use. Ciprofloxacin (1 gm/day) has been used successfully to treat adults with shigellosis. Because of the potential for producing arthropathy, ciprofloxacin is not approved for use in children.

TABLE 1. Antimicrobial Therapy of Shigellosis

Antimicrobial Agent	Dose	
	Children	*Adults*
First choice: Trimethoprim (TMP)-sulfamethoxazole (SMX) (Bactrim, Septra)	TMP (10 mg/kg/24 hr plus SMX (50 mg/kg/24 hr) orally for 5 days; give in 2 divided doses	TMP (160 mg) plus SMX (800 mg) orally for 5 days every 12 hr
Alternates: Ampicillin, only if susceptible strain is known	50–75 mg/kg/24 hr orally for 5 days; give in 4 divided doses	500 mg orally for 5 days; give in 4 divided doses
or Tetracycline	Not recommended	2.5 gm orally in a single dose one time
or Nalidixic acid for resistant organisms	55mg/kg/day orally for 5 days; give in 4 divided doses	4 gm/day
or Ciprofloxacin for resistant organisms	Not recommended for children	1 gm/day

The prognosis for an uneventful recovery from shigellosis is excellent in the majority of infected patients. Mortality in the United States is less than 1 per cent. Complications may include dehydration and electrolyte imbalance or the rare problems of perforation of the colon, generally following a procedure such as sigmoidoscopy; rectal prolapse due to unrelenting diarrhea; Ekiri syndrome; and bacteremia. The extraintestinal complications of Reiter's syndrome and hemolytic-uremic syndrome can be initiated by *Shigella* infections, the latter following infection with *S. dysenteriae* 1.

TYPHOID FEVER

SANDOR FELDMAN, M.D.

Modern sanitation has dramatically reduced the incidence of typhoid fever in this country. In 1989, approximately 460 cases (a 20 per cent increase over the median, 374 for 1984 to 1988) were reported in the United States. However, worldwide, in underdeveloped countries *Salmonella typhi* remains a significant health problem. Typhoid fever is still to be suspected in children with prolonged high fevers (39 to 41°C), headache, nausea, anorexia, malaise, irritability, cough, abdominal pain, leukopenia, splenomegaly, or rose spots. Constipation is common, while diarrhea is relatively uncommon. *S. typhi* can be isolated from blood and bone marrow. Later in the course of infection the organism can be isolated from urine and stool. Elevated O-antigen agglutinating antibody ($\geq$ 1:320) or rising O- and H-antigen agglutinating antibodies to *S. typhi* are suggestive of typhoid fever.

Therapy. Initial therapy should be intravenous chloramphenicol, 50 to 100 mg/kg/day (maximum of 2 gm/day) in four divided doses, or ampicillin, 100 to 200 mg/kg/day in four divided doses. Within 3 to 5 days there will usually be defervescence of fever, and the symptoms will have begun to ameliorate. At that time, if the oral fluid intake is adequate, antibiotic therapy may be changed to the oral route. Amoxicillin, 100 mg/kg/day in three divided doses, may be substituted for ampicillin. Antibiotic therapy should continue for 14 days. Alternatively, trimethoprim-sulfamethoxazole* (TMP-SMZ)—trimethoprim, 10 to 12 mg/kg/day and sulfamethoxazole, 50 to 60 mg/kg/day in two divided doses—has been found to be effective therapy for salmonellosis, including *S. typhi*. Intravenous TMP-SMZ requires 125 ml of diluting fluid for each 80 mg TMP. Children receiving this antibiotic intravenously should have careful monitoring of fluid intake.

Third-generation cephalosporins such as cefotamine have demonstrated in vitro activity against *S. typhi* and the other *Salmonella* serotypes. Recent clinical studies have shown that this group of antibiotics were effective for the treatment. First- and second-generation

---

*This use of trimethoprim-sulfamethoxazole is not listed in the manufacturer's directive.

cephalosporins should not be used in these infections.

Salmonellae, including *S. typhi*, have shown some resistance to ampicillin, chloramphenicol, and TMP-SMZ. Simultaneous resistance to the three antibiotics is increasing. Antibiotic-resistant *Salmonella* species are imported from third world countries. Antibiotic sensitivity to *Salmonella* isolates is required to ensure appropriate therapy.

Treatment for less than 14 days increases the risk of relapse, while treatment for more than 14 days does not decrease this risk. Relapse rates are reported to be from 10 to 20 per cent. Relapse appears to occur less often following treatment with ampicillin (amoxicillin) or TMP-SMZ than with chloramphenicol.

In the United States, children with typhoid fever should be hospitalized for enteric isolation and nursing care. Careful handwashing measures are necessary to decrease the likelihood of intrafamily spread and spread to hospital personnel. During the initial stage of therapy, intravenous fluids may be required, with careful monitoring of fluid and electrolyte balance. The diet should be bland and well balanced and include a generous amount of fluids.

Avoid antipyretic therapy with acetaminophen or salicylates, as they can produce hypothermia. Tepid sponge baths can be used to control fever. Physical activity should be markedly limited during the acute phase of the illness and curtailed during convalescence.

Recently a placebo-controlled trial, jointly undertaken by the United States and Indonesia, revealed that dexamethasone 3 mg/kg initially, followed by 8 doses at 1 mg/kg every 6 hours for 48 hours, significantly reduced the mortality in severely toxic, stuporous, and delirious patients. The routine use of steroids for fever and symptomatic control is not indicated.

Complications. Complications tend to occur during the third and fourth weeks of illness and are more frequent in the untreated or in those whose therapy was started late. Recurrence of fever usually heralds the onset of relapse or other complications. Gastrointestinal hemorrhage and intestinal perforation are the most severe life-threatening complications. Intensive supportive therapy, antibiotics, and blood products are administered as indicated. Failure of medical management to stabilize the patient may require surgical intervention. However, mortality rates after surgical intervention are high. Sound clinical judgment will be necessary to guide the medical and surgical management of this complication.

Acute cholecystitis with gallstones may require surgery. *S. typhi* involving the lungs, liver, bones, joints, and so on will require prolonged antibiotic therapy.

Chronic Carriers. Chronic carriage is defined as fecal excretion of *Salmonella* for at least 1 year. Overall, the carriage rate of *S. typhi* is 2 per cent; however, the rate is much lower in children. The most common source of the organism is the gallbladder with the presence of gallstones. Cholecystectomy should be considered.

Ampicillin, 100 to 200 mg/kg/day, or trimethoprim-sulfamethoxazole* (trimethoprim, 8 mg/kg/day, and sul-

famethoxazole, 40 mg/kg/day) for 3 to 4 weeks has been used successfully to treat *S. typhi* carriers. Failures are common.

Vaccination. For nearly 30 years heat-phenol and acetone-inactivated *S. typhi* vaccines have been available. Protective efficacy with the former has been reported from 51 to 67 per cent and with the latter from 56 to 88 per cent. Duration of protection is usually 3 or more years. A new live oral typhoid vaccine, Ty21a, derived from a mutant strain of *S. typhi* has undergone extensive testing. Field trials suggest that its protective efficacy over a 5-year period is similar or greater than that of the inactivated vaccines. Licensing of this vaccine is imminent. Adverse reactions are minimal. It will be available either as enteric-coated tablets or a suspension with three (or four) doses administered over a week. A parenteral IV polysaccharide vaccine has also undergone extensive field testing in underdeveloped countries. Its efficacy and lack of adverse effects are similar to those of the oral vaccine; licensing is expected in the near future.

Although these older vaccines are protective, they have been generally unsatisfactory for routine immunization because of the high frequency of adverse effects: fever in 20 to 25 per cent and local reactions in 40 to 50 per cent. Until such time as the newer vaccines become available, the standard vaccines are recommended for persons exposed to documented typhoid carriers (household exposure, travelers to endemic areas, and laboratory workers at risk for infection) The heat-phenol–inactivated vaccine is given subcutaneously in two doses: (a) 0.5 ml/dose 3 weeks apart for children 10 years or older, and (b) two doses 0.25 ml/dose 3 weeks apart for those children 6 months to 10 years. A booster dose of either 0.5 ml or 0.25 ml, depending on the child's age, should be given every 3 years for the child at high risk for typhoid fever. Adverse effects are pain at the site of injection, fever, malaise, and headaches and may require dose reduction.

SALMONELLOSIS

SANDOR FELDMAN, M.D.

Despite major local and national public health efforts, nontyphoidal salmonellosis continues to be an important cause of outbreaks and sporadic cases of gastroenteritis in the United States. In 1989 more than 1600 cases with 13 deaths occurred in 49 outbreaks. Man usually acquires the infection through contact with infected domestic animals and pets or food such as poultry, meat, eggs, and milk products. Multiple-drug–resistant *Salmonella* from antimicrobial drug–fed animals had resulted in a four-state outbreak of gastroenteritis. Water-borne salmonellosis is uncommon in this country. There are three primary species: *S. typhi* (one serotype), *S. choleraesuis* (one serotype), and *S. enteritides* (over 1700 serotypes). In the latter group, serotypes *S. typhimurium*, *S. enteritides*, and *S. heidelberg* are the most

---

*This use of trimethoprim-sulfamethoxazole is not listed in the manufacturer's directive.

common isolates. Children less than 5 years of age, particularly those under 1 year of age, have the highest incidence of salmonellosis.

Gastroenteritis (Enterocolitis). This acute-onset syndrome is the most common presentation of *Salmonella* infection. Within 4 to 48 hours of ingestion of the contaminated food there is nausea, vomiting, headache, malaise, and fever. These symptoms usually resolve and are followed by abdominal cramps and diarrhea. The latter may vary from a few loose stools to a fulminant diarrhea. The mainstay of therapy is fluid and electrolyte replacement with either oral (clear liquids) or intravenous fluids, depending on the child's clinical condition. Abdominal cramps may be treated with infrequent doses of paregoric. In general, antispasmodics and analgesics should be avoided, since overdose for this self-limiting symptom has been reported. Over-the-counter antidiarrheals play no role in the management of gastroenteritis. Usually within a week the diarrhea resolves. Once the child's appetite is regained and the stool frequency has decreased, a soft, bland diet can be instituted.

Antimicrobial therapy is not indicated in this self-limiting form of salmonellosis. However, ampicillin, trimethoprim-sulfamethoxazole* (TMP-SMZ), or chloramphenicol therapy should be considered in that order of preference and depending upon in vitro susceptibility tests for patients at increased risk for disseminated infections. Examples are newborns, infants during the first year of life, children with hemoglobinopathies such as sickle cell disease, human immunodeficiency virus infection, or congenital immunodeficiencies, and children receiving prednisone, antimetabolites, and/or radiation therapy. Bacteremia in conjunction with gastroenteritis may occur in 9 per cent or more of infants under 1 year of age. Antibiotic therapy should be administered only during acute phase of the infection.

Enteric Fever. Nontyphoidal enteric fever presents clinical features indistinguishable from typhoid fever. Antibiotic therapy is the same as that discussed in the section entitled typhoid fever. Resistance of nontyphoidal *Salmonella* to ampicillin, chloramphenicol, and TMP-SMZ is increasing, particularly when the strain is imported from outside the United States. Antibiotic sensitivities are required to ensure proper therapy for *Salmonella* infections. As with *S. typhi*, first- and second-generation cephalosporins are not indicated in the treatment of *Salmonella* infections. The newer third-generation cephalosporins such as cefotaxime are effective in vitro for salmonella infections. They are fast becoming the drugs of choice for systemic treatment of salmonellosis. Gastrointestinal hemorrhage and intestinal perforation are uncommon complications following nontyphoidal salmonellosis.

Bacteremia. This is characterized by a hectic fever pattern for days to weeks and chronic bacteremia without the constitutional symptoms of enteric fever or gastroenteritis. *S. choleraesuis* is frequently the causative serotype. Therapy is similar to that for typhoid fever

and requires monitoring with blood cultures. Dissemination to other organ systems can be expected in about 10 per cent of patients. *Salmonella* bacteremia is one of the more common infections in pediatric AIDS.

Local Infections. Localized infections of almost any organ system can occur following salmonellosis. Osteomyelitis in children with sickle cell anemia is well known. Surgical drainage of abscesses is indicated. Intravenous antibiotic therapy with either ampicillin or chloramphenicol may be prolonged, depending on the infected organ. Antibiotic therapy should be continued for at least one week after the signs of infection have disappeared.

As with the treatment of all *Salmonella* infections, antibiotic sensitivities are required because of the increasing resistance. TMP-SMZ* is an alternative to ampicillin and chloramphenicol.

Salmonella meningitis, occurring chiefly in neonates and infants under 1 year of age, has a mortality rate of 85 per cent and relapses occur frequently. The duration of antibiotic therapy in children with meningitis should be at least 14 to 21 days with parenteral ampicillin, 200 to 300 mg/kg/day, or chloramphenicol, 100 mg/kg/day. Several cases have been successfully treated with TMP-SMZ* (trimethoprim, 10 to 20 mg/kg/day, and sulfamethoxazole, 50 to 100 mg/kg/day). Chloramphenicol should be avoided in the newborn because of the high risk of the gray baby syndrome.

Chronic Carriers. Chronic carrying of nontyphoidal *Salmonella* occurs in less than 1 per cent of infected children. Intrafamily spread can usually be prevented by hand-washing measures. Antibiotic therapy is not usually indicated.

---

*This use of trimethoprim-sulfamethoxazole is not listed in the manufacturer's directive.

CAMPYLOBACTER INFECTIONS

MELVIN I. MARKS, M.D.

Campylobacter are vibrio-shaped, gram-negative bacteria that commonly cause gastroenteritis (normally *C. jejuni* or *C. coli*) in young children. Occasionally, the infection extends beyond the gastrointestinal tract, particularly in malnourished and immunocompromised hosts (usually *C. jejuni, C. coli, C. fetus*). The major reservoirs are food (including raw milk), water, and animals (dogs, cats, turtles, and fowl).

GASTROENTERITIS

By far, the most common infections due to *Campylobacter* are confined to the gastrointestinal tract and are self-limited in most normal hosts. Nevertheless, carefully controlled prospective in vivo clinical studies indicate that treatment with erythromycin in dosages of 40 to 50 mg/kg/day, divided four times a day for 5 days, will rapidly eliminate *Campylobacter* from the stools of these patients. The patient should be free of diarrhea and fever for at least 48 hours before discontinuing

---

*This use of trimethoprim-sulfamethoxazole is not listed in the manufacturer's directive.

TABLE 1. In Vitro Susceptibilities of *Campylobacter*

Highly susceptible to:	Erythromycin Gentamicin, amikacin, and tobramycin Tetracycline Furazolidone

Moderately (or variably)
susceptible to:
	Ampicillin (*C. pyloridis* is more
	    susceptible)
	Cefotaxime
	Chloramphenicol
	Clindamycin
	Trimethoprim-sulfamethoxazole
	    (*C. pyloridis* is resistant)

Resistant to:	Penicillins (including cloxacillin, carbenicillin, and ticarcillin) Vancomycin Rifampin Cephalothin Cefamandole Metronidazole (*C. pyloridis* is susceptible)

therapy. Clinically significant effects on diarrhea, fever, abdominal pain, or malaise are noted if treatment is initiated in the earliest stages of illness. Considering the low cost and minimal toxicity of erythromycin, it seems worthwhile to use this drug in confirmed and highly suspected cases of *Campylobacter* gastroenteritis. Erythromycin stearate is often selected because it is acid resistant and is converted to active base in the duodenum before absorption; hence, it is active against *Campylobacter* in the gastrointestinal tract. Erythromycin ethylsuccinate is also of proven efficacy.

The bacteriologic effects of therapy might reduce spread (especially among infants in daycare centers); however, hand washing and hygienic precautions are also important control measures. In-hospital treatment should include careful disposal of excreta, double bagging of bedclothes and bedding, and hand washing and precautions in handling excretion.

The in vitro susceptibilities of *Campylobacter* are outlined in Table 1. On the basis of these data and clinical results, erythromycin is the drug of choice for treatment of gastrointestinal campylobacteriosis. In rare instances, organisms resistant to erythromycin have been reported. Thus, in vitro susceptibility tests are indicated in cases apparently resistant to antibacterial treatment.

GASTRITIS AND PEPTIC ULCER

Considerable evidence has supported a causative role for *C. pyloridis* in gastritis and associated gastric and duodenal ulceration. This species of *Campylobacter* is sensitive to beta-lactam antibiotics, as well as bismuth salts. Both amoxicillin and bismuth have been useful clinically (alone or in combination). Although conclusive data about dosage, duration, and synergy are not yet available, it seems prudent to attempt treatment with both of these for 14 to 21 days in such cases. Prolonged therapy is recommended because of the tendency for this condition to relapse.

EXTRAGASTROINTESTINAL *CAMPYLOBACTER* INFECTIONS

When infection becomes bacteremic or involves joints, urinary tract, fetus, or other extragastrointestinal foci,

aminoglycosides should be used. Gentamicin, in a dose of 5.0 to 7.5 mg/kg (divided every 8 hours) given intravenously (IV), is recommended. Therapy should be continued for at least a week after clinical defervescence and bacteriologic eradication in normal hosts and for 2 weeks in immunocompromised patients. Stool cultures should also be obtained in these patients and, should the stools be positive, appropriate hygiene and isolation procedures carried out. Drainage may also be necessary in certain localized infections.

In the rare case of *Campylobacter* meningitis, chloramphenicol, 75 mg/kg/day, or ampicillin, 400 mg/kg/day (this dose may exceed that recommended by the manufacturer) plus gentamicin, may be used. Other complications, such as encephalopathy and Guillain-Barré syndrome, are apparently immunopathic and are treated supportively.

YERSINIA ENTEROCOLITICA INFECTIONS
MELVIN I. MARKS, M.D.

Yersinia enterocolitica organisms are gram-negative bacilli that frequently cause gastroenteritis in temperate climates in many countries of the world; however, these infections seem to be relatively infrequent in the United States. Several outbreaks in the United States have been associated with contaminated milk products, dogs, and cats. Other gastrointestinal manifestations are seen in children over 5 years of age. These include appendicitis, pseudoappendicitis, terminal ileitis, mesenteric adenitis, and colonic diverticulitis. Pancreatitis and cholecystitis, erythema nodosum, migratory polyarthritis, and myocarditis may accompany, or follow, gastrointestinal infection.

Invasion beyond the gastrointestinal tract is generally restricted to immunocompromised patients, although some persons who are not immunocompromised may occasionally have bacteremia, septic arthritis, osteomyelitis, cellulitis, and focal abscesses. Rarely, deaths have been reported.

TREATMENT
Gastroenteritis

Guidelines for the treatment of yersiniosis are gleaned from in vitro susceptibilities (Table 1) and

TABLE 1. In Vitro Susceptibilities of *Yersinia enterocolitica*

Highly susceptible to:	Trimethoprim-sulfamethoxazole Aminoglycosides (gentamicin, amikacin, and tobramycin) Cefotaxime
Moderately (or variably) susceptible to:	Kanamycin Tetracycline Chloramphenicol Rifampin
Resistant to:	Ampicillin Erythromycin Penicillin Cloxacillin Cephalothin

TABLE 2. Indications for Antibiotic Therapy of
Yersinia enterocolitica Gastroenteritis

Under 3 months of age
Leukemia/lymphoma
Acquired or congenital immunodeficiency disease
Moderate or severe malnutrition
Thalassemia
Iron overload
Appendicitis
Ulcerative colitis or other inflammatory bowel disease
Associated symptomatic intestinal parasitosis

clinical experience. However, a placebo-controlled prospective study showed no clinical or bacteriologic advantage of antibiotic therapy in children with *Yersinia* gastroenteritis. Therefore, as for *Salmonella* gastroenteritis, treatment is generally not recommended for *Y. enterocolitica* infections confined to the gastrointestinal tract. Exceptions are listed in Table 2. In such cases, treatment with trimethoprim-sulfamethoxazole—in a dose of 5 to 10 mg/kg/day of trimethoprim and 25 to 50 mg/kg/day of sulfamethoxazole, divided three times a day—is recommended. This treatment may shorten the course of fever and diarrhea if used early, but this result is only theoretically possible, since in the only controlled clinical study therapy was initiated well into the course of the illness. The intended function of the treatment in these cases is the prevention of extragastrointestinal infection. Hence, treatment should be discontinued when diarrhea and fever subside.

Treatment of *Y. enterocolitica* gastroenteritis should include hygienic instructions about hand washing, particularly in relation to food handling, bathing, and defecation. In the hospital, precautions in regard to excretion and hand washing should be observed.

Extragastrointestinal Yersiniosis

Extragastrointestinal *Y. enterocolitica* infections are rare but can be life threatening. When present, these should be treated aggressively with aminoglycosides or third-generation cephalosporins. My choice is cefotaxime, in a dose of 100 to 150 mg/kg/day divided four times a day. If the patient is able to take oral medication and therapy can be monitored by bacteriologic and microbiologic criteria, trimethoprim-sulfamethoxazole should be used in the higher doses described previously. Chloramphenicol may also be effective. Serum or other body fluid bactericidal activity should be followed to ensure adequate absorption and distribution of antibiotic. In most cases, therapy should be continued for a week after bacteriologic and clinical resolution, although a period of 2 weeks is indicated in immunocompromised patients and in those with infections of the central nervous system. Surgical drainage of abscesses should also be carried out, if possible.

Like salmonellosis, infections in bones and meninges may relapse and recur weeks to months after therapy is discontinued. Thus, I treat these patients for long periods during their initial course of illness. For meningitis, this means at least 2 weeks after bacteriologic and clinical subsidence of disease. In early bone infection, 6 weeks will usually suffice. When radiologic evidence of bone destruction is present at the time of initial therapy, a period of at least 3 months of monitored antibiotic therapy is required. The Wintrobe erythrocyte sedimentation rate should be normal, and clinical and radiologic features favorable, before discontinuing antibiotics. Some detective work should also be carried out to ensure that repeated exposures to infection in animal or food reservoirs can be avoided for the patient and other contacts.

BRUCELLOSIS
MOSES GROSSMAN, M.D.

Brucellosis is a contagious disease of animals, principally ungulates, that is occasionally transmitted to man. The infective organism (a gram-negative bacillus) is transmitted through handling of infected meat (in slaughter houses) and infected placentae (farms, veterinarians) and by ingestion of nonpasteurized milk or milk products from infected animals. Human infection is rare in the United States (less than 200 cases a year) and is particularly rare in children. Brucellosis is often featured in the differential diagnosis of prolonged fever despite its rare occurrence. Diagnosis depends on culturing the organism from blood, bone marrow, or a focal infection site, or on a fourfold increase in agglutination titer measured in paired specimens of sera.

Specific antimicrobial treatment serves to shorten the course of the disease and to prevent complications. The drug of choice by virtue of greatest clinical experience is tetracycline, 30 to 40 mg/kg/24 hr given orally in four divided doses (maximal adult dose 2 gm/24 hr) for a period of some 3 weeks. Seriously ill patients or those with localizing infections (osteomyelitis or endocarditis) do better if they receive streptomycin 20 to 30 mg/kg/day intramuscularly in two divided doses (maximum 1 gm/day) in addition to tetracycline. Children under the age of 9 years should not receive tetracycline. The best alternate drug is probably trimethoprim-sulfamethoxazole* (10 mg/kg/day trimethoprim and 50 mg/kg/day sulfamethoxazole in two divided doses given orally). Ampicillin may also be effective. Response to treatment is apt to be slow. Relapses with a recurrent positive blood culture may occur and require retreatment. Besides specific antimicrobial therapy, children require supportive therapy, attention to nutrition, and an individualized approach to bed rest and school attendance depending on the severity of the disease.

---

*This specific use is not listed by the manufacturer. Also, this drug is not recommended for infants less than 2 months of age.

TULAREMIA
WALTER T. HUGHES, M.D.

Francisella tularensis is one of the most virulent bacteria causing human disease, but it is remarkably susceptible to antibiotics introduced during the acute stage of the infection. Type A strains are found only in North America, are associated with rabbits and tick vectors, account for 70 to 90 per cent of all cases of tularemia, and without treatment 5 to 7 per cent of infected patients will die. Type B strains are less virulent, rarely cause fatal disease, and are associated primarily with rodents and aquatic animals.

Streptomycin, gentamicin, tetracycline, and chloramphenicol have been used successfully for the treatment of tularemia. In most cases streptomycin is the drug of choice, given in the dosage of 20 to 30 mg/kg/day in two equally divided doses intramuscularly for 7 to 10 days. The total daily dose should not exceed 2.0 gm. Ototoxicity, which is primarily vestibular, is the most serious adverse effect; nephrotoxicity is rarely a problem with the usual doses.

Gentamicin is an alternative to streptomycin and may be equally effective, although comparative studies in children have not been done. The dose of gentamicin is 5.0 mg/kg/day in two or three equally divided doses intramuscularly or intravenously. Vestibular and auditory ototoxicity and nephrotoxicity are adverse side effects encountered in a few patients. Both streptomycin and gentamicin are bactericidal for *F. tularensis*, and relapses rarely occur after a course of treatment. Other aminoglycosides have not been adequately tested to judge their effectiveness in tularemia.

Tetracycline and chloramphenicol are also effective in the treatment of this infection; however, they are bacteriostatic, and relapses occasionally occur with courses of treatment of less than 2 weeks. Tetracycline may be given orally in the dose of 30 mg/kg/day in four equally divided doses (not to exceed a total dose of 2.0 gm). The intravenous tetracycline preparation is given in the dose of 20 mg/kg/day in four equal doses (not to exceed a total dose of 2.0 gm). Tetracycline should be avoided in infants and children less than 9 years of age because of the staining effect on developing teeth. Chloramphenicol is given in the dosage of 50 to 100 mg/kg/day in four equally divided doses (not to exceed a total daily dose of 2.0 gm), orally or intravenously. Aplastic anemia is a rare complication of chloramphenicol therapy. The course of treatment with either tetracycline or chloramphenicol is usually about 2 weeks.

Despite the high virulence of *F. tularensis*, man-to-man transmission rarely occurs. The Centers for Disease Control recommends drainage-secretion precautions for open lesions. No isolation is required for pulmonary or other systemic forms of the disease. Laboratory personnel should be forewarned of specimens sent for culture, since once the organism replicates in culture, it is hazardous.

Defervescence occurs in about 48 hours with most cases treated early in the course of the infection. In nonfatal cases in which treatment is started late in the infection, e.g., with chronic draining lesions, little impact of antibiotic therapy may be evident and slow recovery can be expected. Relapses are more likely in patients treated early in the course with bacteriostatic drugs for less than 2 weeks. Lifelong immunity follows the primary infection. The overall mortality rate in treated cases of tularemia is less than 1.0 per cent.

Prevention. Documented cases should be reported to the local health department so that high-risk areas may be identified for the institution of control measures. A live attenuated tularemia vaccine (investigational) is available from the Immunobiologics Branch, Centers for Disease Control, Atlanta, Georgia, for use under special conditions.

Impervious gloves should be used in handling rabbits and other wild animals killed by hunters or found dead of unknown causes. Meat to be consumed should be thoroughly cooked. *F. tularensis* survives freezing. One should avoid drinking raw water from creeks, rivers, or lakes.

Children in tick-infested areas should be disrobed and inspected at least daily for adherent ticks. Hairy portions of the body are prime sites. The tick should be removed with forceps or a gloved hand. An attempt should be made not to burst the tick, since infected tissues and fluids may be expelled, sometimes reaching the eyes. Domestic pets should be regularly inspected and deticked. Tick repellents such as diethyltoluamide or dimethylphthalate may be used for the prevention of tick adherence.

The use of antibiotics prophylactically for tick bites or contact with suspect animals is not warranted and when used may only serve to prolong the incubation time.

PLAGUE

HEINZ F. EICHENWALD, M.D.

Plague, a potentially very severe disease caused by *Yersinia pestis*, continues to occur in various parts of the world, including the western United States and Canada. In its classic form, the infection is transmitted from rats to humans by the flea, a mechanism that still operates in developing countries. In the United States, however, the epidemiologic situation is now far more complex and involves a number of species of wild rodents, household animals such as the cat, various types of fleas, and presumably some environmental factors.

Plague pneumonia is a dangerous complication of bubonic disease and is of considerable epidemiologic interest because patients thus affected become highly contagious, spreading the organism via the air. The inhalation of *Y. pestis* by exposed individuals results in primary pneumonic plague, a rapidly fatal illness.

TREATMENT

Two groups of antimicrobial agents are highly efficacious: the aminoglycosides, such as streptomycin and gentamicin, and the tetracyclines. More information is available about the use of tetracycline and streptomycin than for other drugs; strains resistant to the latter antibiotic occur in Asia. However, they are susceptible to gentamicin. The aminoglycosides are so effective that huge numbers of bacteria are killed within hours after treatment has begun, resulting in the massive release of endotoxin and other bacterial products. This phenomenon has led to an apparent paradox in therapy: to avoid endotoxemia, tetracycline is often used for the first 2 or 3 days of treatment because it is *less* effective than an aminoglycoside. In severely ill patients, however, especially those with hemorrhagic or pneumonic disease, streptomycin or gentamicin should be used for the initial 5 days, followed by tetracycline for an additional 5-day period. Some experts recommend tetracycline as the initial drug even in these severely ill patients.

If streptomycin is employed, the usual daily dosage is 20 to 30 mg/kg in two or three doses administered intramuscularly or infused slowly intravenously. Gentamicin dosage is 5 to 7.5 mg/kg/day given every 8 or 12 hours intramuscularly or intravenously. Dosage of tetracycline is 30 to 50 mg/kg/day, with an initial loading dose of 30 mg/kg. Because of the hazards of intravenous administration of this drug, it is best given orally, but if this is not possible a slow intravenous infusion should be employed in a dosage of 15 mg/kg/day, following a loading dose of 10 mg/kg.

Ten days is the usual duration of therapy; some investigators recommend that medication be continued for a week after body temperature has returned to normal.

Various other antimicrobial agents also have been successfully employed, but there is less experience with their use. Chloramphenicol is administered in a dosage of 50 mg/kg/day orally or intravenously in four equal doses; sulfonamides* in a dosage of 75–100 mg/kg/day have also been reported to be effective, but their use is not recommended at present because resistant strains occur frequently.

In the laboratory, *Y. pestis* is susceptible to third-generation cephalosporins such as cefotaxime, but little clinical experience in their use exists.

Nonspecific therapy consists of the administration of appropriate fluids during the active phase of the illness to prevent the patient from becoming excessively dehydrated, and the management of septic shock.

PREVENTION

Persons in contact with a patient with plague, especially in cases of plague pneumonia, should be quarantined and given prophylactic treatment with tetracycline (20 to 25 mg/kg/day) or sulfonamides* (75 mg/kg/day).

Persons caring for plague patients usually are advised to wear a face mask and goggles, but whether these precautions prevent infection is not known. It seems more prudent to protect these individuals with chemoprophylaxis. Discharges from the patient, including feces, should be handled carefully and decontaminated because they usually contain plague bacilli.

A plague vaccine has been produced, but its efficacy remains in question. In those areas of the world where the chain of transmission includes rats and fleas, flea control followed by eradication of all rats in the community offers the best prospect for the elimination of plague.

---

*Manufacturer's warning: Sulfonamides are not indicated in infants younger than 2 months of age.

TUBERCULOSIS

LAURA S. INSELMAN, M.D.

Although the overall case rate of tuberculosis in the United States has declined in recent years, its incidence has actually increased in many large cities throughout the country. This apparent resurgence is due, in part, to the large influx of foreign-born into the United States in the late 1970s, but it is also recognized in the native-born population. It has occurred in both children and adults and appears to continue on its upward trend at present, at least in New York City. In addition, an increasing proportion of extrapulmonary tuberculosis has been identified in all age groups. Many of these cases have manifestations that differ from earlier classic descriptions of the disease—miliary tuberculosis in a completely asymptomatic child, clinically advanced tuberculous meningitis with repeatedly normal cerebrospinal fluid examinations, and growth of tubercle bacilli in a pleural effusion.

Chemotherapy for tuberculosis is directed toward the eradication of the tubercle bacilli in both extracellular and intracellular sites harboring large and small numbers of organisms, the prevention of the emergence of drug-resistant strains of *Mycobacterium tuberculosis*, and the prevention of the complications of tuberculosis. To accomplish this, in the longer therapeutic regimen previously used extensively, two drugs, at least one of which was bactericidal, were utilized to treat most types of pulmonary and localized extrapulmonary tuberculosis. Three drugs were employed for more intensive initial therapy for widespread pulmonary involvement, as, for example, endobronchial tuberculosis, and for systemic disease. These guidelines were based on the number of bacilli anticipated in a lesion, with more drugs required for larger numbers of organisms.

Short-Course Chemotherapy. Until recently, daily treatment for 1 to 2 years was the recommended therapeutic regimen for pulmonary tuberculosis. Short-course chemotherapy using two bactericidal drugs, isoniazid and rifampin, and supplemented by pyrazinamide, ethambutol, and/or streptomycin either as a daily or an intermittent regimen for 6 to 9 months, appears to be as effective as longer treatment for uncomplicated pulmonary tuberculosis. This regimen results in sputum conversion in more than 90 per cent of patients by the third treatment month (compared to 73 per cent by 6 months in 1981 with the longer regimen), has a reported relapse rate of 1 to 2 per cent after completion (compared to 7 per cent in 1982 with the longer regimen), improves patient compliance, and is less costly.

Short-course chemotherapy should not be used when sterilization of the sputum or clinical response in the early phase of treatment fails to occur; when either isoniazid or rifampin cannot be utilized because of drug toxicity or intolerance; when drug-resistant bacilli are present; or when "complicated" pulmonary disease, such as tuberculous empyema, and other medical conditions, such as diabetes mellitus, silicosis, malignant disease, human immunodeficiency viral infection, and immunosuppression, occur.

There are two possible short-course regimens. In the 9-month regimen, isoniazid and rifampin are prescribed daily for two months and then either daily or twice weekly for the next seven months. In the six-month regimen, isoniazid, rifampin, and pyrazinamide are prescribed daily for two months, with isoniazid and rifampin prescribed either daily or twice weekly for the next four months. Dosage guidelines are listed in Table 1.

Intermittent therapy (twice weekly) is administered only if patient compliance can be ascertained. The drugs are prescribed for a minimum of six months after the sputum culture no longer grows *Mycobacterium tuberculosis*. Therapeutic efficacy is not augmented by use of pyrazinamide for more than two months and is reduced by substituting ethambutol or streptomycin for pyrazinamide. Since pharmacokinetic data are presently unavailable for use of pyrazinamide in children, the nine-month regimen is currently recommended.

Ethambutol is included initially if isoniazid resistance is suspected. If isoniazid resistance does occur, then two new drugs that demonstrate in vitro inhibition of *Mycobacterium tuberculosis* are added or substituted for at least one year. One or both of these drugs should be bactericidal.

The following recommendations for chemotherapy of children with tuberculosis are based on the use of the short-course treatment regimens. These guidelines may be individualized when appropriate, and in certain situations, such as treatment of adolescents with chronic pulmonary tuberculosis or children with human immunodeficiency viral infection, the longer treatment regimen may be advisable (Table 2).

TYPE OF TUBERCULOSIS

PPD Conversion

The presence of a positive reaction to an intermediate-strength Mantoux test and the absence of radiographic changes and physical signs or symptoms suggestive of tuberculosis indicate that exposure to tuberculosis, i.e., infection without disease, has occurred. Pulmonary tuberculous lesions are presumably

TABLE 1. Dosages for Short-Course Chemotherapy

Drug	Daily Regimen	Intermittent Regimen
Isoniazid*	10–20 mg/kg/day†	20–40 mg/kg/dose‡
Rifampin*	15–20 mg/kg/day§	10–20 mg/kg/dose‖
Pyrazinamide	15–30 mg/kg/day††	50–70 mg/kg/dose
Ethambutol**	15–25 mg/kg/day§§	50 mg/kg/dose
Streptomycin	20–40 mg/kg/day△	25–30 mg/kg/dose
Prednisone	1–2 mg/kg/day△△	—

*The hepatic toxicity of isoniazid and/or rifampin may be increased and may cause one or both to be discontinued when administered concomitantly. The Centers for Disease Control recommend that the isoniazid dose not exceed 10 mg/kg/24hr and that the rifampin dose not exceed 15 mg/kg/24hr when these drugs are used concurrently.
**Manufacturer's warning: Ethambutol is not recommended for children under 13 years of age.

†Maximum, 300 mg/day	†† Maximum, 2 gm/day
‡Maximum, 900 mg/dose	§§ Maximum, 1500 mg/day
§Maximum, 600 mg/day	△ Maximum, 1 gm/day
‖ Maximum, 600 mg/dose	△△Maximum, 60 mg/day

TABLE 2. Dosages for Long-Course Chemotherapy

Drug	Daily Regimen	Maximum Dose
Isoniazid*	10–20 mg/kg/day	300 mg/day
Rifampin*	15–20 mg/kg/day	600 mg/day
Pyrazinamide	15–30 mg/kg/day	2 gm/day
Ethambutol†	15–25 mg/kg/day	1500 mg/day
Streptomycin	20–40 mg/kg/day	1 gm/day
Prednisone	1–2 mg/kg/day	60 mg/day

*The hepatic toxicity of isoniazid and/or rifampin may be increased and may cause one or both to be discontinued when administered concomitantly. The Centers for Disease Control recommend that the isoniazid dose not exceed 10 mg/kg/24hr and that the rifampin dose not exceed 15 mg/kg/24hr when these drugs are used concurrently.
**Manufacturer's warning: Ethambutol is not recommended for children under 13 years of age.

present but are too small to be radiographically identified and cause clinical manifestations.

A positive tuberculin skin test in a child indicates recent exposure to tuberculosis. Any child with a positive tuberculin skin test reaction who never received previous therapy for tuberculous infection or disease or previous immunization with the bacillus Calmette-Guérin (BCG) antigen is considered a recent PPD converter and should receive appropriate evaluation and treatment.

Therapy consists of isoniazid, 10 to 15 mg/kg/day (maximum 300 mg), given daily for 9 months in the short-course regimen or 12 months in the longer treatment course. Isoniazid is prescribed prophylactically to prevent the development of widespread extrapulmonary tuberculosis, which could originate from the radiographically unidentifiable pulmonary lesions and spread hematogenously. Such systemic disease, particularly meningitis and miliary tuberculosis, is more likely to occur in children. In addition, prophylactic isoniazid may prevent the further development of pulmonary lesions. Prophylactic treatment extended beyond 1 year does not provide greater protection.

Pulmonary Tuberculosis

Mediastinal Lymphadenopathy. Enlarged tuberculous hilar lymph nodes are present radiographically as part of the primary tuberculous complex, which also consists of the primary tuberculous lesion in the lung parenchyma and its associated lymphatic vessels. If calcification occurs in the primary lesion, the Ghon complex is formed. Mediastinal lymphadenopathy without the radiographically identifiable primary parenchymal lesion is the most frequent type of pulmonary tuberculosis in children.

Treatment consists of isoniazid and rifampin as a daily or intermittent short-course regimen (Table 1). If intermittent or 6-month treatment is utilized or if there is widespread disease or naturally impaired host immunity, pyrazinamide is added for two months (Table 1). If the longer regimen is used, isoniazid and either rifampin or ethambutol are prescribed for 12 months (Table 2).

Pneumonia. A radiographic tuberculous pneumonic process indicates local and/or bronchogenic extension of the primary tuberculous complex. The treatment regimen includes isoniazid, rifampin and pyrazinamide as a daily or intermittent short-course regimen (Table

1). If the longer regimen is used, isoniazid and either rifampin or ethambutol are prescribed for 12 months (Table 2).

Pleural Effusion. A tuberculous pleural effusion can result from extension of a subpleural site of infection but could also represent a hypersensitivity reaction to tuberculin. The effusion usually has small numbers of tubercle bacilli, and therefore cultures may not always indicate the presence of the organisms.

Treatment consists of a combination of isoniazid, rifampin, and pyrazinamide as a daily or intermittent short-course regimen (Table 1). In the longer treatment regimen, isoniazid and either rifampin or ethambutol are prescribed for 12 to 18 months (Table 2). Occasionally, in order to enhance resorption of the fluid, prednisone is given until the effusion has diminished (Tables 1 and 2).

Endobronchial. Endobronchial tuberculosis results from erosion of tuberculous caseous lymph nodes into a bronchus, causing partial or complete airway obstruction. A sinus tract may form, allowing passage of caseous material into the bronchus.

Isoniazid, rifampin and pyrazinamide are prescribed as a daily or intermittent short-course regimen (Table 1). In order to reduce the size of the enlarged caseous lymph nodes and thereby decrease the airway inflammation, prednisone may be added for 6 to 12 weeks or until wheezing and dyspnea subside (Table 1). In the longer treatment regimen, isoniazid and rifampin are prescribed for 12 months, with the optional addition of prednisone (Table 2).

Miliary. Lymphohematogenous dissemination of *Mycobacterium tuberculosis* from a tuberculous pulmonary site can result in diffuse, nodular, millet-sized lesions throughout both lungs and other organs. Treatment consists of isoniazid, rifampin, and pyrazinamide in a daily 9-month regimen (Table 1). Streptomycin may be added for 1 to 3 months (Table 1). In the longer treatment course, isoniazid and rifampin are prescribed for 12 to 18 months, with the addition of pyrazinamide for 2 months, streptomycin for 3 months, or ethambutol for 3 to 6 months (Table 2). If acute respiratory distress occurs, prednisone is added in either regimen until dyspnea or cyanosis resolves (Tables 1 and 2).

Chronic. Chronic pulmonary tuberculosis usually occurs in adolescents and adults but may be manifested in the younger age group. It occurs in individuals who have been previously infected with *Mycobacterium tuberculosis* and may result from either reactivation of the latent infection, i.e., endogenously acquired, or from acquisition of a new infection, i.e., exogenously acquired. Isoniazid and either rifampin or ethambutol are prescribed for 12 to 18 months (Table 2). Use of isoniazid, rifampin, and pyrazinamide in a daily short-course treatment schedule for these unstable pulmonary lesions may be indicated only if compliance can be ensured (Table 1). Otherwise, the longer treatment regimen is preferred.

Extrapulmonary Tuberculosis

Meningitis. Tuberculous meningitis results from hematogenous spread of tubercle bacilli. Like miliary

tuberculosis, it has a 100 per cent mortality rate if untreated and is particularly likely to occur in children under 4 years of age.

Treatment includes isoniazid and rifampin daily for 12 months in the short-course regimen (Table 1) and 12 to 18 months in the longer treatment regimen (Table 2), with the addition of pyrazinamide for 2 months and/ or streptomycin for 1 to 3 months in either therapeutic protocol. Prednisone is utilized for 6 to 12 weeks in order to decrease the intracranial pressure.

Skeletal, Superficial Lymph Nodes, Gastrointestinal, Renal, Pericardial, Dermatologic, Endocrinologic, Genital, Ophthalmologic, and Upper Respiratory Tract. Chemotherapy of each of these forms of extrapulmonary tuberculosis is similar and consists of isoniazid, rifampin, and pyrazinamide in a 9-month short-course regimen (Table 1). Alternatively, isoniazid and either rifampin or ethambutol may be prescribed in the longer treatment regimen (Table 2) for 18 to 24 months for skeletal tuberculosis, 24 months for renal tuberculosis, and 12 to 18 months for the other forms of extrapulmonary disease.

In addition, therapy is directed at the specific organ system involved. For example, in skeletal tuberculosis, accessible abscesses are surgically drained, and such weight-bearing structures as the hip and vertebrae are immobilized. The presence of a paravertebral abscess, spinal cord compression, or progression of the disease process despite chemotherapy is an additional indication for surgery. In tuberculosis of the superficial lymph nodes, surgical excision of the nodes is combined with antituberculous chemotherapy if the size of the nodes is increasing or, in order to prevent spread of tubercle bacilli, if spontaneous drainage will occur. Pericardial surgery may be necessary in tuberculous pericarditis if tamponade or constriction develops. In renal tuberculosis, intravenous pyelography, ureteral calibration, urinalyses, urine cultures, and renal function tests are performed periodically during and for approximately 10 years following chemotherapy to evaluate the development of complications. Follow-up after completion of chemotherapy for the other organ systems is also indicated to detect complications and permanent changes resulting from tuberculosis.

Special Situations

Congenital Tuberculosis. Chemotherapy for a newborn with congenital pulmonary tuberculosis includes isoniazid, 10 mg/kg/day, and rifampin, 15 mg/kg/day, for 12 months. Treatment for congenital systemic and extrapulmonary tuberculosis is directed along the previously mentioned longer treatment guidelines for these conditions, with streptomycin often used as a third antituberculous chemotherapeutic agent, if indicated. Short-course chemotherapy has not been evaluated for congenital tuberculosis and is not currently recommended in this age group. As with any serious infectious disease in the newborn, the presence of central nervous system involvement, even if asymptomatic, must be determined.

Newborn Infant of Tuberculous Mother. The neonate and mother are separated after delivery until the neonate is adequately protected, either with isoniazid prophylaxis or with BCG immunization, and until the mother's treatment renders her noninfectious. These measures are employed to prevent the newborn from acquiring tuberculosis.

If the infant's initial tuberculin skin test reaction and chest radiograph are negative, then either isoniazid prophylaxis or BCG immunization is administered. If isoniazid is used, it is prescribed for 1 year at a dose of 10 mg/kg/day. Conversion of the tuberculin skin test reaction is evaluated every 3 months by Mantoux testing, and, if it occurs, necessitates further investigation for the possible development of tuberculous disease despite isoniazid prophylaxis. If the skin test remains negative, isoniazid is frequently continued for 1 year even if the mother is theoretically noninfectious without bacilli in her sputum. This protection is employed because the mother may still shed bacilli with subsequent respiratory tract infections.

If the initial tuberculin skin test reaction and chest radiograph are negative and BCG immunization is used, the infant and mother are separated until the infant's tuberculin skin test reaction becomes positive. If either the initial tuberculin skin test reaction or chest radiograph are positive, then the infant is evaluated and treated for congenital tuberculosis.

Antituberculous drugs are secreted in breast milk, although in small amounts. Thus, recommendations regarding breast feeding for a noninfectious mother taking antituberculous chemotherapy should be individualized, with evaluation of the advantages of breast feeding and the possible risks of drug toxicity to the infant.

Pregnancy. Although guidelines for chemotherapy of tuberculosis during pregnancy are not well established, two drugs are used for treatment of intrapartum active pulmonary disease. Isoniazid and rifampin are usually prescribed, and, if isoniazid resistance is suspected, ethambutol is added. Either the 9-month short course or the longer treatment regimen may be used. Isoniazid, rifampin, streptomycin, and ethambutol cross the placenta. However, only streptomycin has a definite adverse effect, ototoxicity, on the fetus. The possibility of teratogenicity of pyrazinamide is unknown at present, and this drug should be avoided during pregnancy.

Therapy for other manifestations of tuberculosis during pregnancy varies according to individual circumstances. Isoniazid prophylaxis for a recent tuberculin skin test conversion or antituberculous chemotherapy for untreated, inactive pulmonary disease may be given either during or after pregnancy. The risk of developing tuberculosis is greatest during the first year after infection and may, therefore, necessitate the use of isoniazid prophylaxis in some instances. Isoniazid prophylaxis is often begun after the first trimester. Therapy is not necessary in pregnant women with long-standing tuberculin skin test conversions or with previously treated, inactive pulmonary disease.

The presence of tuberculosis during pregnancy is not an indication for a therapeutic abortion. When the disease is properly treated during pregnancy, the mother and fetus have an excellent prognosis. After

delivery, the mother and newborn are separated, and the infant is evaluated and treated as previously described.

Human Immunodeficiency Viral Infection. The relatively longer chemotherapeutic regimens are recommended for treatment of tuberculosis with human immunodeficiency viral infection because of the presence of profound and extended immunodeficiency. Antituberculous drugs are prescribed for at least 6 months following three negative culture specimens, and total therapy is administered for a minimum of 9 months. However, more prolonged regimens may be used, including the administration of isoniazid indefinitely. If resistance or toxicity is present with isoniazid or rifampin, antituberculous therapy is prescribed for a minimum of 12 months following culture conversion, and total therapy is prescribed for a minimum of 18 months. Isoniazid prophylaxis should be administered for at least one year.

Exposure in the Home. Any child who has been in contact with an adult in the home with active tuberculosis should be evaluated for exposure or disease due to tuberculosis. If the Mantoux intermediate tuberculin skin test reaction and chest radiograph are negative, isoniazid prophylaxis, 10 to 15 mg/kg/day (maximum 300 mg), is prescribed for at least 3 months. Tuberculin skin test conversion may not have occurred yet, and isoniazid is employed to prevent the development of infection. If the skin test reaction remains negative and if exposure to active tuberculosis is no longer present, isoniazid can be discontinued. If the skin test reaction becomes significant, which, in this setting, is interpreted as having at least 5 mm of induration, then additional evaluation and therapy are necessary.

Exposure Outside the Home. Mantoux tuberculin skin testing is sufficient evaluation of a child exposed to active tuberculosis in a school, camp, or day care center. If the tuberculin skin test reaction is negative, no treatment is necessary, provided that the contact with active tuberculosis is broken. If the tuberculin skin test reaction is positive and the chest radiograph is negative, isoniazid prophylaxis is prescribed for 9 to 12 months. Usually an adult, rather than another child, with active tuberculosis is the source of exposure in these settings.

Drug Resistance. Both primary and secondary antituberculous drug resistance have become increasingly important in the United States, particularly with the recently arrived foreign-born from Southeast Asia and the Caribbean. Drug resistance is prevented by the simultaneous use of at least two antituberculous agents, usually isoniazid and rifampin. If resistance to either one occurs, two new drugs to which the tubercle bacillus is sensitive are either substituted or added, and treatment is prescribed for at least 12 to 18 months. One or both of these drugs should be bactericidal. A drug that demonstrates in vitro resistance may still be included because its in vivo activity may differ.

If prophylaxis is prescribed for exposure to an isoniazid-resistant strain of *Mycobacterium tuberculosis*, rifampin, 15 to 20 mg/kg/day (maximum 600 mg), or isoniazid, 10 to 15 mg/kg/day (maximum 300 mg), may be used alone or in combination for one year. However, these regimens have not been evaluated for efficacy in prevention of tuberculous disease.

Characteristics of Antituberculous Drugs

Isoniazid. Since its introduction in 1952, isoniazid has become the primary drug in the treatment of tuberculosis in children. It is a hydrazide of isonicotinic acid, is bactericidal, and affects both intracellular and extracellular organisms. It exerts its action in cavities, caseous tissue, and pulmonary alveolar macrophages by possible inhibition of the biosynthesis of mycolic acids in the mycobacterial cell wall and inhibition of enzymes within the bacilli. Peak plasma concentrations of 3 to 5 $\mu g/ml$ are attained by 2 hours after ingestion, with therapeutic levels persisting until 6 to 8 hours. The drug easily penetrates almost all tissues and fluid collections, including cerebrospinal fluid. It is metabolized by the liver and excreted by the kidney.

Isoniazid is administered orally or, for widespread disease, intramuscularly, as one daily dose, usually in the morning. Dosages of isoniazid for the daily and intermittent short-course regimens differ, with higher doses in the intermittent regimen following the initial 2 month daily treatment, whereas the dose remains unchanged in the daily regimen (Table 1).

Adverse effects of isoniazid include neurotoxicity and hepatotoxicity. Peripheral neuritis associated with isoniazid administration is due to increased pyridoxine excretion and is prevented by the daily ingestion of 10 mg of pyridoxine (maximum 50 mg) for every 100 mg of isoniazid administered. Pyridoxine supplementation is prescribed in adolescents and adults, including pregnant women, but is unnecessary in young children with adequate nutrition and without predisposition to peripheral neuropathy. Isoniazid-induced neurotoxicity may also cause convulsions, optic neuritis, tremors, ataxia, toxic encephalopathy, and memory disturbances.

Hepatotoxicity resulting from isoniazid alone or in combination with rifampin has a much lower incidence in children than adults, even when both drugs are used. The hepatic injury usually occurs within the first 3 months of therapy and is transient, with the elevated liver enzyme levels frequently returning to normal despite continuation of the drug. In general, isoniazid is administered if the serum aspartate aminotransferase (glutamic oxaloacetic transaminase) level is below three times normal and clinical manifestations of liver disease are absent. The risk of isoniazid-associated hepatitis is increased with alcohol ingestion.

Other side effects of isoniazid include hematologic reactions, with anemia, agranulocytosis, and thrombocytopenia; vasculitis, including a lupus erythematosus–like syndrome; hypersensitivity, with skin rashes, fever, and eosinophilia; gastrointestinal disturbances; and arthritic symptoms of arthralgias and joint pains. Isoniazid potentiates the actions of carbamazepine, phenytoin, and barbiturates, resulting in toxicity of the central nervous system (somnolence, confusion, ataxia) and liver. Dosages of these drugs are often decreased during their administration with isoniazid. Metabolic acidosis, hyperglycemia, seizures, and coma can result from isoniazid overdose.

Rifampin. The combination of isoniazid and rifampin has become the most effective treatment of tuberculosis in children. Rifampin is produced by *Streptomyces mediterranei* and was introduced as an antituberculous agent in the 1960s. It is bactericidal to intracellular and extracellular organisms, causing suppression of mycobacterial RNA chain formation by inhibiting the DNA-dependent RNA polymerase. It penetrates easily into most tissues, macrophages, and fluid collections but only across an inflamed blood-brain barrier. Peak serum levels of 7 $\mu g/ml$ are attained by 3 hours following ingestion. The drug is metabolized by the liver and excreted by the kidney and gallbladder.

Rifampin is administered orally in one daily dose, usually in the morning. Its absorption may be delayed by para-aminosalicylic acid, and administration of both drugs should be separated by 8 to 12 hours.

The primary adverse effect of rifampin is hepatotoxicity, as discussed with isoniazid. Rifampin causes secretions, including urine, stool, saliva, sweat, tears, and sputum, to become a benign red-orange color and may discolor contact lenses. It can also cause gastrointestinal disturbances; hematologic reactions, with anemia, thrombocytopenia and leukopenia; hypersensitivity, with dermatitis, fever, eosinophilia, stomatitis, hemolysis, and renal insufficiency; neurotoxicity, consisting of drowsiness, ataxia, confusion, and headache; and cell-mediated immunosuppression. Intermittent therapy may result in the hepatorenal syndrome, thrombocytopenia, or autoimmune anemia.

Rifampin enhances the hepatic metabolism of coumarin, quinidine, digoxin, oral contraceptives, corticosteroids, oral hypoglycemic agents, theophylline, chloramphenicol, and methadone, resulting in a decrease in their serum levels and subsequent effects. Increased serum rifampin concentrations caused by diminished hepatic uptake of rifampin occur with probenecid. Rifampin overdose can result in a red-orange discoloration of skin and secretions but not sclera; gastrointestinal irritation; angioedema; somnolence; diffuse pruritus; and elevated liver enzymes.

Ethambutol. Ethambutol* is sometimes used as an alternative to rifampin in the longer treatment regimen, as an additional antituberculous agent in multidrug regimens, and with rifampin or isoniazid for an 18-month regimen if one of these two drugs cannot be employed because of intolerance or resistance. Ethambutol is a synthetic alcohol that is bacteriostatic to intracellular and extracellular organisms, causing inhibition of RNA synthesis. It attains peak serum levels of 5 $\mu g/ml$ within 4 hours after ingestion; concentrates within erythrocytes, which may act as its storage for entry into the plasma; and is excreted by the kidney.

Ethambutol is administered orally in one daily dose, usually in the morning. It is prescribed in high doses (25 mg/kg/day) for the first 6 to 8 weeks and in low doses (15 mg/kg/day) subsequently. A higher dose (50 mg/kg/dose) is used in the intermittent regimen.

Adverse effects of ethambutol include ocular toxicity,

---

*Manufacturer's warning: Ethambutol is not recommended for children under 13 years of age.

which may result in unilateral or bilateral optic neuritis, diminished visual acuity, central scotoma, absence of red/green color perception, and a defect in the peripheral visual field. The incidence and intensity of the ocular toxicity are related to the dose and duration of therapy, usually not occurring with the lower dosage and subsiding upon discontinuation of the drug. Visual acuity and red/green color perception, even in young children, should be tested before, during, and after administration of ethambutol.

Other side effects of ethambutol include hyperuricemia, which usually occurs by the third week of treatment and results from diminished renal clearance of urate; gastrointestinal irritation; hypersensitivity, with fever, dermatitis, and joint pain; and central nervous system alterations, with headache and mental confusion. Ethambutol has no known drug interactions.

Streptomycin. Streptomycin is often used in multidrug regimens for treatment of severe systemic tuberculosis, such as miliary or meningeal disease. As an aminoglycoside and a product of *Streptomyces griseus*, it inhibits ribosomal protein synthesis. It is bactericidal to extracellular organisms in cavities and, to a lesser degree, to intracellular organisms, where its action is primarily bacteriostatic. It does not easily penetrate fluid collections and crosses the blood-brain barrier only if the barrier is inflamed. Cell membrane transport of streptomycin is oxygen dependent, and the drug's antitubercular activity is markedly diminished in the anerobic milieu of a tuberculous abscess. Peak serum levels of 25 to 50 μg/ml are attained within 2 hours after administration, and the drug is excreted by the kidney.

Streptomycin is administered intramuscularly either once daily or, in severe disease, as a 12-hour regimen initially for a few days and then once a day. Adverse effects of streptomycin include ototoxicity and nephrotoxicity, which are more likely to occur with increased dose and duration of therapy. Ototoxicity may be manifested as vestibular, with vomiting, vertigo, tinnitus, headaches, and nystagmus, and as auditory, with hearing loss, which may be irreversible. Audiograms and tests of vestibular function should be performed before, during, and after therapy with streptomycin.

Although nephrotoxicity is less likely with streptomycin than with other aminoglycosides, albuminuria, cylindruria, and oliguria can occur. Additional side effects of the drug include hypersensitivity, with fever, dermatitis, eosinophilia, and stomatitis; hematologic reactions, with agranulocytosis, anemia, and thrombocytopenia; and peripheral neuritis. Streptomycin may potentiate the effects of neuromuscular blocking agents, ethacrynic acid, and cephalosporins. Elevated serum levels of streptomycin occur with probenecid and result in enhancement of its effects.

Pyrazinamide. Pyrazinamide is utilized as a third drug in short-course chemotherapy of tuberculosis. It is synthesized from nicotinamide, is probably bactericidal to intracellular organisms in an acid environment, and penetrates well into tissue and fluid, including cerebrospinal fluid. Peak serum levels of 45 μg/ml occur within 2 hours after ingestion, and the drug is excreted by the kidney.

Pyrazinamide is administered orally in three to four divided doses per day. Pharmacokinetic data are presently unavailable for its use in children.

Side effects include hepatotoxicity, which is rare even when the drug is given with isoniazid and rifampin, hyperuricemia, gastrointestinal irritation, and arthralgia. Pyrazinamide has no known drug interactions.

Adrenocorticosteroids. Corticosteroids are used in combination with antituberculous drugs to treat tuberculosis in children in certain situations. They are often employed to diminish intracranial pressure in tuberculous meningitis, decrease the alveolocapillary block causing cyanosis in miliary disease, promote fluid absorption in symptomatic pleural and pericardial tuberculous effusions, and enhance shrinkage of tuberculous lymph nodes in endobronchial disease.

The drugs are administered intravenously or intramuscularly in divided doses initially if the patient is seriously ill or orally as one daily dose for less symptomatic disease. Prednisone is frequently used as the oral preparation.

Adverse effects of corticosteroids include pituitary-adrenal suppression, growth inhibition, osteoporosis, behavioral disturbances, cataracts, myopathy, electrolyte imbalance, and peptic ulcer. Corticosteroids enhance the action of neuromuscular blocking agents and decrease the effect of calcium salts. Rifampin, barbiturates, and phenytoin cause suppression of the effects of corticosteroids.

Other Drugs. Para-aminosalicylic acid, capreomycin, kanamycin, cycloserine, and ethionamide are second-line antituberculous drugs used to treat isoniazid- and rifampin-resistant tuberculosis. They are not utilized in short-course chemotherapy. Except for para-aminosalicylic acid, their use in children is limited. Para-aminosalicylic acid is bacteriostatic to extracellular organisms, diffuses readily into tissues but not cerebrospinal fluid or macrophages, and is administered orally in a dose of 200 mg/kg/day (maximum 12 gm) in three divided doses after meals to decrease gastrointestinal irritation. Side effects include hepatotoxicity, pancytopenia, eosinophilia, thyroid imbalance, and hypokalemia.

Capreomycin and kanamycin are bactericidal to extracellular organisms, are prescribed intramuscularly in doses of 15 to 30 mg/kg/day (maximum 1 gm), and can cause nephrotoxicity and vestibular and auditory ototoxicity.

Cycloserine and ethionamide are bacteriostatic to intracellular and extracellular organisms and are prescribed orally in doses of 15 to 20 mg/kg/day (maximum 1 gm). Cycloserine can cause seizures, psychosis, and skin rashes, while gastrointestinal irritation, hepatotoxicity, and hypersensitivity can occur with ethionamide.

Supportive Therapy

General supportive measures, including adequate nutrition and unnecessary exposure to other infections, which may further compromise the body's defense mechanisms, are important in the care of a child with tuberculosis. Unless the child is acutely ill, bed rest is not required.

The need for hospitalization varies according to the type and extent of disease. Ideally, all children with recent PPD conversions or with tuberculous disease should be hospitalized to obtain appropriate culture material, ascertain tolerance and compliance with medications, investigate household contacts for exposure to tuberculosis, identify and initiate treatment of the index case, and remove all sources of active tuberculosis from the environment before returning the child home. In addition, hospitalization provides an opportunity for family education concerning the importance of the medications and follow-up care. However, this may not be practical, and the decision to hospitalize children with recent PPD conversions or asymptomatic pulmonary tuberculosis may have to be individualized. All children with symptomatic pulmonary, extrapulmonary, or systemic tuberculosis should be hospitalized until the previously mentioned goals have been accomplished and the disease is under control.

If acid-fast bacilli are present on sputum smears, isolation is required until further smears are negative, which usually occurs by 2 weeks after antituberculous therapy has begun. Isolation is unnecessary for children without sputum or without an open wound growing tubercle bacilli.

Prevention

The best prevention of tuberculosis is the minimization of exposure by identification and treatment of the index case and chemoprophylaxis of infected individuals. All cases of tuberculosis should be reported to the local health department.

BCG Vaccine. The protection afforded by the BCG vaccine, a derivative of *Mycobacterium bovis*, is controversial. The vaccine varies in potency, efficacy, and immunogenicity and has resulted in serious reactions, including BCG osteomyelitis, dissemination of BCG infection, and death. In addition, conversion of the Mantoux tuberculin skin test reaction caused by the immunization results in loss of negativity of the skin test as an index of subsequent exposure to active tuberculosis.

In the United States, the vaccine is employed when compliance with isoniazid prophylaxis cannot be assured in an individual with a negative Mantoux tuberculin skin test and negative chest radiograph who has repeated exposure to active tuberculosis. The vaccine is also used for asymptomatic children with human immunodeficiency viral infection who are at increased risk of developing tuberculosis. It is administered intradermally at doses of 0.05 ml for neonates and 0.10 ml for older children and adolescents. If the Mantoux tuberculin skin test reaction does not become significant 6 to 8 weeks later, BCG is readministered, and the tuberculin skin test is repeated 6 to 8 weeks after that time. The size of the induration of the skin test reaction resulting from a BCG immunization usually measures 5 to 9 mm in diameter. The vaccine is not used for patients with burns, skin infections, immunosuppression, or children with human immunodeficiency viral infection who are symptomatic or unlikely to develop tuberculosis. The vaccine is also not administered during pregnancy.

LEPROSY
ROBERT H. GELBER, M.D.

Leprosy (Hansen's disease) is a chronic infectious disease caused by *Mycobacterium leprae*. It is only rarely fatal but, owing to the predilection of the causative agent for peripheral nerves, may cause insensitivity, myopathy, and their resultant deformity. The World Health Organization estimates that there are 12 to 15 million cases worldwide.

The successful treatment of leprosy requires long-term compliance with an appropriate antimicrobial regimen, recognition of and considered intervention for a variety of immunologically determined reactional states, patient cooperation in protecting insensitive parts from further damage, and skilled reconstructive and cosmetic surgery for established disabilities and deformities. Compliance in any disease requiring prolonged therapy is often inadequate. This may be an especial problem in leprosy because of the lack of troublesome symptoms both initially and especially after some months or years of treatment and, also, because of reactional symptoms often perceived by the patient to be the result of therapy itself. Because of social stigma, patients and their parents are often fearful of institutionalization and rejection by other family members and friends and do not seek medical attention for a diagnosis that they suspect or reject the diagnosis and therapy when offered by a professional.

Sociocultural fears and expectations decidedly affect patients' lives. Many patients believe their disease is a result of some wrongdoing. Upon diagnosis patients frequently remove themselves from the life of their families. They may begin to use separate dishes and toilet facilities and to sleep alone. Because of the belief in certain cultures that the disease is in the blood and because in some countries it had been the practice to separate children at birth from affected parents, patients frequently believe that they should not parent children. Children with established deformities become stigmatized and often are ridiculed by their peers. Both functional and cosmetic repairs are integral to the success of medical therapy and in allowing patients to live normally in society. Education and counseling are necessary initially and on a continuing basis to help patients comply with therapy and not allow certain cultural and psychosocial aspects of the diagnosis themselves to contribute to the debilitation of the patient.

Chemotherapy

Dapsone. Because of the enormous numbers of *M. leprae* and the lack of cell-mediated immunity, the lepromatous form of leprosy presents the greater therapeutic difficulty. Dapsone (4,4'-diaminodiphenylsulfone, or DDS) is still the agent of choice for treating all forms of leprosy (Table 1). It is the only agent approved for general use as treatment of leprosy in the United States and has the virtues of being relatively safe, effective, and inexpensive. Dapsone is available in 25-mg and 100-mg tablets. In lepromatous leprosy administration of dapsone should be initiated and maintained

TABLE 1. Pediatric Dosage of the Most Important Antimicrobials for Leprosy

	2–5 Years of Age	6–12 Years of Age	13–18 Years of Age
Dapsone	25 mg three times weekly	25 mg/day	50 mg/day
Rifampin*	150 mg/day	300 mg/day	600 mg/day

*Dosage is 10–20 mg/kg, not to exceed 600 mg/day.

as a single adult daily dose of 100 mg for lifetime. Suggested pediatric doses are the following: for ages 2 to 5 years, 25 mg three times weekly; for ages 6 to 12 years, 25 mg daily; and for ages 13 to 18 years, 50 mg daily. Although previously leprologists had built up to the maintenance dose slowly and discontinued dapsone during reaction, particularly erythema nodosum leprosum, these measures no longer appear reasonable. Dapsone is cross-allergenic with sulfonamides and should not be initiated in patients with a history of sulfa allergy. It may cause a hemolytic anemia, particularly in G6PD-deficient patients, and may result in dose-related methemoglobinemia and sulfhemoglobinemia in certain patients. Early in therapy, a syndrome termed the sulfone syndrome, associated with an initially morbilliform rash followed by an exfoliative dermatitis, and at times a mononucleosis-type blood picture, fever, lymphadenopathy, hemolytic anemia, and hepatic dysfunction, uncommonly occurs and may require corticosteroids in addition to discontinuation of dapsone.

Dapsone monotherapy of lepromatous leprosy may result in the development of dapsone-resistant relapse. This becomes clinically apparent with the development of new lesions despite continued dapsone administration at a minimum of 5 years after the initiation of dapsone therapy. The risks of developing dapsone-resistant relapse vary between 2.5 and 40 per cent in different series. It appears that lower dosage regimens and intermittent adherence to therapy predispose to such relapse. Furthermore, even after 10 or more years of dapsone therapy, lepromatous leprosy patients harbor viable dapsone-sensitive *M. leprae* "persisters," capable of causing clinical relapse if therapy is discontinued; hence the recommendation for lifetime antimicrobial therapy of lepromatous disease.

In certain remote regions where patients do not have access to medical facilities and cannot be expected to take medication regularly, the repository sulfone DADDS,* 225 mg intramuscularly every 77 days in adults and proportionally less according to weight in children, might be substituted for dapsone in all forms of leprosy. However, resulting plasma levels of DDS are sufficiently low and the potential for developing dapsone resistance is of sufficient magnitude that treatment of the lepromatous form of the disease with this agent alone should be avoided if at all possible.

Because of the dual problems of bacterial resistance and persistence, borderline and lepromatous leprosy ideally should be treated with at least two agents, generally dapsone and rifampin. On the other hand, tuberculoid leprosy patients, in whom neither dapsone

*DADDS is not available in the United States.

resistance nor persisters are generally problems, require in most instances only monotherapy with dapsone. Tuberculoid leprosy patients may be treated for 5 years with dapsone alone.

Rifampin. Rifampin has proved in both animal and human studies to be significantly more potent than dapsone against *M. leprae*. It is available in 150-mg and 300-mg capsules. A single daily adult dose of 600 mg is recommended, and proportionately less is used for children, generally 150 mg daily for ages 2 to 5 years; 300 mg daily for ages 6 to 12 years; and 600 mg daily for ages 13 to 18 years, depending on body weight (10 to 20 mg/kg, not to exceed 600 mg/day). Rifampin turns the urine an orange-red color. It may be hepatotoxic and should be avoided in all patients with established liver dysfunction. Discontinuation of rifampin followed by reinstitution has been associated with severe and even fatal episodes of thrombocytopenia and renal failure. There is no available information on what duration of rifampin together with dapsone will prevent drug-resistant relapse, and whether such combination chemotherapy for any duration will allow discontinuation of therapy without subsequent relapse from "persisters." Furthermore, the cost of rifampin, about $300 per adult patient-year, is prohibitively expensive in most developing nations where leprosy is a problem. At present, then, it is recommended that in lepromatous leprosy rifampin be administered for at least 2 to 3 years, depending on local financial resources, together with dapsone, which should be continued indefinitely.

Second-Line Drugs. Particularly because of allergy to sulfones and in the therapy of sulfone resistance, other second-line antimicrobial agents may be necessary to treat leprosy.

Clofazimine* (B663, or Lamprene) appears as potent as dapsone against *M. leprae*. In adults 100 mg orally twice or three times weekly is an effective alternative to dapsone administration. Its administration is unfortunately associated with a red-black discoloration, which may be unnoticeable in blacks and other dark-skinned persons but is cosmetically unacceptable to many people with lighter complexions. Clofazimine-induced gastrointestinal side effects of a mild to moderate degree affect some patients.

Ethionamide† is even more active than dapsone against *M. leprae* and, when utilized, should be given in a once-daily adult dosage of 250 to 375 mg and proportionally less in children. Unfortunately, gastrointestinal intolerance to ethionamide is common, as is liver dysfunction, particularly when it is used together with rifampin. Indeed, if such a combination is utilized, liver function tests should be carefully monitored.

Streptomycin in a daily adult dose of 1 gm (and proportionally less in children) intramuscularly is as potent as dapsone against *M. leprae*. However, because of its potential for nephrotoxicity and eighth-nerve damage, no more than 1 year's therapy can be recommended. Hence, streptomycin should be used only with

*Clofazimine is available from the National Hansen's Disease Center, Carville, Louisana.
†This use of ethionamide is not listed by the manufacturer.

another agent that can be administered on a longer-term basis.

On therapy, tuberculoid macules may resolve somewhat, disappear entirely, or remain unchanged. Their anesthesia or hypoesthesia may also variably respond to therapy. Lepromatous infiltration does not begin to show noticeable improvement for a few months. Effective antimicrobial therapy will, however, prevent new lesions from appearing and the progressive neuropathy of untreated disease. It is important that both clinician and patient understand these expectations.

The Chemotherapy Recommendations of the World Health Organization

Because of growing concerns with the emergence of secondary and even primary dapsone resistance, the World Health Organization in 1981 developed some novel treatment recommendations. They suggest triple drug therapy for adults with multibacillary leprosy with rifampin, 600 mg once monthly (supervised); dapsone, 100 mg daily; clofazimine, 300 mg once monthly (supervised) plus 50 mg daily. The WHO recommends this therapy be maintained for at least 2 years, preferably until skin smears are bacteriologically negative for 5 years, and then discontinued. For adult patients with paucibacillary disease, they recommend dapsone, 100 mg daily, and rifampin, 600 mg monthly (supervised), for a total of 6 months. Our own experience suggests that primary dapsone resistance is most uncommon, and what little is found is only partially resistant but sensitive to levels achieved by generally recommended dapsone doses. Furthermore, patients harboring partially dapsone-resistant strains respond clinically to dapsone. We recommend dapsone sensitivity studies be done on newly diagnosed patients, and, if high-level dapsone-resistance is found, multibacillary patients receive rifampin daily and clofazimine three times weekly and paucibacillary patients receive rifampin daily alone.

Monthly rifampin and the reduced duration of therapy recommended by the WHO for both tuberculoid and lepromatous leprosy are largely a result of important economic considerations in developing countries. Because these are not particularly relevant in the United States and Western Europe and because there is limited clinical experience with these reduced durations and none with the WHO-recommended regimens, most authorities in the United States and Europe have not adopted monthly rifampin or these reduced courses of therapy.

Reactions and Their Treatment

About 50 per cent of patients with lepromatous leprosy may develop the syndrome of erythema nodosum leprosum (ENL), generally within the first few years of antimicrobial therapy. This syndrome may consist of one or a number of the following manifestations: crops of erythematous painful skin papules that remain a few days and may pustulate and ulcerate, and are most commonly found on the extensor surface of the extremities; fever that may be as high as 105°F (40.5°C); painful neuritis that may result in further nerve damage; lymphadenitis; uveitis; orchitis; and occasionally large

joint arthritis and glomerulonephritis. Histopathologically, this syndrome is secondary to a vasculitis and is probably the result of immune complexes. The clinical manifestations may be mild and evanescent or severe, recurrent, and occasionally fatal.

Patients with borderline leprosy may develop signs of inflammation, usually within previous skin lesions, and painful neuritis, which may cause further nerve damage and occasionally fever; these are called lepra type 1 reactions. If they occur prior to therapy, they are termed "down-grading reactions"; if they occur during therapy, usually within a few weeks or months of the start of treatment, they are termed "reversal reactions." Therapy is required in the presence of neuritis, with skin inflammation of a sufficient extent that ulceration appears likely, or for cosmetic reasons, especially if lesions involve the face.

Because the majority of cases of childhood leprosy are indeterminant or tuberculoid and because the described reactional states occur in borderline and lepromatous leprosy, reactions are not really as much a problem in affected children as they are in adults.

Corticosteroids are effective in ENL and generally even the most severe cases can be controlled with adult doses of 60 mg prednisone. In this respect we have not found alternate-day steroids useful. Individual ENL papules resolve in a matter of days, and control can be best judged by the assessment of the prevention of new manifestations. When episodes are controlled, steroid doses can be tapered and then discontinued generally in 1 to 4 weeks. If ENL appears to be recurrent, thalidomide is the drug of choice for its control and prevention. The dosage must be individualized, and the minimal amount necessary to control ENL manifestations is advised; generally in adults 100 to 400 mg in a single evening dose is sufficient. In the United States thalidomide is available only through the National Hansen's Disease Center, Carville, Louisiana, and a number of regional Hansen's disease centers. An occasional patient, despite thalidomide therapy, may require small doses of corticosteroids to prevent recurrent ENL.

Because of thalidomide's potential for causing severe birth defects, including phocomelia, it should not be administered to women in the childbearing years. Side effects include tranquilization, to which tolerance generally develops rapidly, leukopenia, and constipation.

Clofazimine, although slow in onset and only moderately effective in adult doses of 300 mg per day, may enable one to reduce the steroid requirement for therapy of ENL.

Thalidomide is of no value for lepra reactions. Corticosteroids are usually effective in controlling these reactions in adult doses of 40 to 60 mg prednisone per day but generally must be maintained at a lowered dose for a few months to prevent recurrence. Clofazimine may be of some value in decreasing the steroid requirement in these reactions in the same dose as for treating ENL but is not as effective in nonlepromatous lepra reactions.

Rehabilitation

Follow-up visits should always include examination of the feet, and plantar ulcers must be vigorously treated with specific antibiotics, débridement, and either bed rest or a total-contact walking cast until healed. Judicious use of extra-depth shoes with molded inserts or specially molded shoes is crucial to prevent recurrence. Tendon transfers to permit substitution of innervated for denervated muscles may provide patients with more functional use of hands, correct foot drop, and enable them to close their eyes so that corneal trauma and its sequelae will not lead to blindness. If maximal results are to be expected, reconstructive surgery should not be initiated until patients have received at least 6 months of therapy directed against *M. leprae* and at least 6 months have passed since signs of reaction have abated. When possible, mechanical devices may help the severely deformed, and special job training may be necessary to prevent trauma and further disability.

Prophylaxis

The close, prolonged intimate contact of household members of lepromatous patients poses some risk for the development of subsequent disease (about 10 per cent in endemic countries and 1 per cent in nonendemic locales). Although tuberculoid leprosy is not contagious, family members of tuberculoid patients may be incubating disease obtained from the same source. We recommend that household contacts of patients be examined annually for 5 to 7 years, preferably by a physician experienced in leprosy. Health workers and casual contacts appear to be at no significant risk. Therefore, when patients are hospitalized, no isolation requirements are necessary.

Trials of chemoprophylaxis with sulfones have at most been marginally effective. Thus, they are not generally recommended. BCG vaccination has been successful in some locales and not in others. It is not generally recommended. However, in the future vaccines utilizing heat-killed *M. leprae* alone and combined with BCG or *M. leprae* products may prove more efficacious in inducing the necessary protective cellular immunity. Specific and sensitive serodiagnosis of leprosy has recently become possible owing to the presence of circulating antibodies, particularly of the IgM class, directed at an *M. leprae*–specific phenolic glycolipid in nearly all lepromatous patients and about two thirds of tuberculoid patients. It is hoped that early serodiagnosis during the long incubation period may soon prove feasible and useful in leprosy control.

NONTUBERCULOUS (ATYPICAL) MYCOBACTERIAL DISEASES*

ANDREW M. MARGILETH, M.D.

In the past decade, nontuberculous mycobacterial (NTM) infections have been diagnosed and reported in

---

*The opinions and assertions contained herein are the private views of the author and are not to be construed as official or as reflecting the views of the Uniformed Services University of the Health Sciences or of the Department of Defense.

the United States more frequently than *Mycobacterium tuberculosis* (tuberculosis, or TB) infections. As the incidence of TB infection in the United States decreases, physicians will become more aware of NTM disease. Of the 19 known species of NTM, three *(M. avium-intracellulare, M. scrofulaceum,* and *M. marinum)* account for the majority of NTM diseases in children. Although NTM disease is rarely observed in daily practice, it is essential to distinguish patients with NTM disease from those with TB infection to avoid unnecessary and prolonged courses of drugs as well as the stigma attached to labeling a child "tuberculous." It is also unnecessary for healthy children with a positive NTM-PPD (purified protein derivative) reaction or a suspected NTM infection to undergo prophylactic isoniazid (INH) therapy. NTM disseminated disease is being reported more frequently in patients with human immunodeficiency virus disease.

DISTINGUISHING TUBERCULOSIS FROM NONTUBERCULOUS MYCOBACTERIAL INFECTIONS

When tuberculosis or NTM infection is suspected and a diagnosis is supported by the history, physical examination, tuberculin testing, roentgenographic evidence, or laboratory test results (acid-fast bacillus [AFB] smear or tissue biopsy), physicians must make some therapeutic decisions while awaiting AFB culture reports. Weeks or months may pass before the organism is finally isolated and identified and its drug susceptibility is known. Often, mycobacteria fail to grow, especially the slow-growing NTM species.

Proper application and accurate measurement of induration by the ballpoint method at 72 hours produced by PPD-T and Mono-Vacc skin tests can be helpful. If the Mono-Vacc test is reactive or a PPD-T reaction gives more than 15 mm of induration, infection with TB is probable (Table 1). If the induration caused by PPD-T is less than 10 mm, NTM infection is more likely, especially if the PPD-T is negative and a Mono-Vacc test is positive (1 mm or more). Other clinical factors to help differentiate NTM from TB infection are noted in Table 1.

INCIDENCE OF NONTUBERCULOUS MYCOBACTERIAL INFECTION IN CHILDREN

Atypical mycobacteria, or NTM, are acid-fast bacilli found in the soil, dust, water, and occasionally food (e.g., eggs, milk, and vegetables). Of the 19 species of NTM, none are pathogenic for guinea pigs, as are the human strains: *M. tuberculosis* and *M. bovis.* Disease or latent infection produced in humans is usually caused by *M. avium-intracellulare* (MAIC), *M. xenopi, M. fortuitum, M. chelonei, M. scrofulaceum, M. kansasii,* and *M. marinum.* NTM isolates obtained from closed aspiration of lymph nodes or abscesses and from tissue (cerebrospinal fluid, blood, pleural, peritoneal) fluids or resected tissue that culture more than a few colonies should be diagnostic.

The most common NTM disease in children is cervical lymphadenitis. During 20 years, our study of 229 patients with TB and NTM lymphadenitis showed a definite age-related difference. Most children, ages 1

TABLE 1. Differentiation of Nontuberculous Mycobacterial (NTM) Infections from *M. tuberculosis* Disease in 124 AFB Culture–Positive Patients

Clinical/PPD/Radiograph	*Mycobacterium tuberculosis*	Nontuberculous Mycobacteria
History of contact*	Common	Rare
Lymphadenitis, cervical	Uncommon, bilateral	Common, unilateral
PPD-T skin test (5 tuberculin units [TU])	15 mm or greater†	0 to 14 mm‡
Chest roentgenogram	Abnormal§	Normal usually§
Tuberculosis chemotherapy	Effective	Ineffective usually

*Person with active *M. tuberculosis* infection.
†In 87 per cent (26/30) of patients on the initial test, *M. tuberculosis* isolated; in 100 per cent (30/30) on PPD-T retest.
‡In 68 per cent (63/93) of patients, results are positive on the initial or repeat PPD-T skin tests; the NTM culture positive in 93.
§Abnormal in 27 per cent (9/33) with TB and in 4.6 per cent (8/172) with NTM disease.

through 12 years, had NTM adenitis, whereas most patients over 12 years of age had TB adenitis. MAIC accounted for 75 per cent of infected nodes; 17 per cent were due to *M. scrofulaceum.* Skin, joint, and bone disease is uncommon, and pulmonary NTM disease is rare in children and adolescents. In contrast, NTM pulmonary disease caused by MAIC and *M. kansasii* occurs almost exclusively in adults.

Human-to-human transmission of NTM infection has not been documented. Most NTM strains are resistant to antituberculous drugs. Therefore, it is essential to perform mycobacterial cultures and drug susceptibility studies to determine appropriate antituberculous therapy (Table 2).

MANAGEMENT OF NONTUBERCULOUS MYCOBACTERIAL INFECTION

Lymphadenitis

Treatment initially depends upon the presumptive diagnosis. The recommended therapy for excellent results is surgical excision of only the larger infected nodes. Incisional biopsy or drainage or excision of all infected nodes is *not* recommended. I prescribe antituberculous drugs, such as INH and rifampin (RMP), when (1) the family refuses surgical excision; (2) the TB contact or family history is positive; (3) the PPD-T skin test of the patient or family is positive, especially if the area of reaction is 15 mm or larger or if the reaction is equal to or larger than the patient's NTM-PPD reaction; (4) the incisional or spontaneous drainage persists; (5) the drainage or prominent adenopathy persists over several months following surgery; or (6) the AFB culture is positive for *M. tuberculosis* or an NTM species susceptible to INH or RMP is isolated.

If prescribed, INH and RMP should be administered until culture results and antibiotic susceptibilities are known or until healing is complete, usually in 2 to 6 months. Data for determination of RMP dosage in children under 5 years are not available. To avoid hepatotoxicity, the recommended daily dose for INH is 10 mg/kg, and when combined with RMP, the daily dose of RMP is 15 mg/kg. If cultures are positive for TB, treatment is continued for 1 year or longer, until healing is complete.

Skin and Soft Tissue Disease

Cutaneous NTM granuloma and abscesses may occur after skin abrasion from barnacles, shrimp, fish, or shellfish or after repeated exposure to fresh or salt water. These benign lesions usually manifest as mildly inflamed nodules, sporotrichoid nodules; small, crusted, wartlike excrescences; abscesses; or deep ulcers. Cutaneous infections caused by the rapidly growing mycobacteria *M. chelonei* and *M. fortuitum* are best treated by surgical excision. Therapy with minocycline, 2 mg/kg daily given orally for several months, can be effective against *M. chelonei* and *M. marinum.* All cultures of aspirated or biopsy material from such patients should be incubated for AFB at 30 to 33°C and at 37°C in a carbon dioxide atmosphere to enhance growth of *M. marinum* or *M. chelonei.* Most NTM skin granulomas are self-limited, with spontaneous healing in several months or more. The rapid growers are generally resistant to antituberculous drugs. Application of local heat may hasten healing because these mycobacteria grow best at 30 to 33°C. The combination of ethambutol, 15 to 20 mg/kg daily, and RMP orally for 6 to 12 months has been used to treat infections with *M. marinum.* (Manu-

TABLE 2. Antibiotic Dosage for Nontuberculous Infection of Lymph Nodes or Skin or for Pulmonary Disease*

Drug	Daily Dosage (per kg/Body Weight)	Maximal Daily Dosage	Number of Doses per Day	Duration of Therapy	Toxicity (Primary)
Isoniazid	10–20 mg	500 mg	1 or 2	≥12 mo	Hepatic, renal
Rifampin†	10–20 mg	600 mg	1 or 2	6–12 mo	Gastric, hepatic
Ansamycin	5 mg	—	1 or 2	6–12 mo	Gastric, hepatic
Ethambutol‡	15–25 mg	—	1	≥12 mo	Neuritis, optic
Ethionamide	15–20 mg	1 gm	1 or 2	6–12 mo	Gastric, hepatic
Minocycline	2 mg	400 mg	2	2–3 mo	Dental, vertigo
Streptomycin§ *or*	20–40 mg	1 gm	1 or 2	2–4 mo	Otic, vestibular, renal
Kanamycin§	10–15 mg	1 gm	1 or 2	2–4 mo	Otic, vestibular, renal
Amikacin	15–30 mg	1 gm	3	2–4 mo	Otic, vestibular, renal
Pyrazinamide	20–30 mg	3 gm	3 or 4	2–4 mo	Hepatic

*Drug treatment to be continued if culture is positive for *M. tuberculosis;* excisional biopsy is recommended only for NTM adenopathy.
†When sputum culture is negative for AFB, ethambutol may be substituted.
‡Ethambutol is not recommended for children under 13 years.
§For streptomycin and kanamycin, a single intramuscular dose is given daily and then 3 times weekly after clinical improvement.

facturer's precaution: Ethambutol is not recommended for children under 13 years of age.) Alternatively, excisional biopsy of the lesion can be effective. Infection produced by *M. kansasii* is usually susceptible to RMP, ethionamide, or streptomycin.

Pulmonary, Joint, Bone, or Disseminated Disease

Pulmonary, joint, bone, or disseminated NTM disease, rare in children, is usually due to *M. avium-intracellulare* or *M. scrofulaceum*. Three or four antituberculous drugs, such as RMP, ethionamide, kanamycin, and possibly ansamycin, based upon susceptibility studies to the NTM isolated, may be effective. Unfortunately, in patients with human immunodeficiency virus infection, traditional drug regimens may fail. Newer drugs (pyrazinamide, ansamycin, clofazimine, and ciprofloxacin) may be tried (Table 2). Use of ciprofloxacin in children is currently limited owing to adverse effects on cartilage. Surgical excision of localized disease, such as endobronchial tuberculous disease, lymphadenopathy, or bone, joint, or bursal lesions, is usually curative. In patients with uncomplicated disease, preoperative or postoperative chemotherapy is unnecessary. Owing to difficulty in testing visual acuity and red-green color discrimination in children under age 3, ethambutol is not recommended. The potential toxicity of antituberculous drugs should be explained to each patient or to the parent or guardian, and written instructions regarding possible untoward reactions should be provided. Patients should be followed closely (monthly or bimonthly) to ensure compliance with chemotherapy. Periodic monitoring of serum glutamic-oxaloacetic transaminase (SGOT) and bilirubin is recommended during the first 6 months of therapy, especially if the patient is taking both RMP and INH.

Isolation of the patient is not necessary. If large amounts of caseous material are being discharged from lesions, or if cavitary pulmonary disease is present, respiratory isolation precautions should be considered until the results of cultures are available or until triple antituberculosis therapy has been given for several weeks.

It is essential to distinguish patients with NTM disease from those with TB infections to avoid unnecessary and prolonged courses of drugs. Prophylactic INH therapy is unnecessary for healthy children with positive NTM-PPD reactions. Until special NTM-PPD antigens are available, repeat PPD-T testing 1 to 3 months after the initial PPD test will usually reveal a larger induration (≥ 5 mm difference) than the initial PPD-T reaction, with an induration greater than 15 mm if the patient has an *M. tuberculosis* infection. If an NTM infection is present, the repeat PPD-T induration will usually be less than 15 mm. Close follow-up for several years is recommended for these patients.

SYPHILIS

HUGH E. EVANS, M.D.

In the past decade, there has been an increase in the prevalence of sexually transmitted diseases. Both con-

genital and acquired syphilis increased in 1987 by 21 per cent and 30 per cent, respectively, compared with 1986. This increase led to the highest incidence of syphilis since 1950. Particularly affected have been sexually active, urban populations, including homosexual or bisexual men. Lethal cases of congenital lues have occurred in many high-risk centers. Some, but not all, of this upsurge appears related to human immunodeficiency virus (HIV) infection.

Health care workers may treat minors with sexually transmitted diseases without parental consent at a given age, which varies in different jurisdictions. In an appropriate environment in which confidentiality is protected, case finding may permit the early treatment of sexual contacts and help to interrupt transmission. This factor is of increased importance in those with HIV coinfection. Accidental contamination with the treponeme may occur during the highly contagious primary and secondary stages as well as with HIV coinfection, and hence the health care worker must be careful in treating such patients.

Penicillin, initially used in 1943, remains the mainstay of treatment, with the *Treponema pallidum* remaining an extremely sensitive organism. Serum concentrations of 0.03 μ/ml assure killing of the spirochete and must be maintained for 7 days in early cases and up to 3 weeks in late disease. Differences of opinion are noted further on regarding the treatment of neurosyphilis. Similarly, standard therapy of syphilis occurring among those with HIV infection may require re-evaluation.

PRIMARY, SECONDARY, OR LATENT SYPHILIS: DURATION OF LESS THAN 1 YEAR

The treatment of choice is benzathine penicillin G, 2.4 million units (1.2 $\times$ 10^6 in each buttock). For those allergic to penicillin, tetracycline hydrochloride, 500 mg orally four times a day for 15 days (not to be used in pregnancy), or erythromycin, 500 mg orally four times a day for 15 days, is an alternative. Treatment of primary syphilis with this regimen should lead to a cure, with reversion of the Venereal Disease Research Laboratory (VDRL) test to negative in nearly all cases. "Failure" may in part be due to reinfection. The Jarisch-Herxheimer reaction occurs within 2 to 12 hours after the initial dose of penicillin. Symptoms include fever, chills, headache, myalgias, and arthralgias, and they last for 24 hours. This reaction may be due to the release of spirochetal antigens when there are large numbers of organisms present, as in early syphilis and in up to 90 per cent of cases of secondary syphilis. Therapy should be continued. Prednisone, 5 mg orally four times a day for 24 hours before the penicillin injection and continuing for 1 or 2 days thereafter, may prevent the reaction. Failure to treat will lead to late syphilis 2 to 20 years later in 20 to 40 per cent of cases.

SYPHILIS OF MORE THAN 1 YEAR'S DURATION (EXCLUDING NEUROSYPHILIS)

Benzathine penicillin G, 50,000 units/kg, given intramuscularly (IM) weekly (to a maximum of 2.4 million units) for 3 consecutive weeks, is the most favored approach. Alternative agents in those allergic to penicillin are erythromycin stearate, ethylsuccinate, and base (500 mg four times a day for 30 days). The cerebrospinal fluid should be examined (VDRL, protein and cell counts) in patients with suspected or symptomatic neurosyphilis or in those receiving antibiotics other than penicillin for more than 1 year.

NEUROSYPHILIS

The treatment of neurosyphilis is controversial. Proposed regimens are cumbersome, and there are no adequate studies of efficacy. The Centers for Disease Control (CDC) recommends 2 to 4 million units of aqueous penicillin intravenously (IV) or procaine penicillin, 2.4 million units daily for 10 days, with oral probenecid (500 mg orally, four times a day). This treatment is followed by benzathine penicillin G, 2.4 million units given IM weekly for 3 weeks.

The administration of three doses of 2.4 million units of benzathine penicillin G at weekly intervals arrests neurosyphilis in most patients, even though levels of penicillin in the cerebrospinal fluid are nearly undetectable and hence not treponemicidal. This approach is acceptable to the CDC but not to the World Health Organization. It is included as an option in the "Red Book" (Committee on Infectious Diseases of the American Academy of Pediatrics, 1988 edition).

Another regimen uses aqueous crystalline penicillin G, 12 to 24 million units/day (2 to 4 million units every 4 hours) IV for 10 days, followed by benzathine penicillin G, 2.4 million units IM for 3 successive weeks. An adaptation of this in children is the administration of aqueous crystalline penicillin G, 50,000 units/kg/day for 10 days (not to exceed the adult dose), followed by benzathine penicillin, 50,000 units/kg per dose in three weekly doses. The use of agents other than penicillin has not been thoroughly studied. Where clinically feasible, as with aggressive, nonthreatening, recent reactions, skin testing and desensitization should be undertaken. If an alternative to penicillin is absolutely required because of life-threatening reactions, chloramphenicol, 1 gm every 6 hours, has been recommended. Third-generation cephalosporins cross the blood-brain barrier and have antitreponemal effect. They may prove helpful.

PREGNANCY

All pregnant women should have a nontreponemal serologic test for syphilis at the first prenatal visit, preferably in the first trimester, with a repeat test prior to delivery recommended in high-risk populations.

The VDRL, if positive in high titer (>1:16), usually signifies active infection. However, it is neither specific nor highly sensitive, and hence treponemal-specific tests should be used, such as the fluorescent treponemal antibody absorption (FTA-ABS) and the microhemagglutination assay (MHA). The *T. pallidum* immobilization (TPI) test is a difficult, expensive test performed in only a few research laboratories. A pregnant woman with serologic evidence of syphilis (with a specific treponemal test), a history of sexual contact with someone with documented syphilis, darkfield microscope confirmation of the presence of spirochetes, or in whom the diagnosis cannot be definitely ruled out should be treated. Similarly, those with previous treatment but current laboratory or clinical evidence of reinfection should be treated. Monitoring therapy during pregnancy and at 3, 6, 9, and 12 months after therapy with quantitative VDRL titers should be carried out.

Treatment is basically the same as in nonpregnant individuals, according to the stage of the disease. Specifically, benzathine penicillin G, given as a single IM dose of 2.4 million units in the first trimester, should prevent fetal infection. In spite of such treatment, congenital infections have occurred. If the mother has early syphilis, aqueous procaine penicillin G, 600,000 units daily IM for 8 days, is recommended. Latent syphilis is treated with either 2.4 million units of benzathine penicillin G weekly for 3 weeks or 600,000 units of parenteral procaine penicillin G daily for 15 days. Neurosyphilis should be treated with procaine penicillin G, 600,000 units twice daily for 2 to 3 weeks.

Tetracycline is hepatotoxic to the mother, has potentially harmful effects (osseous, dental) on the fetus, and hence should not be used. Erythromycin base or stearate should be reserved for those with documented evidence of penicillin allergy by skin test findings or history of anaphylaxis. Erythromycin estolate has potential hepatotoxicity for the mother and adverse effects on the fetus and hence should be avoided. Passage of erythromycin across the placenta is unpredictable, often limited, with low levels achieved in the fetus. Thus, treatment failures occur, and the newborn should be evaluated as though no maternal therapy had been given. Cephalosporins may prove to be an alternative in this setting. Close clinical follow-up of both mother and infant is required. If the disease is untreated, there is a 25 per cent fetal mortality, with postnatal death occurring in another 25 per cent of those infants infected.

The Newborn. In most cases, the newborn of a mother known to have been appropriately treated with penicillin theoretically should not require therapy. However, since congenital syphilis has occurred in spite of such treatment and documentation of maternal therapy may be uncertain, each neonate at risk should be evaluated, and most should be treated. The adverse effects of therapy are negligible and outweighed by the potential benefits. If any drug other than penicillin was used in treatment of the mother, there is then no doubt at all about the need to treat the infant.

If the infant is symptomatic (jaundice, hepatosplenomegaly, skin rashes, snuffles, or bone changes on radiograph), 10 days of treatment with aqueous crystalline penicillin G or procaine penicillin G, in a dose of 50,000 units/kg, in two divided doses or once daily as a single dose, respectively, is required. Recently, a regimen of 100,00 to 150,000 units/kg of aqueous crystalline penicillin G (administered as 50,000 units/kg IV every 8 to 12 hours) has been recommended. If neurosyphilis has been excluded, one IM dose of benzathine penicillin G, 50,000 units/kg, would be sufficient. Since criteria for neurosyphilis vary, one should assume the infant to have neurosyphilis, even though this is a rare manifestation at present.

In theory, an asymptomatic neonate of a penicillin-treated mother, or one whose mother is serofast, need not be treated but should be clinically and serologically re-evaluated at 1, 2, and 4 months. Sequential testing will show a reduction in antibody titer. In practice, many of these infants are born to mothers of lower socioeconomic groups who have had little or no antenatal care. Compliance with a program of multiple follow-up visits is unlikely in this context. Treatment with benzathine penicillin G (as discussed previously) may be the more prudent and cost-effective approach in such cases. If the mother's treatment status is uncertain, the asymptomatic infant with a positive serology should have skeletal radiographs and a cerebrospinal fluid examination. It is rare for a neonate to require antibiotics other than penicillin, which remains the drug of choice in virtually all types of syphilis. The current reports of fetal and neonatal deaths due to congenital syphilis reflect mainly inadequate antenatal care. The latter may be due in turn to socioeconomic factors, cultural differences, and an "attitudinal barrier." Inadequate control programs and surveillance also contribute to this adverse outcome, as may HIV coinfection.

Infancy. The treatment regimen for congenital syphilis diagnosed in infancy, but after the neonatal period, is the same as that recommended for newborns. For older children, calculation of the dose should be modified so that adult levels are not exceeded.

SEXUAL ABUSE AND RAPE

Laboratory examination in the case of rape should include a VDRL determination. Medical prophylaxis in the form of a 7- to 10-day course of tetracycline, 500 mg orally four times a day for 7 days, or doxycycline, 100 mg orally twice a day for 7 days, is effective against gonorrhea, chlamydial infection, or incubating syphilis and should be considered in those over 8 years of age and who are not pregnant. Occasionally, abused children present with symptomatic primary or secondary syphilis, but the incidence in sexual abuse is very low in general.

HUMAN IMMUNODEFICIENCY VIRUS

Testing for syphilis is recommended for persons with HIV infection acquired through sexual contact or intravenous drug abuse. Conversely, HIV testing (with informed consent) is advised for sexually active patients with syphilis. Unusual serologic responses in HIV-infected patients include both high titers on nontreponemal serologic tests for syphilis and the opposite, namely, negative nontreponemal and treponemal tests for syphilis, in those with biopsy-confirmed secondary syphilis.

There is no change recommended in the therapy for early syphilis in HIV-infected patients, although the issue is in dispute. Neurosyphilis, especially meningovascular syphilis, may occur earlier in HIV-infected individuals and may represent a failure of benzathine penicillin. Similarly, erythromycin has failed to cure secondary syphilis in a patient infected with HIV. Coinfection with HIV may increase the risk of neurosyphilis. For these reasons, the CDC recommends that benza-

thine penicillin G *not* be used in the treatment of neurosyphilis in those with HIV infection. Instead, a regimen of 10 days or more of either aqueous crystalline penicillin G, 2.4 million units IV every 4 hours (12 to 24 million units daily), or aqueous procaine penicillin G, 2.4 million units IM daily, plus probenecid, 500 mg orally four times a day, is recommended. Careful follow-up of serologic status is particularly important in these patients.

Unpublished experience suggests an upsurge in the prevalence of severe congenital syphilis associated with the epidemic of HIV infection.

FOLLOW-UP AND RETREATMENT

Careful clinical and serologic follow-up is required in all cases.

Infants should be re-evaluated as part of routine care at 1, 2, 4, 6, and 12 months, with nontreponemal serologic tests repeated at 3, 6, and 12 months after the conclusion of treatment or until they become nonreactive.

Those with early acquired syphilis should undergo repeat nontreponemal testing at 3, 6, and 9 months after the conclusion of treatment. Additional testing at 24 months after treatment is necessary for those with syphilis of more than 1 year's duration. Those with neurosyphilis should have serologic and clinical evaluations at 6-month intervals and repeat cerebrospinal fluid examinations for at least 3 years.

Indications for retreatment include recurrence or persistence of clinical signs, a sustained fourfold rise in nontreponemal test titer, or failure of an initially high nontreponemal titer to decease fourfold within a year or, in pregnancy, within 3 months.

The treatment regimen is that recommended for syphilis of more than 1 year's duration.

LEPTOSPIROSIS
RALPH D. FEIGIN, M.D.

Leptospirosis is a disease caused by a single family of organisms of which there are multiple serogroups and serotypes. In the last decade, the dog has been incriminated as an important vector as well as a reservoir of this disease.

To be of maximum therapeutic benefit an antimicrobial agent must be administered before the invading organisms damage the endothelium of blood vessels and various organs or tissues. One problem in evaluating the efficacy of therapy to date has been that, generally, leptospirosis is a self-limited disease with a favorable prognosis. Even patients with severe icteric leptospirosis may recover without specific treatment.

Most claims of the beneficial value of antimicrobial agents in human leptospirosis are based on the response of individual patients rather than on controlled studies. However, when penicillin therapy was given to 28 patients prior to the fourth day of illness and compared with a control group of 33 patients who were given only supportive care, the duration of fever and the incidence of jaundice, meningismus, renal involvement, and hemorrhagic manifestations were diminished in the treated group. Therefore, when a diagnosis of leptospirosis is considered possible or probable and the patient has been ill for less than 1 week, treatment with penicillin or tetracycline (avoid the latter in children less than 8 years of age) should be initiated. Parenteral aqueous penicillin G (6 to 8 million units/m² of body surface/24 hr in six divided doses) provides optimal blood and tissue concentrations of penicillin. For patients who are sensitive to penicillin, tetracycline (20 to 40 mg/kg/24 hr) should be provided intravenously or orally in four divided doses for 1 week. Do not give tetracycline intravenously in excess of 1 gm total dose.

A sudden increase in body temperature, drop in systemic blood pressure, and exacerbation of other symptoms may accompany the initiation of penicillin therapy (a Herxheimer reaction). This reaction generally subsides spontaneously and is not a contraindication to continued treatment.

The management of leptospirosis requires careful attention to supportive care. Profound fluid and electrolyte changes may be noted, particularly significant hyponatremia. Thus, fluid and electrolyte balance must be accorded meticulous attention. Dehydration, cardiovascular collapse, and acute renal failure require prompt, specific treatment. In some cases, acute renal failure may be prevented by ensuring adequate renal perfusion and appropriate fluid administration early in the disease when prerenal azotemia and shock may be seen. If prerenal azotemia is suspected, diuresis may be attempted with the administration of a fluid or colloid load designed to expand extracellular volume and replace extracellular fluid deficits. In patients who do not respond to such therapy, acute tubular necrosis should be suspected, and appropriate fluid restriction should be initiated. Urine output, urine specific gravity, serum and urine osmolalities, and accurate measurement of body weight should be monitored sequentially. Children should receive sufficient fluid to replace insensible water loss plus their urine output. This may require adjustments of fluid intake on an hourly basis. Generally, a multiple electrolyte solution containing 5 or 10 per cent glucose and 40 mEq of sodium and chloride per liter, 35 mEq of potassium per liter, and 20 mEq of lactate or acetate per liter administered at a rate calculated as above is appropriate fluid therapy. If azotemia is severe or prolonged, peritoneal dialysis or hemodialysis should be instituted. Exchange transfusion has been suggested for patients with marked hyperbilirubinemia.

The use of corticosteroids in the treatment of severe cases has not been evaluated critically. Their use has been suggested in patients with impending hepatic coma. Anecdotal reports also suggest that they may be of value in patients with profound hypotension or shock.

Hemorrhagic manifestations of disease may be related to disseminated intravascular coagulation or thrombocytopenia without disseminated intravascular coagulation or may merely reflect friability of blood vessels due to the severe vasculitis. Platelet transfusions have been used for patients with thrombocytopenia, but generally the lifespan of the infused platelets is short. Heparin has been used for the treatment of disseminated intravascular coagulation, but there is little evidence to suggest that such therapy is beneficial.

When uveitis is present, ophthalmologic consultation should be sought. Conjunctival suffusion is common with leptospirosis and clears without specific topical therapy.

RAT BITE FEVER

MOSES GROSSMAN, M.D.

The clinical term *rat bite fever* refers to two separate and similar syndromes, both induced by bites of infected rodents. The microorganisms involved are *Spirillum minor* and *Streptobacillus moniliformis*. The syndrome caused by the former is also known as sodoku; the latter produces a syndrome also known as Haverhill fever or streptobacillary fever. Specific etiologic diagnosis may be attained by darkfield examination, inoculation of laboratory animals, or serologically.

Antimicrobial therapy is important. Untreated the disease lasts longer and may have a distinct mortality. The drug of choice is penicillin for both microorganisms and for all forms of the disease. The traditionally recommended regimen is 20,000 to 50,000 units of procaine penicillin/kg/24 hours divided into twice-daily doses for 7 days. While there is no published experience with using oral penicillin there is every reason to believe than an oral regimen of penicillin would be effective if compliance could be assured. Patients allergic to penicillin should be given tetracycline as an alternate drug of choice (30 to 50 mg/kg/24 hr) in divided doses. In children younger than 9 years it is inadvisable to use tetracycline. Erythromycin might be a third-choice drug, particularly in the spirillary form of the syndrome.

In addition to antimicrobial therapy, local care of the ulcerated area at the site of the bite and attention to tetanus prophylaxis are important adjuncts to treatment.

Pneumocystis Carinii PNEUMONITIS

WALTER T. HUGHES, M.D.

Pneumonitis caused by *Pneumocystis carinii* is usually fatal if untreated. With specific antimicrobial therapy about 75 per cent of patients can be expected to recover if treatment is begun early. Since the infection usually occurs in immunocompromised patients and a definitive diagnosis requires an invasive procedure, such as bronchoalveolar lavage, open lung biopsy or percutaneous needle aspiration, management requires close attention to complications from the underlying primary disease and the diagnostic procedures. Thus, associated or secondary viral, bacterial, or fungal infections may occur and pneumothorax or pneumomediastinum may complicate the diagnostic procedure. Hypoxia with low arterial oxygen tension (PaO$_2$) is regularly present, while carbon dioxide retention is unusual and the arterial pH is frequently increased. Unlike other infections in the immunosuppressed host, *P. carinii* infection remains localized entirely to the lungs.

When *P. carinii* pneumonitis is recognized as the first illness of an infant or child, careful search should be made for an underlying disease.

Specific Therapy. Trimethoprim-sulfamethoxazole (TMP-SMZ)* and pentamidine isethionate are equally effective in the treatment of *P. carinii* pneumonitis, but TMP-SMZ is the drug of first choice because of its low toxicity and easy availability.

TMP-SMZ may be given orally or intravenously. The oral dose is 20 mg trimethoprim and 100 mg sulfamethoxazole/kg/day, divided into four parts at 6-hour intervals. It is advisable to give half of the calculated daily dose initially as a loading dose when the oral route is used. TMP-SMZ is available in tablet form ("regular size" with 80 mg trimethoprim, 400 mg sulfamethoxazole and as a "double-strength" tablet with twice these amounts). An oral suspension contains 40 mg trimethoprim and 200 mg sulfamethoxazole per 5 ml. The intravenous preparation is available in 5.0-ml ampules containing 80 mg trimethoprim and 400 mg sulfamethoxazole. Each 5.0-ml ampule must be added to 125 ml of 5 per cent dextrose in water. The dosage for intravenous use is 15.0 mg trimethoprim and 75.0 mg sulfamethoxazole/kg/day divided in three to four equal doses. Each dose is infused over a 60-minute period. From available data, peak serum levels of 3 to 5 μg/ml of trimethoprim and 100 to 150 μg/ml of sulfamethoxazole seem to be the optimal ranges.

The adverse and toxic side effects are essentially those of sulfonamides, and although uncommon they include transient maculopapular rash, nausea, vomiting, diarrhea, neutropenia, agranulocytosis, aplastic anemia, megaloblastic anemia, hemolytic anemia, methemoglobinemia, Stevens-Johnson syndrome, allergic reactions, toxic nephrosis, and drug fever. Folic acid deficiency has occurred rarely. It is reversible by folinic acid, 10 to 25 mg daily. Folinic acid does not interfere with the therapeutic effects of the drug. Patients with acquired immune deficiency syndrome (AIDS) have a higher rate of adverse reactions than other patients.

Pentamidine is the drug of second choice because of its high frequency of adverse effects. The drug was approved by the Federal Drug Administration in 1984 and is marketed in the United States by LyphoMed (Melrose Park, IL).

Pentamidine is administered as a single daily dose of 4 mg/kg intravenously infused over a period of 1 hour for 10 to 14 days. If improvement is apparent after 5 days of treatment, this may be reduced to 3 mg/kg/day. The total dosage should not exceed 56 mg/kg. The drug may also be given by intramuscular injection if

use of the intravenous route is not possible. Intramuscular injections should be given deeply into the anterolateral aspect of the thigh.

Adverse effects include induration, abscess formation, and necrosis at injection sites; nephrotoxicity; hypoglycemia or, rarely, hyperglycemia; hypotension; alteration in liver function; tachycardia; hypocalcemia; nausea and vomiting; skin rash; anemia; hyperkalemia; and thrombocytopenia.

Isolation. Recent studies indicate that *P. carinii* is transmitted by the airborne route. It is advisable to use respiratory isolation procedures to separate active cases of *P. carinii* pneumonitis from other compromised individuals at high risk for this infection.

Supportive Measures. Oxygen should be administered by mask as needed to maintain the PaO$_2$ above 70 mm Hg. The fraction of inspired oxygen (FIO$_2$) should be kept below 50 volumes per cent if possible, to avoid oxygen toxicity, since oxygen therapy usually is required for relatively long periods.

Assisted or controlled ventilation is indicated in patients with arterial oxygen tension less than 60 mm Hg at FIO$_2$ of 50 per cent or greater. Those with acutely elevated PaCO$_2$, without pH changes and with or without hypoxemia, should be considered candidates for ventilatory therapy.

Patients receiving immunosuppressive drugs should have these discontinued if the status of the primary disease permits.

Fluid and electrolyte quantities are calculated by the patient's needs, but the solution should contain 5 or 10 per cent glucose to help prevent hypoglycemia during pentamidine therapy. Metabolic acidosis must be corrected.

Bacterial pneumonia or sepsis may occur in association with *P. carinii* pneumonitis, in the seriously ill patient with marked neutropenia (absolute neutrophil count less than 500/cu mm) or evidence of bacterial infection, antibiotics should be given. Oxacillin, 200 mg/kg/day, and gentamicin, 5 to 7 mg/kg/day, are administered intravenously until the results of cultures are known.

Efforts should be made to improve the nutritional status of the patient by dietary means even during the acute stage of the disease. Multivitamins should be given empirically. The value of intravenous alimentation has not been determined.

Give blood transfusion if hemoglobin level is less than normal. The hemoglobin content must be sufficient to result in an arterial oxygen content of 15 to 20 ml/dl of blood at an arterial oxygen tension of 100 mm Hg.

Pneumothorax may be a complication of the diagnostic procedures. If it is less than 15 per cent with no adverse effect on respiration, close observation is adequate. If it is more extensive, insertion of a thoracotomy tube with a water seal drainage system is necessary.

Parameters to Monitor. *Serum immunoglobulins:* At the onset of the illness, administer immune serum globulin (165 mg/ml) 0.66 ml/kg if the immunoglobulin G level is below 300 mg/dl.

Roentgenograms of chest should be done daily until there is clinical evidence of improvement. If needle

---

*Manufacturer's precaution: Not recommended for infants less than 2 months of age.

aspiration of the lung, lung biopsy, or endotracheal brush catheter technique has been used as a diagnostic procedure, chest roentgenograms should be made at 30 minutes, 4 hours, and 12 hours after the procedure to detect pneumothorax.

Hemoglobin, WBC count and differential, and platelet estimate daily.

Measure body weight, intake and output daily.

Arterial blood gases: Measure pH, $PaCO_2$, PaO_2, and base excess or deficit initially and as often as necessary, based on severity of clinical course.

Serum electrolytes: Measure sodium, chloride, potassium, and carbon dioxide content every 3 days, or more frequently if indicated.

Total serum proteins, albumin, and globulin: Monitor every 3 days. Hypoalbuminemia may occur.

Blood pressure, pulse, and respiratory rate: Monitor every 4 hours, or more often if the condition is critical.

For patients receiving pentamidine: Check *blood urea nitrogen (BUN), creatinine, and urinalysis* every 3 days. If the BUN exceeds 30 mg/dl or serum creatinine is greater than 1.5 mg/dl, withhold pentamidine for 1 or 2 days; monitor *blood glucose* 4 to 6 hours after each injection of pentamidine. Administer glucose if blood glucose value is less than 40 mg/dl; monitor *serum glutamic-oxaloacetic transaminase (SGOT)* every 3 days; withhold pentamidine for 1 to 2 days if evidence of hepatic toxicity exists; and monitor *serum calcium and phosphorus* every 3 days. If the serum inorganic phosphate level becomes increased and the calcium level becomes decreased from normal values on the basis of renal insufficiency, give calcium lactate, 15 to 20 gm/day, or calcium carbonate, 5 to 8 gm/day orally. The diet should be low in phosphate, and 25,000 to 50,000 units of vitamin D are given orally. For patients with renal impairment and receiving trimethoprim-sulfamethoxazole, the dosage should be regulated on the basis of serum drug levels. Measurement of serum levels of the sulfonamide is adequate. The level of free sulfonamide should be maintained with peak values between 100 and 150 μg/ml measured 2 hours after the oral dosage.

Experimental studies suggest that diaminodiphyenylsulfone (dapsone), trimetrexate with leucovorin, and fansidar may be effective in *P. carinii* pneumonitis.

Expected Course. Fever, tachypnea, and pulmonary infiltrates usually persist with little change for 4 to 6 days. If no improvement is apparent after a week of therapy, concomitant or secondary infection most likely exists. These infections have included bacterial pneumonia or sepsis, systemic candidiasis, aspergillosis, cryptococcosis, histoplasmosis, and cytomegalovirus inclusion disease, as well as other viral infections. *P. carinii* pneumonitis may recur several months after apparent recovery in 10 to 15 per cent of cases.

Prevention. *P. carinii* pneumonitis can be prevented by chemoprophylaxis with TMP-SMZ.* Dosage is one fourth the therapeutic dose, 5 mg/kg of trimethoprim and 25 mg/kg of sulfamethoxazole per day in two divided doses. The protection is afforded only while

*This use is not listed by the manufacturer.

the patient is receiving the drug. Aerosolized pentamidine has been found to be effective in preventing *P. carinii* pneumonitis in adults with AIDS. However, similar studies in children are lacking.

MEASLES

EDWARD A. MORTIMER, Jr., M.D.

Measles is an acute, systemic viral infection that in the past affected nearly all children in the United States and therefore was classified as one of the usual childhood diseases. A severe disease, it is characterized by a course of approximately 7 days with high fever; moderately severe respiratory symptoms, including coryza, conjunctivitis, and cough; the classic enanthem (Koplik's spots); and a characteristic rash. Besides the severity of the acute illness, the importance of the disease in the United States has been measured by its complications, particularly otitis media, pneumonia, measles encephalitis, and, rarely, subacute sclerosing panencephalitis. In the past in the United States mortality was largely a result of pneumonia; perhaps because of better nutrition, antibiotics, and other factors, deaths from the disease declined remarkably even before widespread use of the vaccine.

Even today, however, the situation in the remainder of the world is very different. WHO estimates for 1980 indicate that of the 120 million babies born in the Third World annually, 1,860,000 (1.6 per cent) succumb to measles before their fifth birthdays. Undoubtedly complicating factors such as low birth weight, malnutrition, recurrent diarrhea, and other infections contribute to this high mortality. Thus, measles remains a severe disease.

Control of Measles

Control of measles and its associated morbidity and mortality depend on timely active immunization of all eligible children. Treatment of the illness is only symptomatic; its bacterial complications are susceptible to therapy, but the more serious neurologic and other sequelae are not. Passive immunization of susceptible children with immune serum globulin is useful only in occasional instances when exposure is recognized early.

Live, Attenuated Measles Vaccine. Isolation and propagation of the measles virus in 1954 led to the development and licensure of inactivated and live, attenuated vaccines in 1963. Since 1967 only the live vaccine has been used. A single dose of properly administered measles vaccine induces seroconversion and clinical immunity in more than 95 per cent of recipients. Available preparations include monovalent measles vaccine, measles vaccine combined with live, attenuated rubella vaccine (MR), and the familiar MMR, which comprises live, attenuated measles, mumps, and rubella vaccines, the preparation of choice for routine immunization since 1971. There is no biologic advantage to administering measles, mumps, or rubella vaccine in monovalent form.

It was originally recommended that measles vaccine be administered at 9 months of age, but the preferred age was raised first to 12 months and in 1976 to 15 months because of interference with the immune response by small amounts of persisting transplacental maternal antibody. From 1976 until 1989 a single dose of MMR at 15 months of age was recommended as a routine policy; in 1989 this policy was changed to include a second dose of MMR.

Rationale for Two-Dose Measles Vaccine Policy. The widespread use of measles vaccine in the U.S. has resulted in a remarkable decline in disease incidence and a shift in the age distribution of cases. Indeed, in 1983 only 1497 cases were reported. Since then, however, there has been a considerable increase with a preliminary estimate of more than 15,000 cases in 1989. The majority of these cases occurred in localized outbreaks rather than being sporadic. These outbreaks have occurred in preschool children and even in school-age populations with vaccination rates of more than 98 per cent. In 1989 college outbreaks also presented problems. Prior to the use of measles vaccine 90 per cent of all measles cases occurred in children less than 10 years and only about 3 per cent in persons 15 years and older. With widespread immunization the incidence decreased markedly in all age groups, and particularly in elementary school children. However, the proportions of cases in adolescents older than 10 years and adults have increased strikingly, now accounting for more than 60 per cent. Indeed, since 1983 there has been an actual increase in rates in all age groups but especially in persons 15 years and older. The reasons for this recrudescence of measles appear to be two: failure to achieve high rates of measles immunization in preschool children who are unaffected by school entry laws, and vaccine failures, either primary (failure of the vaccine to "take") or secondary (waning immunity) in a few instances.

VACCINE FAILURES. Vaccine failures, as evidenced by clinical measles in a previously immunized child (or failure of serologic conversion in studies of efficacy), have been reported in 5 to 10 per cent of children. Many, if not most, of these can be attributed to any one of three factors: improper handling of the vaccine, administration at too young an age, or simultaneous use of immune serum globulin. The vaccine is susceptible to inactivation by light or by warmth during transport or storage (breaks in the "cold chain"); it should always be transported and stored until use at or below 45°F (8°C). The vaccine also should not be directly exposed to bright light unnecessarily.

As noted above, administration of properly stored and handled vaccine may nonetheless be associated with failure to immunize because of persistent maternal antibody; the younger the infant, the higher the proportion of failures. Many of the cases of measles occurring during outbreaks in previously immunized persons are so explained. Accordingly, for some years it was a recommended (and frequently mandatory) policy to re-immunize all children who received measles vaccine prior to their first birthdays, and it was considered acceptable to re-immunize those who were vaccinated between 12 and 14 months.

Some vaccine failures are attributable to the simultaneous administration of immune globulin to many children who received measles vaccine prepared from the less attenuated Edmonston B strain of virus between 1963, when it was first licensed, and 1975, when it was replaced by the further attenuated vaccine. Immune globulin was given to ameliorate the excessive reactions from the Edmonston B vaccine, and, indeed, some physicians continued to use it in conjunction with the further attenuated vaccine. Unfortunately, although the immune serum globulin reduced reaction rates, it also prevented the acquisition of active immunity in some children, particularly those who received the further attenuated vaccine.

Currently there is some suggestive but unproved evidence of vaccine-induced immunity waning to the point of clinical susceptibility to measles in a few individuals. Such might occur because measles vaccine produces lower antibody titers than does natural disease and, more importantly, because the near disappearance of the disease has resulted in lack of a booster effect from casual exposure to the disease (the "street car" booster).

Recommendations for Vaccine Use. In 1989 both the U.S. Public Health Service and the American Academy of Pediatrics recommended adding a second dose of measles vaccine, given as MMR, as part of the routine childhood immunization schedule. The optimal age for reimmunization has not been determined at present. The American Academy of Pediatrics recommends the second dose at about 12 years; the U.S. Public Health Service advises the second dose at the time of kindergarten entry (4 to 6 years). Some communities with high rates of measles have recommended the first dose at 1 year and the second at 18 months. Under any schedule at least one month should elapse between the two doses. It is likely that more general agreement as to the optimal ages for the two doses will occur as experience is gained.

There are certain circumstances, including outbreaks and foreign travel, that require special considerations. For full review of these considerations and all aspects of the changed vaccine policy and its rationale, the reader should consult the recommendations of the U.S. Public Health Service Immunization Practices Advisory Committee (ACIP), published in the *MMWR*, Vol 38, pages S1–S18, December 29, 1989.

Reactions to Measles Vaccine. Because measles vaccine produces a "mild" measles infection, side effects may be anticipated in some recipients. The most frequent of these is fever, usually appearing 6 days after inoculation. Although fever is usually slight and lasts only a few days, in approximately 10 per cent of children it may reach 103° F (39.4° C) or more. Less commonly, transient, nondescript rashes occur. An important question is whether the neurologic sequelae of the disease (acute encephalitis and SSPE) occur following measles vaccine. Although there have been isolated anecdotal reports of acute encephalitis following the vaccine, their rarity suggests that they probably represent coincidence and not causation. Similarly, if measles vaccine causes SSPE, the rate is only a minute fraction of that from natural measles, for the reason that the incidence of SSPE in the United States has declined remarkably following widespread use of the vaccine.

Children with a past or family history of convulsions are at slightly increased risk of a febrile convulsion secondary to vaccine-induced fever. Because short febrile convulsions are considered harmless (though distressing), such a history is not considered a contraindication to measles vaccine on the basis that the disease risk is far greater. Since fever is most likely to occur 5 to 12 days after immunization, some physicians may wish to advise antipyretic prophylaxis with acetaminophen during those days. Unless the child is already receiving anticonvulsant medications, these drugs are probably of little value because of the weeks required to attain satisfactory levels. As with any vaccine or other medication given to children, the benefits and risks should be explained to the parents.

A unique problem is presented by those individuals, now young adults, who received killed measles vaccine during the years it was licensed (1963 to 1967). Up to 1 million children received the killed vaccine. The vaccine was abandoned when it became apparent that protection was transient and that children exposed to measles 2 or more years later experienced a severe type of measles with high fever, unusual rash, edema, pneumonitis, and other findings (atypical measles). Such persons also exhibit greater reactivity to subsequent live measles vaccine; a few have quite severe reactions resembling atypical measles. However, because atypical natural measles is far more severe than the vast majority of reactions to the live vaccine in these persons, most authorities advise administering the live vaccine with adequate warning to the parents. Reimmunization of those who received killed vaccine or vaccine of unknown type is particularly important for those who travel to other countries where measles is common.

Contraindications to Measles Vaccine

Prior Immunization. Prior immunity to measles, mumps, or rubella, whether acquired from disease or by immunization, is *not* associated with untoward reactions to MMR and is therefore of no concern.

Egg Sensitivity. Live measles vaccine is propagated in chick embryo cell culture. In recent years, cases of potentially serious immediate allergic reactions to the vaccine have been unquestionably related to egg sensitivity. Therefore, rare cases of children with a clear history of anaphylactic type of response to egg ingestion should not receive measles vaccine.

Immunocompromised States. Except for children with HIV infection, children with congenital immune deficiencies and those whose immune systems are compromised by immunosuppressive therapy should not receive measles vaccine because of the risk of enhanced infection with the vaccine virus. For most children receiving intense immunosuppressive therapy the vaccine may be delayed until treatment is discontinued. Low-dose therapy is not a contraindication. Because recipients of the vaccine do not transmit the virus, immunodeficient persons are not jeopardized by the immunization of others, including siblings.

MMR is safe for asymptomatic HIV-infected children and should be given. Because incomplete data currently suggest that symptomatic HIV-infected children, including those with AIDS, do not incur serious untoward effects, MMR should be considered, although immune responses may be blunted.

Neomycin Allergy. Measles vaccine contains small amounts of neomycin but no other antibiotic. The rare individual who has experienced an anaphylactic response to topical or systemic neomycin should not receive the vaccine. Contact dermatitis from topical neomycin is not a contraindication, although such persons may develop a small, transient nodule at the injection site.

Pregnancy. Although there is no evidence that measles vaccine (or any live vaccine, including that for rubella) is deleterious to the fetus, pregnant women should not receive measles vaccine on theoretical grounds and to avoid confusion about causation of any adverse outcome of the pregnancy.

Prior Receipt of Immune Serum Globulin. Human immune serum globulin contains substantial amounts of measles antibody, which may interfere with a measles vaccine "take." Therefore, administration of the vaccine to any child who has received immune serum globulin should be deferred for at least 3 months after receipt of the globulin.

Acute Illness. Because children repetitively display evidence of mild, transient respiratory infections with little or no fever and because there is no evidence of deleterious interaction between such illnesses and the receipt of measles vaccine or of interference with acquisition of immunity, whether to administer measles vaccine in the presence of such symptoms should be determined by individual circumstances.

Passive Immunization

Immune serum globulin (ISG) will prevent or modify measles in exposed susceptible individuals, depending on the dose administered and on its administration as soon as possible after exposure (no later than 6 days). Preventive doses of ISG (0.25 ml/kg intramuscularly, maximum dose 15 ml) should be given to all infants between 6 and 24 months of age and to all nonimmune immunodeficient persons exposed to measles, because of the high incidence of complications in such children. An alternative approach for certain susceptible individuals exposed within the previous 72 hours is to administer measles vaccine, because vaccine-induced immunity appears promptly, often prior to the development of the clinical disease.

For unimmunized children older than 2 years who are exposed to measles, a modifying dose of ISG may be given (0.04 ml/kg body weight as a single injection). This dose may be expected to ameliorate the severity of the disease if given within 6 days and nonetheless permit the development of active immunity. Unless such children develop modified (mild) measles, they should receive measles vaccine 3 months after receipt of ISG.

ISG should not be used to control measles outbreaks in schools or communities. Instead, all persons at risk of exposure born since 1957 should receive measles vaccine unless they have proof of physician-diagnosed measles or immunization with live measles vaccine age 12 months or older. In such situations ISG should be given only to individuals for whom the vaccine is contraindicated and to infants 6 to 24 months of age with documented exposure to the disease.

Management of Measles

The treatment of measles is symptomatic only. ISG will not modify the course or prevent complications once symptoms have begun. Prophylactic antibiotics are of no utility in preventing secondary infection. Acetaminophen, 5 mg/kg, may be given as often as every 4 hours for symptomatic relief. Symptoms of the disease are such that bed rest during the febrile stages is not difficult to enforce. Mild cough suppressants may be given but usually appear to have little effect.

A frequent problem that has arisen since the advent of the vaccine is that of misdiagnosis, because an increasing number of physicians have never seen measles. If there is doubt, a quick way to obtain diagnostic help is to have the patient seen by an older physician who had past experience with outbreaks of the disease.

Important in the management of measles is recognition and treatment of complications. The most common of these is bacterial otitis media, which requires appropriate antimicrobial therapy. In the past, mastoiditis frequently ensued. Pulmonary complications include bronchiolitis, especially in infants, and pneumonia, which may be lobar or bronchopneumonic in distribution. Suspicion of pneumonia usually arises when the patient worsens late in the course of the disease or fever fails to subside with full appearance of the rash. A chest radiograph may be required for diagnosis. Pneumonia may be bacterial in origin, especially if lobar, and should be treated with antimicrobial drugs. Rarely, pneumothorax or pneumomediastinum occurs. Occasionally, inflammation of the upper airway progresses to obstructive laryngotracheitis and may require tracheostomy.

Other rare complications include appendicitis, presumably secondary to lymphoid hyperplasia; abdominal pain and vomiting in the course of measles or early in convalescence suggest this possibility. Acute measles encephalitis, estimated to occur in about 1 per 1000 cases, usually appears near the end of the course of the disease or early in convalescence. Persistent or recurring fever, somnolence, irrational behavior, vomiting, and convulsions are frequent manifestations. Treatment is symptomatic; neurologic consultation is advisable.

RUBELLA AND CONGENITAL RUBELLA

PHILIP R. ZIRING, M.D.

The decline in the incidence of rubella and congenital rubella since licensure of live attenuated rubella virus vaccines in 1969 has been one of the most notable achievements of modern medicine. The last major epidemic of rubella in the United States in 1964 was accompanied by rubella infection in one in every 100

pregnancies and the birth of approximately 20,000 infants with rubella-associated defects. More than 100,000,000 doses of rubella vaccine have been administered in the United States since 1969, which brought the predictable 7-year cycles of rubella epidemics to a conclusion. So dramatic has this change been that by 1989 there were only 3 cases of congenital rubella nationwide reported to the Centers for Disease Control.

We will consider rubella and congenital rubella in this section because, despite their low incidence, they are matters for pediatricians to remain concerned about. Sporadic cases of rubella still occur, especially in clusters among older adolescents and young adults who have not had the disease or been immunized and in susceptible persons immigrating to the United States. There is a great need to maintain a high level of awareness about the importance of immunization and the safety and efficacy of rubella vaccine. Furthermore, we have an ongoing concern for the thousands of patients with congenital rubella, many of whom were victims of the 1964 epidemic who are now entering the third decade of life and who are at risk for developing new clinical manifestations of this disorder.

Rubella

In general, rubella (German measles, three-day measles) can be considered among the mildest viral illnesses. In fact, a significant percentage of adults and even larger numbers of children may undergo infection that is completely asymptomatic. Although often pruritic, the rash generally responds to simple antihistamine treatment. There may be an associated sore throat, tender lymphadenopathy, and low-grade fever, which is responsive to analgesics. It is most important to recall that the patient is highly contagious for a period of time beginning a few days prior to the onset of rash until 1 to 2 weeks after the rash clears. During this time it is important to avoid exposure of the patient to a woman who may be in early pregnancy and whose rubella susceptibility status is unknown. The most important common complication of rubella is postinfectious arthralgia or arthritis, principally involving the small joints of the hands and feet. Although these joint symptoms sometimes are quite painful and may recur periodically for an extended period of time, they always clear completely without residua. Thrombocytopenia of mild degree is not uncommon and usually resolves without treatment. Thrombocytopenic purpura is a rare complication, which should prompt thorough hematologic investigation to ensure that there is no other underlying cause. A course of prednisone may be initiated if significant thrombocytopenia is persistent. Postinfectious encephalitis is seen in rubella far less often than in measles and usually responds to simple supportive measures.

Congenital Rubella

It is most useful to consider the clinical manifestations of congenital rubella in three stages: those that are present and identifiable at birth, those that are developmental and appear only as the infant grows older, and those late manifestations that may not be clinically apparent until the second decade of life or beyond.

Disorders Apparent in the Neonatal Period. The rubella-associated birth defects that are apparent at birth are a result of rubella virus interference with cell growth and cell division in the fetus. They include defects of the eye (cataract, glaucoma, and retinopathy), of the heart (stenosis of the main pulmonary artery and/or its branches, patent ductus arteriosus, and other less common heart defects less commonly seen), central nervous system (sensory neural hearing loss and other evidence of brain injury), bone marrow (anemia, thrombocytopenia, and defects of the immune system), and general intrauterine growth retardation. The management of these disorders is little different from that used when such defects result from other diverse etiologies.

A few clinical issues are especially worth remembering. For example, surgery for congenital glaucoma must be performed promptly after diagnosis in the neonatal period to guard against permanent visual loss from high intraocular pressure. Surgery for congenital cataracts, on the other hand, can often be deferred until as late as 1 year of age, when optimum surgical results are often obtained. Surgery for a uniocular rubella cataract has rarely been rewarded by useful vision in the operated eye. Sensorineural hearing loss is the most common clinically significant consequence of rubella infection during the first 4 months of pregnancy and must be ruled out in every infant suspected of having congenital rubella. The hearing loss may be unilateral or bilateral and range in severity from mild to profound and may be manifest in hearing at all frequencies. Early diagnosis through testing of infants by skilled audiologists followed by early amplification with hearing aids and enrollment in auditory training programs can often spell the difference between an individual capable of speech and one unable to communicate orally.

Developmental Disorders. As the infant passes beyond the neonatal period, other disorders of a developmental character may appear. Mental retardation is more likely and more severe the earlier in pregnancy the infection takes place and is often complicated by the presence of impairment of vision and/or hearing. The enrollment of these infants in preschool enrichment programs often helps them to make maximum use of their residual abilities and assists the family with needed training and support.

Symptoms of spastic cerebral palsy are usually not apparent until the first year of life. In such cases, close follow-up by neurologists, orthopedists, physiatrists, and physical, occupational, and speech therapists skilled in the management of physically handicapped children can often be helpful in management related to ambulation, sitting, feeding, and other skills of daily living.

Behavioral disorders occur commonly and are often complicated by the presence of sensory defects or mental retardation. Extreme restlessness and hyperactivity or symptoms of autism often prove difficult to manage. The results of the use of stimulant medication, tranquilizers, or barbiturates have generally been disappointing. More success has followed the use of mild sedatives such as diphenhydramine (Benadryl) or psy-chotropic agents such as thioridazine (Mellaril). Consultation with child psychiatrists and behavioral psychologists may also be helpful.

Late Manifestations of Congenital Rubella. Clinical disturbances of endocrine function in children and young adults with congenital rubella, with onset not until the first or second decade of life, are now well recognized. Patients with hypo- or hyperthyroidism have been described, with identification of rubella virus antigen in the thyroid gland of at least one child with Hashimoto's thyroiditis. The most common endocrine disturbance seems to be insulin-dependent diabetes mellitus, with up to 20 per cent or more of patients having some evidence of this disorder by the second decade of life. Recent interest has been focused on the association of insulin-dependent diabetes mellitus in children with congenital rubella, predominantly with certain HLA phenotypes, especially DR3 and B8. In such cases, the rubella infection of the islet cells in utero seems to have acted as a "trigger" in the expression of insulin-dependent diabetes mellitus in children who are so genetically predisposed. Early diagnosis of these disorders through measurement of antibodies directed against thyroid and islet cells is now becoming more commonplace. The interpretation of such tests and their therapeutic implications may often best be carried out in consultation with a pediatric endocrinologist.

Several patients with congenital rubella were reported a few years ago with progressive rubella panencephalitis, a degenerative disorder of the central nervous system apparently caused by an exacerbation of rubella infection within the brain. Although few patients have been so identified thus far, it is important to be alert to the existence of this entity in patients with congenital rubella who undergo deterioration in behavior, intellectual performance, or motor function or develop seizures.

Prevention of Rubella. As noted, immunization of most children at approximately 15 months of age and selected adults who are shown to be rubella seronegative has resulted in a dramatic decline in the incidence of rubella and congenital rubella. The RA 27/3 strain of virus grown in human diploid cell culture may be given alone or in combination with other live attenuated virus vaccines (measles, mumps). A single inoculation of this vaccine produces durable immunity, although the antibody levels achieved may be lower than that following natural rubella infection. The immunity so induced is protective and may well be lifelong. Ongoing surveillance conducted by the Centers for Disease Control in Atlanta of the risk to the fetus of inadvertent rubella immunization of a susceptible woman in early pregnancy has taken place since the introduction of the vaccine. It has been well established that vaccine virus so inoculated can be recovered from the fetus, but evidence is still lacking that this vaccine virus is teratogenic. Numerous such pregnancies have gone to term with no evidence of congenital rubella birth defects present in the offspring. Pregnant women so exposed should be counseled regarding the *theoretical* risks such vaccination poses; but they may be reassured at this time regarding the lack of known association with congenital rubella birth defects. Side effects of vaccination are similar (although generally milder) than those seen in natural rubella, with transient arthralgias and arthritis being the most common clinical conditions observed.

VARICELLA AND HERPES ZOSTER

PHILIP A. BRUNELL, M.D.

Varicella and zoster in normal children are usually bothersome but rarely life threatening. Thus, we have generally not found treatment with antiviral agents to be necessary. The main objectives of therapy have been to reduce itching and decrease the likelihood of infection in varicella. The latter has been accomplished by daily bathing with pHisoHex-containing soaps. Itching can be controlled by the local application of calamine lotion. Occasionally, oral therapy with trimeprazine is required. Pain accompanying zoster is less commonly a problem than in adults. If treatment is necessary, mild analgesics, such as acetaminophen with codeine, can be given. *Salicylates should not be given to children with varicella zoster (VZ) infections.*

In immunocompromised children, we have used acyclovir intravenously (IV), 500 mg/kg per dose, every 8 hours for at least 5 days, to treat varicella. We do not use oral acyclovir in these cases, as it has not been evaluated. The VZ virus is far less sensitive to acyclovir than is the herpes simplex virus. We observe immunocompromised patients with zoster as outpatients, as most do not require antiviral therapy. Those whose condition is generalizing, as defined by more than 20 lesions remote from the involved dermatome, or those with visceral involvement, such as pneumonia, are treated with the same regimen as described for varicella. The exceptions are children who have received bone marrow transplants, all of whom are treated.

Children who have received experimental varicella vaccine and develop varicella following exposure rarely require therapy with antiviral drugs. We generally count lesions and treat those who have greater than 500, who appear to have no decrease in the appearance of new lesions by the fourth day, or who have evidence of visceral involvement. Recent evidence suggests that stopping anticancer therapy may not influence the prognosis of VZ infections. Passive immunization, when indicated, should be given as soon as possible following exposure. Although one study has shown that the VZ antibody titer after regular intravenous globulin, 4 ml/kg, is similar to that following the recommended dose of VZ immune globulin (VZIG), there are no clinical data to assess efficacy. Intravenous preparations have the advantage of immediate availability of antibody. Absorption of antibody from the intramuscular injection site might take hours or days. At the present time, if passive immunization is indicated, the intramuscular VZIG still is advised.

VZIG is recommended for use in susceptible adult contacts. A delay in serologic testing often makes this impractical. On the other hand, the cost of this preparation, several hundred dollars for the average adult, makes one hesitate to use it unless immune status is ascertained. We have found that about 1 in 10 hospital employees with a negative history of varicella actually was seronegative. The rate of seronegativity for non-hospital workers who say they have not had chickenpox is higher.

Passive immunization is recommended for newborns whose mothers have onset of varicella from 5 days prior to the 2 days following delivery. There are increasing reports of failure of VZIG in this situation. One should be prepared to use acyclovir if necessary. One of the explanations of the poor performance of VZIG may be the low serum antibody levels. We have found that newborns given several times the dose recommended for older children barely attain the lower levels of VZ antibody found in normal immune adults. Indeed, we recommend that whenever VZIG is given for household exposure and a second case occurs 2 weeks later, a second dose be given rather than relying on the dose of VZIG given 2 weeks previously. We have used VZIG for exposures in neonatal intensive care units, as we have found that these infants frequently have lower VZ antibody levels than we had anticipated because of frequent blood drawing. Usually, red blood cells, rather than plasma-containing antibodies, are replaced. We do not recommend VZIG for exposures occurring in full-term nurseries or for exposure in the neonatal period, even if the mother has a negative history of varicella.

HERPES SIMPLEX VIRUS INFECTIONS

TERRY YAMAUCHI, M.D.

The human herpesviruses include herpes simplex virus (HSV), varicella zoster virus, cytomegalovirus, and Epstein-Barr virus. The most prevalent of these herpesviruses is HSV. Approximately 75 per cent of the population has been infected with this virus. Although most of these HSV infections are asymptomatic, multiple clinical syndromes have been recognized.

Two varieties of HSV have been identified: Type 1 (HSV-1) and Type 2 (HSV-2). HSV-1 infections in children can be either primary or recurrent. HSV-2 infections usually, but not exclusively, cause genital infections in the pediatric patient and most of the neonatal infections.

PRIMARY GINGIVOSTOMATITIS

These lesions may persist 7 to 10 days and, because of the pain, lead to dehydration. Lack of oral intake is a reason for hospitalization and intravenous fluid therapy. Topical analgesic preparations, systemic analgesic-antipyretic medications, oral fluids, and soft food have constituted the treatment of choice. Acyclovir and vidarabine have been advocated for several cases. Acyclovir has been the preferred agent because of lower toxicity and ease of administration.

KERATOCONJUNCTIVITIS

Although both HSV-1 and HSV-2 may cause ocular infections, HSV-1 is much more common. Treatment involves a topical ophthalmic drug (3 per cent vidarabine or 1 per cent iododeoxyuridine) in combination with systemic antiviral therapy (acyclovir or vidarabine). Systemic antiviral therapy is usually not necessary with superficial keratitis. Ophthalmologic consultation should be obtained.

GENITAL INFECTION, VULVOVAGINITIS, AND CERVICITIS

Primary Infection. The antiviral agent acyclovir has been demonstrated to decrease both the duration of symptoms and viral shedding in primary genital herpes infections. Topical ointment and oral acyclovir are most effective when given as near to the onset of symptoms as possible. Unfortunately, treatment of the primary infection does not affect subsequent recurrent infections.

Recurrent Infection. Recurrent infections of genital herpes are not usually affected by antiviral therapy. If any benefit is to be obtained, oral acyclovir should be administered as close to onset as possible (within 48 hours). Topical acyclovir may shorten the period of viral shedding but offers little in the reduction of symptoms.

MENINGOENCEPHALITIS

Herpes meningoencephalitis may be mild in nature and may require only supportive management. Analgesics and appropriate hydration are usually sufficient treatment in most cases. However, since herpes encephalitis may progress rapidly and result in severe morbidity or even death, the clinician must consider aggressive antiviral therapy when suspecting herpes simplex virus as the cause.

Only two antiviral agents are approved for treating herpes encephalitis: adenine arabinoside and acyclovir. Since adenine arabinoside may present problems with fluid load in infants and children and has a higher incidence of toxicity, acyclovir is the agent of choice. The appropriate regimen is acyclovir, 30 mg/kg/day divided every 8 hours intravenously for 5 to 10 days.

MUMPS

GREGORY F. HAYDEN, M.D.

No specific therapy is currently available for this self-limited illness. The selection of treatment, if any, depends solely upon the presence and severity of particular signs and symptoms. The spectrum of clinical illness is broad. Many infections are subclinical and require no therapy. Many children with mild clinical cases also benefit from therapeutic restraint. Occasional antipyretic-analgesic therapy with acetaminophen or aspirin may be used for symptomatic fever and general discomfort. Those relatively few children with severe or complicated cases may require more intensive supportive measures, sometimes including hospitalization.

MANAGEMENT OF SPECIFIC FEATURES

Appropriate management varies according to the manifestations of mumps that are encountered.

Parotitis. A regular diet is often well tolerated, but if chewing is painful, a soft diet with generous fluids will be appreciated. If acidic, sour, or highly seasoned foods induce pain, a bland diet is advisable. Analgesic therapy with acetaminophen often relieves parotid discomfort; aspirin can also be helpful but may make matters worse if allowed to dissolve in the mouth. Warm or cold compresses may provide local relief. Anecdotal reports suggest that a short course of corticosteroids may reduce intense parotid swelling and pain, but such therapy has not prevented the development of contralateral parotid involvement. This mode of treatment remains experimental and cannot be recommended.

Meningitis and Encephalitis. The spectrum of central nervous system (CNS) involvement is broad, ranging from asymptomatic lymphocytic pleocytosis in the cerebrospinal fluid (common) to severe encephalitis (rare). Acetaminophen or aspirin may relieve associated headache. Lumbar puncture sometimes relieves the headache associated with mumps but is indicated only for diagnostic purposes. Children with severe CNS involvement may require hospitalization for bed rest, analgesic-antipyretic therapy, and carefully monitored parenteral fluid therapy. Hospitalization is not required for mild, typical CNS involvement as long as the etiology has been established as mumps with reasonable certainty. Limited recent experience in the Soviet Union suggests that interferon therapy can shorten the course of CNS involvement associated with mumps, but these preliminary findings require confirmation in a double-blind clinical trial.

Pancreatitis. Mild elevation of pancreatic enzymes in the absence of symptoms is frequent. Clinically apparent pancreatitis is unusual, but parenteral fluid therapy may be necessary for those children with abdominal pain and severe vomiting associated with pancreatitis. Acetaminophen therapy may sometimes relieve pain adequately. Narcotic agents can be used for severe pain but can potentially induce biliary spasm, with transient elevations of plasma amylase and lipase levels. Antiemetic therapy is not recommended.

Orchitis. About 20 to 30 per cent of postpubertal male patients with mumps develop orchitis, usually unilateral. Analgesia with acetaminophen or aspirin may relieve associated discomfort, but narcotic agents may be required. Bed rest, intermittent application of ice packs, and gentle support of the affected testis may also be helpful. Anesthetic block of the spermatic cord has been reported to relieve pain but should be reserved for severe cases refractory to less extreme measures. Treatment with systemic corticosteroids has been reported to decrease fever associated with orchitis but has not been documented to accelerate the resolution of orchitis or to reduce the incidence of subsequent atrophy. Diethylstilbestrol therapy and surgical incision of the tunica albuginea are likewise of largely unproven benefit and should be used infrequently, if at all.

There is no evidence that bed rest reduces the risk of orchitis. When given after the onset of illness, standard immunoglobulin (Ig) does not prevent orchitis or otherwise modify the clinical course. In previous years, a human hyperimmune globulin (mumps immune globulin, or MIG) was sometimes given to young men with early mumps in the hope of preventing the subsequent development of orchitis. The efficacy of such therapy was controversial, however, and this expensive preparation is no longer commercially available.

Patients and their parents may benefit from reassurance about normal reproductive function following mumps orchitis. Only about 25 per cent of cases of orchitis are bilateral, and only a fraction of young men with such cases develop progressive testicular atrophy. Subnormal sperm counts have occasionally been observed among such patients, but this impairment of fertility is generally partial and may be temporary. Contrary to popular belief, mumps orchitis does not cause impotence and rarely, if ever, results in frank sterility.

Arthritis. Salicylate therapy is often ineffective in treating the arthritis occasionally associated with mumps. A short course of corticosteroids or nonsteroidal anti-inflammatory agents is more likely to be helpful.

Other Manifestations. Other rare manifestations of mumps may include myocarditis, thyroiditis, nephritis, hepatitis, mastitis, epididymitis, oophoritis, and thrombocytopenia. These manifestations may be treated with a combination of careful monitoring, general supportive care, and symptomatic therapy.

Isolation. Hospitalized patients should remain in respiratory isolation until the parotid swelling has subsided or other manifestations have cleared. Attempts to isolate patients at home and in the community are less useful because patients are often contagious before the onset of parotid swelling and because persons with inapparent infection can nevertheless be contagious.

Treatment of Contacts. The comprehensive treatment of a child with mumps includes counseling family members and other close contacts about their risk of developing mumps and informing them what preventive measures are available. In planning a suitable course of action, the first step is to determine whether the exposed persons are likely to be susceptible to mumps. Laboratory testing is unfortunately of only limited value. The presence of mumps-neutralizing antibodies reliably indicates immunity, but this assay is time consuming, expensive, and not generally available. The mumps skin test and the commonly available serologic tests for mumps are not adequately sensitive to be clinically useful.

In most instances, estimation of susceptibility must therefore depend upon simple historical information. A definite history of previous mumps illness or immunization strongly suggests immunity and provides grounds for reassurance. In contrast, a negative history of mumps illness is poorly predictive of mumps susceptibility; approximately 90 per cent of adults with such histories are immune on the basis of previous, unrecognized infection.

If susceptibility to mumps is nevertheless suspected, what can be done? Standard Ig is not effective in preventing mumps infection. The efficacy of even the higher potency MIG in this setting was questionable. It is uncertain whether the administration of live mumps vaccine after exposure can prevent or modify illness. In deciding whether to recommend vaccine, several considerations apply. On the positive side, adverse reactions to mumps vaccine are uncommon, and there is no increased risk of adverse reactions following the vaccination of an immune person. Vaccination after exposure is not known to increase the severity of incubating mumps. If the recognized exposure has not resulted in incubating infection, live mumps vaccination should provide protection against subsequent exposures. On the negative side, vaccination after exposure has never been demonstrated to be effective, and the vaccination (and vaccinator) may wrongly be blamed for the manifestations of mumps illness that develop after the vaccination. Contraindications to live mumps vaccination include immunodeficiency, anaphylactic allergy to neomycin, severe febrile illness, pregnancy, and receipt of Ig or blood products within 3 months. Persons with anaphylactic allergy to eggs should receive mumps vaccine only with extreme caution. If vaccination is considered, these limitations and uncertainties should be described in sufficient detail that the involved persons understand what benefits can reasonably be expected.

INFLUENZA

PAUL F. WEHRLE, M.D.

The clinical symptoms and signs of influenza closely resemble those of many other acute respiratory infections. The specific diagnosis is suspected on epidemiologic grounds, including season, prevalence of similar illnesses, and substantial increases in school absenteeism. Specific information regarding the virus type may be available through national, state, and local health departments.

In the older child, complaints of aching, substernal discomfort, and frontal headache resembling that of acute sinusitis are helpful clinical symptoms, although bacterial causes should be excluded. Antimicrobial therapy is not indicated unless specific bacterial complications are recognized or suspected. Prophylactic immunization against influenza using currently available inactivated vaccines is recommended for infants and children more than 6 months of age, particularly if debilitating disease or chronic health problems are present.

Treatment. Although uncomplicated influenza is a self-limited disease, some relief of symptoms will be appreciated. Bed rest, acetaminophen, sponging or tepid baths for fever relief, cough suppressants if cough is troublesome, and fluids to maintain hydration are usually sufficient. Although aspirin has been recommended previously, its use in influenza has been discouraged, since there is evidence that aspirin may be a factor in the association of at least some cases of Reye syndrome with influenza.

Amantadine hydrochloride (Symmetrel) has been useful in the prophylaxis of influenza A infections among unimmunized individuals at risk. It has also been shown to shorten the course of illnesses resulting from influenza A virus if administered within the first 48 hours after onset of illness. It may be used in children at least 1 year of age in a dose of 4 to 6 mg/kg of body weight per 24 hours in two divided doses each for 5 days. The drug is available in both syrup and tablet form, and the total daily dose should be limited to 150 mg/day for children under 9 years of age. Older children may be given 100 mg twice daily.

Although not recommended for general use, prophylactic therapy with amantadine should be considered for high-risk children who have not been immunized, and dosage should be continued as long as influenza A remains prevalent among potential contacts and immunization against influenza has been completed.

Complications. Complications are primarily related to the respiratory tract. Tracheitis and laryngitis are common and may be helped with steam or mist therapy. If fever persists, complications such as otitis media, sinusitis, or pneumonia must be suspected. The most likely pathogens are those bacteria normally found in the respiratory tract.

Convulsions sometimes occur, and a coexistent bacterial meningitis should be ruled out. Reye syndrome, a serious complication, is found more frequently with influenza B infections; it occurs predominantly among school-aged children and appears to be related to aspirin use in some children. Intensive supportive therapy is required for this complication.

Immunization. Conditions for which influenza immunization may be indicated include (1) cardiac disease, especially with evidence of cardiac insufficiency; (2) chronic bronchopulmonary disease, such as cystic fibrosis, chronic asthma, chronic bronchitis, bronchiectasis, or limited respiratory function due to other causes; (3) severe metabolic disease; (4) chronic renal disease; and (5) chronic neurologic disorders, particularly those involving ventilatory function.

Two doses of inactivated, trivalent, split-virus vaccine administered 4 weeks apart are required for primary immunization. Annual single doses during subsequent years are sufficient to maintain protection, unless major shifts in the antigenic structure of the virus occur. If such a shift should occur, this will be recognized by health authorities, and information will be forthcoming. The vaccine is used in reduced dosage in children who are between 6 months and 3 years of age, and only the split-virus product is used in infants and children.

Although the Guillain-Barré syndrome appeared to follow use of the swine influenza vaccine, no evidence of this problem has been seen since 1978. Since the vaccine is prepared in embryonated eggs, it should not be administered to children with egg allergy without appropriate tests and precautions.

RABIES

ADAM FINN, B.M., B.Ch., M.R.C.P., *and* STANLEY A. PLOTKIN, M.D.

Human rabies is now extremely rare in the United States; there has been an average of less than one reported case per annum since 1980. The incidence of the disease in dogs, previously the main animal vector, has been much reduced by effective vaccination programs. Highly effective pre-exposure and post-exposure immunization schedules for people have also contributed to this rarity. Since the disease itself still has a mortality of very nearly 100 per cent, the most important therapeutic maneuvers are related to prevention of the clinical illness, for which 30,000 people are vaccinated in the United States every year.

The epidemiology of animal rabies varies greatly from one area to another, both internationally and within the United States, and constantly changes with time. Whenever there is uncertainty, local or state health departments should always be consulted for up-to-date information. There is no rabies in Hawaii and in a number of island countries throughout the world. A variety of wild animals frequently have rabies in the United States: more than 90 per cent of reported animal cases are in skunks, racoons, foxes, coyotes, and bats, while only a few domestic animals, generally dogs and cats in approximately equal numbers, are affected. In many tropical countries, the main vector is still dogs, and human rabies is still frequent.

Although the human is classically infected by a bite, leading to inoculation of virus in the saliva of an infected animal, transmission is also thought to have occurred by inhalation of virus in bat-infested caves and in laboratories handling rabies virus. It can occur by contact of virus-containing fluids with broken or abraded skin or with mucous membranes. Documented human-to-human transmission has occurred only by transplantation of infected corneal grafts.

Passive and active immunization both play important roles in rabies prevention. The past 10 years have seen rapid progress in developing agents that are both more effective and less toxic for these purposes, and further work is in progress to design more plentiful and less expensive equivalents for use in poorer countries where rabies is still common.

Human rabies immunoglobulin (HRIG) is now the mainstay of passive immunization therapy. It is prepared from the pooled serum of human donors immunized against rabies, who therefore have high antibody titers. It is very safe, almost devoid of adverse effects, and does not transmit the human immunodeficiency virus (HIV) or any other blood-borne viral infections. Equine antirabies serum (ARS) frequently causes adverse effects; it should be used only when HRIG cannot be obtained.

Since 1980, inactivated virus vaccines prepared from virus grown on in vitro cell lines have become established as the best form of vaccine for active immunization. The human diploid cell vaccine (HDCV), manufactured by Merieux, is the vaccine of this class currently used in the United States. A number of similar vaccines that use animal cell lines, allowing production of larger quantities of vaccine at less expense, have now been developed. The first of these to be licensed in the United States, rhesus diploid cell rabies vaccine, adsorbed (RVA), became available in Michigan in March, 1988, with plans for distribution in other states soon thereafter.

POSTEXPOSURE PROPHYLAXIS

The first and frequently the most difficult part of the physician's task is to decide whether a significant exposure to rabies has occurred. Once that decision is made, the procedure to follow is usually straightforward. Prophylactic therapy should not be given unnecessarily. A number of factors should be considered that pertain to the nature of the attack or contact and injury, the animal, and the current local animal rabies epidemiology.

Bites and exposures of open cuts, abrasions, and mucous membranes to saliva or other body fluids from a potentially rabid animal should be considered significant. Other casual contact should not. Unprovoked attacks in which no attempt was being made to feed or handle the animal are a cause for concern, as are attacks resulting in severe injury, especially those involving the head and neck.

The species of animal is important. Healthy, owned domestic dogs and cats in most parts of the country are unlikely to have rabies. Animals previously immunized against rabies are much less likely to transmit the disease, but such transmission has been recorded. After a bite or significant attack, the animal should be confined and observed for 10 days. A veterinarian should examine the animal before release or at the first sign of illness. If rabies is suspected, the animal should be killed and the head removed and sent, refrigerated, for examination of the brain at a designated rabies laboratory, and prophylactic therapy should be started at once. If results are negative, therapy can be discontinued. In attacks by stray dogs and cats and any animals that elude capture, therapy should be considered in consultation with local or state health departments to determine if rabies is present in the particular geographic area.

Attacks by carnivorous wild animals (skunks, racoons, foxes, coyotes, and bobcats) and bats carry a much higher risk of rabies. Often, the animal is not available for examination, and in such cases full prophylactic therapy will normally be necessary. If the animal is caught, it should be killed and the head sent for testing, as noted previously. If results can be obtained without delay and the animal is not clearly rabid, prophylactic therapy can be withheld until the result is available; otherwise, it should be started and discontinued only if the test result is negative.

Livestock, rodents (squirrels, hamsters, guinea pigs, gerbils, chipmunks, rats, and mice), lagomorphs (rabbits and hares), and birds are rarely or never found to be infected with rabies. Prophylactic therapy is seldom necessary after bites by animals of these species. Local or state health departments should be consulted in such cases.

In cases of human rabies, stringent isolation precautions should be taken with the use of gowns, gloves, masks, and goggles. When bites penetrating the skin occur, and when saliva or other potentially infected body fluids or tissues (including cerebrospinal fluid, nervous tissue, ocular tissue, and other organs, but *not* blood, stool, or unspun urine) come into contact with broken skin or mucous membranes or are involved in needle sticks or scalpel cuts, postexposure prophylaxis should be given. However, it is worthy of emphasis that transmission from a patient with the disease to a care provider or other personal contact has never been documented, and in many parts of the world few precautions are taken in handling rabies cases.

The regimen for postexposure prophylaxis is as follows:

1. The wound should be thoroughly washed with soap and water at once. This step is important in all bites and wounds but has been shown to reduce the risk of rabies transmission substantially. Experiments with animal models suggest that further disinfection with ethyl alcohol or a detergent gives added protection against transmission of the virus. Other measures, including tetanus prophylaxis and antibiotics, should be given as necessary.

2. One dose only of 20 IU/kg of HRIG should be given. Excessive doses may interfere with active immunization. Up to a maximum of half the dose should be infiltrated around the area of the wound, the amount being determined by its size and position. The rest of the dose should be given by intramuscular injection into a different limb from that used for HDCV or RVA inoculation. HRIG should be administered as soon as possible after exposure but should still be given even if there is delay in starting therapy. If immunization with HDCV or RVA alone has been started, HRIG is still of value if given within 8 days of the first dose of HDCV. ARS (40 IU/kg) should be given only as an alternative if HRIG cannot be obtained. Only people who have previously received full pre-exposure or postexposure courses of HDCV or RVA or those who have documented adequate antirabies antibody titers following immunization with other vaccines do not require HRIG.

3. Five doses of 1 ml of HDCV or of RVA should be given by intramuscular injection into a different limb from that injected with HRIG, starting as soon as possible after exposure and on days 3, 7, 14, and 28 thereafter, as recommended by the Centers for Disease Control. If the exposed individual has previously received full pre-exposure or postexposure courses of HDCV or RVA or has documented adequate antirabies antibodies, only two doses at 0 and 3 days are required. Serology need not be tested after vaccination unless the patient is immunocompromised. Infants and children are given the same dose as adults.

PRE-EXPOSURE PROPHYLAXIS

Individuals whose activities put them at increased risk of exposure to rabies relative to the population in general should be immunized. This practice protects them from exposures of which they may be unaware, reduces the risk of any delay in institution of postexposure therapy, and reduces the course of postexposure therapy to two doses of HDCV. The primary course of immunization is either 1 ml of HDCV given by intramuscular injection or 0.1 ml given by intradermal injection on days 0, 7, and 21 or 28 or 1 ml of RVA given by intramuscular injection on days 0, 7, and 28. The intradermal route uses much smaller volumes of vaccine, and the regimen therefore costs less. In persons receiving concurrent malaria prophylaxis with chloroquine, the intramuscular course should be given. RVA should not be given intradermally, as its use by this route has not yet been studied. When booster doses are given, either route may be used (1 ml given intramuscularly or 0.1 ml given intradermally). Doses in infants and children are the same as those in adults.

People who work in laboratories involved in research or in manufacturing rabies virus should receive a primary course and have their serology checked every 6 months and should be given booster doses of vaccine when antibody titers fall below a designated level. Those who work in rabies diagnostic laboratories, those who explore caves, and veterinarians and others who work with animals in areas in which rabies is epizootic should receive a primary course and should either receive boosters every 2 years or have antibody titers checked every 2 years and booster doses given when necessary. Veterinarians and those who work with animals in areas of low rabies endemicity, travelers to areas of foreign countries in which the risk of rabies exposure is high (the only group likely to include children), and veterinary students should receive a primary course, but no booster doses or serologic assessments are necessary.

SPECIAL CIRCUMSTANCES

Local and mild systemic reactions to HDCV are quite common (20 to 25 per cent of recipients). An immune complex–like reaction that is not life threatening sometimes occurs, starting 2 to 21 days after the dose, and may involve joint pain as well as rash and other symptoms. It is more common in recipients of booster doses. Rabies postexposure prophylaxis generally should not be interrupted because of such reactions or a history of hypersensitivity, and aspirin or acetaminophen, antihistamines, and epinephrine should be given as appropriate. Anaphylaxis and other life-threatening reactions are fortunately very rare, as they present serious management dilemmas for the physician in the context of postexposure prophylaxis. Switching to another type of rabies vaccine may be the simplest solution.

Immunocompromised individuals receiving rabies vaccination should have their serology carefully monitored, as they may fail to produce adequate antibody responses and may require further immunization. Pregnancy does not contraindicate postexposure therapy, and pre-exposure prophylaxis may also be considered if the risk of exposure is very high. Needle stick or spray exposure to modified live rabies virus vaccines intended for animals does not usually necessitate postexposure prophylaxis, although persons routinely handling such material should normally be given pre-exposure immunization.

RABIES: THE ILLNESS

Physicians currently practicing in the United States will be extremely unlikely to encounter a single case of human rabies; such is its current rarity that the diagnosis commonly is not made at presentation. The precise mechanism of the progress of the virus from bite to central nervous system is poorly understood but may involve binding to acetylcholine receptors at the neuromuscular junction in the early stages. Once clinical symptoms and signs of rabies are present, the disease is virtually always fatal. Only three patients with well-documented rabies have ever survived, and these had all received some form of antirabies inoculation prior to developing symptoms. Modern intensive care techniques, including respiratory support, hydration, anticonvulsants, vasopressors, antibiotics, and dialysis, have prolonged survival time but not changed mortality. Specific therapy after the onset of symptoms, such as vaccine, antiserum, and antivirals, including interferon, has not been beneficial.

INFECTIOUS MONONUCLEOSIS AND EPSTEIN-BARR VIRUS—RELATED SYNDROMES

ADAM FINN, M.D., M.R.C.P., and STANLEY A. PLOTKIN, M.D.

As with other herpesviruses, infection with Epstein-Barr virus (EBV) is lifelong and almost universal. Nearly all children from underdeveloped nations are infected by the age of 5 years, while the more privileged tend to encounter the virus between the ages of 10 and 30. This has important implications for the pediatrician, as the majority of young children have an asymptomatic or mild illness associated with primary infection, while between a third and a half of those infected in their second and third decades will have the clinical syndrome of infectious mononucleosis, with the characteristic fever, pharyngitis, lymphadenopathy, malaise and lethargy, and, in some, splenomegaly and mild hepatitis.

The diagnosis is confirmed usually by the demonstration of a lymphocytosis on peripheral blood film, often with 10 per cent or more atypical cells, and by the presence of heterophil antibodies. Currently used rapid assays (e.g., Monospot) are as sensitive as the traditional Paul-Bunnell-Davidsohn test and are adequately specific because of the absorption steps included in the test. However, heterophil antibodies are absent in the early days of the illness and remain absent in approximately 10 per cent of cases caused by EBV in teenagers and adults and in a much higher proportion of cases in younger children. A smaller proportion of heterophil-negative cases are due to other agents, such as cytomegalovirus, *Toxoplasma*, and human immunodeficiency virus. Specific EBV serologic testing does not need to be performed in typical infectious mononucleosis and should be reserved for severe or atypical cases, particularly if heterophil antibodies are absent. If the illness is current or recent, there is usually a raised anti–viral capsid antigen (VCA) titer (IgG and/or IgM), there may be a raised anti–early antigen (EA) titer, and the antibody to Epstein-Barr nuclear antigen (EBNA) is usually low or absent.

The diagnosis is a signal to reassure both patient and parents, as the illness usually follows a benign course. A regular dose of acetaminophen may be prescribed for the acute illness, saline gargles may provide symptomatic relief, and the importance of adequate fluid intake should be emphasized. Codeine may be used if discomfort is severe. Penicillin therapy should be reserved for the 5 per cent or fewer of patients with coexistent positive throat culture or antigen test for group A beta-hemolytic streptococci. Ampicillin or amoxicillin should not be given, as they will produce generalized rash in almost all patients with mononucleosis. Rest in bed or at home should be adequate for the severity of symptoms but should not be strictly enforced, although it is important that the 50 per cent of patients who develop transient splenomegaly avoid activities such as contact sports, which expose them to the risk of splenic rupture. The physician should also be alert to the other very rare but potentially life-threatening complication of upper airway obstruction, which causes stridor because of enlarged tonsillar and other lymphoid tissue. Such patients should be admitted for observation and maintenance of hydration and will often be given a course of steroids (such as prednisone, 40 mg/kg/day for 4 to 7 days) in the belief that this may reduce inflammation and soft tissue swelling, although good evidence for this belief is lacking. In trials of intravenous acyclovir in patients with infectious mononucleosis, little or no amelioration in duration or severity of symptoms was demonstrated, and viral shedding was reduced only transiently. Other antiviral agents have not been assessed in vivo.

The acute symptoms and fever usually last between a few days and a month, but it is common for splenomegaly to last for 2 or 3 months and for up to 6 months to elapse before the patient recovers completely from the residual sense of lethargy and malaise, with a recovery course that is often unsteady rather than smooth and progressive.

Other severe manifestations of primary EBV infection are seldom seen and merit attention from a specialist. Pneumonia, hemolytic anemia, bone marrow dysfunction (especially thrombocytopenia), hepatitis and liver failure, renal dysfunction, cardiac arrhythmias, and neurologic involvement all occur occasionally and may be by-products of the vigorous cell-mediated immune response to the virus, which is reflected in the lymphocytosis seen in the typical illness. In some of these cases, the use of steroids may also be warranted.

On the other hand, some individuals, unable to mount this T-cell response, develop overwhelming lymphoproliferative disease owing to unchecked EBV-infected B cells, which may also involve multiple organs. A well-known syndrome occurs in boys with the rare X-linked lymphoproliferative syndrome whose primary EBV infection is usually a fatal illness. However, chil-

dren with a variety of other congenital immunodeficiencies and iatrogenically immunosuppressed children—in particular, those receiving organ transplants—may also suffer abnormally severe and prolonged disease.

Those infected with the human immunodeficiency virus (HIV) pose new problems. EBV may be a cofactor in the pathogenesis of acquired immunodeficiency syndrome (AIDS). It is likely that increased activity of latent EBV resulting from reduced T-cell–mediated immune surveillance plays a part in the pathogenesis of at least some of the lymphomas seen in these children. This observation may have some parallels with the pathogenesis of endemic Burkitt lymphoma seen in African children previously infected with EBV, in whom the virus was first described. Whether EBV plays a role in the pathogenesis of the lymphocytic interstitial pneumonitis seen in children with AIDS is not yet known conclusively. The roles of antiviral agents such as acyclovir and other nucleoside analogues, of cytotoxic agents, of interferon, and of gamma globulin therapy in the treatment of all these severely affected children remain to be elucidated.

Of relevance to the physician in primary care is the question of the role of chronic EBV infection in the chronic fatigue syndrome, also known as chronic mononucleosis, sporadic neurasthenia, myalgic encephalitis, and a number of other pseudonyms. It is clear from the preceding discussion that chronic—in fact, lifelong—latent infection with EBV is the norm, although only a very few children have severe chronic manifestations of infection. These individuals generally have impaired immunity and usually show a characteristic pattern of specific antibodies to EBV, with persistently very high titers of anti-VCA (>1:640) and anti-EA (>1:40). Titers of anti-EBNA may be low (<1:10), and heterophil antibody levels may be chronically intermittently raised. In contrast, patients with chronic fatigue syndrome have subjective complaints of longstanding fatigue, aches and pains, fever, allergies, sore throat, swollen glands, weight loss, and other problems that are unaccompanied by objective signs on physical examination. This poorly defined syndrome probably has a number of causes, and in the majority of cases, the characteristic serologic pattern previously described is absent and there is no reason specifically to indict EBV. In those patients whose serologic pattern is found to resemble the "chronic" pattern, the result is merely suggestive and does not confirm EBV as the cause, so that other causes must be considered and excluded. In any case, specific antiviral therapy is not available; acyclovir appears to produce only temporary relief in cases in which chronic proliferative EBV infection is more clearly present, its beneficial effects disappearing on withdrawal of the drug; neither this agent nor any other has been shown convincingly to have long-term ameliorative effects on chronic fatigue. Patients are often relieved to be told that neither progressive disease nor development of EBV-related malignancies is a feature of this syndrome and that even when symptoms have lasted several months they tend to resolve spontaneously. At present, group therapy and other forms of counseling and education are probably the best available treatment modalities for these patients. As time passes, we are likely to gain a clearer understanding of the infectious and immune mechanisms of this condition or group of conditions.

CAT SCRATCH DISEASE

HUGH A. CARITHERS, M.D.

Controlled studies have never been performed for this nonfatal, usually benign, universally encountered disease. There is evidence, however, that a few patients with cat scratch disease (CSD) have been benefited by infrequently used antibiotics.

Since the first description of the disease in 1950, most antibiotics have been used in treatment, including sulfonamides, penicillin, chloramphenicol (Chloromycetin), erythromycin, and first-generation aminoglycosides. It is the strong impression of investigators that these antibiotics, whether administered orally or parenterally, early or late, singly or in combination, failed to prevent the progression of involved lymph nodes to suppuration, which occurs in about 12 per cent of patients.

Since the discovery of the pleomorphic, gram-negative bacterium in 1983 that almost certainly causes CSD, in vitro studies have shown that the organism may be sensitive to cefoxitin sodium, cefotaxime, three aminoglycosides, netilmicin sulfate, and mezlocillin.

Recently, several reports of systemic CSD, including liver and spleen involvement, have been acknowledged. Unpublished reports have indicated that acutely ill patients benefited from third-generation cephalosporins. Four toxic, acutely ill patients with high fever and liver abscesses attributed to involvement with the CSD bacillus responded within a few days to gentamicin. These studies need confirmation.

If it is confirmed that CSD responds to the newer antibiotics, this does not mean that they should be used in treating this usually benign disease, except in unusual circumstances. Fewer than 5 per cent of more than 1700 patients whom I have seen with the condition were hospitalized, and many of them were admitted for the diagnosis of lymphadenopathy rather than for an acute illness.

In about half the patients with CSD, fever will not be recognized, but in about 10 per cent it may be high. Antipyretics may be comforting, and the prevention of trauma to involved lymph nodes is indicated. Complete resolution of involved lymph nodes may require a few months, and most patients can lead normal lives after swelling of the lymph nodes begins to regress.

In approximately 1 in 10 patients in whom the involved lymph node progresses to suppuration, aspiration with a 16- to 18-gauge needle is indicated. One should wait until pus formation is unquestionable in order to reduce the likelihood of reaspiration, which occurs in almost half of the patients. The degree of pain and discomfort felt by the patient will influence the time of drainage, but delay will not be harmful. By the time the lymph node has "ripened," the skin over it is so thin that intradermal injection of an anesthetic is usually impossible. Spraying the area with ethyl chloride will provide enough anesthesia so that the patient will not be aware of the puncture, which should be made directly over the fluctuant area. Sinus formation is unlikely with this technique, which is not the case when the incision is made with a scalpel.

Surgical removal of lymph nodes is not indicated, except in the rare patient in whom a diagnosis cannot be made and in whom delay might hinder the treatment of malignancy. In tissue diagnosis, entire lymph nodes must be removed, not part of one, and general anesthesia is necessary. Tissue study can only suggest the diagnosis of CSD unless the causative organisms are found. This study requires special stains not available in many laboratories, and interpretation by a pathologist familiar with the organism is necessary. The organism, under the best of circumstances, is not found in all involved lymph nodes; special difficulty is encountered in those affected for more than a short while or when suppuration is present or imminent.

A skin test for the disease, not commercially available, can be invaluable in the study of complicated cases, such as those with encephalopathy. Disease caused by the test has not been reported after its use in thousands of patients, and its sensitivity is probably as accurate as is purified protein derivative (PPD) in the diagnosis of tuberculosis.

Oculoglandular disease of Parinaud is by far the most common unusual manifestation of CSD, occurring in about 0.5 per cent of patients. In this condition, the preauricular lymphadenopathy, with or without regional involvement, requires protection, but no unusual care, as with involvement of lymph nodes elsewhere. The granuloma seen within the eye is, as a rule, soft, not painful, and has indistinct borders, and removal of this tissue is strongly condemned. Secondary infection is rare in this form of CSD, but antibiotic ophthalmic ointments may be used in the event it occurs.

Encephalopathy accompanying CSD is being diagnosed with increasing frequency. Supportive, symptomatic treatment of the condition, which has an excellent prognosis, despite severe manifestations, including convulsions in about half the patients, is all that is recommended.

Discovery of the causative bacillus of CSD may radically modify treatment of the condition in the near future. A commercial skin test may become available. Physicians should consult the current literature when confronted with the patient who has a complicated case.

Most patients inquire about disposal of the cat, usually of immature age, that transmitted the disease. The animal is not ill, and how long it can transmit the disease is not known. Disposal of a cherished pet is not recommended.

LYME DISEASE

LEE TODD MILLER, M.D.

The appropriate treatment of Lyme disease is determined by the clinical stage of presentation. The current mainstay of treatment is antibiotic therapy directed against the etiologic spirochete, *Borrelia burgdorferi*. Clinical studies suggest that initiation of antibiotic therapy early in the clinical course may prevent the late complications of Lyme disease.

The *first stage* of Lyme disease is marked by the onset of the characteristic skin lesion, erythema chronicum migrans. In only approximately one third of patients will there be a positive history of a tick bite at the site of the initial lesion. The primary macule or papule is located most often on the thigh, groin, or axilla and expands as an erythematous annular rash. This unique skin finding may expand to up to 15 cm in diameter, with red borders, and manifests central clearing, induration, discoloration, or even necrosis. This lesion is frequently accompanied by systemic symptoms, including malaise, fatigue, severe headache, stiff neck, myalgias, weakness, and occasionally fever. When administered during the first stage of disease, antibiotics have been shown to decrease the duration of skin disease, to lower the incidence of recurrence, and to reduce the frequency of major complications. Tetracycline has been shown to be somewhat more effective than penicillin in shortening the duration of erythema chronicum migrans and in preventing or minimizing further complications. Both tetracycline and penicillin have been demonstrated to be more effective than erythromycin. Therefore, children more than 8 years of age should receive oral tetracycline at a dose of 40 to 50 mg/kg/day in four divided doses (maximum of 1 gm/day) for 10 days and for up to 30 days if symptoms recur. Children younger than 8 years of age should be treated with phenoxymethyl penicillin at a dose of 50 mg/kg/day orally for the same duration of 10 to 30 days, or alternatively with amoxicillin at a dosage of 20 to 40 mg/kg/day in three divided doses for the same duration. Children less than 8 years of age with suspected drug allergy to penicillin may be treated with erythromycin at an oral dose of 30 mg/kg/day in divided doses for 10 to 30 days, depending on the clinical response. Some patients treated with penicillin or tetracycline have demonstrated the Jarisch-Herxheimer reaction. This accentuation of symptoms during antibiotic therapy is more commonly associated with the treatment of syphilis but may occur in patients infected with *Borrelia burgdorferi*.

The *second stage* of Lyme disease follows the first stage by weeks to months and is characterized by neurologic and cardiac complications. Up to one third of patients may develop meningeal irritation, Bell's palsy or other cranial neuropathies, peripheral radiculoneuropathies, or mild encephalitis. Patients with Lyme meningitis should be treated for a 10- to 14-day course with high-dose intravenous (IV) penicillin G (200,000 to 300,000 units/kg/day, up to a maximum of 20 million units/day). Ceftriaxone (50 to 75 mg/kg/day intravenously, not to exceed 2 gm, given in divided doses every 12 hours) may also be effective, particularly in those patients who have not responded to therapy with penicillin. Patients who present with an isolated cranial nerve VII palsy and have received no prior antibiotic treatment may be managed with the same pharmacologic regimen as that given to patients in the first stage of the disease; how-

ever, patients with cranial nerve palsies in association with other neurologic complications, such as meningitis, should be managed more aggressively with intravenous penicillin or ceftriaxone therapy, as described previously. Approximately 10 per cent of patients will develop cardiac complications, such as myocarditis or disturbances of electrical conduction and rhythm, most often involving varying degrees of atrioventricular block. Some patients with only mild first-degree AV block may be treated with oral antibiotics as in *stage one* of this disease. More significant cardiac complications should be managed with the same antibiotic regimen as for Lyme meningitis, for 10 to 21 days depending on the rapidity of response, with the possible addition of appropriate anti-inflammatory therapy. Aspirin may be administered at a dose of 80 to 100 mg/kg/day (up to a maximum of 3.6 gm/day) or, alternatively, prednisone at 1 to 2 mg/kg/day (up to a maximum of 60 mg/day). The development of complete heart block may necessitate intervention with a temporary pacemaker.

The major manifestation of the *third stage* of Lyme disease is Lyme arthritis, which develops in more than 50 per cent of all patients weeks to months after the development of erythema chronicum migrans. The arthritis is characterized by recurrent episodes of mono-articular or oligoarticular swelling and pain, usually involving the large joints and most frequently affecting the knee. Approximately 10 per cent of patients will subsequently develop chronic destructive joint changes, with erosion of cartilage and bone. Up to 50 per cent of patients with Lyme arthritis have demonstrated significant improvement with the same antibiotic regimen as recommended for Stage 2 meningitis, including high-dose IV penicillin G at 200,000 to 300,000 units/kg/day (up to a maximum of 20 million units/day) for at least 2 weeks, or, alternatively, intravenous ceftriaxone. Symptomatic treatment may also include aspirin, at 80 to 100 mg/kg/day (up to a maximum of 3.5 gm/day); other nonsteroidal anti-inflammatory agents, such as tolmetin sodium (10 to 30 mg/kg/day); or, if necessary, prednisone at 1 to 2 mg/kg/day. Surgery (arthroscopic synovectomy) or intra-articular steroid therapy may be indicated for cases of arthritis refractory to medical management.

Some patients will present with late (i.e., Stage 3) neurologic complications, including chronic fatigue, dementia, intellectual dysfunction, and late peripheral neuropathies. Such patients may not have received any prior antibiotic therapy, as up to 20 to 30 per cent of all patients in the third stage of disease have no history of erythema chronicum migrans. In some cases complicated by these late neurologic findings, ceftriaxone has proved to be useful for disease refractory to treatment with penicillin.

Despite the increasing prevalence of Lyme disease, prophylactic antibiotics are not advised for all patients with a history of tick bites. Treatment should be reserved until initial symptoms suggestive of Lyme disease appear or until laboratory data confirm the diagnosis. Even though all stages of Lyme disease may respond to antibiotic therapy to varying degrees, the long-term efficacy of each treatment regimen is still uncertain.

CYTOMEGALOVIRUS INFECTIONS

JAMES BARRY HANSHAW, M.D.

Congenital Infection. Approximately 90 per cent of congenital cytomegalovirus infections are asymptomatic; the remaining 10 per cent may have mild to severe, even fatal, cytomegalovirus disease. Although several drugs such as adenosine arabinoside and acyclovir have been used experimentally in patients, there is no evidence of any lasting effect on the progression of the disease. The arabinosides can induce a diminution in virus excretion in some patients. However, in view of their unproved efficacy, they cannot be recommended. There is little evidence that acyclovir will be useful in cytomegalovirus infections. Interferon and transfer factor are still regarded as experimental therapeutic modalities.

Most infants with symptomatic infection do not require therapy. Exchange transfusion is rarely necessary for indirect hyperbilirubinemia. Neonatal sepsis, an unusual complication of cytomegalic inclusion disease, is usually due to enteric organisms or a streptococcal infection. Thus, the therapy would not be different from that used in other neonates with sepsis. Since congenital cytomegalic inclusion disease may be a cause of spastic quadriplegia, mental retardation, and obstructive hydrocephalus, long-range measures dealing with these chronic problems must be planned on an individual basis. It is especially important to identify deafness in early life in order to maximize hearing and speech as the child matures.

Acquired Infection. Clinically apparent disease due to cytomegalovirus infection occurs in patients with primary or iatrogenic immune deficiency as well as in individuals who have been previously well. Infection may result in a variety of abnormalities, including an infectious mononucleosis–like illness (cytomegalovirus mononucleosis), infectious polyneuritis, hepatomegaly with abnormal liver function tests, and pneumonitis. The last manifestation is more often associated with a deficiency of cellular immunity such as that induced by immunosuppressive therapy or in patients with AIDS. In the former situation the pneumonitis may be benefited by a temporary reduction of immunosuppressive therapy. Cytomegalovirus retinitis in immunocompromised patients has responded to cytovene (ganciclovir sodium) in a dosage of 5 mg/kg (given intravenously at a constant rate over 1 hour) every 12 hours for 14 to 21 days. Once a day maintenance of 5 mg/kg (given intravenously over 1 hour) is then administered until regression of retinitis occurs. Adverse reactions occur in approximately one third of patients. The safety and efficacy of cytovene has not been established for neonates, nor for treatment of other CMV infections in immunocompromised or nonimmunocompromised persons. Some young adult patients with cytomegalovirus mononucleosis have persistent fatigue over months but rarely for more than a year. Such patients may require 15 or more hours of sleep per day. Although satisfactory controlled studies have not been done, it would appear that improvement is often correlated with

extended periods of bed rest. Conversely, attempts to increase activity level frequently result in clinical relapse.

Prevention. Cytomegalovirus mononucleosis may occur in previously healthy young adults or following the transfusion of fresh blood. The greater the number of transfusion units, the higher the probability of cytomegalovirus transmission. Because of the lability of cytomegalovirus, this complication of transfusion can be diminished significantly by using citrated or deglycerolated blood that has been stored or frozen for more than 72 hours or by using seronegative donors. This is especially important in preterm infants.

Although there is no licensed vaccine for the prevention of cytomegalovirus infection, live virus vaccine trials are currently under way in this country and abroad. Induction of passive immunity using high-titered antibody is now under study and may prove useful in the prevention of disease in immunocompromised patients.

MYCOPLASMA INFECTIONS

GAIL H. CASSELL, M.S., PH.D.,
and KEN B. WAITES, M.D.

Of the 12 species of mycoplasmas isolated from the respiratory or genitourinary tract of humans, three are a significant cause of disease: *Mycoplasma pneumoniae*, *Mycoplasma hominis*, and *Ureaplasma urealyticum*. Concepts regarding the pathogenic potential of all three have changed dramatically during the last decade.

RESPIRATORY DISEASE

Most medical textbooks and reviews in the literature emphasize the benign, often subclinical course of *M. pneumoniae* infection. Indeed, most clinical infections consist of nothing more serious than upper respiratory tract infection. The most frequent clinical presentation of *M. pneumoniae* infection is the syndrome of tracheobronchitis associated with an influenza-like illness. Clinically apparent pneumonia develops in only 3 to 10 per cent of infected persons. Nevertheless, *M. pneumoniae* probably accounts for up to 20 per cent of all pneumonia cases in the general population and for up to 50 per cent in closed populations. It is estimated that 500,000 cases of pneumonia and 11,500,000 cases of tracheobronchitis due to *M. pneumoniae* occur annually in the United States. A mycoplasmal etiology should be considered in the differential diagnosis of pneumonia in any age group (not just in individuals 6 to 21 years of age, as is commonly done). Viral and bacterial pneumonia can occur concomitantly with mycoplasmal infection. Although severe mycoplasmal respiratory disease has been uncommon, recent reports suggest that the disease spectrum is wider than previously thought and that severe pulmonary involvement can occur in otherwise healthy children and adults of all ages. The severe disease, often mimicking necrotizing bacterial pneumonia, can initially cause diagnostic confusion. Lung abscesses, pneumatoceles, extensive lobar consolidation, pleural effusion (up to 20 per cent of cases), and relapsing or recurrent pneumonia may occur. Reduced pulmonary clearance has been observed as late as 1 year after infection. Finally, *M. pneumoniae* has been associated with exacerbations of chronic respiratory disease, in particular, chronic bronchitis and asthma, but the role of this organism in sustaining the chronic state or initiating exacerbation is unknown. A number of nonpulmonary complications occur in association with *M. pneumoniae* infection. These include CNS disease, carditis, mucocutaneous lesions, gastrointestinal symptoms, joint manifestations, nephritis, and hematologic disorders.

Contrary to popular belief, controlled therapy trials indicate treatment with either oral erythromycin (30 to 60 mg/kg/day) or tetracycline* (25 to 50 mg/kg/day) markedly reduces the duration of symptoms of the respiratory disease.

Erythromycin is the drug of choice, especially in children less than 8 years old, owing to the bone and tooth toxicity of tetracycline in young children. It has been noted that patients sometimes relapse following the 5- to 7-day courses of antibiotics that are commonly prescribed. This may be due to the continued presence of the mycoplasma; thus 14 to 21 days of therapy are more appropriate. As yet there are no data available to judge the clinical efficacy of fluoroquinolones in pediatric or adult mycoplasmal respiratory infections. This is due, at least partially, to concern over their potential to induce cartilage damage based on animal studies, thus leading to recommendations that they not be used in children whose skeletal growth is incomplete. In vitro studies suggest that ciprofloxacin possesses intermediate activity against *M. pneumoniae*, with MICs exceeding those for erythromycin.

The effect of antibiotic therapy on extrapulmonary complications is debatable. Since most cases involving complications are not diagnosed until late in the course of disease, the benefit of early treatment is unknown. Corticosteroids in conjunction with antibiotic therapy appear to be helpful in patients with severe pneumonia and erythema multiforme, but controlled, prospective studies are needed before their true value can be assessed.

GENITAL TRACT INFECTION

The pediatrician may be faced with basically three groups of patients in whom disease due to *U. urealyticum* and *M. hominis* is likely to occur; the sexually active adolescent, the neonate, and the child with hypogammaglobulinemia. Genital mycoplasmal colonization of many (up to 70 per cent) sexually active teenagers in good health suggests that after puberty and sexual contact these organisms may exist as commensals in some members of this population; however, both organisms have been associated with specific urogenital and systemic diseases in both males and females. *M. hominis* causes pyelonephritis and pelvic inflammatory disease as well as septicemia in susceptible persons. *U.*

urealyticum is the etiologic agent in over 20 per cent of cases of nongonococcal urethritis and can also be responsible for acute prostatitis and pyelonephritis. Both organisms have been isolated from the lungs of neonates with congenital pneumonia in the absence of other pathogens from the bloodstream and from cerebrospinal fluid of infants with meningitis. Isolation of *U. urealyticum* from the lower respiratory tract of newborn preterm infants with birth weights < 1000 gm has been associated with an increased risk for development of chronic lung disease and death. Infant colonization by genital mycoplasmas at birth tends to be transient, but older children with no history of sexual contact may have prolonged lower genital tract carriage of these organisms.

The final group of patients who are at high risk for systemic mycoplasma infections are individuals with immunodeficiencies, particularly hypogammaglobulinemia. Several mycoplasmal species, including *M. pneumoniae*, *M. hominis*, and *U. urealyticum*, have been isolated from septic joints in both children and adults with this disorder. Owing to the severity of polyarticular joint destruction, prompt diagnostic joint aspiration and antibiotic therapy should be instituted.

Many infections due to mycoplasmas are discovered accidently, either by observing the presence of *M. hominis* growing on blood agar or because of treatment failure with antibiotics directed at common bacterial pathogens but ineffective against mycoplasmas. A positive culture for mycoplasmas is sufficient justification for chemotherapy if the specimen was obtained from a patient with a disease condition for which there is evidence of a mycoplasmal etiology or association. Tetracyclines are the preferred drugs to treat urogenital tract infections in children over 8 years of age. Both *M. hominis* and *U. urealyticum* are generally sensitive to all drugs in the tetracycline group, but in recent years increasing reports of resistant strains of ureaplasmas (approaching 20 per cent) and *M. hominis* (up to 40 per cent) have been reported. Oral tetracycline (25 to 50 mg/kg/day) or doxycycline (4 mg/kg/day) is usually adequate for local urogenital infections with either organism. The duration of therapy necessary to resolve symptoms and eradicate the organism may vary, but an initial treatment for at least 10 days is recommended. Treatment failure with tetracycline may indicate a resistant strain; therefore, repeated cultures with appropriate antibiotic sensitivities should be obtained and alternative drugs employed. *U. urealyticum* is sensitive to erythromycin (although resistant strains have been reported) and resistant to sulfonamides, clindamycin, lincomycin, and often to aminoglycosides. There is variable sensitivity to chloramphenicol. Erythromycin (40 mg/kg/day) is the preferred drug for ureaplasma infections in infants and young children. *M. hominis* is uniformly resistant to erythromycin, sulfonamides, and sensitive to clindamycin and lincomycin. It may be moderately sensitive to chloramphenicol and aminoglycosides. Clindamycin (8 to 16 mg/kg/day) is a useful drug for neonatal *M. hominis* infections or any infection with a tetracycline resistant strain. For the same reasons as for infection with *M. pneumoniae*, information concerning efficacy of quino-

---

*Manufacturer's warning: Tetracycline should not generally be used in children under 8 years of age.

lones in treatment of pediatric infections caused by the genital mycoplasmas is also lacking.

In infants and children, severe systemic infections such as CNS invasion, warrant aggressive antibiotic therapy, preferably guided by antibiotic sensitivity testing of isolates. In view of the potentially life-threatening nature of CNS infections, a 2-week course of parenteral antibiotic is justified. Eradication of *U. urealyticum* from cerebrospinal fluid has been accomplished with either parenteral doxycycline or erythromycin using the same dosage guidelines as for oral therapy. *M. hominis* cerebrospinal fluid infections have been successfully treated with either parenteral doxycycline, tetracycline, or even clindamycin. Despite contraindications, in the case of CNS involvement with *M. hominis*, there may be no realistic therapeutic option other than tetracyclines.

The child with mycoplasmal arthritis or other deep seated infection, especially if immunosuppressed, may require prolonged parenteral antibiotic therapy followed by oral medication for several weeks to months to eradicate the organism.

VIRAL PNEUMONIAS

NANCY C. LEWIS, M.D.

Viruses are the most important and common cause of pneumonia in infants and children less than 5 years old. Thirty to 40 per cent of all outpatient visits are for evaluation of respiratory illnesses, the vast majority of which are viral, self-limited, and not in need of specific therapy. However, respiratory viruses also have the potential for producing respiratory failure and death, as well as more chronic sequelae, such as bronchiectasis, bronchiolitis obliterans, or reactive airway disease.

In most cases, specific viral etiologic agents are not identified, and diagnosis is based on clinical presentation and epidemiologic setting. Respiratory syncytial virus (RSV) is generally recognized as the most frequent cause of lower respiratory tract infections in infants and children, usually causing a mild, self-limited bronchiolitis. Depending on host response factors, however, pneumonia may occur. Parainfluenza Type 3 virus, adenovirus, and influenza A and B viruses are the next most common causes of viral pneumonias. Reinfection rates with RSV and parainfluenza Type 3 virus are high. Measles and varicella zoster may produce pneumonia during the course of a systemic viral disease.

Therapy for viral pneumonia is primarily supportive, including controlling fever, ensuring adequate hydration, and closely monitoring respiratory status. Mild dehydration may occur because of fever and tachypnea, with increased insensible respiratory losses. Children with enough ventilation-perfusion mismatch to cause hypoxemia will require hospitalization for supplemental oxygen. Oxygen via nasal cannula is the most convenient method of delivery and is generally well tolerated by children of all ages. Mist tents have not been shown to be effective at humidifying lower respiratory tract secretions. The benefits of postural drainage and per-

cussion have been debated but may prove helpful when atelectasis has occurred. The course of uncomplicated viral pneumonia is not altered by antibiotics, although they are frequently used, since the clinical, laboratory, and radiographic findings in bacterial infection may be indistinguishable from those in viral infection. With mild disease, especially during fall or winter seasons of known viral epidemics, withholding antibiotics seems reasonable. For severe disease, or in children younger than 1 year of age, antibiotics are appropriate, pending further diagnostic evaluation. The usual bacteria identified are *Streptococcus pneumoniae*, *Haemophilus influenzae*, and *Staphyloccus aureus*, and therapy should be selected to cover these organisms. Rapid diagnostic techniques (for both viral and bacterial etiologies), such as immunofluorescent antibody or antigen detection assays, are increasingly available in clinical laboratories and will provide help in the development of rational treatment plans.

Combined viral-bacterial pneumonias have been reported in 25 to 75 per cent of patients hospitalized with bacterial pneumonia, supporting the hypothesis that viral infection may be important in the pathogenesis of bacterial pneumonia. Viruses may interfere with both cellular and noncellular lung defenses, including increased susceptibility of epithelial cells to adherence by certain bacteria (especially *S. aureus*), impaired ciliokinesis, and altered macrophage function.

Nevertheless, there is no evidence that prophylactic antibiotics are of use in viral pneumonia, and they may predispose to superinfection with more resistant organisms. Evidence of superinfection, such as purulent secretions, organisms on Gram stain, or new infiltrate after a period of improvement, requires appropriate antimicrobial therapy.

Apnea occurs in approximately 20 per cent of infants with RSV infection, particularly in infants with a history of premature birth and apnea of prematurity, and may also occur in infections with parainfluenza and influenza viruses. The use of cardiorespiratory monitors in hospitalized infants under 6 months of age is recommended.

In immunocompromised hosts, viral pneumonias may take a fulminant course, and specific antiviral chemotherapy should be considered. Amantadine is effective for the prophylaxis and treatment of influenza A infection. If given within 24 to 48 hours of the onset of illness, it has been shown to decrease signs, symptoms, and duration of illness. The dose is 5 to 8 mg/kg/day orally, divided every 12 hours, with a maximal dose of 150 mg/day in children less than 9 years old. Treatment should be continued for 5 to 7 days. The major side effects are central nervous system symptoms of insomnia, trouble in concentrating, and nervousness. The drug is excreted in the urine, and a decreased dose is required in the presence of impaired renal function. Ribavirin is a broad-spectrum virustatic agent effective against RSV, influenza A and B virus, parainfluenza virus, and adenovirus. Patients treated with ribavirin have a more prompt improvement in oxygen saturation and a shorter duration of viral shedding. Ribavirin is approved for use and is available only as aerosolized therapy for RSV infection; it should be considered in hospitalized infants younger than 2 months of age and high-risk infants with underlying cardiopulmonary disease (e.g., bronchopulmonary dysplasia and congenital heart disease), immunodeficiency, or prematurity. It is delivered by Oxygen hood or tent 12 to 18 hr/day for 3 to 6 days and appears safe and well tolerated. The role of ribavirin in the treatment of milder RSV infection has yet to be defined, but convincing studies documenting significant objective clinical efficacy are lacking. Acyclovir is effective for treating pulmonary infections caused by varicella zoster virus. Given intravenously or orally, it decreases viral shedding and prevents dissemination. Treatment should begin as early as possible. The intravenous dose is 500 mg/m² every 8 hours. Gancyclovir is an investigational antiviral agent that has shown promising results in the treatment of cytomegalovirus infection in immunocompromised hosts, although cytomegalovirus pneumonia may be more refractory to treatment.

A number of studies have evaluated the role of respiratory viral infection in acute asthma. Respiratory viral infection is the precipitating factor most frequently associated with acute asthma and can be documented in about 30 per cent of children with reversible airway obstruction, particularly in the spring and fall. Although the mechanisms by which acute viral lower respiratory tract infection produce airway obstruction are unknown, likely factors include increases in airway wall thickness because of cellular infiltrates and edema; increased luminal contents from excess secretions, sloughed epithelium, and ciliary dysfunction; and virus-induced changes in airway smooth muscle, resulting in increased contraction and decreased relaxation. Virus-specific immunoglobulin E (IgE) and increased histamine concentrations have been detected in the secretions of children with RSV or parainfluenza virus infection and concomitant airway obstruction. In healthy individuals, viral infections may cause a transient bronchial hyperreactivity lasting as long as 4 to 6 weeks. When wheezing is a prominent part of the clinical picture, a trial of beta-adrenergic bronchodilators is appropriate at any age.

VIRAL HEPATITIS

SAUL KRUGMAN, M.D.

Viral hepatitis is an infectious disease caused by at least five viruses: hepatitis A virus (HAV), hepatitis B virus (HBV), hepatitis C virus (HCV), hepatitis D virus (HDV), and hepatitis E virus (HEV). HDV, formerly called the delta virus, is a defective virus that can cause infection only in the presence of active HBV infection. HCV was formerly designated non-A, non-B virus, the most common cause of post-transfusion hepatitis. HEV was previously designated enterically transmitted non-A, non-B virus, the cause of large water-borne epidemics of hepatitis that have occurred in Asia, Africa, India, and Mexico.

The five types of hepatitis have features that may be similar or distinctive. The incubation period for Type A is about 2 to 6 weeks, that for Type B is 2 to 6 months, and that for Types C and E may be 2 weeks to 4 months. Hepatitis A is usually transmitted via the fecal-oral route. Therefore, infection is associated with close contact (household exposure) or the ingestion of fecally contaminated water or food such as shellfish. Hepatitis B and C may be transmitted by the inoculation of contaminated blood or blood products or by intimate physical contact. Most hepatitis infections in children are asymptomatic; illness, if present is anicteric.

The following specific markers of infection have been identified: hepatitis A antigen (HAAg) and antibody (anti-HAV), hepatitis B surface antigen (HBsAg) and antibody (anti-HBs), hepatitis B core antigen (HBcAg) and antibody (anti-HBc), hepatitis B e antigen (HBeAg) and antibody (anti-HBe), and hepatitis D antigen (HDAg) and antibody (anti-HD). These tests have made it possible to diagnose Types A and B hepatitis specifically and to identify HBV-contaminated units of blood. Tests for the detection of HCV and HEV antibody are not commercially available at the present time.

Each type of hepatitis is followed by homologous, but not heterologous, immunity. In the United States, about 25 to 35 per cent of adults have serologic evidence of immunity to hepatitis A (anti-HAV). In contrast, the prevalence of anti-HBs may range from 5 per cent in healthy blood donors to 20 per cent in health care workers with frequent blood contact to 70 per cent in such high-risk persons as immigrants from areas of high HBV endemicity, residents of institutions for the mentally retarded, intravenous drug abusers, homosexually active men, and household contacts of HBV carriers.

PREVENTION OF TYPE A HEPATITIS

General Measures. Procedures designed to block intestinal-oral pathways should be used for control; these include scrupulous hand washing, proper sterilization of food utensils, reduction of the fly population, and exclusion of potentially infectious food handlers. Although close contact is the most common mode of transmission, common-source epidemics stemming from contaminated food, milk, and water supplies may occur.

Passive Immunization. The efficacy of standard immune globulin (Ig) for prevention has been well established. *Postexposure prophylaxis* is recommended for all individuals who have had intimate exposure to a person with the disease. IG is also indicated for persons living in the same household because they are likely to have contact with the virus. However, routine use of IG in schools, offices, and factories is not warranted; spread of the disease is unlikely under the conditions existing in these open facilities. The recommended dose of IG is 0.02 ml/kg; it should be given within 48 hours, if possible, but not later than 1 week after exposure.

Pre-exposure prophylaxis with standard IG is recommended for persons traveling to or working in areas where Type A hepatitis is highly endemic. The recommended dose is 0.02 ml/kg. A repeat dose should be given if exposure is continuous for more than 4 months. If the serologic test to detect anti-HAV is available, evaluation should be done to determine the immune status of frequent travelers to areas where hepatitis A is prevalent. If antibody is present, IG should be discontinued.

HAV infection is not characterized by a carrier state. In addition, perinatal transmission of HAV does not occur after an acute infection during pregnancy. Therefore, immune prophylaxis is not needed for infants whose mothers had acute hepatitis A during pregnancy.

Active Immunization. A licensed HAV vaccine is not available. Experimental live attenuated and inactivated hepatitis A vaccines are under study.

PREVENTION OF TYPE B HEPATITIS

General Measures. Contaminated blood, blood products, and needles are the most common sources of HBV infection. The most common mode of transmission is parenteral, but the virus can infect via the oral route and by close physical contact with HBV-contaminated body fluids. Hepatitis B is a sexually transmitted disease. Blood obtained from commercial donors carries a 10- to 15-fold greater risk of causing hepatitis than blood obtained from volunteer donors. The indications for administering blood or blood products should be carefully assessed to be sure that the potential advantages warrant the risk.

Immunoprophylaxis. Two types of products are available: hepatitis B immune globulin (HBIG) for passive immunization and inactivated hepatitis B vaccine for active immunization. The vaccine is recommended for both pre-exposure and postexposure prophylaxis. HBIG provides temporary protection, and it is recommended for certain postexposure situations.

Hepatitis B Immune Globulin. HBIG is prepared from human plasma that contains a high titer of anti-HBs. The titer of anti-HBs in HBIG prepared in the United States is greater than 1:100,000 by radioimmunoassay (RIA). The human donor plasma is screened for antibodies to human immunodeficiency virus (HIV). In addition, the Cohn fractionation process used to prepare HBIG inactivates and eliminates HIV from the final product, if present. There is no evidence that acquired immunodeficiency syndrome (AIDS) has been transmitted by HBIG.

In the past, HBIG was recommended after exposure to HBV in the following situations: (1) perinatal exposure of an infant born to an HBsAg-positive mother, (2) accidental percutaneous or mucosal exposure to HBsAg-positive blood, (3) sexual exposure to an HBsAg-positive person, and (4) the presence of an intimate household contact. For accidental percutaneous and sexual exposures, two doses of HBIG, one given after exposure and one a month later, were recommended. For perinatal exposure, three doses of HBIG, given at birth, 3, and 6 months, were recommended.

The two- or three-dose schedule of HBIG previously recommended for postexposure prophylaxis should be replaced by a combined HBIG and hepatitis B vaccine regimen. Under these circumstances, one dose of HBIG

is given as soon as possible after exposure, and the first dose of vaccine is given at a separate site.

Hepatitis B Vaccine. Two types of hepatitis B vaccine are licensed in the United States: plasma-derived and yeast recombinant. Extensive experience to date has confirmed the safety, immunogenicity, and efficacy of these vaccines in adults and in infants.

Primary vaccination consists of three intramuscular doses of vaccine given at 0, 1, and 6 months. An alternate schedule of four doses at 0, 1, 2, and 12 months has also been recommended. Since various hepatitis vaccines are not generic, the age-specific doses may be variable. The recommended dose for a particular product approved by the Food and Drug Administration (FDA) is recorded in the package insert.

All hepatitis B vaccines are inactivated (noninfective) products. There is no evidence of interference with other vaccines administered simultaneously. There has been no evidence of risk to the fetus following vaccine given during pregnancy. In contrast, HBV infection in a pregnant woman may cause a severe disease in the mother and chronic infection of the newborn infant. Therefore, pregnancy and lactation are not contraindications to the use of the vaccine in women who are at high risk of contracting hepatitis B.

Hepatitis B vaccine is recommended for the following individuals who are at increased risk: health care professionals exposed to blood or blood products, patients with hemophilia or thalassemia, children or staff at institutions for the developmentally disabled, promiscuous male homosexuals, intravenous drug abusers, and household contacts of chronic carriers.

Prevention of Neonatal Hepatitis B

Postexposure prophylaxis of perinatal HBV infection with HBIG and hepatitis B vaccine has proved to be effective because (1) intrauterine infection is rare (about 5 per cent), (2) most infants are infected at the time of birth, and (3) the incubation period of hepatitis B may range between 6 weeks and 6 months. Consequently, active immunization with hepatitis B vaccine can induce an antibody response before the onset of infection.

Several studies have confirmed the efficacy of combined passive (HBIG) and active (hepatitis B vaccine) immunization for the prevention of perinatally acquired infection. The hepatitis B vaccine used in these studies was either plasma derived or yeast recombinant. The results of these studies revealed that the following regimen should prevent 85 to 90 per cent of chronic infections in infants born to mothers whose blood is positive for HBsAg and HBeAg: (1) HBIG, 0.5 ml given intramuscularly within the first few hours after birth, and (2) hepatitis B vaccine, given intramuscularly before the baby leaves the hospital, a second dose at 1 month, and a third dose at 6 months. The first dose of vaccine may be given at the same time as HBIG at a separate site.

Combined HBIG and hepatitis B vaccine prophylaxis is recommended for all infants whose mothers are HBsAg positive, regardless of their HBeAg status. Recommendations for the prophylaxis of perinatal hepatitis B infection incorporated into the routine pediatric vac-

TABLE 1. Hepatitis B Viral Prophylaxis for Infants of HBsAg-Positive Mothers, Incorporated into Routine Pediatric Immunization Schedule

Age (mo)	Hepatitis B Prevention Schedule	HBV Marker Screening	Routine Pediatric Schedule
Birth	HBIG* and HB vaccine†	—	—
2	HB vaccine	—	DPT, polio
4	HB vaccine	—	DPT‡, polio
6	—	—	DPT, polio
15	HB vaccine	HBsAg§ and anti-HBs‖	MMR¶
18	—	—	DPT, polio

*Hepatitis B immune globulin, 0.5 ml given intramuscularly within 12 hours of birth.
†Hepatitis B vaccine; see package insert for dose.
‡Diphtheria-tetanus-pertussis.
§HBsAg-positive blood indicates failure of immunization.
‖Anti-HBs–positive blood indicates success of immunization.
¶Measles-mumps-rubella.
The fourth dose of hepatitis B vaccine at 15 months is optional.

cination schedule are summarized in Table 1. As indicated in the table, blood should be tested for HBsAg and anti-HBs at 15 months. The absence of HBsAg and the presence of anti-HBs indicate that the infant is protected and immune. The presence of HBsAg at 15 months confirms a chronic carrier state.

The efficacy of the combined treatment regimen depends in great part on the administration of HBIG shortly after birth. Consequently, it is essential that HBsAg-positive pregnant women be identified during the prenatal period. Notification of the obstetric staff will enable them to protect themselves and other patients from infectious blood or secretions. Notification of the pediatric staff will alert them to institute therapy immediately after birth.

In 1988, the U.S. Public Health Service recommended that *all* pregnant women should be tested routinely for HBsAg. However, routine screening of all pregnant women is neither feasible nor recommended for those living in developing areas of the world where HBV infection is hyperendemic. Under these circumstances, routine immunization of all newborn infants with hepatitis B vaccine is indicated. This strategy should prevent perinatally or postnatally acquired HBV infection.

Hepatitis B Carrier Mothers and Breast Feeding

The breast milk of hepatitis B carrier mothers may contain HBsAg. In addition, serum from cracked nipples may contain infectious HBV. Nevertheless, breast feeding should not be discouraged because HBIG and hepatitis B vaccine are very effective for the prevention of neonatal hepatitis B infection.

TREATMENT

There is no specific treatment for children with hepatitis A or B. The disease is generally so mild that bed rest is unnecessary after the acute stage. The child's diet and return to activity usually are gauged by the child's desire. When anorexia is present, food is rejected; broths and fruit juices should be offered. A normal diet is recommended when appetite returns.

Corticosteroids and other drugs are not indicated for children with uncomplicated hepatitis.

Fulminant Hepatitis. The sudden onset of mental confusion, emotional instability, restlessness, coma, and hemorrhagic manifestations may progress to a fatal outcome within 10 days. Under these extraordinary conditions, the following measures should be considered: (1) corticosteroid therapy; (2) withdrawal of protein from the diet; (3) oral neomycin, 25 mg/kg every 6 hours, to suppress the bacterial flora of the intestinal tract; (4) laxatives and cleansing enemas; and (5) exchange transfusion. There are isolated reports of successful liver transplantation in adults with fulminant hepatitis.

ENTEROVIRUSES

GILBERT M. SCHIFF, M.D.

Approximately 70 specific serotypes of enteroviruses have been detected. They are members of the picornavirus group, are 270 to 300 angströms in size, contain single-stranded RNA, are stable at acid pH and room temperature, and are resistant to lipid solvents. The enteroviruses are classified according to pathogenicity for experimental animals and other biochemical, physical, and molecular criteria. At present three poliovirus, 23 coxsackie A virus, 6 coxsackie B virus, and 32 echovirus serotypes are recognized. In addition, more recently identified viruses are classified as the "newer, higher numbered enteroviruses," i.e., enteroviruses 68 to 72. The newest member, Enterovirus 72, is the hepatitis A virus.

Prevention. Passive immunization with human immune globulin (IG) is effective in the prevention of clinical hepatitis A infection (Enterovirus 72). Use of pooled human IG (0.2 ml/kg intramuscularly) for passive protection against other enteroviruses is possible but would appear to be of value only in certain situations, such as severe enteroviral outbreaks in nurseries.

Widespread use of inactivated poliomyelitis vaccine and oral live, attenuated poliomyelitis vaccine (OPV) has been highly effective for the control of poliomyelitis. An increased danger of paralytic poliomyelitis following administration of OPV to infants with agammaglobulinemia is recognized. Because OPV is given at such a young age, the congenital immune deficiency may not be recognized. Therefore, OPV should not be administered to an infant with a family history of agammaglobulinemia until the condition can be ruled out.

Attenuated viral vaccines for other enteroviruses are not available. Preliminary evaluation of hepatitis A vaccines have started. Other enteroviral vaccines undoubtedly could be developed but require more aggressive efforts to document specific needs and cost effectiveness. The multiplicity of enteroviral serotypes tends to direct attention toward the development of broad-spectrum antiviral therapy to counter the medical problems caused by these viruses.

Treatment. At the present time no specific antienteroviral therapy is available. Supportive therapy is the keystone for treatment and varies according to the clinical manifestations. Passive antibody therapy in severe neonatal enteroviral infections (when specific maternal antibody is absent) and in chronic enteroviral infections in agammaglobulinemic children remains experimental. If nothing else, this type of therapy may terminate viremia and prevent continued seeding of organs. There are a number of newer antiviral agents that have been shown to be effective against a broad spectrum of enteroviruses in tissue culture systems and some animal models. Some of these drugs are ready for evaluation in·well-controlled human studies.

A recurring problem has been the use of corticosteroids as part of the treatment regimen in such illnesses as severe neonatal viral myocarditis and meningoencephalitis, myopericarditis in older children, and acute hemorrhagic conjunctivitis. On the basis of animal experiments, we generally accept the fact that viruses and corticosteroids or other immunosuppressive agents are not good bedfellows. In reality, there have been no well-controlled human studies to suggest that such is the case. However, in general, I recommend avoidance of these agents in the presence of documented active viral diseases whenever possible. In myopericarditis, which we tend to see in active adolescents and young adults, and in cases of myocarditis in infants and older children, the treatment is bed rest, relief of pain, and if congestive failure occurs, the careful use of cardiac glycosides and diuretics. The heart in infants with myocarditis is frequently very sensitive to cardiac glycosides and only low doses are necessary, especially the initial dose. As mentioned, I prefer avoidance of corticosteroids or immunosuppressive agents in acute myocarditis despite some clinical studies that suggest a favorable effect of corticosteroids alone or in combination with azathioprine. These studies lacked proper controls and laboratory diagnosis. Better clinical studies and additional data are needed.

In patients with meningoencephalitis, treatment for cerebral edema is frequently required, and urea, mannitol, or large doses of corticosteroids have been used. Again, I recommend that the latter be avoided because of the potential overall adverse effects of corticosteroids in the presence of acute viral infections.

Acute hemorrhagic conjunctivitis is usually self-limited and is generally an illness that occurs in adolescents and adults. There is the potential for this illness to become a greater problem in children of all ages. The supportive treatment usually includes local application of broad-spectrum antibiotics and sulfonamides to prevent or treat secondary bacterial infection. Corticosteroids have been used to reduce inflammation and relieve pain. However, relapses are four to five times more frequent after their use, and development of chronic conjunctivitis and corneal ulceration has been reported among patients who received corticosteroids. I recommend avoidance of corticosteroids for this condition.

Finally, the role of laboratory diagnosis in relation to treatment should be emphasized. Prompt diagnosis of viral etiology can result in avoiding the unnecessary use of antibiotics in many patients. Aseptic meningitis is a typical example of a situation in which this phenomenon may be operative. Initial examination may not be conclusive, and antibiotics should be intelligently initiated to "cover all fronts." But once an enteroviral etiology has been established, antibiotics should be discontinued.

ASEPTIC MENINGITIS

SHELDON L. KAPLAN, M.D.

Aseptic meningitis is not a specific diagnosis but rather a syndrome that is characterized by an abrupt onset of meningeal irritation and a CSF pleocytosis. It generally has a benign clinical course. Although there are numerous infectious and noninfectious causes of aseptic meningitis, a viral infection is the most common etiology. Enteroviruses account for approximately 80 per cent of the cases of viral meningitis. It is important to recognize that an enterovirus can be isolated from the CSF of infants and children who do not have abnormal CSF white blood cell counts. Once the diagnosis of viral meningitis is suspected, the age of the patient will determine how the physician will approach the managment of this condition. Since in young children, particularly under a year in age, viral meningitis may not be easily distinguished from bacterial meningitis on the basis of historical or physical finding or from the results of cerebrospinal fluid (CSF) examination, antibiotics may be administered intravenously for 48 to 72 hours, at which time CSF culture results are available. Antibiotics administered prior to hospitalization may alter the biochemical, morphological, and cultural results of the CSF examination and confuse its interpretation. In children who have not received antibiotics and who have negative CSF cultures by 72 hours, antibiotics can be discontinued. Although antiviral therapy is not currently recommended for viral meningitis, such treatment is available for herpes encephalitis, which in an early phase may present like viral meningitis. The value of vidarabine or acyclovir in treating aseptic meningitis associated with genital herpes infections is unknown.

Older children with viral meningitis generally do not require hospitalization, but antipyretics and analgesics may allow symptomatic relief. Avoidance of light is helpful if the patient has photophobia, and elevation of the head may help relieve headaches. Infants and children with more severe symptoms are usually admitted to the hospital initially for supportive care. Serum electrolytes may reveal hyponatremia, which can result from the inappropriate secretion of antidiuretic hormone. In such patients, mild fluid restriction is warranted. Intravenous fluids may be required for provision of maintenance fluid rates if the child has persistent nausea and vomiting. Meningitis due to enteroviruses can be associated with a disseminated infection, including myocarditis, pericarditis, hepatitis, and so on, which must be recognized for optimal management of the patient. Intravenous immunoglobulin may be beneficial in these instances as well as in the immunodeficient child with enteroviral meningoencephalitis. Enteric or excretion isolation is recommended for patients with viral meningitis.

The majority of children with viral meningitis appear to recover uneventfully. Some children continue to complain of headaches, weakness, fatigue, dizziness, or other similar problems for variable periods of time after the meningitis. Younger children and especially those under 3 months of age with enteroviral meningitis may suffer neurologic sequelae despite the fact that their general and neurologic examination is completely normal at discharge. Delayed language and speech development, behavior problems, and other developmental abnormalities may become evident years following the episode of meningitis. Therefore such children deserve careful follow-up and psychologic evaluation, if necessary, as they enter the school-age years. Seizures during the acute illness appear to be correlated with an increased risk for these neurologic sequelae.

ENCEPHALITIS INFECTIONS— POSTINFECTIOUS AND POSTVACCINAL

MARVIN L. WEIL, M.D.

Postinfectious and postvaccinal encephalitis refers to a group of immune disorders of the brain and spinal cord that can complicate viral and bacterial infections as well as immunization with live and inactivated viral and bacterial vaccines. Treatment involves relief of specific symptoms and modulation of the immune system in some instances. Although a diverse group of agents and antigens can elicit this type of encephalomyelitis, manifestations of these disorders are limited to a number of symptom complexes, each with its own requirements for therapy.

Acute disseminated encephalomyelitis, which is sometimes hemorrhagic, may occur after rubeola, rubella, varicella, variola, Epstein-Barr virus, mumps, and influenza as well as after vaccinia or rabies immunization. Onset is usually abrupt, with seizures requiring anticonvulsant medication such as lorazepam, dilantin, phenobarbital, or paraldehyde. Somnolence and coma may ensue as the result of either diffuse brain involvement or elevated intracranial pressure. The hemorrhagic encephalomyelitis variant should be treated promptly with steroids (e.g., dexamethasone, 1.5 mg/kg/day), since this may result in prompt improvement. Symptoms of increased intracranial pressure should receive appropriate attention. Supportive therapy is important during the first 7 days, since patients surviving the first week generally recover to a variable degree.

In some cases of postvaccinal encephalomyelitis due to vaccinia, virus can be isolated, suggesting a mixed process involving both the acute infection and the immune response. In such cases, immunosuppressants such as dexamethasone may be contraindicated.

Focal neurologic syndromes associated with these conditions such as transverse myelitis, optic atrophy, or

acute cerebellar ataxia should be treated with appropriate supportive measures. Inappropriate antidiuretic hormone secretion should be treated by limitation of free water. Postencephalomyelitic sequelae such as static neurologic deficits, seizures, and cognitive and psychiatric disturbances require long-term treatment.

Symptoms of acute parainfectious encephalopathy (e.g., Reye's syndrome) should be treated appropriately and not confused with this condition.

Cerebral Edema and Increased Intracranial Pressure

Appropriate therapy for increased intracranial pressure requires almost continuous careful, accurate, and perceptive clinical and technological monitoring. Prompt recognition of changes in clinical status is essential, so that appropriate therapeutic responses can avert added morbidity or mortality. A therapeutic regimen based on physiologic principles is essential, since each patient may present a different array of problems.

The cranial vault of the older child or adult has a fixed volume occupied by brain parenchyma (approximately 80 per cent), cerebrospinal fluid (approximately 10 per cent), and vascular bed (approximately 10 per cent). Space-occupying lesions or brain swelling causes encroachment on the cerebrospinal fluid space and the vascular bed except for more rigid vessels such as the dural sinuses. Small increases in the volume of this encroachment lead to minimal increases in intracranial pressure until there is no further room for expansion and cerebral compliance is lost. Beyond this point, any small increase in intracranial volume, by either enlargement of a space-occupying mass, increase in the size of the edematous brain, or vasodilatation, results in a marked increase in intracranial pressure. Physiologic changes that result in vasoconstriction decrease the volume of the vascular bed and lower intracranial pressure. This can improve cerebral perfusion pressure and cerebral perfusion, provided vasoconstriction does not become excessive and produce ischemia by impedance of cerebral blood flow. Blood supply to cerebral tissue (average value about 50 ml/100 gm/min) is determined by the size of the vascular bed and its resistance to blood flow, and the cerebral perfusion pressure (mean arterial pressure [diastolic blood pressure plus about one third of the pulse pressure] minus the intracranial pressure). Normal cerebral perfusion pressure, about 38 torr for newborns and 50 torr for older children and adults, is maintained by cerebral blood vessel autoregulation. Loss of autoregulation results in the linear transfer of mean arterial pressure to the cerebral vasculature with increased capillary pressure as well as increased intracranial pressure. Once brain compliance is lost, physiologic changes that result in increased blood flow by means of vasodilatation or increased mean arterial pressure result in an elevation of intracranial pressure and a reduction in perfusion pressure.

Therapy of increased intracranial pressure may require surgical reduction of any intracranial mass lesions. Different types of cerebral edema—vasogenic, cytotoxic, interstitial, or a combination—respond to treatment modalities in different ways. Vasogenic edema results from breaks in the tight junctions of the microvasculature with leakage of plasma and plasma proteins into the interstitial spaces of the brain. Steroids, which can cause tightening of these junctions in the cerebral microvasculature, may be of benefit. Hyperosmolar agents such as mannitol and urea are of benefit in that they shrink the remaining normal brain, while they may fail to produce an osmolar gradient at sites of vascular damage. Hyperosmolar agents may prove harmful in the presence of widespread vasogenic edema. Cytotoxic edema involves the accumulation of intracellular water; hence, it is more responsive to mannitol and other hyperosmolar agents. Steroids, which are effective in preventing hypoxic damage to mitochondria, have little benefit in treatment if given after the hypoxic event. Drugs such as furosemide, which reduce cerebrospinal fluid production, may also improve intracranial pressure.

Management. With due regard for the concepts outlined above, the following method is recommended for the management of intracranial hypertension:

Keep the head of the bed elevated to about 30 degrees if this is not contraindicated in order to promote venous drainage and minimize venous back-pressure to the head. Avoid neck flexion and compressive tracheostomy ties, which may impede venous drainage from the brain. Maintain the blood pressure below 140 mm Hg systolic if possible without compromising cerebral perfusion pressure. This assumes importance when autoregulation of cerebral blood flow is lost. Dexamethasone, 1.5 mg/kg/day, is beneficial for tumor or abscess edema. Benefits of steroids in traumatic or posthypoxic cerebral edema have not been clearly established in controlled studies, but many centers continue to use them. It is generally advisable to discontinue their use at the earliest opportunity, especially after about 5 days, in order to minimize complications of steroid therapy. Normovolemic hydration is preferred to partial dehydration in order to avoid iatrogenic hypotension. The initial serum osmolality is maintained at around 300 mOsm.

Controlled hyperventilation to a $PaCO_2$ of 25 to 28 torr may be necessary to keep the intracranial pressure below 20 torr for young children and adults and below about 8 to 12 torr in infants with open fontanels. $PaCO_2$ values below 23 are not recommended, since they are of little additional benefit and may cause added cerebral ischemia. Supplemental oxygen should be used if necessary to keep the PaO_2 above 90 torr. A PaO_2 below 50 torr may result in a severe increase in intracranial hypertension. Even short bouts of hypoventilation may result in severe exacerbations of intracranial hypertension. Positive end-expiratory airway pressure (PEEP) may be increased as needed to keep the FiO_2 below 50 per cent in order to avoid oxygen toxicity; however, PEEP above 3 torr should be avoided unless pulmonary compliance is reduced in order to minimize pulmonary embarrassment of venous return from the brain.

Intracranial pressure monitoring by epidural, subdural, subarachnoid, or intraventricular devices has been an important advance in the management of intracranial hypertension. Patients who achieve a Glasgow Coma Scale score of 7 (Table 1) or less should be considered candidates for intracranial pressure monitors.

TABLE 1. Glasgow Coma Scale

Best Motor Response	
Obeys	6
Localizes	5
Withdraws	4
Abnormal flexion	3
Extensor response	2
Nil	1
Verbal Response	
Oriented	5
Confused conversation	4
Inappropriate words	3
Incomprehensible sounds	2
Nil	1
Eye Opening	
Spontaneous	4
To speech	3
To pain	2
Nil	1

If, despite the above therapy, the intracranial pressure rises above 20 torr; spontaneous waves (of Lundberg) over 20 torr last for more than 5 minutes; waves over 20 torr triggered by turning or suctioning do not subside in 5 minutes; or any pressure occurs over 30 torr, then give furosemide, 0.5 mg/kg IV, and if necessary, mannitol, 0.5 to 1.0 gm/kg IV as a 20 per cent solution. Should combined therapy with mannitol and furosemide be required, the furosemide should be given about 15 minutes after the mannitol bolus for optimal results. If benefits fail to last more than 3 hours, an intravenous drip of mannitol at 0.05 to 0.15 gm/kg/hr may be tried. Serum osmolality should be maintained at 320 mOsm or less to avoid rebound phenomenon. The serum glucose may be maintained at about 200 mg/dl to minimize the amount of mannitol required.

If the intracranial pressure continues to be elevated, hypothermia with a core temperature of 32° C is recommended to lower intracranial pressure and decrease cerebral metabolism. Temperatures below this limit may result in cardiac arrhythmias.

Should the above measures prove ineffective at keeping the intracranial pressure below 20 torr and the cerebral perfusion pressure at about 50 torr, pentobarbital has been recommended, although its use remains controversial. Some centers have been unable to duplicate the beneficial results claimed by others. Should pentobarbital be used, a loading dose of 5 mg/kg is given intravenously as 50 to 100 mg bolus doses, followed by 0.5 to 3.0 mg/kg/hr IV to achieve a blood level of 25 to 40 μg/ml. If the intracranial pressure continues to be elevated, the infusion rate is increased until the pressure is controlled, or the EEG demonstrates burst suppression, or the cardiac index falls below normal (2.7 liters/min/m²). Excessive doses of pentobarbital should be avoided, since they may result in decreased peripheral vascular resistance and excessive cerebral vascular resistance which can augment cerebral ischemia.

The use of hypothermia or pentobarbital may decrease the need for mannitol therapy. Should the intracranial pressure rise during such treatment and the serum osmolality is less than 320 mOsm, mannitol 0.5 gm/kg IV may be given.

The detrimental effects of even transient episodes of elevated intracranial pressure with concomitant reductions in perfusion pressure cannot be overemphasized. Pancuronium (Pavulon), 0.06 to 0.1 mg/kg, can be used in conjunction with pentothal when intubation is required or when suction is necessary in restless, struggling patients or those who develop dystonic posturing during nursing or other procedures.

PSITTACOSIS

CAROL F. PHILLIPS, M.D.

Psittacosis (ornithosis) is a zoonotic disease acquired by inhaling infected particles from bird secretions or droppings. The disease may be transmitted by healthy birds, is rare in children, and has no seasonality. The incubation period is 7 to 14 days.

The clinical picture consists of fever, severe headache, chills, pneumonia, weakness, and myalgia. Rarely, hepatitis, arthritis, endocarditis, severe anemia, pulmonary embolism, erythema nodosum, or disseminated intravascular coagulation occurs. Untreated, severe illness persists for 2 to 3 weeks.

Isolation of the organism should be attempted only in experienced laboratories. The diagnosis is usually made by demonstrating a significant rise in the complement fixation (CF) titer of blood specimens between the time of acute illness and convalescence. There is no prolonged immunity, and reinfections occur despite high CF titers. The chest radiograph usually shows atypical pneumonia, but lobar consolidation can occur.

Tetracycline, 30 to 40 mg/kg/day, is the treatment of choice for patients older than age 8. Erythromycin, 40 mg/kg/day, can be used in younger children, but experience is limited. Therapy should be continued for 3 weeks.

Bed rest, oxygen, adequate fluids, and antipyretics are supplemental therapy. The disease is rarely communicable from person to person; however, hospitalized patients should be placed in respiratory isolation.

RICKETTSIAL DISEASES

PAUL J. HONIG, M.D.

The rickettsial infections are spread by the bites of blood-sucking arthropods. There are four major diseases: (a) typhus, (b) Rocky Mountain spotted fever, (c) scrub typhus, and (d) Q fever. The primary rickettsial disease found in the United States is Rocky Mountain spotted fever (1000 cases/year), with scattered outbreaks of rickettsialpox having been reported recently. The typhus group, which occurs infrequently, and Q fever will not be discussed.

RICKETTSIALPOX

Although the illness is usually mild, the duration of symptoms can be shortened with antibiotic treatment. Patients respond in 1 to 2 days to oral doses of tetracycline (25 to 50 mg/kg/24 hr) every 6 hours (usually given for a total of 5 days). Children under 8 years of age who have mild symptoms should not be treated because of the effects of tetracycline on the teeth. Children with more severe symptoms or high fever who are under 8 years of age may benefit from as little as 2 days of tetracycline therapy, however.

ROCKY MOUNTAIN SPOTTED FEVER

Since no test is available that will confirm the diagnosis of Rocky Mountain spotted fever early in the course of the disease, treatment must be initiated presumptively. The disease can be aborted if antibiotics are started in time (by the first day or two of the exanthem). Oral doses of chloramphenicol, 50 mg/kg/day in children under 8 years of age, or tetracycline, 50 mg/kg/day in older youths, are recommended. (It is important to remember that chloramphenicol and tetracycline will only suppress the growth of the rickettsia. Final eradication of the rickettsia depends upon a normal functioning immune system.)

When the disease is diagnosed late in the course (clinically toxic, obtunded, or hyponatremic), hospitalization is necessary. Supportive measures are in order. Hypovolemic shock due to chronic leakage of fluid from damaged vessels must be watched for closely. Although antibiotics, such as intravenous chloramphenicol, 50 mg/kg/day, will arrest the growth of rickettsia, the natural course of the disease will not be altered when severe vascular damage has already occurred. If the diagnosis is in doubt, broader antibiotic coverage for sepsis is advisable.

Prevention of this disease is important. Children and their dogs should be routinely inspected for ticks if they play in wooded areas. Insect repellents are somewhat effective. If a tick is found attached to the skin, it must be removed so as not to have fragments of the mouth parts in the skin (risk for granuloma formation) or to introduce body fluids containing infectious organisms. Various methods have been recommended for removal of ticks from the skin. However, proper mechanical removal is the only safe procedure. The tick should be gently grasped with a tweezer or forceps as close to the skin surface as possible. A steady, even pulling force perpendicular to the skin surface should be used. Do not squeeze, crush, or puncture the tick. A twisting or jerking motion may cause the mouth parts to break off in the skin. Ticks should not come in direct contact with the skin because infectious agents may enter through breaks in the skin. Prophylactic antibiotic therapy (tetracycline) should be considered when children who live in endemic areas are bitten by ticks, especially if new cases of Rocky Mountain spotted fever are currently being diagnosed. Treatment can be instituted as soon as the biting tick is discovered or following the first signs of illness.

CHLAMYDIA INFECTIONS
CAROL F. PHILLIPS, M.D.

A number of diseases are caused by *Chlamydia trachomatis*, and a newly recognized disease is caused by *Chlamydia pneumoniae.*

The diagnosis can be made by isolation of the organism in tissue culture. Rapid tests using monoclonal antibody or enzyme-linked immunosorbent assay are available for testing for *Chlamydia trachomatis* in cervical or urethral specimens from adults and eye and nasopharyngeal specimens from infants. Cross-reaction with fecal flora makes these tests unreliable for evaluation of rectal, vaginal, or urethral specimens from children. The method of choice for diagnosing *Chlamydia* pneumonia is demonstration of a rise in the antibody titer of sera between the time of acute illness and convalescence, using microimmunofluorescent or complement fixation tests.

CHLAMYDIA PNEUMONIA (TWAR)

The clinical picture of this disease consists of severe pharyngitis, fever, cough, and cervical adenopathy. Illness is prolonged, and sore throat may precede the cough by 1 to 2 weeks.

The disease is caused by a newly recognized strain of *Chlamydia* and is spread from person to person. The peak age of infection is between the ages of 5 and 20 years. Recurrence is common.

Therapy is not well defined. Some patients have been treated with erythromycin, 1 gm/day for 5 to 10 days, with some response, although relapse is common. A longer duration of therapy might be needed. Tetracycline, 2 gm/day for 7 to 10 days or 1 gm/day for 21 days, has also been recommended for patients older than age 8.

EYE INFECTIONS

Neonatal inclusion conjunctivitis develops 5 days to several weeks after birth, with the appearance of edema and congestion in one or both eyes. Discharge is minimal. Trachoma is a follicular keratoconjunctivitis that can lead to blindness.

Inclusion conjunctivitis should be treated with erythromycin, 50 mg/kg/day in four divided doses for 14 days. Topical therapy is not as effective and will not eliminate nasopharyngeal colonization. Treatment of trachoma is difficult and requires prolonged therapy. Topical tetracycline twice daily, plus doxycycline, 50 mg once daily for 5 days monthly times 6 months, has been shown to be effective. In this circumstance, systemic therapy with tetracyclines is indicated even in children younger than 8 years.

CHLAMYDIAL PNEUMONIA

Patients with chlamydial pneumonia are usually between 1 and 5 months of age and afebrile, and they present with staccato cough and tachypnea. Wheezing is rare, but rales may be heard. The chest radiograph shows hyperinflation with diffuse infiltrates.

Erythromycin, 40 mg/kg/day, or sulfisoxazole, 150 mg/kg/day in four divided doses for 2 weeks, is effective therapy. Chest physical therapy may be helpful. Occasionally, oxygen therapy may be necessary.

UNCOMPLICATED URETHRAL, CERVICAL, AND RECTAL INFECTIONS

Infection may be asymptomatic, acute, or chronic. Reinfection is common. Chronic pelvic inflammatory disease may cause infertility.

Tetracycline, 500 mg four times a day for 7 days, is the treatment of choice. Alternative therapy is sulfisoxazole, 1 gm four times a day. The sexual partner should be treated concurrently.

LYMPHOGRANULOMA VENEREUM

Lymphogranuloma venereum is caused by an agent related to *Chlamydia trachomatis* and is spread sexually. It occurs worldwide and is much more frequent in men than women.

Clinical illness begins with a small erosion or papule on the genitalia. In women, the lesion can be missed. Inguinal adenitis, usually unilateral, develops, and eventually the nodes drain. Rectal stricture can develop in women or homosexual men.

Tetracycline, 500 mg four times a day, should be given for 3 to 6 weeks. Sulfisoxazole, 1 gm four times a day, can be substituted, although some organisms are resistant to this drug. The complement fixation titer should be followed. If there is an increase in titer after therapy is finished, the patient should be re-treated.

LEGIONELLA INFECTIONS
MICHAEL E. RYAN, D.O.

The causative agent of legionnaires' disease, *Legionella pneumophila*, is a fastidious, gram-negative, aerobic bacillus with 12 serogroups. There are 23 other species of *Legionella,* with a total of 39 serogroups, of which 14 of these species have caused infections in humans. *L. pneumophila* is the cause of the majority of cases of legionnaires' disease. This disease is a rare cause of pneumonia in otherwise healthy children. Legionnaires' disease should be considered in all immunocompromised children with pneumonia of undetermined etiology.

SUPPORTIVE THERAPY

The elements of supportive therapy include adequate hydration, maintenance of oxygenation, mobilization of lower respiratory secretions, and careful monitoring of respirations. Because of increased losses of fluids in children with pneumonia, mild dehydration is frequently observed, and continuing losses are expected early in the disease process. Thus, one should replace fluid deficits and provide adequate maintenance fluids. In the child with respiratory distress, noninvasive monitoring with ear oximetry can reduce the need for frequent blood gas sampling and arterial lines. Oxygen-

TABLE 1. Therapy for *Legionella* Infections

	Drug	Route	Doses per Day	Total Daily Doses
Mild illness with no respiratory compromise	Erythromycin	Oral	4	30–50 mg/kg/day
	Alternative—doxycycline*	Oral	1–2	5 mg/kg/day first day, followed by 2.5 mg/kg/day
Moderate-to-severe illness	Erythromycin	Intravenous (IV)	4	30–50 mg/kg/day for children under 50 kg; 4 gm/day maximum
	Alternative—erythromycin with rifampin†	IV	4 1–2	As above 10–20 mg/kg/day for children over 5 years, not to exceed 600 mg/day‡
	Alternative—doxycycline*	IV	1–2	5 mg/kg first day, 2–4 mg/kg/day 12 hours later, and then daily for children under 50 kg; 200 mg first day and then 100–200 mg daily for children over 50 kg
	With rifampin†	Oral	1–2	Doses as above

*Tetracyclines may not be effective in all cases; tetracyclines should not be used in children younger than 8 years of age for even short courses unless clearly indicated.

†Rifampin should not be used as a single agent; erythromycin with rifampin is preferred for pulmonary abscess.

‡Not FDA approved for children under 5 years of age.

ation should be maintained with supplemental oxygen or mechanical ventilation if required. Acetaminophen should be used to control high fever. Immunosuppressive agents should be omitted if possible. Corticosteroids do not seem to be of benefit as a primary treatment. No isolation precautions are recommended for the hospitalized patient, as the major environmental reservoir appears to be water, and person-to-person transmission has not been reported. Pleural effusion, with or without parenchymal infiltrates, can occur, and drainage for empyema may be necessary.

CHEMOTHERAPY

On the basis of retrospective reviews and experimental studies, erythromycin remains the drug of choice for the treatment of legionnaires' disease. There is evidence that erythromycin and other macrolide antibiotics penetrate well into the phagocytes, which appears to be necessary for adequate therapy. Erythromycin, in doses described in Table 1, is usually given intravenously and then is switched to oral administration as the patient's clinical condition improves. Therapy should be continued for a minimum of 21 days. Relapses and treatment failures have been reported. Rifampin, given in combination with erythromycin for the first week of therapy, is indicated for severe disease, especially in the immunocompromised patient. If patients are unable to tolerate oral rifampin, intravenous rifampin is commercially available. The recommendation for use of rifampin is based on experimental animal models, as rifampin for the treatment of legionnaires' disease is not an indication approved by the U.S. Food and Drug Administration (FDA). Alternative therapeutic agents with demonstrated clinical activity include tetracycline and trimethoprim-sulfamethoxazole. Use of tetracyclines is contraindicated in children less than 8 years of age. New quinolone derivatives are impressive in experimental infections, but clinical efficacy has not been demonstrated, and these agents have not been approved for use in children.

The majority of children with legionnaires' disease show prompt clinical improvement after initiation of erythromycin therapy. Fever usually will subside over the first week of therapy, although the chest roentgenogram may worsen despite this clinical improvement. Resolution of infiltrates on the chest roentgenogram may take from 3 weeks to 3 months after the initiation of therapy. The early institution of therapy is most important in this serious infection, which has an overall case fatality rate of 5 to 25 per cent and a mortality of up to 80 per cent in immunocompromised patients.

SYSTEMIC MYCOSES

GARY D. OVERTURF, M.D.

Amphotericin B remains the primary antifungal agent for most systemic mycoses, including disseminated candidiasis, cryptococcosis, blastomycosis, histoplasmosis, coccidioidomycosis, and aspergillosis. Specific details of the treatment of histoplasmosis and coccidioidomycosis are reviewed in other articles. For serious or disseminated infections due to blastomycosis, cryptococcosis, candidiasis, aspergillosis, and sporotrichosis, amphotericin B is the central focus of therapy. Other agents may be added or substituted for less severe forms or for those patients who are unresponsive to, or intolerant of, amphotericin B; these exceptions will be discussed further on. Serious toxicity can be minimized if appropriate precautions and monitoring are employed.

Amphotericin B is primarily fungistatic but may be fungicidal, depending upon the concentration obtained in body fluids at the site of the infection and the susceptibility of the fungal agent. The drug probably acts by binding to sterols in the fungus cell membrane, with a resultant change in membrane permeability.

ADVERSE REACTIONS TO AMPHOTERICIN B

Hematology. Self-limited anemia of mild severity may occur during the course of amphotericin B therapy. Anemia is not an indication for discontinuance. The normocytic-normochromic anemia is usually the result of mild hemolysis and a shortened half-life of erythrocytes resulting directly from systemic fungal infection plus suppression of erythrocyte production by amphotericin B. In addition, amphotericin B may bind to normal-occurring sterols in red blood cell walls. Neutropenia and thrombocytopenia may also occasionally be observed.

Fever, Nausea, and Vomiting. Fever (up to 40° C) and chills occurring during the administration of amphotericin B are frequent. Therapy includes aspirin or acetaminophen and the usual antipyretic measures. Fever is so common and expected that it should not necessitate the interruption of therapy. Nausea and vomiting are as common as fever but vary considerably in severity from patient to patient. Headache may also be a frequent complaint.

Thrombophlebitis. If the same vein is used continuously for the administration of amphotericin B, thrombophlebitis will inevitably result. Small doses of steroids in the intravenous fluid should not be used because of the uncertainty of interdrug reactions. Provision of liberal fluids to flush the vein may be helpful. When administration of repetitive doses is to be given over many weeks, the use of a surgically placed central venous catheter (e.g., Broviac or Hickman) should be considered.

Systemic Adverse Effects. Seizures, apnea, and cyanosis rarely occur during intravenous administration of amphotericin B. In addition, hypotension and cardiovascular collapse may occur. The exact mechanism by which these severe reactions take place is not known. These reactions are particularly common with the first few doses of amphotericin B or in seriously ill patients, but these effects can be minimized by ensuring optimal volume repletion and good electrolyte balance (particularly sodium repletion) prior to beginning therapy.

Nephrotoxicity. Four effects on renal anatomy in association with amphotericin B therapy have been described; these effects are at least partially reversible and include glomerular thickening and epithelial proliferation, cortical tubular atrophy with necrosis, degeneration and thickening of tubular epithelium, and intratubular and interstitial calcification. The clinical and laboratory manifestations of these changes include proteinuria, increases in blood urea nitrogen, decreases in renal concentrating ability, renal tubular acidosis, decreases in renal blood flow and glomerular filtration rate, and hypokalemia. Hypokalemia is the most common complication, resulting from defective tubular reabsorption; it may be heralded by lethargy, severe muscular weakness or partial paralysis, or cardiac arrhythmias. Each patient's renal and electrolyte status should be monitored at least weekly, with determinations of serum blood urea nitrogen (BUN), creatinine, and electrolyte levels, as well as urinalysis.

Prophylactic Premedication. The usual side effects (fever, nausea, and vomiting) of amphotericin B administration may be eliminated or diminished by careful preparation with antipyretics or antihistaminics or both. Aspirin or acetaminophen, in usual doses, and promethazine (Phenergan) or chlorpromazine may be given 30 to 60 minutes before amphotericin B infusions. Subsequent doses may be necessary for up to 24 hours after a single dose to control fever, myalgia, headache, or vomiting.

ADMINISTRATION OF AMPHOTERICIN B

Intravenous Administration. The first doses of amphotericin B should be administered intravenously to a hospitalized patient for whom adequate medical supervision and nursing care are available. The drug is very irritating, and care must be taken to secure the needle within the vein so that no perivascular or subcutaneous leakage occurs. Each dose of antibiotic should be prepared in a concentration of 0.1 mg/ml (1 mg/10 ml) or less and diluted in 5 per cent dextrose in water (not saline); light shielding of the infusion bottle is unnecessary, since infusion times of 1 to 6 hours do not lead to light inactivation of conventional doses. Patients may vary in their tolerance of amphotericin B and thus in their tolerance of the rate at which it may be administered. Subsequent doses may be administered at a more rapid rate, if tolerated, but usually not in less than 1 to 2 hours per infusion.

Dosage. Although the total dosage for the treatment of systemic fungal infections has not been well established, a total dose of 30 to 40 mg/kg (i.e., equivalent to 2.0 to 2.5 gm in a 70-kg adult) of the antibiotic over a 6- to 8-week period is usually considered a therapeutic maximal dose. Therapy is usually initiated with a test dose of 0.1 mg/kg (maximum of 1.0 mg) infused over a period of 6 hours. Subsequently, the dose may be gradually increased in daily increments (e.g., 0.1 to 0.5 mg/kg/day) over a period of 5 to 7 days, until a maximal daily dose of 1.0 to 1.5 mg/kg is attained. The speed of incremental increase will depend upon both the severity of infection and the patient's tolerance of the drug. However, larger doses are commonly tolerated by infants and younger children. The excretion of the drug is very slow, and since renal toxicity, manifested by increasing BUN levels, invariably occurs, it is usually possible to maintain "therapeutic" levels of amphotericin B by administering the drug 3 days per week or every other day. Thus, after the clinical response and tolerance to doses is established, therapy may be maintained on an outpatient basis or in an office setting, with 1- to 2-hour infusions completed two or three times per week.

OTHER ANTIFUNGAL AGENTS

Although amphotericin B is the treatment of choice for most systemic mycoses, several additional agents may be considered in special circumstances.

Flucytosine. Flucytosine (5-FC) is indicated specifically in the treatment of cryptococcosis, in combination with amphotericin B. A dosage of 50 to 150 mg/kg/day is given in four divided doses. When combined with 5-FC, amphotericin B doses may be lowered to 0.3 mg/kg/day, and both drugs may be administered for 6 weeks for cryptococcal meningitis. Bone marrow suppression, nausea, vomiting, and hepatotoxicity (signaled by an elevation in serum transaminase levels) may occur. Severe bone marrow suppression may necessitate discontinuance of 5-FC. The dosage should be reduced in accordance with the manufacturer's recommendations if there is an increasing BUN level or abnormal creatinine clearance. 5-FC may be combined with amphotericin B in selected cases of systemic *Candida* infections. However, emerging resistance to 5-FC among *Candida* populations is frequent, and continued use of 5-FC should be guided by in vitro susceptibilities.

Imidazoles. Miconazole or ketoconazole may be used as an adjunct to amphotericin B for the treatment of candidiasis. In the case of the syndrome of chronic mucocutaneous candidiasis, ketoconazole frequently is successful when used alone. The ketoconazole dosage is 5 to 10 mg/kg/day, administered orally in two or three daily divided doses for 5 to 6 weeks. Adverse reactions include rash, nausea, vomiting, rare hyperlipidemia, or hyponatremia and abnormalities of liver function. In addition, ketoconazole suppresses testosterone production. There has been little experience with this drug in pubertal children, but children in this age group who are receiving large doses of ketoconazole should be followed by a pediatric endocrinologist. The success of ketoconazole has largely supplanted the use of miconazole, which is an intravenously administered imidazole.

Other imidazoles, fluconazole and itraconazole, are undergoing current evaluations. Fluconazole penetrates the meninges well and may prove useful in some cases of fungal meningitis (candidal and cryptococcosis). Itraconazole has marked in vitro activity against aspergillosis and may be effective in some clinical infections caused by this fungus. Miconazole and ketoconazole (5 to 10 mg/kg/day) have been used with success in occasional patients with *Blastomyces dermatitidis* infection, particularly in nonmeningeal diseases; when used, either drug has been administered for at least 6 months.

TREATMENT OF SPOROTRICHOSIS

Cutaneous sporotrichosis is treated with iodides. A saturated solution of potassium iodide is initiated at a dosage of 1 to 2 drops per year of age three times per day and incrementally increased up to a maximum of 90 to 120 drops per day or until toxicity occurs. The drops may be added to milk or juice. Toxicity is expressed as increased lacrimation or salivation, swelling of salivary glands, nausea, vomiting, abdominal discomfort, or diarrhea. A pustular, acneiform rash may occur but should not necessitate discontinuance of the drug. Allergic rashes may occur rarely. Therapy is usually given until 1 to 2 weeks following the resolution of lymphocutaneous lesions. In extracutaneous (i.e., systemic) sporotrichosis, amphotericin B is the treatment of choice, given in regimens comparable to those that have been previously described.

TREATMENT OF CANDIDIASIS

Candidal infections, as reviewed previously, will often respond to lower doses (5 to 15 mg/kg, total dose) of amphotericin B. Flucytosine or ketoconazole may be added to facilitate a synergistic action. Combined regimens should be reserved for disseminated infection, often observed in premature infants, immunocompromised or neutropenic hosts, and complicated nosocomial infections. In candidiasis limited to the urinary tract, a 7-day course of 5-FC alone may be effective. Alternatively, amphotericin B, provided as daily infu-

sions into the bladder via a triple-lumen cather, may be successful for cystitis (1000 ml/day with 50 mg of amphotericin in 5 per cent dextrose in water for 5 days). Candidal esophagitis may respond to intravenous 5-FC or to oral ketoconazole or clotrimazole (10-mg troche given orally every 4 hours for 7 days).

HISTOPLASMOSIS

CYNTHIA BLACK-PAYNE, M.D.,
and JOSEPH A. BOCCHINI, Jr., M.D.

The majority of childhood infections with *Histoplasma capsulatum* are benign and self-limited. The polyene antibiotic amphotericin B is the most effective drug available for patients who require therapy. Since amphotericin B is commonly associated with uncomfortable side effects and a high incidence of renal and hematologic toxicities, prudence in candidate selection is mandatory. The drug is reserved for those with presumed or documented serious or life-threatening histoplasmal infections. These include children with disseminated histoplasmosis, meningitis, acute symptomatic disease complicated by underlying immunosuppression or immunodeficiency, or histoplasmal lymphadenitis resulting in compression of vital organs. Infants experiencing acute progressive primary histoplasmosis and children with severe or prolonged pulmonary symptoms should also be considered for therapy.

Amphotericin B is a bile salt and buffer complex that forms a colloidal suspension upon hydration. The physician should be fully aware of the specific preparation and infusion details before administration of the drug. Amphotericin B must be suspended in an electrolyte-free solution (water or D5W) at a concentration not to exceed 0.1 mg/ml. One unit of heparin per milliliter is traditionally combined with the suspension to decrease the incidence of thrombophlebitis, although the efficacy of this practice remains unknown. The final suspension is stable for 24 hours and does not need protection from light.

Therapy is initiated with a test dose of 0.1 mg/kg of amphotericin B (not to exceed 1.0 mg) infused over 1 to 2 hours. The pulse, respirations, blood pressure, and temperature are monitored every 15 to 30 minutes. The child's condition is constantly observed. If the test dose is tolerated, 0.25 mg/kg is administered the following day, 0.5 mg/kg on the third, and 1.0 mg/kg up to a maximum dose of 35 mg on the fourth and subsequent days. Amphotericin B should be administered over 4 to 6 hours. Accelerated dosing schedules, including giving the first dose 2 to 4 hours following the test dose, should be considered in the critically ill child. In urgent situations, the dose of amphotericin B may be increased at the rate of 0.25 mg/kg every 12 hours until the optimal dose is reached. The intervals between monitoring vital signs may be increased as the child demonstrates tolerance to the therapy.

Toxic symptoms such as chills, fever, nausea, and/or

vomiting are commonly experienced during the infusion. While adverse effects tend to occur more variably in pediatric patients, usually amphotericin B is better tolerated by infants and children than by adults given comparable doses. Side effects may be minimized by premedication and/or lengthening the infusion time. Acetaminophen (10 to 15 mg/kg, maximum 1000 mg) and diphenhydramine hydrochloride (1.25 mg/kg, maximum 50 mg) given orally 30 minutes prior to the infusion are generally helpful in ameliorating these adverse symptoms. The acetaminophen should be repeated in 4 hours if the infusion is incomplete. Should symptoms persist, hydrocortisone (0.5 to 0.7 mg/kg, maximum 50 mg) may be included in the infusate or given as an intravenous bolus before the amphotericin B. If severe reactions continue, intravenous meperidine hydrochloride (1.0 to 1.5 mg/kg, maximum 50 mg) immediately before the infusion may be helpful. Fortunately, some tolerance to adverse effects usually develops with time allowing premedication to be reduced or discontinued.

Before therapy a complete blood count, serum potassium, blood urea nitrogen (BUN), and serum creatinine should be obtained. These are followed biweekly for the first 4 weeks and weekly thereafter. Significant renal toxicity in children is rarely a problem; however, in case of rising BUN and creatinine, the amphotericin dosage may need to be decreased or the treatment interval increased. Therapy should be interrupted if the BUN exceeds 40 mg/dl or the creatinine 3.0 mg/dl. Significant urinary potassium wasting often occurs during therapy and can usually be treated with oral replacement. A mild anemia also develops which seldom requires intervention. Hepatotoxicity and neutropenia occur rarely.

A universally accepted treatment schedule for histoplasmosis with amphotericin B does not exist for children or adults. In fulminating cases and in the immunosuppressed host, therapy should extend for a minimum of 4 weeks. Clinical improvement is usually apparent within the first week of therapy. If improvement is rapid, amphotericin B may be given on an alternate-day or thrice-weekly schedule after the initial 10 to 14 days of daily therapy. When clinical parameters permit an alternate-day or thrice-weekly interval, the dose may be increased to 1.5 mg/kg/day, up to a maximum dose of 50 mg. Even though most children recover from progressive primary and acute pulmonary histoplasmosis without specific therapy, those who remain symptomatic and have abnormal chest radiographs, anemia, and an elevated erythrocyte sedimentation rate for longer than 3 weeks may benefit from a 2-week course of amphotericin. Intrathecal amphotericin B is rarely required in pediatric patients for central nervous system disease because intravenous therapy is usually sufficient.

Cessation of treatment is based on clinical improvement, hematologic values that normalize, and, if feasible, negative cultures. Established signs of clinical improvement in pediatric patients with disseminated histoplasmosis are improved appetite, playfulness, weight gain, defervescence, and lessening hepatosplenomegaly. Relapses are uncommon; but when they

occur, retreatment with amphotericin B for a longer course is necessary. Relapses are less frequent in immunocompetent adults if the total cumulative dose of amphotericin B is at least 30 mg/kg.

In 1981, ketoconazole, a comparatively safe oral antifungal agent, was licensed for use in several mycotic diseases and has been used to a limited extent in children. Experience to date with ketoconazole indicates that it has a place in the treatment of systemic histoplasmosis, but sufficient controlled trials are lacking. Its use should be reserved for infected children who are immunocompetent and in whom an observation period for response will not be hazardous. Ketoconazole is administered at 5 to 10 mg/kg/day divided in two doses (maximum 400 mg daily). Gastric distress (nausea, vomiting) is the most frequently reported adverse effect. Liver function must be monitored. In more severely ill patients, initial therapy with amphotericin B (2 to 4 weeks) followed by ketoconazole is a consideration. Although the optimal duration of ketoconazole therapy is unknown, from 3 to 12 months has been suggested. Ketoconazole and amphotericin B should not be administered simultaneously.

Currently, liposomal amphotericin B (liposomal encapsulated amphotericin B) has entered clinical trials. This new formulation may be more effective, may produce fewer infusion-related adversities, and may be less nephrotoxic.

In addition, two conazoles, fluconazole and itraconazole, are presently undergoing intensive clinical evaluation and offer promise in the parenteral and oral treatment of systemic mycoses. Fluconazole was approved in 1990 for several mycoses in adults.

Surgery is rarely required for the diagnosis or therapy of childhood histoplasmosis. Surgical intervention may become necessary in rare cases when sclerosing mediastinitis or mediastinal granulomas result in compression of the vena cava, pulmonary vessels, esophagus, or tracheobronchial tree, the last-mentioned being particularly common in children due to the soft, elastic nature of the airways. In general, only children with concomitant neoplastic disease require amphotericin B in addition to surgery. We advocate a course of ketoconazole in histoplasma-infected immunocompetent children who have undergone diagnostic or therapeutic chest surgery if significant spillage of purulent material within the mediastinum occurred.

COCCIDIOIDOMYCOSIS

H. ROBERT HARRISON, Ph.D., M.D., M.P.H.

Most human coccidioidal infection is either asymptomatic or mildly symptomatic, is self-limited, goes undiagnosed, and by definition is thus not treated. This article deals with the types of pediatric coccidioidal infection that require therapy, which I classify as follows: (1) chronic nonresolving or progressive pulmonary infection in "normal" children, (2) acute pulmonary infection (either primary or relapse) in children whose immune function is compromised (by illness and/or therapy), (3) acute pulmonary infection in infants, and (4) disseminated infection (outside the lungs), including skin, bone, mediastinal mass, and meningitis.

The two options for medical therapy are amphotericin B, and the imidazole and triazole antifungals miconazole, ketoconazole, itraconazole, and fluconazole. Amphotericin B is parenteral, fungicidal, and unpleasant and has many serious side effects but acts relatively rapidly. Ketoconazole is given orally, is probably primarily fungistatic, is relatively well-tolerated, and appears to have few side effects. Early enthusiasm for this drug's efficacy has lessened, but our results in children continue to be good. Itraconazole and fluconazole have been successful in nonmeningeal coccidioidomycosis in adults; fluconazole has shown promise in meningitis. Neither has been well studied in children. Thus amphotericin B should be used in overwhelming, rapidly progressive coccidioidal disease in which quick action is desired and the side effects are justified. Such cases include *all infants* with category 3 disease and some in categories 1 and 2 (note that coccidioidal meninigitis is not included).

Categories 1, 2, and 3: Pulmonary Disease. Most patients except infants can be treated with oral ketoconazole. Although experience is limited, we have successfully treated pneumonia in Hodgkin's disease, systemic lupus erythematosus, and renal transplants on immunosuppressive therapy.

We aim for a maintenance dose of 10 to 20 mg/kg/day in one dose, higher than that used for adults. Each tablet is scored and contains 200 mg of drug. The parent is instructed to cut the tablet with a razor blade *perpendicular* to the score, and then, if necessary, break each half in two again along the score. This allows dosing in 50-mg quarter-tablet increments.

Therapy is started at as close as possible to 5 mg/kg once daily 1 to 2 hours before breakfast. In young children the pieces of tablet can be crushed into applesauce or juice. The dose is doubled after 1 week (to approximately 10 mg/kg) and can, if necessary, be further increased after another week.

We have not yet encountered in children a therapeutic failure or progressive disease on treatment. Such cases, as well as infants and those with immediate life-threatening illness (overwhelming pneumonia) require amphotericin B. This drug is administered, if necessary, intravenously beginning at 0.25 mg/kg/day and is increased by 0.3 mg/kg/day to a maximum of 1 mg/kg/day. It is usually administered daily for 10 to 14 days and then gradually decreased in frequency to once weekly or less depending upon the patient's clinical response and the degree of renal and hematologic toxicity present. The drug is diluted 1 mg to 10 ml of 5 per cent glucose in water and infused over 4 to 6 hours. Adding 1 mg/kg hydrocortisone equivalent and 2 U/cc heparin to the IV as well as premedication with 1 mg/kg IV demerol 30 min before infusion ameliorates such effects as fever and vomiting.

In the earlier literature surgical excision of localized granulomas has been recommended. We have not found this to be necessary in children, although it is conceivable that in refractory or localized cavitary disease that is not improving, excision may be desirable.

Category 4: Disseminated Infection

SKIN AND BONE. Such disease may be treated with high-dose ketoconazole as already described. Response of bone disease has been more variable than other types of disease in the few children whom we have treated. Amphotericin B and surgical excision are alternatives to be considered in unresponsive cases.

MEDIASTINAL MASSES. We have seen two children with chronic fever, weight loss, fatigue, cough, supraclavicular node enlargement, and mediastinal mass on x-ray in whom the presumptive diagnosis was lymphoma until biopsy confirmed massive lymphadenopathy with coccidioidal granulomata. Both were successfully treated with ketoconazole at 10 to 20 mg/kg/day.

MENINGITIS. The life-threatening aspect of this illness is hydrocephalus due to blockage of cerebrospinal fluid flow and/or resorption and brain stem herniation due to increased intracranial pressure. The infection itself is chronic and *not* acutely lethal.

Emergency therapy requires placement of a ventriculoperitoneal shunt with relief of excess pressure. It is important that the diagnosis be suspected prior to the neurosurgical procedure so that an occluder reservoir and on-off valve device can be placed subcutaneously on the skull in the shunt line. This device is essential for disease monitoring and therapy. We have had great success with the Heyer-Schulte assembly (V. Meuller, distributor, Chicago, Illinois), but others are available.

Ongoing therapy is long-term, usually years, and both patient and physician must become adjusted to a close relationship. The most frequent long-term life-threatening complications encountered are shunt obstruction and infection. Thus the pediatrician caring for the child and administering medical therapy must be alert and responsive to signs of either disorder and must develop a close working relationship with a pediatric neurosurgeon. Any combination of headache, fever, vomiting, change in mental status, gait disturbance, and abdominal pain with peritoneal findings should prompt an immediate shunt tap through the reservoir, assessment of shunt hydrodynamics, with cell count, Gram's stain, and culture of the fluid. Pediatric neurosurgical care must be easily and quickly available. Shunt obstructions occur most commonly in the first 6 months of therapy due to the ventriculitis of the disease. The ventriculitis produces high protein, cell count, and general debris, all of which can clog the valve mechanism.

Medical therapy consists of intraventricular therapy with miconazole plus oral ketoconazole. No cisternal or intrathecal drug administration is necessary. Intraventricular therapy is performed with the rigor of a surgical procedure. The on-off valve is closed, preventing drainage of ventricular fluid, gloves and mask are put on, and the skin site over the device is shaved, prepped three times with povidone-iodine, and cleaned with alcohol. The subcutaneous reservoir is then punctured with a 27-gauge "butterfly"-type needle and 2 to 5 ml of cerebrospinal fluid are withdrawn. Next, 3 to 5 mg (depending on the age of the patient) of miconazole in 2 ml of 5 per cent glucose in water is injected into the reservoir, and followed with 1 ml of glucose water "flush." The valve is left closed for 1 hour following instillation or until headache occurs, whichever occurs first. Intraventricular therapy is given initially on a daily basis, usually for 2 to 3 weeks, and is gradually tapered, over months, to once weekly or less often depending on the child's clinical and laboratory response.

This is an essentially painless, well-tolerated procedure. Even children of 2 rapidly learn to climb upon the examining table and lie quietly without restraint throughout the procedure, which requires 5 to 10 minutes. Parents are taught to open the shunt valve themselves. The shunt reservoirs normally last for 2 to 3 years without leakage if a small-gauge needle is used. In 9 years of experience involving 7 children and hundreds of ventricular injections, we have encountered only one documented iatrogenic shunt infection.

Oral therapy employs ketoconazole at a maintenance dose of 20 mg/kg/day. This is reached as discussed above. Pathologic evidence based on tissue obtained from our patients at the time of neurosurgical procedures indicates that, at this dosage, effective levels of drug penetrate into tissue.

Side Effects

The hematologic and renal toxicity of amphotericin B is well-known. This toxicity must be monitored carefully as therapy progresses. Infusions of drug are often associated with fever, chills, and vomiting. These have been treated with various combinations of preinfusion aspirin, diphenhydramine, promethazine hydrochloride, and, if necessary, intravenous meperidine.

We have observed no side effects with the intraventricular administration of miconazole. The most common side effects of oral doses of ketoconazole have been abdominal pain and emesis 1 to 6 hours after administration. These symptoms resolved within 6 months of initiation of therapy in all patients. We have advised parents to repeat the dose if vomiting occurs within 1 hour of ingestion. Mild urticarial reactions occurred in one patient after 1 month of treatment; these resolved when the drug dose was split and given twice daily. Two months later she was returned to her once-daily dose without recurrence of urticaria. No patient has had clinical hepatitis, elevation in liver function tests, or decreased serum cholesterol levels. The long-term side effects of ketoconazole and miconazole in children are unknown. Ketoconazole has been found to suppress ACTH-induced cortisol release and to block testosterone synthesis, although the clinical consequences of these actions are not clear.

Disease Monitoring and Duration of Therapy

Almost all patients requiring therapy have positive serum CF titers at ≥1:16 and negative skin tests. Patients with progressive pulmonary disease and meningitis have very high serum titers. Patients with meningitis most often have positive ventricular fluid fungal cultures, elevated protein and cell count, decreased sugar, and positive ventricular fluid CF titers.

The best way to monitor disease activity in nonmeningeal disease is to follow the appearance of the lesions (chest or bone radiographs, observation of the skin) and the CF titer. Both disease activity and titer change slowly, so that we usually use monthly CF titers for the first 3 months and then every 2 or 3 months thereafter. A skin test with 1:100 coccidioidin is performed every 6 months. It is of utmost importance to perform the CF test *consistently*—that is, always in the same proven and reliable laboratory. The error in the test itself is generally thought to be one twofold dilution. Thus, wildly varying titers from month to month should make one question the competence of the laboratory. Another serologic test that is of use, particularly if sera are anticomplementary, is quantitative immunodiffusion. Titers are generally similar to those obtained with the CF test. In meningitis, the above parameters plus the ventricular fluid cell count, sugar, protein, bacterial and fungal culture, and CF titer are followed on the same schedule.

Duration of treatment is unclear for ketoconazole and is generally limited by toxicity for amphotericin B. Relapses of disease have been observed in adults following cessation of ketoconazole therapy.

Our results with ketoconazole have been so favorable and the medication has been so well tolerated, that we have treated patients until their clinical disease has disappeared, serum CF titers were <1:16, and skin tests were positive. For meningitis cases, we continue miconazole intraventricularly until the ventricular fluid culture, if initially positive, is negative for 1 year *and* the ventricular fluid CF titer is 1:2 or less. These guidelines have resulted in courses of ketoconazole therapy as short as 3 months in some pneumonia patients to 1 to 2 years in other more severe cases and over 6 years in meningitis cases. Miconazole has been discontinued successfully in several meningitis cases without ventricular relapse, and our first meningitis case, diagnosed in 1976, now has a positive skin test. All patients have had steady decline in ventricular and serum CF titers.

CYSTICERCOSIS

LOUIS M. WEISS, M.D., M.P.H., *and* MURRAY WITTNER, M.D., Ph.D.

The pork tapeworm, *Taenia solium*, is one of the most common tapeworms of humans. Infection with its larval form, or *Cysticercus*, is a common cause of central nervous system (CNS) disease in endemic areas. When humans (or hogs) ingest mature eggs, the embryos hatch (stimulated by gastric juice, intestinal enzymes, and bile), enter the circulation, and are transported throughout the body. They then enter and encyst in striated muscle and other tissues, where, in 10 to 11 weeks, they become infective larvae termed *Cysticercus cellulosae*. Cysticerci are bladder-like cysts in which protoscolex has developed. Symptomatic disease can result when these larvae become encysted in the CNS, eye, or heart. Often, symptoms occur when the cysts die and are believed to be due in part to the host's inflammatory response.

Human infection with cysticerci is found wherever adult *T. solium* infection is common. Thus, human cysticercosis is often encountered in Mexico, South and Central America, Africa, India, and parts of China. In Mexico, autopsy studies have demonstrated this parasite in 3.5 per cent of the population. Although the usual onset of symptoms is within 7 years of acquiring the infection, the onset of symptomatic disease has occurred in patients out of endemic areas for 30 years or more. In some cases, disease has occurred within 6 months of exposure.

The clinical manifestations depend on the number, anatomic localization, swelling, and expansion of the cysts, as well as the inflammatory response of the host. Cysticerci have been found in almost every tissue and organ of the body. Except in eye lesions, the cyst often provokes the development of a fibrotic capsule. CNS lesions often provoke seizures and in endemic areas may be the leading cause of seizure disorders. A cyst located in the ventricles may cause noncommunicating hydrocephalus; rarely, a ball-valve mechanism can occur, causing sudden blockage and syncope. In the basilar cisterns, cysts may cause communicating hydrocephalus and cranial nerve palsy. A proliferating or racemose form may develop in this location and has a poor prognosis. Heavy cyst burdens may be associated with dementia and personality changes. Ocular cysticercosis can manifest as disturbances of vision, scotoma, free-floating parasites in the vitreous, or retinal detachment. In some cases, the retinal lesion has been misdiagnosed as retinoblastoma, and the eye has been enucleated. Rarely, myositis may also develop, although skeletal muscle involvement is usually asymptomatic.

In any person with CNS manifestations who is from an endemic area, the diagnosis of CNS cysticercosis should be considered. Computed tomographic scanning should help demonstrate active cysts with edema, old calcified cysts, or hydrocephalus in 70 to 80 per cent of cases. Magnetic resonance imaging (MRI) may be more sensitive to active lesions with edema but is less sensitive to old calcified lesions. At present, no comparative studies are available that assess which is the more useful imaging modality. Calcified cysticerci can often be seen by roentgenographic examination; thus, multiple comma-shaped or arc-like calcifications in the brain or soft tissues are suggestive of cysticerci. Careful physical examination may reveal subcutaneous cysticerci, which can be biopsied for diagnosis. In selected patients—that is, those with hydrocephalus or aseptic meningitis—myelography to demonstrate extraventricular cysts may be useful.

Serologic studies are useful for the diagnosis of this infection. Specimens of cerebrospinal fluid (CSF) and serum should be examined in suspected cases, although CSF is often more sensitive than serum in establishing the diagnosis. In addition, the presence of an active meningitic profile in the CSF is an indication to treat the infection. CSF eosinophilia is present in a small number of cases. Recently, a western blot technique has replaced the indirect hemagglutination (IHA) test as the diagnostic test at the Centers for Disease Control (CDC). This procedure has essentially precluded previous problems of cross-reactivity with *Echinococcus*. The reported sensitivity and specificity of the western blot are 98 per cent and 99 per cent or more, respectively. These tests are available from the CDC.

Even though the yield is low, patients with cysticercosis should have stool examinations for *T. solium*. Family members should also be screened. Heavy CNS infections in children may possibly be due to autoinfection in children harboring adult *T. solium*.

With the advent of praziquantel, the treatment of CNS cysticercosis has changed dramatically. Praziquantel, at 50 mg/kg/day in three divided doses for 14 days, in controlled studies has been shown to be successful in reducing the number of cysts and the CNS symptoms. However, severe reactions, including death, with this therapy, probably resulting from the death of the cysticerci and subsequent host inflammatory response, have been reported. For this reason, treatment is indicated only in patients with symptomatic neurologic disease, active meningitis, or hydrocephalus. Ocular cysticercosis is a contraindication to therapy. Steroids should be administered to reduce inflammation—prednisone, 1 to 3 mg/kg/day, starting 2 to 3 days before therapy. Praziquantel is of no benefit when all of the cysticerci are calcified. As the natural history of an isolated, asymptomatic cyst is usually benign, there is debate about the use of praziquantel in this setting. Presently, we do not routinely treat patients with parenchymal cysts whose symptoms can be controlled with appropriate medication such as antiseizure drugs or medication for headaches.

Alternative drugs with reported success in CNS cysticercosis are albendazole (15 mg/kg for 30 days), metrifonate (7.5 mg/kg for 5 days), and flubendazole. Metrifonate has also been reported to be effective for ocular disease.

Patients with hydrocephalus often require shunts. If intraventricular cysts are present, shunt obstruction may occur. This obstruction can be treated by simple ventriculostomy with cyst removal. Resection of parenchymal cysts should be reserved for intractable seizures unresponsive to medical therapy, so that an epileptic focus may be removed. Basilar cistern adhesions may require lysis if involvement of the optic chiasm has resulted in compromised vision.

Prevention of this infection is the same as that for any parasitic infection transmitted by the fecal-oral route.

MUCORMYCOSIS

JOHN F. BROWN, Jr., M.D.

Mucormycosis is a disease caused by saprophytic fungi. It almost always occurs in a compromised host. Broad nonseptate hyphae are found in the tissues, usually growing into the arteries, producing thrombosis, infarction, and necrosis, and resulting in the most rapidly progressive fungal disease known.

The portal of entry of the fungus and the type of previous debility of the patient largely determine whether the form of infection will be rhinocerebral, pulmonary, gastrointestinal, disseminated, cutaneous, or focal. Rhinocerebral and focal infections are more often associated with the acidosis of uncontrolled diabetes. Pulmonary and disseminated forms occur more often in patients with blood diseases, particularly leukemia and lymphoma.

Unfortunately many cases of mucormycosis are diagnosed after death. Although mucormycosis is rare, the diagnosis must be considered in patients who are immunosuppressed or in those with diabetic acidosis. It is most urgent that scrapings and tissue biopsies of suspicious lesions be obtained and examined.

The general management is determined by the extent of the associated disease and the pattern of organ involvement. General measures include the prompt and vigorous control of the diabetes if present and the treatment of any dehydration or acidosis. One must consider reducing or temporarily withholding immunosuppressive therapy.

Surgery plays a vital role. The drainage of sinuses or abscesses, the removal of devitalized tissue, and/or the débridement of infected tissues must not be delayed.

When there is destruction of the hard palate, a prosthesis should be fitted immediately so that the patient will be able to swallow and satisfy nutritional needs. Later plastic repair of residual defects in the mucous membranes, bone, and craniofacial structures may be required.

Baseline studies should be obtained before amphotericin B therapy, the antibiotic of choice, is started. These studies are hemoglobin, hematocrit, serum potassium and creatine, and creatinine clearance. They should be monitored three times a week until stable. There should then be weekly follow-ups of serum creatinine and potassium plus hematocrit.

Premedications such as oral acetaminophen (10 to 15 mg/kg) and diphenhydramine hydrochloride (1.25 mg/kg) given 30 minutes prior to the amphotericin B infusion often reduce or eliminate the toxic effects, which include fever, chills, headache, nausea, and vomiting. If toxic symptoms persist, 10 to 15 mg of intravenous hydrocortisone may be given at the same time. Extreme chills usually can be stopped immediately with intravenous meperidine.

Amphotericin B should be prepared according to the package insert. The concentration infused should be no more than 0.1 mg/ml in 5 per cent dextrose in water (never saline). The infusion does not need to be protected from light. The experience of many clinicians has been that there are fewer side effects if the infusion is given within 1 to 3 hours instead of the usual 6 hours.

In this rapidly progressive disease one cannot take 7 to 10 days to reach a 1 mg/kg daily dose. A more reasonable program is an initial dose of 0.25 mg/kg followed by a 0.25 mg/kg increase daily until 1.0 mg/kg daily is reached. It may be necessary to hold the same dosage level or resort to alternate-day therapy until the patient develops tolerance to a given dose. When the clinical picture improves, the dosage may be dropped to three times a week and later to twice a week. The total dose is dependent on the clinical improvement and the toxic effects of the amphotericin B; 35 to 40 mg/kg is the average total dose required.

The amphotericin B dose should be cut in half or the dose schedule reduced to two or three times a week if the hematocrit drops to 25 per cent or the creatinine rises to 3.0 mg/dl (or 1.5 mg/dl when the child is less than 10 years of age). Daily oral potassium supplementation usually prevents the hypokalemia that develops with daily amphotericin therapy.

Wound infections may be treated with 3 per cent topical amphotericin B ointment, and débrided bony lesions may be irrigated with 10 per cent amphotericin B solution.

TOXOCARA CANIS INFECTIONS, INCLUDING VISCERAL LARVA MIGRANS

DOUGLAS C. HEINER, M.D., Ph.D.

Visceral larva migrans is most common in young children who have a habit of eating dirt. If there is a high density of the ova of dog or cat ascarids in the soil, the risk is proportionately increased. Larvae released into the child's intestinal tract may migrate to the liver, lungs, heart, brain, or eye, where their presence can cause local inflammation, granulomas, and impaired organ function as a result of larval invasion or a hypersensitivity response to larval antigens. The constellation of abdominal pain, hepatosplenomegaly, cough, wheezing, pulmonary infiltrates, urticaria or papular skin eruptions, marked absolute eosinophilia (usually over 5,000 per cubic millimeter), anti-A and/or anti-B isoagglutinin titers in excess of 1:256, hypergammaglobulinemia, and a high serum level of immunoglobulin E (IgE) justifies the clinical diagnosis of visceral larva migrans in a child with a history of dirt ingestion. Confirmation of the diagnosis is made by finding an elevated titer of antibodies to larval *T. canis* by enzyme-linked immunosorbent assay (ELISA) or by demonstrating circulating larval antigen or immune complexes containing larval antigen. An absolute diagnosis is made only on finding characteristic larvae by biopsy, but this is possible in a very small percentage of cases, since the larvae are difficult to locate and often have degenerated beyond recognition.

The diagnosis of ocular larva migrans is often made by an ophthalmologist after removal of an involved eye for presumed retinal tumor. The usual signs of visceral larva migrans may be absent. Fortunately, it is now possible to make a presumptive diagnosis on the basis of ocular findings aided by suggestive ultrasonographic, computed tomographic, or magnetic resonance imaging findings in association with elevated titers of anti–*T. canis* larval antibodies in the serum. Additional support for the diagnosis is present, of course, if there is eosinophilia, a high serum level of IgE, other signs of active visceral larva migrans, a prior history of visceral larva migrans or pica, or a close association with dogs, particularly puppies.

It is important to remember the specific risk factors for *T. canis* infestation. The greatest risk exists in a household that has newborn pups and a toddler who plays with the pups. If the child happens to have pica—that is, a tendency to eat dirt from the yard—or frequently puts contaminated hands and objects into his or her mouth, the risk becomes greater. If there is an infant or toddler in a household with a dog or pups, it is important to deworm the pups as well as the pups' mother. This deworming is best done under the direction of a veterinarian. An effective drug is fenbendazole (50 mg/kg/day) for the last 2 weeks of gestation and the final 2 weeks of nursing. This practice greatly diminishes or prevents infection in the pups. Vertical transmission to pups is almost universal, and infected pups have a heavy worm burden, presenting a major hazard to infants. If this type of preventive deworming is not accomplished, single-day treatments of pups at 2, 5, and 11 weeks of age and of their mother at the same intervals with piperazine (100 mg/kg) is effective in diminishing worm burdens. For weaned pups (or kittens, which often harbor similar ascarids), two treatments with piperazine, 10 to 14 days apart, or fenbendazole, 50 mg/kg/day for 3 days, have been recommended. Older dogs and cats in households without pups or kittens should be dewormed once or twice a year if there are small children in the household or in the neighborhood. Indeed, because of the occasional occurrence of serious disease in infants and the slight danger of insidious acquisition of ocular or central nervous system disease later in childhood or adult life, optimal pet management suggests that all domestic dogs and cats should be dewormed once or twice each year. Because of the high percentage of dogs (especially pups) that are infested with *T. canis*, it is reasonable to schedule deworming even without testing for the presence of ova in the stools. Expelled worms should be promptly disposed of by being flushed down a toilet—not simply by being covered with a small amount of dirt in the yard. However, the turning over of topsoil and buried dog feces at intervals will help decrease the likelihood of toxocariasis.

It is equally important to prevent, insofar as possible, the ingestion of ova by infants and small children. This means that infants and small children should not play with pups or kittens that have not been properly dewormed until they are old enough to learn they are to wash their hands after petting these animals. If there is a habit of eating dirt, the child must be told not to eat dirt, and he or she should be given frequent offerings of cookies, crackers, chewing gum, and so on, to help break the habit. Ideally, pets should be removed from the household and yard until a child has given up the habit of eating dirt.

The child who is not seen until he or she has symptoms or until a markedly elevated eosinophil count is discovered should be treated according to the severity of symptoms. If there are no symptoms, nothing need be done other than minimizing the sources of infection. If there is significant respiratory distress with broncho-spasm, the child may be treated with 1:1000 epinephrine, 0.01 mg/kg twice at 20-minute intervals; nebulized beta-adrenergic agents; theophylline, 5 to 6 mg/kg four times daily; and diphenhydramine (Benadryl), 25 to 50 mg four times a day. For the patient with severe symptoms, corticosteroids may be lifesaving. Methylprednisolone is given intravenously in a dose of 2 mg/kg every 6 hours until symptoms have subsided, and then oral prednisone, 2 mg/kg every 6 hours, is given until the patient has been symptom free for 2 days, after which the dose can be tapered over the ensuing 2 to 3 weeks and then stopped.

Once acute symptoms are under control, the patient is covered with corticosteroids, and theophylline has been discontinued for at least 48 hours, treatment with thiabendazole, 25 mg/kg/twice a day for 7 days may hasten destruction of the larvae. It should be noted that thiabendazole prolongs the metabolism of theophylline and may lead to theophylline toxicity if the two are given concurrently. Treatment with anthelmintics without corticosteroid coverage occasionally causes dangerous exacerbations of bronchospasm, seizures, or ocular manifestations of toxocariasis, presumably because of the killing of larvae and the increased release of antigen.

An alternative drug to thiabendazole may be prescribed if there is a history of prior allergic reactions in the patient or members of the family. We observed two siblings in one family who developed Stevens-Johnson syndrome following thiabendazole therapy for ascariasis. Diethylcarbamazine (Hetrazan), 6 mg/kg/day in three divided doses for 3 weeks, is recommended.

In addition to the preceding measures, some patients with ocular larva migrans have been reported to benefit from vitrectomy or, if the larvae are visualized, from photocoagulation. All such patients must be managed jointly with an experienced ophthalmologist.

MALARIA

LOUIS M. WEISS, M.D., M.P.H.,
and MURRAY WITTNER, M.D., Ph.D.

Malaria continues to be a major disease in tropical climates, despite major efforts to control it through vector control measures. It has been established that as many as 200 million people are infected and that 2 million deaths per year are directly attributable to malaria. Malaria is an important health risk to individuals who travel to the areas of the world endemic for malaria. In addition, the continued extension of chloroquine-resistant *Plasmodium falciparum* (CRPF) in Africa, South America, Southeast Asia, and Oceania has effectively reduced the available drugs for prophylaxis.

Malaria is caused by infection with one of four species of *Plasmodium*: *P. vivax*, *P. ovale*, *P. malariae*, and *P. falciparum*, all of which are transmitted by the bites of infected female *Anopheles* mosquitoes. Transmission by blood transfusion, shared needles, or congenital means is possible. The most severe infections in travelers have been due to *P. falciparum* (PF). In addition, PF is responsible for all cases of cerebral malaria brought into this country.

Clinically, the disease should be suspected in individuals returning from endemic areas with fever and influenza-like symptoms (chills, headache, myalgia, and malaise). The fever pattern may assume classic periodicity in some patients, but especially early in the infection, the fever pattern can be irregular. PF malaria may cause kidney failure, coma, and death. Identification of the particular malaria-producing species may be accomplished by examination of Giemsa-stained thick and thin blood smears.

In cases of low-level parasitemia, examination of smears at 6-hour intervals may be necessary to establish the diagnosis. Recently described DNA probes may improve the diagnostic capabilities in low-level parasitemias in the future. In vitro culture techniques and drug sensitivity testing are not useful in most patients because of the time required to perform such studies. More important in deciding on appropriate therapy is the travel history of the affected patient. Serologic studies for malaria are available from the Centers for Disease Control (CDC) but are not useful in making a diagnosis on an acute basis.

TREATMENT

If adequate parasitologic facilities are available and determining the species of the malaria parasite is possible, treatment should be species specific, as outlined further on. If a smear is nondiagnostic (i.e., a ring forms only) or speciation is in doubt, treatment should be given for PF infection, as it may be fatal, if left untreated. In addition, a travel history is helpful to establish the risk of CRPF. Presently only the Middle East, Mexico, North Africa, Central America (North of Panama), and Haiti have chloroquine-sensitive *Plasmodium falciparum*. Help with CRPF risk can be obtained from Health Information for International Travel (U.S. Department of Health and Human Services, HHS Publication No. [CDC] 85–8280), the CDC Parasitology Branch (404–329–3670), or the recently available CDC Malaria Hotline (404–639–1610). If the travel history is unobtainable or information on CRPF is not available, it is best to treat the patient as if the infection is due to CRPF.

P. vivax, P. ovale, and P. malariae Infections

Generally, chloroquine resistance has not been described for these species; however, recently *P. vivax* resistant to chloroquine has been reported from Papua, New Guinea. Resistance to dihydrofolate reductase inhibitors (e.g., pyrimethamine) is known to occur. Suspected infection should be treated with oral chloroquine phosphate, 10 mg of base per kilogram (adult or maximal dose of 600 mg of chloroquine base or 1 gm of chloroquine phosphate), followed by 5 mg of base per kilogram in 6 hours (maximal dose of 300 mg of base) and then 5 mg/kg daily for the next 2 days. Chloroquine can also be given intramuscularly (IM), or subcutaneously (SQ), 200 mg of base (3.5 mg of base/kg every 6 hours) or 250 mg of chloroquine phosphate every 6 hours, but the injection is painful, and abscesses at

injection sites often develop. In severe infections or when oral therapy is not possible, we use a continuous infusion of chloroquine HCl of 0.83 mg of base/kg/hr for 30 hours. Electrocardiographic monitoring is essential with these drugs.

Both chloroquine and quinidine or quinine are highly effective against intraerythrocytic parasites but have no effect on extraerythrocytic parasites in the liver, which are responsible for the relapses in *P. vivax* and *P. ovale* malaria. In these infections, radical cure can be achieved by administering primaquine phosphate, 0.3 mg of base per kilogram per day for 14 days (maximal dose of 15 mg of base per day), following primary therapy. Since this drug causes severe hemolysis in patients with glucose-6-phosphate dehydrogenase deficiency (G-6-PD), especially in the Mediterranean variant, screening for G-6-PD should precede therapy. In G-6-PD–affected individuals, primaquine should not be used, since the resultant hemolysis may be fatal, but, rather, the patients should be treated again with chloroquine if malaria relapses. Usually, most cases will no longer relapse after 6 years, and ordinarily only two or three relapses occur.

P. falciparum Infections

Infection from areas without chloroquine resistance should be treated with chloroquine, as described for *P. vivax* infections. Radical cure with primaquine is not required. Serial blood smears at least every 8 hours are essential. Response to therapy usually is seen by 48 to 72 hours. If the parasitemia fails to diminish or increases, CRPF should be suspected, and the therapy should be adjusted accordingly.

In CRPF infections, treatment should be initiated orally with quinine sulfate for 3 days (25 mg/kg/day in three doses, with a maximal or adult dosage of 650 mg every 8 hours), combined with pyrimethamine for 3 days (>20 kg or adult, 25 mg/day; 10 to 20 kg, 12.5 mg/day; 10 kg, 6.25 mg/day) and sulfadiazine for 5 days (100 to 200 mg/kg/day in four doses, maximal dose of 2 gm/day). In children more than 7 years of age, tetracycline (5 mg/kg every 6 hours for 7 days) can be substituted for pyrimethamine and sulfadiazine. In infections acquired in Thailand, quinine and tetracycline should be given for 7 days in the dosages described previously. Mefloquine 1250 mg once is an effective alternative. Although this drug has not been approved by the FDA for pediatric use, for children above 15 kg body weight it has been used at 25 mg/kg once. It is not recommended in pregnancy as it is teratogenic. In children under 7 or in pregnant women, quinine alone for 7 days is often effective.

In severe infections or cerebral malaria (coma), treatment should begin with intravenous quinidine or quinine. Quinidine gluconate, 10 mg of base/kg loading dose (maximum dose 600 mg) in normal saline administered over 1 hour followed by a continuous infusion of 0.02 mg/kg/min for 3 days or until oral therapy is possible. Electrocardiographic monitoring is essential with these drugs. When oral therapy is possible, pyrimethamine and sulfadiazine should be added to the intravenous quinidine or quinine therapy. Supportive care is essential, and often an intensive care unit setting is required. The following problems are often encountered: renal dysfunction (5 per cent of cases require hemodialysis), shock (responsive to volume expansion), anemia (transfusion is often needed for a hematocrit <20 per cent), convulsions (responsive to phenobarbital or diazepam), hypoglycemia (responsive to 50 per cent glucose), and pulmonary edema (may not be responsive to diuretics). In cases of high-level parasitemia—higher than 10 per cent with the previously cited complications or higher than 50 per cent in the absence of complications—exchange transfusion is of benefit. Corticosteroids are contraindicated in cerebral malaria, as they increase secondary infections and the length of coma without beneficial effects on the parasitemia.

In pregnancy, severe malaria is often complicated by hypoglycemia, and intravenous 5 per cent glucose is recommended, as well as frequent blood glucose monitoring. Quinine should not be withheld in severe malaria in pregnancy for concerns regarding its abortifacient effects in the third trimester. In fact, uterine contractions often return to normal with quinine therapy because of the decrease in parasitemia. Fetal monitoring is essential during therapy, as fetal bradycardia is common. Cesarean section may be required in late pregnancy. Chloroquine is usually used during pregnancy without untoward effects. In CRPF malaria, pyrimethamine can be used. Despite concerns regarding the administration of pyrimethamine in pregnancy, few adverse experiences have been reported. An overall guiding principle is that untreated malaria in the immunocompromised state of pregnancy is often fatal and induces abortion, so therapy should not be withheld.

PREVENTION

All travelers to areas endemic for malaria should use an appropriate drug treatment regimen and personal protection measures to prevent acquisition of infection. Travelers should be advised to seek medical therapy for febrile illness, as even with chemoprophylaxis, malaria can occur.

Anopheles mosquitoes primarily are nocturnal feeders, and most transmission occurs between dusk and dawn. Travelers should thus reduce mosquito contact during these hours through the use of mosquito nets and clothing covering most of the body. In addition, travelers should use a mosquito repellent. The most effective repellents contain *N,N*-dimethylmetatoluamide (DEET); the percentage of this compound in the preparation correlates with duration of effectiveness. There have been reports of central nervous system side effects in infants treated with high-concentration DEET preparations.

Chemoprophylaxis should begin 1 to 2 weeks before travel to endemic areas and should continue for 6 weeks after departure to "treat" any latent infections. The exception to this rule is doxycycline, which, because of its short half-life, can be started 1 to 2 days before travel and continued for 4 weeks after returning. In choosing therapy, the risk of CRPF infection is the primary consideration. The specific risk can be assessed from the information sources mentioned earlier in this article. Insufficient concentrations of antimalarials are present in breast milk to provide chemoprophylaxis for breastfeeding infants. Such infants should receive medication as indicated below.

In areas with low CRPF risk, chloroquine phosphate (5 mg of base per kilogram per week; maximal or adult dose, 300 mg base/wk) is sufficient for the prevention of malaria produced by all species. In areas of CRPF, mefloquine prophylaxis is recommended. The adult dose is 250 mg weekly beginning 1 week before travel. It is taken every other week after the 4th dose. For a stay of 2 weeks or less, 4 weekly doses followed by one more dose 2 weeks later is recommended. The pediatric dose is ¼ tablet for children 15 to 19 kg, ½ tablet for children 20 to 30 kg, ¾ tablet for children 31 to 45 kg, and 1 tablet (250 mg) for children >45 kg (the pediatric dose is not FDA approved). Mefloquine is contraindicated for patients on beta-blockers, calcium channel blockers, or other drugs that may prolong or alter cardiac conduction. Individuals with a history of seizures or psychiatric disorders and those whose occupations require fine coordination or spacial discrimination probably should avoid mefloquine. Alternatively, if mefloquine is not available or contraindicated, chloroquine should still be administered (to prevent infection with chloroquine-sensitive malaria species and PF strains), along with the following: in Africa (below the Sahara), proguanil given daily (2 years, 50 mg/day; 2 to 6 years, 100 mg/day; 7 to 10 years, 150 mg/day; 10 years to adult, 200 mg/day); or in Southeast Asia or the Amazon Basin, doxycycline daily (≥7 years, 2 mg/kg/day, up to the adult dose of 100 mg/day). Proguanil is available overseas but not in the United States. Patients taking doxycycline should be advised regarding photosensitivity reactions and should wear sunscreen (a sun protection factor [SPF] ≥15).

In addition to the regimen just described, we provide all patients with a treatment regimen of Fansidar (25 mg of pyrimethamine and 500 mg of sulfadoxine), which is self-administered for febrile illness if medical care is not available (dosages: 2 to 12 months, 1/4 tablet; 1 to 3 years, 1/2 tablet; 4 to 8 years, 1 tablet; 9 to 14 years, 2 tablets; 14 years to adult, 3 tablets administered once and then medical care sought). Patients are told to continue chemoprophylaxis through Fansidar treatment. Patients with sulfa allergy should not take Fansidar. Rashes occurring after therapy require prompt medical evaluation, as fatal Stevens-Johnson reactions have been recorded.

If travel was to an area with endemic *P. vivax* or *P. ovale*, we administer a course of primaquine, as previously described, as no prophylaxis regimen prevents relapse. Before administration (often before travel), we routinely screen for G-6-PD deficiency.

In pregnancy, chloroquine prophylaxis is safe. Mefloquine is not approved for prophylaxis in pregnancy. Women taking mefloquine should practice birth control for two months following the last dose due to the long half-life of mefloquine and its reported teratogenicity. Primaquine, however, should not be used. Doxycycline is contraindicated. In general, we advise pregnant women against travel to areas endemic for CRPF.

BABESIOSIS

LOUIS M. WEISS, M.D., M.P.H.,
and MURRAY WITTNER, M.D., Ph.D.

Babesiosis is a worldwide tick-borne hemolytic disease of wild and domestic animals caused by intraerythrocytic protozoan parasites of the genus *Babesia*. Human infection with several species of *Babesia* may cause a broad spectrum of clinical manifestations similar to those produced by malaria: from severe and rarely fatal hemolytic anemia, with fever, jaundice, and splenomegaly, to an entirely asymptomatic infection. The most severe infections have been reported in immunocompromised, that is, asplenic, hosts. Immunosuppression with corticosteroids or human immunodeficiency (HIV) virus (acquired immunodeficiency syndrome [AIDS]) does not appear to be a risk factor for severe disease, although there are case reports of inability to clear *B. microti* infection with concomitant HIV infection. Untreated, clinically symptomatic *B. microti* infections in immunocompetent individuals are usually clinically self-limited. Symptomatic infections in the pediatric age group are rare.

B. microti infections have been reported with increasing frequency, especially along the northeastern coast of the United States. The most highly endemic areas are the islands off the coast of Massachusetts (Nantucket and Martha's Vineyard) and Long Island (Shelter and Fire Island), New York. In these areas, a 4 to 7 per cent seroprevalence rate among residents has been reported. Most European and African cases have been caused by bovine and other nonmurine strains. *B. microti* infection is transmitted by the bite of the northern deer tick, *Ixodes dammini*, as is Lyme disease (*Borrelia burgdorferi*).

The diagnosis of babesiosis should be considered in anyone with fever or a malaria-like illness who has been to an endemic area or has had a blood transfusion, particularly in those who have been splenectomized. The diagnosis can be established by finding the characteristic intraerythrocytic parasite on Giemsa- or Wright-stained blood smears. The parasite resembles the signet ring stage of *P. falciparum*, except no residual hemozoin pigment is present. In some cases, pathognomonic cruciate, maltese cross, or tetrad forms may be present. It may be necessary to examine several smears made at frequent intervals to make the diagnosis in patients with low levels of parasitemia. An indirect immunofluorescent test may be helpful in selected cases (Centers for Disease Control [CDC]). High titers (>1024) are present during acute disease. If 1 ml of a patient's blood is inoculated into a hamster or gerbil, parasitemia becomes evident within 12 to 14 days. Lyme serology should also be done on suspected cases, as both diseases are transmitted by *Ixodes dammini*.

As shown both in experimental studies in hamsters and in clinical trials, *B. microti* infection responds to the combination of clindamycin, 20 to 40 mg/kg/day divided into four doses (maximal dose of 600 mg every 6 hours), and quinine, 25 mg/kg/day divided into three doses (maximal dose of 650 mg every 8 hours) given for 7 days. In patients with very high levels of parasitemia (>40 per cent), exchange transfusion may be beneficial. Pentamidine isethionate (Lymphomed, Rosedale, Illinois), at 4 mg/kg/day for 14 days, will also reduce the level of parasitemia, but clearance of parasitemia does not occur.

In *B. bovis* and *B. divergens* infections, the clinical disease is often severe. Transfusion therapy in these cases has proved useful. In addition, there are case reports in adults of successful therapy with trimethoprim-sulfamethoxazole, 3 gm/day orally for 28 days, combined with pentamidine, 240 mg/day for 18 days.

TOXOPLASMOSIS

JAMES W. BASS, M.D.*

Pyrimethamine (Daraprim), an antimalarial drug, is highly effective in destroying the proliferative forms (tachyzoites) of toxoplasmosis, but it is not effective in eradicating the intracellular or encysted form of the parasite. Although both pyrimethamine and sulfonamides are individually active against toxoplasmosis, an eightfold synergistic activity is achieved when pyrimethamine is given in combination with a sulfonamide drug. Sulfadiazine and triple sulfonamide (trisulfapyrimadines) are both highly effective, while other sulfonamide drugs, including sulfisoxazole, are much less effective. Since renal toxicity is less with triple sulfa, this may be the sulfonamide of choice to use with pyrimethamine in the treatment of toxoplasmosis. Successful treatment depends on functional humoral immunity to maintain suppression of parasitemia and functional cell-mediated immunity to keep the encysted forms in an inactive or latent state. In fact, asymptomatic primary acquired infection followed by lifelong asymptomatic latent infection is the usual response in the immunocompetent host. Symptomatic infection with progressive disease occurs most commonly in individuals with congenital or acquired defects in these immune systems. Examples are the pregnant female, the congenitally infected infant, individuals who have primary immunodeficiency diseases with defects in humoral or cell-mediated immunity, or more commonly in both systems.

Normal individuals with latent infection who develop cancer, particularly lymphoma, and those who receive chemotherapy, which further compromises cell-mediated immunity, frequently have problems with reactivated toxoplasmosis with progressive disease. Patients with the acquired immune deficiency syndrome (AIDS) who have a severe acquired defect in cell-mediated immunity and a defect in ability to produce specific humoral antibodies to new antigens develop progressive local (cerebral toxoplasmosis) and systemic toxoplasmosis. Individuals with ocular and central nervous system infection may have locally progressive disease, as

---

*The opinions or assertions contained herein are the private views of the author and are not to be construed as official or as reflecting the views of the Department of the Army or the Department of Defense.

humoral antibodies do not permeate these tissues well. These infections are particularly more prone to progression when the host experiences transient or persistent impairment of cell-mediated immunity, as may be caused by other infections, such as hepatitis B, herpes, and cytomegalovirus, or due to other host factors such as malnutrition. These facts must be taken into consideration in the treatment of patients with toxoplasmosis. The mature immunocompetent host may require no specific treatment, while aggressive chemotherapy for extended periods is nearly always required to control infection in immunocompromised individuals. Treatment in these individuals is aimed at controlling the infection with specific chemotherapy as well as treating the underlying defect in immunity.

Specific Therapy

The recommended dosage of pyrimethamine for treatment of toxoplasmosis in infants and children is 1 mg/kg/day orally, divided into two equal doses; after 2 to 4 days, this dose may be reduced by one half and continued for 1 month. Some authorities recommend higher dosages, with loading doses of 2 mg/kg/day* for 1 to 2 days followed by a continued dosage of 1 mg/kg/day for periods varying from only 21 days to as long as a year, depending on the type of infection and the presence or absence of immune defects in the host. The total daily dose of pyrimethamine should not exceed 25 mg/day.

A sulfonamide should always be used in conjunction with pyrimethamine for maximal effectiveness. Triple sulfa or sulfadiazine, 100 to 120 mg/kg/day, orally in four equally divided doses is recommended.

Both pyrimethamine and sulfonamide are potentially toxic drugs, so patients receiving these drugs should be monitored for untoward reactions associated with each. Crystalluria, hematuria, and hypersensitivity skin rashes are associated with sulfonamide toxicity, and a dose-related reversible bone marrow depression occurs frequently with the relatively high dosages of pyrimethamine that are required for treatment of toxoplasmosis compared with the smaller dosages used for the treatment of malaria. Additionally, absorption of pyrimethamine varies, so that toxicity may occur in some patients on relatively small dosages, and favorable treatment response may fail to occur in others receiving relatively large dosages. All patients who are treated with pyrimethamine should have blood cell counts and platelet counts twice a week. Severe thrombocytopenia, leukopenia, or anemia may require a downward adjustment in the pyrimethamine dosage or temporary discontinuance of the drug. Bone marrow depression by pyrimethamine may be prevented or minimized by the daily administration of folinic acid (leucovorin calcium injection), which may be given parenterally or by ingestion. Leucovorin will not interfere with the antiparasitic activity of pyrimethamine, but it will counteract its hemotologic effects. The dosage recommended for children and adults is 5 to 10 mg daily or every other day. There are no data to establish the optimal dosage of folinic acid in newborns or very young infants, but 1 mg along with 100 mg of fresh bakers' yeast daily has been recommended by some authorities.

Other drugs that are effective in the treatment of toxoplasmosis are spiramycin, clindamycin, and trimethoprim-sulfamethoxazole, but they are less active than pyrimethamine-sulfa combination therapy. Spiramycin has been shown to be effective in the treatment of pregnant women with toxoplasmosis. It is less toxic than pyrimethamine-sulfa therapy, and it has not been shown to be teratogenic, a problem that has caused concern with the use of pyrimethamine, particularly during the first trimester before organogenesis is completed. Spiramycin can be used in this circumstance as soon as the diagnosis is made. Unfortunately, it is not available in the United States. Clindamycin is concentrated in the ocular choroid, and encouraging results have been reported with the use of this drug in the treatment of ocular toxoplasmosis, but comparative studies are needed to establish if it is as effective as or more effective than pyrimethamine-sulfa treatment of ocular toxoplasmosis. Although trimethoprim-sulfamethoxazole is effective in the treatment of toxoplasmosis, it is significantly less effective than pyrimethamine-sulfa, so it is not recommended for treatment of this disease.

Corticosteroid treatment is recommended only in conjunction with antitoxoplasmosis chemotherapy in patients with active inflammatory lesions such as central nervous system infection with marked elevation of the cerebrospinal fluid protein or progressive choroidoretinitis, particularly with involvement of the macula or the optic nerve. The dosage recommended is 1 to 2 mg/kg/day (maximum 80 mg/kg/day) of prednisone or the equivalent dosage of another corticosteroid. Corticosteroid therapy should be continued until signs of the abatement of acute inflammation, such as a significant decrease of cerebrospinal fluid protein levels, or evidence of arrest of choroidoretinitis lesions, occurs. The dosage should then be tapered and the drug discontinued.

Congenital Toxoplasmosis

All infants suspected of having congenital toxoplasmosis should be treated immediately pending confirmation of the diagnosis. Asymptomatic normally appearing infants may suffer further serious neurologic damage if treatment is delayed. Immediate treatment of infants with obvious far-advanced disease may arrest progression of the infection and minimize further tissue injury and neurologic damage. Optimal duration of treatment is not known. A minimum of 21 days is recommended, but some authorities recommend that treatment be continued for 1 year.

Acquired Toxoplasmosis

Acquired toxoplasmosis in immunocompetent individuals is most often asymptomatic. A mild transient infectious mononucleosis–like illness is seen most often in patients who have symptomatic infections, and these patients rarely require treatment except in exceptional

---

*The dosage of 2 mg/kg/day is higher than that recommended by the manufacturer.

instances in which symptoms are severe and persistent. Rarely, a severe life-threatening fulminating disease occurs, and these patients frequently have meningoencephalitis pneumonia and a florid typhus-like skin rash. Early diagnosis and treatment of these patients may be lifesaving.

Ocular Toxoplasmosis

Hypersensitivity to products of the *Toxoplasma* organism appears to be responsible for most of the inflammatory reaction that occurs with relapse or reactivation of ocular toxoplasmosis. For this reason, corticosteroids have been used and shown to be beneficial as adjunctive therapy along with antitoxoplasmosis chemotherapy. Duration of treatment is determined by clinical response and tolerance of therapy.

Congenital or Acquired Immunodeficiency

Treatment of patients with congenital or acquired immunodeficiency who develop acquired toxoplasmosis or reactivation of latent toxoplasmosis often requires long-term antitoxoplasmosis chemotherapy. Duration of therapy is usually determined by response to treatment directed at restoring or treating the underlying immunodeficiency disease.

CHOLERA
VENUSTO H. SAN JOAQUIN, M.D.

Cholera continues to be a major cause of diarrheal illness worldwide, particularly in Asia and Africa. The present cholera pandemic, which began in 1961, is the seventh since 1817. In the United States, the Gulf Coast is an endemic locale. Although there is a spectrum of clinical severity in cholera, the severe form of the disease results in the most copious infection-induced diarrhea in humans. If replacement therapy is being given, the volume of the watery stools passed in 24 to 48 hours can be the equivalent of the patient's body weight. Death results from severe dehydration and its complications. The mortality in untreated cases is 50 to 70 per cent. All the same, the principle of managing cholera is simple, and with early and appropriate therapeutic intervention, mortality should be negligible.

PATHOPHYSIOLOGY

Vibrio cholerae is a noninvasive enteropathogen that elaborates an enterotoxin (cholera toxin) that acts topically on enterocytes, stimulating them to secrete large amounts of fluid and electrolytes. After ingestion, the vibrios that survive the acidity of the stomach penetrate the mucous coat of the small intestines and adhere to the enterocytes of the crypts and villi. By itself, the adherence to the intestinal mucosa is a benign event. No identifiable structural injury or inflammatory reaction results from the membrane-to-membrane attachment. At the mucosal surface, the vibrios multiply and actively elaborate an enterotoxin. The cholera toxin is composed of one A subunit, which is further subdivided

into A_1 and A_2, and five identical B subunits. The B subunits bind the cholera toxin irreversibly to the monosialosyl ganglioside (GM-1) receptors on enterocytes, allowing the A subunit to be transferred across the plasma membrane into the cell. The nonenzymatic A_2 is believed to hold A_1 and the B subunits together. In the enterocyte, A_1 causes a sustained increase in adenyl cyclase activity, resulting in intracellular accumulation of cyclic adenosine monophosphate (AMP). The increase in cyclic AMP causes active secretion of fluid and salt by the crypt and villi cells and overwhelms the absorptive capacity of the intestinal mucosa. In adults, isotonic fluid losses of up to 1 L/hr may occur.

The secreted fluid is rich in sodium, potassium, chloride, and bicarbonate and contains a small amount of proteins. The copious production and subsequent loss of this fluid can rapidly cause severe dehydration, electrolyte disturbances, metabolic acidosis, shock, renal shutdown, and death unless replacement measures are instituted promptly. In children, probably because of low reserve, hypoglycemia may develop and manifest as loss of consciousness and convulsions.

Despite the massive secretory activity, the enterocytes are not damaged and are functionally intact. In particular, the glucose-facilitated cotransport of sodium and chloride in the small intestines is not affected.

THERAPY

The primary aim of therapy is the replacement of fluid and electrolyte losses; antibiotic treatment is of secondary importance. Cholera is a self-limited illness that may last up to 6 days. If water and salt are replaced as they are secreted and lost in the stools, mortality from cholera could be almost completely prevented. Minimizing nutritional insult during the illness is a corollary objective of the management plan. The latter is particularly germane for children in the Third World, where malnutrition of varying degree is rampant.

Patients who are in shock, are unconscious, have ileus, or otherwise are severely dehydrated (≥ 10 per cent dehydrated) should receive rapid intravenous rehydration. Ringer's lactated or a similar polyelectrolyte solution is given at a rate of 40 ml/kg/hr until blood pressure, state of consciousness, pulse rate, and bowel sounds return to normal. Colloidal plasma expanders, vasopressors, and steroids are not indicated. The patient's state of hydration is reassessed, and management for mild or moderate dehydration is instituted, as suggested below.

Unless vomiting is intractable, oral rehydration with a glucose-electrolyte solution is preferred. Experience in the Third World shows that vomiting per se need not be a contraindication to oral hydration. In such instances, the solution can be given by spoon or through a nipple; usually, only a small fraction of what the child can tolerate is lost by emesis. The success of oral rehydration is predicated on the continued absorption of sodium (and water) associated with active glucose transport in the enterocytes, even in the presence of enterotoxin-induced diarrhea.

Rehydration, or the correction of the existing dehydration, constitutes the first phase of treatment. An oral rehydration solution containing 2.0 to 2.5 per cent glucose, 75 to 90 mEq/L of sodium, and 20 mEq/L of potassium is appropriate (a solution with a similar composition can be used intravenously when indicated). An amount from 40 to 75 ml/kg, depending on the estimated deficit, should be given in 4 hours. After rehydration, the second phase of treatment—that is, the replacement of ongoing fluid and salt losses—is begun, using an oral maintenance solution. The maintenance solution differs from the rehydration solution (Table 1) in its lower sodium concentration (40 to 60 mEq/L). The administered volume of the maintenance solution should not exceed 150 ml/kg/24 hr. If additional fluid is needed, water, breast milk, or other low-solute fluids should be used. Oral solutions with a composition similar to the rehydrating solution cited previously have been used in Third World countries for both rehydration and maintenance. Hypernatremia, which is a theoretical risk with this regimen, has not been a problem, although some children develop transient periorbital edema. If, by necessity, such a solution is used for maintenance therapy, it is probably best given with free water at a 1:1 ratio.

Altered sensorium and convulsions should prompt investigation and management of hypoglycemia, hypernatremia, or cerebral edema. Replacement of potassium may be indicated even in the presence of anuria to prevent hypokalemia-induced cardiac arrhythmias. Conservative treatment of renal failure is appropriate.

Antibiotic treatment shortens morbidity, reduces the amount of fluid and electrolytes needed for replacement therapy, and decreases the period of vibrio shedding. Tetracycline, 30 mg/kg/day, given every 6 hours for 2 to 3 days, is the antibiotic of choice, although occasional strains of *V. cholerae* have been found to be resistant to tetracycline. The relatively small amount of drug used in this setting is unlikely to result in dental or skeletal side effects. *V. cholerae* is also generally sensitive to trimethoprim-sulfamethoxazole, chloramphenicol, furazolidone, and aminoglycosides.

Oral feeding should be reinstituted as early as possible, that is, as soon as vomiting is controlled. Breast milk or lactose-free formula is preferred for unweaned babies; a regular diet may be resumed in older children. Preventing the aggravation of a pre-existing malnourished state or the development of diarrhea-induced malnutrition is the goal of early feeding. In Asia, where rice is the staple food, a rice-based oral rehydration

TABLE 1. Composition of Oral Rehydration and Maintenance Solutions for Pediatric Patients

	Rehydration Solution	Maintenance Solution
Glucose	2.0–2.5% (110–140 mM/L)	2.0–2.5% (110–140 mM/L)
Sodium	75–90 mEq/L	40–60 mEq/L
Potassium	20 mEq/L	20 mEq/L
Anions	20–30% as base (acetate, lactate, citrate, or bicarbonate); remainder as chloride	20–30% as base (acetate, lactate, citrate, or bicarbonate); remainder as chloride

Adapted from the American Academy of Pediatrics Committee on Nutrition. Use of oral fluid therapy and posttreatment feeding following enteritis in children in a developed country. Pediatrics 75:358, 1985.

solution has been used with results that are as good, if not better, than those achieved with the glucose-electrolyte preparation. In the rice-based solution, rice powder (30 to 80 gm/L) replaces glucose; electrolyte contents are the same. At the highest concentration of rice (80 gm of rice powder boiled in 1 L of water, before electrolytes are added), the solution provides four times more calories than does the glucose-electrolyte preparation. In addition, rice is 7 to 10 per cent protein. The use of rice-based oral rehydration solution may meet the needs for rehydration and early feeding in developing countries.

PREVENTION

Good hygiene practices and sanitation are of primary importance in controlling cholera, but these measures are difficult to implement in poor, developing countries.

Immunity to cholera stems from the development of local vibriocidal antibody and antitoxin, which appear to be synergistic. Hence, the ideal vaccine should stimulate the production of both types of antibody in the intestinal mucosa. The currently available killed whole-cell vaccines, which are parenterally administered, induce a short-lived (≤6 months) immunity in approximately half of those vaccinated. A search for a more effective, orally administered vaccine is ongoing. One of the more promising vaccines being evaluated is an oral preparation consisting of purified B subunits from cholera toxin and killed cholera vibrios. This vaccine has been shown to stimulate mucosal immunoglobulin A (IgA) antibody responses to cholera toxin and bacteria in the intestines and to induce local immunologic memory. Recombinant live oral vaccines are also being tested. The gene encoding for the A subunit has been deleted from the vaccine strains.

THE MANAGEMENT OF SEPTIC SHOCK

D. H. SHAFFNER, Jr., M.D.
and S. C. ARONOFF, M.D.

Septic shock is a state of generalized hypoperfusion that accompanies systemic infection. Although gram-negative bacteria are most frequently implicated etiologically, other bacteria, fungi, protozoa, and viruses may give rise to the syndrome.

The early stage of septic shock is characterized by vasodilation. The child appears flushed and febrile. The reduction in peripheral vascular resistance coupled with increased metabolic demand results in tachycardia and a subsequent increase in cardiac output. Blood pressure is frequently low owing to a relative hypovolemia. This stage has been labeled "warm shock."

With the release of endogenous catecholamines, blood pressure may normalize; however, with intense vasoconstriction, tissue hypoperfusion results. The patient appears cold and clammy and has a decrease in capillary refill. The complications of septic shock relate to multiple organ system failure following prolonged hypoxia.

The management of the child with septic shock requires aggressive monitoring, antimicrobial therapy, and support of the cardiovascular, respiratory, and renal systems. Successful management of these patients is accomplished best in an intensive care setting.

Monitoring

Since therapy needs to be individualized, constant monitoring of cardiovascular, respiratory, and renal function is necessary. Frequent periodic evaluation of neurologic status, cardiac rhythm, and peripheral perfusion is needed in all cases.

The placement of an intra-arterial catheter allows for continuous measurement of systolic, diastolic, and mean arterial pressures. This line also provides a sampling port for arterial blood gas determinations, electrolytes, and other necessary parameters.

Measurement of preload (ventricular filling pressure) is accomplished with a central venous catheter or a Swan-Ganz catheter. In most cases, the former is adequate and safer. Frequent measurement of central venous pressure allows for precision in fluid management. Calculation of cardiac output from arterial oxygen saturation and mixed venous oxygen saturation provides a guide in the use of cardiotonic agents and vasodilators.

An indwelling urinary bladder catheter allows for the collection of urine cultures initially and monitoring of urine output. Collections of urine for creatinine determination over 4- to 8-hour intervals provide an estimate of glomerular filtration rate.

Anti-infective Therapy

Anti-infective therapy can be applied most specifically when the invading organism is identified and the source of the infection is known. Identification of the organism is accomplished by bacterial cultures of available body fluids. Additional information can be gained by Gram-stained smears of material from petechiae, wounds, sputum, urine, and buffy coats. Indirect determinations of bacterial antigens also provide useful information in identifying the causative pathogen.

The goal of anti-infective therapy is elimination of the pathogen and is accomplished by the removal of contaminated foreign bodies, incision and drainage of abscesses, and antibiotic administration. Without sterilization, hemodynamic stabilization may not be possible.

Antibiotic administration is based on the clinical setting and the suspected pathogens (Tables 1 and 2). Failure of effective antibiotic therapy to clear the pathogen results from bacterial drug tolerance, inadequate dosage, or inadequate drainage of a localized site of infection. Since renal impairment is common in septic shock, close monitoring of serum aminoglycoside concentrations and alteration of dosing schedules are often needed.

Fluid Therapy

Septic shock is associated with hypovolemia caused by extravasation of intravascular fluid and peripheral vasodilation. Fluid is required to meet maintenance requirements, to correct the deficit, and to replace ongoing fluid losses. The goal of therapy is to maximize tissue perfusion without producing pulmonary edema or hyperviscosity.

The fluids available for replacement therapy include crystalloids (lactated Ringer's solution and normal saline), colloids (albumin and hetastarch), and blood components. Crystalloid solutions have the advantages of being less expensive, easier to store, and more readily available. Lactated Ringer's and normal saline are equally effective. The disadvantages of these solutions are the need for larger volumes to restore hemodynamic stabilization and the possibility of producing pulmonary edema.

Colloid administration requires less volume for hemodynamic stabilization than crystalloids and maintains intravascular oncotic pressure. The disadvantages of colloids include an increase in extravascular extravasation seen with severe capillary leak and decreased perfusion due to hyperviscosity.

Packed red blood cells are administered to maintain a hemoglobin that maximizes oxygen delivery and minimizes viscosity. A hematocrit range of 30 to 45 per cent (hemoglobin 10 to 15 gm/dl) is suggested, while higher levels may be required when cardiac or respiratory contributions to oxygen delivery are compromised. Platelets, fresh frozen plasma, cryoprecipitate, and vitamin K should be administered as needed to maintain normal coagulation.

Careful replacement of fluid deficit is necessary to maintain tissue perfusion without fluid overload. The fluid challenge is a technique used to determine fluid requirements. A volume of fluid (10 ml/kg) is given over a brief period of time and measurement of left ventricular filling pressure (CVP or pulmonary artery wedge pressure) is monitored. In the face of a large deficit, the increase in filling pressure will be minimal or transient. When the deficit is small or absent, sustained elevations of filling pressure will occur. Further information can be gained by including serial assessments of cardiac output. A fluid challenge producing a decrease in cardiac output suggests that the left ventricle is maximally dilated, and diuretics or vasodilatory therapy may be more appropriate than additional fluid. A fluid challenge that produces a rise in cardiac output indicates that additional volume may be given safely.

The major complication of fluid administration is overload, which results in increased hydrostatic pressure and pulmonary edema. Pulmonary edema is best avoided by adequate monitoring of blood pressure, central venous pressure, cardiac output, renal output, and arterial oxygen saturation.

Acid-Base Status. The metabolic acidosis that occurs with septic shock is caused by tissue hypoperfusion and lactic acid production. When acidosis is severe (pH <7.2) and metabolic in nature, parenteral sodium bicarbonate (1 to 2 mEq/kg/dose) will improve cardiac function. Only partial correction of the acidosis should be attempted, since the complications of overcorrection include hypernatremia, hyperosmolarity, hypokalemia, hypocalcemia, alkalosis, and resultant decreased oxygen delivery to the tissues, paradoxical CNS acidosis, and worsening respiratory acidosis.

TABLE 1. Bacterial Pathogens Associated with Septic Shock Based on Clinical Settings

Setting	Pathogens	Therapy
Neonatal period	Group B streptococci	Ampicillin and gentamicin
	Enterobacteriaceae	Ampicillin and cefotaxime
	Haemophilus influenzae	Oxacillin or vancomycin and gentamicin if
	Listeria monocytogenes	suspect line colonization
	Staphylococci (with invasive monitoring)	Cefotaxime and ampicillin
Older children	*Streptococcus pneumoniae*	
With source from community setting	*Neisseria meningitidis*	
	Staphylococcus aureus	
	Enterobacteriaceae	Ampicillin and gentamicin
With suspected genitourinary tract source	Enterococcus	
	Gram-positive organisms	Ampicillin and cefotaxime
With suspected respiratory tract source	*H. influenzae*	
	Enterobacteriaceae	Aminoglycoside and clindamycin
With suspected abdominal source	Anaerobic organisms	
	S. aureus	Ticarcillin, nafcillin, and gentamicin
With immune compromise	Enterobacteriaceae	
	Pseudomonas species	Vancomycin and ceftazidime

Cardiovascular Pharmacotherapy

Tissue oxygen delivery can be maximized by improving cardiac output. Cardiac output is dependent on heart rate, preload, peripheral vascular resistance, and myocardial contractility. Each of these factors needs to be considered individually.

Heart rate is usually elevated in septic shock. A 50 per cent elevation in heart rate is well tolerated in children. If the heart rate is not elevated or bradycardia exists, isoproterenol or atropine can be used to augment cardiac output.

Preload augmentation is discussed under fluid therapy.

Afterload has many components, although peripheral vascular resistance to left ventricular outflow is the most important. In the early stages of septic shock, peripheral vascular resistance is low. Blood flow is often maldistributed and needs to be redirected. Dopamine* (<5 μg/kg/min) increases cerebral, coronary, splanchnic, and renal blood flow. In late septic shock, vasocon-

striction occurs and may be reversed with vasodilatory therapy (see below).

Myocardial contractility, which is decreased in septic shock, may be improved pharmacologically. Because of the rapid onset of action, ease of titration, short half-life, and readily reversible toxicities, sympathomimetic amines are more useful in this situation than cardiac glycosides. These agents should be used cautiously to avoid arrhythmias, vasoconstriction, and increased myocardial oxygen consumption.

The use of individual drugs needs to be tailored to each patient. For example, when adequate perfusion is established, it may be better to accept a slightly low blood pressure than to push pressor therapy further. High dosages of many of these agents cause vasoconstriction, which increases blood pressure at the expense of perfusion.

Dopamine is a sympathomimetic amine that has different effects at different dosages. Low dosages (2 to 4 μg/kg/min) yield a dopaminergic response with increased flow to cerebral, coronary, splanchnic, and renal vascular beds. At higher dosages (4 to 8 μg/kg/min), chronotropic and inotropic responses result in an in-

---

*Safety and efficacy of dopamine in children have not been established.

TABLE 2. Antimicrobial Dosages (Intravenous)

Ampicillin	Neonate	<7 day	100–200 mg/kg/day given q12h
		>7 day	given q8h
	Child		200–400 mg/kg/day given q4–6h
Gentamicin	Neonate	<7 day	5 mg/kg/day given q12h
		>7 day	7.5 mg/kg/day given q8h
	Child		5–7.5 mg/kg/day given q8h
Cefotaxime		<7 day	100 mg/kg/day given q12h
		>7 day	150 mg/kg/day given q8h
Oxacillin	Neonate	<7 day	40 mg/kg/day given q12h
		>day	60 mg/kg/day given q8h
	Child		100 mg/kg/day given q4–6h
Vancomycin		<7 day	30 mg/kg/day given q12h
		>7 day	60 mg/kg/day given q6h
Cefuroxime			50–100 mg/kg/day given q6
Clindamycin			15–40 mg/kg/day given q6–8h
Ticarcillin			200–300 mg/kg/day given q4–6h
Nafcillin	Neonate	<7 day	40 mg/kg/day given q12h
		>7 day	60 mg/kg/day given q8h
	Child		150–200 mg/kg/day given q4h
Ceftazidime	Child	—	50–75 g/kg/dose q8h
Ceftriaxone	Child	—	75–100 g/kg/day q12h

creased cardiac output. Even higher doses (>10 μg/kg/min) give an alpha-adrenergic response and peripheral vasoconstriction.

Dobutamine, in dosages ranging from 2 to 20 μg/kg/min, is a beta agonist that improves cardiac output by increasing contractility without raising the heart rate in older children. Dobutamine and low-dose dopamine may be used in combination to increase cardiac output and direct flow to important tissues while avoiding vasoconstriction.

Isoproterenol is used at dosages of 0.05 to 0.4 μg/kg/min, is a pure beta-adrenergic agonist, and causes more tachycardia and vasodilation than dobutamine. Because of the vasodilation, additional fluid administration may be required to maintain adequate preload during drug administration. Isoproterenol is used in situations in which augmentation of heart rate or further vasodilation is desired. Drug-associated complications include increased myocardial oxygen demands, arrhythmias, and dilatation of skeletal vasculature ("splanchnic steal"). To avoid this last problem, isoproterenol should be used in conjunction with low-dose dopamine.

Epinephrine or norepinephrine may be required when fluids and less potent inotropes have failed to maintain perfusion. The inotropic and alpha-agonist effects of these agents may be necessary to counteract retractory hypotension. Unfortunately, the associated vasoconstriction may worsen perfusion to compromised tissues. These agents should be used as briefly as possible.

Vasodilators are useful when left ventricular filling pressure is high, blood pressure is adequate, and the patient is peripherally vasoconstricted. Vasodilators increase cardiac output and tissue perfusion by decreasing afterload. Nitroprusside (0.5 to 10 μg/kg/min) is titrated to achieve maximal tissue perfusion and urine output without inducing hypotension.

Respiratory Support

Oxygen delivery can be addressed in terms of respiratory, cardiac, and hematologic factors. Early intervention with mechanical ventilation is required to decrease metabolic demands. Additionally, the early application of positive end-expiratory pressure has been advocated as a means of reducing adult respiratory distress syndrome.

Pulmonary edema is one of the major respiratory complications seen in septic shock and results from one of three mechanisms. First, left ventricular dysfunction with its incumbent increase in pulmonary capillary hydrostatic pressure drives fluid into the alveolar space. Second, capillary leakage caused by damaged endothelium allows the escape of proteinaceous fluid into the pulmonary interstitium. Finally, overaggressive fluid therapy causes increased intravascular pressure and adds to pulmonary fluid accumulation.

The other major pulmonary complication of septic shock is adult respiratory distress syndrome. In this disease, type II alveolar cells are damaged; decreased surfactant production results in atelectasis, hypoxemia, and diffuse alveolar infiltrates. Since treatment is difficult and mortality is high, adequate ventilatory pressures are required to distend alveoli yet must be balanced against compromising cardiac output and the risk of barotrauma.

Ventilatory support in septic shock should include supplemental oxygen delivered under pressure to keep alveoli open. Pulmonary physiotherapy and drainage may be used to avoid secretion accumulation and atelectasis. Careful attention to fluid therapy and appropriate monitoring are needed to control pulmonary edema.

Renal Support

Acute renal failure is a frequent complication of septic shock. Oliguria is defined as a urine output of less than 0.5 ml/kg/hour. Determination of the cause of oliguria requires measurement of serum and urinary creatinine, urea nitrogen, electrolytes, and osmolalities. A low fractional excretion of sodium (<1 per cent) is suggestive of a prerenal cause of oliguria (hypovolemia). A high fractional excretion of sodium indicates oliguria of renal origin.

Therapy is designed to convert renal insufficiency from oliguria to nonoliguric failure in order to reduce morbidity and decrease the need for dialysis. Treatment with furosemide or mannitol is usually the first step. Diuretic therapy also causes compartmental fluid shifts, volume loss, and electrolyte abnormalities. Patients resistant to diuretics should receive a trial of low-dose dopamine to increase renal perfusion.

The indications for dialysis include excesses of fluid, sodium, potassium, or acid that cannot be managed medically. Hemodialysis has a theoretical advantage over peritoneal dialysis, since splanchnic perfusion in septic shock is often inadequate to produce good fluid or solute clearance. When indicated, dialysis should be implemented promptly. A complication of dialysis is removal of dialyzable drugs needed in management.

Additional Modalities

Corticosteroids given early and in high doses have been advocated previously to reduce morbidity in adults with septic shock. More recent experience in adults gives conflicting results and there remains a paucity of experience in pediatric patients. Clearly, steroids in stress doses should be given to patients suspected of adrenal insufficiency. If given solely to improve outcome from septic shock, a large dose (30 mg/kg methylprednisolone) should be given early and for only a few doses.

Naloxone infusions to reduce hypotension from beta-endorphins, prostaglandin inhibitors, and anticachetin antibodies are some of the modalities that show promise but remain experimental.

IMMUNIZATION

PHILIP A. BRUNELL, M.D.

In recent years, a number of new vaccine preparations have been licensed for use. Diphtheria conjugated *Haemophilus influenzae* type b vaccine is now available for use in children as young as 18 months of age. It is recommended routinely at this age and for children up to 60 months of age, particularly for those in daycare. It is recommended beyond this age for patients with sickle cell disease, asplenia, and malignancies. As the vaccine does not prevent colonization, vaccinees who have had an exposure requiring rifampin prophylaxis should receive it. Reimmunization of children who received the original *Haemophilus* type b polysaccharide vaccine prior to their second birthday is advised.

An improved inactivated polio vaccine has replaced the older Salk-type vaccine. The indications for the use of this vaccine—namely, for immunization of adults and for immunocompromised patients and their household contacts—remain the same. Consideration is being given to using this vaccine routinely prior to giving oral polio vaccine (OPV).

Two doses of oral polio vaccine, followed by a third 6 to 12 months later, are considered adequate for routine immunization for infants in the United States. One dose prior to school entry still is recommended. Previously, a third dose was given at 6 months of age—this is not necessary.

Hepatitis B vaccine, which is genetically engineered from plasma, has replaced the preparation. The dose is half that recommended for the plasma-derived vaccine. Routine testing of all pregnant women for hepatitis B surface antigen (HB_sAg) is now recommended. Infants of positive mothers should receive 0.5 ml of hepatitis B immune globulin as soon as possible after birth, as well as hepatitis B vaccine. Additional doses of vaccine are recommended for these infants 1 and 6 months later.

A family history of seizures is not a contraindication to the use of measles or diphtheria-tetanus-pertussis (DTP) vaccine. Contraindications to pertussis vaccine include a seizure, persistent crying for 3 hours that cannot be appeased, unusual crying after immunization, unexplained fever of 105°F, greater hypotonic-hyporesponsive state within 3 days following administration of the DTP vaccine, or encephalopathy within a week after administration of the pertussis-containing vaccine.

Measles vaccine is recommended for all those born after 1956 who have not received live measles vaccine after their first birthday or had measles diagnosed clinically or documented serologically. Particular attention should be paid to college students and foreign travelers. It is recommended for human immunodeficiency virus (HIV)–positive individuals, even those with minimal clinical signs of acquired immunodeficiency syndrome (AIDS).

Under the vaccine compensation law, it is necessary that parents of patients be made aware of the side effects of vaccines their children are to receive. The lot number of the vaccine, the manufacturer, and the site of injection are to be recorded. Reporting of certain reactions also is mandated.

It has been suggested that OPV, measles-mumps-rubella (MMR), and DTP may be given simultaneously when the child is 15 months of age. The current schedule for routine immunization is as follows:

Vaccine	Age
OPV, DTP	2 months
OPV, DTP	4 months
DTP	6 months
MMR	15 months
Hib-D, DTP, and OPV	18 months
DTP, OPV	4–6 years

19

Allergy

TREATMENT OF ALLERGIC RHINITIS

BERNARD A. BERMAN, M.D.

Rapid advances in basic immunology are contributing new insights to the clinical management of allergic rhinitis. Studies of IgE production by peripheral blood lymphocytes, binding of IgE to membrane receptors on the surface of mast cells and basophils, degranulation of mast cells and basophils, and the effects of the preformed and newly formed mediators released by activated mast cells and basophils are all changing our understanding of seasonal and perennial allergic rhinitis. The concentration of IgE, IgG, and albumin is elevated in nasal secretions of allergic rhinitis patients. The identification of histamine, TAME-esterase, prostaglandins (PGD_2), and leukotrienes (LTC, LTD, and LTE) in nasal secretions from ragweed-sensitive patients challenged intranasally with ragweed pollen has confirmed the role of mediator release in allergic rhinitis.

Release of histamine and other preformed mediators from mast cells and basophils accounts for the immediate anaphylactic response of the nasal mucosa in allergic rhinitis—rhinorrhea, itching, sneezing, and congestion. Production and release of the newly formed prostaglandins, leukotrienes, and other powerful mediator substances also account for a more severe and longer-acting late-phase reaction. This late-phase reaction of the nasal mucosa typically begins 2 to 4 hours after allergen challenge and persists for 12 to 24 hours or longer.

The presence of newly formed mediator substances associated with the late-phase reaction may also account for the "priming" effect. Even when no late-phase reaction is clinically observable, a nasal allergic response lowers the threshold for succeeding allergic nasal responses. Any complete treatment of allergic rhinitis must therefore address signs and symptoms of both the immediate and the late-phase reaction.

The conventional approaches to the management of allergic rhinitis are antihistaminics, decongestants, cromolyn sodium, corticosteroids, immunotherapy, and environmental control.

PHARMACOTHERAPY

In addition to the difficulties associated with treating any patient with allergic rhinitis (incomplete elimination of symptoms, problems of tailoring the medication and dose to the individual patient, and the many idiosyncrasies of the disease), treatment of children presents special problems. Compliance is always an issue. Children stalwartly defend their turf, so that getting medication into a child's nose is no simple matter. Parents require love, patience, and more patience to administer drops or sprays. Physicians must always consider this simple fact before writing a prescription for nasal medication.

Another important point to remember is that what looks like an adverse drug reaction may in fact be a reflection of the disease process itself. The fatigue, malaise, inability to concentrate, irritability, and drowsiness can be part of the disease. These symptoms can be more disabling than the itchiness, sneezing, and stuffy nose—especially for children. Physicians should bear this in mind when patients (or their parents) complain of adverse reactions to medications.

Antihistaminics

Antihistaminics block histamine receptors on arterioles and postcapillary venules by competing with histamine for binding sites. Because antihistaminics work by competitive binding to receptor sites, however, high concentrations of histamine can displace antihistaminics from the receptor site. Consequently, antihistaminics cannot give full protection. The effectiveness of antihistaminics is reduced during peak pollen season—precisely when patients most need their protection. Furthermore, tolerable doses of antihistaminic drugs may be limited so that it is difficult to bring tissue concentrations of the drug to clinically effective levels.

The major adverse side effects of antihistaminics are drowsiness, irritability, and tachyphylaxis with repeated use. The half-life of most antihistaminics is short. Finally, antihistaminics block the effects of histamine but have no effect on pathophysiologic mechanisms triggered by the many other mediator substances released by mast cells and basophils.

For years our prescribing habits were dictated by our understanding of the structure of antihistaminics. Five major classes of antihistaminics have been identified on the basis of their chemical structure. Studies have shown, however, that there are no rules with antihistaminics. In fact, there is at least as much functional variation within the five classes of antihistaminics as between them. Because it is impossible to predict how a particular patient will react to an antihistaminic, the physician is forced to rely upon his experience in prescribing. It is advisable, therefore, for a physician to be familiar with several antihistaminics, changing from one to another as dictated by the patient's response.

Antihistaminics have important pharmacologic actions other than competitive inhibition of the actions of histamine. Central nervous system stimulation and sedation are unwanted effects, whereas the anticholinergic action of antihistaminics may or may not be helpful.

Finding the most effective and best-tolerated antihistaminic sometimes requires careful evaluation of the options, trials, and even a bit of luck. To determine the right medication and the proper dose, it is advisable to start at a low dose and increase gradually. Children should be started on a new medication after school or during the weekend in an effort to minimize the consequences of drowsiness, irritability, or personality changes that may be part of a reaction to antihistaminics.

Intensive research is being carried out throughout the world in pursuit of antihistaminics that are long-acting, are not readily displaced from binding sites, and because they have limited access to the brain, usually are nonsedating and lack anticholinergic effects (dryness of the mouth). Both terfenadine and astemizole are antihistaminics that have the properties just described. Astemizole (Hismanal) and terfenadine (Seldane) are equipotent. Their antihistaminic activity is equivalent to low-dose chlorpheniramine. (They both should be given to children 12 years and older.) Astemizole, with a prolonged elimination half-life, needs be given once a day (10 mg), while terfenadine, with a somewhat shorter half-life, is prescribed twice a day (60 mg). More than half of all patients taking astemizole are likely to gain weight—in one study as much as 1 to 2 kg over an 8-week period. Neither terfenadine nor astemizole is effective in relieving the congestion component of allergic rhinitis. To combat stuffiness, these antihistaminics should be combined with a decongestant. For the child attending school, and to minimize the risk of tiredness, irritability, and diminished cognitive function, terfenadine can be prescribed along with a decongestant in the morning and the traditional long-acting antihistaminic-decongestant combination at bedtime.

Decongestants

Oral sympathomimetic decongestants (Table 1) with alpha-adrenergic activity can constrict blood vessels of the nasal mucosa and relieve the nasal congestion associated with allergic rhinitis. Preparations of pseudoephedrine, phenylpropanolamine, and phenylephrine are used widely for immediate relief from nasal congestion. Physicians must be careful to avoid the unwanted effects of these drugs—headache, nervousness, restlessness, insomnia, and loss of appetite.

Topical decongestants are useful for opening the nasal airway so that the topical corticosteroid or cromolyn that follows can reach the target tissue of the nasal mucosa. Second, the topical decongestants are extremely effective in reducing the potential complications of aero-otitis. Children or adults with a stuffy nose derived from allergic rhinitis or a viral upper respiratory infection are at risk, when flying, of developing obstruction of the eustachian tube. Symptoms may relate to a feeling of fullness, diminished hearing, discomfort, pain, or (rarely) rupture of the eardrum. Administration of topical decongestants before, during, and immediately after flight usually provides dramatic relief.

Cromolyn sodium

Cromolyn sodium 4 per cent nasal solution (Nasalcrom), one spray to each nostril four to six times daily, reduces the rhinorrhea, stuffiness, nose blowing, and sneezing as well as the conjunctivitis often associated with allergic rhinitis. It has also been shown to reduce consumption of antihistaminics. Cromolyn sodium may be more effective in patients with higher serum IgE levels than in patients with only moderately elevated serum IgE levels. Cromolyn sodium has been found to be effective in the treatment of both seasonal and perennial allergic rhinitis. The protective effect of cromolyn sodium has been shown to be at least 4 hours, and demonstrable protection has been shown to last for 8 hours in some.

The mechanism of action for cromolyn sodium has not been fully explained. Its primary action, however, is to stabilize the membrane of the mast cell against degranulation when allergen is presented to the mast cell membrane–bound IgE antibodies. By inhibiting mast cell degranulation, cromolyn sodium prevents the immediate allergic reaction associated with the release of histamine and the late-phase reaction associated with the production and release of leukotrienes, prostaglandins, and other products of arachidonic acid metabolism. Thus cromolyn sodium is most effectively used as a prophylactic agent, protecting the mast cell membrane before allergenic challenge. Although cromolyn sodium is a first-line drug for the management of allergic rhinitis, it should always be administered with an antihistaminic-decongestant, particularly at bedtime.

Cromolyn sodium is the safest medication for the treatment of allergic rhinitis. There is no concern about overdose. Whatever rate side effects have been observed are readily reversible when the drug is stopped. No deaths have been reported.

The strategy in prescribing cromolyn sodium is to start with frequent applications. Once the condition is brought under reasonably good control, reduce the frequency of application to twice daily for better compliance.

Corticosteroids

The topical nasal agents flunisolide (Nasalide) and beclomethasone (Beconase, Vancenase) are available in

TABLE 1. Examples of Long-Acting Antihistamine/Decongestants

Trinalin Repetabs tablets (Schering)		
Azatadine maleate	1 mg	
Pseudoephedrine hydrochloride	120 mg	
Sig: 1 tablet q12h	For children 12 years and older	
*Bromfed Capsule (Muro Pharmaceutical)		
Brompheniramine maleate	12 mg	
Pseudoephedrine hydrochloride	120 mg	
Sig: 1 tablet q12h	For children 12 years and older	
*Bromfed-PD Capsules (Muro Pharmaceuticals)		
Brompheniramine	6 mg	
Pseudoephedrine hydrochloride	60 mg	
Sig: 1 tablet q12h	For children 6 to 12 years	
Rynatan Tablets (Wallace Laboratories)		
Phenylephrine tannate	25 mg	
Chlorpheniramine tannate	8 mg	
Pyrilamine tannate	25 mg	
Sig: 1 or 2 tablets q12h	For children 12 years and older	
*Kronofed-A-Jr Kronocaps (Ferndale Laboratories)		
Chlorpheniramine maleate	4 mg	
Pseudoephedrine hydrochloride	60 mg	
Sig: 1 tablet q12h	For children 6 to 12 years	
*Extendryl T. D. Capsules Jr. (Fleming & Company)		
Chlorpheniramine maleate	4 mg	
Methscopolamine nitrate	1.25 mg	
Phenylephrine hydrochloride	10 mg	
Sig: 1 tablet q12h	For children 6 to 12 years	

*Capsules contain beads. If the child cannot swallow a capsule, the contents can be sprinkled on food, such as applesauce, and then ingested.

the United States. Triamcinolone acetonide is not yet available for use in the nose. Topical intranasal corticosteroids inhibit every step of the inflammatory component of the allergic response without inducing the side effects often associated with systemic corticosteroids. Toxicity is low and the cushingoid appearance, glucose intolerance, hypertension, and other signs and symptoms of hypocortisonism have not been reported when an appropriate dose is prescribed. To maximize the effectiveness of medication, corticosteroids should be given along with an antihistaminic-decongestant.

Annoying side effects of topical corticosteroid therapy include nosebleeds and crusting. Rarely, topical corticosteroids may cause septal perforation. In my own experience, I find the beclomethasone aqueous nasal spray (Beconase aqueous and Vancenase aqueous) in a metered-dose, manual pump spray unit preferable to a metered-dose aerosol unit with the same medication. Aqueous beclomethasone appears to be more effective and less irritating than the same medication in a metered-dose aerosol.

Systemic Corticosteroid Hormones

For the child with severe, self-limited pollen disease of eyes and nose who is unresponsive to conventional medication, a pulse dose of oral prednisone, given in

TABLE 2. Liquid Delta-1 Steroid Preparations

Pediapred Oral Liquid (Fisons)
 Prednisolone sodium phosphate, USP, oral liquid, 5 mg/5 ml
Prelone syrup (Muro Pharmaceuticals)
 Prednisolone, 15 mg/5 ml

conjunction with an antihistaminic-decongestant medication, usually reverses acute symptoms within several days.

As soon as there appears to be an adequate nasal passageway, quickly introduce nasal preparations of either cromolyn sodium, beclomethasone, or both. The prednisone pulse dose that I find effective is as follows: 30 to 40 mg/day in divided doses, usually two to three times per day. On the morning of the fourth or fifth day, change to alternate-day schedule; that is, administer 10 to 15 mg every other day after breakfast as a single dose. I usually continue the alternate-day program for a total of four doses (8 days).

IMMUNOTHERAPY

The beneficial clinical effect of immunotherapy depends upon more than just the production of IgG "blocking" antibody. Serum IgG concentrations do rise with immunotherapy; but serum IgE concentrations are reduced, IgA and IgG concentrations rise in secretions, and basophil and mast cell sensitivity and reactivity are reduced, as is lymphocyte responsiveness to allergens. Contrary to earlier understanding of how immunotherapy works, its major effect may be on the late-phase, rather than the immediate, allergic response.

Patients with perennial allergic rhinitis and patients with severe seasonal allergic rhinitis with multiple symptoms are candidates for immunotherapy. Patients with less severe perennial or seasonal allergic rhinitis, whose symptoms are tolerably controlled by conventional pharmacotherapy and environmental control, are ordinarily not candidates for immunotherapy.

Gradually increasing doses of allergen extract are administered over the course of months until the maximal effective dose of allergen extract has been attained. This dose is then administered every week to a month. How quickly a clinical effect of immunotherapy is observed depends on many factors. If there is no clinical improvement during the second pollen season, the immunotherapy program should be re-evaluated. It may be necessary to discontinue immunotherapy injections. If clinical improvement has been observed, experience has shown that a 3- to 5-year course of immunotherapy is the usual duration.

ENVIRONMENTAL CONTROL

If possible, the most effective means of managing allergic rhinitis is to avoid exposure to offending allergens. Although avoidance is simple in theory, putting theory into practice is often far more complicated. For instance, patients sensitive to animal danders could easily avoid exposure by removing the dog or cat from the home. Emotional factors often outweigh the practical ones, however, and the offending allergens remain.

Indoor allergens can be controlled somewhat. House dust and the allergenic fragments of house dust mites can be reduced by meticulous cleaning, especially in the bedroom. The mattress can be covered with a plastic material to control exposure to dust mites. Dust-collecting blankets and quilts can be covered with material that can be removed easily and washed. Air conditioners, high-efficiency particle assimilators (HEPAs), and electrostatic filters all remove particles from indoor air but are not efficient for removing dust mite allergens. Growth of mold may be inhibited somewhat by dehumidifiers.

Exposure to outdoor allergens (pollens and molds) is a matter of common sense. Use of air conditioners in the car and house allows the patient to keep windows closed during the pollen season. Exposure to ragweed and other allergenic pollen cannot be reduced by controlling the growth of ragweed or other potentially allergenic plants. Exposure to molds and mold spores can be reduced by avoiding damp indoor environments in which the molds grow.

There is considerable controversy relating to the use of home cool mist humidifiers and vaporizers. Home humidity can drop to as low as 8 to 10 per cent during prolonged cold spells. Although supplemental humidification results in some patients feeling better, no studies indicate any medical benefits accruing from their use. When vaporizers are used, they should be cleaned and rinsed regularly with any household detergent to prevent the growth or dissemination of any potentially harmful particulate matter. Furthermore, excessive humidity, greater than 50 per cent, fosters the growth of the dust mite, an extremely potent allergen.

Finally, the "priming" effect associated with the continuing phase of the anaphylactic response can make the nasal mucosa sensitive to a variety of irritants, even though the initial precipitating factors are strictly allergenic. Consequently, avoidance of tobacco smoke, certain irritating fumes, and other irritants of the nasal mucosa help alleviate the symptoms of allergic rhinitis.

SUMMARY

Several points bear repeating in conclusion:

1. Allergic rhinitis has no standard treatment.
2. Repeated trials are necessary to discover the proper medication (typically a combination of medications) and dosages for each patient.
3. Start antihistaminic dosages low and build up to the maximum tolerable dose during the pollen season.
4. Traditional antihistaminics should be started at night or during the weekend to avoid side effects that might interfere with school, work, or accustomed activity.
5. Cromolyn sodium and corticosteroids do not usually give immediate relief. Patients must be encouraged to continue the program. If a regimen of topical corticosteroids does not show positive results within 2 weeks, discontinue the medication.
6. Cromolyn sodium and corticosteroids are effectively used prophylactically. This, too, requires considerable patient education because patients are often reluctant to take medications in the absence of bothersome symptoms.
7. Pharmacotherapy is only part of a total allergy program. Controlling the environment and immunotherapy (if needed) are essential ingredients for a successful outcome.

ASTHMA

R. MICHAEL SLY, M.D.

Asthma is a chronic pulmonary disease characterized by increased irritability of the airways and manifested by recurrent episodes of generalized airway obstruction that is usually reversible. One can prevent or interrupt the chain of events that leads to allergic asthma by elimination of allergens, prevention or modification of release of mediators, inhibition of the actions of mediators, or reversal of their actions. Cromolyn prevents movement of calcium ions into the cell, inhibits both immediate and late phase asthmatic responses to challenge with inhaled allergen, and can reduce bronchial hyperreactivity. Cholinergic agents such as acetylcholine or methacholine increase the formation of cyclic guanosine monophosphate from guanosine triphosphate, enhancing antigen-induced mediator release. Cholinergic agents also cause bronchoconstriction by direct action on smooth muscle. Thus, an anticholinergic agent such as atropine or ipratropium bromide can cause inhibition of mediator release and bronchodilation.

Beta-adrenergic stimulation with an agent such as isoproterenol increases formation of cyclic adenosine monophosphate from adenosine triphosphate through interaction with adenylate cyclase. An increase in the concentration of cyclic AMP before allergen challenge of the mast cell inhibits release of mediators, and increased cyclic AMP concentrations in smooth muscle cause bronchodilation by augmenting sequestration of calcium.

The chief mode of action of theophylline is unknown,

but it enhances contractility of fatigued diaphragm and can inhibit the bronchoconstrictive effect of inhaled adenosine, which is released by allergenic challenge. Therapeutic doses of theophylline cause only 10 per cent inhibition of phosphodiesterase, insufficient to ascribe the beneficial effect of theophylline to an increase in cyclic AMP due to inhibition of the phosphodiesterase responsible for its degradation.

One of the chief beneficial effects of adrenal corticosteroids is probably induction of plasma proteins that inhibit activation of phospholipase A_2, one of the enzymes responsible for liberation of arachidonic acid from membrane phospholipids. Corticosteroids can also prevent and reverse the beta-adrenergic receptor uncoupling from the adenylate cyclase system that can follow continual treatment with beta-adrenergic agonists and is partly responsible for the tolerance or subsensitivity that ensues. Corticosteroids also have many other potentially beneficial effects, including a decrease in vascular permeability and inhibition of resynthesis of histamine. Corticosteroids inhibit the late asthmatic response to allergen inhalation but are much less effective in inhibiting the immediate response.

Elimination of Allergens and Irritants

The most effective treatment for allergy is elimination of exposure to the allergen. House dust mites and other components of house dust are the allergens identified most commonly in patients with allergy to inhalants. Precautions that limit exposure to these allergens can help control asthma in such patients (Table 1). Cats and dogs are sources of potent allergens and should be

TABLE 1. Preparation of a Dust-Free Bedroom*

1. Remove all carpet, rugs, curtains, and venetian blinds. Use only a plain, wooden floor or tile. Small cotton throw rugs may be acceptable if washed at least weekly with hot water in a washing machine. Use permanent press curtains that can be laundered weekly or no curtains at all. Shades are acceptable at the windows.
2. Clean the room and closet thoroughly and wax the floor.
3. Close and seal hot air vents unless there is a central high-efficiency particulate air (HEPA) filter or an electronic air filter. As an alternative, fiberglass or cheesecloth filters may be placed over the air vents, but do not place flammable material in contact with metal that may become hot.
4. Encase all mattresses, box springs, and pillows in air tight, dustproof covers, sealing with adhesive tape where the zipper ends. Durable covers are available from Allergy Control Products, 89 Danbury Road, Ridgefield, Ct. 06877.
5. Use comforters, quilts, mattress pads, and pillows filled only with Dacron or polyester. Replace pillows each year unless encased in allergen-proof covers. Launder blankets and bedspreads weekly in hot water.
6. Permit use of stuffed toys only if filled with polyester or other synthetic stuffing.
7. Minimize furniture and eliminate upholstered furniture.
8. Dust the room daily and clean thoroughly at least weekly, including window sills, tops of window frames, and tops of doors. Vacuum the covered mattress at least weekly.
9. Air the room thoroughly during and after cleaning; otherwise keep doors and windows closed. Keep the allergic patient out of the room for at least 1 hour after vacuuming or cleaning.
10. Keep only clothing currently in use in the closet, and keep the closet door closed.

*Modified from Sly RM: Textbook of Pediatric Allergy. New Hyde Park, NY, Medical Examination Publishing Co, 1985, p 307.

eliminated completely from the houses of patients with allergy to them.

Exposure to allergenic fungi can occur both outdoors and indoors. Patients with allergy to fungi should avoid dead leaves, mulch, hay, and ensilage. Fastidious cleaning of bathrooms, kitchens, and laundry rooms is necessary, with special attention to shower curtains, sinks, refrigerator drip trays, and garbage pails. Use of a dehumidifier may be required to prevent growth of fungi in a damp basement or a damp room.

Complete avoidance of allergenic pollens is impossible, and there is virtually no habitable region where some do not abound. Air conditioning can reduce exposure to pollens and other inhalant allergens substantially, and central HEPA filters or electronic air filters are even more effective.

Irritants can cause bronchoconstriction in asthmatics whether there is also allergy or not. Cigarette smoking is the most common source of local air pollution. Both active and passive smoking can cause airway obstruction. Maternal smoking increases the frequency as well as the severity of asthma among children. Cigarette, cigar, and pipe smoking should be prohibited in the house of an asthmatic patient.

Wood-burning stoves, gas ranges, kerosene heaters, and fireplaces can be sources of irritants. Proper venting and adjustment are essential when exposure to these is unavoidable. Use of an exhaust fan during cooking can minimize inhalation of irritating cooking fumes.

During periods of intense air pollution from industry or motor vehicles asthmatic patients should avoid strenuous exercise and if possible should remain indoors, breathing filtered air.

Pharmacologic Treatment

Theophylline. Although the major mode of action of theophylline is still unknown, extensive investigation has established a sound basis for safe and effective use of this drug. There is a log linear relationship between bronchodilation and serum theophylline concentration over the range of 5 to 20 μg/ml. Most children require serum concentrations of at least 10 μg/ml to approach optimal response, but most experience adverse side effects at concentrations that exceed 20 μg/ml. Furthermore, there is substantial variation in rates of metabolism and elimination of theophylline from patient to patient, with serum half-lives ranging from 1 to 10 hours. Serum half-life in a healthy, young adult can vary by as much as 55 per cent within 3 to 4 days.

Ninety per cent of the drug is usually eliminated by metabolism in the liver by cytochrome P450 enzymes. Accordingly liver disease can substantially reduce clearance of the drug, increasing serum concentrations from a given dose. Other factors that can decrease theophylline clearance include heart failure, viral respiratory diseases, and concurrent treatment with erythromycin, troleandomycin, norfloxacin, ciprofloxacin, oral contraceptives, allopurinol, and cimetidine. Ranitidine has less effect than cimetidine on theophylline clearance. Propranolol also decreases theophylline clearance, but its use is generally contraindicated in asthmatics. Dietary xanthines found in chocolate, coffee, tea, and colas can cause modest decreases in clearance, and so can high-carbohydrate diets. Renal failure has a negligible effect because only 10 per cent of the drug is excreted without prior biotransformation.

Factors that can increase clearance of theophylline, decreasing the serum concentration, include smoking tobacco or marijuana, including passive smoking; ingestion of charcoal-broiled beef; high-protein diets; and treatment with phenobarbital, phenytoin, carbamazepine, rifampicin, nifedipine, or intravenous isoproterenol.

Rates of elimination also vary with age. Average doses are shown in Table 2, but because of individual variations in rates of clearance and variations in the serum concentration at which adverse effects occur from patient to patient, I recommend starting at approximately two-thirds the average dose and later increasing the dose gradually if necessary to the average dose. Factors known to alter theophylline clearance require modification of the dosage, and signs or symptoms of possible theophylline toxicity may necessitate a reduction in dosage. Maintenance dosage should be based upon ideal body weight for obese patients.

Determination of serum theophylline concentrations is often necessary to ensure optimal therapy. Peak concentrations are most helpful in assuring administration of safe doses. Peak concentrations usually occur ½ to 1½ hours after administration of liquid theophylline preparations and 1½ to 2½ hours after administration of a plain tablet or capsule. Peak concentrations that follow administration of a slow-release preparation are more difficult to predict but usually occur 4 to 8 hours after administration of most products and 6 to 10 hours after Theo-Dur, Sustaire, or Uniphyl. Absorption of slow-release preparations is delayed at night, possibly owing to the recumbent position, and the peak concentration may not occur until the following morning. Administration of a slow-release preparation with a meal usually delays attainment of the peak concentration by 1 to 2 hours but causes much more extreme delays for products such as Theolair-SR with pH-dependent dissolution. Administration of Theo-Dur Sprinkle (but not Theo-Dur tablets) with meals not only delays the peak but also substantially reduces bioavailability. Theo-Dur Sprinkle should be administered at least 1 hour before or 2 hours after meals. Slow-release preparations are helpful even in children too young to swallow capsules because the beads from the capsule can be sprinkled on a teaspoonful of applesauce and swallowed without alteration in the slow-release properties. The child must not chew the beads, however, and slow-release tablets must be broken only where scored. Decreasing the number of doses required daily enhances compliance. Capsules cannot be divided accurately because many beads may contain no theophylline.

Table 3 shows recommended changes in dosage for various peak serum theophylline concentrations at steady state after five half-lives of the drug (usually within 20 to 36 hours after regular dosing has started) for patients in whom inadequate control of symptoms suggests a need for an increase in dosage. Changes in

TABLE 2. Average Doses of Theophylline by Age

<1 year old	0.3 × age (weeks) + 8 mg/kg/day
1–9 years old	24 mg/kg/day
9–12 years old	20 mg/kg/day
12–18 years old	16 mg/kg/day
>18 years old	12 mg/kg/day

dosage should be cautious near concentrations of 10 to 20 µg/ml, because a change of 10 per cent in dosage may cause a greater change in the serum concentration.

Signs and symptoms of theophylline toxicity include restlessness, nausea, vomiting, irritability, headache, abdominal pain, hematemesis, twitching, convulsions, pallor, fever, and coma. Most children have adverse side effects if the serum concentration exceeds 20 µg/ml, but some have side effects at concentrations as low as 15 µg/ml, and rare children cannot tolerate concentrations of 10 µg/ml. Convulsions are rare at concentrations less than 30 µg/ml.

Treatment of serious toxicity from oral administration of the drug includes induction of vomiting or gastric lavage followed by administration of a slurry of 30 gm activated charcoal. If ipecac has been administered to induce vomiting, one should delay administration of the charcoal until after emesis because charcoal adsorbs ipecac. Administration of charcoal several times at intervals of 2 hours or less can be of further benefit, especially after ingestion of a slow-release preparation. The charcoal can even remove theophylline that has already been absorbed. A saline cathartic is also indicated. Hemoperfusion with resin or activated charcoal cartridges may be indicated for concentrations of 60 µg/ml or more 4 hours after ingestion and may merit consideration for serum concentrations of 40 to 60 µg/ml if clearance is unusually slow or if there are symptoms of toxicity.

Beta-Adrenergic Agonists. Although isoproterenol is one of the most effective bronchodilators, it has a short duration of action of only 1 to 2 hours. Another limitation is the decrease in arterial PO_2 of a few torr that can follow its inhalation despite lessening of airway obstruction. This phenomenon, also observed after subcutaneous administration of epinephrine or treatment with intravenous aminophylline, is probably due to

TABLE 3. Theophylline Dosage Adjustments Recommended for Various Peak Serum Concentrations*

Serum Concentration (µg/ml)	Adjustment in Total Daily Dosage
<5	100% increase in 2–4 equal increments at intervals of 2 days
5–7.5	50% increase in 2 equal increments at intervals of 2 days
8–10	20% increase
11–13	10% increase if necessary for control of symptoms
14–20	10% decrease if side effects present
21–25	10% decrease
26–30	25% decrease after omitting next dose
31–35	33% decrease after omitting next dose
>35	50% decrease or more after omitting next 2 doses

*From Hendeles L, et al: Am J Dis Child 132:876, 1978; and Sly RM: Textbook of Pediatric Allergy. New Hyde Park, NY, Medical Examination Publishing Co, 1985, p 115.

aggravation of the ventilation-perfusion imbalance typical of acute asthma. It can be prevented by simultaneous administration of supplemental oxygen.

Efforts to develop safer drugs with longer durations of action have led to the introduction of metaproterenol, bitolterol mesylate, terbutaline, albuterol, fenoterol, and pirbuterol, which elicit longer lasting bronchodilation than isoproterenol (5 to 6 hours or more after inhalation for the last four; 6 to 8 hours for bitolterol) and most are effective after oral administration. Inhalation is the route of choice for their administration because of rapid bronchodilation after very small doses that cause minimal side effects, including very little cardiac stimulation at doses usually recommended. Oral or intravenous administration does cause cardiac stimulation.

Metered-dose inhalers usually deliver drugs as effectively as powered nebulizers, which may require six to eight times as much drug for the same bronchodilating effect. The bronchodilator is best delivered from a metered-dose inhaler during a slow inhalation from functional residual capacity (the end of a quiet exhalation) to total lung capacity followed by breathholding for 10 seconds. Intervals of several minutes between inhalations enhance response to two or three inhalations. Use of a spacer tube or cone can increase pulmonary deposition of aerosol by permitting evaporation of the large propellant particle that surrounds the bronchodilator particle, reducing the particle size to one more consistent with delivery to the lower airway, and by allowing a decrease in the speed of the particles before they reach the patient, reducing deposition in the pharynx by impaction. Use of a chamber such as the Inhal-Aid, InspirEase, or Aerochamber obviates the need for synchronization of inhalation with actuation of the canister, enabling children as young as 3 years of age to receive effective treatment with metered-dose inhalers.

Continual treatment with either inhaled or oral beta-agonist drugs can elicit tolerance or subsensitivity manifested by some decrease in the peak and duration of bronchodilation that follows each dose. Regular treatment with terbutaline, albuterol, or fenoterol for 12 to 13 weeks may reduce peak improvement in parameters of airway obstruction and duration of bronchodilation after a given dose by 30 to 60 per cent. When tolerance occurs, it has usually become maximal within the first 2 weeks of continual treatment and may apply to all beta-adrenergic drugs, not just the drug that induced the tolerance. Adrenal corticosteroids administered by intravenous injection can restore beta-adrenergic responsiveness within 1 hour in such patients, however, and oral or inhaled corticosteroids can minimize tolerance induced by concurrent treatment with a beta-agonist. Continual treatment with a beta-agonist can induce tolerance to tachycardia and tremor as well as to bronchodilation.

Beta-adrenergic agonists and theophylline can have additive effects on bronchodilation when used together. Combined therapy can sometimes minimize adverse side effects by reducing the dose of each drug required for the same bronchodilating effect. Administration of bronchodilators concurrently by both inhaled and systemic routes may also enhance bronchodilation.

Concurrent treatment with theophylline and an oral beta-agonist has caused chest pain with electrocardiographic changes in a few asthmatic children in whom symptoms and electrocardiographic abnormalities resolved after discontinuation of the beta-agonist. Orally administered beta-agonists can cause premature ventricular contractions in susceptible adults with chronic obstructive pulmonary disease. Administration even by inhalation can cause chest pain with electrocardiographic changes in rare asthmatic adults with cardiovascular disease. In general these drugs seem quite safe at recommended doses, however. The chief potential hazard of their use may be overdependence in a patient who may use larger and larger doses at shorter and shorter intervals, not recognizing the loss of effectiveness of the drug and the need for other therapy. Tolerance is less likely to remain unrecognized with the more recent drugs than with isoproterenol because of their longer duration of action. When it occurs, however, the patient must know whom to contact for adjunctive therapy. Accordingly, completely unsupervised use of these drugs may be dangerous.

Cromolyn. Cromolyn is a prophylactic drug that can inhibit both immediate and late bronchoconstrictive effects of allergen, exercise-induced asthma, bronchoconstriction induced by inhalation of ultrasonically nebulized distilled water, and the decrease in tracheal mucus velocity induced by allergen challenge in asthmatics. It can also inhibit bronchoconstriction induced by toluene diisocyanate, sulfur dioxide, and methacholine or histamine in some patients. It may prevent seasonal increases in bronchial reactivity or may reduce bronchial reactivity within 8 weeks of treatment.

Improvement has occurred in 60 to 89 per cent of asthmatics treated with cromolyn. Improvement is sometimes dramatic, but treatment for 12 weeks may be necessary for maximal response at times. The usual initial dose is 20 mg four times a day. After improvement this can usually be decreased to 20 mg three times a day without loss of control. If response is inadequate, a larger dose of 40 mg three or four times a day may be helpful. Adequate bronchodilation to permit satisfactory delivery to the lower airways is necessary and may require an initial increase in use of bronchodilators or even adrenal corticosteroids to ensure an adequate trial of cromolyn.

Children less than 5 years old are usually unable to inhale cromolyn effectively from the Spinhaler, but the cromolyn nebulizer solution permits treatment of these young children as well as the few older children in whom inhalation of cromolyn powder may trigger coughing or wheezing. The solution can be nebulized by an air compressor such as the DeVilbiss No. 561 compressor and nebulizer. The nebulizer solution is compatible with metaproterenol inhalant solution, albuterol solution, and terbutaline solution, and both cromolyn and the bronchodilators are stable in such solutions for at least 1 hour. Thus the cromolyn and bronchodilator can be nebulized simultaneously for patients who need both. Coughing and wheezing after inhalation of cromolyn powder are often inhibited by pretreatment with an inhaled bronchodilator.

Significant adverse reactions are extremely rare, occurring in only 1 to 2 per cent of patients treated. The most common minor side effect is throat irritation due to deposition of the powder. Swallowing a liquid after treatment prevents this annoyance.

Adrenal Corticosteroids. Adrenal corticosteroids are very effective in the treatment of asthma, but their use is limited by numerous possible adverse side effects. Suppression of linear growth and the most common side effect, suppression of the hypothalamic-pituitary-adrenal axis, depend upon dose, the duration of treatment, and the corticosteroid selected. Some adrenal suppression can follow even a single dose, and as little as 2.5 mg daily of prednisone can maintain adrenal suppression.

Adrenal function has usually returned to normal within 9 months after discontinuation of continual therapy, and plasma cortisol concentrations may become normal within 2 weeks after discontinuation of daily prednisone in children. Children at risk for adrenal insufficiency who encounter stress, such as the stress of a severe asthmatic episode unresponsive to usual therapy with bronchodilators, should receive parenteral corticosteroids.

Use of the smallest dose necessary for the shortest time possible can minimize adverse effects. Prednisone, prednisolone, or methylprednisolone, 2 mg/kg/day divided into three or four equal doses (total daily dose 20 to 80 mg), usually controls asthma adequately within 3 days. One can then discontinue the corticosteroid, or it can be tapered over several days. When a corticosteroid is necessary, the dose should be adequate to control symptoms, and occasionally treatment for more than 3 days may be necessary.

If continual treatment with a corticosteroid is necessary, inhaled beclomethasone, triamcinolone acetonide, or flunisolide is least likely to cause adverse side effects. The recommended dose of inhaled beclomethasone is 100 μg three or four times a day (maximum total daily dose 500 μg for children). Inhaled beclomethasone probably induces adrenal suppression only at doses that exceed 14 μg/kg/day. The recommended dose of triamcinolone acetonide aerosol for children 6 to 12 years old is 100 to 200 μg three or four times a day (maximum 1200 μg/day for children or 1600 μg/day for adults). An advantage of this preparation over other inhaled corticosteroids is the delivery device, which includes a spacer tube that minimizes deposition of drug in the pharynx and may thus minimize the side effect of pharyngeal or laryngeal candidiasis. This has not been a frequent or serious side effect of inhaled corticosteroids, however. The dose of flunisolide recommended for children 6 to 15 years old is 500 μg twice daily (maximum daily dose for adults is 2 mg). Larger than usual doses of inhaled corticosteroids are necessary occasionally for adequate control of asthma. The small risk of pharyngeal candidiasis can be minimized by rinsing the mouth after inhalation of beclomethasone or flunisolide or by inhalation from a chamber.

If continual treatment with an oral corticosteroid

becomes necessary, use of prednisone, prednisolone, or methylprednisolone as a single morning dose on alternate days reduces the risk of adrenal suppression, at least at small or modest doses. Dexamethasone is not a suitable choice for therapy on alternate days because of its longer biologic half-life.

Immunotherapy

At least 15 published, placebo-controlled studies attest to the beneficial effect of immunotherapy in patients with allergic asthma due to allergy to inhalant allergens, including ragweed pollen, grass pollen, mountain cedar pollen, cat allergen, house dust, and *Dermatophagoides pteronyssimus*. Immunotherapy induces specific IgG blocking antibody; suppresses the usual seasonal increase in specific IgE antibody that follows environmental exposure and decreases specific IgE concentrations in the serum over several years; reduces basophil reactivity and sensitivity to allergen; induces increases in specific IgG and IgA antibodies in secretions; and reduces in vitro lymphocyte responses to allergen. Immunotherapy may inhibit late-phase asthmatic responses to inhaled allergen.

Response to therapy is specific for allergens included in the allergy extract and dependent upon the dose administered. Small doses are ineffective, but treatment must begin with small doses to avoid systemic reactions to the injections of the extract. The dose is gradually increased over several weeks or months with weekly or more frequent injections to the maximal dose tolerated. The interval between injections can then often be increased to 4 weeks, and therapy is continued until the patient has been free of significant symptoms or substantially improved for 1 to 1½ years. Periodic renewal of the extract is necessary to maintain potency. Symptoms may recur a few months or a few years after discontinuation of therapy. Improvement usually occurs in 80 to 90 per cent of patients appropriately treated for allergy to unavoidable inhalant allergens such as pollens or mites. That improvement usually occurs during the first year of therapy, but some who do not improve during the first year improve during the second year.

Immunotherapy can induce hypersensitivity where previously there was none; accordingly, treatment extracts should contain only allergens to which the patient has demonstrable allergy. Results of skin testing should correlate with the clinical history.

Immunotherapy with bacterial vaccines is not of demonstrable benefit.

Immunotherapy is indicated for most patients with allergic asthma and allergy to unavoidable inhalant allergens. It is not appropriate for those who have recently failed to respond to an adequate trial of immunotherapy with large doses of potent extracts that have included all relevant allergens.

Intermittent Asthma

Most patients with asthma experience episodes of mild or moderate airway obstruction fewer than six times each year. These patients need treatment that will afford rapid relief of symptoms. An inhaled beta-adrenergic agonist is most rapidly effective. The best choice is albuterol or fenoterol because of sustained bronchodilation and long-lasting inhibition of exercise-induced asthma. Dosage is indicated in Table 4. For children 3 to 6 years old an InspirEase, Inhal-Aid, or Aerochamber permits effective delivery of the drug from the metered-dose inhaler. Such a chamber is also helpful for older children unable to coordinate actuation of the canister with inhalation. Children younger than 3 years old and older children unable to use the metered-dose inhaler with the chamber during moderately severe airway obstruction require nebulization of the beta-adrenergic agonist by an air compressor. Albuterol solution, metaproterenol inhalant solution, and terbutaline are available for nebulization. All three solutions are free of sulfites, which can provoke bronchoconstriction in some asthmatics.

Because airway obstruction is likely to persist for several days after relief of symptoms, the patient should receive treatment with a bronchodilator for 4 or 5 days after resolution of coughing or wheezing. A slow-release theophylline or slow-release albuterol preparation is most convenient because of the possibility of dosing at intervals of 8 or 12 hours. I prefer Theo-Dur tablets

TABLE 4. Beta-Adrenergic Agonist Drugs

Drug	Route	Dose
Albuterol	Inh	0.15 mg/kg q4h or stat and 0.05–0.15 mg/kg q 20–30 min prn acute asthma (0.5% or 0.083% solution, maximum dose 5 mg)
	Inh	180 μg q4–6h (MDI)
	Oral	0.1 mg/kg tid or 2–4 mg tid-qid (>12 years old)
Bitolterol mesylate*	Inh	740–1110 μg q8h (MDI)
Ephedrine	Oral	0.5–1 mg/kg q4–6h
Epinephrine, 1:1000, aqueous	SC	0.01 ml/kg (max. 0.3 ml) q 20 min × 3 if necessary; may repeat in 4 hr
Epinephrine, 1:200, aqueous suspension (Sus-Phrine)	SC	0.005 ml/kg (max. 0.3 ml); may repeat in 8 hr
Ethylnorepinephrine (Bronkephrine)	SC	0.01–0.02 ml/kg (max. 0.5 ml); may repeat in 20 minutes
Fenoterol†	Inh	160–320 μg q4–6h (MDI)
Metaproterenol‡	Inh	0.1–0.3 ml q4–6h (inhalant solution, 5%, diluted in 3 ml saline and nebulized)
	Inh	1.3–1.95 mg q4–6h (MDI)
	Oral	0.5 mg/kg q6–8h (max. 20 mg qid)
Pirbuterol	Inh	400 g q4–6h (MDI)
Terbutaline§	Inh	400 μg q4–6h (MDI)
	Inh	0.1 mg/kg q4–6h (max 6 mg, nebulized)
	SC	0.01 mg/kg (max. 0.25 mg); may repeat in 20 min (max. 0.5 mg in 4 h)
	Oral	0.075 mg/kg or 2.5 mg q6h tid (max. 5 mg q6h tid)

Inh = by inhalation; SC = by subcutaneous injection; MDI = metered-dose inhaler.

*Bitolterol mesylate is not recommended for children under 12 years of age.

†Fenoterol is an experimental drug and is not yet approved for use by the FDA. It is not recommended for children under 12 years of age.

‡Inhaler dose of metaproterenol is not recommended for use in children under 12 years of age.

§Terbutaline is not recommended for children under 12 years of age.

(200 or 300 mg) for children who can swallow tablets. The 100-mg tablets do not have quite the same sustained release as the larger tablets. For younger children who cannot swallow tablets, I recommend sprinkling the slow-release beads from a capsule such as Slo-bid Gyrocaps or Somophylline-CRT on applesauce every 8 hours. Both the initial dose of the inhaled beta-adrenergic drug and the slow-release theophylline are started at the first sign of symptoms, but the theophylline is continued for 4 to 5 days after resolution of symptoms. Administration of theophylline once daily in a preparation such as Uniphyl tablets may be appropriate for children at least 12 years of age, and use of this convenient preparation may further enhance compliance, but meals can enhance its bioavailability.

Infants and toddlers who will not swallow slow-release beads require liquid preparations of theophylline or albuterol or metaproterenol at intervals of 6 hours.

Frequent Asthma

Patients with airway obstruction several times each month or somewhat less frequently if episodes are severe require continual drug therapy when avoidance of allergens is impossible or insufficient. Use of a slow-release theophylline preparation is most practical. Such a patient also requires treatment of acute asthma that may recur despite continual treatment with theophylline, and an inhaled beta-agonist is most appropriate for this purpose.

If continual treatment with theophylline at optimal doses does not afford adequate control of symptoms and restoration of pulmonary function to normal, a trial of cromolyn is indicated. Some recommend a trial of cromolyn before continual treatment with theophylline because of the remarkable paucity of side effects from cromolyn.

When even the combination of bronchodilators and cromolyn afford inadequate control, one should add inhaled beclomethasone, triamcinolone acetonide, or flunisolide. Both cromolyn and inhaled corticosteroids are effective only when delivered adequately to the lower airways. Airway obstruction should be controlled if necessary with oral corticosteroids when one initiates therapy with these inhaled drugs. If attempts to discontinue the oral corticosteroid are unsuccessful, it may be necessary to continue treatment with prednisone, prednisolone, or methylprednisolone as single doses in the morning on alternate days.

Evidence is accumulating that patients with frequently recurrent or chronic asthma may require cromolyn or an inhaled corticosteroid to inhibit late-phase reactions and to attenuate airway hyperresponsiveness.

Exercise-Induced Asthma

Nasal breathing or use of a muffler or scarf wrapped around the nose and mouth or a cold weather mask can minimize the airway obstruction induced by strenuous exercise. When these measures are inadequate, pretreatment with inhaled albuterol or fenoterol can inhibit exercise-induced asthma for 4 to 6 hours. Cromolyn is most effective in inhibiting exercise-induced asthma only during the first hour after treatment, although it has some effect for 4 hours. A slow-release theophylline preparation may be most convenient for inhibition of this abnormal response to exercise in a youngster who may be exercising unpredictably at any time of day, but optimal effectiveness would require continual treatment or administration of an unusually large dose to maintain the serum concentration at 15 to 20 μg/ml if tolerated. When a single drug does not afford adequate protection, combinations of an inhaled beta-agonist with cromolyn or theophylline or all three may be more effective.

A warm-up period before strenuous exercise may be helpful by causing brief, exercise-induced asthma that is followed by a refractory period that may persist 60 to 90 minutes.

For asthmatic children in whom 1 to 2 minutes of strenuous exercise causes bronchodilation while exercise for 5 to 6 minutes causes airway obstruction, activities that require only intermittent, brief intervals of exercise may be more tolerable than those that require more prolonged exercise. Swimming is usually tolerated especially well, partly because of inhibition of exercise-induced asthma by ventilation with air fully saturated with water. Appropriate pretreatment with medication enables most children with asthma to tolerate whatever activities they choose, however.

Prophylaxis

Pretreatment with cromolyn is the method of choice for prevention of asthma due to unavoidable exposure to allergen when this is predictable.

Status Asthmaticus

The treatment for acute, severe asthma administered most frequently at emergency rooms in the United States has been 1:1000 aqueous epinephrine by subcutaneous injection followed by epinephrine 1:200 (Sus-Phrine) when there has been a satisfactory response (Table 4). Terbutaline by subcutaneous injection is at least equally effective and often reduces the number of injections required. An inhaled beta-agonist is also as effective as injected epinephrine but may require somewhat more prolonged observation for possible recurrence of airway obstruction. Administration by nebulization may deliver the drug to the lower airways better than use of a metered-dose inhaler during severe airway obstruction.

Failure of adequate response to the beta-agonist establishes the diagnosis of status asthmaticus. Some also require failure of response to intravenous theophylline or aminophylline for this diagnosis.

The indicated treatment is summarized in Table 5. Correct dehydration with 5 or 10 per cent glucose in one-third normal saline or 5 per cent glucose in saline followed after establishment of renal flow by a polyionic, hypotonic solution containing potassium, but do not overhydrate when there is no dehydration.

Intravenous theophylline (Travenol Laboratories) is the drug of choice, which avoids the risk of rare allergic reactions to the ethylenediamine of aminophylline and obviates the need for calculating the theophylline equivalence of aminophylline, which is only 78.9 per cent

TABLE 5. Treatment of Status Asthmaticus

1. Intravenous fluids: 360–400 ml/M² during first hour; then 1500–3000 ml/m²/24 hours when dehydration is present.
2. Aminophylline: 5 mg/kg diluted and infused intravenously over 20 minutes; follow with constant infusion of 0.5–1.1 mg/kg/hr to maintain serum concentration of 10–20 μg/ml (preferably 14–18 μg/ml if necessary and tolerated).
3. Oxygen. Maintain arterial PO₂ > 65 torr and <100 torr.
4. Sodium bicarbonate: 1.5–2.0 mEq/kg diluted and infused intravenously over 10–20 minutes when there is metabolic acidosis. Repeat same dose over next 45 minutes and every hour if arterial pH remains less than 7.25 and serum sodium less than 145 mEq/liter.
5. Albuterol solution by inhalation after nebulization q20–30 min until improved, then q3–4 h as required (see Table 4).
6. Adrenal corticosteroids: hydrocortisone, 4 mg/kg, or methylprednisolone, 1 mg/kg, q4h by intravenous injection.
7. SEDATIVES, TRANQUILIZERS, MORPHINE, and ANTIHISTAMINES CONTRAINDICATED.
8. Endotracheal intubation and controlled ventilation for progression to respiratory failure despite these measures.

*Metaproterenol and terbutaline are not recommended for children under 12 years of age.

anhydrous theophylline when assayed as the dihydrate. Nevertheless, aminophylline is still used more widely than intravenous theophylline in the United States.

The initial infusion of aminophylline, 5 mg/kg, is safe for patients with serum theophylline concentrations expected to be less than 3 μg/ml (Table 5). Each dose of 1 mg/kg increases the serum concentration by approximately 2 μg/ml, but the rate at which the concentration then falls depends upon the rate of clearance for the particular patient. Determination of the serum concentration one-half hour after completion of infusion of the loading dose indicates whether an additional small bolus may be required to obtain a serum concentration of 14 to 18 μg/ml. Determination of another serum concentration approximately 6 hours after completion of the infusion of the initial loading dose indicates whether the rate of constant infusion of theophylline is adequate or excessive, and any required correction can be made. Subsequent determinations of theophylline concentrations 12 hours later and then at intervals of 12 to 24 hours assure continued safe, effective therapy. Some patients cannot tolerate concen-

TABLE 6. Clinical Scoring System for Children with Status Asthmaticus*

	Score†		
	0	**1**	**2**
PO₂ or	70–110 in air	≤70 in air	≤70 in 40% O₂
Cyanosis	None	In air	In 40% O₂
Inspiratory breath sounds	Normal	Unequal	Decreased or absent
Use of accessory muscles of respiration	None	Moderate	Maximal
Expiratory wheezing	None	Moderate	Extreme or none because of poor air exchange
Cerebral function	Normal	Depressed or agitated	Coma

*From Wood DW, et al: Am J Dis Child 123:227, 1972.
†Total score of 5 suggests impending respiratory failure. Score of 7 with arterial PCO₂ ≥ 65 torr indicates respiratory failure.

trations of 14 µg/ml without adverse side effects and should be maintained at lower concentrations that do not cause side effects. Lower concentrations are satisfactory whether or not there are side effects if airway obstruction has been relieved adequately.

If the patient has already received theophylline within the previous 24 hours (36 hours for Theo-24 or Uniphyl), it is safest to determine the serum concentration before administration of the initial loading dose. That concentration must be interpreted with consideration of the type of preparation administered and the anticipated time and duration of peak response to avoid overdosing a patient who may still be absorbing a slow-release preparation.

If necessary the inhaled beta-agonist can be administered more frequently than at intervals of 4 hours with continual cardiac monitoring for arrhythmias or electrocardiographic signs of ischemia. Tachycardia and other adverse effects of beta-agonist drugs are more frequent with intravenous administration than with inhalation, and response to intravenous treatment is no better than to inhalation therapy.

Inhalation of nebulized atropine sulfate (0.01 mg/kg, maximum 1 mg, diluted to 3 ml in normal saline) can cause further bronchodilation and can be given at intervals of 4 hours. Use of inhaled atropine has not been studied extensively in children, however.

Progression to respiratory failure despite the measures listed in Table 5 indicates a need for intubation and mechanical ventilation. Use of a clinical scoring system facilitates diagnosis of respiratory failure (Table 6).

Allergic Rhinitis

Control of allergic rhinitis to facilitate filtration and conditioning of inspired air is especially important in patients with asthma. Antihistamines are helpful for most patients with allergic rhinitis but may cause bronchoconstriction in a small proportion of asthmatics and are contraindicated in status asthmaticus. Nasalcrom or intranasal beclomethasone or flunisolide is often effective.

Unlabeled Use of Approved Drugs

Many of the drugs safest and most effective in the treatment of asthma are not labeled for use in children. The United States Food and Drug Administration regulates industry rather than physicians, however. Lack of approval does not indicate disapproval. Choice of therapy should be determined by all information available regarding safety and effectiveness in children. Use of a drug not labeled for use in children, however, must be distinguished from use of a drug contraindicated in children because investigation has shown it to be unsafe or ineffective in children.

SERUM SICKNESS

LEONARD BIELORY, M.D.

Serum sickness as classically described in 1905 by von Pirquet and Schick consisted of a spectrum of clinical findings that included fever, malaise, cutaneous eruptions, primarily urticaria, arthralgias, lymphadenopathy, edema, and albuminuria. Their patients consisted mainly of children who developed one or a combination of these symptoms 6 to 10 days after their first exposure to heterologous antisera for the treatment of various infectious diseases. The administration of heterologous antisera remained the major cause of serum sickness until the advent of modern drug therapy. Currently the most frequently encountered medications producing serum sickness include the penicillins, streptomycin, cephalosporins, sulfonamides, thiouracils, and hydantoins. Penicillin-induced serum sickness is the most common agent, unusual with dosages under 2 gm/day, followed by the use of sulfa-based medications in human immunodeficiency virus infected patients. The medications producing serum sickness with the highest consistent frequency are still the heterologous proteins that are currently being used for crotalid and arachnid envenomation, specific clostridial infections, and rabies and as immunosuppressant agents for organ allograft rejection or preconditioning agents for organ transplantation.

The treatment of serum sickness is either prophylactic or symptomatic. Prophylactically, all physicians should maintain up-to-date vaccinations of their patients as recommended by the American College of Physicians Committee's Guide for Adult Immunization and the Red Book of the American Academy of Pediatrics in order to immunize their patients against those diseases still treated with heterologous antisera. Heterologous antisera are still in use in several underdeveloped countries for acute infections such as diphtheria. All individuals traveling to underdeveloped countries should be vaccinated for endemic infectious agents as recommended by the Centers for Disease Control in their Morbidity and Mortality Weekly Reports. Individuals may contact their local or state health departments to locate the closest "certified" immunization center. Most cases of serum sickness are probably never seen by the physician, since the clinical spectrum of complaints is very similar to what the public perceives as the "flu" and patients are apt to treat themselves with fluids, aspirin, and bedrest. It is only the unusual circumstance of a frightening cutaneous eruption or severe arthralgias that usually brings a person to the attention of a physician for medical treatment.

Symptomatic treatment of serum sickness is based upon the severity and extent of the patient's complaints. First, if possible, the offending antigen should be eliminated. It is known from animal models that elimination of antigen will lead to rapid resolution of immunopathologic damage. Symptomatic treatment usually involves the use of combinations of antipyretics, analgesics, antihistamines, and glucocorticosteroids.

Antipyretic medications such as the salicylates, as noted by von Pirquet and Schick, are of some benefit in ameliorating the febrile response but have relatively little effect on the arthralgias or the various cutaneous eruptions. In addition, the use of salicylates must be considered in the light of their effect on platelet function, since some serum sickness patients develop thrombocytopenia. Acetaminophen (Tylenol) as an antipyretic is a better choice in thrombocytopenic individuals.

Other symptoms, particularly those associated with proteinuria or arthralgias, usually warrant treatment with a "burst" of glucocorticosteroids. "Burst" glucocorticoid therapy involves the use of 1 to 2 mg/kg/day of prednisone in divided doses for 7 to 10 days. This is followed by consolidation to once-a-day doses coinciding with the normal diurnal (A.M.) variation of cortisol levels and then tapering the drug by 10 mg decrements to 30 mg and then 5 mg decrements to 10 mg and then by 2.5 mg decrements until the prednisone is discontinued within a period of about 3 to 4 weeks.

Antihistamines have proved to be of value in the treatment of generalized urticaria and pruritus with such medications as diphenhydramine (Benadryl) 50 mg every 4 hours (1 mg/kg in children) or alternatively hydroxyzine (Atarax, Vistaril) 25 mg every 4 hours (0.3 mg/kg in children). The prophylactic value of antihistamines in serum sickness has not been proved, but these drugs may be useful. Doses of diphenhydramine or cyproheptadine are started 4 days prior to the expected onset of serum sickness and continued for a period of 1 to 2 weeks. Marked urticarial eruptions or angioedema is usually treated with aqueous epinephrine, 1:1000, 0.01 ml/kg subcutaneously with a maximum of 0.3 to 0.5 ml every 15 minutes for three doses. If attacks of angioedema recur after using the preceding treatment, intramuscular aqueous epinephrine suspension (Sus-Phrine) can be used at a dose of 1:200, 0.005 ml/kg with a maximum of 0.2 ml every 6 hours.

In the event that large amounts of heterologous antisera are required over a course of days the usual precautions as recommended by the pharmaceutical company for its administration should be strictly followed. Skin testing with the antigen and appropriate controls should be done prior to the administration of the heterologous protein. If there is an immediate hypersensitivity reaction, desensitization may be required to prevent anaphylaxis. This will not prevent the occurrence of serum sickness.

Glucocorticosteroids in the form of prednisone (or intravenous methylprednisolone) at a dose of 1 mg/kg/day in three or four divided doses should be started concomitantly with the first dose of heterologous antisera. This dose should be increased to 1.5 mg/kg/day at the first sign of serum sickness, maintained for 3 or 4 days or as long as the heterologous protein must be given, and then tapered by 10-mg decrements every 2 or 3 days to 30 mg and then tapered by 5-mg decrements every 2 or 3 days to 10 mg and then tapered using 2.5-mg decrements over the course of a week. If the antigen persists longer than expected and the patient has a breakthrough of symptoms while glucocorticosteroids are being tapered, the dose at which the symptoms reappeared (usually between 10 and 20 mg prednisone) should be doubled. The glucocorticosteroids may then be decreased on alternate days rather than daily in 10-mg decrements every two or three cycles until a dose of 30 mg is reached and then tapered by 5-mg decrements every two or three cycles until 20 mg and then tapered by 2.5-mg decrements every two

or three cycles until the alternate-day dose has been discontinued. If exacerbations occur on the off days one should increase the dose to a previous level that controlled the symptoms and then taper even more slowly. When the alternate-day therapy is achieved, it is maintained for 2 to 4 weeks to permit the hypothalamic-pituitary-adrenal (HPA) axis to recover and then tapered 5 mg a week. The alternate-day regimen has been shown to cause far less HPA axis suppression and to result in fewer opportunistic infections.

In cases requiring the readministration of heterologous antisera where the "accelerated" form of serum sickness is expected within 24 to 72 hours after administration, the concomitant use of glucocorticoids as described above is recommended. One should also be extremely careful of the possibility of anaphylaxis, since the patient has had a previous exposure to the heterologous protein.

Local reactions at the site of intramuscular injections of heterologous antisera during the course of serum sickness can range from a mild urticarial eruption to a severely indurated granulomatous lesion. Treatment usually involves the use of oral antihistamines for the mild reaction and systemic "burst" of glucocorticosteroids for the severe reaction.

ALLERGIC GASTROINTESTINAL DISORDERS

WARREN RICHARDS, M.D.

The cornerstone of therapy of allergic gastrointestinal disorders is identification of the offending food followed by avoidance. A number of diagnostic approaches can be used in an effort to find the causes of gastrointestinal allergy, including history, diet diary, laboratory tests, elimination diets, and open and blind food challenges. The history should include a complete description of the chronology of the reactions, treatment, the amount of food necessary to provoke the reactions, and preparation of other foods ingested in close proximity to the reaction. If the symptoms are intermittent, a food symptom diary recording the symptomatology associated with food intake may be useful in identifying offending foods.

Skin and in vitro tests for the presence of specific IgE may be helpful in identifying the causes of allergic gastrointestinal symptoms. In vitro tests such as RAST are probably less sensitive than skin tests. Unfortunately, these tests are often abused or their results overinterpreted and an overly restrictive diet instituted. With a negative test, there is only a small likelihood that the food tested is responsible for the allergic symptoms. If a food test is positive, there is approximately a 50 per cent probability that the allergen in question will be found by challenge to be a definite trigger. Interpretation of the significance of the test results should be based on (1) correlation with the history and (2) the results of blind food challenge. If the patient's history, diet diary, or tests suggest a symptomatic association with ingestion of a suspected food or foods, a short period of elimination of the foods should be considered, provided that the symptoms are sufficiently severe to warrant the inconvenience and discomfort attendant upon a trial diet. If the decision is made to proceed, all forms of the suspected offending foods are removed from the diet for 4 weeks and a daily symptom diet diary is kept and compared with baseline symptoms. If significant improvement is observed, the patient should be challenged sequentially with the removed foods. If there is a positive response, the suspect food should again be removed from the diet and further challenges delayed until the child's condition has stabilized for at least 1 week. Food challenges are most effectively performed double blind, in which neither the child nor the observer is aware of the food being consumed. In young children, the food in question can be hidden in some other tolerated food; in older children, foods can be placed in capsules after having been crushed or dried. Challenges should never be conducted if the original reaction was anaphylactic in nature or otherwise very severe.

If the avoidance of one or two foods from the diet is not successful in eliminating clinical symptoms, a short trial of a severely limited diet may be justified in selected cases. In no case should extreme dietary measures such as this be carried out for minor problems, nor should they be conducted for more than 2 or 3 weeks. Care must be taken to ensure adequate nutrition while on the diet. Following a brief period on the elimination regimen, usually consisting of Vivonex, Nutramigen, or Pregestimil, foods are then added to the diet in an orderly fashion to see whether symptoms are provoked. In general, challenge testing and elimination diets are best carried out by an experienced subspecialist.

DRUGS

Antihistamines, cromolyn sodium, and corticosteroids have been used to treat gastrointestinal allergy. Antihistamines have not been shown to be efficacious for use in subjects with food sensitivity, and recent evidence suggests that cromolyn sodium given orally in large doses is likewise ineffective. Steroids are used rarely in the treatment of gastrointestinal allergy and then only for the most severe cases. Eosinophilic gastroenteritis and protein-losing gastroenteropathy associated with food allergy are two conditions in which steroid use may be instituted and tapered as symptoms resolve. Subcutaneous and oral desensitization/neutralization have been advocated by some investigators. However, there is insufficient evidence to support the usefulness of these procedures, and they should be avoided. Other unproven procedures are cytotoxic testing, IgG4 assays, basophil-histamine release assays, and measurements of circulating IgG and IgE food immune complexes. Indeed, there are insufficient data to support the pathogenic role for IgG or IgG subclass antibodies in food hypersensitivity reactions.

PREVENTION

Infants are considered to be at high risk for food sensitivity, probably because of increased intestinal mucosal permeability to incompletely digested macromolecules and the lack of adequate protection by secretory IgA at the mucosal membrane surface. Breast feeding has been advocated as a means of reducing the risk of sensitivity in the infant, but the results of clinical studies have been conflicting and the benefits not conclusively established. The usefulness of hypoallergenic formulas containing soybean or casein hydrolysate for long-term prophylaxis of food allergy has also not yet been adequately studied. Since it has been established that intrauterine sensitization of the fetus does occur, limiting the allergens ingested by the mother in her last trimester of pregnancy has been advocated as a possible means of avoiding sensitization of the infant, but the efficacy of this approach is still unclear. On the other hand, since it is well established that allergens ingested by the mother can be transmitted in her breast milk, limiting the allergen in her diet is useful in reducing allergen exposure of the nursing infant.

REFERRAL

Consultation with a subspecialist should be sought when symptoms are particularly severe or resistant to simple therapeutic approaches.

ADVERSE REACTIONS TO DRUGS
H. JAMES WEDNER, M.D.

Adverse reactions to drugs may be classified into three broad groups: dose-related toxic effects, idiosyncratic reactions, and hypersensitivity reactions. The toxic reactions are unwanted pharmacologic effects of the drug in question. They will occur, to a greater or lesser extent, in all patients if sufficient quantities of the drug are given. They are "normal" properties of the drug.

Side Effects

Toxic reactions may be subdivided into those that occur within the therapeutic dose range, commonly referred to as side effects, and those that occur when doses of the drugs produce blood or tissue concentrations in excess of therapeutic levels. In some cases these two classifications will merge, since the sensitivity of individuals to side effects varies widely and one individual can tolerate high levels of a given drug without observable side effects while another is unable to tolerate the drug at all. Patient perception is also of great significance. The same degree of a given symptom, nausea for example, may be severely compromising to one patient and largely overlooked by another. This phenomenon is seen with many drug side effects, including the somnolence associated with antihistaminics. This is a true side effect, since many individuals become sleepy within the true therapeutic dose range. With the same blood level the somnolence may be mild or it may be overwhelming and necessitate discontinuance of the drug.

With antihistaminics, as is the case with a number of

drug groups, switching from one chemical class of drug to another may allow one to maximize the therapeutic potential while minimizing the side effect. Another approach to side effects is to simply continue the drug. The undesirable side effects may disappear, and therapeutic potential is maintained. It is also possible to minimize side effects by starting at relatively low doses of a drug and increasing the dose gradually over a period of time. This is effective not only with antihistaminics but also with such diverse groups as beta-adrenergic agonists or antihypersensitive agents. It is important in all cases to explain to patients that there is a potential for an undesirable side effect and that this effect may indeed disappear if they will persevere in taking the drug.

Toxic Effects

In contrast to undesirable side effects, toxic reactions to drugs occur at dosages that yield blood levels in excess of the therapeutic range. Toxic reactions are still, however, intimately related to the chemical nature of the agent and amount of drug that is given. Examples of this type of reaction include cardiac toxicity with digitalis; postural hypotension with antihypertensive agents; and nausea, vomiting, and, if sufficient drug is given, convulsions with theophylline or its salts. It is important to remember that the gap between therapeutic and toxic levels of a given drug varies greatly with the type of pharmacologic agent. It may be quite broad, giving the physician a great deal of latitude in prescribing the drug, or narrow, requiring careful monitoring of blood levels to assure maximum benefit with minimum chance for a toxic side effect. A notable example of this phenomenon occurs in the use of theophylline for the treatment of asthma. With theophylline, the therapeutic range is generally considered to be 10 to 20 μg/ml, while the toxic range, beginning with mild anorexia and progressing through nausea and vomiting, generally starts between 18 and 20 μg/ml. The toxic effects become progressively worse at higher blood levels. Because the ability to transform theophylline biologically varies widely from patient to patient, it is impossible to predict with any degree of certainty the blood level that will be achieved by a given dose. Therefore, it is recommended that measuring the exact blood level is the only way to achieve maximum therapeutic benefit while minimizing side effects. It should also be noted that with theophylline, as with a number of other drugs, some patients may experience a degree of discomfort at blood levels that are in the relatively low range and that may be as low as 10 to 15 μg/ml in a small percentage of patients. In this instance one can still achieve therapeutic benefit by carefully adjusting the dose to achieve a blood level that reduces the majority of unwanted toxic effects while remaining in the low end of the therapeutic range. Similar considerations should be taken into account with any drug for which the toxic and therapeutic ranges approximate one another.

It is also important to remember that with some classes of drugs the toxic effects are related to the total amount of drug given and not to the absolute blood level achieved. In these instances one must keep in mind the progressive amount of drug (dose × duration) and discontinue use of that particular agent prior to reaching a level that is associated with toxic side effects. Excellent examples of this phenomenon are found with gold salts and a number of antibiotics. The aminoglycoside antibiotics cause renal and ototoxicity based on the total amount of drug given; chloramphenicol also has a toxic effect, bone marrow depression, which is related to the total cumulative dose.

Idiosyncratic Reactions

In contrast to dose-related toxic side effects, idiosyncratic reactions to drugs bear no relation to the amount or duration of therapy. They may occur with the initial introduction of the drug or may occur after long periods of time on an adequate therapeutic dose. They are impossible to predict, with the exception that a patient who has had one idiosyncratic reaction to a drug is likely to have a second if the drug is reinstituted. It is also important to remember that some idiosyncratic reactions to drugs are relatively benign while others are life threatening. Fortunately the majority of idiosyncratic reactions, to a greater or lesser extent, fall into the former category. One must always be aware of the potential for an idiosyncratic reaction. In those instances in which the idiosyncratic reaction may be life threatening, the physician must balance the potential for idiosyncratic reactions with the potential therapeutic benefit. This should take into account the frequency at which idiosyncratic reactions occur and the severity of those reactions. For example, although the aplastic anemia seen with chloramphenicol is disastrous, the percentage of treated patients actually experiencing this idiosyncratic reaction is significantly less, for example, than the chance of a penicillin reaction. For this reason it would be inappropriate to withhold this drug in cases in which it would life saving for fear of an idiosyncratic reaction. On the other hand, the use of this drug in instances in which another antibiotic with significantly less potential toxicity is available would be inappropriate.

Toxic effects of drugs and idiosyncratic reactions to drugs most probably have different underlying biochemical bases. However, in some instances toxic effects and idiosyncratic effects are very similar. And when an adverse effect occurs, such as bone marrow depression with chloramphenicol, it is important to differentiate the dose-related toxic effects from the idiosyncratic reactions. A patient who has had an idiosyncratic reaction to a drug should not be given the drug again unless one is faced with dire consequences. On the other hand, in instances in which overdosages occur, the toxic effects can be prevented with appropriate dose regimens, and this does not prevent the patient from receiving that drug or a drug of the same class again.

Hypersensitivity Reactions

Hypersensitivity reactions can occur with virtually any drug in the pharmacopeia. These reactions can be differentiated into three basic types: immediate hypersensitivity (Type I), delayed antibody-mediated of the

Arthus type (IgG Types II and III), and cell-mediated (Type IV). Immediate type reactions may be further subdivided into anaphylactic and anaphylactoid reactions. *Anaphylactic* reactions refer to those in which the drug induces the production of IgE antibody directed against the drug or more appropriately against a drug-protein complex; the reaction occurs on subsequent administration of the drug following interaction of the agent with specific IgE molecules bound to tissue mast cells or circulating basophils. In contrast, *anaphylactoid* reactions refer to those instances in which release of mast cell mediators is accomplished through a non–IgE-mediated mechanism. This may be the result of direct interaction of a drug with the mast cell membrane, with the release of chemical mediators by the drug polymyxin B; or it may occur secondarily, as with interaction of a drug with the complement system, generating the anaphylatoxins C5a and C3a. These anaphylatoxins are capable of inducing the release of mediators from mast cells and or basophils. In either case the net result is the same, since the mediators released are identical.

A complete discussion of the chemical mediators of anaphylaxis is beyond the scope of this review. Suffice it to say that there are a diverse number of chemical entities, including (1) biogenic amines, histamine, and to a lesser extent serotonin; (2) lipoxygenase products of arachidonic acid, leukotrienes C, D, and E (also called slow-reacting substance of anaphylaxis, SRSA); (3) cyclooxygenase products of arachidonic acid, largely prostaglandin D_2; (4) platelet-activating factor (acetyl glyceral ether phosphorylcholine); (5) a number of enzymes, including a trypsin-like enzyme; (6) *chemoattractants* for both eosinophils and polymorphonuclear leukocytes; (7) the matrix component heparin. These factors, alone or in combination, are responsible for the symptoms of immediate hypersensitivity reactions, skin pruritus, urticaria, angioedema, laryngeal edema, wheezing, and hypotension. The severity of the reaction will depend on the location of the activated mast cells and the number of mast cells activated. Hypersensitivity reactions may be extremely mild (mild pruritus or hives) or may be an overwhelming, life-threatening, severe systemic allergic reaction (anaphylaxis).

Since anaphylactoid reactions do not require the production of IgE antibody they may occur on the initial use of a given drug, although in some instances they do occur after prolonged exposure. An example of this type of hypersensitivity is the severe reaction seen with various radiocontrast dyes. In this instance current evidence would suggest that, in susceptible individuals, injection of radiocontrast media results in the activation of complement with release of anaphylatoxins and subsequent stimulation of mediator release from mast cells. The reactions that are seen to radiocontrast material suggest two other major points concerning anaphylactoid reactions. First, not all individuals will experience this type of reaction when presented with the drug. In the majority of cases the factors that determine those patients who will react to a given drug are at the present time unknown. Secondly, although not all individuals will have a reaction on their initial

exposure to the drug, in general, patients who have one anaphylactoid reaction to a given agent will continue to have anaphylactoid reactions unless some intervention is taken. In the case of radiocontrast materials, pretreatment of patients with corticosteroids and an H_1 type antihistaminic as well as an H_2 antihistaminic is sufficient to decrease the severity of or completely abrogate the reaction in more than 90 per cent of the cases. The protocol we utilize at Washington University is shown in Table 1.

Another group of agents that frequently cause anaphylactoid-type reactions, either local or systemic, are local anesthetics. Although a small minority of reactions to local anesthetics represent true anaphylactic sensitivity, in the majority of cases it would appear that mediator release is the result of direct interaction of the drug with the plasma membrane of mast cells. As in many other reactions, the reaction to local anesthetics is highly class-specific. Thus, it is possible, using appropriate skin testing and provocative dose challenge protocols, to find a local anesthetic to which the patient does not react. At Washington University School of Medicine we generally test to three non–cross-reacting local anesthetics: lidocaine, carbocaine, and tetracain. We use 1 or 2 per cent solutions diluted 1:100 and 1:10. Scratch or prick tests are done starting with the most dilute concentration. If the patient does not react, intradermal skin tests are performed, again starting with the lowest concentration. Of the three local anesthetics, the one that caused no reaction is selected and 0.1 ml followed by 0.5 ml is given subcutaneously. If no local or systemic reaction is seen in 20 to 30 minutes, the agent can be utilized.

Another point that must be considered when dealing with local anesthetics and many other drugs is the fact that in some instances the patient may not be reacting to the drug per se but rather to a constituent of the drug preparation. This is particularly true with preservatives such as metabisulfites or parabens. Indeed, several patients seen by the author for sensitivity to local anesthetics turned out in fact to be highly sensitive to sodium metabisulfite and methyl paraben and had no reaction when tested with a metabisulfite- and paraben-

TABLE 1. Protocol for Pretreatment of Patients with Radiocontrast Media Sensitivity

Time Before Procedure	Drug	Dose*	Route
25 hr	Cimetidine†	300 mg	PO/IV or IM‡
19 hr	Cimetidine	300 mg	PO/IV or IM‡
13 hr	Cimetidine	300 mg	PO/IV or IM‡
	Prednisone	50 mg	PO/IV§
7 hr	Cimetidine	300 mg	PO/IV‡
	Prednisone	50 mg	PO/IV
1 hr	Cimetidine	300 mg	PO/IV or IM‡
	Prednisone	50 mg	PO/IV§
	Diphen-hydramine	50 mg	PO/IV‡

*Usual adult dosage. Equivalent pediatric dosage:
  Cimetidine 5–10 mg/kg.
  Prednisone 0.8–1.75 mg/kg.
  Diphenhydramine 1.25 mg/kg.
†Not recommended for patients under 16 years of age. If protocol without cimetidine has failed, then cimetidine 5–10 mg/kg may be added.
‡Oral route is preferred unless patient is unable to take oral medication.
§For intravenous route give 40 mg methyl prednisolone.

free preparation of a number of local anesthetics. One patient was subsequently able to undergo extensive dental work under local anesthesia using a preservative-free preparation.

A number of drugs cause immediate hypersensitivity reactions by mechanisms that do not involve IgE formation or direct or indirect mediator release. The classic example is aspirin and all of the large group of nonsteroidal anti-inflammatory agents (NSAI). These compounds have been studied extensively; however, the mechanism for reactions to aspirin and NSAI, either aspirin-sensitive asthma or rhinitis, remains obscure. Neither IgE-mediated nor direct mast cell activation seems to be present. Since aspirin is a potent inhibitor of the enzyme fatty acid cyclooxygenase, it inhibits prostaglandin synthesis and it has been suggested that individuals sensitive to aspirin may have a marked inhibition of a necessary prostaglandin such as PGE_2 or enhanced secretion of detrimental lipoxygenase products such as the leukotrienes. However, efforts to identify these metabolites have proved unsuccessful to date. Aspirin and NSAI are not unique, and there are many other drugs in which the differentiation between anaphylactic and anaphylactoid reactions is difficult.

Anaphylactic reactions, as pointed out above, are the result of the generation of IgE (and perhaps IgG_4) type antibodies. As such, the drug must serve as a hapten and be conjugated to tissue proteins to be immunogenic. For this reason the ability of any drug to induce anaphylactic-type reactions is related to its ability to bind covalently (or in some cases noncovalently) to appropriate tissue proteins. The classic example of this type of reaction is seen in penicillin-allergic individuals.

In the majority of patients penicillin is coupled to protein via an amide bond, forming a penicilloyl protein derivative. In some patients penicillin couples by other means such as disulfide formation between penicillenic acid and cysteine or methionine. These derivatives, in susceptible individuals, are highly immunogenic. The great ability of penicillin to interact with protein most probably accounts for the large number of patients sensitive to penicillin or its semisynthetic derivatives. It is important to remember that in the case of penicillin the major offending agent is not penicillin itself but rather the penicilloyl moiety, which is generated by cleavage of the beta-lactam ring.

A significant percentage of individuals (15 to 18 per cent) do not react to the penicilloyl moiety; rather, they react to a group of "minor determinants," the result of other types of penicillin-protein conjugations, which can be detected by skin testing using penicilloic acid or penicillin G itself. In these instances the exact immunogen is not known, and one relies on rapid conjugation of penicillin G or penicilloic acid to tissue proteins, which then interact with cell-bound IgE. It is important to remember that antibodies to penicillin are directed against the core of the molecule, i.e., the sulfur-containing thiozolidone (five-membered) and the beta-lactam (four-membered) rings. For this reason a patient sensitive to one penicillin should be considered sensitive to any penicillin derivative. Indeed, even the newer, highly modified semisynthetic penicillins and cephalosporins cannot be excluded, as evidenced by recent reports of allergic reactions to piperacillin and moxalactam. There are some rare exceptions to this rule. At Washington University we have seen three patients sensitive to carbenicillin but no other penicillin, but this is exceedingly unusual (also see below). In addition to penicillin, the cephalosporins are also potential problems: a small proportion of individuals produce a true anti-cephalosporin IgE. A much larger percentage, between 5 and 15 per cent of penicillin-allergic patients, have an anti-penicillin IgE that cross-reacts with cephalosporins. Thus, although some authors consider cephalosporins to be a suitable alternative in penicillin-sensitive individuals, we do not, and due care, such as provocative dose challenge (see below), must be taken when treating penicillin-sensitive individuals with cephalosporins.

Because the appropriate immunogens have been elucidated, patients with suspected penicillin allergy can be skin tested. Studies by our group and others have shown that penicillin skin testing can determine with a high degree of confidence whether a patient is or is not at risk for a severe systemic reaction upon receiving the drug. Unfortunately only the major determinant is available commercially at present (penicilloyl-polylysine, Pre-Pen, Kremers Urban). This will still identify 85 per cent or more of patients at risk for anaphylaxis to penicillins. We strongly recommend that skin testing be performed in all patients with suspected penicillin allergy when penicillin or cephalosporins are the drug of choice. Moreover, as demonstrated by our group, it is possible to desensitize highly sensitive individuals with penicillin, using a protocol of increasing amounts of oral penicillin followed by parenteral penicillin and subsequent administration of the drug in full therapeutic doses. This procedure is of significant benefit and allows acutely ill patients who require penicillin for a life-threatening illness to be treated appropriately. In general, similar studies on desensitization have not been carried out with other drugs, with the exception of insulin, for which desensitization is also of great value.

In the case of penicillin the exact chemistry of the immunogen has been elegantly described. However, with the majority of drugs, the exact chemistry of the immunogen is largely unknown, although evidence would suggest that an IgE antibody directed against the drug is present. As a result, in contrast to penicillin, one must rely almost solely on the historical evaluation of the patient to determine that a drug-related immediate hypersensitivity reaction is present, since adequate skin test reagents are not available and simple skin testing with the drug in question may yield spurious results.

Recently, allergic sensitivity to trimethoprim-sulfamethoxazole (Bactrim, Septra) has become an increasing problem, particularly in patients with the acquired immune deficiency syndrome (AIDS) and other states in which immunity is compromised. This is most likely due to the widespread use of this combination as a prophylactic measure, particularly for *Pneumocystis*. We have skin tested several of these patients and have seen positive skin reactivity at concentrations that do not cause a wheal and flare reaction in normal individuals.

This suggests that this is a true IgE-mediated reaction. In addition we have desensitized two patients without difficulty, one to sulfonamide alone and the other to the combination drug. We do not, however, recommend this procedure at the present time, as adequate studies have not been performed to indicate the efficacy of the skin testing or the effectiveness of the oral desensitization procedure.

In instances in which one suspects, from historical evaluation, that the patient does have a true allergy two procedures are available. Obviously, the most logical is to find an alternative therapeutic modality. In the majority of instances it is possible to find an alternative non–cross-reacting drug. If a non–cross-reacting drug is unavailable or would not provide sufficient therapeutic benefit because of the severity of the patient's illness, a procedure similar to that which has been described for penicillin can be utilized. Begin with extremely small doses and administer increasingly larger amounts of the drug until therapeutic levels are obtained. The patient should be monitored closely for signs of allergic reactions and the protocol either modified or discontinued if these occur. We suggest that if possible the initial stages of the desensitization should be done orally to reduce the chance of a severe reaction.

When there is some degree of doubt as to the allergic nature of the patient's reaction, one can use the "provocative dose challenge" technique. In this technique a subtherapeutic dose of the drug is given, preferably by the oral route, and the patient is observed for allergic symptoms for 20 to 60 minutes. If no reaction occurs, a second and perhaps third and fourth challenge with increasingly larger doses can be given; if no adverse reaction occurs, the drug can be given in full therapeutic doses.

It is important to remember that these techniques, either progressive desensitization or provocative dose challenge, are designed merely to circumvent or prevent a severe systemic allergic reaction (anaphylaxis). They are not designed to prevent any allergic reaction at all, and once desensitized, patients are still capable of exhibiting mild allergic reactions, usually evidenced by generalized pruritus or hives. These patients should be maintained on the drug as long as is necessary and the minor allergic manifestations treated with an appropriate antihistamine in adequate doses. Once a patient with proven drug hypersensitivity has been adequately desensitized it is important that the drug be maintained for as long as is necessary. It is not clear at present how long the desensitized state remains. In some instances it may be as long as several days; on the other hand, it may be relatively short, on the order of 6 to 12 hours. In this case stopping therapy would necessitate reinstitution of the desensitization protocol, which could be difficult since the patients tend to be somewhat hyperreactive for a period of time after the desensitized state is lost.

In addition to inducing IgE-type antibodies, drugs are also capable of inducing IgG-type antibodies. In many instances IgG-type antibodies are relatively innocuous and neither affect the bioavailability of the drug nor cause any significant side reaction. For example, greater than 90 per cent of patients who receive parenteral penicillin develop IgG antipenicillin antibodies. This, however, does not mean that they will have any subsequent difficulties when penicillin therapy is reinstituted. On the other hand, IgG antibodies may lead to significant drug reactions. Several types of reactions have been recognized. All are the result of antibodies that are directed against the drug itself and haptenized on tissue proteins or antibodies that are directed against tissue proteins which are altered by interaction with the drug and are thus recognized as foreign. Drug-protein conjugates may interreact with antibody in the fluid phase, yielding significant amounts of antigen-antibody complexes. This then results in a serum sickness–like picture. In addition, if the complex is of the appropriate size, specific organs may be affected, for example, kidneys in drug-induced lupus erythematosus or Henoch-Schönlein purpura. In addition, drugs may be bound only to a specific organ, yielding diseases that are organ specific. Perhaps the best example of such a drug reaction is the production of antibodies that react with quinine (quinidine) bound to platelets, resulting in quinine-induced severe thrombocytopenia. Similarly drugs may bind to the liver, yielding a drug-induced hepatitis, or to a variety of other specific organs. Although these diseases may in many ways mimic autoimmune-type phenomena, they are generally self-limited and respond well simply to removal of the drug. The use of corticosteroids in these types of drug reactions is controversial and in the majority of instances there is rapid clearing of drug and drug-protein conjugates by antibody, and the use of steroids neither hinders nor helps.

A variety of drugs are also associated with the development of cell-mediated immunity or delayed-type hypersensitivity. In this instance the drug-protein conjugate results in the production of "effector" or cytotoxic T cells. Delayed sensitivity has been associated with a large number of drugs. Whether given orally or parenterally or applied to the skin, the major organ affected is the skin. When the drug is applied locally, the classic picture is a pruritic papulopustular eruption limited to the areas of application. In cases of a systemic reaction the most common reaction is a generalized eczematoid dermatitis. Other forms include erythema multiforme and in rare cases erythema nodosum. Although many drugs have been implicated in Type IV reactions, in many instances actual proof has been lacking. Reapplication of a drug to the skin (patch testing) can be done to identify reactions; on the other hand, drugs given parenterally or orally may require more sophisticated studies, such as in vitro blast transformation. In this instance simple incubation of the drug with white cells in vitro may be inappropriate, since, as already discussed for Type I reactions, the true immunogen is a drug-protein conjugate. In the case of a "fixed drug eruption" (a skin reaction that occurs in the same limited area of the skin each time the drug is introduced) a serum factor has been described that transforms lymphocytes, suggesting that this is a Type IV reaction. Although patch testing or other laboratory studies can be performed in most instances, sophisticated laboratory studies are not necessary and sufficient information can be obtained from a careful history.

For all of the hypersensitivity states it is important to remember that immunogenicity or lack thereof, or the type of response that is stimulated, is related not only to the drug and its chemical properties but also to the route of administration. For example, many drugs are much less immunogenic when given orally than when given parenterally. A drug applied to the skin may induce a Type IV reaction while the same drug in oral or parenteral form may be relatively nonimmunogenic. A case in point is the antihistaminics, which are infrequent producers of hypersensitivity unless applied topically, when they commonly produce delayed hypersensitivity reactions. These considerations are not without practical benefit. Selection of the appropriate dosage form, avoiding those associated with the induction of hypersensitivity states, may help to prevent hypersensitivity reactions.

While by no means complete, the list of drug-related adverse effects presented here does indicate the broad diversity of such reactions. Drugs may have side effects that represent pharmacologic actions other than those that are actually desired. These toxic effects may occur at blood levels within the therapeutic range or at supratherapeutic blood levels or may be related to the cumulative dose given. The adverse reaction may be idiosyncratic in nature or may result from a hypersensitivity state. Hypersensitivity reactions of the anaphylactoid type may represent a pharmacological effect of the drug on an unknown enzyme system (e.g., aspirin), interaction with complement system, or direct action of the drug on the surface of the mast cell or basophil. In addition, those drugs capable of conjugating with tissue proteins may generate an immune response against the drug-protein complex. The immune response may be a Type I anaphylactic-type reaction by production of specific IgE, a Type II or III response due to the production of IgG and subsequent formation of either antigen-antibody complexes or cytotoxic antibodies, or a Type IV cell-mediated response.

Finally, one must always remember that a single drug can be associated with all three types of adverse reactions noted above. And it may be as critically important to differentiate the type of adverse reaction as to recognize the reaction itself. For example, thrombocytopenia may be seen with certain semisynthetic penicillins as a toxic effect or on an immunologic basis. Similarly, nephritis in patients treated with semisynthetic penicillins may be part of a serum sickness reaction or may be the interstitial nephritis associated with several semisynthetic penicillins; the most recently described being mezlocillin and piperacillin. The differentiation of immunologic from a nonimmunologic basis may allow the use of an alternative beta-lactam antibiotic in the latter case while an immunologically based reaction precludes further use of this class of antibiotic. Similar considerations are important for many other classes of drug. Thus, when possible, the type of adverse reaction—toxic, idiosyncratic or immunologic—should be determined.

It is imperative that the physician be aware of the broad diversity of adverse reactions to drugs that can occur. In the majority of cases a detailed drug history will be sufficient to alert the physician to the potential of an adverse reaction to a drug, and this can then be handled either by use of an alternative therapeutic modality, by appropriate treatment of the patient to block the effects of mediator release, or by appropriate desensitization procedures. It is also important that the patient as well as the physician be apprised of the potential for side effects, the nature of these side effects, and the methods that will be utilized to decrease or circumvent them. In this way the problem of drug-related adverse reactions can be minimized, and when they occur, they can be treated appropriately. No drug is free of adverse effects and as long as physicians continue to utilize drug therapy adverse reactions will continue to be a major problem. This should not lead to therapeutic nihilism but rather to the utilization of measures to minimize or circumvent these reactions.

PHYSICAL ALLERGY
JOHN A. ANDERSON, M.D.

Physical factors, such as mechanical pressure, light, heat, cold, water, and exercise, may result in urticaria, angioedema, or systemic signs and symptoms usually associated with allergic reactions. As a group, these reactions are referred to as physical allergies. The exact incidence of physical factors resulting in "allergic" reactions in children is unknown, but urticaria caused by physical factors accounts for approximately 3 per cent of all patients with urticaria and 10 per cent of patients with chronic urticaria (mostly adults). Cold-induced urticaria followed by cholinergic urticaria is the most common physical urticaria seen in children.

The therapy used in physical allergy involves either avoidance of the physical agent or pharmacologic therapy designed to combat the effects of chemical mediators released by exposure to these agents.

GENERAL PRINCIPLES OF PHARMACOTHERAPY

Table 1 lists the antihistamines used for the treatment of physical allergy and the usual doses for children, beginning with the most commonly used drug. Table 2 lists the emergency and adjuvant drugs used in the treatment of these conditions.

The prime drug used in the emergency treatment of urticaria and angioedema is Adrenalin. In the usual case of urticaria/angioedema and exercise-induced anaphylaxis seen in the emergency situation, a systemically administered antihistamine, such as intramuscular Benadryl, is also given. Follow-up treatment could include Sus-Phrine, a long-acting form of epinephrine (4 to 6 hours), and antihistamines to be taken at home, such as Benadryl, 25 mg three times daily, or Chlor-Trimeton, 4 to 8 mg three times daily.

For prophylactic treatment of any of the physical urticaria/angioedema conditions or exercise-induced anaphylaxis, the use of a single antihistamine listed in

TABLE 1. Antihistamines for Treatment of Physical Allergy

Antihistamine Class (*Histamine Receptor*)	Drug (*Trade Name*)	Usual Dose, 27-kg Child (*Dose by Weight*)
Ethanolamine (H_1)	Diphenhydramine (Benadryl) (more sedative)	12.5–50 mg 3 × daily (5 mg/kg/24 hr—not to exceed 300 mg/24 hr)
Ataractic (H_1)	Hydroxyzine (Atarax, Vistaril) (more sedative)	10–25 mg 3 × daily
Alkylamine (H_1)	1. Chlorpheniramine (Chlor-Trimeton, Teldrin) 2. Brompheniramine (Dimetane) (less sedative)	2–8 mg 3 × daily
Piperidine (H_1)	1. Cyproheptadine (Periactin)	2–4 mg 3–4 × daily (0.25 mg/kg/24 hr)
	2. Azatadine (Optimine)	1–2 mg 2 × daily; not recommended under 12 yr of age
Phenothiazine (H_1)	Promethazine (Phenergan)	6.25–12.5 mg 3 × daily
Ethylenediamine (H_1)	Tripelennamine (PBZ)	25–50 mg 3 × daily (5 mg/kg/24 hr—not to exceed 300 mg/24 hr)
Benzhydryl ether (H_1)	Clemastine fumarate (Tavist)	1.34 mg 2 × daily; not recommended under 12 yr of age
Piperidinebutanol (H_1)	Terfenadine (Seldane) (less sedative)	60 mg 2 × daily for 12 yr of age or older; not recommended below this age
Benzimidazol-Amine (H_1)	Astemizole (Hismanal) (less sedative, long acting)	10 mg 1 × daily for 12 yr of age or older. ½ life: 1 day; appetite, weight gain (4%); not recommended under 12 yr of age
Thioguanidine (H_2)	Cimetidine (Tagamet)	20–40 mg/kg/24 hr; very limited experience in children under 16 yr of age
Ethenediamine (H_2)	Ranitidine (Zantac)	Dosage not established in children; see manufacturer's recommendations
Ataractics (H_1, H_2?)	Doxepin (Sinequan)	10–25 mg 2 × daily for 12 yr of age or older as a single drug; not to exceed 75 mg/24 hr; not recommended below this age

TABLE 2. Emergency and Adjuvant Drugs for Treatment of Physical Allergy

Drug Type	Drug (*Trade Name*)	Usual Children's Dosage
Sympathomimetics and beta-agonists	Epinephrine HCl 1:1000 (Adrenalin)	0.1–0.3 ml/dose SC (0.005–0.01 ml/kg/dose)
	Epinephrine 1:200 in thioglycolate (Sus-Phrine)	0.05–0.15 ml/dose SC (0.005 ml/kg/dose)
	Epinephrine HCl 1:1000 (Adrenalin) in Ana-Kit (Hollister-Stier Labs.)	0.3 ml/dose; 2 doses possible
	Epinephrine HCl 1:1000 (Adrenalin) in Epi-Pen and Epi-Pen Jr. (Center Labs.)	0.3 ml and 0.15 ml (Epi-Pen and Epi-Pen Jr., respectively) in automatic doser
	Metaproterenol (Alupent, Metaprel)	1–3 puffs by inhalation; not recommended under 12 yr of age
	Terbutaline (Bricanyl, Brethine)	2.5–5.0 mg 3 × daily; not recommended under 12 yr of age
	Albuterol (Proventil, Ventoline)	1–2 puffs by inhalation 3 × daily or 2–4 mg 3 × daily; not recommended under 12 yr of age
Methylxanthine	Theophylline (Slo-bid 50, 75, 100, 125, 200, 300 mg) (Theo-Dur 100, 200, 300 mg)	Therapeutic blood levels, 10–20 µg/ml
Corticosteroid	Prednisone (Prednisone 5 mg tab) (Pediapred, 5 mg prednisolone/tsp)	As needed
Other	Cromolyn Sodium (Intal)	20-mg powder by inhalation per dose; not recommended under 5 yr of age

Table 1 might be tried, but hydroxyzine (Atarax) usually is most effective. Because Benadryl and Atarax are likely to produce drowsiness, other antihistamines, such as either terfenadine (Seldane) or the chlorphenira-mines, might be tried. Cyproheptadine (Periactin) is most efficacious in the treatment of cold urticaria. In resistant cases of cold urticaria/angioedema, various combinations of antihistamines might be tried, including Benadryl, Atarax, or Chlor-Trimeton during the day, plus Phenergan or PBZ at night. Azatadine (Optim-ine*) and clemastine fumarate (Tavist†), terfenadine (Seldane) and astemizole (Hismanal)‡ are newer, longer-acting antihistamines usually used for the treatment of allergic rhinitis. Terfenadine and astemizole have the least effect on the central nervous system. However, in some cases of pruritus-urticaria/angio-edema, these drugs might be tried if other antihista-mines have failed to control the condition.

Recently, there have been reports of successful use of the combination of an H_2 histamine receptor drug, cimetidine (Tagamet§) or ranitidine (Zantac§), with one of the H_1 antihistamines, such as hydroxyzine, in the treatment of chronic urticaria. Experience has shown the effect to be variable among patients. In some resis-tant cases of chronic urticaria, doxepin (Sinequan†), which has been shown to exhibit some H_2 and H_2 antihistamine-like activity, has been used as a single drug. The experience in children is limited, and any drug trial should be cautious in nature.

In addition, terbutaline (Bricanyl) and theophylline compounds have been shown to decrease histamine release in hypersensitivity states. Both drugs decreased chronic urticaria/angioedema in some studies, in spite of the fact that neither drug has been shown to signifi-cantly alter the antigen-induced immediate-reacting skin test. From experience, we have found that some resistant cases of chronic urticaria/angioedema (physi-cally induced or idiopathic) respond to the addition of either terbutaline‖ (2.5 mg three times a day) or a theophylline compound (enough Slo-Phyllin given three times a day to maintain a theophylline level between 10 and 20 µg/ml) to one of the single or multiple antihis-tamine regimens.

Corticosteroids may be used in the treatment of severe emergency urticaria/angioedema or anaphylaxis. These drugs may be helpful on a short-term basis for exacerbation of the problem but are not a substitute for the antihistamines. Corticosteroids have not been help-ful on a long-term basis in the routine treatment of physical allergies.

SPECIFIC THERAPY

Dermographia. Treatment of dermographia consists of avoiding trauma and, when necessary, the use of an

antihistamine. Hydroxyzine (Atarax) is the most likely drug to be helpful in this condition (on an as-needed basis), although other antihistamines and drug combi-nations may be tried.

Pressure Urticaria/Angioedema. Treatment consists of avoiding sustained pressures as much as possible. Antihistamines, and even corticosteroids, can be tried but are usually not helpful.

Vibratory Angioedema. Treatment consists of avoid-ing vibrating stimuli. Usually the condition is mild and does not require medications. However, prophylactic antihistamines and corticosteroids have been used suc-cessfully in one case in which the condition was serious and avoidance was not possible (e.g., dental work).

Urticaria/Angioedema Secondary to Light Exposure. Drug ingestion combined with sunlight exposure may result in either a direct toxic rash (phototoxic reaction) or an immunologic contact dermatitis (photoallergic reaction). Drugs implicated in causing a phototoxic reaction include psoralens, topical coal tar, and dimeth-ylchlortetracycline. Drugs implicated in photoallergic reactions include phenothiazines, sulfonamides, and griseofulvin. Bacteriostatic agents like bithionol and halogenated salicylamides, used in soaps and topical medications, can also induce reactions.

Light can also produce sunburn and exacerbate pri-mary dermatologic and systemic diseases, including the polymorphic light eruption and systemic lupus erythe-matosus.

Management of this condition is often difficult and consists primarily of avoiding the reaction-producing light wavelength. In the case of drug sensitivity, the treatment consists of correctly identifying and then avoiding the causative drug or chemical.

Repeated exposure to small, increasing doses of sun-light may induce tolerance in some patients. It is advis-able to wear protective garments whenever possible. Sunscreens or sun-blocking agents can be used to help protect skin exposed to sun in susceptible individuals.

Chemical sunscreens act by absorbing a specific por-tion of the ultraviolet light spectrum. Chemical sun-screens include agents such as para-aminobenzoic acid (PABA), esters of PABA, the benzophenones, digalloyl trioleate, the cinnamates, the anthranilates, the pyrones, and the salicylates. For an agent to be effective, it must have the ability to absorb ultraviolet light in the 290- to 320-nm range—the range at which virtually all sun-burns occur. Five per cent PABA in 50 to 70 per cent ethanol provides an excellent protection against sun-burn. The benzophenones, unlike the other sunscreens, also absorb long-wave ultraviolet light in the 320- to 400-nm range.

Recently, criteria for sun protection have been estab-lished. Sun protective factors (SPF)—the ratio of the amount of exposure necessary to produce a minimal erythematous response with a sunscreen in place di-vided by the amount of exposure needed to produce the same reaction without the sunscreen—now serves as a measure of the sunscreen's protection. Any com-mercial sunscreen with an SPF value of 15 should be an excellent protective agent. Examples include Pre-Sun 15, Pabanol, Supershade 15, Total Eclipse, Sun-down 15, Ti Screen, and Piz Buin 8.

---

*Manufacturer's Precaution: Clinical experience in children is lim-ited. Drug cannot be recommended below age 16 years.

†Manufacturer's Precaution: Safety and efficacy in children have not been established.

‡Manufacturer's Precaution: Not recommended for children below the age of 12 years.

§Manufacturer's Precaution: Safety and efficacy in children have not been established.

‖Manufacturer's Precaution: Not recommended for use in children under 12 years of age.

Sensitivity to wavelengths of light above 320 nm may be avoided by the use of physical sunscreens or sunblocking agents, even though they are less cosmetically acceptable than the chemical sunscreens. Some available agents include zinc oxide paste (RVPaque), titanium dioxide (A-Fil Cream or Solar Cream), and red veterinary petrolatum (RVP Cream or RV Plus).

The 280- to 320-nm UV light (sunburn range) is filtered by window glass. The higher wavelengths, which can still produce light sensitivity in some patients, are not filtered by ordinary glass.

Antihistamines and corticosteroids given orally may reduce the reactions to light. Although the antimalarial drug chloroquine has been used in resistant cases of light sensitivity, the results are disappointing.

Cholinergic Urticaria. "Keeping cool" is a good rule when one is considering the management of cholinergic urticaria. Antihistamines are usually helpful, beginning with hydroxyzine (Atarax) or diphenhydramine (Benadryl), and progressing to combination therapies. A trial on anticholinergic medications has been advised, but this type of treatment has not been helpful in this condition in our experience.

Another method, that of deliberately producing the rash (such as taking a warm shower) in order to produce a short refractory period, is also not a helpful treatment method in our opinion.

Localized Heat Urticaria. This rare disorder can be confirmed by placing a carefully heated Erlenmeyer flask of water on an area of skin. The hive reaction usually occurs within minutes. Antihistamines have been reported to block the heat challenge.

Cold-Induced Urticaria/Angioedema. The mainstay of treatment in cold-induced conditions is to avoid chilling the body. During the summer, one should be careful about sudden changes in temperature, especially swimming in cold water. During the winter, one should be certain to wear good gloves and warm footgear, since the skin of the extremities is already at a lower ambient temperature. A hat is important since the head is a major source of heat loss from the body. A mask can be helpful for protecting the exposed area of the face.

In one study, cyproheptadine (Periactin) was the superior antihistamine in preventing cold reactions, but hydroxyzine (Atarax) and other antihistamines and antihistamine-theophylline or -terbutaline combinations should be tried in stubborn cases.

Gradual "desensitization" to cold by taking serial baths with increasingly cold water has been advocated as a therapy for this condition. In our opinion, the therapy is generally unsuccessful.

Exercise- and Cold-Induced Asthma. Most children with asthma have some degree of bronchoconstriction when they exercise; in some asthmatics, exercise is the major reason for wheezing. Children may also wheeze when exposed to cold air. Running is the exercise most likely to produce wheezing, and swimming is the exercise least likely to do so. The therapy in exercise-induced asthma involves avoidance of that type of exercise and the degree of exercise that produces significant difficulty, when possible. To restrict otherwise normal children, however, from all exercise, especially running, is not practical in our society.

In some cases, children can "run through" their exercise-induced asthma. Breathing through the nose rather than the mouth while exercising, thus allowing the inhaled air to become properly heated and humidified, reduces exercise-induced asthma. Recently, the use of an inexpensive, disposable, hard-paper surgical mask that fits over the nose and mouth has been found to reduce exercise-induced asthma significantly. The mask works by allowing the patient to "rebreathe" a reservoir of warm, humidified air when exercising.

Medication also can be used to reduce or prevent an exercise-induced asthma (Table 2). Cromolyn sodium* (Intal) by inhalation one-half hour before exercise provides significant help in 60 per cent of children up to 2 to 4 hours. Sympathomimetics and beta-agonists taken immediately before exercising, such as albuterol (Proventil, Ventolin), terbutaline (Bricanyl, Brethine), and metaproterenol† (Alupent, Metaprel), are most efficacious in reducing the incidence of exercise-induced asthma, but there are some potential cardiovascular side effects with these drugs, as opposed to essentially no side effects with cromolyn sodium. Oral sympathomimetic agents and oral theophylline agents are helpful but not as efficacious as metaproterenol, albuterol, or cromolyn sodium. Inhaled atropine-like compounds are helpful in this condition in about one third of the cases.

The treatment of cold-induced asthma is similar to that of exercise-induced asthma.

Exercise-Induced Anaphylaxis. Recently, a group of young adults have been described who develop symptoms of anaphylaxis, including pruritus, generalized urticaria, angioedema, nasal stuffiness, and, on occasion, abdominal colic, dizziness, and collapse while exercising, particularly jogging. These patients were found not to have exercise-induced asthma or cholinergic urticaria. The mechanism of action in this condition is not clear, although some patients are atopic and may be experiencing increased exposure during jogging to environmental allergens, such as pollen. Case reports have also described patients who have anaphylaxis only after exercising following a meal of shrimp or celery or—in one patient—following any meal.

The therapy for this condition involves the avoidance of strenuous exercises like jogging. In some instances, this is not acceptable to the patient. The use of antihistamines, such as hydroxyzine (Atarax), or other drug combinations prior to exercise may be helpful. On an emergency basis, Adrenalin is the prime mode of therapy for anaphylaxis. Since some patients may have a history of a potential life-threatening episode of exercise-induced anaphylaxis and may refuse to discontinue the practice of strenuous exercise, they should be supplied with Adrenalin in a loaded syringe and taught to use this drug in an emergency situation. Ana-Kit (supplied primarily for patients allergic to stinging insects) contains such a conveniently loaded syringe of Adrenalin. The dose may be varied but usually is 0.3 ml,

---

*Cromolyn sodium is not recommended for children under 5 years of age.

†Inhalation form is not recommended for children under 5 years of age.

which is suitable for an older teenager and adult but not a young child. An automatically administered Adrenalin device that will penetrate clothing (i.e., of the thigh) is also available (Epi-Pen and Epi-Pen Jr.). The doses are fixed at 0.3 ml and 0.15 ml respectively and are suitable for different age children. See Table 2 for recommended pediatric doses of epinephrine.

ANAPHYLAXIS

DOUGLAS C. HEINER, M.D.

Anaphylaxis refers to a severe acute reaction following exposure to an allergen. It usually involves smooth muscle contraction, vasodilation, and increased capillary permeability secondary to the widespread release of chemical mediators. It generally is IgE-mediated, but in a few instances involvement of IgE cannot be demonstrated. If it is impossible to demonstrate any abnormal immunologic response to the offending substance, this type of reaction is termed an "anaphylactoid" reaction. If there is associated hypotension, the term "anaphylactic shock" or "anaphylactoid shock" may be used.

The symptoms of anaphylaxis include itching, urticaria, vomiting, diarrhea, sneezing, wheezing, difficult breathing, abdominal pain, tachycardia, weak pulse, lightheadedness, hypotension, a feeling of impending doom, cyanosis, convulsions, coma, and occasionally death. Usually several symptoms occur simultaneously. Similar symptoms are seen in anaphylactoid reactions, presumably due to nonimmunologic release of the same mediators. The treatment for either is the same.

Most instances of anaphylactic or anaphylactoid reactions are due to exposure to a specific food, drug, chemical, or insect sting. The most common foods to cause anaphylaxis are nuts, fish, and egg, although any food is capable of inducing anaphylaxis in a subject with a high degree of specific sensitivity. Penicillin and aspirin are the two most common drugs to cause anaphylaxis, probably because they are so commonly administered. A variety of penicillin metabolic products have been implicated in anaphylactic reactions. When testing for penicillin sensitivity, one must use both the major (penicilloyl) and minor determinants (metabolites) as antigen. Unfortunately, it is not yet possible to identify IgE antibodies to most other drugs that cause anaphylactic reactions, probably because the drugs, or their metabolites, act as haptens and do not cause immunologic reactions until they are combined with protein carriers in the body. Since both the protein carrier and the offending drug metabolite often are unknown, it is difficult to devise effective skin or in vitro tests for sensitivity.

Symptoms usually occur within a few seconds or minutes of exposure to the offending substance. Rarely does the first symptom begin after more than an hour. On the other hand, the symptoms may persist for hours and may recur any time during the ensuing 24 to 48 hours, after the effects of medications have waned.

Thus, treatment must be instituted without delay and should be continued for a minimum of 24 hours—better still, 48. It should be individualized according to the patient's response because of the variable severity of clinical manifestations. Principles of treatment are outlined below.

SEQUENTIAL MANAGEMENT OF ACUTE ANAPHYLAXIS

1. Establish a clear airway with adequate gas exchange using mouth-to-mouth respiration, oxygen, intubation, positive-pressure ventilation, cricothyrotomy, and cardiac resuscitation as needed.

2. Administer aqueous epinephrine, 1:1000, 0.1 to 0.5 ml (0.01 ml/kg, or 0.1 ml/20 lbs) to a maximum of 0.5 ml intramuscularly or intravenously. If there is cardiac standstill, this should be given into the heart, followed by external cardiac massage. The same dose may be repeated at 5- to 20-minute intervals to a total of three doses. Susphrine, 1:200, 0.008 ml/kg, or 0.08 ml/20 lbs, may be used if there is a response to the aqueous epinephrine. Aqueous epinephrine may also be given by slow intravenous infusion, titrating the rate according to blood pressure, heart rate, and symptomatology.

3. When applicable, place a venous tourniquet above the site of entry of the offending agent (such as an insect bite or antigen injection) to slow its absorption. Half the intramuscular dose of aqueous epinephrine is diluted in 2 ml of normal saline and infiltrated proximal to and surrounding the site of entrance of the foreign antigen.

4. If anaphylaxis is severe, or if epinephrine results in incomplete clearing of respiratory and cardiac symptoms, give aminophylline (7 mg/kg, or 70 mg/20 lbs) intravenously slowly over 10 minutes. This may be repeated after 6 hours.

5. Diphenhydramine (Benadryl), 1.25 mg/kg; chlorpheniramine (Chlor-Trimeton), 0.25 mg/kg; or promethazine (Phenergan), 1 mg/kg is given intravenously immediately after the initial dose of epinephrine (or after aminophylline in severe forms of anaphylaxis). Hydroxyzine (Vistaril), 1.0 mg/kg, may be used intramuscularly but not intravenously. One of the antihistamines should be given every 6 hours for 48 hours to minimize late recurrences of symptoms. On leaving the hospital, patients may be given a single dose of astemizole (Hismanal), 0.5 mg/kg to a maximum of 20 mg, to provide antihistamine coverage for the ensuing 48 hours. Ranitidine (Zantac), an H_2-blocking antihistamine, may be given intramuscularly or intravenously in a dose of 1 mg/kg every 6 hours. Care should be taken to administer it slowly (over 5 minutes) if given intravenously, since rapid administration may cause or aggravate bradycardia. An H_2 antagonist is recommended only after an H_1 antihistamine has been administered and the patient has not responded well to this and the other measures listed above over a period of 30 to 60 minutes.

6. Oxygen is administered by mask or endotracheal tube as long as there is clinical hypoventilation or cyanosis or the arterial Po_2 is below 70 mm Hg in room air.

7. An intravenous drip of normal saline is maintained as long as there are symptoms of anaphylaxis. Twenty ml/kg up to 1 L is given rapidly if there is hypotension. Following this, the fluid is changed to 5 per cent dextrose or half-normal saline in 5 per cent dextrose. Volume expanders, fluid and electrolyte replacement of losses, intravenous medications, and other supportive measures, are administered as indicated.

8. If hypotension, heart failure, arrhythmia, or anoxia is a problem, continuous monitoring of peripheral blood pressure, central venous pressure, pulmonary capillary pressure, electrocardiogram, and blood gases may be needed.

9. For persistent hypotension use an intravenous vasopressor such as norepinephrine (Levophed), 4 ml (4 mg) in 1 L of 5 per cent dextrose, not to exceed a rate of 1 to 2 ml/min, regulating the speed of administration according to the arterial pressure. An alternative to norepinephrine is dopamine (dilute a 5-ml ampule containing 200 mg in 200 ml normal saline [1 mg or 1000 μg/ml]). This may be given at a rate of 5 μg/kg/min, titrated to a maximum of 50 μg/kg/min as needed to maintain blood pressure. Plasma (or 5 per cent human serum albumin), 10 ml/kg up to 300 ml, may also be given intravenously.

10. Corticosteroids; hydrocortisone (Solu-Cortef), 2 mg/kg; methylprednisolone succinate (Solu-Medrol), 1 mg/kg; or dexamethasone sodium phosphate (Decadron), 0.2 mg/kg should be given intravenously initially and every 6 hours for 2 days in patients with severe anaphylaxis to forestall a recurrence. Oral corticosteroids may be used in place of intravenous once shock is under control and oral fluids are well tolerated. Steroid action is optimal only after 1 to 2 hours; hence these are *not* the drugs of choice for initial therapy.

11. Isoproterenol (Isuprel) by intravenous drip, 0.2 mg/100 ml of 5 per cent dextrose in water, is a useful drug should epinephrine not be available or if the patient is resistant to other therapy. One must be cautious when using this drug in conjunction with epinephrine, especially in adults, because of the synergistic effect of the two in causing tachycardia, arrhythmia, or myocardial ischemia. Continuous cardiovascular monitoring is essential whenever the two drugs are used within an hour of one another or when isoproterenol is given by intravenous drip. Isuprel and epinephrine (Medihaler) can also be given by inhalation.

The above outline may be followed in managing the various clinical manifestations encountered in human anaphylaxis. The severity and type of symptoms dictate the specific approach. Intravenous or, if necessary, intracardiac administration of epinephrine is recommended when alarming symptoms must be reversed immediately (severe shock or cardiac standstill). Deep intramuscular administration is sufficient in most instances of moderately severe anaphylaxis. The subcutaneous route is somewhat less rapid and is satisfactory for mild reactions. If the patient fails to respond to the initial dose of aqueous epinephrine, the same dose may be repeated within a minute or two in life-threatening situations. The minimal lethal dose of epinephrine is probably about 0.1 mg/kg or, in an adult, 4 mg (4 ml of 1:1000 aqueous). This is six to ten times the recommended therapeutic dose. In the rare case in which it may be necessary, phenotolamine (Regitine) in a dose of 1 mg per 20 lbs, up to 5 mg for an adult, may be given intravenously or intramuscularly to counteract the untoward effects of epinephrine overdosage.

The second most valuable drug in the therapy of severe anaphylactic reactions is aminophylline, an agent that has received too little attention for this purpose. While it is true that mild systemic anaphylaxis can be managed effectively with epinephrine and antihistaminics alone, it is equally true that many lives could be saved if the treatment of severe reactions included early administration of aminophylline in proper dose as well as its subsequent use to prevent and treat relapses.

Anaphylactic reactions following hyposensitization injections with pollen extracts are more likely to occur when the pollen season is at its peak, when a new lot of allergen is used, or when an excessive dose is mistakenly given. Injections should be low enough in the arm to permit the use of a tourniquet to slow absorption in the event that an anaphylactogenic dose is unwittingly administered.

If there has been a prior systemic anaphylactic response to a bee sting, one should quickly administer epinephrine both systemically and by local infiltration when a repeat sting is experienced. Bee sting kits are available commercially and should be carried at all times when outdoors by those who have had systemic reactions to hymenoptera. Hyposensitization of patients known to have had venom-induced anaphylaxis is recommended.

Persons who have had a systemic reaction to a specific food should be cautioned to read the labels on all food products to be certain that the offending food is not included. They also should be aware of the danger that may accompany prepared foods in restaurants. Patients should carry epinephrine for self-injection whenever they eat out and cannot be sure that an offending food is excluded from their food or drink. Fortunately, the patient with anaphylaxis generally has a good prognosis if skilled treatment is promptly undertaken. Children seldom have simultaneous heart disease and therefore are less likely than adults to have a myocardial infarction or cardiac arrest in association with an anaphylactic reaction.

Anaphylaxis following ingestion of an allergenic food or drug may begin within minutes or may be manifest only after an hour or more has passed. A certain time is required for absorption of intact food molecules or for their conversion to allergenic metabolic products in the gastrointestinal tract. The size of the molecule, its susceptibility to acid or proteolytic degradation, gastric emptying time, intestinal motility, the presence of unrelated food, and emesis or diarrhea may contribute to the time that elapses prior to the onset of symptoms. Sublingual or oropharyngeal absorption may account for a rapid systemic reaction to a low molecular weight allergen. Symptoms of anaphylaxis vary widely owing to individual differences in chemical mediator release and in the reactivity of target organs in different subjects.

Prevention of anaphylactic reactions is as important as an effective plan of treatment. There must be awareness of the potential hazards of antibiotics and other medicines, immunizations, allergy shots, intravenous radiographic dyes, insect stings, and so forth. A knowledge of the signs and symptoms that may be encountered, prompt judicious therapy for 48 hours, and careful identification and avoidance of the offending allergen can be life-saving. Subjects with exercise- or cold-induced anaphylaxis or cold urticaria must be cautious when running or swimming. They also should avoid food, drinks, and medications for 4 to 6 hours prior to these activities. Any substance previously known or thought to have caused an anaphylactic reaction in the past should be used again only when essential to the life or health of the patient. Skin tests, oral or injection desensitization, and premedication with antihistamines, adrenergic drugs, and corticosteroids all have a place in managing the patient who will be reexposed to a known offending substance.

These procedures are best carried out by, or in consultation with, an experienced allergist or clinical immunologist. Patients with frequent recurrent idiopathic anaphylaxis often remit when placed on prednisone prophylaxis, 2 mg/kg every other day. Some patients may be managed on chronic antihistamine therapy alone. Others may require both prednisone and antihistamines. Acute episodes should be treated as any other acute anaphylaxis. Care should be taken to avoid the use of beta-blocking agents in patients who have experienced anaphylaxis, since these agents may predispose to severe allergic reactions and lessen the effectiveness of treatment.

An emergency kit should be kept in each physician's office or should be available for immediate use if he or she deals with patients who might require treatment of anaphylactic reactions. Suggested contents of a kit are listed below:

DRUGS

Epinephrine hydrochloride solution 1:1000, 1-ml ampules or 30-ml vials

Injectable H₁ antihistamines—two of the following:
  Diphenhydramine (Benadryl), 50-mg ampules
  Chlorpheniramine (Chlor-Trimeton), 10-mg vials
  Hydroxyzine (Vistaril), 10-ml vials (25 mg/ml)
  Promethazine hydrochloride (Phenergan), 25-mg ampules
Injectable H₂ antihistamine
  Ranitidine (Zantac), 25 mg in 1-ml vials
  Injectable aminophylline, 250-mg ampules
Water-soluble corticosteroids
  Hydrocortisone (Solu-Cortef or Hydrocortone), 100-mg vials
  Methylprednisolone (Solu-Medrol), 40-mg vials
  Dexamethasone (Decadron), 4-mg vials
Injectable adrenergic agents (2)
  Metaraminol (Aramine), ampules or vials (10 mg/ml or 10 ml)
  Levarterenol (Levophed), 4-ml ampules (2 mg/ml)
  Isoproterenol hydrochloride, 1-ml ampules (1:5000 solution, 0.2 mg/ml)
Dopamine (Intropin) in 5-ml ampules, each containing 100 mg
Parenteral fluids
  Normal saline
  Dextrose 5 per cent in normal saline
  Dextrose 5 per cent in half-normal saline
  Salt-poor serum albumin, 20-ml vials
Injectable anticonvulsant drugs
  Amobarbital sodium (Amytal), 65-mg ampules
  Diazepam (Valium), 10- and 50-mg ampules
Sodium bicarbonate, 50-ml ampules (45 mEq)

EQUIPMENT

Tourniquets
Equipment for intravenous infusions
Sterile syringes and needles
Several sizes of airway and endotracheal tubes
Ambu bag
Aspirator or suction bulb
Surgical instruments for venous cut-down

20

Accidents and Emergencies

BOTULINAL FOOD POISONING

BARRY H. RUMACK, M.D.

Botulism is most frequently due to improperly home-processed foods such as vegetables, meats, fruits, pickles, and seafood. Rarely, commercial products are involved and recently these have been fish and meat products, especially in soups. Simple cooking for 6 to 10 minutes is capable of destroying the formed toxin.

Treatment. Empty the stomach, being careful to protect the airway. Administer activated charcoal and a cathartic. Hospitalize if there are *any* symptoms (paralysis, ptosis, blurred vision, diplopia, sore throat, other). Administration of antitoxin should be done under the supervision of the Centers for Disease Control or state health department. Guanidine therapy has been used in some cases, as has penicillin. The value of either of these drugs is questionable. Treatment consists primarily of antitoxin and respiratory support. Patients with minimal findings, usually mild neurologic, that do not progress will not require therapy. Treatment for the supportive and other needs of the patient is similar to treatment of any serious neurologic problem. Recovery is the rule with modern therapy.

ACUTE POISONING

HOWARD C. MOFENSON, M.D.,
and THOMAS R. CARACCIO, Pharm. D.

The ingestion of household products by a child is the most common medical emergency encountered in pediatric practice. Over 900,000 of these patients are treated in emergency departments annually. There is a biphasic curve to the incidence of pediatric poisonings, with the age groups peaking at 1 to 5 years and in adolescence.

IDENTIFICATION OF THE SUBSTANCE AND TELEPHONE MANAGEMENT

Information about the condition of the patient is obtained, and if there are no life-threatening manifestations, a telephone history is obtained by asking the reporter's questions: who, what, when, where, how much, and action taken and why?

If symptoms are already present, the patient should be referred to a medical care facility for further evaluation. Always remind the caller to **bring the container** or substance that may have been involved. It is recommended that the physician consult the regional poison control center for updates on the ingredients and management (see Table 43, p. 662, for telephone numbers). The "antidote" labels on products are notoriously inaccurate. Proper phone management, including callbacks, can reduce hospital emergency visits.

ASSESSMENT AND MAINTENANCE OF VITAL FUNCTIONS

1. *The first priority* is to establish and maintain vital functions. Immobilize the cervical spine. Establish and secure an airway and administer 100 per cent oxygen. Any patient with impaired airway protective reflexes should have an endotracheal tube. Adult pressure-cuffed endotracheal tubes are not recommended for children under 8 years of age.

2. *Cardiopulmonary resuscitative measures* should be initiated, if necessary, and 100 per cent oxygen is administered. Establish vascular access and obtain blood specimens for arterial gases and pH, glucose, electrolytes, BUN, creatinine, complete blood count, and 5 to 10 ml for toxicologic studies. Obtain urine for urinalysis; 50 to 100 ml of urine and gastric contents should be sent for toxicologic analysis. Save a portion of blood and urine for additional studies or in case of breakage or loss.

3. *Manage hypotension and shock* by positioning, a bolus of isotonic fluids at 20 ml/kg over 5 minutes, repeated as necessary, and if these measures fail, vasopressors. Shock may be caused by heart failure due to myocardial

depression, hypovolemia, and decreased peripheral vascular tone from CNS depression or adrenergic blockade.

4. *Hypertensive crisis* (encephalopathy, heart failure), usually from sympathomimetics, is treated with intravenous therapy such as diazoxide or nitroprusside and continuous arterial pressure monitoring.

5. *Pulmonary edema*, both cardiac and noncardiac, may develop. Noncardiac pulmonary edema may be produced by inhalation or ingestion of substances that may damage the alveolar-capillary membrane. Substances with antidiuretic activity are likely to cause this complication with fluid overload. Other agents increase pulmonary permeability or cause a massive sympathetic discharge, resulting in neurogenic pulmonary edema. Management consists of minimizing fluid administration, diuretics, and oxygen and may require respiratory support with mechanical ventilation and positive end-expiratory pressure.

6. Obtain an ECG and treat *dysrhythmias* if the patient's condition is unstable. Correction of hypoxia and metabolic derangement spontaneously corrects many dysrhythmias. Obtain a 12-lead ECG as soon as possible.

7. *Renal failure* due to tubular necrosis may occur as a result of hypotension, hypoxia, or the direct effect of the toxin on the tubular cells. Hemoglobin, myoglobin, and metabolites of ethylene glycol may precipitate in the renal tubules. Dialysis may be required.

8. *Cerebral edema* in intoxications may be produced by many causes and computed tomography (CT) may aid in the diagnosis. Management consists of reducing the increased intracranial pressure by hyperventilation to a Pco_2 of 25 mm Hg, 20 per cent mannitol 0.5 gm/kg run in over 30 minutes, and head elevation.

9. *Metabolic acidosis with increased anion gap* is present in many intoxications. Mnemonic MUDPILES: M—methanol, U—uremia, D—diabetic ketoacidosis, P—paraldehyde and phenformin, I—iron and isoniazid, L—lactic acidosis, E—ethylene glycol and ethanol, S—salicylates, starvation, and solvents such as toluene. Intravenous sodium bicarbonate may be needed if the patient persists with a pH less than 7.1 after correction of hypoxia and establishment of perfusion.

10. *Temperature control.* Manage hypothermia or hyperthermia. In hyperpyrexia due to intoxications, antipyretics are not indicated.

11. *Chest and abdominal radiographs* may be useful in evaluation for aspiration, foreign bodies, and radiopaque substances. Mnemonic CHIPES: C—chloral hydrate, H—heavy metals, I—iodine, P—Playdoh, Pepto-bismol, phenothiazines, and packets of contraband, E—enteric-coated tablets, S—chlorinated solvents.

12. *Classify the state of consciousness* and record it with the time of assessment. The Glasgow Coma Score, originally designed for estimating the prognosis in head trauma, overestimates the depth of coma in intoxications.

EMERGENCY TREATMENT OF THE COMATOSE OR CONVULSING PATIENT

Poisoning is the largest single cause of stupor and coma of unknown etiology. Obtain specimens for determinations listed above and immediately perform glucose reagent strip testing and confirmation by laboratory glucose analysis. Administer 10 per cent glucose 2 ml/kg in an infant or 25 per cent glucose 1 ml/kg in a child or 50 per cent glucose 1 ml/kg in an adolescent or adult and record response. If no response, administer naloxone every 2 to 3 minutes (antidote 25) and chart response (change in level of consciousness, pupillary response, and improvement in respirations). If an adolescent has a history of chronic alcoholism, administer intravenous thiamine 50 to 100 mg to avoid thiamine depletion encephalopathy. Anaphylactoid reactions to intravenous thiamine may occur, so be prepared to treat this rare occurrence.

Convulsions are controlled with diazepam intravenously, 0.2 to 0.5 mg/kg/dose slowly at rate of less than 2 mg/min up to maximum of 10 mg in children or 30 mg in adults and phenytoin 15 to 20 mg/kg up to a maximum of 1000 mg administered slowly at a rate of less than 30 mg/min while monitoring for dysrhythmias and hypotension.

PREVENTION OF ABSORPTION AND REDUCTION OF LOCAL DAMAGE

Use appropriate protection for rescuers, attendants, and the environment.

1. **Ocular** exposure is managed by immediate irrigation with water for 15 to 20 minutes with the eyelids fully retracted. Avoid neutralizing agents. All caustic and corrosive injuries should be evaluated by an ophthalmologist.

2. **Dermal** exposure is treated immediately by rinsing, not forceful flushing, which could result in deeper penetration.

3. **Injected** toxins such as intramuscular or subcutaneous needle injections or envenomation may require a proximal constriction band if there is delay in reaching a medical facility.

4. **Inhalation** exposure patients are immediately removed from the contaminated environment and administered 100 per cent oxygen. Evaluation may include arterial blood gases, chest radiography, and tests for bronchospasm.

5. **Gastrointestinal** exposures are the most common route of poisoning. If there is the possibility of potential intoxication, gastrointestinal decontamination (unless contraindicated) should be performed rather than waiting for symptoms to develop.

Dilutional and Neutralization Treatment

Dilutional treatment is indicated for the immediate management of the ingestion of caustics and corrosives (if the patient has no signs of airway obstruction, esophageal perforation, or shock and can swallow). It is otherwise not useful. Only small quantities of diluting fluid, 60 ml in small children and 250 ml in adults, should be used because of the danger of inducing vomiting. Neutralizing solutions are not recommended because of an exothermic reaction.

Gastrointestinal Decontamination

In small children emesis in the home or activated charcoal orally or via nasogastric tube in a medical care

TABLE 1. Contraindications to the Induction of Emesis

1. Ingestion of a caustic or corrosive.
2. Loss of protective airway reflexes* such as in coma or convulsions.
3. Ingestion of substances that are likely to produce rapid depression of consciousness, e.g., ethanol, tricyclic antidepressants, short-acting barbiturates.
4. Ingestion of substances that are likely to produce an early onset of seizures, e.g., camphor, isoniazid, strychnine, tricyclic antidepressants.
5. Ingestion of petroleum distillates. See *Hydrocarbons*.
6. Prior significant vomiting or hematemesis.
7. Age under 6 months because of possible immature protective airway reflex and the lack of data to establish the safe and effective dose.
8. If the patient ingested a foreign body, emesis is ineffective and risks aspiration and obstruction of the airway.
9. Neurologically impaired individuals with possible impaired airway protective reflexes.
10. Absence of bowel sounds. When no bowel sounds are present gastric lavage is preferred.

*The gag reflex may be absent in some normal individuals and does not mean that the airway protective reflexes are lost.

facility is preferred to gastric lavage, especially in cases of ingestion of particulate matter, because of the difficulty in inserting a large enough orogastric tube. In older children and adolescents, gastric lavage is preferred if they are in a medical facility, because it may be accomplished without lag time and will not interfere with retention of activated charcoal or oral antidotes. Both emesis and gastric lavage should be used with caution in patients with dysrhythmias or in ingestions of cardiotoxic drugs, since the vagal response may result in serious dysrhythmias or cardiac arrest. Neither emesis nor lavage is completely effective, removing only 30 to 50 per cent of the ingested substance.

Emesis. Syrup of ipecac is the method of inducing emesis. The contraindications to the induction of emesis are listed in Table 1 and the dosage of syrup of ipecac in Table 2. Some studies have safely used larger doses of ipecac syrup. The dose may be repeated once if the child does not vomit in 15 to 20 minutes. The vomitus should be inspected for fragments of pills or the toxin and saved for toxicologic analysis. The appearance, color, and odor of the gastric contents should be noted.

Gastric Aspiration and Lavage. Plants and large pills are not readily removed by gastric lavage. The best results are obtained with the largest possible orogastric hose that can be reasonably passed. Nasogastric tubes are not large enough for this purpose. In adolescents and adults a Lavacuator hose or a No. 36 Fr Ewald tube should be used. In young children use a No. 22 to 28 Fr orogastric tube. Aspirate first and save contents. The amount of fluid used varies with the size. In children

TABLE 2. Dose of Syrup of Ipecac

Age	Amount
6 to 9 months	5 ml
9 to 12 months	10 ml
1 to 12 years	15 ml
over 12 years	30 ml

TABLE 3. Contraindications to Gastric Lavage

1. Caustic or corrosive ingestions because of the danger of perforation
2. Uncontrolled convulsions because of the danger of aspiration or injury during the procedure
3. Petroleum products without endotracheal intubation
4. Comatose patients or patients with absent protective airway reflexes require insertion of endotracheal tube to protect against aspiration.
5. Cardiac dysrhythmias must be controlled first because the insertion of the tube may create a vagal response and cause a life-threatening dysrhythmia.

use 15 ml/kg of 0.9 per cent saline per wash until returns are clear; in adolescents and adults use 300 ml per wash of 0.9 per cent saline until returns are clear. Contraindications to gastric lavage are listed in Table 3.

Activated Charcoal (AC). In the emergency department, where compliance can be assured, AC may be used alone or after emesis and gastric lavage for substances adsorbed by it. Some emergency departments use AC as the lavage fluid after initial aspiration. This has the advantage of adsorbing any toxin and also serves as a marker for completion of lavage "until clear."

The initial oral dose of AC is 1 to 2 gm/kg or 15 to 30 gm in children and 60 to 100 gm in adults. It is administered as a soupy slurry suspension in at least 100 ml of water with a cathartic to avoid forming "briquettes" in the bowel. If the patient vomits, the dose may be repeated. If AC is used concomitantly with the oral antidote *N*-acetylcysteine, two loading doses of 140 mg/kg of *N*-acetylcysteine are recommended, or the antidote may be separated from the charcoal by 1 to 2 hours. The substances AC does not adsorb are more easily remembered than the multitude of agents it does. They are listed in Table 4.

Repeated doses of 0.5 gm/kg of AC may be administered orally every 2 to 6 hours, and an initial cathartic may be given. Repeated doses of AC appear to facilitate the passage of substances from the blood plasma into the intestinal fluid, presumably by creating a concentration gradient. There are a number of studies showing that repeated doses of oral AC are effective in reducing the nonrenal half-life of substances and their metabolites even when the substances were administered intravenously. This has been referred to as "gastrointestinal dialysis." Table 5 lists some of the products for which repeated doses of AC have been studied and recommended as effective therapy. The patient should have gastrointestinal (GI) motility monitored during therapy. Table 6 lists the contraindications to oral AC.

Cathartics. Despite the lack of scientific data that

TABLE 4. Substances That Activated Charcoal Does Not Adsorb

Alcohols	Cyanide
Aliphatic hydrocarbons	Glycols
Boric acid	Metals—iron, lead, lithium,
Caustics and corrosives	mercury
Drugs insoluble in aqueous solutions	Saline cathartics—sodium, magnesium

TABLE 5. Substances with Shortened Half-Lives by Repetitive Dosing of Oral Activated Charcoal

Acetaminophen	Nadolol
Carbamazepine	Phenobarbital
Chlordecone	Phenylbutazone
Dapsone	Phenytoin (controversial)
Digoxin	Salicylates
Digitoxin	Theophylline
Glutethimide	Tricyclic antidepressants
Methotrexate	Valproate

cathartics are useful in poisonings, they continue to be used by most authorities. The saline-type cathartics are recommended in children. Oil-based cathartics are not. Sorbitol, a very potent cathartic, is not recommended under 1 year of age and should be used with caution in children under 3 years of age because of possible severe electrolyte disturbances. The dosage is listed in Table 7. The contraindications to cathartics are listed in Table 8.

Whole Bowel Washout. This procedure has been used successfully with iron overdose when abdominal radiography identified incomplete emptying of ingested iron. It has additional implications for gastrointestinal decontamination in other ingestions. It consists of using a colonic irrigation solution (GoLytely), 0.5 L/hr in children under 5 years of age (not FDA-approved) and 2 L/hr in adolescents and adults. The end-point is a rectal effluent with the appearance of the infusate. This takes approximately 2 to 4 hours. These measures should not be used if there is extensive hematemesis, ileus, signs of bowel perforation, or peritonitis.

ANTIDOTES

Systemic antidotes should be highly specific and efficacious with relatively low toxicity. A small number of antidotes have these characteristics. In some cases the physician may start antidotal therapy on the basis of the history and clinical picture while awaiting laboratory confirmation. Antidotes are not used prophylactically. **The antidote formulary** (Table 9) is an alphabetical list of commonly used antidotes, their indications, and methods of administration. It is useful to contact your regional poison control center (see Table 43) for additional advice and guidance when using an antidote.

ENHANCEMENT OF ELIMINATION

The methods for elimination of the absorbed toxic substances or their toxic metabolites are forced diuresis and osmotic diuresis with or without ion trapping, peritoneal dialysis, hemodialysis, hemoperfusion, exchange transfusion, plasmapheresis, and enzyme induc-

TABLE 7. Doses of Cathartics

Cathartic	Pediatric	Adolescent/adult
Sodium sulfate (Glauber's salt)	250 mg/kg/dose	15–30 gm/dose
Magnesium sulfate (Epsom salt)	250 mg/kg/dose	15–30 gm/dose
Magnesium citrate	5 ml/kg/dose	240 ml (8 oz)/dose
Sorbitol Conc.	35% (diluted)	70% (standard)
Age	>3 year	
Dose	1.4–2.1 ml/kg	2.8–4.3 ml/kg
Maximum	143 ml	214 ml
Frequency	Once only	Once only

tion and inhibition. The methods to increase the renal excretion have been fairly extensively studied, but the others have not been well evaluated. In general, the supportive *indications for dialysis* are the mnemonic AEIOU: A—acidosis and alkalosis (refractory), E—electrolyte imbalance (refractory), I—intoxications by a dialyzable poison, O—overhydration, U—uremia. The use of these modalities will be discussed in the management of the specific poisons.

THE TOXICOLOGY LABORATORY

If legality is involved, establish a "chain of custody" to ensure the security of the specimen. The physician must always ascertain the units used in the laboratory report.

MANAGEMENT OF COMMON DRUG OVERDOSES AND POISONS*

These agents will be presented alphabetically in the following scheme: generic name (common name), toxicity, kinetic data (pharmacokinetic or toxicokinetic) and mechanism of toxicity that has relevance to management, major manifestations, and management with referral to the antidote in Table 9.

Acetaminophen (ARAP, Tylenol, many brands). See chapter on Acetaminophen poisoning.

Acetone (dimethyl ketone 2-propanone). Nail polish remover, solvents.

Text continued on page 633

Abbreviations used in the text: $t_{1/2}$ = Half life, the time required for the blood concentration to fall by 50 per cent.

S.G. = specific gravity.

Vd = Apparent volume distribution, the theoretical portion of the body mass in which the drug is distributed, or the body burden.

MAC = Maximum allowable concentration.

TWA = Time-weighed allowance. Allows excursions above stated value provided that they are compensated by equivalent values below stated values during the workday. Presented as parts per million. 1 mg/L = 1 ppm.

TABLE 6. Contraindications to Oral Activated Charcoal

1. Caustics or corrosives—charcoal ineffective and may obscure or look like a burn
2. Absence of bowel sounds (adynamic ileus)
3. Intestinal obstruction or evidence of peritonitis
4. Unable to confirm location of gastric tube
5. Lack of adequate airway protection, in which case an endotracheal tube should be inserted first.

TABLE 8. Contraindications to Cathartics

1. Absence of bowel sounds (adynamic ileus)
2. Evidence of intestinal obstruction
3. Pre-existing electrolyte disturbances
4. Magnesium sulfate in renal impairment
5. Sodium sulfate in conditions requiring salt restriction
6. Evidence of gastrointestinal perforation or peritonitis
7. Evidence of gastrointestinal bleeding

TABLE 9. Antidote Formulary*

Medication	Indications and Adverse Reaction (AR)	Comments
1. **N-Acetylcysteine** (NAC, *Mucomyst*), Mead Johnson. Glutathione precursor that prevents accumulation and helps detoxify acetaminophen metabolites. **Dose:** *Adult,* 140 mg/kg PO of 5% solution as loading dose, then 70 mg/kg PO every 4 hr for 17 doses as maintenance dose. *Child,* same as adult. **Packaged:** 10 and 20% solution in 4, 10, and 30 ml vials.	Acetaminophen toxicity. Most effective within first 8 hr (to make more palatable, administer through a straw inserted into closed container of citrus juice). AR: Stomatitis, nausea, vomiting. See Acetaminophen. The full course of therapy is required in any patient whose level falls in the toxic range.	IV preparation experimental. The dose of NAC should be repeated if the patient vomits within 1 hr after administration. Methods to stop vomiting of the NAC are (a) placement of a tube in the duodenum, (b) slow administration over 1 hr, (c) one half hour before NAC dose use metoclopramide (*Reglan*) 1 mg/kg intravenously over 15 min. (Max dose 10 mg) every 6 hrs. In infants 0.1 mg/kg/dose Im, IV or droperidol (*Inapsine*) 1.25 mg IV; for extrapyramidal reactions use diphenhydramine (antidote 18).
2. **Ammonium chloride** USP, usually given via nasogastric tube. **Dose:** *Adult,* 2 gm every 6 hr in 60 ml dose to maximum of 12 gm/day or 1.5 gm as 1–2% IV q6h up to 6 gm/day. *Child,* 75 mg/kg (2.75 mEq/kg) 4 times/day to maximum of 2–6 gm IV or PO. **Packaged:** 325, 500, and 1000 mg tablets: 2.14% in 500 ml, 21.4% in 30 ml, 26.75% in 20 ml	Acidification of urine may enhance the elimination of phencyclidine and other weak bases (amphetamines and strychnine), but the danger of rhabdomyolysis and precipitation of myoglobin in the renal tubules in an acid milieu indicates that this therapy is too dangerous to recommend routinely.	Goal in acid diuresis is to keep urine pH 4.5–5.5 and output 3–6 ml kg/hr. Monitor blood pH, keep at 7.2–7.3. A diuretic may be used to enhance acid diuresis. Contraindications: weak acid drugs, rhabdomyolysis and myoglobinuria, liver dysfunction, renal dysfunction, closed head injury.
3. **Amyl nitrite**	See 14, Cyanide kit	
4. **Antivenin Black Widow Spider** (*Latrodectus mactans*) **Dose:** 1–2 vials infused over 1 hr. **Packaged:** 6000 units/vial with 2.5 ml sterile watering and 1 ml horse serum 1:10 dilution.	Black widow spider; all *Latrodectus* species with severe symptoms. Most healthy adults will survive with supportive care. Used in elderly or infants or if underlying medical condition causing hemodynamic instability. AR: Same as antivenin polyvalent because derived from horse serum.	Preliminary sensitivity test. Supportive care alone is standard management.
5. **Antivenin Polyvalent** for Crotalidae (pit vipers), Wyeth. IV only. **Dose:** depends on degree of envenomation—minimal: 5–8 vials, moderate: 8–12 vials, severe: 13–30 vials. Dilute in 500–2000 ml of crystalloid solution and start IV at a slow rate, increasing after the first 10 minutes, if no reaction occurs. **Packaged:** 1 vial (10 ml) lyophilized serum, 1 vial (10 ml) bacteriostatic water for injection, 1 vial (1 ml) normal horse serum.	Venoms of crotalids (pit vipers) of North and South America. AR: (Shock anaphylaxis) Reaction occurs within 30 min. Serum sickness usually occurs 5–44 days after administration. It may occur less than 5 days, especially in those who have received horse serum products in the past. Symptoms include fever, edema, arthralgia, nausea, and vomiting, as well as pain and muscle weakness.	Consider consulting with regional poison control center and herpetologist. Administer IV. Preliminary sensitivity test. Never inject in fingers, toes, or bite site.
6. **Antivenin,** North American coral snake. Wyeth. IV only. **Dose:** 3–5 vials (30–50 ml) by slow IV injection. First 1–2 ml should be injected over 3–5 min. **Packaged:** 1 vial antivenin, 10 ml, 1 vial bacteriostatic water 10 ml for injection.	*Micrurus fulvius* (Eastern coral snake); *Micurus tenere* (Texas coral snake) AR: Anaphylaxis (sensitivity reaction). Usually 30 min after administration. Signs/Symptoms: Flushing, itching, edema of face, cough, dyspnea, cyanosis. Neurologic manifestations—usually involve the shoulders and arms. Pain and muscle weakness are frequently present and permanent atrophy may develop.	Same as for Antivenin polyvalent: for Crotalidae. Will not neutralize the venom of *Micrurus euryxanthus* (Arizona or sonoran coral snake)
7. **Atropine** (various manufacturers). Antagonizes cholinergic stimuli at muscarinic receptors. **Dose:** *Adult,* initial dose 2–4 mg IV. Dose every 2–5 min as necessary until cessation of secretions. Severe poisoning may require doses up to 2000 mg. *Child,* initial dose of 0.02 mg/kg to a max of 2 mg every 10–15 min as necessary until cessation of secretions. **Packaged:** 0.3 mg/ml in 30 ml; 0.4 mg/mi in 0.5, 1, 20, and 30 ml vials; 1 mg/ml in 1 and 10 ml vials.	Therapy in carbamate and organophosphate insecticide poisonings. Rarely needed in cholinergic mushroom intoxication (*Amanita, Muscaria, Clitocybe, Inocybe* spp.) Lack of signs of atropinization confirms diagnosis of cholinesterase inhibition. AR: Flushing and dryness of skin, blurred vision, rapid and irregular pulse, fever, and loss of neuromuscular co-ordination. Diagnostic test: child–0.01 mg/kg IV; adult–1 mg total	If cyanosis—establish respiration first because atropine in cyanotic patients may cause ventricular fibrillation. If severe signs of atropinization, may correct with Physostigmine in doses equal to one-half dose of atropine. If symptomatic administer until the endpoint of drying secretions and clearing of lungs. Hallucinations, flushing of the skin, dilated pupils, tachycardia, and elevation of body temperature are not endpoints and do not preclude atropine administration. Atropinization should be maintained for 12 to 24 hours, then taper dose and observe for relapse.

*This is for informational purposes and is not intended to substitute for independent judgment. It is always advisable to review the package insert for the most up-to-date information. Contact Regional Poison Control Center for additional details on use.

Abbreviations: AR = adverse reactions to antidotes; MP = monitor parameters; FDA = U.S. Food and Drug Administration; ECG = electrocardiogram; CNS = central nervous system; GI = gastrointestinal.

Table continued on following page

TABLE 9. Antidote Formulary *Continued*

Medication	Indications and Adverse Reaction (AR)	Comments
		Atropine has successfully been administered by IV infusion although this method has not received FDA approval. **Dose:** Place 8 mg of atropine in 100 ml D5W or saline. Conc. = 0.08 mg/ml Dose range = 0.02–0.08 mg/kg/hr or 0.25–1 ml/kg/hr. Severe poisoning may require supplemental doses of intravenous atropine intermittently in doses of 2–4 mg until drying of secretions occurs.
8. **BAL**	See 17, Dimercaprol	
9. **Bicarbonate**	See 35, Sodium bicarbonate	
10. **Botulism antitoxin,** Connaught Med. Research Labs. **Dose:** *Adults,* 1 vial IV stat then 1 vial IM repeat in 2–4 hr if symptoms appear in 12–24 hr. *Child,* Check with State Health Dept.	Prevention or treatment of botulism.	Contact local or state health department for full management guidelines.
11. **Calcium disodium edetate** (EDTA), *Versenate,* Riker. **Dose:** *Adult,* max 4 gm. *Child,* 1 gm max. Moderate toxicity, IM or IV, 50 mg/kg day for 3–5 days. Severe toxicity, IV or IM, 75 mg/kg/day for 4–5 days, divided into 3–6 doses daily. Dilute 1 gm in 250–500 ml saline or D5W, infuse over 4 hr twice daily for 5–7 days. For lead levels over 69 μg/dl or if symptoms of lead poisoning or encephalopathy, add BAL alone initially, 4 mg/kg, then combination BAL and EDTA at different sites. EDTA dose: 12.5 mg/kg IM. (See lead text for latest recommendations.) Modify dose in renal failure. **Packaged:** 200 mg/ml. 5 ml amps.	For chelation in cadmium, chromium cobalt, copper, lead, magnesium, nickel, selenium, tellurium, tungsten, uranium, vanadium, and zinc poisoning. **AR:** 1. Thrombophlebitis. 2. Nausea, vomiting. 3. Hypotension. 4. Transient bone marrow suppression. 5. Nephrotoxicity, reversible tubular necrosis (particularly in acid urine). 6. Fever 4–8 hours after infusion. 7. Increased prothrombin time.	Hydrate first and establish renal flow. Avoid plain sodium EDTA since hypocalcemia may result. Procaine 0.25–1 ml of 0.5% for each ml of IM EDTA to reduce pain. Do not use EDTA orally. Limit use to 7 days (otherwise loss of other ions and cardiac dysrhythmias may occur). MP: Calcium levels, urinalysis, renal profile, erythrocyte protoporphyrin, blood lead, and liver profile. Contraindicated in iron intoxication, hepatic impairment, and renal failure.
12. (A) **Calcium gluconate** Various manufacturers. **Dose:** *Adult:* 10 gm in 250 ml of water PO or by NG tube. 30 gm max daily dose. **Packaged:** 500, 650 mg, 1 gm tabs.	To precipitate fluorides, magnesium, salts, and oxalates after oral ingestion.	
(B) **Calcium gluconate** 10% **Dose:** IV 0.2 to 0.5 ml/kg of elemental calcium to max 10 ml (1 gm) over 5–10 min with continuous ECG monitoring. Titrate to adequate response. **Packaged:** 10% in 10 ml vial.	Calcium-channel blocker poisoning, e.g., nifedipine (Procardia), verapamil (Calan), diltiazem (Cardiazem). It improves the blood pressure but does not affect the dysrhythmias. Hypocalcemia as result of poisonings. Black widow spider envenomation.	Repeat dose as needed. Monitor calcium levels. Contraindicated with digitalis poisoning.
(C) **Calcium chloride** **Dose:** IV 0.2 ml/kg to max 10 ml (1 gm) with continuous IV monitoring. Titrate to adequate response.	Hydrofluoric acid (HF) (if irrigation with cool water fails to control the pain). **AR:** IV bradycardia, asystole, necrosis with extravasation.	Infiltration with calcium gluconate should be considered if HF exposure results in immediate tissue damage and erythema and pain persists following adequate irrigation.
(D) **Infiltration of calcium gluconate.** **Dose:** Infiltrate each square cm of the affected dermis and subcutaneous tissue with about 0.5 ml of 10% calcium gluconate using a 30 gauge needle. Repeat as needed to control pain. **Packaged:** 10% in 10 ml vial.		
(E) **Calcium Gel** 3.5 gm USP calcium gluconate powder added to 5 oz of KY jelly.	Dermal exposures of hydrofluoric acid less than 20%.	Gel must have direct access to burn area; if pain persists then calcium gluconate injection may be needed. Placing a loose fitting surgical glove over the gel when the fingers are involved helps to keep preparation in contact with burn area.
13. **Chlorpromazine,** various manufacturers. Phenothiazine derivative. **Dose:** *Adult,* 1 mg/kg dose IV/IM or 0.5 mg/kg dose if taken with barbiturate or if exhausted. **Packaged:** 25 mg/ml in 1, 2, and 10 ml vials.	Only in *pure* amphetamine OD with life-threatening manifestations. (Diazepam [Valium] is preferred.) Toxicity: CNS depression, coma, hypotension, extrapyramidal syndrome, agitation, fever, convulsions, dry mouth, cardiac arrhythmias, ECG changes.	Do not use if any signs of atropinization are present or "street drug" amphetamines. Watch for hypotension. In general it is safer to use diazepam (Valium) or haloperidol (Haldol).

628

TABLE 9. Antidote Formulary *Continued*

Medication	Indications and Adverse Reaction (AR)	Comments
14. **Cyanide antidote kit** Lilly. Nitrite-induced methemoglobinemia attracts cyanide off cytochrome oxidase and thiosulfate forms nontoxic thiocyanate. **Doses:** *Adult*, amyl nitrite. Inhale for 30 sec of every min. Use a new ampule every 3 min. Reapply until Na nitrite can be given. Then inject IV 300 mg (10 ml of 3% solution of Na nitrite at a rate of 2.5 to 5 ml/min. Then inject 12.5 gm (50 ml of 25% sol.) of Na thiosulfate. *Child*, use the following chart for children's dosage. **Packaged:** 2–10 ml ampules Na nitrite injection: 2–50 ml ampules Na thiosulfate injection: 0.3 ml amyl nitrite inhalant.	Cyanide poisoning. **AR:** Hypotension, methemoglobinemia.	*Note:* If a child is given the adult dose of Na nitrite a fatal methemoglobinemia may result. *Do not use methylene blue* for methemoglobinemia in cyanide therapy. Observe for hypotension and have epinephrine available. Cyanide kits should have amyl nitrite changed annually. Administer oxygen 100% between inhalations of amyl nitrite. Monitor hemoglobin, arterial blood gases, methemoglobin concentration (nitrite given to obtain a methemoglobin of 25%). Some add cyanide ampul to resuscitation bag.

Hemoglobin

	Initial Child Dose of Sodium Nitrite 3% (do not exceed 10 ml)	*Initial Child Dose of Sodium Thiosulfate (do not exceed 12.5 gm)*
8 gm	0.22 ml/kg (6.6 mg/kg)	1.10 ml/kg
10 gm	0.27 ml/kg (8.7 mg/kg)	1.35 ml/kg
12 gm	0.33 ml/kg (10 mg/kg)	1.65 ml/kg
14 gm	0.39 ml/kg (11.6 mg/kg)	1.95 ml/kg

If signs of poisoning reappear repeat above procedure at one-half the above doses.

Medication	Indications and Adverse Reaction (AR)	Comments
15. **Deferoxamine mesylate** (DFOM, *Desferal* Ciba). Has a remarkable affinity for ferric iron and chelates it. **Therapeutic Dose:** *Adult*, 90 mg/kg* IM or IV every 8 hr to max 1 gm/inj. May repeat to max 6 gm in 24 hr. *Child*, same as adult. IM or IV. IV administration should be given by slow infusion at rate not exceeding 15 mg/kg/hr. **Packaged:** 500 mg/amp (powder).	DFOM is useful in the treatment of symptomatic iron poisoning or serum iron levels greater than 350–500 µg/dl. If the DFOM challenge test is positive it is not a definite indication that therapy is necessary in the asymptomatic patient. Oral DFOM is not recommended. Iron intoxication. Therapeutic—see dose in left column. *Diagnostic trial.* Give deferoxamine, 50 mg/kg IM (up to 1 gm). If serum iron exceeds TIBC unbound iron is excreted in urine, producing a "vin rose" color of chelated iron complex in the urine (pink orange). However, may be negative with high serum iron exceeding TIBC. **AR:** Flushing of the skin, generalized erythema, urticaria, hypotension, and shock may occur. Blindness has occurred rarely in patients receiving long-term, high dose DFOM therapy. Contraindicated in patients with renal disease or anuria.	Therapy is usually continued until urine color and/or iron levels are normal. Therapy is rarely required over 24 hr. Establish a good renal flow. To be effective, DFOM should be administered in first 12–16 hr. In mild to moderate iron intoxication, IM or IV route. In severe intoxication or shock, IV route only. Monitor serum iron levels, urine output, and urine color.
16. **Diazepam** (*Valium*). Roche. **Dose:** *Adult*, 5–10 mg IV (max 20 mg) at a rate of 5 mg/min until seizure is controlled. May be repeated 2 or 3 times. *Child*, 0.1–0.3 mg/kg up to 10 mg IV slowly over 2 min. **Packaged:** 5 mg/ml, 2 ml, 10 ml vials.	Any intoxication that provokes seizures when specific therapy is *not* available, e.g., amphetamines, PCP, barbiturate and alcohol withdrawal. Chloroquine poisoning. **AR:** Confusion, somnolence, coma, hypotension.	Intramuscular absorption is erratic. Establish airway and administer 100% oxygen and glucose.
17. **Dimercaprol** (BAL). Hynson, Westcott, and Dunning. **Dose:** Recommendations vary, contact regional poison control center. Prevents inhibition of sulfhydryl enzymes. Given deep IM only. For *severe lead poisoning*—see 11, EDTA. For *mild arsenic or gold*—2.5 mg/kg every 6 hr for 2 days, then every 12 hr on the third day, and once daily thereafter for 10 days. For *severe arsenic or gold*—3–5 mg/kg every 6 hr for 3 days, then every 12 hr for 10 days. For *mercury*—5 mg/kg initially, followed by 2.5 mg/kg 1 or 2 times daily for 10 days. **Packaged:** 100 mg/ml 10% in oil in 3 ml amp.	For chelation of antimony, arsenic, bismuth, chromates, copper, gold, lead, and mercury nickel. **AR:** 30% of patients have reactions: fever (30% of children), hypertension, tachycardia, may cause hemolysis in G-6-PD deficiency patients. Doses greater than recommended may cause various adverse effects: nausea, vomiting, headache, chest pain, tachycardia, and hypertension.	Contraindicated in instances of hepatic insufficiency, with the exception of postarsenic jaundice. Should be discontinued or used only with extreme caution if acute renal insufficiency is present. Monitor blood pressure and heart rate (both may increase), urinalysis, qualitative urine excretion of heavy metal. Contraindicated in iron, silver, uranium, selenium, and cadmium poisoning.

*This dose may exceed the manufacturer's recommendation.

Table continued on following page

TABLE 9. Antidote Formulary *Continued*

Medication	Indications and Adverse Reaction (AR)	Comments
18. **Diphenhydramine** (*Benadryl*), Parke Davis. Antiparkinsonian action. **Dose:** *Adult,* 10–50 mg IV over 2 min. *Child,* 1–2 mg/kg IV up to 50 mg over 2 min. Maximum in 24 hr, 400 mg. **Packaged:** 10 mg/ml in 10 and 30 ml vials. 50 mg/ml in 1, 5, 10, and 30 ml vials. Caps, tab 25 mg. Elixir, syrup 12.5 mg/5 ml.	Used to treat extrapyramidal symptoms and dystonia induced by phenothiazines and related drugs. **AR:** Fatal dose, 20–40 mg/kg. Dry mouth, drowsiness.	Continue with oral diphenhydramine 5 mg/kg/day to 25 mg 3 times a day for 72 hours to avoid recurrence.
19. **EDTA**	See 11, Calcium disodium edetate	
20. **Ethanol** (ETOH) Competitively inhibits alcohol dehydrogenase. **Dose:** *Loading*—Administer 7.6–10.0 ml/kg of 10% ETOH in D5W over 30 min IV or 0.8–1.0 ml/kg 95% ETOH PO in 6 oz of orange juice over 30 min. While administering loading dose, start maintenance. **Maintenance Dose:** Volume of 10% ETOH needed IV or 95% oral solution (not on dialysis). [See table of maintenance dose below.] If patient is on dialysis, add 91 ml/hr in addition to regular maintenance dose. See comments to prepare 10% solution if not commercially available. **Packaged:** 10% ethanol in D5W 1000 ml; 95% ethanol. May be given as 50% solution orally.	Methanol, ethylene glycol **Ethanol infusion** therapy may be started in cases of suspected **methanol** and **ethylene glycol** poisoning presenting with increased anion gap and osmolal gap, or if the urine shows the crystalluria of ethylene glycol poisoning or the hyperemia of the optic disc of methanol intoxication. **AR:** CNS depression, hypoglycemia.	Monitor blood ethanol 1 hr after starting infusion and every 4–6 hr. Maintain a blood ethanol concentration of 100–200 mg/dl. Monitor blood glucose, electrolytes, blood gases, urinalysis, and renal profile at least daily. Continue infusion until safe concentration of ethylene glycol or methanol is reached. Ethanol-induced hypoglycemia may occur. Dialysis, preferably hemodialysis, should be considered in severe intoxication not controlled by ethanol alone. To prepare 10% ethanol for infusion therapy, remove 100 ml from a liter D5W and replace with 100 ml of tax free bulk absolute alcohol after passing through 0.22 micron filter. 50 ml vials of pyrogen-free absolute ethanol for injection are available from Pharm-Serve 218–20 96th Avenue, Queens Village, NY 11429. Telephone 718–475–1601.

Maintenance Dose:

Patient Category	ml/kg/hr using 10% IV	ml/kg/hr using 50% oral
Nondrinker	0.83	0.17
Occasional drinker	1.40	0.28
Alcoholic	1.96	0.39

Medication	Indications and Adverse Reaction (AR)	Comments
21. **Fab** (antibody fragment) (*Digibind*). **Dose:** The average dose used during clinical testing was 10 vials. Dosage details are specified by the manufacturer. It should be administered by the IV route over 30 min. Calculate out on basis of body burden either by known amount ingested or by serum digoxin concentration. Calculation of dose of Fab: 1. Known amount ingested multiplied by bioavailability (0.8) = body burden. Body burden divided by 0.6 = number of vials. 2. Known serum digoxin (obtained 6 hr postingestion) multiplied by volume distribution (5.6 L/kg) and weight in kg divided by 1000 = body burden. Body burden divided by 0.6 = number of vials.	Digoxin, digitoxin, oleander tea with life-threatening intoxications, refractory dysrhythmias, hyperkalemia. 40 mg binds 0.6 mg digoxin.	Contact regional poison control center. Preliminary sensitivity test. Administer through a 0.22 micron filter. It causes a rise in measured bound digoxin but a fall in free digoxin.
22. **Glucagon.** Works by stimulating production of cyclic adenyl monophosphate. **Dose:** 50–150 µg/kg over 1 min IV followed by a continuous infusion of 1–5 mg/hr in dextrose and then taper over 5–12 hr. **Packaged:** 1 mg (1 unit) vial with 1 ml diluent with glycerine and phenol; also in 10 ml size.	Propranolol and other beta-blocker intoxication. **AR:** Generally well tolerated—most frequent are nausea, vomiting.	Do not dissolve the lyophilized glucagon in the solvent packaged with it when administering IV infusion because of possible phenol toxicity. Effects of single dose observed in 5–10 min and last for 15–30 min. A constant infusion may be necessary to sustain desired effects.
23. **Labetalol hydrochloride** (*Normodyne*) Schering; (*Trandate*) Glaxo. Nonselective beta and mild alpha blocker. **Dose:** IV 20 mg over 2 min. Additional injections of 40 or 80 mg can be given at 10-min intervals until desired supine blood pressure achieved. Max dose, 300 mg Alternative: Slow IV infusion: 200 mg (40 ml) is added to 160 or 250 ml of D5W and given at 2 mg/min. Titrate infusion according to response. **Packaged:** Solution 5 mg/ml in 20 ml.	Hypertensive crises secondary to cocaine. **AR:** GI disturbances; orthostatic hypotension; bronchospasm; congestive heart failure, AV conduction disturbances, and peripheral vascular reactions.	Concomitant diuretic enhances therapeutic response. Patient should be kept in a supine position during infusion. **MP:** monitor blood pressure during and after administration.

TABLE 9. Antidote Formulary *Continued*

Medication	Indications and Adverse Reaction (AR)	Comments
24. **Methylene blue,** Harvey and others. Physiologically transformed to reduced form leukomethylene blue, which is then oxidized to methylene blue in the presence of methemoglobin which is converted to hemoglobin. **Dose:** *Adult,* 0.1–0.2 ml/kg of 2% solution (1–2 mg/kg over 5 min IV). *Child,* same as Adult. **Packaged:** 1% 10 ml ampules. May repeat in 1 hr if necessary.	Methemoglobinemia **AR:** GI (nausea, vomiting), headache, hypertension, dizziness, mental confusion, restlessness, dyspnea when IV dose exceeds 7 mg/kg. Treatment is unnecessary unless methemoglobin is over 30% or respiratory distress.	Saliva, urine, and other body fluids may turn blue. *Contraindications:* Renal insufficiency, cyanide poisonings when sodium nitrite is used to induce methemoglobinemia in G-6-PD deficiency patients. Monitor hemolysis, methemoglobin level, and arterial blood gases. Avoid extravasation because of local necrosis.
25. **Naloxone** (*Narcan*) Pure opioid antagonist. **Dose:** *Adult,* 0.4–2.0 mg IV and repeat at 3 minute intervals until respiratory function is stable. Before excluding opioid intoxication on the basis of a lack of naloxone response, a minimum of 2 mg in a child or 10 mg in an adult should be administered. *Child,* initial dose is 0.1 mg/kg IV. **Packaged:** 0.02 mg/ml. 0.4 mg/ml ampule, and 10 ml multidose vial.	Narcotic, opiate, CNS depression. This drug is relatively free of adverse reactions. Rare report of pulmonary edema. Should be administered with caution in pregnancy. It is used only to reverse depression and hypoxia.	Naloxone infusion therapy should be used if a large initial dose was required, repeated bolus are necessary, or a long-acting opiate is involved. In infusion therapy the initial response dose is administered every hour and may need to be boostered one-half hour after starting. The infusion may be tapered after 12 hours of therapy. Naloxone infusion: Calculate out daily fluid requirements, add initial response dose of naloxone multiplied by 24 to the solution. Divide fluid by 24 = ml/hr of naloxone infusion. Does not cause CNS depression Routes: IV or endotracheal are preferred routes. Pentazocine (Talwin), dextramethorphan, propoxyphene (Darvon), and codeine may require larger doses.
26. **Nicotinamide,** various manufacturers. **Doses:** *Adult,* 500 mg IM or IV slowly, then 200–400 mg q4h. If symptoms develop, the frequency of injections should be increased to every 2 hr (max 3 gm day). *Child,* one-half suggested adult dose. **Packaged:** 100 mg/ml: 2, 5, 10, 30 ml vials; 25 and 50 mg tablets.	Vacor poisoning: phenylurea pesticide intoxication. *Note:* Vacor 2% is now available only to professional exterminators. 0.5% Vacor is available to the general public and can be toxic to children if swallowed. **AR:** Large doses—flushing, pruritus, sensation of burning, nausea, vomiting, anaphylactic shock.	Nicotinamide is most effective when given within 1 hr of ingestion. Do not use niacin or nicotinic acid in place of nicotinamide. Monitor liver profile.
27. **Oxygen** 100% **Dose:** *Adult,* 100% oxygen by inhalation or 100% oxygen in hyperbaric chamber at 2–3 atm. *Child,* same as adult.	Carbon monoxide, cyanide, methemoglobinemia. Any inhalation intoxication.	Half-life of carboxyhemoglobin is 240 min in room air 21% oxygen; if a patient is hyperventilated with 100% oxygen, the half-life of carboxyhemoglobin is 90 min, in chamber at 2 atm, half-life is 25–30 min.
28. **Pancuronium bromide** (*Pavulon*) Nondepolarizing (competitive) blocking agent. **Dose:** *Adults and children,* initially, 0.1 mg/kg IV; for intubation, 0.1 mg/kg IV, repeated as required (generally every 40–60 min). **Packaged:** Sol 1 mg/ml in 10 ml 2 mg/ml in 2 and 5 ml containers.	Neuromuscular blocking agent. Used for intubation and seizure control. Acts in 2 min, lasts 40–60 min. **AR:** Main hazard is inadequate postoperative ventilation. Tachycardia and slight increase in arterial pressure may occur due to vagolytic action.	The required dose varies greatly and a peripheral nerve stimulator aids in determining appropriate amount. Should monitor EEG since motor effect may be abolished without decreasing electrical discharge from brain.
29. **D-Penicillamine** (*Cuprimine*) Merck; (*Depen*) Wallace. Effective chelator and promotes excretion in urine. **Dose:** 250 mg 4 times daily PO for up to 5 days for long-term (20–40 days) therapy: 30–40 mg/kg/day in children. Max 1 gm/day. For chronic therapy 25 mg/kg/day in 4 doses. **Packaged:** 125 and 250 mg capsules.	Heavy metals, arsenic, cadium, chromates, cobalt, copper, lead, mercury, nickel, and zinc. **MP:** Routine urinalysis, white differential blood count, hemoglobin determination, direct platelet count, renal and hepatic profiles. Collect 24-hr urine, quantify for heavy metal. **AR:** Leukopenia (2%); thrombocytopenia (4%); GI—nausea, vomiting, anaphylactic shock, diarrhea (17%); fever, rash, lupus syndrome, renal and hepatic injury.	This is not considered standard therapy for lead poisoning after chelation therapy. May produce ampicillin-like rash, allergic reactions, neutropenia, and nephropathy. Contraindication: Hypersensitivity to penicillin.

Table continued on following page

TABLE 9. Antidote Formulary *Continued*

Medication	Indications and Adverse Reaction (AR)	Comments
30. **Physostigmine salicylate** (*Antilirium*), O'Neil. Cholinesterase inhibitor, a diagnostic trial is not recommended. **Dose:** *Adult,* 1–2 mg IV over 2 min: may repeat every 5 min to max dose of 6 mg *Child,* IV, 0.02 mg/kg over 2 min to a max dose of 2 mg. Once effect accomplished give lowest effective dose every 30–60 min if symptoms recur. **Packaged:** 1 mg/ml 2 ml/amp.	Used if conventional therapy fails for coma, convulsions, severe cardiac dysrhythmias, severe hypertension, hallucinations secondary to anticholinergics, antihistamines, and anticholinergic plants. **AR:** Death—respiratory paralysis, hypertension/hypotension, bradycardia/tachycardia/asystole, hypersalivation, respiratory difficulties/convulsions (cholinergic crisis).	Do not consider for the following: antidepressants, amoxapine, maprotiline, nomifensine, bupropion, trazadone, imipramine. IV administration should be at a slow controlled rate, not more than 1 mg/min. Rapid administration can cause adverse reactions. Can be reversed by atropine. Lasts only 30 min. Contraindicated in asthma, cardiovascular disease, intestinal obstruction.
31. **Pralidoxime chloride** (2-PAM, *Protopam*), Ayerst. Cholinesterase reactivator by removing phosphate. **Dose:** *Adult,* 1–2 gm IV infused in 100–250 ml saline over 30 min. In severe cases may repeat in 1 hr. Repeat every 8–12 hr when needed; if severe, can give 0.5 gm/hr infusion. *Child,* 25–50 mg/kg IV over 30 min, no faster than 10 mg/kg/min; max 12 gm/24 hr. **Packaged:** 1 gm/20 ml vials.	Organophosphate insecticide (OPI) poisoning. Not usually needed in carbamate insecticide poisoning. Most effective if started in first 24 hours before bonding of phosphate. **AR:** Rapid IV injection has produced tachycardia, muscle rigidity, transient neuromuscular blockade. IM: conjunctival hyperemia, subconjunctival hemorrhage, especially if concentrations exceed 5%. *Oral:* nausea, vomiting, diarrhea, malaise.	Should be used only after initial treatment with atropine. Draw blood for RBC cholinesterase level prior to giving 2-PAM. The use of 2-PAM may require a reduction in the dose of atropine. **MP:** Monitor renal profile and reduce dose accordingly. (t½ = 1–2 hours; reversal of OPI effects at 4 μg/ml of 2-PAM. Start early because "aging" of PO_4 on AChE makes it more difficult to reverse.
32. **Propranolol** (Inderal). Nonselective beta blocker. **Dose:** *Adult,* 0.1–0.15 mg/kg IV, administered in increments of 0.5 to 0.75 mg every 1–2 min with continuous ECG and blood pressure monitoring up to 10 mg. *Child,* 0.01–0.15 mg/kg dose slow IV with repeat dose q 6–8h as needed. **Packaged:** 1 mg/ml: tab: 10, 20, 40, 60, 80, 90 mg: cap: 20, 80, 160 mg.	Cocaine intoxication. Has not been scientifically proved to be safe and effective. Anecdotal reports only. Labetolol is theoretically preferred agent for cocaine intoxication. **AR:** Bradycardia, hypotension, pallor; neurologic effects include hallucinations, coma, and seizures.	Not a specific antidote: used for catecholamine storm and dysrhythmias. Increased mortality has been reported in animals that received propranolol for cocaine poisoning and hypertension has occurred in humans following its use in cocaine intoxication.
33. **Protamine Sulfate** **Dose:** 1 mg neutralizes 90–115 units of heparin. Maximum dose = 50 mg IV over 5 min at 10 mg/ml. **Packaged:** 5 ml = 50 mg; 25 ml = 250 mg.	Heparin overdose. **AR:** Rapid administration causes anaphylactoid reactions.	**MP:** Monitor thromboplastin times. Doses of up to 200 mg have been tolerated over 2 hours in an adult.
34. **Pyridoxine (Vitamin B$_6$)** Gamma-aminobutyric acid agonist. **Dose:** *Unknown amount ingested:* 5 gm over 5 min IV. *Known amount:* Add 1 gm of pyridoxine for each gram of INH ingested IV over 5 min. **Packaged:** 50 and 100 mg/ml; 10, 30 ml.	Isoniazid (INH), Monomethylhydrazine mushrooms. **AR:** Unlikely owing to the fact that vitamin B$_6$ is water soluble. However, nausea, vomiting, somnolence, and paresthesia have been reported from chronic high doses.	Pyridoxine is given as 5–10% solution IV mixed with water. It may be repeated every 5–20 min until seizures cease. Some administer pyridoxine over 30–60 min. **MP:** Correct acidosis, monitor liver profile, acid-base parameters. Lethal dose pyridoxine 1 gm/kg.
35. **Sodium bicarbonate** **Dose:** IV 1–3 mEq/kg as needed to keep pH 7.5 (generally 2 mEq/kg every 6 hr). When alkalinization is desired to correct acidosis to a pH of 7.3, use 2 mEq/kg to raise pH 0.1 unit. **Packaged:** 50 ml. 44.6 mEq, 50 mEq ampule.	To promote urinary alkalinization for salicylates, phenobarbital (weak acids with low volume of distribution excreted in urine unchanged). To correct severe acidosis. To promote protein-binding and supply sodium ions into Purkinje cells in cyclic antidepressant intoxication. **AR:** Large doses in patients with renal insufficiency may cause metabolic alkalosis. In patients with ketoacidosis, rapid alkalinization with sodium bicarbonate may result in clouding of consciousness, cerebral dysfunction, seizures, hypoxia, and lactic acidosis.	Alkaline diuresis. The assessment of the need for bicarbonate should be based on both the blood and urine pH. Maintain the blood pH at 7.5. Keep the urinary output at 3–6 ml/kg/hr. May use a diuretic to enhance diuresis. Potassium is necessary to produce alkaline diuresis. Monitor electrolytes, calcium, pH of both urine and blood, arterial blood gases.
36. **Sodium nitrite**	See 14, Cyanide kit	
37. **Sodium thiosulfate**	See 14, Cyanide kit	
38. **Vitamin K** (Aqua MEPHYTON) Merck. Promotes hepatic biosynthesis of prothrombin and other coagulation factors. Competitive antagonist of warfarin. It may be administered orally in the absence of vomiting.	Warfarin (coumarin), salicylate intoxication.	Fatalities from anaphylactic reaction have been reported following IV route. It takes 24 hr for vitamin K to be effective. The need for further vitamin K is determined by the prothrombin time test. If severe bleeding, fresh blood or plasma transfusion may be needed.

TABLE 9. Antidote Formulary* *Continued*

Medication	Indications and Adverse Reaction (AR)	Comments

Dose: *Adult,* 2.5–10 mg IV, depending on potential for hemorrhage. Oral dose is 15–25 mg/day. Severe bleeding, 5–25 mg slow IV push. Rate 1 mg/min. Repeat q4–8h depending on prothrombin time.
Child, 1–5 mg IV, may be given orally when vomiting ceases at a dose of 5–10 mg/day.
  Packaged: 2 mg/ml in 0.5 ml ampules. 2.5 or 5 ml vials.

*This is for informational purposes and is not intended to substitute for independent judgment. It is always advisable to review the package insert for the most up-to-date information. Contact Regional Poison Control Center for additional details on use.

Abbreviations: AR = adverse reactions to antidotes; MP = monitor parameters; FDA = U.S. Food and Drug Administration; ECG = electrocardiogram; CNS = central nervous system; GI = gastrointestinal.

Toxicity. Ingestion of 2 to 3 ml/kg in children, 200 ml in adults has caused CNS depression. TWA is 1000 ppm.

Manifestations. Drowsiness, coma, and bronchopulmonary irritation if inhaled.

Management. (1) GI decontamination if over 2 ml/kg ingested. Avoid emesis because of rapid onset of coma. (2) Administer 100 per cent oxygen if comatose and correct acidosis.

Alcohols

ETHANOL (GRAIN ALCOHOL, COLOGNE, PERFUMES)
Toxicity and Kinetics. In general, 1 ml/kg 100 per cent ethanol produces a blood ethanol concentration (BEC) of 100 mg/dl. The proof is double the per cent. Ethanol is metabolized by hepatic alcohol dehydrogenase at a constant rate of 15 to 30 mg/dl by zero-order kinetics. Peak action occurs at 30 to 60 minutes depending on last meal. Vd is 0.6 L/kg. S.G. is 0.789. Equation to determine possible blood ethanol concentration (BEC) from an approximate amount ingested:

$$BEC = \frac{Amount\ ingested\ (ML) \times \% \times SG\ 0.789}{Vd\ (0.6\ L/kg) \times body\ wt\ kg}$$

Manifestations. If there is no sign of intoxication by 3 hours, it is unlikely to occur. In small children, BEC greater than 50 mg/dl may produce toxicity and hypoglycemia (Table 10).

Management. (1) GI decontamination. **Caution**: The rapid onset of CNS depression may preclude the induction of emesis. If a child consumes more than 1 ml/kg of 50 per cent (100 proof), it is recommended that the child be evaluated for hypoglycemia. However,

TABLE 10. Manifestations of Alcohol Intoxication

Blood Ethanol Levels (mg/dl)	Manifestations
over 30	Euphoria
over 50	Incoordination and intoxication
over 100	Ataxia (legal toxic level)
over 300	Stupor
over 500	Flaccid coma, respiratory failure
500 to 700	May be fatal

a recent report indicated that the ingestion of up to 105 ml of cologne or perfume, 50 to 90 per cent ethanol, did not produce serious symptoms. Activated charcoal and cathartics are **not** indicated unless other drugs are ingested. (2) Treat hypoglycemia and hypothermia, and correct ketoacidosis. (3) Thiamine, 100 mg intravenously, if chronic alcoholism is suspected, to prevent Wernicke-Korsakoff syndrome. (4) Hemodialysis is considered at potentially fatal blood ethanol concentrations when conventional therapy is ineffective (rarely needed). (5) Treat nonhypoglycemic seizures with intravenous diazepam followed by intravenous phenytoin if needed. Repeated seizures, focal neurologic findings, or head trauma warrants computed tomography.

Laboratory. Blood ethanol concentrations: determine anion and osmolar gap; each 1 mg/dl of ethanol increases the serum osmolality 0.22 mOsm/kg water.

ISOPROPANOL (RUBBING ALCOHOL)
Toxicity. Twice as toxic as ethanol. Potentially fatal blood concentration in adults is 120 to 300 mg/dl.

Kinetics. It is metabolized by hepatic alcohol dehydrogenase to acetone. Peak action is 30 to 60 minutes. Vd is 0.6 L/kg. Use the same equation as for ethanol to calculate blood isopropyl alcohol concentration, substituting S.G. 0.785 of isopropanol.

Manifestations. Ethanol-like intoxication with acetone odor to breath, acetonuria, hyperglycemia, occasionally hypoglycemia, acetonemia often without systemic acidosis, gastritis with hematemesis.

Management. (1) GI decontamination as listed for ethanol. (2) Hemodialysis in life-threatening overdose (rarely needed).

Laboratory. Osmolal gap 1 mg/dl of isopropyl alcohol increases the serum 0.176 mOsm/kg water; serum isopropyl alcohol levels; serum acetone.

METHANOL (WOOD ALCOHOL, NONPERMANENT ANTIFREEZE, WINDSHIELD WIPER FLUID)
Toxicity. One teaspoonful, 100 per cent, is potentially lethal for a 2-year-old and can cause blindness in an adult. The toxic blood level of methanol is above 20 mg/dl; the potentially fatal level is over 50 mg/dl. It is six times more toxic than ethanol.

Kinetics. Methanol is oxidized by alcohol dehydrogenase (ADH) into formaldehyde, which is quickly converted into formic acid, the toxic metabolite, which is further oxidized by a folate-dependent pathway to carbon dioxide and water. Peak methanol blood concentration occurs in 1 to 2 hours; Vd is 0.6 L/kg. Use the same equation as for ethanol for calculating the blood methanol concentration, substituting S.G. 0.719 of methanol.

Manifestations. Metabolism may delay onset for 12 to 18 hours or longer if there is concomitant ethanol ingestion. It produces violent abdominal pain (pancreatitis), blurred vision, and hyperemia of optic disc, and within 3 to 24 hours, blindness and "feeling like being in a snow storm" and shock. The odor of formaldehyde on the breath or from the urine may be a clue.

Management. (1) GI decontamination. Activated charcoal and cathartics are **not** indicated. (2) Treat acidosis with intravenous sodium bicarbonate. (3) If methanol is suspected because of a metabolic acidosis with an anion or blood methanol concentration greater than 20 mg/dl, immediately treat with intravenous ethanol or orally to produce blood ethanol concentration (BEC) of 100 to 150 mg/dl (antidote 20). Ethanol has 10 to 20 times the affinity for ADH of methanol. Monitor BEC every 4 to 6 hours. (4) Folinic acid and folic acid have been used successfully in animal investigations. Leucovorin 1 mg/kg up to 50 mg IV every 4 hours for six doses. (5) Consider hemodialysis if the blood methanol level is greater than 50 mg/dl or blood formate greater than 20 mEq/L, refractory metabolic acidosis, or visual or mental symptoms are present. *Note*: The ethanol dose has to be increased during dialysis therapy. (6) Continue therapy (ethanol and hemodialysis) until blood methanol is below 20 mg/dl and preferably undetectable, there is no acidosis, and there are no mental or visual disturbances. This may require 2 to 5 days. (7) Ophthalmology consultation. (8) 4-methyl-pyrazole, an ADH inhibitor, is being investigated as therapy.

Laboratory. Each 1 mg/dl of methanol increases the serum osmolality 0.337 mOsm/kg water. It causes a delayed metabolic acidosis with anion gap in 12 to 24 hours. Blood methanol and ethanol concentrations every 4 to 6 hours. Blood formate level is better indication of toxicity if it can be obtained.

Amphetamines. These include diet pills and various trade and street names, such as "speed."

Toxicity. Child, 5 mg/kg; adult, 20 mg/kg has been reported as lethal.

Kinetics. Peak time of action is 2 to 4 hours. Route of elimination is the liver. Stimulates endogenous catecholamines.

Manifestations. (1) Cardiovascular effects: tachycardia, dysrhythmias, hypertension. (2) CNS effects: argumentative behavior, hyperpyrexia, convulsions, paranoia, and violence. (3) Other: reactive mydriasis, flushed moist skin, hyperactive bowel sounds. The symptoms last four to eight times longer than cocaine. The sequelae may be myocardial infarction, cerebral hemorrhage, or hypertensive encephalopathy. Rhabdomyolysis and myoglobinuria. Chronic use produces dependency and addiction.

Management. (1) GI decontamination if less than 1 hour post ingestion. Avoid induction of emesis. (2)

Control extreme agitation or convulsions with diazepam. **Avoid** chlorpromazine (antidote 13), which may be dangerous in impure "street" amphetamine analogues (STP, MDA, DMT). (3) Treat hypertensive crisis with intravenous nitroprusside. (4) Acidification diuresis with ammonium chloride (antidote 2) is dangerous because of myoglobinuria. (5) Treat hyperpyrexia with physical cooling, not antipyretics. (6) If there are unusual neurologic symptoms, obtain computed tomography scan. (7) Observe for suicidal depression that may follow intoxication. (8) If there is toxic psychosis, treat with haloperidol (Haldol). (9) Significant life-threatening tachydysrhythmia may respond to an alpha- and beta-blocker (antidote 23) or other appropriate antidysrhythmic agents. In the severely hemodynamically compromised patient (hypotension, shock, ischemic chest pain), immediate synchronized cardioversion is necessary.

Laboratory. Monitor for rhabdomyolysis (creatine phosphokinase), myoglobinuria, hyperkalemia, and disseminated intravascular coagulation. Toxic blood concentration is greater than 0.1 μg/ml.

Anticholinergic Agents. Examples include antihistamines; antipsychotics—phenothiazines; antidepressants—tricyclic antidepressants; antiparkinson drugs; over-the-counter sleep and cold medicine; ophthalmic products; plants (see plant section) and bowel antispasmodic agents.

Toxicity. Potential fatal dose of atropine: 10 to 20 mg in child, 100 mg in adult. Toxic dose: 0.05 mg/kg in child, 2 mg in adult.

Kinetics. Atropine: Peak action in 1 to 3 hours, $t_{1/2}$ is 2 to 3 hours. Elimination is hepatic; duration of action is only 4 to 6 hours unless very large amounts were ingested.

Manifestations. (1) Anticholinergic descriptive quotation: "red as a beet (vasodilation), dry as a bone (anhidrotic), blind as a bat (nonreactive mydriasis), hot as a hare (anhidrotic), and mad as a hatter." (2) Cardiac: tachycardia may be preceded by bradycardia, supraventricular tachycardia, hypertension, rarely life-threatening dysrhythmias. ECG: wide QRS, prolonged QT interval. (3) CNS: hallucinations, coma, convulsions, and organic brain syndrome. (4) Other: hyperpyrexia, nonreactive mydriasis, flushed skin, dry mucosa, hypoactive or absent bowel sounds, urinary retention, delirium, and leukocytosis.

Management. (1) GI decontamination up to 12 hours post ingestion. **Avoid** activated charcoal and cathartics if there are no bowel sounds. (2) Control seizures with diazepam. (3) Monitor ECG. Control dysrhythmias. Treat atrial dysrhythmias only if patient is not perfusing tissues adequately or is hypotensive. (4) **Avoid** physostigmine as a diagnostic test or for routine treatment (antidote 30). Consider it only for life-threatening anticholinergic effects refractory to conventional treatments. (5) Relieve urinary retention by catheterization to avoid reabsorption. (6) Control hyperpyrexia by external cooling. **No** antipyretics. (7) Hemodialysis is ineffective.

Anticoagulants. Used as rodenticides. A very large single dose or repeated small doses of warfarin are

TABLE 11. Management of Anticoagulant Ingestion

Product	Contents	Emesis, Activated Charcoal Prothrombin time at 48 hrs
Warfarins		
D-Con Ready Mix	Warfarin 0.025%	>50 gm
D-Con Concentrate	Warfarin 0.33%	>5 gm
Superwarfarins		
4-Hydroxycoumarins	Brodifacoum 0.005%	>25 gm
Talon, Havoc	Bromodialone 0.005%	>25 gm
Super-caid, Maki		
Indanediones		
Caid, Drat, Rozol	Chlorophacinone 0.005%	>25 gm
	Solution 0.25%	
	Concentrate 2.5%	
Pival, Triban, Pivalyn	Pindone 0.025%	>25 gm
	Powder 0.025, 0.1, 0.2, 0.5%	
	Concentrate 0.5%, 1.5%, 2.0%	
Diphacin, Ramik	Diphacinone 0.005%	>25 gm
	0.05%, 9.1%, 0.2%	
	Concentrate 2%	

Modified from Jaeger and DeCastro: Poisoning Emergencies. St. Louis, MO, Catholic Health Assoc, 1986, p. 120; Smolinske, SC, et al: Superwarfarin Poisoning in Children: A Prospective Study. Pediatr 84:490–494, 1989; and Katona, B, Wason, S: Superwarfarin poisoning. J Emerg Med 7:627–631, 1989.

necessary to produce toxicity. The more toxic anticoagulant rodenticides referred to as "superwarfarins" are 40 or more times more potent and have a prolonged anticoagulant effect that may last weeks to months.

Toxicity. Doses greater than 50 gm of 0.025 per cent warfarin or 25 gm 0.005 per cent brodifacoum as a single dose are estimated to be toxic. Mechanism of toxicity: inhibition of regeneration of vitamin K_1 and damage to capillary endothelial integrity.

Kinetics. Action continues for 2 to 3 days. Peak hypoprothrombinemia at 36 to 48 hours. Half-life varies—warfarin 42 hours, brodifacoum 156 hours or longer in humans.

Manifestations. Hematomas and bleeding. Hypoprothrombinemia may occur without symptoms.

Management. (1) GI decontamination of over 50 gm of 0.025 per cent warfarin, over 25 gm or 10 pellets (Talon) of brodifacoum or mouthful of indandione. (2) For GI decontamination, obtain prothrombin time at 24 to 48 hr. Prothombin times at 24 hr may not detect defects. (3) If bleeding or prothrombin time is 10 seconds over control, administer vitamin K_1 (Antidote 38) until normal. Vitamin K takes 24 hours to be effective. Do not use vitamin K_3 or K_4. (4) For severe bleeding, give fresh frozen plasma or blood. (5) Give ascorbic acid 50 mg for a child, 100 mg for an adult to limit capillary damage.

Anticonvulsants

Toxicity. In general, the ingestion of five times the daily therapeutic dose is expected to have the potential for toxicity and ten times the daily therapeutic dose the potential for fatality (Table 12).

Manifestations. Nystagmus, ataxia, mental confusion, vertigo, slurred speech, hypotension, hypothermia, alteration of state of consciousness, and respiratory depression. Carbamazepine and intravenous phenytoin may cause dysrhythmias. Phenytoin overdose patients may experience nystagmus at blood levels greater than 20 µg/ml, ataxia at 30 to 40 µg/ml, and convulsions at over 40 µg/ml.

Management. (1) GI decontamination. Repeated doses of oral activated charcoal shorten $t_{1/2}$ of carbamazepine, phenobarbital, primidone, phenytoin, and possibly others. (2) Monitor specific anticonvulsant blood levels. (3) The effectiveness of hemoperfusion and dialysis has not been established.

Antihistamines or H_1 Histamine Receptor Antagonists. H_1 receptor antagonists have anticholinergic properties. Onset of action is 30 minutes; duration of action is 4 to 8 hours, unless they are slow-release preparations; elimination is hepatic.

Toxicity. Potential toxic dose is four times the therapeutic daily dose (Table 13). Manifestations are anticholinergic, GI upset, tachycardia, drowsiness, ataxia, and hallucinations. In children CNS stimulation occurs initially and may produce convulsions followed by depression. Caladryl (diphenhydramine, camphor, ethyl alcohol) has been absorbed through the skin and has produced toxic encephalitis.

Management. (1) If asymptomatic and less than three times the therapeutic daily dose has been ingested, observe at home. If between three and four times the daily therapeutic dose has been ingested, GI decontamination using emesis at home is sufficient. If greater than four times the therapeutic daily dose was ingested or the patient is symptomatic, evaluation in a medical facility is advised. GI decontamination with activated charcoal and a cathartic may be useful but **caution** is suggested when inducing emesis with large ingestions because of the early onset of seizures. (2) Management as for anticholinergic poisoning. (3) Dialysis and hemoperfusion are not effective.

Arsenic and Arsine Gas (some ant traps, rodenticides)

Toxicity. The toxic dose of arsenic trioxide is 5 to 50

TABLE 12. Anticonvulsants

Drug Name	Peak (hr)	Vd (L/kg)	T$_{1/2}$ (hrs)	Elimination Route	Protein Binding	Therapeutic Dose	Therapeutic Blood Concentration (μg/ml)	Comments
Carbamazepine (Tegretol)	8–24	1.0	18–54	Hepatic	70	10–20 mg/kg/day (max 1600 mg/day)	5–12	
Ethosuximide (Zarontin)	24–48	0.8	36–55	Hepatic	0	20–30 mg/kg/day (max 1500 mg/day)	40–100	
Phenytoin oral (Dilantin)	6–12	1.0	24	Hepatic	90	4–7 mg/kg/day (max 1200 mg/day)	10–20	Has zero-order kinetics above therapeutic concentrations
Primidone	3–4	0.6	3–12	Hepatic	60		8–12	Massive overdose produces white crystalluria
Phenobarbital metabolite (Mysoline)			30–36		1	<8 yr—125 mg/day >8 yr—250 mg/day		
Valproic acid (Depakene)	1–2	0.4	5–15	Hepatic	20	10–15 mg/kg/day (max 1500 mg/day)	84–96	
Clonazepam (Klonopin)	?		20–60	Hepatic	90	0.05–0.2 mg/kg/day (max 20 mg/day)	0.025–0.075	
Phenobarbital	3–6	0.75	50–100	Hepatic	30		14–40	

mg; the potential fatal dose is 120 mg, or 1 to 2 mg/kg. Sodium arsenite is nine times as toxic as trioxide. Organic arsenic, e.g., alkyl arsonates in weeding agents, is less soluble and less toxic. Arsine gas forms when an acid comes in contact with arsenic and releases fumes.

TABLE 13. Common H$_1$ Antihistamines

Generic Name	Trade Name	Dose—Therapeutic and Toxic
Ethanolamine (diphenhydramine) Caps 25, 50 mg Tabs 50 mg Elixir 12.5 mg/5 ml	Benadryl	Therap 5 mg/kg/day (max 300 mg) Toxic 20–40 mg/kg/dose 2 ounces fatal in 2 year old. Toxic blood conc >5 μg/ml Fatal adult dose 2.8 gm
Ethylenediamine (tripelennamine) Tabs 25, 50 mg	Pyribenzamine	Therap 5 mg/kg/day (max 300 mg) Toxic 20–40 mg/kg/dose
Piperidine (cyproheptadine) Caps 25, 50 mg	Periactin	Therap 0.25 mg/kg/day (max 12 mg)
Phenothiazines (promethazine) Tabs 12.5, 25, 50 mg Syrup 6.25 mg/5 ml	Phenergan	Therap 0.5 mg/kg/day (max 40 mg) Not for use under 2 years 200 mg in 2 year old fatal
Alkylamines (chlorpheniramine) Tabs 4 mg Slow release 8, 12 mg Syrup 2 mg/5 ml	Chlor-Trimeton	Therap 0.35 mg/kg/day (max 12 mg) Toxic 5–10 mg/kg/dose
Piperazine (hydroxyzine) Caps 25, 50, 100 mg Susp 25 mg/5 ml Syrup 10 mg/5 ml Tabs 10, 25, 50, 100 mg	Atarax	Therap <6 yrs 50 mg/day >6 yrs 50–100 mg/day
Miscellaneous Terfenadine	Seldane	Therap 3–5 yr 30 mg/day

Kinetics. Elimination is renal.

Manifestations. (1) Acute poisoning: onset 1 to 3 hours. Initially garlic odor to breath, severe abdominal pain, radiopaque material in bowel, hematemesis, diarrhea with "rice water stools" often bloody, hypotension, shock, seizures, coma, later exfoliative dermatitis, cardiac abnormalities, subsequent hepatorenal involvement. (2) Chronic and subacute: prolonged low-level exposure produces stomatitis, a pigmented "rain drop" or scaly rash, and sensory "glove and stocking" peripheral neuropathy, alopecia, Mee's white lines in the fingernails, encephalopathy, cirrhosis of liver, nephritis. (3) Arsine inhalation is characterized by a latent period of 2 to 48 hours and a triad of abdominal pain, hematuria, and jaundice (due to hemolysis).

Management. (1) GI decontamination followed by abdominal radiographs for radiopaque arsenic. Consider whole bowel washout if usual methods fail to remove radiopaque arsenic. (2) Intravenous fluids to correct dehydration and electrolyte deficiencies. (3) Treat shock with oxygen, blood, and fluids. BAL is ineffective against shock. (4) Administer BAL (dimercaprol) (antidote 17). Indications for its use are unknown amount or 1 mg/kg of arsenic trioxide ingested if symptoms of arsenic intoxication or toxic concentrations are present. Liquid arsenic ingestion should be treated until the laboratory tests prove it is not necessary. The BAL-arsenic complex is dialyzable. (5) In chronic poisoning, D-penicillamine (antidote 29) may be used to chelate arsenic. Therapy should be continued in 5-day cycles until the urine arsenic is less than 50 μg/24 hours. (6) Hemodialysis is effective in acute poisoning and can be used concurrently with chelation therapy in severe cases, especially if renal failure develops. Treat renal and liver impairment. (7) Arsine intoxication is treated by exchange transfusion and hemodialysis if renal failure occurs. BAL is ineffective.

Laboratory. Blood arsenic level greater than 1 μg/ml is toxic. Urine arsenic concentrations greater than 50 μg/L may indicate excessive exposure.

Barbiturates

Manifestations. Barbiturates are the prototype of CNS depressants producing ataxia, horizontal nystagmus (plasma phenobarbital greater than 40 μg/ml), slurred speech, pupil size variations, absent oculovestibular reflexes, depressed respiration, hypotension, pulmonary edema, and flaccid coma. Plasma phenobarbital greater than 120 μg/ml usually produces coma and interferes with cardiorespiratory function. Subcutaneous bullae and dermatographia may be present. Duration of action has no relationship to the duration of coma.

Toxicity. Table 14 lists toxic doses unless the patient is tolerant.

Management. (1) GI decontamination up to 8 to 12 hours. **Avoid** emesis in short-acting barbiturates. Activated charcoal with a cathartic initially and in repeated doses has been shown to reduce the serum half-life and increase the nonrenal clearance of phenobarbital over 50 per cent. Give repeated doses of activated charcoal every 4 hours while signs of toxicity are present. (2) Supportive and symptomatic care is all that is necessary in the majority of cases. (3) Alkalinization with intravenous sodium bicarbonate 2 mEq/kg during the first hour followed by sufficient NaHCO₃ (antidote 35) to keep the urinary pH at 7.5 to 8.0 enhances excretion of long-acting barbiturates. Forced diuresis must be used with caution considering the danger of fluid overload and pulmonary edema. (4) In severe cases with

pulmonary edema or high blood barbiturate concentrations not responding to conservative measures, consider hemodialysis (useful in long-acting and intermediate barbiturates) or hemoperfusion. (5) Treat any bullae as local second-degree skin burns.

Laboratory. Emergency plasma barbiturate concentrations rarely alter management.

Batteries (disc type). They usually measure 8 by 23 mm in diameter. They are marked with imprint codes allowing identification of manufacturer and contents. The content of the batteries varies but usually consists of magnesium, silver, or mercury as the cathode and zinc as the anode. An alkali, usually 26 to 45 per cent sodium or potassium hydroxide, may be present. Lithium may occasionally be present.

Toxicity. Most negotiate the GI tract without difficulty, although they may take 14 days to pass. Complications occur with the larger diameter batteries or if the battery lodges in the esophagus or a Meckel's diverticulum. Complication rate is less than 2 per cent. Mechanism of injury is related to leakage of the alkali and/or direct current electrolysis.

Manifestations. All reported complicated cases have been associated with overt symptoms of dysphagia, vomiting, and abdominal pain.

Management. (1) Relief of airway obstruction is the first priority. (2) **Avoid** GI decontamination procedures. (3) Locate the battery on radiograph of the chest and abdomen. Contact the regional poison control center to identify the ingredients. (a) If the battery is in the esophagus or respiratory tract, undertake immediate endoscopic removal. (b) If the battery appears lodged

TABLE 14. Toxic Doses of Barbiturates

Feature	Long Acting (LA)		Intermediate (IA)		Short (SA)
Barbiturate	*Barbital*	*Phenobarbital*	*Amobarbital*	*Pentobarbital*	*Secobarbital*
Trade name	Veronal	Luminal	Amytal	Nembutal	Seconal
Slang name	—	Purple hearts	Blues	Yellows	Red devils
pKₐ	7.74	7.24	7.25	7.96	7.9
Elimination route	Renal 20%	Renal 30%	Hepatic	Hepatic	Hepatic
	Hepatic 80%	Hepatic 70%	98%	>90%	>90%
Onset IV	22 min	12 min	—	0.1 min	0.1 min
Onset oral	1 hr	20–60 min	15–30 min	15–30 min	10–30 min
Peak conc oral	12–18 hr	6–18 hr	3–4 hr	2–4 hr	1–2 hr
Protein-bound	6%	20–40%	40–50%	40–60%	40–60%
Oral doses					
Fatal dose	10 gm	8 gm	5 gm	3 gm	3 gm
	75 mg/kg	65 mg/kg	40 mg/kg	50 mg/kg	30 mg/kg
Toxic dose	>8 mg/kg	15–35 mg/kg	>6 mg/kg	>6 mg/kg	>6 mg/kg
Adult nontol.*		300 mg	200–300 mg	200–300 mg	200 mg
Therap dose	2–6 mg/kg	2–6 mg/kg	2–6 mg/kg	2–6 mg/kg	6 mg/kg
Adult dose	300–500 mg	100–200 mg	100–200 mg	100–200 mg	100–200 mg
Blood concentrations					
Therap	5–8 μg/mL	15–40 μg/mL	5–6 μg/mL	1–5 μg/mL	1–5 μg/mL
Toxic	>30 μg/mL	>40 μg/mL	10–30 μg/mL	>10 μg/mL	>10 μg/mL
Lethal	>100 μg/mL	>100 μg/mL	>50 μg/mL	>35 μg/mL	>35 μg/mL
Duration	16 hr	6–8 hr	6 hr	6 hr	6 hr
T₁/₂ elim	56–96 hr	50–120 hr	8–42 hr	15–48 hr	19–34 hr
Vd	—	0.75 L/kg	0.5 L/kg	0.65 L/kg	1.5 L/kg
Available	Cap mg	16	65, 200	50, 100	50, 100
	Tab mg	16, 32, 65, 100	15, 30, 50, 100	—	100
	Elixir mg/5 mL	15, 20	—	20	—
	Supp mg	—	—	30, 60, 120, 200	—

* = nontolerant.

in a Meckel's diverticulum, surgical removal is indicated. (c) If the battery has passed beyond the esophagus, observe at home for vomiting, tarry or bloody stools, or abdominal pain. All stools should be examined to retrieve the battery. Repeat radiography is done in 7 days if the battery has not passed. Lack of movement of the battery is not an indication for immediate surgical intervention. (d) Asymptomatic patients may receive a cathartic. (e) If the battery opens, monitor the blood and urine concentrations for contents of battery, i.e., mercury, lithium. Mercuric oxide in batteries is converted into elemental mercury in the GI tract and is poorly absorbed. (f) If the patient develops symptoms of peritoneal irritation, surgical intervention is necessary. (4) Batteries in ears, nose, or other orifices should be removed immediately. Magnetic screwdrivers may aid in removal.

Benzodiazepines (BZP)

Classification by Duration of Action. (1) Long-acting (>24 hr): chlordiazepoxide (Librium), chlorazepate (Tranzene), clonazepam (Clonopin), diazepam (Valium), flurazepam (Dalmane), prazepam (Centrex), quazepam (Dormalin). (2) Short-acting (3–20 hr): alprazolam (Xanax), lorazepam (Ativan). (3) Ultrashort (< 10 hr): temazepam (Restoril), triazolam (Halcion), midazolam (Versed), oxazepam (Serax).

Toxicity. Low toxic potential. Benzodiazepines have an additive CNS depressant effect with other sedatives. Most patients intoxicated with BZP alone recover within 24 hours. Therapeutic dose of diazepam is 0.2 or 0.8 mg/kg oral to maximum 10 mg total in adolescents. Five times the therapeutic dose is considered toxic.

Kinetics. Elimination is hepatic. Peak blood concentrations occur 1 to 4 hours after oral administration. Long-acting forms are metabolized into active metabolites.

Manifestations. CNS depression; can cause psychosis. Deep coma with respiratory depression and/or cardiac disturbances suggests presence of other drugs or another cause.

Management. (1) GI decontamination. (2) Supportive and symptomatic care.

Laboratory. Document benzodiazepines in urine.

Beta-Blockers. See *Propranolol and beta-blockers.*

Bleach

Toxicity. Household laundry bleach (Clorox, Dazzle) is usually 5.25 per cent hypochlorite, which is not caustic. Commercial types of "caustic soda" 10 to 20 per cent could cause caustic injuries. Other bleach products may be hydrogen peroxide (see *Hydrogen peroxide*) or perborates (see *Boric acid*). Oxalic acid in some rust removers, metal cleaners, and ink eradicators may cause caustic injuries (see *Caustics*).

Manifestations. Household hypochlorite bleach does not produce esophageal burns unless vomiting occurs or very large quantities are ingested. Gases produced by mixing hypochlorite bleach with acids or ammonia are irritating to mucous membranes, eyes, and upper respiratory tract. Ocular injuries may occur from concentrated or undiluted swimming pool hypochlorite. They usually heal in 3 weeks.

Management. (1) Ingestion: **Avoid** GI decontamination procedures. Dilute with water or milk if the patient can swallow. (2) Esophagoscopy only if symptomatic or if the product is stronger than the household hypochlorite bleach. (3) Inhalation: Remove from the contaminated area and if symptoms persist, observe for pulmonary edema (very unlikely). (4) Ocular exposure requires immediate gentle irrigation with water for at least 15 minutes followed by fluorescein dye stain for damage. If pain persists, an ophthalmologic consultation should be obtained.

Boric Acid. One teaspoonful of 100 per cent boric acid powder equals 2.9 to 4.4 gm. Borax cleaners contain 21.5 per cent boron by dry weight.

Toxicity. The potential fatal dose is much higher than the quoted values of 20 gm in adults and 5 gm in children. The majority of exposures are probably nontoxic. There have been no deaths since 1928.

Kinetics. Elimination is renal.

Manifestations. Acute gastroenteritis with blue-green vomitus and feces. CNS stimulation and in severe cases seizures and coma. Renal failure may develop. An erythematous rash may develop in 3 to 5 days postingestion and desquamates, giving the "boiled lobster" appearance.

Management. (1) For initial management and GI decontamination, see Table 15. (2) Activated charcoal is not useful. (3) Treat seizures with diazepam. (4) Hemodialysis if renal failure occurs. Monitor renal function.

Botulism. See article on botulinal food poisoning.

Calcium-Channel Blockers (Antihypertensives, antianginals, antidysrhythmics)

Toxicity. In adults 3 gm and in children 40 mg/kg may produce serious intoxication. Digitalis increases the risk of toxicity.

Kinetics. Elimination is hepatic; $t_{1/2}$ varies from 3 to 7 hours. Vd is 3 to 7 L/kg.

Manifestations. Hypotension, bradycardia within 1 to 5 hours postingestion, mental status changes, seizures, CNS depression, gastric distress, conduction disturbances, pulmonary edema, and hyperglycemia (insulin inhibition). The first action of verapamil is slowing of conduction through the AV node seen on ECG as an increase in the PR interval, whereas nifedipine increases AV nodal conduction (Table 16).

Management. (1) GI decontamination. (2) Treat hypotension with intravenous calcium gluconate or chloride (antidote 12A) slowly under ECG monitoring. Cal-

TABLE 15. Management of Boric Acid Ingestion

Body Weight	Amount Ingested	Management
<30 kg	<200 mg/kg	Observe at home
	200–400 mg/kg	Syrup of ipecac to induce emesis
	>400 mg/kg	Emergency department for GI decontamination and evaluation
>30 kg	<6 gm	Observe at home
	6–12 gm	Syrup of ipecac to induce emesis
	>12 gm	Emergency department for GI decontamination and evaluation

TABLE 16. Properties of Calcium-Channel Blockers

Feature	Generic Name (Trade Name)		
	Nifedipine (Procardia)	Verapamil (Calan, Isoptin)	Diltiazem (Cardiazem)
Preparations	10, 20 mg tabs	80, 120 mg tabs	30, 60, 90, 120 mg tabs
Onset oral	<20 min	<30 min	<30 min
Peak oral	1–2 hr	5 hr	30 min
Peak blood conc	30–60 min	90–120 min	120–180 min
Toxic blood conc	>100 ng/ml	>300 ng/ml	>200 ng/ml
Coronary vasodilation	+ + +	+ +	+ + +
Peripheral vasodilation	+ + +	+ +	+
Negative inotropy	–	+	+
Slow AV conduction	–	+ +	+
Slow SA conduction	–	+	+ +
Preload	Decreased	–	Decreased
Heart rate	Increased	Decreased	Decreased
Contractility	—	Decreased +	Decreased

cium elevates the blood pressure but does not affect the tachydysrhythmias. If this fails, use positioning, fluids, and vasopressors (dopamine, norepinephrine). (3) Treat bradydysrhythmias and conduction defects with intravenous calcium gluconate or chloride (antidote 12A) slowly under ECG monitoring. If no response, try atropine sulfate or isoproterenol (may aggravate the hypotension) or a pacemaker. If unstable, use a pacemaker immediately. (4) Tachydysrhythmias are infrequent and require appropriate antidysrhythmic management. (5) Hyperglycemia does not require insulin therapy.

Camphor. Vicks Vaporub 4.8 per cent, Campho-Phenique 11 per cent. Five ml of camphorated oil (20 per cent camphor, banned in 1982) or 20 ml of Vicks Vaporub equals 1 gm of camphor.

Toxicity. Over 10 mg/kg may cause a seizure. Mean fatal dose is 200 mg/kg. Adult 5 gm, child 1 gm has been fatal.

Kinetics. Elimination is hepatic. Pulmonary excretion causes a distinctive odor on the breath.

Manifestations. Onset in 5 to 90 minutes. Specific odor, nausea, vomiting, and burning epigastric pain. Seizures may occur suddenly and without warning within 5 minutes of ingestion. Apnea and vision disturbances may occur.

Management. (1) **Avoid** the induction of emesis because of early seizures. Take patient immediately to a medical care facility. (2) Remove residual drug by gastric lavage until there is no odor of camphor in the aspirate. (3) Administer activated charcoal and a saline cathartic, although there are no scientific data to support this. **Avoid** oils or alcohol. (4) Treat seizures with intravenous diazepam. (5) Hemoperfusion with Amberlite XAD-4 may rarely be needed in cases unresponsive to conventional therapy.

Carbon Monoxide (CO). This is an odorless, nonirritating gas produced from incomplete combustion; it is found as an in vivo metabolic breakdown product of inhaled methylene chloride (paint stripper, solvent). CO binds 210 times more avidly to hemoglobin than does oxygen and also interferes with cellular cytochrome oxidase.

Kinetics. Elimination through the lungs. The $t_{1/2}$ in room air is 5 to 6 hours; in 100 per cent oxygen 90 minutes; and in hyperbaric oxygen at 2 atmospheres 20 minutes.

Manifestations. Time of exposure, oxygen administration, and mental status are important to analyzing the risk of serious intoxication (Table 17). The skin rarely shows a cherry red color in the live patient. A frequent clinical complaint is flu-like symptoms. Leukoencephalopathy (poor judgment and concentration) may occur within 3 weeks post exposure, and myocardial infarction may occur 1 week after significant exposure. The carboxyhemoglobin (COHb) value in the emergency de-

TABLE 17. CO Exposure and Possible Manifestations

CO in Atmosphere	Duration of Exposure (hr)	COHb Saturation (%)	Manifestations
up to 0.01	Indefinite	1–10	Minimal
0.01–0.02	Indefinite	10–20	Moderate dyspnea on exertion, throbbing headache
0.02–0.03	5–6	20–30	Marked headache, weakness, altered judgment
0.04–0.06	4–5	30–40	Vertigo, weakness, blurred vision
0.07–0.10	3–4	40–50	Confusion, tachycardia, tachypnea, syncope
0.11–0.15	1.5–3	50–60	Above plus Cheyne Stokes, coma, convulsions
0.16–0.30	1.0–1.5	60–70	Coma, convulsions, respiratory and heart failure, death
>0.40	1–2 minutes	70–80	Death

partment may not represent the true insult or peak concentration. **Severe poisoning may have only mild to moderate COHb levels.**

Management. (1) Remove from contaminated area. Establish vital functions. (2) 100 per cent oxygen is administered to **all** patients until the COHb is 5 per cent or less. Assisted ventilation may be necessary. The exposed pregnant woman should be kept in 100 per cent oxygen for several hours after her COHb is zero because CO concentrates in the fetus, and oxygen is needed five times longer to ensure elimination of CO from fetal circulation. CO or hypoxia may be teratogenic. (3) Monitor arterial blood gases and COHb. (4) If pH remains below 7.0 after correction of hypoxia and adequate ventilation, give sodium bicarbonate cautiously. Avoid overcorrecting because alkalosis and COHb shifts the oxygen-hemoglobin dissociation curve to the left, decreasing tissue oxygen. (5) Indications to consider for admission and possible therapy with hyperbaric oxygen (controversial): (a) COHb greater than 25 per cent. (b) COHb greater than 15 per cent in a child or a patient with cardiovascular disease. (c) COHb greater than 10 per cent in a pregnant female and monitor the fetus. (d) Abnormal or ischemic chest pain or ECG abnormalities. (e) Abnormal neuropsychiatric examination. (f) Presence of hypoxia, myoglobinuria, or abnormal renal function. (g) Abnormal chest radiograph. (h) History of unconsciousness, syncope, or neuropsychiatric symptoms. A list of hyperbaric chambers may be obtained from Duke University (919-684-8111). The most important indicator for hyperbaric chamber is altered mental state. (6) Treat seizures with intravenous diazepam. (7) Treat cerebral edema with elevation of the patient's head, minimizing intravenous fluid, hyperventilation, and, if needed, mannitol and intracranial pressure monitoring. (8) Follow closely and reevaluate after recovery for cardiac, pulmonary, and neuropsychiatric sequelae.

Laboratory. Arterial blood gases show metabolic acidosis and normal oxygen tension but reduced oxygen saturation: monitor electrocardiogram, chest radiograph, and serum creatine phosphokinase (CPK).

Caustics and Corrosives (alkalis and acids). Acid and alkali are grouped together, but their pathophysiology differs. *Alkalis* produce liquefaction necrosis and saponification and penetrate deeply. In 80 per cent of the alkali injuries the esophagus is damaged, and the stomach is involved in 20 per cent, usually with liquids. *Acids* produce coagulation necrosis and form an eschar, preventing further penetration. They usually do not penetrate deeply (exception: hydrofluoric acid). In 80 per cent of the acid injuries the gastric mucosa is damaged, and the esophagus is involved in 20 per cent.

Manifestations. (1) *Alkalis:* Oropharyngeal burns, drooling, pain, dysphagia, stridor or dyspnea if the respiratory tract is involved. The absence of oral burns does not exclude the possibility of esophageal burns. Esophageal perforation and mediastinitis and shock may develop. The late sequelae are esophageal strictures, usually 1 to 3 weeks post ingestion. Carcinoma of the esophagus has occurred years after original injury. (2) *Acids:* May produce symptoms similar to alkalis but

more frequently damage the stomach and may produce a "silent" asymptomatic perforation and peritonitis.

Management. (1) If ingested and the patient can swallow, has no signs of respiratory obstruction, perforation or shock, dilute with small amounts of milk or water immediately (up to 60 ml in children or 250 ml in adults) to avoid emesis. **Avoid** the induction of emesis, neutralization with acidic or alkalinic agents, gastric lavage, and activated charcoal. (2) Dermal and ocular decontamination should be carried out immediately by gentle irrigation with copious amounts of water for at least 15 minutes. (3) In acid ingestions some advocate nasogastric intubation with a small, well-lubricated tube, preferably inserted under direct endoscopic vision and aspiration of the stomach contents within the first half hour post ingestion. This timing is very difficult to accomplish. (4) Patients should receive only intravenous fluids following dilution until endoscopic consultation. (5) Esophagoscopy at 12 to 48 hours post ingestion may be indicated to assess severity of the burn. The scope is introduced to the level of the first lesion. (6) Steroids are controversial. Some recommend that steroids be administered if a second-degree (transmucosal) or circumferential burn is found or esophagoscopy is not performed but a transmucosal burn is suspected. Steroids are not used in superficial burns because they do not develop strictures and are avoided in a transmural burn or if perforation is suspected. The dose is prednisone 2 mg/kg/day for 3 weeks or more. (7) Antibiotics are not useful prophylactically. They are used if there is evidence of perforation. (8) Esophagrams are not as reliable but may be used after several days. An esophagram and upper GI series at 10 days to 3 weeks post ingestion may be necessary to assess severity of damage. (9) Esophageal dilation may need to be performed at 2- to 4-week intervals if there is evidence of a stricture. (10) Severe strictures may require surgical replacement if dilation fails to provide an esophagus of adequate size to consume appropriate nutrients. (11) Inhalation requires immediate removal from the environment and clinical, radiographic, and arterial blood gas evaluation when appropriate. Oxygen and respiratory support may be required.

Clonidine (Catapres). An antihypertensive, sometimes used in opiate withdrawal. Tablets 0.1 and 0.2 mg and transdermal preparation.

Toxicity. Toxic amount in children is 0.025 mg/kg, in adults 4 to 5 mg.

Kinetics. Onset within 30 to 60 minutes, peak in 3 to 5 hours, and duration of 8 hours but in overdose may last up to 96 hours. Elimination is hepatic.

Manifestations. (1) CNS depression, hypotonia, hypothermia, miosis. Apnea and seizures may occur within 8 hours post ingestion in significant poisonings. (2) Cardiovascular effect occurs within 1 to 3 hours post ingestion and consists of bradycardia and hypotension. A transient initial hypertension may occur. AV block occurs with severe poisonings.

Management. (1) ECG and blood pressure monitoring. Be prepared for intubation and ventilation. (2) GI decontamination with charcoal/cathartic. **Avoid** emesis induction because of rapid onset of coma. (3) **Caution:**

Naloxone may reverse toxicity; however, it has been reported to produce hypertension and may be dangerous to hypertensive patients being treated with clonidine. (4) Treat convulsions with diazepam; bradycardia with hemodynamic instability with atropine; hypotension with positioning, fluids, and vasopressors; hypertensive crisis with intravenous antihypertensive agents. Phentolamine 5 mg/kg/day orally in four divided doses or 0.1 mg/kg IV may be used to treat rebound hypertension after clonidine withdrawal.

Cocaine (benzoylmethylecgonine)

Toxicity. The potential fatal adult dose is 1200 mg, but death has occurred with 20 mg parenterally. Its mechanism of action is interference with reuptake of norepinephrine and dopamine.

Kinetics (Table 18). It is metabolized in liver to mostly inactive metabolites excreted in urine which serve for detection.

Manifestations. (1) Low dose—euphoria and central nervous system stimulation. (2) High dose—anxiety, agitation, paranoid delusions, hypertension, convulsions, hyperthermia, tachycardia, and cardiac dysrhythmias. CNS stimulation is followed by CNS depression. (3) Sequelae—paranoid psychosis, perforation of nasal septum (rare), myocardial infarction, intracranial hemorrhage, intestinal ischemia, suicidal depression, sudden death. (4) Perinatal complications are spontaneous abortion, abruptio placentae, prematurity, teratogenicity (prune belly syndrome), and neonatal cerebral infarction. Cocaine is found in breast milk and has caused adverse reactions in nursing infants. (5) Unusual ingestion types are the "body packer" (illicit transport) and the "body stuffer" (hiding evidence). The packages may leak or rupture and cause sudden death.

Management. (1) GI decontamination with activated charcoal/cathartic if ingested. **Avoid** induction of emesis or gastric lavage because of rapid onset. Do not flush cocaine in the nose but remove with applicator dipped in non–water-soluble product (lubricating jelly). (2) Cardiac and thermal monitoring. Phenytoin may be effective for ventricular dysrhythmias, whereas lidocaine may be ineffective and enhance toxicity, since lidocaine is often an adulterant. (3) Alpha- and beta-blockers (antidote 23) and calcium-channel blockers (Netredipine in Europe) are being evaluated to control life-threatening hypertension and tachycardia. Nitroprusside, 0.5 μg/kg/min, may be used in severe hypertension. **Avoid** propranolol. (4) Control seizures with diazepam and if needed phenytoin. Neuromuscular blockers may be needed. (5) Treat the hyperthermia with vigorous external cooling. **No** antipyretics. (6) In pregnancy monitor the fetus and prepare for spontaneous abortion, abruptio placentae, and prematurity. (7) Suicide precautions. Imipramine and dopamine agonists (bromocriptine, amantadine) may aid withdrawal. Establish the patient in a treatment program. (8) The management of the "body packer" and "body stuffer" is to administer repeated doses of activated charcoal (except with plastic vials), secure venous access, and have drugs readily available at the bedside for treating life-threatening manifestations until contraband cocaine is passed in the stool. Surgical removal may be indicated if material does not pass the pylorus. **No** emesis or lavage, but endoscopy may be used to remove hard plastic vials containing crack, but not the bags.

Laboratory. Cocaine is detected in urine up to 12 hours; its metabolite benzylecognine may be detected for 48 to 144 hours depending on method.

Cosmetics

For *colognes, perfumes, aftershave lotions, oral hygiene products, suntan lotions,* toxicity depends on the concentration of alcohol (see *Alcohols*).

Deodorants (personal) of aluminum and zinc are of low toxicity.

Depilatory preparations are usually sulfides or thioglycolates. They are usually irritants to skin and GI tract. Large doses may produce hypoglycemia and convulsions.

Fingernail polish removers are usually acetone but may contain toluene and aliphatic acetates (see *Acetone*). Artificial nail remover may contain acetonitrile which forms cyanide in the body (see *Cyanide*).

HAIR PRODUCTS. *Dyes and bleaches* contain hydrogen peroxide bleach (See *Hydrogen peroxide*). Metallic hair dyes usually contain small amounts of toxic metals; large ingestions may require treatment. Vegetable dyes are nontoxic. *Permanent wave neutralizers* may contain perborates (see *Boric acid*) or rarely the nephrotoxic bromates. Plain *shampoos* are nontoxic. Dry shampoos can be dangerous and contain methyl or isopropyl alcohol (see *Alcohols*). *Sprays* that are chronically inhaled may cause hilar adenopathy and pulmonary infiltrates (thesaurosis). *Straightening and hair-waving preparations* may contain 1 to 3 per cent sodium or ammonium hydroxide (see *Caustics*). *Ointments, creams, and plain soaps* are usually nontoxic.

Cyanide.

Cyanides occur in fumigants (hydrogen cyanide), in some silver and furniture polishes, in the seeds of fruit stones (harmful only if the capsule is broken), and in the antihypertensive nitroprusside. Cyanide is released in fires involving the decomposition of silk, wool, polyurethane, and acrylonitrile.

Toxicity. The ingestion of 1 mg/kg or 50 mg of potassium or hydrogen cyanide can produce death within 15 minutes. Volatile hydrocyanic acid MAC is 10 ppm; 300 ppm is fatal in minutes. Ferriferrocyanide (Prussian blue) is of low toxicity; over 50 gm is toxic in adults.

Kinetics. Elimination is hepatic via the thiosulfate-rhodanese pathway.

Manifestations. (1) Early symptoms may mimic the hyperventilation syndrome. The patient may taste bitter almonds and/or the odor may be on the breath or be emitted from gastric contents (the threshold of odor is 0.2 to 5 ppm, and only 50 per cent of the population can perceive the odor). If no symptoms by 2 hours, exclude *acute* cyanide intoxication. (2) Later respiratory depression and hypoxic symptoms without cyanosis. The following may be present: vomiting, seizures, coma, cardiac dysrhythmias, dilated pupils with red retinal veins, bright red venous blood, pulmonary edema, lactic acidemia, normal arterial blood Po_2 and high venous

TABLE 18. Pharmacokinetics of Cocaine

Type	Route	T$_{1/2}$ (min)	Onset	Peak	Duration
Hydrochloride	Insufflation	75	t<5 min	30–60 min	60–90 min
	Ingested	49	Delayed	50–90 min	Sustained
	Intravenous	54	<2 min	15–30 min	60–90 min
Free base and crack	Smoked	—	Seconds	10–15 min	<20 min
Coca paste	Smoked	—	Unknown		

PO$_2$ with decreased arterial-venous oxygen difference. (3) Late cyanosis unresponsive to oxygen. (4) Subacute poisoning may produce neuropathies and thyroid dysfunction.

Management. (1) **Do not perform mouth-to-mouth resuscitation** (cyanide is released in the patient's breath). If inhaled, remove patient from contaminated atmosphere. Immediately administer 100 per cent oxygen and, if needed, assisted ventilation. Continue oxygen and respiratory support during and after antidote therapy. (2) Cyanide antidote kit (antidote 14). **Caution: Children require special doses**. If symptoms recur, repeat antidotes in 30 minutes as one-half of the initial dose. Use the antidotes if suspicious of diagnosis, as in urethane, plastic, or upholstery fires with (a) impairment of consciousness, (b) manifestations not corrected by oxygen and out of proportion to carboxyhemoglobin level, (c) lactic acidosis and bright red venous blood with high PO$_2$. **Never** use methylene blue to reverse methemoglobinemia in cyanide poisoning because it will release the cyanide ion. Use exchange transfusion if the methemoglobin concentration exceeds 50 per cent. (3) GI decontamination by gastric lavage. **Avoid** emesis. Activated charcoal is not a very effective adsorbant. (4) Treat seizures with intravenous diazepam. (5) Hydroxycobalamin, vitamin B$_{12a}$, which forms vitamin B$_{12}$ cyanocobalamin (investigational) may be a useful antidote if given early after exposure and in very large doses. (7) Hyperbaric oxygen effectiveness is not documented.

Laboratory. If on nitroprusside infusion and thiocyanate concentration is greater than 10 mg/dl, discontinue; if between 5 and 10 mg/dl, discontinue if associated with metabolic acidosis or symptoms.

Detergents

Soaps are salts of fatty acids and are nontoxic. *Anionic* detergents (Ajax Cleanser, Comet Cleanser, Oxydol, Tide Laundry) and *nonionic* detergents (Ivory Snow liquid, Joy Dish Detergent) contain sodium phosphates as a water softener and are nontoxic unless they contain more than 50 per cent carbonates, phosphates, or silicates, which may produce alkaline damage to esophagus and stomach. Polyphosphates ingested in large amounts may produce hypocalcemic tetany. Granular dishwashing detergents (Cascade, Calgonite, Electrosol) may have the potential of caustic properties (see *Caustics*).

Management. (1) Immediately dilute with milk or water. Avoid emesis. Irrigate eyes and skin and observe for dysphagia, drooling, dyspnea, and stridor with agents that have the potential for caustic injury. Soaps and anionic and nonionic detergents require only home observation. (2) If tetany develops, administer calcium gluconate (antidote 12A).

Cationic detergents are quaternary ammonia compounds such as hexachlorphene (Phisohex), benzalkonium (Zephiran), and cetylpyridium (Creepryn). In concentrations greater than 2 per cent they may cause systemic toxicity with convulsions. In concentrations over 7.5 per cent they may be caustic. Most of these are low concentration (2 per cent or less) and are not toxic unless large quantites are ingested.

Management. (1) If less than a 7.5 per cent, treat by home observation. Over 7.5 per cent, dilution with milk or water. **Avoid** emesis (see *Caustics*). At present there are no data to support that soap will absorb the unabsorbed cationic detergent, and it may produce emesis. (2) Supportive and symptomatic therapy.

Digitalis Preparations. Cardiac glycosides are found in medication and plants (Table 19).

Manifestations. May be delayed 9 to 18 hours. (1) GI: abdominal pain, nausea, vomiting, diarrhea. (2) CNS: depression, colored-halo vision, delerium, hallucinations. (3) Cardiovascular: acute poisoning—more likely bradycardia, blocks, atrial dysrhythmia, and hyperkalemia. Chronic intoxication—more likely tachycardia, serious premature ventricular contractions, ventricular dysrhythmias, and hypokalemia. (4) ECG: no dysrhythmia is characteristic of digitalis toxicity.

Management. (1) GI decontamination. **Avoid** syrup of ipecac, which may increase vagal effect. With gastric lavage pretreatment with atropine to avoid vagal effect has been suggested. Activated charcoal is useful and repeated doses of activated charcoal may interrupt enterohepatic recirculation in digitoxin. (2) **Avoid** quinidine, bretylium, carotid sinus massage, calcium, and calcium-channel blockers. **Caution**: Use direct current countershock only as a last resort in life-threatening

TABLE 19. Common Digitalis Preparations: Toxicity and Kinetics

Generic Name	Digoxin	Digitoxin
Trade name	Lanoxin	Crystodigin
Onset time oral	1.5–6 hr	3–6 hr
Toxic dose	0.07 mg/kg	
GI absorption	50–80%	90–100%
Peak oral	1.5–6 hr	6–12 hr
Protein bound	25%	90%
Vd In neonate	7–8 L/kg	0.6 L/kg
In children	16 L/kg	
Half-life	30–45 hr	>100 hr
Elimination	Renal 75%	Liver 80%
Therap plasma conc	0.5–2.0 ng/ml	15–30 ng/ml
Toxic plasma conc	>2.4 ng/ml	>30 ng/ml
young infants	>4 ng/ml	
Enterohepatic	30%	14%
Recirculation		
Available tablets mg	0.125, 0.250, 0.50	0.05, 0.1, 0.15, 0.2
elixir mg/ml	0.05	0.05

dysrhythmias because of the tendency to produce ventricular fibrillation in digitalis intoxication. Treat ventricular premature contractions, including bigeminy, trigeminy, quadrigeminy, ventricular tachycardia, and atrial tachycardia with phenytoin, loading dose 2 to 4 mg/kg IV slowly at a rate of less than 30 mg/min, with ECG and BP monitoring. Lidocaine also may be administered for ventricular dysrhythmias. Magnesium sulfate has been successful in treating serious dysrhythmias, 20 ml 20 per cent solution IV over 20 minutes. (3) Treat hemodynamically unstable bradycardia and second- and third-degree AV block with atropine, 0.01 mg/kg up to 0.6 mg, or low-dose phenytoin 1 mg/kg up to 25 mg. Insertion of a pacemaker may be needed. (4) Treat hyperkalemia (above 6 mEq/L). **Avoid calcium**. *If hyperkalemia is present (ominous sign), the availability of fragment-binding antibody for treatment should be assured.* (5) Specific Fab antibody fragments (FAB; Digibind) (antidote 21) have been used for life-threatening cardiac dysrhythmias refractory to conventional measures and hyperkalemia.

Laboratory. Monitor electrocardiogram and potassium. Draw digoxin levels 6 to 8 hours after ingestion. An endogenous digoxin-like substance that cross-reacts with most common immunoassay antibodies has been reported in newborns, chronic renal failure patients, and abnormal immunoglobin patients.

Disinfectants. See *Detergents* (cationic), *Pine oil, Mercury, Herbicides.*

IODINES AND IODOPHORS. See *Iodine.*

PHENOL AND ITS DERIVATIVES. These have local caustic properties as well as systemic toxicity.

Toxicity. Oral lethal dose 10 to 30 gm.

Kinetics. Elimination is hepatic.

Manifestations. (1) Systemic: Symptoms develop in 5 to 30 minutes post ingestion and involve the CNS, liver, kidney, and lungs and may produce early convulsions, coma, acidosis, and shock. Some phenols may produce methemoglobinemia (see *Nitrites*). Pentachlorophenol has produced transdermal intoxication in infants with perfuse diaphoresis. Phenol disinfectants have caused hyperbilirubinemia in infants. (2) Local: Phenol denatures protein and produces dermal and mucosal burns with a coagulum. No esophageal strictures have been reported.

Management. Immediate medical evaluation and immediate administration of activated charcoal are necessary. (1) **Avoid** emesis, alcohol, and oral mineral oil. Immediate dermal decontamination by copious irrigation with water followed by olive oil to allow for the formation of a coagulum. (2) Control convulsions with diazepam and phenytoin.

Laboratory. Monitor renal and liver function.

Ethylene Glycol (Solvent, Permanent Antifreeze, Brake Fluid)

Toxic Dose. Death has occurred after a 60-ml ingestion; potential fatal dose is 1.4 ml/kg of 100 per cent solution. May use the same equation as ethanol (see *Alcohols*) for calculating blood ethylene glycol concentration, substituting S.G. 1.12 and Vd 0.65 L/kg.

Kinetics. Peak blood concentrations occur in 1 to 2 hours. Elimination is hepatic 80 to 90 per cent. It is metabolized by alcohol dehydrogenase (ADH) and other enzymes to the toxic metabolites oxalate (1 per cent), glycolic acid, and glycoaldehyde by pathways that depend upon cofactors thiamine and pyridoxine.

Manifestations. (1) *Phase I*: CNS depression begins 30 minutes to 12 hours post ingestion with symptoms of drunkenness, coma, or convulsions and metabolic abnormalities of lactic acidosis and hypocalcemia. (2) *Phase II*: Cardiopulmonary depression within 12 to 36 hours post ingestion, resulting in pulmonary edema and congestive heart failure. (3) *Phase III*: Renal failure may develop 1 to 3 days post ingestion. (4) Urine oxalate or monohydrate crystals may be seen 4 to 8 hours post ingestion.

Management. (1) GI decontamination up to 2 hours post ingestion. Activated charcoal and cathartics are not indicated. (2) Treat nonhypocalcemic seizures with intravenous diazepam followed by phenytoin if unresponsive. Treat hypocalcemia. (3) Correct acidosis with intravenous sodium bicarbonate. (4) Initiate ethanol therapy to block metabolism if ingested and blood ethylene glycol is greater than 20 mg/dl, or if symptomatic but acidotic with increased anion gap or osmolar gap. Administer ethanol similar to the management of methanol. Ethanol has 100 times the affinity for ADH as ethylene glycol (antidote 20). (5) Early hemodialysis is indicated if the ingestion is greater than 1.4 ml/kg, if the plasma ethylene glycol is greater than 50 mg/dl, if severe acid-base or electrolyte abnormalities occur despite conventional therapy, or if renal failure occurs. (6) Thiamine 100 mg and pyridoxine 50 mg intravenously four times a day for 48 hours have been recommended but have not been extensively studied. (7) Continue therapy (ethanol and hemodialysis) until plasma ethylene glycol is below 10 mg/dl, the acidosis has cleared, creatinine is normal, and urinary output is adequate. (8) Monitor the calcium and treat hypocalcemia if it occurs.

Laboratory. Urinalysis for oxalate "envelope" crystals and monohydrate "hemp seed" crystals. Obtain plasma ethylene glycol and ethanol levels; each 1 mg/dl of ethylene glycol in the blood raises the serum osmolality 0.17 mOsm/kg water. An ethylene glycol level of 20 mg/dl is toxic. (Levels are difficult to obtain.)

Fertilizers. They contain small quantities of minerals in nontoxic amounts but may contain insecticides and herbicides. In general, noncontaminated fertilizers are of very low toxicity.

Fluoride (Caries Preventative, Insecticide, Rodenticide). One mg elemental fluoride equals 2.2 mg sodium fluoride or 4.0 mg stannous fluoride or 7.6 mg of monophosphate fluoride.

Toxicity. Toxic at greater than 16 mg/kg; potential lethal dose is 32 mg/kg of elemental fluoride. Fluoride is a protoplasmic poison that binds with calcium and inhibits enzyme systems.

Kinetics. Peak plasma concentration in 30 to 60 minutes.

Manifestations. (1) Low overdose—intoxication with

local gastrointestinal upset, salivation, and metallic taste. (2) High overdose, in addition to more severe local manifestations, produces systemic symptoms of convulsions, dysrhythmias, acidosis, paresthesias, and coagulation disturbances. (3) Hypocalcemia may occur.

Management. (1) Caries preventative: Less than 16 mg/kg elemental fluoride—administer milk and observe at home. If symptoms develop, or in excess of 16 mg/kg has been ingested, administer milk and refer for medical evaluation. (2) Insecticide or rodenticide exposure: Administer milk and refer for medical evaluation. Gastric lavage with 0.15 per cent calcium hydroxide 5 ml/L of water or aluminium hydroxide gel (Maalox). (3) If tetany occurs, use calcium gluconate (antidote 12A).

Laboratory. Monitor calcium, ECG, electrolytes, and magnesium.

Hallucinogens

1. LSD (LYSERGIC ACID DIETHYLAMIDE). An antiserotonin ergot-like alkaloid. Toxic dose is 35 μg.

Kinetics. Peak effect, 1 to 2 hours. Duration, 12 to 24 hours. $t_{1/2}$ is 3 hours. Elimination is hepatic.

2. MESCALINE/PEYOTE (*Lophophora williamsii*). Toxic dose is 5 mg/kg. Peyote is a species of cactus containing mescaline, an epinephrine-like compound.

Kinetics. Peak effect, 4 to 6 hours. Duration, 14 hours.

3. PSILOCYBIN. Psilocybin, an antiserotonin tryptamine derivative, is found in the "magic mushroom of Mexico," *Psilocybe mexicana*. Similar in effect to LSD but short-acting.

Kinetics. Peak effect, 90 minutes. Duration, 6 hours.

4. MARIJUANA (*Cannabis sativa*) (9-tetrahydrocannabinol, THC). Marijuana contains 1 per cent THC, but seedless sinsemilla type is 6 per cent THC; when smoked, 50 per cent is destroyed.

Kinetics. Oral bioavailability is 5 to 10 times lower than inhalation. Onset, 2 to 3 minutes (smoked), 30 to 60 minutes (ingested). Duration, 2 to 3 hours (smoked), greater than 5 hours (ingested); $t_{1/2}$ is 28 to 47 hours (shorter for chronic user). Elimination is hepatic. Enterohepatic recirculation is 15 per cent. Vd is 10 L/kg. It concentrates in the breast milk and is absorbed by the nursing infant.

Manifestations. Visual illusions, sensory perceptual distortions, depersonalization, and derealization. The degree of impairment does not correlate with the blood concentration. Conjunctival injection occurs at THC blood concentrations of 5 ng/ml and coma at 180 ng/ml.

Laboratory. A single cigarette allows the metabolite to be detected in the urine for 1 week by screening measures. Chronic use may be detected for a month or longer after cessation.

5. INHALANTS. See *Nitrites* and *Hydrocarbons*.

Management. If vital signs are stable, attempt "talk down" rather than using drugs. Most episodes are over within 12 hours.

Hydrocarbons. These are grouped toxicologically into six categories.

PETROLEUM DISTILLATES. Gasoline (petroleum spirit), 2 to 5 per cent benzene; kerosene (coal oil, charcoal lighter fluid); petroleum naphtha (cigarette lighter fluid, ligroin, racing fuel); petroleum ether (ben-

zine); turpentine (pine oil, oil of turpentine); and mineral spirits (Stoddard solvent, white spirits, varasol, petroleum spirit).

Toxicity and Kinetics. Absorption from GI tract is poor. Can tolerate 300 ml in stomach, but 0.05 ml in trachea could be fatal. Elimination is hepatic.

Manifestations. Materials aspirated during the process of ingestion produce pneumonitis. Hypoxia is the cause of CNS depression, not absorption. Myocardial sensitivity to dysrhythmias is produced by inhalation. If chest radiography demonstrates pneumonitis, it is usually present within 6 hours post ingestion.

Management. It is unlikely that a child accidentally or an adolescent siphoning would ingest a sufficient quantity to warrant the induction of emesis. An extremely large amount, over 2 ml/kg as in suicide attempts, or a product containing a dangerous additive warrants emesis, under medical supervision, within 2 hours post ingestion.

AROMATIC HYDROCARBONS. *Benzene*, a solvent used in manufacturing dyes, phenol, and nitrobenzene. The ingested toxic dose for adults is 15 ml. Chronic exposure may cause leukemia. *Toluene*, used in plastic cements. The adult ingested toxic dose is 50 ml. *Xylene*, used in the manufacture of perfumes. The adult ingested toxic dose is 50 ml.

Manifestations. They are absorbed from the GI tract and produce CNS depression and asphyxiation, defatting dermatitis, and aspiration pneumonitis. Chronic inhalation of toluene has produced renal tubular acidosis.

Management. A bite into a tube of household plastic cement by a young child does not warrant the induction of emesis. Ingestion of aromatic hydrocarbon over 1 ml/kg warrants induction of emesis, under medical supervision, within 2 hours post ingestion.

ALIPHATIC (Straight-Chained) HALOGENATED HYDROCARBONS AND SOLVENTS (Table 20)

Manifestations. Myocardial sensitization and irritability, hepatorenal toxicity, and CNS depression. Dichloromethane (methylene chloride) may be converted into carbon monoxide in the body.

Management. With ingestion of any amount, induce emesis under medical supervision.

DANGEROUS ADDITIVES. Dangerous additives to the hydrocarbons, such as heavy metals, nitrobenzene, aniline dyes, insecticides, demothing agents, and methylene chloride warrant the induction of emesis.

HEAVY HYDROCARBONS. These have high viscosity, low volatility, and minimal absorption, so emesis is unwarranted. Examples are asphalt (tar), machine oil, motor oil (lubricating oil, engine oil), diesel oil (engine fuel, home heating oil), petrolatum liquid (mineral oil, suntan oils), petrolatum jelly (Vaseline), paraffin wax, transmission oil, cutting oil, and greases and glues. No treatment is necessary.

SPECIAL PRODUCTS. Essential oils (e.g., turpentine, pine oil) are treated as petroleum distillates and do not warrant emesis unless large amounts or highly concentrated solutions are ingested. Mineral seal oil (signal oil), found in some furniture polishes, is a heavy, viscous

TABLE 20. Common Examples of Aliphatic Halogenated Hydrocarbons

	Estimated Fatal Dose (Ingested)	TLV-TWA (PPM)	Synonyms
Trichloroethane 1,1,1	15.7 gm/kg	50	Methylchloroform, Triethane, Glamorene Spot Remover, Scotchgard
Trichloroethane 1,1,2	580 mg/kg	10	Vinyl trichloride
Trichloroethylene	3–5 ml/kg ?	50	
Tetrachloroethane	Not known	5	Acetylene tetrachloride
Dichloromethane	25 ml	100	Methylene chloride
Tetrachloroethylene Perchloroethylene	5 ml	50	Tetrachloroethene
Dichloroethane	0.5 ml/kg	200	
Carbon tetrachloride	3–5 ml		

oil that *never* warrants emesis; it can produce severe pneumonia if aspirated. It has minimal absorption from the GI tract.

Management (Table 21). (1) Initial management: If needed, induction of emesis under medical supervision is the method of GI decontamination. **Avoid** gastric lavage without endotracheal tubes, activated charcoal, oils, and cathartics. In the asymptomatic patient, observe for several hours (at least 6) for development of respiratory distress. Dermal decontamination. (2) In the sympto-matic patient: Supportive respiratory care for hypoxia and bronchospasm may be treated with intravenous aminophylline. **Avoid** epinephrine because of danger of dysrhythmias with sensitized myocardium. (3) If cyanosis is present that does not respond to oxygen or the arterial PaO_2 is normal, suspect methemoglobinemia, which may require therapy with methylene blue. See *Nitrites*. (4) Steroids have not been shown to be beneficial. (5) Antimicrobials are not useful in prophylaxis. Fever or leukocytosis may be produced by the chemical pneumonitis itself. (6) Most pneumonic infiltrations resolve spontaneously in 1 week, except for lipoid pneumonia of mineral seal oil aspiration, which may last for weeks. It is not necessary to treat pneumatoceles, which may develop after the pneumonitis subsides; they clear spontaneously.

Hydrogen Peroxide. Available as household strength 3 per cent, industrial strength 10 to 20 per cent.
Toxicity. Household strength is nontoxic; industrial strength may be toxic.
Kinetics. Liberation of large amounts of oxygen causes gastric distention.
Manifestations. Industrial strength can result in burns of the exposed tissues and distention.
Management. GI decontamination is not indicated. Administer water to dilute. Gastric distention may require decompression via nasogastric tube.

Insecticides

PYRETHINS/PIPERONYL (CYPERMETHRIN, DELTA-METHRIN, FENVALERATE). These are obtained from chrysanthemums and mixed with piperonyl butoxide, which is synergistic. It is a common household spray. Toxicity is low, greater than 1 gm/kg. Manifestations usually result from the allergic properties, although CNS excitation could result from very large overdoses.
Management. GI decontamination if very large amounts were ingested. Treat convulsions and allergic reactions.

ORGANOCHLORINE. See *Organochlorides*.
ORGANOPHOSPHATES AND CARBAMATES. See *Organophosphates*.

TABLE 21. Initial Management of Hydrocarbon Ingestions

Symptoms	Contents	Amount	Initial Management
None	Petroleum distillate only	<2 ml/kg	None
None	Heavy hydrocarbon	Any amount	None
	Mineral seal oil		None
	Petroleum distillate	>2 ml/kg	? Emesis
None	Petroleum distillate with dangerous additive (heavy metals, pesticide)	Depends on additives' toxicity	Emesis
	Aromatic	>1 mL/kg	Emesis
	Halogenated hydrocarbons		
	A. Trichlor- compound	>1 mL/kg	Emesis
	B. Tetrachlor- compound	Any amount ingested	Emesis
Loss of protective airway relexes, comatose, seizures	Petroleum distillate with dangerous additive, aromatic, or halogenated hydrocarbon	Gastric lavage	ET tube before gastric lavage

ROTENONE. This is derived from the derris plant roots. Toxicity is 50 to 3000 mg/kg. Manifestations of oral ingestion are gastrointestinal irritation, conjunctivitism, rhinitis, and dermatitis. One death has been reported. Management is symptomatic and supportive.

Insect Repellents. These are generally nontoxic with the exception of diethyltoluamide (DET) found in Off, Repel, and Deep Woods Off. DET in high concentrations or sprayed repeatedly on children has resulted in toxic encephalopathy.

Iodine. USP tincture is 2 per cent iodine and 2.4 per cent sodium iodide in bottles of 15 ml; Lugol's solution is 5 per cent iodine and 10 per cent potassium iodide; organic bound iodide such as providone iodine (Betadine 1 per cent).

Toxicity. Potential fatal dose is 2 to 4 gm of free iodine. Food in GI tract inactivates it to harmless iodide salts. Organic bound iodide has one-fifth the toxicity of its iodine base. Mechanism of toxicity is similar to that of an acid corrosive.

Kinetics. Elimination is renal.

Manifestations. Brown stain to mucosa. GI irritation and burns, renal failure, shock, and hypersensitivity reactions. One case of pyloric stenosis has been reported. Enlargement of the parotid glands has been reported with chronic use.

Management. (1) Milk is given immediately and may be followed by 15 gm of cornstarch or flour in 500 ml of water. Milk may be repeated every 15 min to relieve gastric irritation. **Avoid** GI decontamination. Most household ingestions of tincture or providone require only milk and observation. (2) If there are signs of esophageal or gastric damage, perform endoscopy. (3) If anaphylactoid reaction occurs, treat with epinephrine. (4) Monitor urinary output and renal profile if toxicity develops.

Iron. See chapter on Iron Poisoning.

Isoniazid (INH, Nydrazid). This is an antituberculosis drug.

Toxicity. 35 to 40 mg/kg, produces convulsions; severe toxicity is seen at 80 to 150 mg/kg. Mechanism of toxicity: It produces pyridoxine deficiency and inhibits the formation of GABA in the brain.

Kinetics. Peak in 1 to 2 hours. Elimination is hepatic.

Manifestations. Visual disturbances, convulsions (90 per cent multiple seizures) that often start within 30 minutes, coma, resistant severe acidosis.

Management. (1) Control seizures with large doses of pyridoxine (antidote 34). Repeat until seizures cease. Diazepam should be administered with pyridoxine, as they act synergistically. **Caution**: INH-phenytoin interaction. (2) Correct acidosis. Control of the seizures may spontaneously correct the acidosis. (3) **Avoid** emesis because of rapid onset of seizures. After patient is stabilized or if asymptomatic, other GI decontamination procedures may be carried out; asymptomatic patients should be observed for 6 hours. (4) Hemodialysis is rarely needed but may be used as an adjunct for uncontrollable acidosis and seizures. Hemoperfusion has not been adequately evaluated.

Laboratory. Plasma isoniazid levels above 8 μg/ml are toxic. Monitor the blood glucose (often hyperglycemic),

electrolytes (often hyperkalemic), and liver function tests. Monitor the temperature closely (often hyperpyrexic).

Lead. See chapter on Increased Lead Absorption and Acute Lead Poisoning.

Lidocaine. This is a cardiac antidysrhythmic agent and local anesthetic (2 per cent Xylocaine).

Toxicity. Oral ingestion over 5 mg/kg may produce toxicity.

Kinetics. Peak blood concentration occurs 1 hour post ingestion; oral mucosal kinetics are similar to intravenous but GI bioavailability is about 35 per cent. Duration is 10 to 20 minutes intravenously. Elimination is hepatic. Has active toxic metabolite.

Manifestations. (1) Mild—vertigo, drowsiness, dysarthria, perioral numbness, muscle twitching, confusion, and tinnitus (blood concentrations 5 to 9 μg/ml). (2) Serious—psychosis, convulsions, severe bradycardia, sinus arrest, arteriovenous block, respiratory depression (blood concentration greater than 9 μg/ml). (3) Methemoglobinemia.

Management. (1) Treat the seizures with diazepam initially followed by phenobarbital and neuromuscular blocking agents, intubation, and ventilation if needed. **Avoid** phenytoin because of its possible synergistic cardiac side effects. Convulsions may continue with low blood concentrations of lidocaine owing to its toxic metabolite. (2) The dysrhythmias may require pacing or cardioversion. (3) Methemoglobinemia. See *Nitrites*. (4) GI decontamination, if ingested, with activated charcoal and a cathartic. **Avoid** emesis because of rapid onset of symptoms.

Laboratory. Lidocaine blood concentrations (therapeutic 1.5 to 6 μg/ml). Methemoglobin levels if brown blood or cyanosis occurs.

Lomotil. See *Opioids*. Has the potential for serious intoxication in children.

Mercury (Table 22)

Toxicity. Elemental mercury is toxic by inhalation. The fatal dose of inorganic mercury salts in adults is 1 gm. Ingested elemental mercury in thermometers is poorly absorbed and is nontoxic.

Kinetics. Elemental mercury absorption 89 per cent by inhalation, 0.01 per cent of ingested dose. Elimination is renal.

Manifestations. (1) Acute poisoning: Mercuric salts act as a corrosive, producing stomatitis and gastroenteritis with bloody, bluish vomitus within 15 minutes. Within 1 to 3 days the victims develop foul breath, metallic taste, and evidence of hepatic and renal dysfunction. Inhalation produces similar symptoms and a pneumonitis. (2) Chronic poisoning produces acrodynia (rashes, painful limbs, hypotonia, and hypertension in infants), erethethism (memory loss, emotional disturbances, renal dysfunction in adults), and organic mercury intoxications (ataxia, dysarthria, tunnel vision, and teratogenesis).

Management. (1) Ingestion of mercuric salts is managed by the routine GI decontamination procedures. (2) Dimercaprol (BAL) (antidote 17) enhances mercury excretion through the bile as well as the urine and is

TABLE 22. Types of Mercury and Mercury Poisonings

Classification	Product Exposure	Absorption and Route	Distribution	T$_{1/2}$ (Days)	Elimination	Manifestations and Comments
Elemental	Thermometers Amalgan	Ingestion	—	—	—	Nontoxic unless delayed GI passage
	Industry TLV = 0.05 ppm	Inhalation Rapid Chronic poisoning	Large	58	Renal	Pulmonary, neurologic psychologic
	Abuse	Injection Chronic poisoning	Large	Long	Renal	Pulmonary, neurologic, psychologic, local abscess
Inorganic mercuric salts (HgCl$_2$)	Disinfectant	Ingestion Acute and chronic poisoning	Large	40	Renal	Corrosive, nephrotoxic, acrodynia
Mercurous salts (HgCl)	Teething lotion, laxatives	Ingestion mucosal Chronic poisoning	Large	—	Renal	Acrodynia
Organic						
Alkyl short chained	Methyl: Bioaccumulation Fungicide	Ingestion rapid, complete 100% Chronic poisoning	Large Passes placenta	52–70	Liver enterohepatic	Neurosensory, Developmental, (Minamata disease)
(fish-food chain)	Ethyl: Fungicides	Ingestion rapid Chronic poisoning	Large	—	Renal	GI, renal, neurologic
Aryl phenyl Methoxyethyl	Diaper rinse	Ingestion Very rapid Acute and chronic poisoning	Large	—	Renal	Forms inorganic salts in body
Long-chain thimerosal	Diuretics, antiseptics, fungicide	Ingestion poorly	Large	—	Renal	Low toxicity

the treatment of choice if there is renal impairment. D-Penicillamine (antidote 29) is useful in less severe poisonings or chronic mercury poisonings. BAL in methyl mercury intoxication increases the brain mercury and is contraindicated; penicillamine decreases brain mercury and should be used. An investigational chelator, 2,3-dimercaptosuccinic acid, holds promise of less toxicity and more specificity. (3) Obtain and monitor blood and urine mercury levels. (Use proper collection technique and containers.) (4) Hemodialysis early in the symptomatic patient is useful. (5) Surgical excision of local injection sites.

Laboratory. (1) Blood levels above 4 μg/dl and urine levels above 20 μg/L probably should be considered abnormal in unexposed populations. Blood levels are not reliable after the first few hours because of tissue binding. (2) Methyl mercury is excreted mainly through the feces, so urine mercury would not be a reliable measurement.

Methemoglobinemia. See *Nitrites.*

Mothballs (Table 23). See *Camphor* [discontinued], *Naphthalene, Paradichlorobenzene.*

Naphthalene. This is found in mothballs, repellent cakes, and deodorant cakes.

Toxicity. Ingestion of 250 to 500 mg of pure naphthalene may cause hemolysis in patients with glucose-6-phosphate dehydrogenase (G-6-PD) deficiency. Persons without this deficiency require several grams to produce toxicity.

Kinetics. Oil enhances absorption. Skin absorption occurs from clothes stored in naphthalene, particularly if baby oil is applied. Oxidative metabolites, naphthols, are responsible for hemolysis. Elimination is hepatic.

Manifestations. Hemolysis starts on day 1 to 3 post exposure, nausea, vomiting, diarrhea, fever, jaundice, dark urine, renal failure, coma, and convulsions. Rare hepatocellular damage may occur. Recovery begins in 7 to 10 days.

Management. (1) GI decontamination, including activated charcoal and cathartic. Decontaminate the skin and discard contaminated clothing. Washing does not completely remove naphthalene from clothes. Monitor the hemoglobin or hematocrit and blood smear for 1 week after exposure. (2) If transfusion is needed in G-6-PD deficiency patients, use blood from a donor with normal G-6-PD. Transfuse to 80 per cent of normal G-6-PD value. If there is methemoglobinemia, consider methylene blue (antidote 24). See *Nitrites.* (3) Establish good hydration, alkalinize, and create a diuresis with furosemide to avoid precipitation of hemoglobin in the renal tubules. Monitor urinary output and renal profile. If there is renal shutdown, use dialysis. (4) Corticoste-

TABLE 23. Mothing Agents: Differentiation

	Paradichlorobenzene Crystals, Nuggets	Naphthalene Balls, Flakes
Appearance	Wet	Dry
Turpentine dissolution test	Slowly dissolves in 60 minutes	Slowly dissolves; 25% remains in 60 minutes
Copper wire test	Produces fleeting but intense green flame in minutes	No green flame

roids have been reported as helpful in limiting the hemolysis.

Laboratory. Heinz bodies signify impending hemolysis, eccentrocytes (a dense asymmetric distribution of hemoglobin in the red blood cell) are found in active hemolysis. Reticulocyte counts greater than 7 per cent yield normal G-6-PD even if deficiency exists; therefore if hemolysis is active check the parents for G-6-PD deficiency.

Nicotine. This occurs in insecticides (Black leaf 40 per cent solution), tobacco products, and plants; i.e., *Nicotiana tabacum* has 1 to 6 per cent nicotine content.

Toxicity. Fatal dose is 10 mg/kg of pure nicotine. A cigarette contains 15 to 25 mg and a cigar has 15 to 40 mg nicotine. When ingested, tobacco is much less toxic because of poor absorption. Only about one fourth of the total nicotine is recovered from cigarette butts.

Kinetics. Route of elimination is hepatic. Onset of action is within 1 hour.

Manifestations. (1) Phase I: adrenergic and cholinergic—tobacco odor on breath, vomiting (2 to 5 mg nicotine may cause nausea), tachypnea, bradycardia, miosis, hypertension, salivation, abdominal pain, and diarrhea. Early excitation, tremors, and seizures may occur within 30 minutes. (2) Phase II: Tachycardia, mydriasis, hypotension (ganglionic blockade). Late respiratory muscle paralysis and coma. Ileus and urinary retention may occur. If fatal dose is ingested, patients may die within 1 hour.

Management. (1) Children who ingest less than one cigarette or 3 butts require only observation at home. If larger amounts of nicotine insecticide are ingested, use GI decontamination with lavage and activated charcoal. **Avoid** emesis because of the rapid onset of convulsions. (2) Control convulsions with diazepam and phenytoin. (3) Atropine for cholinergic crisis. Beta- and alpha-blockers, like labetolol, for sympathetic stimulation. (4) Acid diuresis is not recommended. (5) Be prepared for intubation and respiratory support.

Nitrites and Nitrates. Available in both inorganic and organic forms. Inorganic nitrates and nitrites occur in well water and certain foods (spinach, carrots, cabbage, beets) and may produce methemoglobinemia in infants.

Toxicity. The potential fatal adult doses are nitrite, 1 gm; nitrate, 10 gm; nitrobenzene, 2 ml; nitroglycerin, 0.2 gm; and aniline dye (pure), 5 to 30 gm.

Kinetics. Onset with nitroglycerin sublingually is 1 to 3 minutes, with a peak action of 3 to 15 minutes and a duration of 20 to 30 minutes. Other routes have a slower onset (2 to 5 minutes) and longer duration of action (1.5 to 6 hours). Nitrites are potent oxidizing agents and may produce methemoglobinemia. Elimination is hepatic.

Manifestations (Table 24). (1) Vasodilatory: headache, flushing of the skin, sweating, hypotension, tachycardia, and syncope. (2) Methemoglobinemia: slate gray cyanosis with chocolate-colored lips and mucosa, refractory to oxygen therapy, brown-colored blood that fails to turn red on exposure to oxygen, normal PaO_2 and venous PO_2 with low oxygen saturation. Other causes of methemoglobinemia are congenital, medications (antimalarials, some local anesthetics, dapsone, nitrites, sul-

TABLE 24. Manifestations of Methemoglobinemia

Methemoglobin (%)	Manifestations
10	"Chocolate cyanosis," brown blood
10 to 20	Headache, dizziness, tachypnea
50	Mental alterations, coma, convulsions
above 50	Metabolic acidosis and ECG changes
70	Pulmonary edema, encephalopathy, shock

fonamides), and some chemicals (aniline derivates, chlorates, nitrites).

Management. (1) Dermal decontamination, if indicated. Aniline dyes may be removed with 5 per cent acetic acid (vinegar). (2) GI decontamination if acutely ingested. (3) Hypotension can be treated by positioning and fluids. Vasoconstrictors (dopamine or norepinephrine) are rarely needed. (4) If methemoglobinemia occurs, administer 100 per cent oxygen during and after antidotal therapy. Methylene blue (antidote 24) is indicated for methemoglobin levels above 30 per cent, dyspnea, lactic acidosis, or an altered mental state. Methylene blue reduces the $t_{1/2}$ of methemoglobin from 15 to 20 hours to less than 60 minutes. Ascorbic acid is ineffective. **Avoid** methylene blue in G-6-PD deficiency patients because it is ineffective and may precipitate hemolysis. A hyperbaric chamber and/or exchange transfusion should be used in symptomatic patients if methylene blue is not effective or is contraindicated.

Laboratory. Methemoglobin levels, ADG, and oxygen saturation.

Nonsteroidal Anti-inflammatory Agents (NSAIDs) (Table 25)

Kinetics. Peak blood concentration in 1 to 2 hours. Hepatic elimination.

Manifestations. (1) Gastrointestinal: nausea, vomiting, abdominal pain, GI bleeding. (2) Central nervous system: drowsiness, tinnitus, headache, lethargy. Renal failure with chronic use or massive overdose. Specific manifestations of various NSAIDs: Indomethacin—neurologic effects. Meclofenamate and mefenamic acid—bloody diarrhea and seizures. Phenylbutazone and oxyphenbutazone—agranulocytosis, aplastic anemia, and thrombocytopenia; exfoliative dermatitis. Sulindac—hypersensitive hepatitis.

Management (Table 26). (1) Observe for GI symptoms and CNS symptoms. If no GI symptoms in 6 hours, intoxication is unlikely. (2) Monitor vital signs and biochemical, liver, and renal profiles. A metabolic acidosis has been reported in humans with ibuprofen and diflunisal. Test the vomitus and/or gastric aspirate and stools for blood. (3) Initial and repeated doses of activated charcoal have been effective in phenylbutazone overdose and merit consideration, although the data are limited with other NSAIDs. (4) Gastrointestinal bleeding is managed with iced saline lavage and H_2 blockers and/or antacids. (5) Alkaline diuresis with sodium bicarbonate may be useful (antidote 35). Hemodialysis is not useful. Hemoperfusion was successful in one case of phenylbutazone. (6) Treat convulsions with diazepam and phenytoin.

TABLE 25. Pharmacokinetics of Nonsteroidal Anti-inflammatory Agents (NSAIDs)

Drug (Trade Name)	Therap Dose (mg)	Peak (Hours)	Elimination Route	T$_{1/2}$ (Hours)	Comments
Diflunisal (Dolobid)	250	1–2	Hepatic	8–12	Preparations 250 mg
Fenoprofen (Nalfon)	600	1–2	Hepatic	1.5–3	Preparations 300, 600 mg
Ibuprofen (Motrin, Advil, Rufen)	400	0.5–1.5	Hepatic	2–2.5	Preparations 200, 300, 400, 800 mg
Indomethacin (Indocin)	25	1–2	Hepatic	4.5–6.0	Preparations 25, 50 mg; enterohepatic recirculation
Mefenamic acid* (Ponstel)	500	1–3	Hepatic	3–4	Preparations 250 mg
Meclofenamate* (Meclomen)	50	0.5–2	Hepatic	3–4	Preparations 50, 100 mg; active metabolite
Naproxen (Anaprox, Naprosyn)	250	1–2	Hepatic	12–15	Preparations 250, 375, 500 mg
Oxyphenbutazone* (Oxalid, Tandearil)	200		Hepatic	72	Preparations 200, 400 mg
Phenylbutazone* (Azolid, Butazolidin)	75	2	Hepatic	50–100	Preparations 100 mg; active metabolite
Piroxicam* (Feldene)	20	2–5	Hepatic	45	Preparations 10, 20 mg; enterohepatic recirculation
Sulindac (Clinoril)	150	1	Hepatic	7–8	Preparations 150, 200 mg; active metabolite
Suprofen* (Suprol)	200	1	Hepatic	2–4	Preparation 200 mg
Tolmetin (Tolectin)	330 Child 15–30 mg/kg	1–2	Hepatic	1	Preparations 200, 400 mg
Zomepirac* (Zomax) 50, 100 mg	50				Removed from the market 1983

*Potentially more serious ingestion.

Nontoxic Ingestion (Table 27). Criteria for nontoxic ingestion: (1) absolute identification of the product; (2) absolute assurance that a single product was ingested; (3) assurance that there is no signal word on the container; (4) a good approximation of the amount ingested; (5) the ability to call back at frequent intervals to determine if symptoms have developed. (6) a satisfactory explanation of the circumstances is necessary to exclude chemical maltreatment under 1 year and to exclude a "cry for help" over 6 years.

TABLE 26. Management of Overdose of NSAIDs

Amount	Management
Ibuprofen, Indomethacin, Naproxen, Sulindac, Tolmetin, Diflunisal	
Child	
<3 times therapeutic doses (<100 mg/kg ibuprofen)	Observation for symptoms
3–5 times therapeutic doses (100–200 mg/kg ibuprofen)	Induce emesis if <2 hr PI* Observation only >2 hr PI
>5 times therapeutic doses (>200 mg/kg ibuprofen)	Gastric lavage Activated charcoal Observation and monitor for >6 hr
Adolescent	
>10 times therapeutic doses	Gastric lavage Activated charcoal Observation and monitor for >6 hr
Phenylbutazone, Oxyphenbutazone, Piroxicam, Mefenamic acid, Suprofen	
Child	
>2 therapeutic doses	Induce emesis if <2 hr PI Gastric lavage >2 hr PI Activated charcoal Observation and monitor for >6 hr
Adolescent	
>5 times therapeutic doses	Gastric lavage Activated charcoal Observation and monitor for >6 hr

*PI = post ingestion.

Opioids (Narcotic Opiates)

Toxicity. Codeine may produce minor signs of toxicity at 1 mg/kg and respiratory arrest at 5 mg/kg. Propoxyphene (Darvon) 10 mg/kg is toxic, and 35 mg/kg causes cardiopulmonary arrest. Dextromethorphan 10 mg/kg or 90 to 180 mg has produced symptoms; however, no fatalities have been reported.

Kinetics. The onset of action of most opioids varies between 10 and 60 minutes, and the peak between 30 minutes and 2 hours. The usual therapeutic duration of action is 4 to 6 hours. Elimination is hepatic. Meperidine is metabolized into normeperidine, an active CNS stimulant. The t$_{1/2}$ of meperidine is between 0.5 and 5 hours, normeperidine 22 to 97 hours, methadone 15 to 30 hours, and propoxyphene 2 to 4 hours.

Manifestations. The classic triad is coma, slow respirations, and pinpoint pupils. (1) CNS depression, bradycardia and hypotension; (2) seizures may occur with propoxyphene, codeine, meperidine, and lomotil; (3) pulmonary edema, particularly a complication of mainlining (intravenous use); (4) most opiate agonists produce miotic pupils; however, mydriatic pupils are seen with meperidine, dextromethorphan, and rarely Lomotil; (5) physical dependence and withdrawal; (6) dextromethorphan overdose with long-acting preparations causes ataxia, hypertension, tachycardia, restlessness, nystagmus, and lethargy, and naloxone may not be completely successful in reversing these manifestations;

TABLE 27. The Usually Nontoxic Ingestion
(Unless Ingested in Very Large Quantity)

Abrasives	Laxatives
Adhesives	Lipstick
Antacids	Lubricants
Antibiotics	Lysol brand disinfectant (not the
Baby product cosmetics	bowl cleaner)
Ballpoint pen inks	Magic marker
Bathtub floating toys	Makeup (eye, liquid facial)
Bath oil (castor oil and	Matches (book type)
perfume)	Mineral oil
Bleach less than 5%	Newspaper
Body conditioners	Paints (indoor latax acrylic)
Bubble bath soaps (detergents)	Pencil lead (graphite)
Calamine lotion	Perfumes (depends on alcohol
Candles	content)
Caps (for toy pistols)	Petroleum jelly (Vaseline)
Chalk (calcium carbonate)	Plaster (non–lead containing)
Cigarettes (less than one)	Play-doh
Clay (modeling)	Polaroid picture coating
Colognes	Porous tip ink marking pens
Contraceptive pills (without	Prussian blue (ferricyanide)
iron)	Putty
Corticosteroids	Rouge
Crayons (marked A.P., C.P.,	Rubber cements
C.S.-140)	Sackets (essential oils)
Dehumidifying packets (silica or	Shampoo (liquid)
charcoal)	Shaving creams
Detergents (phosphate type,	Soaps and soap products
anionic)	Spackles
Deodorants (spray and	Suntan preparations
refrigerator)	Sweetening agents
Elmer's glue	Teething rings
Etch-A-Sketch	Thermometers (mercury)
Eye makeup	Toilet water
Fabric softner	Toothpaste (even fluoride)
Fertilizer	Vaseline
Fish bowl additives	Vitamins (even flouride)
Fluoride—caries preventative	Warfarin (single dose)
Glues and pastes	Water colors
Golf ball core (may cause	Zinc oxide
mechanical injury)	Zirconium oxide
Grease	
Hair products (dyes, sprays,	
tonics)	
Hand lotions and creams	
Indelible markers	
Ink (blue, Black)	
Iodophor disinfectant	

(7) Lomotil (atropine and diphenoxylate). Atropine toxicity may rarely occur in 1 to 2 hours post ingestion with diphenoxylate toxicity delayed to 2 to 5 hours. It is extremely toxic in children and they should always be admitted for close observation.

Management. (1) If there is severe CNS depression, establish an airway with an endotracheal tube and administer assisted ventilation. (2) Naloxone (Narcan) (antidote 25) is given as an initial bolus intravenously and followed by continuous infusion. Naloxone must be titrated against the clinical response and withdrawal in narcotic addicts. It should be repeated or used to supplement the infusion as necessary, since many opioids in overdose can last 24 to 48 hours, whereas the duration of action of naloxone is only 0.5 to 2 hours. Larger doses are often needed for codeine, pentazocine, and propoxyphene. The signs of naloxone effect are

dilation of pupils, increased rate and depth of respirations, reversal of hypotension, and improvement of obtunded or comatose state. Indications for naloxone infusion are (a) the need for a large initial bolus, (b) the need for repeated boluses, (c) a very large overdose, or (d) an overdose with a long-acting preparation. (3) GI decontamination up to 8 hours post ingestion. **Avoid** induced emesis in overdose because CNS depression and convulsions occur early. (4) If the patient is comatose, obtain a blood specimen and administer 50 per cent glucose (3 to 4 per cent of comatose narcotic opioid overdose patients have hypoglycemia). Naloxone and intravenous glucose should be tried first to control seizures. If these fail, diazepam may be tried. (5) Pulmonary edema does not respond to naloxone and needs respiratory supportive care. Fluids should be given cautiously in opioid overdose, because of antidiuretic hormone effect and pulmonary edema. (6) If the patient is agitated, consider hypoxia before withdrawal. (7) Observe for withdrawal (nausea, vomiting, cramps, diarrhea, dilated pupils, rhinorrhea, piloerection). If these occur, stop naloxone.

Laboratory. For drug abuser, consider testing for hepatitis B, syphilis, HIV antibody tests (HIV usually requires consent).

Organochlorine Insecticides (DDT Derivatives). (Table 28). The groups are (1) cyclodienes used in termite control—chlordane, dieldrin, aldrin; (2) Chlorinated ethane derivatives of chlorophenothane (DDT), which are less acutely toxic than the cyclodienes. (3) Benzene hexachloride (BHC) isomers—lindane, kepone, mirex. They are also used topically for scabies and lice.

Toxicity. Varies. Lindane (Kwell) ingestion of less than 5 ml in a child or less than 15 ml in adult has not been associated with toxicity. Prolonged or excessively frequent topical application has been associated with seizures.

Kinetics. They resist degradation in human tissue and the environment. They accumulate in adipose tissue. Elimination is hepatic.

Manifestations. Usually develop within 1 to 2 hours. CNS stimulation, convulsions, late respiratory depression, increased myocardial irritability. Symptoms may last for 1 week or more. Chronic exposure may cause liver and kidney damage.

Management. (1) Protective garb for personnel. Dermal decontamination, remove contaminated clothing and discard contaminated leather goods. GI decontamination with activated charcoal. **Caution** with emesis because of rapid onset, no oils. Many are dissolved in petroleum distillates, presenting an aspiration hazard. (2) No adrenergic stimulants (epinephrine) because of myocardial irritability. (3) Cholestyramine, 4 gm every 8 hours, has been reported to increase the fecal excretion in chronic exposures. (4) Anticonvulsants, if needed.

Organophosphate and Carbamate Insecticides (Table 29). Biodegradable cholinesterase inhibitors may cause (a) irreversible inhibition of cholinesterase, either direct (TEPP) or delayed (parathion or malathion), or

TABLE 28. Organochlorine Pesticides (DDT Derivatives)

Clinical Name (Trade Name)	Toxicity Rating	Elimination Time	Comment
Endrin (Hexadrin)	Highest	Hours to days	Banned
Lindane (1% in Kwell; Benesan; Isotox; Gamene)	Moderate to high	Hours to days	Scabicide; general garden insecticide
Endosulfan (Thiodan)	Moderate	Hours to days	
Benzene hexachloride (BHC, HCH)	Moderate	Weeks to months	Banned, produces porphyria cutanea tarda
Dieldrin (Dieldrite)	High	Weeks to months	
Aldrin (Aldrite)	High	Weeks to months	
Chlordane (Chlordan) (10% is Heptachlor)	High	Weeks to months	Restricted; termiticide
Toxophene (Toxakil, Strobane-T)	High	Hours to days	
Heptachlor	Moderate	Weeks to months	Malignancy in rats
Chlorophenothane (DDT)	Moderate	Months to years	Banned in 1972
Mirex	Moderate	Months to years	Banned; red anticide
Chlordecone (Kepone)	Moderate	Months to years	Tidewater, Virginia, contamination
Methoxychlor (Marlate)	Low	Hours to days	
Perthane	Low	Hours to days	
Dicofol (Kelthane)	Low	Hours to days	
Chlorobenzilate (Acaraben)	Low	Hours to days	Banned

(b) partially reversible inhibition of cholinesterase (carbamates).

Toxicity. The mechanism of toxicity is the phosphorylation of acetylcholinesterase so that it loses its ability to inactivate acetylcholine.

Kinetics. The onset is usually before 12 hours unless they are absorbed by the dermal route or are lipid-soluble (fenthion), which may delay onset for 24 hours. Inhalation produces intoxication within minutes.

Manifestations. Garlic breath odor or from gastric contents or container may be a clue. (1) Early muscarinic cholinergic crisis: cramps, diarrhea, excess secretion, bronchospasms, bradycardia. Mydriasis may occur early, miosis later. (2) Later, sympathetic and nicotine effects occur: twitching, fasciculations, weakness, tachycardia and hypertension, and convulsions. (3) CNS effects are anxiety, headache, confusion, emotional lability, convulsion, and coma. (4) Hypo- or hypergly-

TABLE 29. Examples of Organophosphate Insecticides (OPI)

Common Name	Synonym	EFD*
Agricultural products (highly toxic; LD$_{50}$ is 1 to 50 mg/kg)		
Tetraethyl pyrophosphate	TEPP, Tetron	0.05
Phorate	Thimet	
Disulfoton	Di-Syston	0.2
Demeton	Systox	
Terbufos	Counter	
Chlortriphos	Calathion	
Mevinphos	Phosdrin	0.15
Parathion	Thiophos	0.10
Methamidophos	Monitor	Delayed neuropathy
Monocrotophos	Azodrin	
Octamethyldiphosphoramide	OMPA, Schradan	
Azinphosmethyl	Guthion	0.2
Ethyl-nitrophenyl thiobenzene	PO4, EPN	
Animal insecticides (moderately toxic; LD$_{50}$ is 50 to 500 mg/kg)		
DEF	DeGreen	
Dichlorvos	DDVP, Vapona	
Coumaphos	Co-ral	
Trichlorfon	Dylox	
Ronnel	Korlan	10.0
Dimethoate	Cygon, De-fend	
Fenthion	Baytex	Long-acting
Leptophos	Phosvel	
Chlorfenvinophos (tick dip)	Supona, Demaron	
Household and garden pest control (low toxicity; LD$_{50}$ is 500 to 5000 mg/kg)		
Malathion	Cythion	60.0
Diazinon	Spectracide, Dimpylate	25.0
Chlorpyrifos	Losban, Dursban	
Temephos	Abate	

*EFD = estimated fatal dose (gm/70 kg)

cemia. (5) An intermediate syndrome of respiratory paralysis, a few days after successful treatment that does not respond to the antidotes and may necessitate ventilatory support. (6) Chronic delayed toxicity that clinically mimics Guillain-Barré syndrome with merphos (Folex) and fenthion (Baytex) in humans and chloropyrifos (Dursban) in animals. (7) In children the scenerio is usually insecticide house spraying and in a few hours miosis, salivation with tachycardia, and seizures predominating.

Management. (1) Protective garb for personnel. Correct hypoxia (suction, 100 per cent oxygen, intubation, and ventilation) and dermal decontamination. Suction until atropinization drying of secretions is achieved. (2) **If the diagnosis is probable, do not delay therapy while awaiting confirmation.** Atropine sulfate (antidote 7) is the cornerstone of acute therapy. It is administered **after** cyanosis is corrected. If symptomatic, atropine is administered every 5 to 10 minutes until drying of secretions and clearing of lungs. Atropine infusions have been used successfully with the addition of supplemental atropine to the infusion, as needed, to keep the secretions dried. Long periods of atropinization may be necessary. Maintain for 12 to 24 hours, then taper the dose observing for relapse. Atropine is both a diagnostic and a therapeutic agent. (3) Intravenous pralidoxime (2-Pam, Protopam) (antidote 31) is required after atropinization. It should be used early before the phosphate bond becomes stable. Its use may require a reduction in the dose of atropine. It is not recommended in mild reversible carbamate poisoning such as with carbaryl (Sevin); however, its use is suggested in life-threatening carbamate poisoning. The end-point is absence of fasciculations and a return of muscle strength. Its effects are usually noted in 0.5 to 1 hour. (4) **Avoid** morphine, aminophylline, phenothiazines, reserpine-like drugs, and succinylcholine. (5) CNS depression may require respiratory support. (6) **Do not** administer atropine or pralidoxime prophylactically to workers exposed to organophosphates.

Laboratory. Obtain blood for red blood cell acetylcholinesterase before giving pralidoxime. Levels are usually depressed more than 75 per cent for severe symptoms. Monitor acetylcholinesterase weekly if depressed. **Carbamates** cause partially reversible carbamylation of cholinesterase (Table 30). The major differences between carbamates and OPI are (1) toxicity is less and of shorter duration; (2) they rarely produce overt central nervous system effects because of poor penetration; and (3) cholinesterase returns to normal rapidly so that blood values are not useful in confirming diagnosis.

Paradichlorobenzene. Available as deodorant and diaper pail cakes and moth repellents, sometimes combined with naphthalene.

Toxic Dose. 500 to 5000 mg/kg.

Kinetics. Elimination is hepatic.

Manifestations. Only one report in the literature of acute toxicity (3-year-old boy who developed methemoglobinemia and hemolysis). Large amounts may produce GI upset. No fatal cases of human poisoning.

Management. GI decontamination is recommended only if large amounts are ingested such as entire moth-

TABLE 30. Toxicity of Carbamates

Common Name	Synonym
Highly toxic (1 to 5 mg/kg)	
Ziram	
Temik*	Aldicarb
Matacil	Aminocarb, carazol
Vydate	Oxamyl
Isolan	Isolan
Furadan	Carbofuran
Lannate	Methomyl, Nudrin
Zectran	Mexacarbate
Mesurol	Methiocarb
Moderately toxic (50 to 500 mg/kg)	
Baygon	Propoxur
Sevin	Carbaryl
Ficam	Methylcarbamate

Some of these may be formulated in wood alcohol and have the added toxicity of methyl alcohol.

ball or over 1 bite of a cake deodorant. Avoid milk and oily foods for at least 2 hours post ingestion because they increase absorption.

Paraquat, Diquat. Paraquat is a herbicide rapidly inactivated in the soil. Preparations of 0.2 per cent are unlikely to cause serious intoxications.

Toxicity. With preparations of 20 per cent, such as Gramoxone, 10 ml has produced death. Ingestion of 20 mg/kg causes vomiting and diarrhea; 20 to 40 mg/kg reversible renal failure, pulmonary fibrosis, and death in days to weeks; and over 40 mg/kg multiple organ failure and death in days. Aerosol droplets are too large to produce systemic toxicity. Paraquat on marijuana leaves is pyrolyzed to nontoxic dipyridyl.

Kinetics. Less than 20 per cent of ingested dose is absorbed. The peak is 1 hour post ingestion. The paraquat concentrates in the lung. Elimination is renal. Toxicity results from the formation of superoxide radicals that destroy the pulmonary cells, resulting in fibrosis.

Manifestations. (1) Local corrosive effect on skin and mucous membranes, renal failure in 48 hours (often reversible). (2) Pulmonary effects occur as early as 72 hours and are progressive. Oxygen aggravates the pulmonary effects. (3) Diquat does not produce effects on the lungs but produces convulsions and GI distention. Long-term exposure may give cataracts.

Management. (1) **Avoid** emesis induction. GI decontamination is by administration of oral absorbent such as activated charcoal and a cathartic. Repeated doses of activated charcoal are recommended. Total bowel irrigation has been used, but proof of its effectiveness is not available. Dermal and ocular decontamination may be needed. (2) Hemoperfusion with charcoal until blood paraquat cannot be detected is the present choice; however, the results are still poor. (3) Avoid oxygen unless absolutely necessary because this aggravates pulmonary fibrosis. Some use hypoxic air, FiO_2 10 to 20 per cent. (4) Corticosteroids may help prevent adrenocortical necrosis and suppress superoxide ions. Dexamethasone 8 mg every 8 hours IV for 2 weeks, then orally 0.5 mg every 8 hours for 2 weeks and cyclophosphamide 5 mg/kg daily IV in three doses to a maximum of 4 gm in 2 weeks reduced the mortality in one series. No studies of effectiveness. (5) Sepsis often develops in 7 to 10 days post ingestion and should be treated appropriately.

Laboratory. Plasma paraquat above 2 μg/ml at 4 hours or above 0.1 μg/ml at 48 hours is fatal. Plasma analysis and advice may be obtained from the ICI America (800-327-8633). Crude plasma concentrations and urine detection may be approximated by adding sodium dithionite. A blue-green color develops when paraquat is present. Negative results early do not exclude paraquat contamination; repeat the tests.

Phencyclidine (Angel Dust, PCP, Peace Pill, Hog). "The drug of deceit" is substituted for many other hallucinogens. Intoxication by inhalation of PCP in a room where adults were smoking has been reported in children.

Toxicity. Two to 5 mg (20 to 30 μg/ml) causes CNS excitement and paranoid behavior, 5 to 10 mg (30 to 100 μg/ml) coma and convulsions, and 10 to 25 mg (100 to 250 μg/ml) prolonged coma and respiratory failure; > 25 mg (> 250 μg/ml) is usually fatal. These values do not always correlate.

Kinetics. Ingested, snorted, and smoked. Enterohepatic recirculation. The onset smoked is 2 to 5 minutes (peak in 15 to 30 minutes); orally, 30 to 60 minutes. The duration at low doses is 4 to 6 hours and normality returns in 24 hours. At large overdoses coma may last 6 to 10 days (waxes and wanes). The adverse manifestations of overdose usually occur within 1 to 2 hours. Elimination is hepatic.

Manifestations. Early CNS stimulation, later depression. Violent behavior (often self-destructive), paranoid schizophrenia. Clues to diagnosis are usually miosis with bursts of horizontal, vertical, and rotary nystagmus and coma with eyes open.

Management. Avoid overtreatment of mild intoxications: (1) GI decontamination post ingestion: Emesis and gastric lavage may not be effective because PCP is rapidly absorbed. Repeated doses of activated charcoal and nasogastric suction may help to remove the drug, which has enterohepatic recirculation even if smoked

or snorted. (2) Protect patient and others from harm. "Talk down" is usually ineffective. Low sensory environment. Diazepam (Valium) may be used orally or intravenously. (3) For behavioral disorders and toxic psychosis, use haloperidol, diazepam, or both. (4) Seizures and muscle spasm are controlled with diazepam. (5) Dystonia reaction: diphenhydramine (Benadryl) intravenously (antidote 18). (6) Hyperthermia: external cooling. (7) Hypertensive crisis: Use nitroprusside or diazoxide. (8) Acid diuresis ion trapping with ammonium chloride (antidote 2) is not routinely recommended because of rhabdomyolysis and the danger of myoglobin precipitation in renal tubules. (9) Myoglobinemia: fluid diuresis and alkalinization. (10) **Avoid** phenothiazines in the acute phase of intoxication because they lower the convulsive threshold. May be needed later for psychosis.

Laboratory. Elevation of CPK is a clue to rhabdomyolysis and myoglobinuria. Test urine for myoglobin and pigmented casts. Plasma phencyclidine. Blood glucose (20 per cent have hypoglycemia). PCP in gastric juice is 40 to 50 times higher than in blood.

Complications and Sequelae. Chronic brain syndrome, intracranial hemorrhage, malignant hyperthermia, schizophrenic paranoid psychosis, and loss of memory for months. Delayed toxicity and "flash backs" occur.

Phenothiazines (PTZ) and Nonphenothiazine Neuroleptics (NPTZ). Neuroleptics have similar pharmacologic properties (Table 31).

Toxicity. Chlorpromazine 20 mg/kg in children, 2 gm in adults.

Kinetics. Varies. The phenothiazines are eliminated by the hepatic route into many metabolites, some of which remain in the body for months.

Manifestations. **Acute poisonings:** (1) Anticholinergic actions but miosis (> 80 per cent), bradycardia and hypotension, hypothermia or hyperthermia, and convulsions. (2) Quinidine effect on heart produces depression of the myocardial contractility and may produce life-threatening dysrhythmias, including torsades de pointes. (3) Impaired catecholamine re-uptake produces transient hypertension followed by peripheral alpha-

TABLE 31. Pharmacokinetics of Phenothiazines and Related Compounds*

Representative Drug Classification	Metabolism	Dose Equivalent	Absorption	Extrapyramidal Signs	Sedation	Hypotension	Vd (L/kg)	$t_{1/2}$ (hr)
Aliphatic: Chlorpromazine (Thorazine)	Hepatic	100 mg	Rapid	Moderate	High	High	10–20	16–30
Piperidine: Thioridazine (Mellaril)	Hepatic	100 mg	Slow	Low	High	Moderate	3.5	9–10
Piperazine: Prochlorperazine (Compazine)	Hepatic	15 mg	Slow	Moderate	Moderate to low	Low	10–35	8–12
Butyrophenone: Haloperidol (Haldol)	Hepatic	2–15 mg	Rapid	High	Low	Low	20–30	12–22
Thioxanthine: Thiothixene (Navane)	Hepatic	2 mg	N/A	High	Low	Low	N/A	34
Dibenzorazepine: Loxapine (Loxitane)	Hepatic	5 mg	Rapid	High	Low	Low	N/A	3–4
Dihydroindolones: Molindone (Moban)	Hepatic	10 mg	Rapid	High	Low	Low	N/A	1.5

*Peak levels occur 1 to 2 hours post ingestion, and they have enterohepatic recirculation.
N/A = not available
Acute fatal dose 15 to 150 mg/kg; reported lethal in oral dose as low as 350 mg in 4-year-old child and 2 gm in adult female.

adrenergic blockade producing severe hypotension. (4) CNS stimulation or sedation. Lowers convulsive threshold, causes neurotransmitter imbalance to produce dystonic reactions. **Idiosyncratic dystonic reaction:**. May occur at therapeutic levels. It begins 5 to 30 hours after start of medication and consists of opisthotonos, torticollis, orolingual dyskinesia, akathisia, and oculogyric crisis (painful upward gaze). **Malignant neuroleptic syndrome:** Characterized by hyperthermia, muscle rigidity, autonomic dysfunction.

Management. (1) GI decontamination. If symptoms are already present, some of these agents have antiemetic action, so lavage may be required. (2) Monitor ECG for dysrhythmias and treat with antidysrhythmic agents. (3) Hypotension is treated with positioning and fluid. Vasopressors are used if these fail. **Avoid** beta-adrenergic agents because of danger of provoking dysrhythmias. If a pressor agent is needed, use norepinephrine. **Avoid** dopamine (Intropin) because PTZ drugs are antidopaminogenic. (4) Physostigmine is used only as a last resort for life-threatening anticholinergic symptoms. (5) Treat hypo- or hyperthermia with external physical measures (not antipyretic drugs). (6) Idiosyncratic dystonic reaction can be treated with diphenhydramine (Benadryl) (antidote 18) or benztropine (Cogentin), 1 to 2 mg intravenously slowly in adolescents. These drugs should be continued orally for 2 to 3 days. This is not the treatment of overdose, only of this reaction. (7) The malignant neuroleptic syndrome may be treated with dantrolene sodium or dopamine agonists bromcriptine mesylate or amantadine.

Laboratory. Two drops of 10 per cent ferric chloride to 1 ml of boiled urine may produce a purple color if there is a sufficient blood level. Nonphenothiazine neuroleptics give a negative test. Salicylates are excluded if concentrated sulfuric acid causes blanching of the color.

Pine Oil. Pine Sol (19.9 per cent pine oil) is the most common ingested household cleaner that results in hospitalizations.

Toxicity. Death from ingestion of 15 ml of 100 per cent solution in a child, although pine oil is alleged to be one fifth as toxic as turpentine.

Manifestations. (1) GI—odor of violets on the breath, irritation, and occasionally hematemesis. (2) CNS—depression, weakness, lethargy, and respiratory depression. (3) Renal—anuria.

Management. (1) Referral to a medical facility for supervised GI decontamination by emesis and several hours observation is recommended in children who ingest 30 ml or more of a 20 per cent solution. More concentrated solutions should be referred for proportionately smaller amounts. (2) Supportive care.

Plants. See Table 32.

Propranolol and Beta-Blockers (Table 33). Antihypertensive, antianginal, antiglaucoma, antimigraine.

Toxicity. Over 1 mg/kg of ingested propranolol or a single adult dose may be toxic in a small child, and more than the maximum daily dose (propranolol 480 mg) in an adolescent.

Toxicokinetics. Elimination is hepatic for lipophilic agents and renal for hydrophilic agents. Duration is 24 to 48 hours; however, long half-lives prolong toxicity.

Manifestations. Bradycardia, hypotension, bronchospasm, apnea, convulsions. Hypoglycemia may occur in children. Fat-soluble drugs have more CNS effects. Partial agonists may produce tachycardia and hypertension (pindolol).

Management. (1) GI decontamination with activated charcoal. **Avoid** emesis because of apnea and seizures. (2) Treat hypoglycemia, hyperkalemia, convulsions. (3) Monitor ECG for cardiovascular manifestations. If they develop, glucagon reverses the negative inotropic effects more effectively than the chronotropic effects (antidote 22). (a) Bradycardia: If unstable or second- or third-degree AV block, use glucagon. If no response, use atropine. **Caution:** Isoproterenol may increase hypotension. A pacemaker may be required if bradycardia is not easily managed by medication. (b) For ventricular tachycardia or serious premature ventricular contractions, use lidocaine or phenytoin. Cardioversion if patient is unstable. (c) Myocardial depression and hypotension: correct dysrhythmias, positioning and fluids. May require hemodynamic monitoring. **Avoid** quinidine, procainamide, and disopyramide (Norpace). (4) For bronchospasm, administer aminophylline. (5) Hemodialysis or hemoperfusion may be considered for unresponsive water-soluble agents, particularly if there is evidence of renal failure. There is limited documentation of effectiveness.

Quinidine and Quinine. Antidysrhythmic and antimalarial agents.

Toxicity. Child—greater than 60 mg/kg; adult—2 to 8 gm.

Kinetics. The quinidine sulfate peak action is 2 to 4 hours, the polygalacturonate is 5 to 6 hours, and the gluconate is 3 to 4 hours. Sulfate half-life is 3 to 4 hours, and gluconate 8 to 12 hours. Elimination is hepatic.

Manifestations. (1) Cinchonism (headache, nausea, vomiting, tinnitus, deafness, diplopia, dilated pupils), confusion, dementia, psychosis, and blindness. (2) Myocardial depression and dysrhythmias. (3) Skin rashes and flushing. Hemolysis may occur in G-6-PD deficiency patients. (4) Respiratory depression, convulsions, coma, acidosis, and hypoglycemia.

Management. (1) GI decontamination with repeated doses of activated charcoal. (2) Monitor ECG. May need antidysrhythmic drugs, pacemaker, and alkalinization. Glucagon may be useful but has not been evaluated. (3) Acid diuresis is not recommended.

Laboratory. Plasma quinidine over 8 μg/ml—cinchonism; over 14 μg/ml—cardiac toxicity.

Rodenticides. See Table 34.

Sedative-Hypnotics, Nonbarbiturate. See Table 35.

Management. Primarily supportive. **Avoid** emesis if rapid onset of convulsions, apnea, and coma. Concretions may form in the stomach and may require mechanical or surgical removal (meprobamate and glutethimide). Vasopressors may be preferable to large quantities of fluids when pulmonary edema is anticipated. Hemoperfusion or hemodialysis should be considered in severe intoxications failing to respond.

1. **Chloral Hydrate:** GI decontamination if ingested over 25 mg/kg or 1 gm in adults. **Avoid** emesis because

TABLE 32. Toxic Plant List*

Common Name/Latin Name	Toxic Class and Parts	Manifestations	Management
Akee (Blighia sapida)	Hypoglycin A: seed, unripe aril, rind	GI upset, hypoglycemia, acidosis biphasic course	S/S†, vigorous hypoglycemic therapy
Apple (Malus sylvestris) Apricot (Prunus armeniaca)	Cyanogenic seeds	See Cyanide	
Arum family Caladium (Coladium) Dumbcane (Diefenbacia) Elephant's Ear (Colocasia) Philodendrum (Philodendrum)	Oxalates: Insoluble, all parts	Mouth burning, GI upset, no systemic effects, airway obstruction	Rinse out mouth, cold pack to mouth
Atropa (Atropa belladonna)	Anticholinergic: all parts, especially black berries	See Anticholinergic Agents	
Autumn crocus (Colchicum atumnale)	Colchicine: all parts	GI upset, coma, convulsions, bone marrow depression	S/S, repeated doses of charcoal
Azalea (Rhododendron sp)	Grayanotoxin I: roots, leaves, honey from flower	GI upset, bradycardia, hypotension, paresthesias, ataxia, convulsions	S/S
Baneberry (Actea pachypoda)	Protoanemonin: all parts	Coumarin-like toxicity	See Anticoagulants
Black locust (Robina pseudoacacia)	Phylotoxin (Toxalbumin): seeds, shoots, bark	Delayed GI upset, 1–3 days, hemolysis, convulsions, renal failure	S/S, alkaline diuresis
Bleeding heart (Diecenta cucullaria)	Isoquinolone: all	Ataxia, convulsions	S/S
Bittersweet, European (Solanum duleanum)	Solanine: all	GI upset, bradycardia, diaphoresis, delayed anticholinergic	S/S
Buckeye (horsechestnut) (Aesculis sp)	Coumarin: nuts, twigs	See Anticoagulants	
Buttercup (Ranunculus)	See Baneberry		
Caladium (Caladium sp)	Oxalates: insoluble, all	See Arum family plants	
Castor bean (Ricinus communis)	Phylotoxin (Toxalbumin): bean	See Black locust plant	
Cassava bean (Manihot Esculenla)	Cyanogenic: bean	See Cyanide	
Cherry, wild (Prunus sp)	Cyanogenic	See Cyanide	
Chinaberry tree (Melia azedarach)	Neurotoxin: seeds, berries, bark, flowers	GI upset, hallucinations, paresis, seizures, CP arrest	S/S
Christmas rose (Helleborus niger)	Digitalis, saponins, protoanemonim: all parts	GI upset, cardiac toxicity, coumarin-like toxicity	S/S See Anticoagulants and Digitalis
Climbing lilly (Gloriosa superba)	Colchicine: bulb	See Autumn crocus plant	
Cocaine (Erythroxylon coca)	Cocaine alkaloid: leaves	See Cocaine	
Crowfoot	See Buttercup		
Daphne (Daphne mezereum)	Daphnetoxin, mezerein: all parts	GI upset, coumarin-like toxicity	See Anticoagulants
Death camas (Zygadenus venenosus)	Zygadenine: all parts	Burning in mouth, bradycardia, shock	S/S
Deadly nightshade (Atropa belladonna)	Anticholinergic: berry, leaves	See Anticholinergic Agents	
Dumbcane (Dieffenbachia sp)	Oxalates, insoluble: root, leaves	See Arum family plants	
Dutchman's breeches	Another name for bleeding heart		
Elderberry (Sambucus canadensis)	Cyanogenic: unripe berries, roots, leaves, bark	See Cyanide	
Elephant ear (Colocasia antiquorum)	Oxalates, insoluble: all parts	See Arum family plants	
English ivy (Hedera helix)	Hederin, saponin	Burning in throat, GI upset	S/S
Ergot (Clavipus purpura)	Ergot fungus on grains	GI upset, gangrene of limbs, convulsions, abortifacient	S/S, vasodilators, e.g., nitroprusside
False hellebore (Veratrum veride)	Veratrum: all parts	GI upset, hypotension, bradycardia, shock	S/S
Foxglove (Digitalis purpura)	Digitalis: all parts	See Digitalis	
Golden chain (Laburnum anagyrodes)	Nicotine: all parts	See Nicotine	
Green hellebore (Veratrum veride)	Veratrum	See False hellebore plant	
Heliotrope (Heliotropopum arborescens)	Pyrrolizidine: all parts	Hepatoxic, GI upset, onset delayed up to weeks (carcinogenic)	S/S
Hemlock, poison (Conium maculatum)	Coniune alkoids, nicotine-like: all parts	Resp. paralysis, GI distress, convulsions	S/S, intensive care

Table continued on following page

TABLE 32. Toxic Plant List* *Continued*

Common Name/Latin Name	Toxic Class and Parts	Manifestations	Management
Hemlock, water (Cicuta maculata)	Cicutoxin, strychnine-like: all parts	Convulsions	Anticonvulsants See *Rodenticides*
Henbane (Hyoscyanus niger)	Anticholinergic: all parts	See *Anticholingeric Agents*	
Holly Tree, bush (Ilex spp)	Ilicin: berries, leaves	GI upset	S/S
Horse nettle (Solanum carolinense)	Solanine	See *Bittersweet* plant	
Hyacinth (Hyacinth orientalis)	Narcissine: bulb	GI upset	S/S
Hydrangea (Hydrangea sp)	Cyanogenic: all parts	See *Cyanide*	
Indian tobacco (Lobelia inflata)	Lobeline	See *Nicotine*	S/S
Iris (Iris sp)	Irisin: all parts	GI upset	S/S
Ivy, English (Hedera helix)	See *English Ivy* plant		
Ivy, German (Senecio milinoides)	Pyrrolizdine: all parts	GI upset, hepatotoxic	S/S
Ivy, ground (Nepeta hederacea)	Essential oils: all parts	Mucous membrane irritants, CNS depression or CNS stimulation	S/S
Jack in the pulpit (Arisaema triphyllum)	Oxalates: fruit, leaves, root	See *Arum family* plant	S/S
Jequirity bean (Abrus precatorius)	Abric acid (Toxalbumins): all parts, especially seeds	See *Black locust* plant	S/S
Jimson weed (Datura stramonium)	Anticholinergic: all parts	See *Anticholinergic Agents*	
Jessamine, yellow (Gelseminum sempervirens)	Gelsemine, solanine: all parts	See *Bittersweet* plant. Gelsemine related to strychnine	
Jerusalem cherry (Solanum pseudocapsicum)	Solanine	See *Bittersweet* plant	
Lantana (Lantana camara)	Lantanine	GI upset, muscle weakness, shock	S/S
Larkspur (Delphinium)	Diterpenoid: leaves, seed	Onset in minutes, paralysis, bradycardia, seizures	S/S
Laurel, mountain (Kalmia latifolia)	Grayanotoxin I: all parts	See *Azalea* plant	
Lily of the valley (Convallaria majalis)	Digitalis: all parts	See *Digitalis*	
Lima beans (Phaseolus limensis)	Cyanogenic: raw bean	See *Cyanide*	
Marijuana (Cannabis sativa)	Cannabinol: all parts	See *Marijuana* in *Hallucinogens*	
Mayapple (Mandrake) (Podophyllum peltatum)	Podophyllum: leaves, stem, fruit	Severe GI upset, tachycardia, hypotension	S/S
Mistletoe (Phoradendron flavescens)	Unknown: all parts	Bradycardia, GI upset, shock, seizures	S/S
Monkshood (Aconite nappelus)	Aconite: all parts	Paralysis, cardiac dysrhythmias, ataxia, convulsions	S/S
Morning glory (Ipomea tricolor)	Unknown	See *LSD* in *Hallucinogens*	
Mountain laurel	See *Laurel, mountain*		
Nightshade, black (Solanum nigram)	Solanine	See *Bittersweet* plant	
Nightshade, climbing (Solanum dulcamara)	Solanine	See *Bittersweet* plant	
Nightshade, deadly	See *Deadly nightshade* plant		
Oleander (Nerium indicum)	Digitalis	See *Digitalis*	
Peach, pear tree (Prunus persica)	Cyanogenic: pit, leaves, sap	See *Cyanide*	
Pennyroyal oil (Mentha pulegium)	Essential oil, pyrrolizidine	Shock, seizures, hepatotoxic, abortifacient	S/S
Philodendron (Philodendrum spp)	Oxalates, insoluble: all parts	See *Arum family* plant	
Poinsettia (Euphorbia pulcherrima)	All parts	Nontoxic unless very large amounts ingested, GI upset	
Pokeweed (Phytolacca americana)	Saponin, phytolacine: roots, berries, leaves	Severe gastroenteritis	S/S
Potato (Solanum tuberosum)	Solanine: sprouts, green tubers, vines	See *Bittersweet* plant	
Privet hedge (Ligustrum sp)	Andromedotoxin: seeds, berries, leaves	GI upset	S/S
Rhododendron (Rhododendron spp)	Grayanotoxin I: leaves, honey from flowers	See *Azalea* plant	
Rhubarb (Rheum rhaponticum)	Oxalates, soluble: leaves, root, stem if eaten raw	Tetany, renal damage, seizures	S/S, calcium
Rosary pea (Abrus precatorius)	Abric acid (Toxalbumins): seeds, stems, leaves	See *Black locust* plant	
Skunk cabbage (Veratrum californicum)	Oxalates, insoluble	See *Arum family* plant	

TABLE 32. Toxic Plant List* Continued

Common Name/Latin Name	Toxic Class and Parts	Manifestations	Management
Star of Bethlehem (Ornithogalum umbellattum)	Digitalis	See *Digitalis*	
Sweet pea (Lathyrus odoratus)	Curare-like	Weakness, paralysis	S/S
Taxus (Taxus sp)	Taxine alkaloid: all except red aril	GI upset, bradycardia, hypotension	S/S
Thornberry (Datura stramonium)	Anticholinergic: all parts	See *Anticholinergic Agents*	
Tobacco (Nicotiana sp)	Nicotinic: all parts	See *Nicotine*	
Tomato (Lycopersicum esculentum)	Solanine: stem, leaves, green fruit	See *Bittersweet* plant	
Wandering Jew (Tradescantia sp)	All parts	Rash, blisters	S/S
Water hemlock	See *Hemlock, water*		
Wisteria (Wisteria sp)	Unknown: seeds, pods, leaves	GI upset (severe)	S/S
Yew (Taxus sp)	See *Taxus*		

*Note: All victims who ingest plants should be observed for airway obstruction. Morbidity and mortality are low from most plant ingestions. The most severe manifestations are generally listed for these plants.
†S/S = Symptomatic and supportive care.
Key: Names of plants are listed alphabetically.

TABLE 33. Pharmacokinetics of Beta-Adrenergic Blockers

Agent	Solubility	$T_{1/2}$ (hr)	Peak (hr)	Elimination	Specificity	Dose	Maximum Daily Dose
Atenolol (Tenormin)	Water	6–9	6–9	Renal	Beta-1	50 mg	200 mg
Labetalol (Normodyne)	Water	3–6		Hepatic	Alpha and beta	400 mg	1–2 gm
Metoprolol (Lopressor)	Fat	3–4		Hepatic	Beta-1	50 mg	450 mg
Nadolol (Corgard)	Water	17–23	3–4	Renal	Beta-1	40 mg	320 mg
Oxprenolol (Traiscor)	Fat	1.5–3	1–2	Hepatic	0	80 mg	480 mg
Pindolol (Visken)	Fat	3–4	1¼	Hepatic	Partial agonist	20 mg	60 mg
Propranolol (Inderal)	Fat	2–3	1½	Hepatic	0	40 mg	480 mg
Timolol (Blocadren)	Fat	3	3	Hepatic	0	20 mg	60 mg

TABLE 34. Toxicity of Rodenticides

Agent	Mechanism of Action	Manifestations	Onset	Management
Highly toxic LD_{50} less than 50 mg/kg				
Thallium PFD 12 mg/kg Gizmo Rat Killer	Combines with —SH groups. Interferes with oxidative phosphorylation	GI upset, alopecia, neuropathy, delirium, convulsions	12–24 hr delayed	Oral Prussian blue, hemoperfusion
Strychnine PFD 5 mg/kg El ROY Mouse Bait	Interferes with glycine inhibition of CNS	Convulsions	10–20 min	Anticonvulsants, neuromuscular blockers
ZN phosphide PFD 40 mg/kg Field Rat Powder	Releases phosphine gas	Fish breath odor, black vomitus, cardiac pulmonary edema, hepatorenal damage	2–3 hr	Milk, avoid water lavage
Yellow phosphorus PFD 1 mg/kg Yellow, waxy Blue Death Rat Killer	Local burns, hepatorenal damage	Garlic odor, luminescent vomitus and stools, cardiac toxicity, coma, "smoking stool syndrome"	1–2 hr	GI decontamination, anticonvulsants

TABLE 35. Toxicity and Kinetics of Nonbarbiturate Sedative-Hypnotics

Drug	Absorption Toxic dose (TD) Fatal dose (FD)	Peak (hr)	Vd (L/kg)	Elimination Route	$T_{1/2}$ (hr)	Toxic Blood Concentration (μg/mL)	Comments*
Chloral hydrate (Noctec) Therapeutic dose: 8 mg/kg child, 250 mg adult Onset 30–60 min	Rapid TD 2 gm FD 4–10 gm	1–2	0.6	Hepatic; active toxic trichloroethanol (TCE) metabolite	8–12	100 (TCE 80)	Pear-like odor, ventricular dysrhythmias, hepatotoxic, GI irritant, radiopaque capsules
Ethchlorvynol (Placidyl) Onset 15–30 min	Rapid TD 2.5 gm FD 5.0 gm	2–4	3–4	Hepatic 90%; lung elimination gives vinyl odor to breath	10–25 >100 in overdose	20–80	Prolonged coma (up to 200 hr), apnea, hypothermia, pulmonary edema, pink gastric contents, odor of vinyl shower curtain
Glutethimide (Doriden)	Slow TD 5 gm FD 10 gm or 150 mg/kg	6	10–12	Hepatic; active toxic 4-hydroxyglutanimide metabolite (?)	10	20–80	Prolonged coma cyclic (up to 120 hr), apnea, convulsions, anticholinergic signs, hyperthermia, coma
Meprobamate (Equanil, Miltown)	Rapid TD 10 gm FD 12–40 gm	4–8	10	Hepatic	6–16	30–100	Coma, convulsions, pulmonary edema, apnea, gastric concretions
Methaqualone (Quaaludes, "love drug")	Rapid TD 0.8 gm	1–3	6	Hepatic	10–40	8–10	Hypertonia, hyperreflexia convulsions, apnea, bleeding tendency
Methyprylon (Noludar)	Rapid TD 3 gm FD 8–20 gm	2–4	1–2	Hepatic	3–6	30	Hyperactive coma (up to 30 hr), miosis, persistent hypotension, pulmonary edema, rare mortality

*Comments include other features besides the typical manifestations of all these agents: respiratory depression, hypotension, hypothermia (except glutethimide hyperthermia), psychological and physiologic withdrawal.

of rapid onset. Activated charcoal/cathartic. Insert gastric tubes with caution because of corrosive action. **Avoid** use of catecholamines that may produce dysrhythmias. Hemodialysis and charcoal hemoperfusion may effectively remove the chloral hydrate and its metabolite in patients who fail to respond and have fatal plasma value 250 μg/ml or greater. Toxic level is 100 μg/ml.

2. **Ethchlorvynol:** GI decontamination up to 12 hours post ingestion. **Avoid** emesis induction because of rapid onset. Has a biphasic course as it redistributes from fat stores. Resin hemoperfusion (Amberlite XAD-4) is the method of extracorporeal removal when other measures fail in a life-threatening situation with ingestion of over 10 gm or 100 mg/kg, and plasma level over 100 μg/ml in the first 12 hours or 70 μg/ml after 12 hours. Toxic plasma level is 20 μg/ml or greater.

3. **Glutethimide:** Highest mortality of all nonbarbiturate sedative hypnotics. GI decontamination up to 24 hours post ingestion but **avoid** emesis because of seizures, apnea, and coma. Repeated doses of activated charcoal may be useful for enterohepatic recirculation. Has a biphasic course, as it redistributes from the fat stores. Resin hemoperfusion removal in life-threatening protracted coma when the patient has ingested over 5 to 10 gm and has a plasma level of over 30 μg/ml. Treat hyperthermia with external cooling.

4. **Meprobamate:** GI decontamination up to 12 hours post ingestion. Failure to respond to supportive therapy, prolonged coma with life-threatening complications, or blood concentrations greater than 100 μg/ml require consideration of extracorporeal removal with charcoal hemoperfusion. Toxic blood level is 5 to 30 μg/ml, levels over 200 μg/ml have more fatalities than survivals.

5. **Methaqualone:** This is no longer manufactured in the United States but is imported. GI decontamination. Forced diuresis, dialysis, and hemoperfusion are not indicated.

6. **Methyprylon:** GI decontamination. The hypotension usually does not respond to position or fluids alone and may require treatment of the hypotension with norepinephrine. This is a dialyzable drug, but usually dialysis is not necessary. Ingestions of greater than 6 gm or blood levels greater than 30 to 60 μg/ml have been associated with serious intoxications.

Stimulants. See *Sympathomimetics.*

Sulfonylurea Agents. These are oral hypoglycemic agents.

Toxicity. Hypoglycemia may occur with therapeutic doses.

Kinetics. Chlorpropamide has the longest half-life and is most commonly reported in accidental and suicidal hypoglycemia.

Mechanism. Stimulates the release of insulin.

Manifestations. Alteration in consciousness, seizures and coma, gastrointestinal upset, inappropriate secretion of antidiuretic hormone (chlorpropamide and tolbutamide). The hypoglycemia may persist for several days, particularly with chlorpropamide.

Management. (1) GI decontamination with repeated doses of activated charcoal has reduced the $t_{1/2}$ of chlorpropamide. (2) If the hypoglycemia is severe or the patient is unconscious, immediately obtain blood for glucose analysis and administer an intravenous bolus of glucose 1.0 ml/kg 25 per cent to a child and 1.0 ml/kg 50 per cent to adolescents. Also start an intravenous infusion of 10 per cent glucose and administer at a sufficient rate (10 mg/kg/min or 0.1 ml/kg/min of 10 per cent), with adjustments made to maintain a blood glucose over 100 mg/dl. The infusion should not be stopped abruptly because of rebound hypoglycemia. Potassium should be administered if there is likelihood of long-term infusion. The symptoms are usually easily reversed unless postictal depression is present. (3) Glucagon is of limited value. (4) Diazoxide in severe hyperinsulinemia 3 to 20 mg/kg/day up to 300 mg in two divided doses orally (Proglycem); the intravenous use is investigational. Corticosteroids have no immediate effect. (5) Alkalinization of the urine with sodium bicarbonate reduces the $t_{1/2}$ of chlorpropamide. (6) Monitor until the blood glucose has been normal for 24 hours on oral intake. Delayed, prolonged, and relapsing manifestations may occur even after apparent recovery.

Laboratory. Glucose reagent strips are inaccurate at low blood glucose concentrations.

Sympathomimetics. Includes the amphetamines, adrenergic beta-agonists (isoethraine, metaproterenol, terbutaline, albuterol), catecholamines, cocaine, ephedrine, phenylpropanolamine (PPA) (Table 36).

Manifestations. Nausea, vomiting, hypertension, pallor, tachycardia (initially PPA produces a reflex bradycardia), dysrhythmias, CNS excitation, tremors, convulsions, and coma. Toxic psychosis, anginal pain,

myocardial infarction, rhabdomyolysis, and intracranial hemorrhage have been reported sequelae with PPA.

Management. (1) GI decontamination for single ingestions of 17.5 mg/kg of PPA in children or if 10 mg/kg are ingested combined with caffeine and ephedrine, or greater than 150 mg in adolescents. Control agitation and seizures with diazepam. (2) Dysrhythmias are treated with appropriate antidysrhythmic agent. (3) Hypertensive crisis with nitroprusside intravenously. (4) Acid diuresis is not recommended.

Theophylline. Theophylline (1,3 dimethylxanthine) is widely used to relieve bronchospasm in asthma and is frequently involved in iatrogenic overdose.

Toxicity. Approximately 1 mg/kg of theophylline increases serum theophylline 2 µg/ml.

Kinetics. Peak levels occur within 1 hour after ingestion of liquid preparations, 1 to 3 hours after regular tablets, and 3 to 10 hours after slow-release preparations. $T_{1/2}$: 3.5 hours average in a child and 4.5 hours in an adolescent (3 to 9 hours). In neonates and young infants the $t_{1/2}$ is much longer. Overdose increases the $t_{1/2}$. Elimination is hepatic.

Manifestations (Table 37). Acute toxicity generally correlates with blood levels; chronic toxicity does not. Metabolic disturbances: dehydration, metabolic acidosis, respiratory alkalosis, hypokalemia (diuretic action), hypophosphatemia, hypocalcemia, hyperglycemia, elevation of amylase and uric acid, rhabdomyolysis, and myoglobinuria. Differences in slow-release preparations from regular preparations: few or no GI symptoms with high levels; peak concentration times may be 10 to 24 hours post ingestion; and onset of seizures may occur 10 to 12 hours post ingestion.

Management. Chronic intoxication is more serious and difficult to treat. (1) GI decontamination in acute overdose, up to 4 hours with regular preparations and up to 8 to 12 hours with slow-release preparations. Test aspirate or vomitus for blood. Give activated charcoal initially with a cathartic, then every 4 hours until serum

TABLE 36. Sympathomimetics: Kinetics and Actions

	Therapeutic Dose (mg)	Toxic Dose (mg)	Onset (min)	Duration (hr)	$T_{1/2}$ (hr)	Elimination Route
Phenylpropanolamine (diet and decongestant over-the-counter drugs) (PPA)						
	37.5	>85 15 mg/kg	15–60	3	3–6	Renal
Ephedrine	30	>60	15–30	4–8	3–6	Renal
Pseudoephedrine (Sudafed)	60	180	15–30	4–8	7	Renal
Terbutaline (Brethine, Bricanyl)						
Oral	2.5–5.0		30–60	4–8	3	Hepatic
Metered	0.2/puff		5–10	5		
Metaproterenol (Alupent, Metaprel)						
Oral	10–20		15–30	4		Hepatic
Metered	0.65/puff		1–5	3		
Albuterol (Proventil, Ventolin)						
Oral	2–4		30	6–8	6.5	Hepatic
Metered	0.65/puff			4–6		
Caffeine	100/cup	500–1000	15–30	3–4	3–10	Hepatic
Phenylephrine (NeoSynephrine)	15	60 mg	1–5	3–6		
Naphazoline (Privine)			1–5	3–6		
Oxymetazoline (Afrin)			1–5	6–12		
Tetrahydrozoline (Tyzine)			1–5	3–6		
Xylometazoline (Otrivin)			1–5	6–12		

TABLE 37. Theophylline Toxicity

Plasma Concentration (μg/ml)	Toxicity	Manifestations
10 to 20	Mild	Therapeutic range, nausea, vomiting, insomnia, nervousness, and irritability.
20 to 40	Moderate	Gastrointestinal complaints and CNS stimulation, agitation, restless, and convulsions. Transient hypertension, hyperthermia, tachypnea.
Over 50	Severe	Convulsions and dysrhythmias may occur at lower levels and without GI symptoms. Children tolerate higher serum levels.

TABLE 38. Factors That Increase Serum Theophylline

Age and Disease	Medication, Substances
Under 6 months	Macrolid antimicrobials, e.g., erythromycin
Over 60 years	
Liver disease, heart failure	Oral contraceptives
Viral infections with respiratory syncytial virus	Cimetidine
	Beta-blockers
Pneumonia	Carbamazepine
Sustained fever	Caffeine

theophylline is less than 20 μg/ml. **Avoid** inducing emesis (interferes with charcoal administration). If intractable vomiting occurs, use antiemetic droperidol, 2.5 mg IV every 6 to 8 hours for two doses (may cause extrapyramidal symptoms), or ranitidine 50 mg IV (never cimetidine). (2) Obtain theophylline levels every 4 hours until below 20 μg/ml. (3) Control seizures with diazepam. (4) Dysrhythmias are treated by appropriate antidysrhythmic agents but **avoid** nonselective beta-blockers in asthmatic patients because of bronchospasm (e.g., propranolol). (5) Treat hypotension with positioning and fluids and, if necessary, vasopressors. Correct fluid and metabolic disturbances. (6) Massive hematemesis is managed with iced saline lavage and blood replacement if needed. (7) Charcoal hemoperfusion is the management of choice in life-threatening convulsions, dysrhythmias, hematemesis, or intractable vomiting refractory to conventional antiemetic measures, so activated charcoal cannot be retained. It is recommended for acute intoxications with serum theophylline concentrations greater than 100 μg/ml and chronic intoxications over 60 μg/ml, especially if factors are present that increase theophylline concentrations (Table 38).

Thyroid

Toxicity. See Table 39.
Kinetics. Elimination is hepatic.
Manifestations. (1) CNS stimulation—fever, agitation, irritability, insomnia, convulsions. (2) Adrenergic—tachycardia, hypertension, cardiac dysrhythmias. (3) Nonspecific—vomiting, diarrhea, abdominal pain, flushing, fever. (4) Symptoms may last 2 weeks or longer.

Management (Table 39). (1) Repeated doses of activated charcoal may be useful for large ingestions or if symptoms occur because of enterohepatic recirculation. (2) Hyperactivity and insomnia: treat with mild sedative. (3) Beta-blocker propranolol interferes with T_4 to T_3 conversion: 0.5 to 1 mg/kg/24 hr oral and increase to control adverse manifestations up to 2 mg/kg/24 hr. Adolescent dose is 40 to 160 mg/24 hr. (4) Control hyperthermia with external cooling.

Laboratory. T_4 at 6 hours post ingestion greater than 12 μg/ml suggests daily assessment for 10 days. The T_3 may not rise for 2 to 3 days.

Tricyclic and Cyclic Antidepressants (TCAD). TCAD cause the greatest number of deaths in overdose.

Toxicity. The toxic dose of imipramine is 10 mg/kg in a child, and in adults as little as 500 to 750 mg has been fatal. The dosages of imipramine in Table 40 may serve as a guide to the degree of toxicity, although the amount ingested correlates poorly with toxicity.

Kinetics. The onset varies from less than 1 hour to 6 hours after ingestion. Protein binding is high and decreases with decreasing pH. The $t_{1/2}$ varies from 10 hours for imipramine to 100 hours for nortriptyline. In an overdose, the $t_{1/2}$ may be much longer. Elimination is hepatic to active secondary amine metabolites, then hydroxylation over a period of days to give rise to inactive metabolites.

Manifestations. Onset rarely after 24 hours, but sudden death has infrequently been reported up to 6 days post ingestion. The phases of intoxication are the following: (1) Initially effects are anticholinergic: dry mouth, mydriasis, ataxia, increased deep tendon reflexes, hyperthermia, and tachycardia; CNS effects occur early, and seizures occur in 20 per cent, often just before cardiac arrest. (2) Coma with hypertension, tachycardia above 160, mydriasis, and supraventricular tachycardia. (3) Coma with hypotension, heart rate under 120, respiratory depression, tonic-clonic seizures, and ventricular

TABLE 39. Management of Children Ingesting Thyroid Preparations

Amount	Management
Levothyroxine (T_4 thyroxine)	
<2 mg	Home observation
2–4 mg	Emesis, home observation, follow-up contact for 10 days
>4 mg	Emesis, activated charcoal, cathartic; follow-up visits for 10 days, thyroid tests
Triiodothyronine (T_3), any amount	Emesis, activated charcoal, cathartic; hospitalize and monitor for 24 hrs
Dessicated thyroid <600 mg	Emesis, activated charcoal, cathartic; follow-up contact for 10 days

TABLE 40. Imipramine Toxicity

Amount Ingested (mg/kg)	Manifestations
10	Light coma, mydriasis, and tachycardia
20	dysrhythmias, respiratory depression, convulsions, usually survive
30	Fatalities may result
50	High mortality rate
Over 70	Rarely survive

dysrhythmias. Some studies have shown that ECG with QRS greater than 0.1 sec is associated with a major overdose and seizures and greater than 0.16 sec is associated with life-threatening dysrhythmias and seizures. The newer cyclic antidepressants such as amoxapine (Ascendin) allegedly have less cardiotoxicity. However, overdose with this agent causes the syndrome of seizures, rhabdomyolysis, and renal tubular necrosis. Maprotiline (Ludiomil), a tetracyclic, has similar cardiotoxicity to tricyclics. Trazodone (Desyrel) may have less toxicity, although orthostatic hypotension, vertigo, and priapism have been reported.

Management. (1) In significant ingestions intensive care should be continued until patients are asymptomatic and there are no ECG abnormalities for at least 24 hours, although some studies suggest that 6 hours postingestion monitoring may be sufficient. (2) GI decontamination. **Avoid** emesis because of the rapid onset convulsions and cardiotoxicity. Gastric lavage should be carried out with caution and after correction of any dysrhythmia. Intact pills have been recovered up to 18 hours. Activated charcoal is recommended initially with a cathartic and repeated every 4 to 6 hours. (3) At risk are the elderly, children, patients with pre-existing heart disease, or patients showing sinus tachycardia or any other sign of overdose. Any potential pediatric overdose should be examined, observed, and monitored for 24 hours. (4) ECG monitoring with the QRS measured periodically on a 12-lead print-out. (5) Control convulsions with intravenous diazepam and phenytoin. (6) Physostigmine is not recommended. (7) Cardiovascular effects (dysrhythmias, blocks, and hypotension) usually begin within 6 hours and are rare after 24 hours. They should be treated with alkalinization by sodium bicarbonate (antidote 35) over 10 to 15 minutes or by hyperventilation or both to a blood pH of 7.5. Alkalinization is believed to increase the protein binding of the cyclic antidepressants, and the sodium ion may inhibit TCAD effect on the rapid sodium channel. Specific management of cardiovascular complications: **Avoid** type Ia antidysrhythmics (procainamide, quinidine, disopyramide), beta-adrenergic blockers, and physostig-

mine. (a) Hypotension that fails to respond to positioning, intravenous fluids, and alkalinization has significant mortality. It should be treated with norepinephrine. If it fails, inotropic agents such as dobutamine may be tried. Hypertension may occur early and usually should not be treated. (b) Bradydysrhythmias and serious conduction defects are managed with phenytoin, which improves conduction; however, phenytoin's usefulness requires further confirmation. A temporary transvenous pacemaker may be used in unresponsive second- and third-degree heart block. **Avoid** atropine. (c) Ventricular tachycardia may require synchronized cardioversion if alkalinization, lidocaine (for one dose only), or phenytoin fails or if the patient is unstable. (d) Supraventricular tachycardia (SVT) with hemodynamic instability (shock, ischemic chest pain, hypotension, or pulmonary edema) requires immediate synchronized cardioversion, 0.25 to 1.0 watt-sec/kg, after sedation. (e) Torsades de pointes is treated with isoproterenol, lidocaine, phenytoin, and atrial or ventricular overdrive pacing to shorten the QT interval. (8) The serum potassium should be followed because the alkalinization may aggravate or precipitate hypokalemia. (9) Dialysis and hemoperfusion are not recommended.

Laboratory. A blood level of 500 ng/ml is usually associated with toxic symptoms, and 1000 ng/ml or greater is generally associated with serious toxicity and a QRS interval usually greater than 100 msec.

Vitamin Ingestions and Intoxications. The toxicity is largely due to their iron content, which in chewable children's vitamins does not usually constitute a risk. Water-soluble vitamins are readily excreted by the kidneys, but fat-soluble vitamins are stored and are more likely to cause toxicity when taken in excess. The excessive doses are usually ten times the daily recommended allowance (Tables 41 and 42). In general, vitamins B, E, C, and K and minerals can be considered benign.

Management. (1) GI decontamination by emesis if over 50 to 100 chewable children's multivitamins were consumed. The fillers and the sugars in the vitamins act as a cathartic. (2) Vitamin D: Severe hypercalcemia can develop. Low calcium diet, salmon calcitonin, prednisolone, mithramycin, and saline infusions are used. Monitor fluids, serum calcium, and ECG. Treat cardiac arrhythmias. Use dialysis if renal failure occurs. (3) Hypervitaminosis A producing increased intracranial pressure may require treatment with mannitol and dexamethasone. (4) Niacin overdose should be monitored for hypotension, which may require positioning and rarely fluids. Usually the symptoms resolve spontaneously in a few hours. (5) Discontinue vitamins, since they are stored in the body.

TABLE 41. Recommended Daily Allowances of Vitamins and Minerals

	Infants 0–12 mo	Children <4 years	Children >4 years and Adults	Pregnant and Lactating
Vitamin A (IU)	1500	2500	5000	8000
Vitamin D (IU)	400	400	400	400
Vitamin E (IU)	5	10	30	30
Vitamin C (mg)	35	40	60	60
Folic acid (mg)	0.1	0.2	0.4	0.8

TABLE 42. Toxic Doses of Vitamins

Vitamin	Dosage	Manifestations
Vitamin A	Acute: >12,000 IU/kg child; 1.5 million IU units adult	Increased intracranial pressure in 8–12 hr, desquamation of skin, hepatosplenomegaly, stomatitis, bone pain in few days
	Chronic: >10,000 IU for months child; >25,000 IU for 8 months adult	Increased intracranial pressure, bone pain, alopecia, hyperostosis, hypercalcemia, edema of lower limbs. orange discoloration of skin
Vitamin D	10,000 IU for 4 months or 200,000 IU for 2 weeks, child; 60,000 IU for weeks to months adult	Hypercalcemia, muscle weakness, apathy, nausea, vomiting, diarrhea, bone pain, ectopic calcification, polyuria, hypertension, renal failure, nephrocalcinosis, cardiac dysrhythmias
Vitamin E	300–800 IU/day adult	Muscle weakness, headache, nausea, intestinal cramps, large doses antagonize vitamin K, hypertension; intravenous preparation— death in premature newborns
Niacin	100 mg adult	Flushing, burning of the face and upper trunk; 3 gm increases uric acid and blood glucose and may produce hepatic damage

TABLE 43. Regional Poison Control Centers in the United States*

State	Name	Phone Number
Alabama	Alabama	800–462–0800; 205–345–0600
	Children's Hospital	800–292–6678; 205–939–9201
Arizona	Arizona (Tucson)	602–626–6016
	Samaritan (Phoenix)	602–253–3334
California	Los Angeles County	213–484–5151
	San Diego	800–576–4766; 619–543–6000
	San Francisco	800–523–2222; 415–476–6600
	Univ. Calif Sacramento	800–342–9293; 916–453–3692
Colorado	Rocky Mountain	800–332–3073; 303–629–1123
District of Columbia	National Capital	202–625–3333
Florida	Tampa Bay	800–282–3171; 813–253–4444
Georgia	Georgia	800–282–5846; 404–589–4400
Kentucky	Kosair Children's Hosp	800–722–5725; 502–589–8222
Louisiana	Louisiana	800–535–0525; 318–425–1524
Maryland	Maryland	800–492–2414; 301–528–7701
Massachusetts	Massachusetts	800–682–9211; 617–232–2120
Michigan	Blodgett	800–632–2727; 616–774–7851
	Children's Hosp	800–462–6642; 313–745–5711
Minnesota	Hennepin	612–347–3141
	Minnesota	800–222–1222; 612–221–2113
Missouri	Cardinal Glennon Children's Hosp	800–392–9111; 314–772–8300
Nebraska	Mid Plains	800–642–9999; 402–390–5400
New Jersey	New Jersey	800–962–1253; 201–923–0764
New Mexico	New Mexico	800–432–6866; 505–843–2551
New York	Long Island	516–542–2323
	New York City	212–340–4494
North Carolina	Duke Univ.	800–672–1697; 919–681–4574
Ohio	Central	800–682–7625; 614–228–1323
	Southwest	800–872–5111; 513–538–5111
Oregon	Oregon	800–452–7165; 503–279–8968
Pennsylvania	Delaware Valley	215–386–2100
	Pittsburgh	412–681–6669
Rhode Island	Rhode Island	401–277–5727
Texas	North Texas	800–441–0040; 214–590–5000
	Texas State Houston	800–392–8548; 713–654–1701
	Austin	800–392–8548; 409–765–1420
Utah	Intermountain	800–662–0062; 801–581–2151
West Virginia	West Virginia	800–642–3625; 304–348–4211

*List of centers obtained from American Association of Poison Control Centers.

SALICYLATE POISONING

HOWARD C. MOFENSON, M.D.,
and THOMAS R. CARACCIO, PHARM. D.

Salicylates are nonsteroidal anti-inflammatory agents with analgesic and antipyretic properties. Methylsalicylate is used topically. They are available as regular-acting and slow-release tablets (65 to 650 mg), chewable tablets (81 mg), regular and enteric-coated capsules (325 to 800 mg), and suppositories (60 to 1200 mg). Oil of wintergreen liniment is 98 to 99 per cent methylsalicylate. Diflunisal is a salicylic acid derivative that is not metabolized to salicylic acid.

Types of salicylates are acetylsalicylic acid (e.g., ASA, aspirin), choline magnesium tricyclicate (e.g., Arthropan), magnesium salicylate (e.g., Mobidin), methyl salicylate (oil of wintergreen), salsalate (e.g., Disalcid), and salicylic acid (e.g., SA, Mediplast).

TOXICITY

See Table 1. The usual analgesic and antipyretic dose of ASA for adults is 650 mg, for children 10 to 15 mg/kg. The maximum single dose is 1 gm, and the maximum daily dose is 4.0 gm. Single doses are not anti-inflammatory. The effect is achieved when plasma concentrations are 150 to 250 μg/ml (15 to 25 mg/dl). The toxic single amount of ASA for adults is usually over 10 gm, and for children over 150 mg/kg, or approximately two 81-mg tablets per kilogram or one half of a 325 mg tablet per kilogram.

Methyl salicylate 98 to 99 per cent (oil of wintergreen): 1 ml equals 1.4 gm of salicylate and one 5-ml teaspoonful equals 7 gm of salicylate, or 21.5 adult aspirins.

Acetylsalicylic acid, unlike other nonsteroidal anti-inflammatory agents, produces irreversible interference with platelet function lasting the life of the cell (8 to 11 days). Salicylates without the acetyl group have no antiplatelet effect.

Chronic intoxication, because of cumulative kinetics, occurs when more than 100 mg/kg have been administered for 2 to 3 days.

KINETICS

The oral absorption of regular ASA is complete and rapid in therapeutic doses (except in patients with Kawasaki disease). In overdose, absorption may be delayed because large amounts interfere with gastric emptying, cause possible pylorospasm, and may form concretions. Absorption of enteric-coated tablets is delayed and incomplete. Absorption of suppositories is slow and erratic. Methylsalicylate, which is highly viscous, may have absorption delayed for 6 to 8 hours.

The onset of action post ingestion is 30 minutes, with peak in 60 to 120 minutes and duration of 4 to 6 hours. ASA is a weak acid with a Pka of 3.5. Plasma concentration is significant in 30 minutes and peaks in 1 to 2 hours but may be delayed 6 hours or more in overdose and with enteric-coated preparations.

The apparent volume of distribution (Vd) is 0.15 to 0.2 l/kg for ASA and 0.13 L/kg for salicylic acid (SA). The spinal fluid (CSF) concentrations may reach 1.5 times the blood concentrations. The lower the blood pH, the higher the CSF concentration. The protein binding is 80 to 90 per cent. In toxic concentrations, the Vd may be 0.6 L/kg owing to decreased protein binding.

Acetylsalicylic acid is rapidly deacetylated to salicylic acid, an active metabolite. Salicylate is metabolized in the liver mainly by the saturable glycine and phenolic pathways and follows zero-order kinetics in overdose.

The half-life ($t_{1/2}$) of a therapeutic dose of 300 mg is 15 minutes for the ASA and 3 hours for SA. The amount ingested increases the $t_{1/2}$; at 1000 mg, the $t_{1/2}$ is 5 to 6 hours; at 10,000 mg, $t_{1/2}$ is 20 hours. Chronic administration, as in arthritic conditions and in toxic overdose, lengthens the $t_{1/2}$ considerably owing to saturation of the enzymes for conjugation.

The amount excreted in the urine is influenced by the urine pH. At acid urine pH (<6.5), 10 per cent free salicylate is excreted; at alkaline urine pH (>7.5), ion trapping inhibits tubular reabsorption and 80 per cent may be excreted. A change of the urinary pH from 6.5 to 7.5 may increase the salicylate excretion 10-fold.

The mechanisms of the manifestations in toxicity are (1) CNS respiratory center stimulation, (2) prostaglandin synthesis inhibition, (3) uncoupling of oxidative phosphorylation, (4) interference with Krebs cycle, (5) stimulation of lipolysis, (6) irreversible interference with platelet function, and, (7) bronchospasm.

MANIFESTATIONS

Mild manifestations are similar to "cinchonism" after ingestion of large doses of quinine, resulting in tinnitus (plasma SA 200 to 300 μg/ml), vertigo, headache, and mental confusion.

In more severe intoxication, *vomiting* is usually present within 3 hours after ingestion of a single overdose.

CNS manifestations are tinnitus (may be present even at the higher therapeutic concentrations), hyperventilation, seizures, and coma. Convulsions need a thorough

TABLE 1. Quantities of Aspirin Ingested: Deposition and Manifestations

Toxicity	Amount Ingested (mg/kg)	Toxicity Expected	Gastrointestinal Decontamination Site*	Manifestation Anticipated
Nontoxic	<150	No	No	None
Often nontoxic	150	No	Yes (Home)	None, tinnitus
Mild	150–200	Yes	Yes (ECF)	Vomiting, tinnitus, hyperventilation
Moderate	200–300	Yes	Yes (ECF)	Hyperpnea, lethargy, excitability
Severe	300–500	Yes	Yes (ECF)	Coma, convulsions
Very severe	>500	Yes	Yes (ECF)	Potentially fatal

ECF = emergency care facility. Intentional ingestions are always sent to ECF.

investigation, since they may be caused in salicylate intoxication by hypoglycemia, decreased ionized calcium with alkalosis, cerebral edema, intracranial hemorrhage, or hypoxia. Convulsions and coma are indications of serious intoxication. Coma is much more common in chronic salicylism. **Altered consciousness is the most important sign of severe intoxication**.

Hyperventilation is also present early (usually within 2 to 8 hours at plasma concentrations greater than 400 µg/ml) with respiratory alkalosis and later in compensation for metabolic acidosis. The lower the PCO_2, the more serious the intoxication. PCO_2 of 10 to 20 torr indicates severe intoxication.

The validity of *fever* is difficult to assess if the patient has been ill. Hyperthermia in a previously healthy person with overdose is a sign of serious intoxication.

Hemorrhagic manifestations are due to interference with platelet function for the life of the cell. In larger doses, salicylate decreases the production of prothrombin clotting factors II, VII, IX, and X and factor VIII and increases capillary fragility. Hemorrhagic manifestations (<1 per cent) other than GI bleeding indicate serious intoxication and a plasma SA greater than 700 µg/ml.

Metabolic disturbances occur. (a) The *acid-base disturbance* in adults and older children is usually respiratory alkalosis for 12 to 24 hours with compensatory loss of sodium, potassium, and bicarbonate in the urine. The acutely mild and moderate adult intoxication does not usually progress to metabolic acidosis. The respiratory alkalosis may be blunted by CNS depression or if CNS depressants are concomitantly ingested. In children under 5 years of age, the initial respiratory alkalosis usually changes to metabolic or mixed metabolic acidosis and respiratory alkalosis within a few hours. Metabolic acidosis increases the severity of the salicylate intoxication by allowing for earlier and easier volume distribution. (b) *Alterations in glucose metabolism* may cause hyperglycemia early in the intoxication owing to decreased tissue utilization and hypoglycemia late in the course of intoxication. Hypoglycemia occurs in chronic salicylism and in small children when the glycogen stores are depleted. (c) *Dehydration and electrolyte disturbances* are due to hyperventilation, vomiting, compensation for metabolic disturbances, diaphoresis, and uncoupling of oxidative phosphorylation.

Pulmonary edema is more frequent in adults over 30 years of age. *Cerebral edema* also may occur in serious intoxications. The mechanisms are not clear, but they may be aggravated by fluid overload in alkaline forced diuresis.

Chronic salicylism is more serious than acute intoxication, and the salicylate plasma concentration does not correlate with the manifestations. A plasma concentration within the therapeutic range does not exclude chronic salicylism because it may have already been distributed to the tissues. Chronic salicylism is associated with exaggerated CNS findings, hypoglycemia, mixed acid-base derangements, hemorrhagic manifestations, renal failure, and pulmonary edema.

There is an association of salicylate administration with *Reye syndrome*. Aspirin may increase the risk of Reye syndrome following an acute febrile illness, especially with influenza and varicella.

MANAGEMENT

Establish and maintain the vital functions.

GI decontamination is necessary if ingestion is greater than 150 to 160 mg/kg or 10 gm in adults. It is useful up to 12 hours post ingestion because some factors delay absorption (food, enteric-coated tablets, other drugs); pylorospasm may delay gastric emptying; and concretions may form. Emesis may be induced in the alert patient, gastric lavage instituted, and activated charcoal/cathartic should be administered. Activated charcoal should be repeated every 4 hours. Concretions and enteric-coated tablets may cause perforation or rising plasma salicylate concentrations and may be removed by lavage, whole body irrigation, endoscopy, or gastrostomy.

Intravenous fluid should be given as an 0.89 per cent saline or Ringer's lactate challenge, 20 ml/kg up 1000 ml over 1 hour, if necessary, then 5 per cent to 10 per cent glucose in 0.45 per cent saline. As soon as the patient voids, potassium should be added 1 to 2 mEq/kg/day or 30 to 40 mEq/L (more than 40 mEq/L if the potassium is below 3.5 mEq/L). If rapid correction of potassium is necessary, administer potassium chloride, 0.25 mEq/kg/hr up to 10 mEq/hr with ECG monitoring for 2 hours and recheck potassium. There is controversy as to whether to produce a *forced diuresis* or just correct the fluid deficit and administer maintenance fluids because of the danger of pulmonary and cerebral edema. The present recommendation is to administer fluids for repair and maintenance and **avoid** diuresis. However, fluid loss may be extensive, up to 200 to 300 ml/kg. Carefully monitor for fluid overload.

Alkalinization (antidote 35 in the article on acute poisoning) enhances salicylate excretion. Bicarbonate is administered to keep blood pH 7.5 and urine pH 7.5 to 8.0. Potassium is essential to produce adequate alkalinization of the urine. Monitor both the urine and blood pH. Paradoxic acid urine and alkaline blood may indicate potassium depletion. Do not use the urine pH alone to assess the need for alkalinization. In general, 2 mEq/kg of sodium bicarbonate raises the blood pH 0.1 unit. Alkalinization should be accomplished if salicylate concentration is greater than 300 µg/ml (30 mg/dl). Severe acidosis pH (7.10) may require 1 to 2 mEq/kg every 1 to 2 hours. Potassium may be needed in excess of 40 mEq/L to adequately alkalinize the urine. **Caution**: Over alkalinization may worsen hypokalemia, precipitate tetany, and cause cardiac dysrhythmias. **Avoid** acetazolamide, the carbonic anhydrase inhibitor, because it causes systemic metabolic acidosis as it alkalinizes the urine. It also alkalinizes CSF and traps salicylate in the CNS. Animal studies show increased mortality when this is used in treatment of salicylism.

Pulmonary edema may require hemodynamic monitoring and assisted ventilation with positive end-expiratory pressure. Fluid retention can be treated with mannitol (20 per cent), 0.5 gm/kg over 30 minutes, or furosemide, 1 mg/kg intravenously.

Hyperpyrexia should be treated with external cooling, not antipyretics.

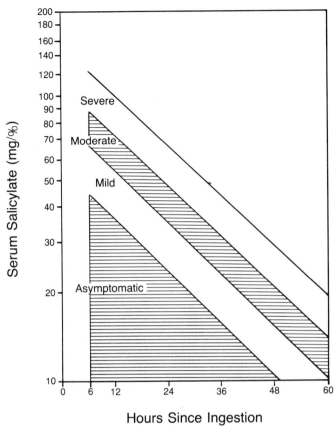

Figure 1. Done nomogram for salicylate poisoning. (From Done AK: Salicylate intoxication: Significance of measurements of salicylate in blood in cases of acute ingestion. Pediatrics 26:800–807, 1960. Reproduced by permission of Pediatrics.)

Abnormal bleeding or hypoprothrombinemia needs vitamin K, 10 to 50 mg intravenously (antidote 38) and, if bleeding continues, fresh blood or platelet transfusion.

Dialysis, preferably hemodialysis, or hemoperfusion is indicated if there is (a) persistent severe acidosis (pH <7.0) and lack of response to fluid and alkali therapy in 6 hours; (b) persistent severe electrolyte abnormalities and lack of response; (c) serum salicylate level initially greater than 160 mg/dl or greater than 130 mg/dl at 6 hours post ingestion (do **not** use the salicylate level as the sole criterion for dialysis); lower serum salicylate levels may be an indication for dialysis in chronic salicylism; (d) coma and uncontrollable seizures, congestive heart failure, pulmonary edema, cerebral edema, or acute renal failure; (e) progressive deterioration despite good management.

Chronic toxicity is usually a more severe intoxication because of the cumulative pharmacokinetics of salicylates and increased tissue distributions, so low plasma salicylate concentration may occur with severe poisoning.

LABORATORY

Monitor the following: (a) Blood: CBC, arterial blood gases, serum electrolytes, blood glucose, coagulation tests (platelets, prothrombin time, partial thromboplastin time), renal function, serum salicylate concentra-

tions. (b) Urine: urine pH and urinalysis, urinary output, urine 10 per cent ferric chloride test.

Laboratory abnormalities: (1) The metabolic acidosis of salicylism has a moderately elevated anion gap. Hyper- or hypoglycemia may exist. (2) Serum salicylate values used in conjunction with the *Done nomogram* (Fig. 1) are useful predictors of expected severity following *acute* single ingestions. The Done Nomogram is not useful (a) in chronic intoxications; (b) in delayed absorption such as in methyl salicylate, phenyl salicylate, or homomethyl salicylate ingestions, enteric-coated tablets; (c) less than 6 hours post ingestion. The salicylate level for use in the Done nomogram should be obtained 6 hours post ingestion, after the distribution phase of the medication. Before 6 hours, levels in the toxic range should be treated and levels below the toxic range should be monitored if a potentially toxic dose was ingested. A delayed peak plasma salicylate concentration until 24 hours or failure to decline may indicate the presence of concretions or something delaying passage of the salicylate through the GI tract. (3) The ferric chloride test. Add 1 to 2 drops of ferric chloride 10 per cent solution to an acidified urine. A purple color develops in 30 to 60 seconds if salicylate has been present in the body for over 30 minutes. The test is nonspecific and will be positive with aminoacidurias, acetoacetic acid, phenothiazines, and other products. The addition of concentrated sulfuric acid causes the salicylate coloration to blanch or disappear, but it remains or itensifies if the color is caused by phenothiazine. The Phenistix reagent strip may be used in a similar manner, and the degree of discoloration by salicylate in the serum allows an approximation of the amount present.

PROGNOSIS

Persistent vigorous treatment of salicylate ingestion is essential, as recovery has occurred despite decerebrate rigidity. The manifestations of serious intoxication are altered consciousness, metabolic acidosis, hyperthermia, hemorrhagic manifestations, and low PCO_2. Death is usually from pulmonary edema, cerebral edema, and cardiac dysfunction.

ACETAMINOPHEN POISONING

HOWARD C. MOFENSON, M.D.,
and THOMAS R. CARACCIO, PHARM. D.

Acetaminophen is also known as APAP, Tylenol, paracetamol in the United Kingdom, and many other brand names.

TOXICITY

Therapeutic dose is 10 to 15 mg/kg up to 2.6 gm/24 hr. The toxic amount is approximately 3 gm or more or 140 mg/kg in a child and 7.5 gm or more in an adult. Liver toxicity usually occurs in amounts greater than 15 gm in adults, but the 7.5 gm value includes those who have liver disease or depleted glutathione stores.

Table 1 calculates the amounts of the different commonly used preparations that equal the toxic amount of 140 mg/kg.

KINETICS

Oral absorption time is 0.5 to 1 hour. The peak plasma concentration following an oral therapeutic dose is 60 to 120 minutes. Following an overdose, the peak plasma concentration may not be reached for 4 hours after ingestion. The apparent volume of distribution (Vd) is 0.9 L/kg. The $t_{1/2}$ is 1 to 3 hours and may increase with overdose to greater than 4 hours. The $t_{1/2}$ over 4 hours is no longer used as a prognostic indicator as it was in the past. Elimination occurs in the liver (90 per cent), where APAP is metabolized to inactive glucuronide metabolite (65 per cent) and inactive sulfate metabolite (30 per cent) in adults by two saturable pathways. In infants and children under 9 to 12 years, elimination is more by conjugation with sulfate than glucuronide, and this may be hepatoprotective. APAP undergoes minor metabolism by the P-450 mixed function oxidase to a highly active arylating intermediate metabolite (5 to 8 per cent).

MANIFESTATIONS

Phase I. Occurs within the first few hours after ingestion and consists of malaise, diaphoresis, nausea, vomiting, and drowsiness for several hours. This is more frequent in children and may be delayed for 12 to 24 hours in adults. Loss of consciousness is *not* a feature and, if present, means either another cause or another drug has been taken concomitantly or in place of APAP.

Phase II. An asymptomatic latent period or a period of diminished symptoms of 24 to 72 hours' duration, occasionally up to 5 days. Hepatic damage begins at this time as indicated by increases in the liver enzymes, serum bilirubin, prothrombin time, pain in the right upper abdominal quadrant, and oliguria.

Phase III. Occurs 72 to 96 hours post ingestion with peak liver function abnormalities. Although liver enzyme tests do not correlate with outcome, values greater than 1000 units indicate hepatotoxicity. If the hepatic damage is extensive, hepatic failure develops about the fourth to fifth day with altered consciousness, hypoglycemia, and coagulation abnormalities. Jaundice does not usually become obvious before the fourth or fifth day.

Phase IV. Occurs at 7 to 10 days. Regeneration or, if extensive, liver damage, sepsis, and disseminated vascular coagulation may occur and the patient dies in 7 to 10 days.

Other organ systems involved include transient renal failure, which develops about 5 to 7 days post ingestion. The renal damage occurs in some patients without evidence of hepatic damage. Back pain, proteinuria, and hematuria may occur at 36 to 48 hours and are reported to herald renal failure. Myocardial necrosis, hemolytic anemia, methemoglobinemia, skin rashes, and pancreatitis have been reported but are quite rare.

MANAGEMENT

The early symptoms of overdose may be minimal or absent so the opportunity to suspect clinically and administer the antidote *N*-acetylcysteine (NAC) may be missed on a purely clinical basis. It is important that an appropriately timed plasma acetaminophen concentration be obtained for diagnostic evaluation and effective management of the overdosed patient. If the plasma APAP concentrations cannot be obtained and a significant overdose is suspected, ingestion therapy should be started within the first 8 to 10 hours. The plasma APAP value should be obtained *after 4 hours post ingestion* (after the distribution phase) and should be plotted on the modified Rumack-Matthew nomogram (Fig. 1) to assess toxicity. The nomogram is based on the plasma acetaminophen concentrations occurring after an *acute single ingestion*. The nomogram line to assess toxicity begins at a peak concentration of 4 hours post ingestion and follows the elimination phase of APAP for 24 hours. The modification of the Rumack-Matthew nomogram has a "probable hepatic toxicity risk line" joining 200 μg/ml at 4 hours to 50 μg/ml at 12 hours and a "possible hepatic toxicity line" from 150 μg/ml at 4 hours to 35 μg/ml at 12 hours (lowered 25 per cent) to account for errors in historical time of ingestion or discrepancies in laboratory determinations. Concomitantly ingested drugs or foods may change the gastric emptying time

TABLE 1. Toxic Amounts of Acetaminophen Packaging

Age	Weight (kg)	Drops 15 ml 100 mg/ml	Elixir 60 & 120 ml 160 mg/5 ml	Chewable Tablets 80 mg	Tablets 160 mg	Tablets 325 mg	Caplets 500 mg
<1 mo	3.5	4.9 ml	15.4 ml	6 tabs	3 tabs	1.5 tabs	1 cap
1 mo	4.0	5.6	17.6	7	3.5	1.72	1.12
6 mo	7.0	9.8	30.8	12.8	6.4	3.0	1.96
1 yr	10.0	14.0	44.0	17.5	8.8	4.3	2.8
2 yrs	12.0	16.8	52.8	21	10.5	5.16	3.36
3 yrs	14.0	19.6	61.6	24.5	12.3	6.02	3.92
5 yrs	18.0	25.2	79.2	31.5	15.8	7.74	5.04
6 yrs	20.0	26.2	88.0	35	17.5	8.6	5.60
9 yrs	28.0	39.2	123.2	49	24.5	12.1	7.84
10 yrs	32.0	44.8	140.8	56	28	13.8	8.96
12 yrs	34.0	47.6	149.6	59.5	30	14.6	9.52
14 yrs	40.0	56.0	176.0	70.0	35	17.2	11.20
15 yrs	50.0	70.0	220.0	87.5	44	21.5	14.00
Adult	60.0	84.0	264.0	105.0	52.5	25.8	16.80
Adult	70.0	98.0	308.0	122.0	61	30.1	19.60

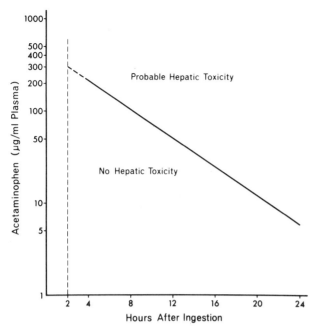

Figure 1. Rumack-Matthew nomogram to assess acetaminophen toxicity. (Adapted from Rumack BH, Matthew H: Acetaminophen poisoning and toxicity. Pediatrics 55:871, 1975.)

and the peak time. In these cases, additional concentrations may be needed to determine the peak. It is recommended that NAC (Mucomyst) be administered if the concentrations and time co-ordinates are above the lower line and the course of therapy be completed *even if the subsequent values fall below the toxic zone.*

Gastrointestinal Decontamination. Emesis is best **avoided** in the emergency department because it may interfere with the retention of activated charcoal and NAC. Gastric lavage is preferred. Studies have indicated that activated charcoal effectively absorbs acetaminophen. Activated charcoal may even be administered concomitantly with NAC if the loading dose of the antidote is administered twice. If activated charcoal administration is separated from NAC administration by 1 to 2 hours, the usual dosing schedule of NAC may be used. (*Note*: In the past, activated charcoal was believed to be contraindicated and, if administered, it was removed by lavage when oral NAC was contem-

plated.) Saline sulfate cathartics are preferred because they may enhance the sulfate metabolic pathway and provide hepatic protection.

Oral N-Acetylcysteine. NAC is used for hepatotoxic overdose (see antidote 1 in the article on acute poisoning). The oral loading dose is 140 mg/kg followed by 70 mg/kg every 4 hours for 17 additional doses, for a total of 72 hours of therapy. The original 20 per cent solution is administered as a 5 per cent solution diluted in a fruit juice or noncarbonated soft drink. (An intravenous preparation is used in Europe and Canada but is not FDA-approved in the United States).

Administer and complete an entire course of NAC if a toxic dose has been ingested or if initial plasma concentration (specimen obtained after 4 hours post ingestion) is above the toxic line (greater than 150 µg/ml at 4 hours or greater than 35 µg/ml at 12 hours) on the nomogram shown in Figure 1, regardless of subsequent plasma concentrations. NAC is most effective when administered in the first 16 hours. After 24 hours, NAC may not be effective. NAC should be stopped if hepatic encephalopathy develops. NAC should be offered orally in a covered "takeout beverage container" through a straw, preferably diluted with tomato juice. If the antidote is vomited within 1 hour after administration, it should be repeated. If vomiting occurs, check to be sure the dilution is correct. Table 2 calculates the amount of antidote and the dilution to make a less irritating 5 per cent solution for oral administration.

If the correct dilution is vomited, it may be necessary to place a radiopaque nasogastric tube in the duodenum and administer the antidote by a slow drip over an hour. Finally, if these measures are unsuccessful, an antiemetic drug such as metoclopramide (Reglan) 1 mg/kg IV up to 10 mg over 1 to 2 minutes or droperidol (Inapsine) 1.25 mg IV given before the dose of NAC may be required. (*Note*: Manufacturer states that metoclopramide may increase APAP absorption.)

Dialysis. Peritoneal dialysis or hemodialysis may be considered in severe cases or if persistent renal failure that lasts over 48 hours develops. Hemodialysis reduces the $t_{1/2}$ of acetaminophen, but there is no evidence that it alters the clinical course.

Agents to Avoid. The following agents may compete with acetaminophen for the conjugation pathway or

TABLE 2. NAC Dilutions

| Body Weight (kg) | Mycomyst (ml) | | Grams | Diluent (ml) | | 5% Solution (ml) |
	20%	10%		20%	10%	
140–149	105	210	21	315	210	420
130–139	95	190	19	285	190	380
120–129	90	180	18	270	180	360
110–119	80	160	16	240	160	320
100–110	75	150	15	225	150	300
90–99	70	140	14	210	140	280
80–89	65	130	13	195	130	260
70–79	55	110	11	165	110	220
60–69	50	100	10	150	100	200
50–59	40	80	8	120	80	160
40–49	35	70	7	105	70	140
30–39	30	60	6	90	60	120
20–29	20	40	4	60	40	80
10–19	15	30	3	45	30	60

stimulate enzyme induction and increase the toxic metabolite.

Agents that Decrease Conjugation	Enzyme Inducers
Phenolphthalein	Barbiturates
Dicumoral	Chronic alcoholism
Testosterone	Phenytoin
Hydroxyzine	Imipramine
Morphine	Chloral hydrate
Chloramphenicol	Ethchlorvynol
Prednisolone	Glutethimide
Tetracycline	Haloperidol
Estrogens	Meprobamate
Salicylamide	Phenylbutazone
Vitamin C	Tolbutamide
Immaturity	
Salicylate	

LABORATORY

Acetaminophen plasma concentrations should be determined at or after 4 hours post ingestion (after the distribution phase) or in any patient when the overdose substance is unknown so as not to miss the "golden first 8 postingestion hours" for antidotal therapy. Acetaminophen plasma concentrations after 24 hours document the presence of the medication but are not useful in therapeutic decisions. Monitor liver and renal profiles, including bilirubin, prothrombin time, serum amylase, coagulation tests, and blood glucose. CBC, platelet count, electrolytes, HCO_3, ECG, and urinalysis should be obtained in toxic cases. Fatal cases usually have a bilirubin level greater than 4 mg/dl and a prothrombin time greater than twice the control or a prothrombin time ratio of 2.2 or greater on the third to the fifth days. Some authorities start prophylaxis against hepatic encephalopathy if the prothrombin ratio rises above 3.0. Monitor blood glucose because, in toxic cases, hypoglycemia and hyperglycemia have been reported. The plasma creatinine rises more rapidly than the BUN when renal failure is present. Liver failure may keep the BUN low.

INCREASED LEAD ABSORPTION AND ACUTE LEAD POISONING

J. JULIAN CHISOLM, Jr., M.D.

The vast majority of children with increased lead absorption now referred to pediatricians by screening clinics are asymptomatic. Acute lead encephalopathy is now rare. Increased lead absorption (with or without symptoms) is a reportable condition. The Centers for Disease Control 1985 guidelines list four risk categories according to the following blood lead groups: class I ("normal"), blood lead values (PbB)* found in healthy populations without undue exposure to lead, PbB <25 μg; class II (moderate risk), PbB = 25 to 49 μg; class III (high risk), PbB = 50 to 69 μg; class IV (urgent risk), PbB ≤ 70 μg. In light of more recent evidence that lead can cause long-lasting neurobehavioral deficits

---

*PbB = μg lead/dl of whole blood.

in children at PbB levels <25 μg, it is anticipated that the Centers for Disease Control will soon issue new guidelines lowering "normal" PbB to 15 μg or less as well as redefining the other risk classifications.

When based on a confirmatory venous sample for PbB, this classification is useful as an initial guide to therapy; however, the trend of PbB and free erythrocyte protoporphyrin (FEP)* values is far more important than single values in the long-term management of this chronic condition. In classes III and IV the risk of symptoms and impairment of central nervous system (CNS) function is distinctly increased, particularly if venous PbB in excess of 45 to 50 μg is long sustained.

In all cases, first priority is given to identification of the important source of excess lead in the child's environment and to prompt separation of the child from the source. Chelating agents are useful in children in classes III and IV, the higher risk categories.

These agents should be used in the asymptomatic phase of lead poisoning, as institution of chelation therapy *after* the onset of acute encephalopathy does not reduce the incidence of severe CNS sequelae. A team approach involving public health personnel, physician, pediatric nurse-practitioner, medical-social worker, and behavioral psychologist is likely to be the most effective. If possible, children should be referred to a special lead clinic for long-term follow-up.

Identification and Abatement of Lead Sources

A thorough history can facilitate the identification and abatement of the most important sources of lead. This crucial part of therapy is usually performed by health department personnel, to whom all information should be reported. Environmental history should include a list of all dwellings visited by the child: primary residence, homes of relatives and babysitters, schools, and day care centers and the age and state of repair of each building. In the United States virtually all such buildings built before 1950 have lead-bearing paints on exposed exterior and/or interior surfaces. Structures in poor repair often have lead-containing chips or pulverized fragments in the household dust. Play areas, especially dirt playgrounds and dirt yards, painted metal fences and walls, and vacant lots formerly containing lead-painted structures should be identified.

Occupational histories for all adults in the various dwellings should be taken to ascertain whether any are exposed to lead-bearing dusts. "Dusty" lead trades include, but are not limited to, the following occupations: secondary lead smelting (recovery of lead from old storage batteries), lead scrap smelting, storage battery manufacturing and repair, metal founding, ship breaking, automobile assembly and body and radiator repair, demolition of painted metal structures (bridges), and demolition and renovation of old housing and other structures. In the renovation and maintenance of older housing, the grinding, sanding, and burning of old

---

*FEP = μg "free" protoporphyrin/dl erythrocytes. Analogous terms include zinc protoporphyrin (ZnP) and erythrocyte protoporphyrin (EP). Values are sometimes stated as concentration in whole blood rather than in erythrocytes.

paint poses an extremely serious hazard. If such workers wear their work clothing home, they contaminate their vehicles and the floors, carpets, and furniture of their homes with fine lead-bearing dusts. When such clothing is mixed with other clothing in the washing machine, lead may be transferred to the uncontaminated clothing. Workers should change their shoes and clothing and leave them for proper cleaning at their place of employment and should shower before coming home.

It is now recognized that exposure to lead-contaminated household dust and soil in outside play areas can account for most cases in which PbB is sustained in a range of 15 to 50 μg and that normal hand-to-mouth activity is the major route of entry of lead into the body. In old housing areas, weekly or more frequent scrubbing not only of floors but also of all woodwork (windows, doors, porches), as well as daily damp dusting of all surfaces a child can touch, is often effective in lowering a young child's PbB. Vacuuming, particularly wet vacuuming, is also helpful, but dry sweeping should be avoided, as it does not remove fine particulates. When lead in paint is found in the dwelling, many local ordinances require its removal. Although this is commonly done by burning with a gas torch and mechanical sanding, these procedures are contraindicated because they generate much dust, thus presenting an acute and potentially serious hazard not only to the worker but also to any infant or young child remaining in the house during the process. Under such conditions, it is not uncommon for a child's PbB to rise within a short time from <30 μg to >90 μg. Removal of lead paint with hot air guns, scrapers, and, wherever feasible, chemical removers presents a lesser hazard and is preferable. Even so, all infants and young children and pregnant and nursing women should find temporary "safe" residence elsewhere *day and night* until the entire "deleading" process is completed, the debris thoroughly removed by repeated wet cleaning, and the areas repainted with "lead-free" paint. All scaling old paint should also be removed. The use of a high-efficiency particle accumulator (HEPA) vacuum, if available, is highly effective in the clean-up process for removal of particulate lead. PbB should be determined frequently in the exposed child until the hazard is abated, since incomplete abatement, a common occurrence, is detected most often by a rise in the child's PbB. It is sometimes appropriate to determine PbB in all family members; if it is elevated in all, a common source, such as contamination of food, should be suspected.

In addition to ingestion of lead-bearing paint, severe symptomatic lead poisoning has been associated with the following: ingestion and retention in the stomach of metallic lead (fishing weights, curtain weights, shot); contamination of acidic foods and beverages from improperly lead-glazed ceramic pitchers, pots, and cups; burning of battery casings or lead-painted wood in the home; Asiatic cosmetics (Surma, Al Kohl); oriental folk medicines; Mexican folk remedies (azarcon, greta). Inhalation of fumes of leaded gasoline, which has been reported in American Indians, can cause a potentially fatal acute toxic encephalopathy.

Dietary Factors

Deficient dietary intake of calcium, magnesium, zinc, iron, and copper, as well as excessive dietary fat, increases the absorption, retention, and toxicity of lead. A diet adequate in these minerals and limited in fat should be assured. For those intolerant of cow's milk (sensitivity, intestinal lactase deficiency), "lactose-free" milk products or an alternative source is necessary to ensure adequate calcium intake. The use of low fat milk and the avoidance of fried foods and fatback should limit excessive dietary fat. Acidic foods such as fruits, fruit juices, tomatoes, sodas, and cola drinks may leach lead from the lead-soldered seams of cans. Dietary lead intake may be reduced if the above items are purchased fresh, frozen, or packaged in aluminum cans, other metal cans with welded seams, or glass, cardboard, or plastic containers. These dietary recommendations are used in all children with increased lead absorption (classes II, III, and IV). *Despite regulation of dietary factors, dust control is of much greater importance.* Children with sickle cell disease (hemoglobin SS) may have secondary zinc deficiency; in such cases, transfer to a safe housing area is likely to be the only effective measure.

Precautions in the Use of Chelating Agents

Edetate (EDTA) is not metabolized in the body but rather is excreted unchanged exclusively by glomerular filtration in the kidney. Calcium (Ca) EDTA but not dimercaprol (BAL) must be withheld during periods of anuria. Administration of CaEDTA at the dosage levels given (Table 1) must not exceed 5 successive days. Dosage should be reduced when glomerular filtration

---

TABLE 1. Dosage Schedule for Chelating Agents in Children

BAL-CaEDTA in Combination

Dosage: BAL* 83 mg/m² of body surface area/dose (IM)
CaEDTA† 250 mg/m² of body surface area/dose (IM)

Administration: For the first dose, inject BAL (IM) only; beginning 4 hours later and every 4 hours thereafter for 5 days, inject BAL and CaEDTA simultaneously at separate and deep IM sites; rotate injection sites.

CaEDTA Only

Dosage: 500 mg/m² of body surface/dose q12h (IM)

Administration: IM injection simpler in young children, but if IV route preferred, as in adults, infuse each dose over a 6-hour period; allow 1 week between each 5-day course of therapy.

D-Penicillamine‡

Dosage: 500 mg/m² of body surface area/day for long-term oral therapy

Administration: Give entire daily dose on empty stomach 2 hours before breakfast; contents of capsule may be mixed in a small amount of chilled fruit or fruit juice immediately prior to administration. Give 25 mg pyridoxine daily concurrently.

---

*BAL. The dosage recommended for adults by the FDA is 2.5 mg/kg of body weight/dose every 4 hours, which in "standard man" (70 kg, 1.73 m²) is equivalent to approximately 100 mg/m² of body surface area/dose, or about 20% higher than the dose recommended for children.

†CaEDTA. Edathamil calcium-disodium (Versenate) is available in 20% solution. For IM use, add sufficient procaine to yield a final concentration of 0.5% procaine. IM injection is more convenient in children and permits better control of IV fluids, a vital consideration in cases of encephalopathy. It has been used in this clinic for 35 years without untoward incident. If given IV in combination with BAL, infuse the total daily dose (1500 mg/m² of body surface area) over 24 hours and monitor ECG continuously.

‡D-Penicillamine. β, β-dimethylcysteine is available as Cuprimine in 125- and 250-mg capsules. It is approved for several uses, but is not approved for use in lead poisoning; see recommendations of AMA Council on Drugs.

rate (GFR) is reduced, and the drug should probably be withheld in non–life-threatening situations when acute renal disease not due to lead is present. Untoward reactions to CaEDTA include the following: local reactions at injection site, hypercalcemia, elevated BUN, proteinuria, microscopic hematuria, and fever. If pretreatment serum chemistries show evidence of hepatocellular injury (elevated SGPT, SGOT) or impaired renal function (elevated serum creatinine, urea nitrogen), chelation therapy should probably be withheld in asymptomatic cases. Carry out pretreatment and on the fifth day monitor serum creatinine, serum urea nitrogen, serum calcium, serum phosphorus, morning fasting plasma zinc and copper, and routine urinalysis. If any abnormalities are found, repeat this 2 and 3 days after a 5-day course of CaEDTA. Patients receiving CaEDTA IV should also be monitored by ECG for irregularities of cardiac rhythm. CaEDTA causes a substantial diuresis of zinc. If morning fasting plasma zinc has not rebounded to the normal range 3 days after therapy, consider oral zinc supplementation.

D-Penicillamine is contraindicated in children with renal disease and in those with a history of sensitivity to penicillin. Reactions to this drug can be minimized if oral dosage is restricted to ≤500 mg/m^2 of body surface/day. Patients who react to D-penicillamine usually do so within the first month. Neutropenia, proteinuria, and hypersensitivity reactions (angioedema, Stevens-Johnson syndrome, thrombocytopenia, acute hemolysis) as well as erythematous rashes are contraindications to its further use. Since it also causes a modest diuresis of iron, zinc, and copper, these metals should be replaced by oral supplements not exceeding the recommended daily dietary allowances for these metals. Pyridoxine (25 mg/day) should be given concurrently.

BAL, which is limited to the treatment of acute encephalopathy and to those patients with PbB >100 µg, should not be given in the presence of severe hepatocellular injury. It is judicious to place patients receiving BAL on parenteral fluids, at least during the first 24 to 48 hours, and then advance them cautiously to clear oral liquids, in order to minimize vomiting, one of the troublesome side-effects of BAL. BAL may induce moderate to severe intravascular hemolysis in children with glucose-6-phosphate dehydrogenase (G6PD) deficiency. BAL may not be given concurrently with medicinal iron. Medicinal iron may be given concurrently with CaEDTA and D-penicillamine.

DMSA, meso-2,3-dimercaptosuccinic acid (Succimer) is a most promising investigational oral chelating agent for lead. Clinical trials in children to date have shown this drug to be apparently safe and efficacious. When it is approved by the FDA, it is likely to become the drug of choice for the treatment of lead poisoning.

Management of Asymptomatic Cases with Increased Lead Absorption

Before treatment PbB and FEP values should be confirmed on a sample of venous blood, as 10 per cent or more of fingerprick screening samples may be seriously contaminated by exogenous lead. For children in class II, dietary correction, vigorous treatment of iron deficiency, stringent dust control, separation of the child from circumscribed environmental lead sources, and close follow-up will suffice. Chelating agents are rarely used to treat this group. PbB and FEP are measured serially every 3 months for at least 18 months to determine responses to medicinal iron and whether the level of lead absorption is increasing, stable, or decreasing.

Indications for chelation therapy in children in class III are not firmly established. We have limited chelation therapy with CaEDTA or D-penicillamine in cases of daily urinary output of coproporphyrin >250 µg/day, urinary delta-aminolevulinic acid output ≥3 mg/m^2/day; or behavioral changes and mild nonspecific symptoms suggestive of early clinical plumbism. FEP is of no value in making decisions regarding chelation therapy. The initial 5-day course of CaEDTA only (Table 1) is given in a hospital or a convalescent pediatric facility, followed by either oral D-penicillamine or one to three additional 5-day courses of CaEDTA only. Discharge from the pediatric convalescent facility is keyed to the availability of "safe" housing for the child. PbB and FEP are always checked 2 to 3 weeks following discharge, and at 1- to 3-month intervals during the next 18 months or longer, including at least one summer during which PbB remains <20 µg or declines to the normal range. Administration of chelating agents to outpatients is rarely appropriate unless safe housing is available. It will not counteract the effects of continued excessive intake of lead and indeed may increase the absorption and retention of lead.

For children in class IV, the risk of serious acute toxicity is unacceptable. As the administration of the diagnostic CaEDTA mobilization test may be hazardous in these children, they are always treated with CaEDTA only (Table 1) for 5 days, and the first day's urinary output is used to determine the chelatable lead (µg Pb excreted/mg CaEDTA administered/day). BAL is not given to such patients unless symptoms are clearly evident or PbB is >100 µg. Further chelation therapy in this group is the same as that described for children in class III.

Treatment of Symptomatic Cases

Children with one or more of the following—persistent vomiting, ataxic gait, gross irritability, severe anemia, seizures, and alterations in the state of consciousness—are treated as potential cases of acute encephalopathy. Symptomatic patients are maintained on parenteral fluids until symptoms abate.

Chelation therapy is started as soon as adequate urine flow is established. Initially, 10 per cent dextrose in water (10 to 20 ml/kg of body weight) is given over a period of 1 to 2 hours. If this fails to initiate urination, mannitol* (1 to 2 gm/kg body weight) is infused intravenously in 20 per cent solution at a rate of 1 ml/min. As soon as urine flow is established, further intravenous fluid therapy is restricted to basal water and electrolyte requirements, to a minimal estimate of the quantities required for replacement of deficits due to vomiting

---

*Manufacturer's precaution: Use of mannitol in pediatric patients has not been studied comprehensively.

and dehydration and to increased requirements resulting from convulsive activity or intercurrent fever. Proper fluid therapy is vital to survival in encephalopathy and is best monitored by placing an indwelling catheter and measuring the rate of urine flow. The rate of infusion is adjusted hourly until a rate is found that maintains the urine flow rate within basal metabolic limits (0.35 to 0.5 ml urine secreted/calorie metabolized/24 hr). This is equivalent to a daily urinary output of 350 to 500 ml/m²/day. Seizures are controlled initially with diazepam (Valium)* and thereafter with running doses of paraldehyde during the first few days. Long-term anticonvulsive drugs, such as phenytoin sodium (Dilantin) and barbiturates, are begun toward the end of the first week of therapy while paraldehyde is being reduced. During the acute phase, one should not await the development of frank seizures; better control can be achieved if doses of paraldehyde are given whenever there is a palpable increase in muscle tone or muscle twitching. Body temperature is maintained at normal but not at hypothermic levels.

Chelation therapy with BAL and CaEDTA is given according to the dosage schedule for combined therapy in Table 1. The usual 5-day course may be cautiously extended to 7 days if clinical evidence of encephalopathy persists beyond 4 days. Serial PbB measurements should be made after the last doses of BAL and Ca-EDTA and at 7, 14, and 21 days thereafter, as PbB generally rebounds following brief courses of chelation therapy. If PbB rebounds to >35 μg Pb, one or more additional 5-day course of CaEDTA only is indicated. If a convalescent pediatric facility is available, rebound may sometimes be minimized if the initial course of BAL and CaEDTA is followed by oral D-penicillamine daily and CaEDTA (500 mg/m²/dose) every other day.

In symptomatic cases, no time is wasted in attempts to evacuate residual lead from the bowel by enema, as enemas are often ineffectual, and the attendant delay may further jeopardize the child's life. Surgical decompression for relief of increased intracranial pressure is contraindicated. The role of steroids in combating cerebral edema in acute lead encephalopathy is not clear. Asymptomatic cases with PbB ≥100 μg are treated for the first 3 days with a BAL-CaEDTA combination, after which BAL is dropped, and CaEDTA only is continued in reduced dosage (500 mg/m² of body surface q12h IM) for an additional 2 days. For those with PbB <100 μg and mild or questionable symptoms, treatment with CaEDTA only (Table 1) should suffice.

Long-term Management

At the outset of treatment a long-term plan of management is developed to meet the needs of each specific child. Age, the intensity of hand-to-mouth activity, pica, and family composition and resources, as well as environmental exposure and laboratory data, are taken into account in developing such a plan. The aim is to minimize recurrences, to curb pica, and if paint is the major problem, to find a safe dwelling for the family. When the child's principal guardian is highly motivated and has the time, the behavioral psychologist may be able to devise a plan that will minimize pica and other highly repetitive hand-to-mouth activity. All pediatric housemates of index cases should be examined. Class III and IV cases should be reported to the medical-social service for assistance in the housing, financial, and emotional problems that such families usually have. Ideally, the level of lead absorption should be reduced so that PbB falls within a few months to 20 μg Pb. In old, dilapidated housing areas in the United States this is beyond the practical realm. Very poor families simply cannot afford "safe" housing. At the very least, PbB should be maintained at <35 to 40 μg Pb to reduce the degree of impairment that subsequently may impede the child's progress in school.

For children with long-sustained PbB in excess of 30 μg Pb or recurrent episodes of clinical plumbism, and survivors of encephalopathy, prolonged follow-up for at least 6 years is mandatory. Phenobarbital and phenytoin are generally adequate for control of seizures; recurrence of seizures without recurrent excess lead ingestion is usually indicative of a lapse in medication or failure to increase the dose in accordance with growth. For children with earlier sustained PbB >30 to 35 μg, follow-up psychometric evaluation should be carried out between 4 and 6 years of age to facilitate appropriate school placement for those in whom learning impediments are identified. When clinical evaluation and follow-up psychometric testing indicate no significant long-lasting impediments, parents should be reassured.

IRON POISONING
ARNOLD H. EINHORN, M.D.

Childhood poisonings due to the accidental ingestion of iron-containing hematinics or vitamin preparations remain common despite increased public awareness and improved safety packaging. Such medications are widely used and readily available without prescription, not only at pharmacies but also at food and discount stores. Many are marketed in the form of brightly colored and dangerously attractive pills or tablets suggesting candies.

The toxicity of any medicinal iron-containing compound is directly related to its elemental iron composition, which may differ widely among various products. Ferrous sulfate, the salt most widely prescribed and the ingredient most often involved in childhood poisonings, contains 20 per cent of elemental iron; preparations with gluconate (12 per cent of elemental iron) or fumarate (33 per cent of elemental iron) salts are also used frequently. Ferric salts (phosphate, pyrophosphate, ammonium citrate) are less commonly prescribed and are less dangerous.

Toxicity

Normally the mucosal cells of the small intestine effectively control both the absorption and the elimi-

*Manufacturer's precaution: The safety and efficacy of injectable diazepam in children under 12 years of age have not been established. Oral diazepam is not to be used in children under 6 months of age.

nation of dietary iron or small excesses of iron intake. Incorporated into ferritin, nutritional iron surpluses are either eliminated in the stools or absorbed after conversion from ferrous (divalent) to ferric (trivalent) iron that combines with apoferritin to form ferritin. This physiologic regulatory mechanism is inoperative when overwhelmed by excessive amounts of iron.

The massive ingestion of iron may be fatal in untreated patients; in survivors it may cause both early and delayed morbidity. Toxic effects are primarily gastrointestinal, circulatory, hepatic, cerebral, and metabolic. Minimal toxic dose and minimal lethal dose of iron for a child have not been clearly determined. The toxic dose has been estimated at 25–50 mg/kg of elemental iron, but toddlers have died after ingesting as little as 200 mg of elemental iron (less than five tablets of ferrous sulfate); on the other hand, recoveries have been reported in children from as much as 15 gm (3000 mg of elemental iron). Both mortality and morbidity have been reduced considerably in the last decades as a result of the institution of improved therapy.

The clinical manifestations characteristically progress in three phases:

The first phase of hemorrhagic gastroenteritis and acidemia usually begins within 30 to 60 minutes after ingestion, with emesis frequently bloody and diarrhea also often hemorrhagic. Hemoconcentration with blood hyperviscosity, metabolic acidemia, dehydration, and circulatory collapse may develop concurrently or may follow the hemorrhagic gastroenteritis within 4 to 6 hours. The patient with severe clinical toxicity who receives no specific treatment and who survives may improve either spontaneously or in response to supportive therapy.

If no symptoms appear within the first 6 to 12 hours after toxic iron ingestion or are limited to very mild gastrointestinal disturbances, it is unlikely that the course will progress further. Such patients may be discharged, provided peripheral white blood count and serum glucose are normal, abdominal radiography shows no residual iron tablets, and good follow-up can be assured.

The second "asymptomatic" phase is one of relative improvement, which is frequently misleading, lasting for 6 to 24 hours, during which symptoms subside or are minimal.

A critical third phase may develop about 24 to 48 hours after ingestion, characterized by progressive or rapid onset of shock, jaundice, and hepatic failure, bleeding diathesis, coma, or convulsions. Appropriate supportive and specific treatment during the first phase may prevent this delayed third phase, which may be fatal.

There may be a fourth phase of delayed gastrointestinal complication with pyloric stenosis or obstruction secondary to gastric scarring, which may develop within 1 to 2 months after recovery from the acute illness. Postintoxication liver cirrhosis is not seen in children.

Treatment

Treatment includes prompt emptying of gastric contents and measures minimizing further absorption of ingested iron; supportive therapy for preventing and correcting shock, dehydration, acidemia, and blood loss; maintaining airway ventilation and oxygenation; sustaining renal function; and chelation with deferoxamine (DFO) in severe intoxications.

Gastric Evacuation and Neutralization. Pharmacologic induction of vomiting with 15 ml of Ipecac Syrup should be limited to the first 2 hours after ingestion provided the child has had no bloody vomitus. Induced emesis should be followed by gastric lavage through a large-bore orogastric tube of sufficient size to permit passage of any undissolved tablets. Beyond the first 2 hours after ingestion, induction of emesis may be dangerous because of the corrosive effects of iron on the gastrointestinal mucosa; lavage without emesis is then preferable using a 1 per cent sodium bicarbonate solution.

Gastric lavage should be followed by a radiographic examination of the abdomen to ascertain whether the procedure has been successful in removing the tablets. In exceptional instances in which repeated gastric lavages proved fruitless to eliminate clumps of imbedded tablets, endoscopic removal or even gastrostomy have been necessary. Alkalinization of the gastric contents binds the iron salt into a noncorrosive, insoluble nonabsorbable ferrous carbonate precipitate. After the lavage is complete, 150 ml of 1 per cent sodium bicarbonate should be left in the stomach to neutralize any residual iron. Iron salts are not absorbed effectively by activated charcoal. Intragastric instillation of disodium phosphate dihydrate (Fleet phosphate) solution is contraindicated because of the potential danger of hyperphosphatemic convulsions.

If there is profuse diarrhea, rectal lavage with the bicarbonate solution may prevent further damage to the rectal sigmoid mucosa by the iron fragments.

Supportive Therapy. Whether the patient is symptomatic or not, if the number of tablets ingested is five or more, or unknown, intravenous fluids should be started to prevent or correct acidemia and dehydration and to maintain renal function. The hydrating solution should contain at least 1 to 2 mEq/kg of sodium bicarbonate. Colloid solutions, plasma analogues, blood, and catecholamines may be required to combat peripheral vascular collapse. Fresh frozen plasma or plasma components, platelets, and vitamin K may be essential in the presence of disseminated intravascular coagulopathy. If there are any nervous system manifestations or threat thereof, measures to ensure airway patency and maintain ventilation and oxygenation must be instituted at once. Excretion of ferrioxamine, the end product of chelated iron, depends upon maintenance of a satisfactory urine output, which will not take place without adequate correction of the hypovolemia and the acidemia.

Chelation. Deferoxamine (DFO) is a highly effective iron-binding compound that has been used with good results in severe iron intoxication. The chelating agent, specific for iron, is a siderochrome of microbial origin. In vitro its iron-binding capacity exceeds that of transferrin. Deferoxamine combines with iron to form ferrioxamine, which is excreted largely in the urine except for a small proportion that is metabolized in the body. The soluble DFO hydrochloride or mesylate salt binds 9.3 mg of trivalent iron per 100 mg of chelate. Whereas iron salts do not dialyse well, extracorporeal hemodialysis will remove effectively ferrioxamine in the presence of inadequate renal function.

Parenteral treatment with DFO should be restricted to instances of severe iron intoxication because of the potential toxicity of the iron complex ferrioxamine. The iron toxicity should be regarded as severe if the amount of ingested iron is known to exceed 25 mg/kg of elemental iron, that is, five tablets or more of ferrous sulfate tablets by a toddler, or the serum iron concentration (normally 65 to 75 μg/dl) exceeds 350 μg/dl within 4 to 6 hours after the ingestion or exceeds the total iron-binding capacity by 50 μg. Serum iron levels tend to decline from 4 to 6 hours after ingestion regardless of the amount taken; a serum iron level less than 300 μg/dl in a sample obtained beyond this time interval does not rule out serious intoxication.

Other clinical and laboratory clues that indicate severity of intoxication include severe or bloody emesis, bloody diarrhea, persistence of radiographic opacities after emesis and lavage, fever and leukocytosis exceeding 15,000, hemoconcentration, hypotension and hypoperfusion, hematologic evidence of coagulopathy, clinical and laboratory evidence of liver failure, including jaundice, hypoglycemia and abnormal liver function tests, and evidence of obtundation or convulsions. All patients who manifest features reflecting potential severity within the first 6 hours after ingestions require gross monitoring of the circulatory, neurologic, hepatic, renal, hematologic, and acid-base status based on clinical and laboratory parameters.

An intravenous DFO challenge of 15 mg/kg/hr (maximum: 250 mg) infused over 1 hour in 50 ml of 5 per cent dextrose in water should be administered to all patients who have ingested either an unknown quantity of iron salts or are known to have ingested five tablets of the ferrous salt or more, have been symptomatic in the first 6 hours of ingestion or are either seen after 6 hours of ingestion or in a situation in which iron levels and total iron-binding capacity are not readily available. After fluids are given to ensure adequate renal function and the bladder is emptied of all residual urine, the passage of a urine of vin rosé, orange, or reddish brown color signals the presence of iron as ferrioxamine in the urine and is an indication for instituting parenteral DFO therapy at once.

For chelation therapy the recommended intravenous dose of DFO is 15 mg/kg/hr to be given for 6 hours in a solution of 300 ml of 5 per cent dextrose in water. As long as the color of the urine continues to be vin rosé, orange, or reddish brown, additional intravenous courses of 15 mg/kg of DFO are to be given, usually in 6-hour courses separated by an interval of several hours. The DFO is not to be administered more rapidly than 15 mg/kg/hr; adverse reactions from the drug such as hypotension, irritability, and convulsions were reported in the past when the drug was given rapidly or in combination with large amounts of oral deferoxamine. These untoward effects virtually disappeared when

both the oral therapy and the rapid infusion of the chelating agents were discontinued. In less severe poisoning the intramuscular route is also effective, provided the patient is normotensive and presents only mild manifestations of poisoning. The recommended IM dose of DFO is 10 mg/kg/hr up to a total of 1.0 gm every 4 to 6 hours for a total of 4 gm/24 hr. Oral therapy with deferoxamine is contraindicated except when the serum iron level exceeds several thousand micrograms and the need to remove with extreme speed all residual iron from the stomach outweighs by far the inherent toxicity of oral DFO. When given orally, DFO does not prevent the absorption of iron from the intestinal tract; toxicity may result from the passage into the circulation of large quantities of the chelate complex ferrioxamine. However, when serum iron levels exceed several thousand micrograms per deciliter, gastric lavage has been recommended with a solution containing 2 gm of DFO mesylate per liter of water and sufficient sodium bicarbonate to alkalinize the gastric contents and increase the DFO complexation of iron. We do not recommend, however, that after lavage DFO be left in the stomach. In the patient with oliguria and anuria secondary to hypotension and circulatory collapse, hemodialysis or exchange transfusion may be required to remove the chelated iron complex ferrioxamine.

Prevention

The most effective means of reducing the needless morbidity and potential fatalities from iron poisoning is prevention rather than treatment. Iron preparations often find their way into the home, as prenatal therapy, as a mineral supplement of an elderly member of the household, or incorporated in vitamin preparations, some of which are fruit flavored, animal shaped, and chewable. Especially attractive to small children are chewable vitamin wafers that represent popular cartoon characters. Marketed in bottles containing as many as 250 tablets and available without prescription and without a danger warning, they are usually considered safe by parents. Proper labeling and educational measures directed to physicians, pharmacists, and parents are necessary to counteract the problem created by the attractive formulation and accessibility of iron-containing medications, which combined with the natural curiosity of children, are the major factors that create this serious problem. As has been emphasized by Robotham and Lietman (1980) "an ounce of prevention is worth more than a pound of deferoxamine."

INSECT STINGS

DAVID F. GRAFT, M.D.

Systemic anaphylaxis resulting from the stings of insects of the order Hymenoptera (honeybees, yellow jackets, hornets, and wasps) affects 1 per cent of children and may be mild, with only cutaneous symptoms (pruritus, urticaria, angioedema), or severe, with potentially life-threatening symptoms (laryngeal edema, bronchospasm, hypotension). Of the 50 deaths per year attributed to insect stings in this country, only one or two occur in children. Large local reactions occur in 10 per cent of individuals and consist of swelling greater than 2 inches (5 cm) in diameter that persists for longer than 1 day.

ACUTE MANAGEMENT

Individuals presenting with anaphylaxis require careful observation. A subcutaneous injection of epinephrine (1:1000) at a dose of 0.01 ml/kg (maximum 0.3 ml) is the cornerstone of management and often is sufficient to terminate a reaction. This may be repeated in 10 to 15 minutes if necessary. Oral antihistamines such as diphenhydramine hydrochloride (Benadryl, 12.5 to 50 mg) or chlorpheniramine (2 to 4 mg) are also usually given. They may lessen urticaria or other cutaneous symptoms, but in more serious or progressive reactions, their use should not retard the administration of epinephrine.

Inhaled sympathomimetic agents such as isoproterenol may decrease bronchoconstriction but do not address other systemic manifestations such as shock. Aminophylline is the drug of choice if bronchoconstriction persists following epinephrine. Severe reactions may require treatment with oxygen, volume expanders, and pressor agents. Corticosteroids such as prednisone (0.5 to 1 mg/kg/day) are often used, but their delayed onset of action (4 to 6 hours) limits their effectiveness in the early stages of treatment.

Systemic reactions commencing more than several hours after a sting usually manifest only cutaneous symptoms. Most are easily managed with oral antihistamines and observation. Treatment recommendations for large local reactions include ice, elevation, and antihistamines. A short course of prednisone (0.5 to 1 mg/kg/day for 5 days), especially if initiated immediately after the sting, may be the best treatment for massive large local reactions.

DECREASING FUTURE REACTIONS

Preventing Stings

Since many stings occur when a child steps on a bee, shoes should always be worn outside. Hives and nests around the home should be exterminated. Good sanitation should be practiced, since garbage and outdoor food, especially canned drinks, attract yellow jackets. Brightly colored clothing and perfumes should be avoided.

Emergency Epinephrine

To encourage prompt treatment, epinephrine is available in emergency kits for self-administration (Table 1). These are used immediately after the sting to "buy time" to get to a medical facility. The Ana-Kit contains a preloaded syringe that can deliver two 0.3-ml doses of epinephrine. Smaller doses may also be given. The physician who prescribes this kit must provide thorough instruction and must be confident that the patient can perform the injection procedure. These kits can be

TABLE 1. Epinephrine Injection Kits for Emergency Self-Treatment of Systemic Reactions to Insect Stings

Injection Kit	Dosage
EpiPen*	Delivers 0.3 ml 1:1000 (0.3 mg epinephrine)
EpiPen Jr*	Delivers 0.3 ml 1:2000 (0.15 mg epinephrine)
Ana-Kit†	Delivers two doses of 0.3 ml 1:1000 (total 0.6 mg epinephrine)

*The EpiPen and EpiPen Jr are spring-loaded automatic injectors and are distributed by Center Laboratories, Port Washington, NY.

†Ana-Kit is capable of delivering fractional doses and is distributed by Hollister-Stier Laboratories, Spokane, WA.

confusing to nonmedical personnel, and some patients have a tremendous fear of needles. A practice self-injection with saline will resolve this question. The newer EpiPen (0.3 mg epinephrine) and EpiPen Jr. (equivalent of 0.15 mg epinephrine, 1:1000) offer a concealed needle and a pressure-sensitive spring-loaded injection device that make them suited for children and families who are uncomfortable with the injection process.

In general, a child who is stung should receive an antihistamine and be watched for 1 hour. If any signs of generalized (systemic) reaction occur, epinephrine should be administered, and the child should be seen by a physician. If no systemic signs occur in the first hour, the child may resume regular activities. Children who are receiving maintenance injections of venom immunotherapy are advised that emergency self-treatment will probably not be required; however, they should have the kit available if they are far from medical facilities.

Venom Immunotherapy (Table 2)

A child who has experienced a sting-induced systemic reaction should be referred to an allergist, who will perform skin tests with dilute solutions of honeybee,

TABLE 2. Selection of Patients for Venom Immunotherapy

Sting Reaction	Skin Test/RAST	Venom Immunotherapy
1. Systemic, non–life-threatening (child): immediate, generalized, confined to skin (urticaria, angioedema, erythema, pruritus)	+ or −	No
2. Systemic, life-threatening (child): immediate, generalized, may involve cutaneous symptoms but also has respiratory (laryngeal edema or bronchospasm) or cardiovascular symptoms (hypotension/shock)	+	Yes
3. Systemic (adult)	+	Yes
4. Systemic	−	No
5. Large local >2 inches (5 cm) in diameter >24 hours	+ or −	No
6. Normal <2 inches (5 cm) in diameter <24 hours	+ or −	No

yellow jacket, yellow hornet, white-faced hornet, and Polistes wasp venoms. Radioallergosorbent testing (RAST) cannot replace venom skin testing but may provide additional information. If the reaction was severe (life-threatening—bronchospasm, laryngeal edema, shock) and the venom testing is positive, immunotherapy with the appropriate venom is commenced. Since children with milder cutaneous reactions have only a 10 per cent recurrence rate, venom treatment is not required. Children with large local reactions or negative skin tests also are not candidates for venom therapy.

Increasing amounts of venom are given weekly for several months until the 100-μg dose (equals two stings) is reached. Maintenance injections are given every 6 weeks after the first year of treatment. Venom therapy is highly effective, protecting 97 per cent of patients from reactions to in-hospital challenge stings. The disadvantages of venom treatment include cost, systemic and local reactions to injections, and the unknown length of therapy. No long-term side effects have been reported. About 25 per cent of patients develop negative skin tests after 3 to 5 years of treatment and may be candidates for discontinuing therapy. Duration of treatment (e.g., 5 years) may constitute another criterion for stopping treatment.

ARTHROPOD BITES AND STINGS

BERNARD A. COHEN, M.D.

Arthropod bites and stings are a major cause of morbidity in infants and children and account for 65 per cent of all deaths from venomous animals in this country. These ubiquitous organisms are elongated invertebrates with segmented bodies, true appendages, and chitinous exoskeletons. Arthropods of importance to physicians include millipedes and centipedes, the eight-legged arachnids (scorpions, spiders, ticks, and mites), and six-legged insects (lice, blister beetles, bed bugs, bees, wasps, ants, fleas, moths, butterflies, flies, and mosquitoes).

MILLIPEDES (DIPLOPODA) AND CENTIPEDES (CHILOPODA)

Although superficially similar, millipedes are vegetarian feeders and centipedes are carnivorous. When handled, millipedes exude a defensive fluid, which may produce immediate burning, erythema, and edema that progresses to vesicles, bullae, and erosions.

Although all centipedes contain poison glands, and some bites result in severe systemic symptoms, in the United States reactions to envenomation are limited to a transient sharp pain at the site. *Treatment*: Irritant reactions and bites can be treated with cool tap water compresses or topical steroids. In severe reactions, prednisone 1 mg/kg/day tapered over 10 to 14 days, can be used.

ARACHNIDS

Arthropods of this class are recognized by their fused cephalothorax and four pairs of legs. Medically important orders include scorpions, spiders, ticks, and mites.

Scorpions. Scorpions are nocturnal tropical arachnids and are readily identified by their stout pinching claws, elongated abdomen, and narrow tail, which ends in a conspicuous bulblike stinger that it swings over the head to attack prey. Poisonous species in North America are restricted to the deserts of the American Southwest and Mexico. They remain hidden in garages, basements, closets, crevices, and gravel. When accidentally provoked, they will bite, producing a hemolytic reaction consisting of localized burning, swelling, purpura, necrosis, and lymphadenitis. Occasionally a more severe neurotoxic reaction results in nausea, lacrimation, diaphoresis, abdominal cramps, restlessness, and rarely, in small children shock, seizures, and death. Children under 3 years of age account for 75 per cent of all deaths from scorpion stings.

TREATMENT. In mild reactions, cool compresses, topical steroids, and antihistamines will provide symptomatic relief. In severe reactions, local measures, including the application of ice to the bite and a tourniquet proximal to the sting, may be helpful until a specific antiserum can be administered. In infested areas, creosote or other repellants may be applied to basements, garages, and out buildings; and shoes, boots, and clothing should be inspected carefully before dressing.

Spiders (Araneae). Spiders are distinguished from other anthropods by their compact cephalothorax and large baglike abdomen. The majority of encounters in North America occur with the black widow (*Latrodectus mactans*), a web spinner that prepares its trap across privy seats and cool dark sites in vacant buildings. The female is very aggressive, attacking humans with little provocation, and may be recognized by her red ventral hourglass markings. Local reactions to bites may be painful but are often unnoticed and sometimes followed within 30 minutes by dizziness, nausea, diaphoresis, lacrimation, muscular rigidity, tremors, paresthesias, and headaches. The number of bites is estimated at 500 each year, with a mortality rate of 1 per cent overall and approaching 5 per cent in small children. Symptoms in nonfatal cases increase in severity for several hours, perhaps a day, and slowly dissipate in 2 to 3 days.

TREATMENT. Prompt treatment with specific antiserum is required for relief of symptoms, especially in children (Antivenin, Merck Sharp & Dohme). After a skin or conjunctival test for horse serum sensitivity, one vial of antivenom reconstituted in 2.5 ml of diluent is administered intramuscularly, or the antivenom may be given intravenously in 10 to 50 ml of saline over 15 minutes.

Other supportive measures include warm baths, intravenous injections of 10 ml of 10 per cent calcium gluconate, morphine, and barbiturates as needed for control of muscle pain and cramps. In healthy adults and older children antivenom may be deferred pending results of therapy with muscle relaxants and analgesics. Methocarbamol* (Robaxin injectable and tablets) is a useful alternative muscle relaxant, and 10 ml should be

---

*Safety and efficacy for use in children under 12 years of age have not been established except in tetanus.

administered over 5 minutes followed by 10 ml in 250 ml of 5 per cent dextrose in water at 1 ml per minute. When the patient is improved or if the reaction is mild, methocarbamol, 800 mg every 6 hours, may be given orally.

Brown Recluse (*Loxosceles reclusa*). Slightly smaller than the black widow, the brown recluse spans an overall diameter of 3 to 4 cm with a body 10 to 12 mm long and 4 mm wide. It abounds in the south central United States, where it can be distinguished from other brown spiders by its characteristic dark brown violin-shaped band extending from the eyes to the end of the cephalothorax. Although occasionally producing a fatal systemic reaction in young children, loxoscelism is characterized by a gangrenous slough at the bite site. Local pain appears 2 to 8 hours after the attack followed by an area of erythema, which develops a necrotic central bulla surrounded by an irregular area of purpura. Over 7 to 14 days necrosis progresses from a well-demarcated eschar to ulceration up to 20 cm in diameter.

TREATMENT. No specific antivenom is available in the United States for treatment of brown recluse spider bites. Antihistamines should be used to treat urticarial reactions, and antibiotics may be initiated if secondary infection develops. The use of steroids is controversial, but some experts recommend immediate administration of systemic corticosteroids as soon as the diagnosis is entertained. Intralesional steroids (4 mg of dexamethasone) may be helpful and can be repeated if the lesion continues to increase in size. Large ulcers usually require excision and skin grafting. Semipermeable or occlusive dressings (Duoderm, Vigilon, Opsite) may be applied to facilitate healing.

Ticks (*Acari*). Ticks are blood-sucking arachnids with short legs and a leathery integument. They are important vectors for a number of rickettsial and viral disorders and erythema chronicum migrans. Tick bite pyrexia and tick paralysis are produced by a toxin elaborated by the female tick and are promptly relieved by removal of the tick.

Typically tick bites go unnoticed for several days until a pruritic red papule with a red halo develops at the site. These lesions may resolve in several weeks unless the tick mouth parts are left in place, resulting in a foreign body reaction, which may persist for months. Erythema chronicum migrans is a peculiar eruption produced by a spirochete transmitted by the bite of the *Ixodes dammini* tick. Three to 20 days after a bite from an infected tick, an expanding indurated annular red plaque with central clearing up to 20 cm in diameter appears at the site. Lesions may be multiple and widely disseminated by hematogenous spread from the primary lesion. The rash occurs most commonly in children and may be associated with a rhematoid factor–negative oligoarticular arthritis (Lyme arthritis), meningoencephalitis, and myocarditis.

TREATMENT. Individuals who have spent time in infested wooded and grassy areas should be carefully inspected daily and all ticks removed immediately. Once the ticks have become embedded in the skin, techniques for removal include application of a hot unlighted match, petrolatum, liquid nitrogen, chloroform, nail polish remover, ethyl chloride spray, and mineral oil. Residual mouth parts are readily removed by skin punch biopsy.

Persistent symptomatic bite reactions will improve with intralesional steroid injections of triamcinolone 0.1 ml of 5 to 10 mg/ml. Erythema chronicum migrans and its associated symptoms may be aborted with oral penicillin or tetracycline,* 250 mg four times daily for 2 weeks.

Insect repellants, particularly those containing diethyltolumide (DEET), may provide some protection in endemic areas. However, toxic side effects have been reported with repeated applications to the skin, especially in young children. This risk may be minimized by applying the product only to clothing.

Mites (*Acari*). Infestations with the human *Sarcoptes scabiei* mite have reached epidemic proportions in some communities. The mite spares no age or socioeconomic group and has been identified as a significant medical problem in schools and day care centers and among promiscuous teenagers and adults. The eruption is asymptomatic for weeks to months until the individual becomes sensitized to the mite or its waste products. Papules, vesicles, pustules, and burrows are characteristically found on the wrists, finger webs, axillae, genitals, breasts, and buttocks. The scalp, palms, and soles are also involved in infants and toddlers. A generalized eczematous eruption may occur in sensitized individuals and overshadow the characteristic lesion, making diagnosis difficult. Diagnosis requires demonstration of mites, eggs, or fecal material from skin scrapings.

TREATMENT. The treatment of choice is 1 per cent gamma benzene hexachloride (Scabene, Kwell), but its use in young children is controversial. Percutaneous absorption of the drug can be reduced by restricting therapy to a single 6- to 8-hour application without a preceding bath and followed by thorough cleansing. Therapy should be repeated in 1 week only if live mites can still be demonstrated. All members of the household should be treated, but prescriptions must be limited to 1 ounce per person per treatment. Alternative therapies for pregnant individuals and infants include 6 per cent precipitated sulfur in petrolatum and 10 per cent crotamiton (Eurax) cream or lotion applied daily for 3 days. Although sulfur appears to be quite effective, the product is messy (malodorous, stains clothing) and must be applied daily for 3 to 5 consecutive days. Several hospital-based studies demonstrate that the failure rate with Crotamiton may exceed one third of those treated. Moreover, studies on toxicity and percutaneous penetration of Crotamiton are lacking.

A new product for treating scabies, permethrin 5 per cent cream (Elimite Cream), will shortly be released. The agent is highly effective and is approved for use in infants as young as 2 months. However, its safety in pregnant women, nursing mothers, and newborns has not been demonstrated.

Clothing and bedsheets should be laundered in hot water, but extensive treatment of fomites is not neces-

---

*Use of tetracycline in children less than 8 years of age may cause discoloration of permanent teeth.

sary, because the mites are dormant at room temperature.

Pruritus, which may last for weeks despite adequate therapy, should be treated with cool baths, emollients, and antihistamines such as hydroxyzine 2 to 5 mg/kg/day divided every 6 hours, or diphenhydramine 5 mg/kg/day divided every 6 hours.

Other Mites. Children are also commonly infested with animal mites from dogs, cats, mice, and birds. A self-limited itchy papular eruption appears on exposed areas of the arms, legs, and trunk. Harvest mites (red bugs, chiggers) are frequently encountered in parks and grassy areas. Pruritic red papules and nodules with central hemorrhagic puncta appear at sites where the mite larvae are caught in clothing, such as at the waist band, sock bands, and underwear. The larvae are removed inadvertently by scratching, and pruritus wanes over 5 to 7 days.

TREATMENT. Symptomatic therapy includes topical corticosteroids, shake lotions (calamine), cool compresses, antihistamines, and in severe cases systemic corticosteroids (prednisone 0.5 to 1 mg/kg/day tapered over 10 to 14 days).

Effective prophylaxis can be achieved with insect repellants sprayed onto clothing, including diethyltoluamide (DEET), ethyl hexanediol, dimethyl phthalate, dimethyl carbate, and benzyl benzoate.

INSECTS

Insects are ubiquitous six-legged arthropods with well-defined body segments, including a head, thorax, and abdomen. Organisms of medical significance include bees, wasps, and ants (Hymenoptera), lice (Anoplura), blister beetles (Coleoptera), bed bugs and kissing bugs (Heteroptera), fleas (Siphonaptera), moths and butterflies (Lepidoptera), and flies and mosquitoes (Diptera).

Pediculosis. Human lice are a major public health problem, especially in areas of overcrowding or where facilities are inadequate for keeping people and clothing clean. Pediculosis occurs in three clinical forms: head and body lice infestations produced by two interbreeding varieties of *Pediculus humanus* with characteristic elongated abdomens, and pubic lice caused by *Phthirus pubis*, or the crab louse, which has a short hairy abdomen and two pairs of crablike claws anteriorly. Lice are acquired through close contact with infested individuals or fomites.

PEDICULUS HUMANUS CAPITIS. Head lice are seen almost exclusively in girls and women. Lice may be identified on the scalp, and nits are seen about 1 inch from the surface, particularly in the postauricular and occipital areas. Pruritus is intense, and secondary infection is common.

Treatment. Patients should be instructed to vigorously lather the scalp and adjacent hairy areas with 1 per cent gamma benzene hexachloride (Kwell) shampoo for 5 minutes and then rinse thoroughly. Remaining nits may be removed with a fine-tooth comb. The nits may be loosened by application of a solution of equal parts white vinegar and water. Retreatment may be necessary in 1 week because some nits may survive the initial

application. Pyrethrins (Rid, R & C shampoo) are effective over-the-counter alternatives, and generally retreatment is not required.

In 1986 a prescription 1 per cent permethrin cream rinse (Nix) was released for treatment of head lice. Permethrin should be applied to the hair after shampooing and left in place for 10 minutes before being rinsed out. Although it is at least as effective as lindane and has a superior safety profile, the safety of permethrin in pregnant women, nursing mothers, and infants under 2 years has not been established.

Earlier this year a prescription 0.5 per cent Malathion product (Ovide Lotion) became available in the United States. This is a highly effective agent with marked ovicidal activity. The preparation binds to the hair shaft after application for up to four weeks, permitting extended residual activity. As a result, while other pediculocides may require a second treatment 7 to 10 days later, only one application is necessary. Patients should be cautioned to avoid hair dryers, open flames, and other heat sources because the product is prepared in a flammable base. As with other pediculocides, its safety in pregnant women, nursing mothers, and young infants has not been established. A new product called Step 2 (formic acid) has been released for use after treatment with Malathion. Formic acid loosens the nits and facilitates easy removal with a fine-tooth comb.

PEDICULUS HUMANUS HUMANUS. The body louse hides in the seams of clothing and produces tiny itchy papules and wheals, particularly in the interscapular, shoulder, and wrist regions.

Treatment. Infestation is effectively treated by laundering of clothing and bedding with hot water.

PHTHIRUS PUBIS. Crab louse infestation has become epidemic among promiscuous teenagers and adults. The insects are readily identified as grayish spots clinging to the skin in the genital area. Lice and nits may also spread to other hair-bearing areas, including the chest, axillae, and eyelashes. Maculae caeruleae are greenish-blue patches produced by bites on the chest, abdomen, and thighs of infested individuals.

Treatment. A 1 per cent gamma benzene hexachloride lotion should be applied to involved areas, except for the eyelashes, left on for 8 to 12 hours, and then thoroughly rinsed. Pyrethrin lotions should be massaged onto infested areas and then rinsed after 10 minutes. Pediculosis of the eyelashes can be safely treated with petrolatum applied twice daily for 7 to 10 days followed by mechanical removal of nits.

Blister Beetles (Meloidae). Blister beetles contain cantharidin, a volatile substance that produces an intraepidermal vesicle when the insects alight on the skin or are inadvertently crushed. Blister beetle dermatosis consisting of a linear vesicular eruption is common during the summer months when the insects are most plentiful.

TREATMENT. Lesions should be left intact to heal spontaneously in 3 to 4 days. Large lesions (greater than 1 cm) may be drained and dressed with a compressive bandage soaked with aluminum acetate (Burow's, Blueboro) solution.

Bedbugs (*Cimex lectularius*). Bedbugs are reddish-brown blood-sucking insects that hide in crevices in floors and walls and feed on unsuspecting victims at night. Although they are a disappearing nuisance, they are still seen occasionally in older, less affluent areas. Although most individuals sleep through the attack, sensitive victims awaken during the bloodmeal, which lasts 5 to 10 minutes. The bite is followed by an urticarial plaque, which may persist for weeks and become reactivated by subsequent bites at other sites. Lesions appear most commonly on the face and other areas not protected by clothing.

TREATMENT. The bugs are effectively eradicated from the home with insecticides such as chlordane, gamma benzene hexachloride, or hexachlorocyclohexane. Symptomatic relief may be obtained from cool compresses, topical corticosteroids, and oral antihistamines.

Kissing Bugs (Reduviidae). Although most of these insects prey upon other insects, earning them the name "assassin bug," 75 species attack man. Bites occur frequently on the face, particularly at a mucocutaneous juncture, and result in various reactions, including red papules, giant urticaria, grouped vesicles, and hemorrhagic nodular lesions.

TREATMENT. Treatment is symptomatic. Insecticides and repellants are not effective.

Fleas (Siphonaptera). Fleas are a common nuisance for humans and animals. Although there are only two parasites that are consistently associated with man, *Pulex irritans* and *Tunga penetrans*, fleas are only partially host specific, and cat and dog ectoparasites commonly attack man. The bite may go unnoticed, but sensitized individuals may discover pruritic urticarial wheals with a central hemorrhagic punctum. Multiple lesions in a linear or roseate pattern are typical.

Papular urticaria, a pruritic urticarial eruption at sites of fresh and old reactivated flea bites, occurs almost exclusively in children. Individual papules persist for 1 to 2 weeks and are found on exposed areas of the arms, legs, and trunk, sparing the buttocks and genitals. Lesions tend to recur in spring and summer but may persist year round for 3 to 4 years.

TREATMENT. Acute reactions are relieved with shake lotions (calamine), topical steroids, cool tap water compresses, and oral antihistamines. Impetiginized lesions should be treated with topical or oral antibiotics if necessary. Fleas may be eliminated by the removal or treatment of infested pets and vacuuming and spraying of carpets, floors, and other infested areas with 5 per cent malathion powder or 1 per cent lindane dust. Despite these measures fleas may survive in the household for months.

Moths and Butterflies (Lepidoptera). Contact with the hairs of the brown-tail moth indigenous to the Northeastern United States and the puss caterpillar found in the Southeastern states from Virginia to the Gulf of Mexico may produce a burning papular eruption and occasionally a severe systemic reaction.

TREATMENT. Tape stripping to remove embedded hair reduces local reactions. Systemic reactions with symptoms such as muscle cramps, headache, tachycardia, restlessness, and rarely shock and seizures require supportive therapy with antihistamines, systemic steroids, and parenteral calcium gluconate.

Flies and Mosquitoes (Diptera). These ubiquitous insects are important vectors in the transmission of viral and parasitic diseases. Mosquitoes (Culicidae) attack exposed sites on the face and extremities, producing pruritic urticarial plaques that persist for hours. Sandflies, moth flies, or owl flies (Psychodidae) bite silently, seeking out the ankles, wrist, knees, and elbows, and produce white wheals, which resolve over several days. Black flies (Simuliidae), horseflies (Tabanidae), and houseflies (Muscidae) attack silently and inflict a painful bite.

TREATMENT. Bite reactions are relieved with antihistamines, cool tap water compresses, and topical steroids. Sensitive individuals should wear protective clothing and insect repellants (Cutter, 6-12, Off).

ANIMAL AND HUMAN BITES AND BITE-RELATED INFECTIONS

JEROME A. PAULSON, M.D.

Bite wounds are very common. Mammalian bites account for 1 per cent of all emergency room visits. There are an estimated 300 reported bites per 100,000 people per year in the United States, and children are over-represented. There are probably fewer than 50 deaths per year due to mammalian bites. Snake bites are relatively common, but only 20 per cent are due to poisonous snakes. Fewer than 20 deaths per year result from snake bites among people of all ages. The frequency of spider bites is unknown. Many bites of all types never come to medical attention.

MAMMALIAN BITES

Types of Injuries

The most common mammalian bites are those caused by humans (to self or others), dogs, cats, and, at least in urban areas, rats. The injuries include scratches, abrasions, lacerations, puncture wounds, crush injuries, and avulsions. Most are minor.

Human bites may include a crush injury or an avulsion because of the strength of the jaw muscles. When the fist of one person strikes the teeth of another person, a clenched-fist injury results, usually involving the third metacarpophalangeal joint of the dominant hand. It may be associated with a phalangeal or metacarpal fracture, a laceration of the tendon, or a perforation of the joint capsule. When the joint is subsequently extended after the injury, perforation of the joint capsule may be obscured by the dorsal expansion hood of the metacarpophalangeal joint, potentially sealing in an infection.

Dog bites may also include a component of crush injury. Cats' teeth produce deep puncture wounds. Rats cause puncture wounds, small lacerations, abrasions, and hematomas without breaks in the skin.

The consideration beyond mechanical trauma is inoculation of bacteria from the mammal's mouth into the wound. Plaque on teeth is primarily bacteria at a concentration of 10^{11} organisms/gm, and saliva has approximately 10^6 organisms/ml. It requires an inoculum of approximately 10^6 organisms to cause infection.

Wound Management

If the wounds are extensive, as might be the case with a large or vicious dog or a larger wild animal, first attention must be given to *Airway*, *Breathing*, and *Circulation*.

Obtain a detailed history of the bite injury. With animal bites, the condition of the animal, whether it is a pet or a stray, and whether it is available for quarantine are all important. Important patient information includes drug allergies, prior tetanus and rabies immunizations, history of cardiac defect susceptible to subacute bacterial endocarditis, immunocompromise, and the presence of prosthetic material in the body.

Control bleeding; then check the injured area for neurovascular status and motor function. Obtain radiographs to identify retained foreign bodies, especially tooth chips, or associated fractures, especially in clenched-fist injuries.

Anesthetize the wound with 1 per cent lidocaine without epinephrine; explore it and irrigate it with a minimum of 1 L of normal saline or povidone-iodine solution. Pressure sufficient to irrigate the wound is achieved using a 35-ml syringe and a 19-gauge needle. Debride all crushed, devitalized tissue.

Bite wound lacerations should be closed, except those of the hand or foot, seen less than 2 hours after injury; those of the face may be closed up to 6 hours after injury. Wounds seen late, or grossly contaminated, or appearing clinically infected are allowed to close by secondary intent with subsequent scar revision. Puncture wounds are not sutured. With facial wounds, consideration should be given to having the wound closed by a plastic surgeon for best cosmetic results; and with hand wounds, consideration should be given to management by an orthopedic surgeon. All patients with hand wounds involving joints are managed on an inpatient basis, as are patients with osteomyelitis, septic arthritis, cellulitis, signs of systemic illness, or history of immunocompromise.

Wounds that are inflamed and/or have a purulent discharge are cultured aerobically and anaerobically. Culture of wounds that appear clean is not helpful. Human bite wounds frequently grow aerobic and anaerobic organisms, with streptococci and staphylococci being the most frequent. *Eikenella corrodens* is often found in clenched-fist wounds. Dog and cat bites become infected with many organisms, including streptococci, staphylococci, and *Pasteurella* sp. (Table 1). *P. multocida* is found in about 25 per cent of dog bite wounds and in some cat bite wounds.

The use of antibiotics for clinically infected wounds is clear cut; the use of prophylactic antibiotics is not. Infected wounds should be cultured and, pending those results, amoxicillin/clavulenate (40 mg/kg/day as amoxicillin) is a good first-choice antibiotic. Tetracyclines (40 mg/kg/day) can be used in those who are allergic to penicillins and are over 8 years and not pregnant or nursing. Cefoxitin (80 to 160 mg/kg/day in divided

TABLE 1. Bite Wound Contamination

Aerobic and Anaerobic Bacteria Isolated from Animal Bite Wounds	Bacteria in Occlusional Human Bite Wounds and Clenched-Fist Injuries
Aerobic bacteria	Aerobic bacteria
Streptococcus species	*Streptococcus* species
Alpha-hemolytic	Alpha-hemolytic
Beta-hemolytic	Beta-hemolytic
Gamma-hemolytic	Gamma-hemolytic
Staphylococcus aureus	*Staphylococcus aureus*
Staphylococcus epidermidis	*Staphylococcus epidermidis*
Staphylococcus saprophyticus	*Acinetobacter* species
Micrococcus luteus	*Eikenella corrodens*
Micrococcus species	*Neisseria gonorrhoeae*
Moraxella species	*Neisseria* species
Corynebacterium species	*Branhamella catarrhalis*
Pasteurella multocida	*Moraxella* species
Pasteurella pestis	*Micrococcus* species
Pasteurella species	*Haemophilus influenzae*
Proteus mirabilis	*Haemophilus parainfluenzae*
Bacillus species	*Haemophilus aphrophilus*
Enterobacter cloacae	*Enterobacter cloacae*
Neisseria species	*Enterobacter* species
Pseudomonas fluorescens	*Klebsiella pneumoniae*
Actinobacillus	*Nocardia* species
actinomycetemcomitans	*Corynebacterium* species
Eikenella corrodens	
Haemophilus aphrophilus	Anaerobic bacteria
Flavobacterium species	*Acidaminococcus* species
Chromobacterium species	*Actinomyces* species
M-5	*Arachnia propionica*
IIj	*Bacteroides melaninogenicus*
Streptobacillus moniliformis	*Bacteroides intermedius*
EF-4	*Bacteroides ruminicola*
DF-2	*Bacteroides disiens*
Spirillum minor	*Bacteroides oralis*
	Bacteroides ureolyticus
Anaerobic bacteria	*Bacteroides* species
Actinomyces species	*Clostridium* species
Bacteroides melaninogenicus	*Eubacterium* species
Bacteroides asaccharolyticus	*Fusobacterium nucleatum*
Bacteroides species	*Peptostreptococcus anaerobius*
Fusobacterium nucleatum	*Peptostreptococcus prevotii*
Fusobacterium russi	*Peptostreptococcus magnus*
Fusobacterium species	*Peptostreptococcus* species
Peptostreptococcus prevotii	
Peptostreptococcus magnus	
Peptostreptococcus species	
Veillonella parvula	
Proprionibacterium acnes	
Proprionibacterium granulosum	
Propionibacterium species	
Eubacterium species	
Leptotrichia buccalis	

From Goldstein & Richwald: Human and animal bite wounds. Am Fam Phys 36:101–109, 1987, published by the American Academy of Family Physicians.

doses intravenously or intramuscularly) is used to cover expected flora in patients in whom tetracyclines are also contraindicated.

The wound is dressed and the extremity is placed in a position of function and elevated.

Give a tetanus toxoid booster if the patient is more than 5 years past the last tetanus immunization, and give 250 units of human immune tetanus globulin if the patient is totally unimmunized.

Potential Complications (Including Rabies)

Infection is the most common complication of bite wounds that have been closed or that presented late for treatment. With clenched-fist injuries and other bites near joints, septic arthritis may occur. Cat bites, because of their depth, and other bites over superficial bones may lead to osteomyelitis. Initial antibiotic management is as suggested above, with definitive management depending on culture results.

In patients with certain cardiac lesions, subacute bacterial endocarditis may develop; and in patients with implanted prosthetic devices, infection at the prosthesis may develop. Patients who are immunocompromised, e.g., an infant infected with HIV living in poor housing and sustaining a rat bite, may develop systemic infection. Antibiotic coverage in these situations should be guided by an infectious disease expert.

Rat bites may develop delayed infections within 1 to 3 weeks due to *Spirillum minus* or *Streptobacillus moniliformis*. The former presents with an indurated lesion at the bite site, regional adenopathy, a diffuse macular erythematous or purple rash, intermittent fever, and myalgias. The latter manifests with fevers, rigors, and severe headache along with a dull red maculopapular rash on the limbs and polyarthritis. Treat both infections with intravenous or intramuscular penicillin (100,000 to 250,000 U/kg/day), or tetracycline (10 to 20 mg/kg/day) for the penicillin-allergic.

Rabies may occur after a bite or a nonbite exposure (a scratch, abrasion, open wound, or mucous membrane contaminated with animal saliva or other potentially infected material such as brain). In the United States, most domestic animals are rabies-free, but those most likely to be rabid are cows, cats, and dogs. Rodents and lagomorphs (rabbits) rarely have rabies. Humans are most likely to be exposed to rabies by wild animals: skunks, raccoons, bats, foxes, coyotes, and bobcats.

Capture all biting animals if possible. Observe domestic animals for 10 days. If the bite was unprovoked or the animal manifests abnormal behavior during observation, it is sacrificed and its brain processed for fluorescent antibody examination. Wild animals are sacrificed and examined immediately. Prior prophylactic vaccination of the animal to prevent rabies is not an absolute guarantee that the animal is not rabid.

Obtain advice regarding the need for rabies immunization from the state health department, a decision on immunization must be made quickly because the longer treatment is postponed, the less likely it is to be effective. Wash the wound with soap and water. If the bite or nonbite exposure came from an animal known to be rabid or an animal likely to be rabid which was not captured, immunization is started. The patient receives 1 ml of human diploid cell rabies vaccine (HDCV) intramuscularly as soon as possible after exposure and 3, 7, 14, and 28 days later. (The World Health Organization recommends a sixth dose at 90 days.) Give rabies immune globulin, human (RIG) at 20 international units/kg. Up to half the dose is infiltrated into the area around the wound (do not compromise circulation) and the remainder is given intramuscularly in a different extremity than the HDCV. RIG may be given up to the eighth day after the first dose of HDCV, if it is delayed for some reason.

VENOMOUS ANIMAL BITES
Snake Bites

Types of Snakes. There are two families of poisonous snakes in the United States: (1) *Crotalidae* or pit vipers, including rattlesnakes, copperheads, and cottonmouths, and (2) *Elapidae*, of which only the coral snake is poisonous. *Crotalidae* are widely distributed in the United States, although primarily in the South and Southwest. Coral snakes are found in the South.

The following identifies pit vipers: a pit midway between the eye and the nostril on both sides of a triangular head, an elliptical pupil, the presence of fangs, and a single row of subcaudal plates. Nonvenomous snakes have no pit, a rounded head, a round pupil, no fangs, and a double row of subcaudal plates. Coral snakes are identified by their color pattern: The nose is black and the red and yellow bands are adjacent. A nonvenomous kingsnake has its red and yellow bands separated by a black band.

Snake venoms are mixtures of glycoproteins, polypeptides, low molecular weight compounds, and enzymes, giving them cytotoxic, hemotoxic, neurotoxic, and cardiotoxic effects. Prognostic factors in individual snake bites include whether venom was injected (up to one fifth of pit viper bites and up to one half of coral snake bites are dry); the character and amount of clothing between the snake and the skin; the size of the snake; the species of the snake; the length of time the fangs were in the victim; the number of bites; the age of the victim (younger, worse); and the proximity of the bite to the trunk.

First Aid. Do the following: (1) put the victim at rest; (2) calm the victim and give reassurance; (3) immobilize the affected extremity; (4) observe for signs of shock; (5) if possible, identify the snake or kill it and bring it in with the victim (transport it in a bag or at the end of a stick, as dead snakes can cause envenomation); (6) transport the patient to the hospital as soon as possible.

Do *not* do the following: (1) immerse the extremity in ice; (2) apply a tourniquet; or (3) excise the bite area. Incision and suction are not recommended because it is useless for *Elapidae* bites and useful in *Crotalidae* bites only if performed within 5 minutes of the bite.

Definitive Management. Initial hospital management consists of identification of the snake and determination of whether envenomation occurred. The latter is heralded by the presence of fang marks and local signs and symptoms: swelling, discoloration, and pain. Mojave rattlesnake venom may cause only slight local reaction. Coral snake bites may have no swelling, only minimal pain, and local numbness and/or weakness.

If the snake was a pit viper, start a large-bore intravenous line, perform a base-line physical examination—pulse, respiration, blood pressure, and circumference of the affected extremity, and laboratory studies—typing and cross-matching of blood, bleeding time, clotting time, clot retraction time, partial thromboplastin time, fibrinogen, fibrin split products, CBC and red cell morphology, platelet count, urinalysis, BUN, and electrolytes. For severe envenomation, also do electrocardiography, arterial blood gases, and pH. Because the venom of a coral snake is primarily a neurotoxin, the clotting studies and most other blood studies are not needed.

Evaluate the severity of pit viper envenomation as follows:

Minimal—Puncture wound. 1 to 6 inches of edema and erythema in the first 12 hours. Moderate pain. No systemic signs.

Moderate—Puncture wound. 6 to 12 inches of edema and erythema in the first 12 hours. Severe pain. Petechiae and ecchymosis. Weakness, nausea, and vomiting. Bloody ooze from fang marks.

Severe—Puncture wound. Greater than 12 inches of edema and erythema. Rapid onset of systemic signs and symptoms noted above.

Very severe—Sudden pain. Rapid local swelling spreading proximally. Ecchymoses, progressive edema, bleb formation, rupture of skin, decreased venous and arterial blood flow. Weakness, vertigo, numbness, fasciculations, painful muscle cramps, tingling of face and head. Yellow vision or blindness. Shock, nausea, vomiting, incontinence, bleeding, and renal, hepatic, and cardiac dysfunction. Seizures. Coma and death.

Envenomation by the pit viper is treated with antivenin (Crotalidae) polyvalent (Wyeth), a horse serum product. Perform a skin test prior to using the antivenin by injecting intradermally 0.02 ml of 1:10 dilution of the serum. Use 0.02 ml of normal saline as the control.

With a negative test, start a second intravenous line and give the antivenin within 4 hours of, and no more than 24 hours after, the bite. Give 5 vials for a minimal envenomation, 10 vials for moderate, and 15 vials for severe. Children and small adults require larger doses of antivenin, as does the treatment of the bite of C. scutulatus (Mojave rattlesnake). Dilute antivenin in D5W or normal saline and give quickly, but no more than 20 ml/kg/hr. Additional antivenin (1 to 5 vials every 2 hours) must be given if swelling of the extremity continues or if systemic signs or symptoms increase or new ones develop. An airway, oxygen, epinephrine, an injectable pressor amine, and corticosteroids must be available to treat a hypersensitivity reaction to the antivenin, even if the skin test was negative. Prednisone 2 mg/kg/day in four divided doses or its equivalent is the agent of choice for treating delayed (1 to 2 weeks) reactions to antivenin.

Coral snake envenomation is treated with 5 vials of Micrurus fulvius antivenin (Wyeth) diluted in 250 ml of intravenous fluid and given rapidly (maximum 20 ml/kg/hr).

Closely monitor vital signs, central venous pressure, and respiratory and cardiac status. Give colloids as needed to treat shock and blood or blood products to treat hemolysis or bleeding. Give clotting factors, fresh frozen plasma, or platelets as needed to treat clotting problems. Exchange transfusion is indicated for severe coagulopathy. Pain is managed with acetaminophen. Because coral snake venom and Mojave rattlesnake venom are neurotoxic, mechanical ventilation is indicated for respiratory failure.

Skin lesions are treated as burns with daily cleaning and débridement. Splint the extremity in a position of function slightly lower than the heart. Antibiotics are indicated if incision and suction were erroneously used in the field or if there is secondary infection of the skin lesions. Monitor renal status with urine output, urinalysis, and serum chemistries. Adjust intravenous fluids accordingly.

Rehabilitation of the affected extremity can begin within 4 to 5 days.

Spider and Scorpion Bites

Types of Spiders and Scorpions. The following are the types of spiders and scorpions in the United States which can cause systemic reactions. Spiders: members of the *Latrodectus* genus, especially *L. mactans mactans* (black widow) and members of the *Loxosceles* genus, especially *L. reclusa* (brown recluse). Scorpions: *Centruroides sculpturatus* and *C. gertschi*. The sting of *Hadrurus arizonensis*, a scorpion, and of tarantulas native to the United States cause only local reactions.

Latrodectus Bites. Black widow spiders are found throughout the United States. They spin disorganized webs in closed spaces. They are black, and the female has a red hourglass-shaped mark on the ventral abdomen. When a child is bitten, the spider should be captured for identification, if possible.

The initial bite is like a sharp pin prick or is painless, leaving two tiny puncture wounds. Within several minutes, there is local erythema and edema. Over the next hour, regional symptoms develop: dull crampy pains followed by severe muscle pains and numbness spreading from the bite. The abdomen may become rigid. There is associated anxiety, headache, dizziness, fever, salivation, nausea, vomiting, speech disturbance, priapism, urinary retention, and muscle fasciculations. There may be associated renal compromise, seizures, shock, cardiac and respiratory failure, and brain hemorrhage.

Hospitalize symptomatic children and those under 5 and monitor them closely in an ICU setting. Perform a CBC, electrolyte, BUN, and clotting studies, urinalysis, and ECG. Give *Latrodectus* antivenin (Merck, Sharp and Dohme): 1 vial in 50 ml normal saline intravenously over 15 minutes after appropriately testing for sensitivity to horse serum (see snake bite antivenin above). Give propranolol for hypertension. Use calcium gluconate, 10 ml of 10 per cent solution intravenously, for symptomatic treatment and repeat every 2 to 4 hours. Morphine is used for analgesia. Methocarbamol and other muscle relaxants are ineffective. Give tetanus prophylaxis as described above and antibiotics to cover skin flora if evidence of infection develops.

***Loxoscles* Bites.** Brown recluse spiders occur throughout the central and southern United States and are identified by a brown violin-shaped mark on the body. They live in abandoned houses, cellars, wood piles, and trash heaps. When a child is bitten, the spider should be captured for identification if possible.

Loxoscles venom causes endothelial damage leading to thrombocytopenia, decreased fibrinogen, and prolonged thromboplastin time. The bite is initially painless but is followed by local pruritus, pain, and erythema. A blister forms, and over several days the local area becomes necrotic secondary to the vascular damage. An ulcer develops which, if larger than 1 cm, may last for weeks and become secondarily infected. A diffuse scarletiniform, morbilliform, urticarial, or petechial rash may develop on the trunk and in the flexural creases and is associated with a poor prognosis. Other systemic signs, known as viscerocutaneous loxosclism, may develop within 72 hours, especially in children: malaise, restlessness, jaundice, generalized urticaria, arthritis, myalgias, headache, seizures, fever, vomiting, diarrhea, hematuria, hemoglobinuria, proteinuria, anuria, shock, and coma.

There is no antivenin for *Loxosecles* bites. Treat local reactions of less than 2 cm with oral analgesics and sterile dressings. Treat larger local reactions with débridement and give oral prednisone (1 to 2 mg/kg/day) or its equivalent for 5 days. Treat viscerocutaneous loxosclism with supportive therapy in an ICU as described above for serious black widow spider bites. Give special attention to renal function because of the hemoglobinuria. Give prednisone at 1 to 2 mg/kg/day or its equivalent. Treat large ulcers with excision and skin grafting. Dapsone (100 mg/day in divided doses) has been described as decreasing the size of the ulcer, speeding healing, and obviating the need for surgery in adults. Give tetanus prophylaxis as indicated by current status and use antibiotics if the wound becomes secondarily infected.

Scorpion Bites. *C. sculpturatus* and *C. gertschi* are nocturnal and found in the desert southwest. *C. sculpturatus*, small, yellow and lacking stripes, is the more dangerous scorpion. The venom contains neurotoxins and other substances, but usually causes only local reactions: severe local pain and paresthesias. Systemic symptoms, if they develop, usually do so within 3 hours: itchy mouth, eyes, and throat; impaired speech, numbness, drowsiness, agitation, roving eye movements, stridor, nausea, vomiting, and incontinence. Local treatment consists of ice or injectable local anesthetic for pain relief. Give acetaminophen orally, but narcotic analgesics are contraindicated. Give barbiturates for seizures; paraldehyde is contraindicated. Antivenin should be given for systemic reactions and is available from the Antivenom Production Laboratory, Arizona State University. Call the regional poison control center at 602-253-3334. Give tetanus prophylaxis as indicated.

BURNS

LAURIE S. AHLGREN, M.D.

Each year one million Americans are burned. One third of these burn victims are children less than 15 years of age. Although many of the burns children sustain require minimal medical attention, over 30,000 of these injuries require hospitalization, and 3000 are fatal. Scald injury is the most prevalent burn in childhood, and accounts for 45 per cent of burn admissions in children under 4 years of age. While clothing ignition is now a rare cause of death in childhood, it is responsible for 10 per cent of all nonfatal hospital burn admissions. Seventy-five per cent of pediatric burn fatalities occur in housefires in which the child is unable to escape.

The ABC's of life support are of utmost importance to burn victims. If inhalation injury is suspected, humidified oxygen should be administered immediately by mask or nasal prongs. An adequate airway must be established. Early nasotracheal intubation is indicated for progressive airway edema or unmanageable secretions. Intubation is also indicated if hypoxemia persists despite supplemental oxygen therapy. This is seen most commonly in inhalation injuries and full-thickness burns of the chest.

Children with burns greater than 20 per cent of the body surface area (BSA) and infants with burns greater than 15 per cent of the BSA require intravenous fluids to maintain adequate perfusion. Management of less extensive burns associated with inhalation injury or burns resulting from chemicals or electricity also requires venous access. These patients must have a large-bore intravenous line placed in an unburned area and maintenance Ringer's lactate solution infused until proper fluid replacement can be calculated. Cut-down and central venous cannulation, which have higher rates of septic and technical complications, should be avoided unless percutaneous venous access is impossible or central venous pressure monitoring is imperative.

Fluid Resuscitation

Estimates of fluid needs for the first 24 hours after the burn are based on the depth and extent of BSA injured. Lund and Bowder charts, which allow for the inversely changing proportionate size of children's heads and extremities, aid in estimating the percentage of surface area burned to the second or third degree. Areas of first degree burn are not used in fluid therapy calculations.

For most children the Parkland formula, infusing 4 ml of Ringer's lactate/kg/per cent BSA burned, offers the best fluid resuscitation. One half of the calculated fluid is given over the first 8 hours of therapy. The patient's response to therapy, however, determines the rate of infusion. Pulse and blood pressure must be restored. Once vital signs, acid-base balance, and mental status are within normal limits, urine output becomes a sensitive indicator of adequate perfusion. Fluid therapy is modified to maintain the patient's urine output at 1 to 2 ml/kg/hr. This modification usually results in older children receiving 3 ml/kg/per cent BSA burned and in infants receiving 5 ml/kg/per cent BSA burned for the first 24 hours.

During the second 24 hours after the burn, the patient will begin to resorb edema fluid and diurese. Consequently, only one half to three fourths of the first day's fluid requirement is infused as 5 per cent dextrose in 0.5 normal saline. Colloid, in the form of albumin or fresh frozen plasma, is administered at a rate of 0.5 ml/kg/per cent BSA burned. After 48 hours the evaporative fluid loss is 85 per cent free water and is replaced at a rate of 1 to 2 ml/kg/per cent BSA burned using 5 per cent dextrose in 0.25 normal saline. Potassium supplementation and red blood cell transfusion may also be needed.

Patients with burns less than 20 per cent BSA can be managed by increasing their oral fluid intake an average of 1 per cent for each per cent BSA burned. Care must be taken to prevent the child from preferentially imbibing excess free water, since this can rapidly lead to hyponatremia. Infants should continue their regular formula. Older children should be offered full liquids or dietary supplements that provide calories as well as salt and water. A return to a normal diet in 1 to 2 days is advisable, with continued surveillance of free water intake. Teenagers especially have become hyponatremic after water and soft drinks are allowed ad lib.

Wound Care and Triage

Emergency room physicians must triage burns into one of three groups: minor, major, critical.

Minor Burns. Minor burns are those covering less than 10 per cent BSA and involving less than 2 per cent full-thickness injury. They are generally treated on an out-patient basis. First aid to minor burns includes cooling the burn with water or ice. The burn is then gently cleansed with saline. Blebs and blisters are left intact. Closed bulky dressings are applied after a thin coating of silver sulfadiazine. Tetanus prophylaxis is given if needed, but no antibiotics are prescribed. Parents are instructed to return the child for a dressing change in 2 days or immediately if the dressing falls off or if the child's temperature rises above 39°C (102°F).

Major Burns. Patients with major burns encompassing greater than 10 per cent BSA or more than 2 per cent third-degree injury require inpatient care. Hospitalization should also be considered in children less than 2 years of age and in children with burns to the hands, feet, face, or perineum; in those with flame burns or electrical burns; and in children who are suspected victims of child abuse. It is often desirable to admit children with lesser burns who come from questionable social situations and observe parental care of the wound for 1 to 2 days before beginning out-patient treatment.

Initial care to major burns differs from minor burn care in that the wound is débrided of all loose skin and blisters using strict sterile technique. Analgesia, using 0.05 mg/kg morphine sulfate or 0.5 mg/kg meperidine hydrochloride intravenous push, can be given during wound débridement.

Escharotomies may be needed to enhance blood flow to extremities with circumferential burns or to allow ventilation in extensive chest burns. Loss of Doppler flow pulsations in digital arteries is a reliable indication for performing escharotomies. Incisions are made through the entire thickness of the burn on the lateral aspects of the extremity. Escharotomies to the chest are along the lower costal margin. Since the burns that necessitate escharotomies are full-thickness burns, local anesthesia is not needed.

Following burn débridement, the application of silver sulfadiazine is quite soothing. Occlusive bulky dressings complete the initial wound care. Baseline weights, serum electrolytes, glucose and osmolality, CBC, arterial blood gas levels, and nasopharyngeal cultures are obtained. Carbon monoxide levels are determined if the child was burned in an enclosed space. Tetanus prophylaxis is given as needed. Penicillin is administered prophylactically only if the patient has a known cardiac anomaly or a concomitant streptococcal infection.

Critical Burns. Critical burns are those that cover more than 30 per cent BSA or involve electrical, "crush" type, or inhalation injuries. These children should be transferred to regional burn centers. Prior to transport, the airway must be assured, a reliable intravenous line must be established, fluid resuscitation must be instituted, and a nasogastric tube and a bladder catheter must be placed. The burn should be wrapped in dry sterile dressings, and if vital signs allow, the patient may have mild intravenous sedation.

Special Problems

Ileus. Ileus following extensive burns is not uncommon, and gastric dilatation with vomiting and aspiration may occur. The subsequent chemical pneumonitis superimposed on the pulmonary response to burn injury may be lethal. Nasogastric decompression is, therefore, mandatory until the intestinal tract is known to be working.

Fever. Fevers up to 39°C (102°F) are routinely seen in burn victims, especially in burned children. This febrile response is not completely understood but is thought to represent pyrogens released during the body's natural inflammatory response to injury. The fevers often persist until the eschar is removed. Antipyretics are usually not efficacious. Tympanic membranes, throats, and burn wounds should be inspected, but extensive septic work-ups are not indicated unless the temperature exceeds 40°C (104°F).

Sepsis. Sepsis is the major cause of death in critically burned patients who survive to hospitalization. *Pseudomonas aeruginosa* is now the main lethal bacterial invader. Topical burn therapy is geared toward local control. One-half per cent silver nitrate solution, the original topical antibiotic, is not used in children because of the hyponatremia that can occur, sometimes within hours. Mafenide acetate 10 per cent cream (Sulfamylon) penetrates eschar well and kills *Pseudomonas*. Unfortunately, because of its carbonic anhydrase inhibition, it causes a metabolic acidosis that makes it unsuitable for use in children. Silver sulfadiazine 1 per cent cream penetrates eschar moderately well and kills *Pseudomonas*. Unlike both silver nitrate and mafenide acetate, it is not painful when applied. Although leukopenia following silver sulfadiazine therapy has been seen, the clinical significance of this side effect has not been well established. It is, therefore, the topical antibiotic of choice in children.

Despite topical therapy, wound surveillance is imperative to ensure early recognition of burn wound sepsis. Quantitative wound cultures growing more than 10^6 organisms/cm^2 demand additional wound débridement and appropriate systemic antibiotic administration. Antistreptococcal prophylaxis (penicillin) is recommended only for patients with valvular heart disease, patients with concomitant or recent streptococcal infection, and patients whose admission throat cultures are positive for hemolytic *Streptococcus*. Tetanus prophylaxis is indicated if the patient has not been adequately immunized.

Inhalation Injuries. Inhalation injuries may not be readily apparent. Burns on the face, singed nasal hairs, and carbonaceous sputum all suggest inhalation injury, but just as their presence does not confirm inhalation injury, neither does their absence exclude it. Early flexible bronchoscopy may be necessary to establish the diagnosis. Once the presence of inhalation injury is established, the treatment consists of the administration of 100 per cent oxygen and observation for one of the following clinical phases.

The first phase occurs 1 to 12 hours after the burn and is characterized by laryngeal edema, bronchospasm, or acute lung consolidation. Laryngeal edema produces a prolonged inspiratory phase and is best treated by endotracheal intubation. Bronchospasm has a prolonged expiratory phase with wheezing and is best treated by a croup tent and a single large intravenous dose of corticosteroids. Acute lung consolidation is characterized by progressive hypoxemia, and its fulminant course is rarely moderated by full ventilatory support.

Phase two occurs 6 to 72 hours after the burn and manifests as pulmonary edema. Leaky pulmonary capillaries and fluid overload account for this clinical picture. Standard medical management of pulmonary edema, including fluid restriction and diuretics, is effective in most cases.

Phase three occurs in children with severe inhalation injuries who manage to survive 3 days after the burn. They almost universally acquire a staphylococcal or gram-negative bronchopneumonia. Good pulmonary toilet and bacteria-specific systemic antibiotics give the best chance of survival for this third clinical phase of inhalation injuries.

Nutrition. Nutrition is a common problem in children with burns of greater than 30 per cent BSA. Burn ileus, fever, and pain reduce appetite. The hypermetabolic state associated with large burns may require up to four times basal caloric needs. In addition, heat calories are lost through evaporation unless the ambient temperature is near 34°C (101°F) with high humidity. It may be physically impossible for the child to eat enough to supply the necessary calories. Supplemental enteral nutrition via nocturnal nasogastric tube feeding remedies this problem with minimal patient discomfort. Rarely, total parenteral nutrition is necessary to provide adequate calories, but it is recommended that the total parenteral nutrition catheter be changed every 3 days over a guide wire to reduce the risk of catheter sepsis.

Facial Burns. Facial burns in children fortunately are rarely full-thickness burns. Because it is difficult to dress the face occlusively, the burns are gently cleansed, débrided, thinly coated with an antibiotic ointment, and left open. The ointment should be reapplied as needed to keep the wound covered. The eyes should be examined by an ophthalmologist before soft-tissue swelling obscures the view. Occasionally, full-thickness burns to the eyelids require tarsorrhaphy to protect the eyes during healing.

NEAR-DROWNING

J. MICHAEL DEAN, M.D.

Drowning is a leading cause of death in children, and near-drowning is associated with significant morbidity.

Near-drowning is strictly defined as an immersion accident in which the victim does not die within 24 hours. For our purposes here, however, the term near-drowning will be used for all patients who survive the accident long enough to reach the hospital.

Emergency management consists of immediate ventilation and restoration, if necessary, of circulation. The airway should be cleared of debris and vomitus, and mouth-to-mouth ventilation should be started as quickly as possible (even while the patient is still in the water). If cardiac arrest has occurred, it is secondary to respiratory arrest, and ventilation and oxygenation may restore spontaneous cardiac activity. If the child requires cardiopulmonary resuscitation, he should be transported to a hospital, and resuscitation should be continued (i.e., he should not be pronounced dead at the scene under any circumstances). If the child is hypothermic, the resuscitation efforts must continue until the child's temperature exceeds 30 to 31°C (86 to 87.8°F); with temperatures below this level, cardiac resuscitation may be impossible. In addition, profound hypothermia (under 31°C or 87.8°F) will depress the neurologic system, and lack of findings on examination of the child may be incorrectly suggestive of brain death. Thus, unless it is known that the child was under water for an extremely long time (several hours), resuscitation efforts must continue until the temperature is relatively normal. Following restoration of the heart beat, hypothermia should be corrected slowly, at a rate not to exceed 1°C (1.8°F) per hour.

Respiratory failure often occurs in these victims. Children who are breathing should be placed on 100 per cent oxygen by mask, and after stabilization, they may be weaned according to arterial blood gas measurements. If the PO_2 cannot be maintained above 100 mm Hg in 50 per cent or less oxygen, then continuous positive airway pressure should be employed, which requires endotracheal intubation. Children who cannot maintain normal carbon dioxide tension (35 to 40 mm Hg) should also be intubated and must be mechanically ventilated. While setting up for intubation, the physician must ventilate the child with a bag and mask and maintain the patency of the airway. If mask ventilation is used, this will increase gastric distention, and the risk of aspiration is increased. Therefore, nasogastric tubes should be placed in these children early in their management to prevent the potentially disastrous complications of aspiration pneumonia.

By far the most difficult problem in near-drowning is the insult to the central nervous system. An estimate of the severity of injury is possible from the first hospital evaluation using the Glasgow coma scale (Table 1).

Children who have *initial* Glasgow scores under 8 are at high risk of neurologic sequelae and intracranial hypertension; children who have a better Glasgow coma score at the first hospital evaluation have a uniformly good outcome. Children with Glasgow coma scores of 7 or less should be monitored for intracranial hypertension and treated appropriately if it occurs. Children in this category (Glasgow score <8) should be intubated, hyperventilated moderately (carbon dioxide tension 25 to 35 mm Hg), and kept on a fluid-restricted diet. The

TABLE 1. The Glasgow Coma Scale

	Points
Eye Opening	
No response	1
Response to pain	2
Response to voice	3
Spontaneously	4
Verbal Response	
No response	1
Incomprehensible sounds	2
Inappropriate words	3
Disoriented conversation	4
Oriented and appropriate	5
Motor Response	
No response	1
Decerebrate posturing	2
Decorticate posturing	3
Flexion withdrawal	4
Localizes pain	5
Obeys commands	6
Maximum Score	15

head should be elevated 30 degrees and kept in the midline (to avoid jugular venous obstruction). Endotracheal suctioning should be minimized if there is intracranial hypertension.

Intracranial pressure monitoring is accomplished with a subarachnoid bolt or an intraventricular drain, which is inserted by a neurosurgeon. Cerebral perfusion pressure is maintained above 50 mm Hg and is calculated as mean arterial pressure minus the mean intracranial pressure. In order to do this calculation, the transducers must be referenced to the same level (i.e., the heart). If the intracranial pressure exceeds 20 mm Hg or if the cerebral perfusion pressure drops below 50 mm Hg, mannitol 0.25 gm/kg is administered to lower intracranial pressure. Hyperventilation may be increased (decreasing PCO_2 to 20 mm Hg). Fever should be aggressively prevented, but hypothermia is dangerous and without proven benefit. If seizures occur, they should be very aggressively treated, since seizure activity will exacerbate the primary neuronal injury. If an intraventricular drain has been used for monitoring pressure, cerebrospinal fluid may be drained, thus lowering intracranial pressure. If intracranial pressure continues to be elevated despite normothermia, absence of seizures, hyperventilation, and mannitol therapy, then barbiturate coma may be instituted. This is accomplished with a loading dose of 5 mg/kg pentobarbital, followed by 1 to 5 mg/kg/hr continuous intravenous infusion. This therapy will lead to cardiac depression, often requires sophisticated hemodynamic support, and should not be attempted in the absence of a Swan-Ganz catheter. While barbiturates are often effective in lowering intracranial pressure, their benefit on long-term outcome is doubtful.

The prognosis of children who arrive at the hospital awake is excellent, and careful attention to pulmonary disease will result in normal survival. Children who are comatose on presentation have a poor outcome if they do not start to awaken within 6 hours. Children who on the first hospital evaluation have a Glasgow coma score less than 8 are at high risk of neurologic sequelae or death. Children in this category who survive with normal outcomes generally have not suffered persistent intracranial hypertension at any time in their hospital course; the occurrence of refractory intracranial hypertension is an extremely grim prognostic sign. The origin of sufficient cerebral edema to lead to intracranial hypertension is primarily cytotoxic, owing to neuronal death, and it is doubtful that any measures will salvage children with this degree of injury. Intracranial pressure monitoring *may* be of value in two respects. One, efforts can be made to avoid the development of intracranial hypertension, and an increase of intracranial pressure can alert the clinician to take further steps in its treatment. Two, if the child develops persistent intracranial hypertension (above 20 to 30 mm Hg despite treatment), consideration may be given to limiting further resuscitative efforts.

In contrast to earlier reports, near-drowning is a lethal disease in cold or warm water, and severely brain-injured children have a grim prognosis. With all these limitations, however, one can expect to salvage (with good neurologic outcome) about 10 to 15 per cent of all children who present to the hospital without any neurologic function (Glasgow coma score = 3) in full cardiac arrest. This is similar to the other populations of children who have suffered cardiac arrest outside the hospital. Intracranial pressure monitoring or other brain resuscitative measures appear to have had minimal impact on this survival rate. However, 15 per cent salvage justifies continued recommendations to resuscitate all children involved in immersion accidents.

21

Unclassified Diseases

LANGERHANS CELL HISTIOCYTOSIS (THE HISTIOCYTOSIS SYNDROMES)

NORMAN JAFFE, M.D., D.Sc.

Histiocytosis X is an eponym for a spectrum of rare disorders with protean manifestations. Histologically, they are characterized by the formation of granulomata and infiltration and proliferation by histiocytes. Traditionally, as originally proposed by Lichtenstein, the disorders were classified as eosinophilic granuloma, Hand-Schüller-Christian disease, and Letterer-Siwe disease, and it was believed that transition occurred unidirectionally from eosinophilic granuloma through Hand-Schüller-Christian to Letterer-Siwe disease. The current nomenclature, Langerhans cell histiocytosis, is derived from the abnormal accumulation or proliferation of cells bearing a Langerhans cell phenotype. Included in the latter is an expression of HLA-DR Antigens, T-6 surface antigen, S-100 intracellular protein, and Birbeck granules detected by electron microscopy. The disease is not necessarily malignant in the classic pathologic sense, but it is generally treated by oncologists.

Patients with Langerhans cell histiocytosis characteristically present with infiltrations of the abnormal cell in the bone, skin, liver, spleen, lung, brain, and other organs. The disease may be localized or diffuse. Consequently, in an effort to systematize the manifestations and provide specific therapy, it is still convenient to discuss the diagnosis and management according to the classification originally proposed by Lichtenstein.

EOSINOPHILIC GRANULOMA

The disorder is most frequently seen in children and adolescents. It is characterized by a lytic lesion in bone manifesting as pain and swelling with a predilection for the skull, femur, rib, pelvis, vertebra, and mandible. The majority of cases are solitary, but two or more lesions are not rare. Investigations to define the extent of disease include radiographic examination of the affected bone, a skeletal survey, chest radiography, hemogram, and liver function studies. Radionuclide

bone studies may occasionally demonstrate the existence of silent lesions. The diagnosis is generally established by surgical biopsy, and cure can invariably be achieved by curettage. In isolated circumstances in which the lesion is considered inoperable, radiation therapy (300 cGy/day for 3 days) has been utilized. The latter may also be considered for multiple lesions. Spontaneous healing, particularly following surgical biopsy, is a well-established entity.

At The University of Texas M. D. Anderson Cancer Center, tissue is generally obtained by needle biopsy under fluoroscopic guidance. Concurrently, following cytologic demonstration of the diagnosis, the disease is treated with instillation of methylprednisolone (Solu-Medrol 150 mg). Because transient expansion of the medullary cavity may cause extreme pain, in patients under 10 years of age, treatment is implemented under general anesthesia. The procedure is extremely useful for lesions located adjacent to the epiphyseal plate which, if damaged by radiation therapy or surgical trauma, may affect normal growth. With cortisone instillation, lesions generally heal within 2 to 3 months.

Follow-up radiographic studies at monthly intervals for 6 to 12 months are required to confirm the healing process. A localized extraosseous form of eosinophilic granuloma involving the lung has also been described. It is characterized by spontaneous pneumothorax, occasional cough, fatigue, and weight loss. The disease is probably related to the Hand-Schüller-Christian or Letterer-Siwe variety and is more appropriately treated with combination chemotherapy (see below).

HAND-SCHÜLLER-CHRISTIAN DISEASE

The disease is characterized by a triad of signs: lytic skull lesions, exophthalmos, and diabetes insipidus. The complete spectrum is rarely seen, and patients usually present with one or more of the triad in association with extracranial bone, cutaneous, or pulmonary lesions. The cutaneous lesions are of the seborrheic or eczematoid variety. Hepatosplenomegaly and lymphadenopathy occur infrequently. Investigations to determine the extent of disease include a skeletal survey, bone marrow examination, hemogram, and liver function studies. Radionuclide bone studies may infrequently reveal the full (silent) extent of bone involvement. The hemogram is generally normal, although occasionally a slightly elevated erythrocyte sedimentation rate and mild leukocytosis may be observed.

Treatment usually involves cytotoxic agents. The vinca alkaloid velban (0.1 mg/kg), administered concurrently with prednisone (60 mg/m² daily in divided dose), is a preferred combination. The latter is administered on a 3-week cycle: velban on days 1 and 4, and prednisone alternate days for 14 days, followed by a rest interval of 1 week. Treatment is usually maintained for 1 year. These agents have not been associated with delayed permanent sequelae.

Responses usually occur within several weeks of initiation of treatment. This manifests as improvement in the clinical status; however, radiographic healing of bone lesions is usually delayed, and complete resolution may be noted only 2 to 3 years later. Cure of diabetes insipidus is rare, but it may occasionally be achieved with radiation therapy (2000 cGy).

LETTERER-SIWE DISEASE

This usually manifests as an acute or subacute disorder with fever, hepatosplenomegaly, lymphadenopathy, rash, and anemia. Bone lesions may not necessarily be detected. Clinical symptomatology includes irritability, fever, earache, pain, cough, lymphadenopathy, hepatosplenomegaly, dyspnea, pallor, petechiae, and otitis media with chronically draining ears. Typically, the skin eruption occurs behind the ears on the scalp and in the diaper area. Initially, the lesions may be diagnosed as cradle cap, seborrheic dermatitis, or diaper rash. Widespread petechiae and purpura are common. Involvement of the liver, spleen, and lymph nodes is in direct proportion to the degree of diffuse infiltration.

Blood and bone marrow findings reflect the degree of infiltration. Radiographic examination of the lungs may reveal diffuse bilateral interstitial pneumonitis or a "honey-combed" lung. The picture may be complicated by spontaneous pneumothorax. A variety of neurologic disturbances, including incoordination, dysarthria, hyper-reflexia, weakness, and impairment of intellectual capacity, have been noted. Involvement of the jaws and teeth may occur. The latter manifests initially as erosion of the lamina dura, after which the teeth become loose and appear to "float" on the dental radiograph.

Lahey has published a linear relationship correlating the extent of disease (Lahey score) and mortality. There is zero mortality for a score of 1 to 2, with increasing mortality of 50 to 75 per cent for a score of 5 or 6. The score comprises evidence of involvement of each of the following: skin, liver, spleen, lung, pituitary, skeleton, and hematopoietic system. The latter comprises anemia (hemoglobin less than 10.5 gm/dl), an abnormal leukocyte count (less than 3,000 or greater than 14,000 WBC/mm³) or thrombocytopenia (less than 200,000/mm³), and/or hemorrhagic skin lesions. Organ dysfunction appears to be a more significant determinant of mortality (66 per cent) than absence of these abnormalities (4 per cent). Children under the age of 3 years carry a greater mortality. The disease may occasionally recur several years after apparent cure.

Many chemotherapeutic agents are utilized for Letterer-Siwe disease. Initially, a vinca alkaloid and corticosteroid as described for Hand-Schüller-Christian disease are administered. These are usually successful in producing improvement and probably cure in a majority of affected children. As long as improvement is apparent, treatment is maintained. However, occasionally the disease appears stationary and quiescent; treatment may then be discontinued and complete resolution will probably be noted several months later. Most therapeutic protocols recommend treatment for 1 to 2 years with discontinuation 6 to 12 months later if the clinical manifestations appear under control or are in the process of abating.

Radiographic evidence of bone involvement does not necessarily disappear once clinical manifestations have become quiescent. Follow-up radiographic studies of the lesions at 2- to 3-month intervals after discontinuation of therapy may be required. This determines if the disease has become stationary or has remitted and will eventually heal.

Patients who fail to respond to a vinca alkaloid and corticosteroid or who relapse are treated with alkylating agents or antimetabolites. The doses are similar to those employed in the treatment of their malignant hematopoietic counterparts (leukemia and Hodgkin's and non-Hodgkin's lymphoma). Other forms of treatment for recalcitrant disease include etoposide, allogeneic bone marrow transplantation, and thymic extract. Supportive care is a major component of treatment.

SARCOIDOSIS

EDWIN L. KENDIG, Jr., M.D.

Sarcoidosis is a multisystem granulomatous disease of unknown cause. It is relatively rare in children. Since the disease process displaces normal tissue by sarcoid tissue, symptoms and signs depend on the organ or tissue involved. Most commonly affected are the lungs, lymph nodes, eyes, skin, liver, and spleen. Bones may also be involved, although this occurs less often; indeed, any organ or tissue may be affected.

Since the causative agent of sarcoidosis is not known, there is no recognized specific therapy. Adrenocorticosteroids are the only agents currently available that can suppress the acute manifestations of the disease. These agents are utilized only during acute and dangerous episodes.

Adrenocorticosteroid therapy is indicated in patients with intrinsic ocular disease, diffuse pulmonary lesions, central nervous system lesions, myocardial involvement, hypersplenism, and persistent hypercalcemia. Relative indications include progressive or symptomatic pulmonary disease, constitutional symptoms, joint involvement, disfiguring skin and lymph node lesions, persistent facial nerve palsy, and lesions of the nasal, laryngeal, and bronchial mucosa.

Fresh lesions appear to be more responsive to adrenocorticosteroid therapy than older ones. Although the suppressive action is often temporary, it is beneficial when the unremitting course of the disease will result in loss of organ function. For example, adrenocorticosteroid therapy can reduce the level of serum calcium and may thus help prevent nephrocalcinosis, renal insufficiency, and, possibly, band keratitis. The use of adrenocorticosteroids in the treatment of patients with only asymptomatic miliary nodules or bronchopneumonic patches in the lung fields is debatable.

Prednisone or prednisolone, 1 mg/kg/day in three or four divided doses, is continued until clinical manifestations of the disease disappear. A maintenance dose (15 mg every other day) is then given until a course of at least 6 months' treatment has been carried out.

Temporary relapse may occur following the discontinuation of adrenocorticosteroid treatment, but improvement usually follows without resumption of therapy. In the management of ocular disease, adrenocorticosteroids in the form of either ointment or drops (0.5 to 1 per cent) are utilized in conjunction with systemic treatment. During the course of local therapy, the pupils are continuously dilated by use of an atropine ointment (1 per cent).

Adrenocorticosteroid ointment may also be used in the treatment of cutaneous lesions, but only in conjunction with systemic therapy; better results are obtained with the latter.

Other drugs occasionally used in the treatment of sarcoidosis in adults (oxyphenbutazone, chloroquine, potassium para-aminobenzoate, azathioprine, and chlorambucil), as well as transfer factor, have seldom been used in children.

FAMILIAL MEDITERRANEAN FEVER

THOMAS J. A. LEHMAN, M.D.

The emphasis of current therapy for familial Mediterranean fever is on prophylactic colchicine administration to suppress the febrile attacks and possibly prevent amyloidosis. Children with familial Mediterranean fever who are of Sephardic Jewish or Arab origin or who have a family history of amyloidosis should receive continuous colchicine therapy. However, the physician caring for a child with familial Mediterranean fever who is of some other ethnic background must carefully weigh the benefits of ongoing colchicine administration against the knowledge that the febrile paroxysms are transitory and resolve without sequelae. Therapy should be restricted to those who are experiencing an unacceptable level of absenteeism from school or whose lives are otherwise significantly disrupted by the disease.

Colchicine* is administered in 0.6-mg tablets. A dosage of 0.6 mg bid is usually required to suppress the attacks in children 4 to 12 years of age, while 0.6 mg tid is often required for older children. These dosages have been utilized without toxicity in a large number of children. Transient diarrhea is often reported at the initiation of therapy but resolves spontaneously in most cases. Families in which the patient is young or in which there are young siblings should be specifically warned about the risk of accidental ingestion. Ingestion of as few as 8 mg (14 pills) of colchicine has led to death.

Patients at risk for the development of amyloidosis should receive colchicine continuously. The necessary duration of colchicine therapy for others is unclear. Although the disease is inherited, there are marked variations in the frequency of attacks without treatment. Once the attacks are initially controlled, colchicine may be gradually withdrawn. However, the episodes often recur when the dosage is decreased, and most patients require continuing therapy.

There is no specific therapy for the acute febrile attack once it has begun. A large hourly dose of colchicine at the first indication of an attack has been recommended for adults who are not receiving ongoing colchicine therapy, but this has not proven satisfactory in children. The fever and pleuritis or peritonitis will resolve spontaneously within 72 hours and should be treated with conservative measures of bed rest and hydration. Aspirin or acetaminophen may provide mild relief. Routine usage of narcotics should be avoided because of the recurrent nature of the attacks and the resultant potential for addiction. If the patient presents with peritonitis and primarily right lower quadrant pain, it may be impossible to exclude the possibility of appendicitis; appropriate surgery should be performed.

The arthritis of familial Mediterranean fever may be treated with appropriate dosages of nonsteroidal anti-inflammatory drugs. It is usually self-limited and ceases when the paroxysmal attacks are controlled. The chronic arthritis of the hip or sacroiliac joints that occurs may be treated symptomatically with anti-inflammatory drugs but does not respond well. Prophylactic colchicine administration is of uncertain benefit for these patients, who may ultimately require joint replacement.

---

*This use of colchicine is not listed by the manufacturer.

22

Special Problems in the Fetus and Neonate

DISTURBANCES OF INTRAUTERINE GROWTH

JOSEPH L. KENNEDY, Jr., M.D.

Infants with birth weights more than two standard deviations from the mean for gestational age are arbitrarily defined as having disturbances of growth. Overnutrition of the fetus (large for dates), while classically associated with large parents or with diabetic mothers, is also seen with transposition of the great vessels and in some syndromes (cerebral gigantism, Beckwith's syndrome). Some of these infants are susceptible to hypoglycemia; screening tests for glucose should be done early.

Infants with birth weights two standard deviations below the mean for gestational age or with birth weights less than the tenth percentile have intrauterine growth retardation. Various factors can affect birth weight. Maternal size, family stature, and altitude should be taken into account when assessing the infant.

There are two types of intrauterine growth retardation. In the first there is an altered growth potential with a fetus that is small throughout the pregnancy. Small size associated with small maternal or familial stature and some infants with syndromes or multiple cogenital anomalies are found in this type.

A second type is associated with impaired support for growth due to placental, maternal, or environmental factors. This type is associated with intrauterine infection, placental insufficiency secondary to hypertension, chronic abruption or placental infarct, and fetal crowding associated with intrauterine anomalies, oligohydramnios, or multiple gestation. Maternal illness, substance abuse, and perhaps socioeconomic factors affect growth support. Fetuses with impaired growth generally fall further below the norm as pregnancy progresses and are often said to have third trimester growth retardation.

Management of intrauterine growth retardation should begin during the pregnancy with screening for poor growth, frequent examinations, and ultrasound evaluation of fetal size and amount of amniotic fluid. Non-stress testing should begin at 26 weeks and contraction stress testing should be done as indicated together with evaluation of the biophysical profile (ultrasound evaluation of fetal movement, amount of amniotic fluid, and fetal breathing movements together with fetal heart rate and posture/tone).

During the pregnancy, bed rest on the left side may be effective when it is thought that there may be impaired placental blood flow, as with hypertensive disorders. Diuretics should be avoided, since they tend to diminish placental blood flow. A mother thought to be at risk of delivering an infant with severe growth retardation or chronic asphyxia should be transferred to a high-risk center. Early delivery may be indicated to remove the infant from a less than optimal environment. During labor and delivery, problems with hypoxia may be minimized by careful fetal monitoring. Asphyxia, if it occurs, should be promptly treated with effective resuscitation. Meconium aspiration should be prevented by aspirating the nasopharynx or trachea as indicated.

In the newborn nursery, the infant should be observed for birth defects and signs and symptoms of chronic or acute hypoxia: seizures, brain edema, irritability, altered consciousness, diminished urine output, respiratory failure, persistent fetal circulation, and cardiac dilatation with mitral insufficiency. Early feedings should be begun by mouth or by gavage, or if the infant has been seriously hypoxic or is also immature or otherwise impaired, by the intravenous administration of glucose.

The infant is examined for minor anomalies that lead to the diagnosis of unsuspected major anomalies. Examination of the placenta is important and often helpful in ruling out intrauterine infection. TORCH screening of cord blood serum is often unrewarding. If intrauter-

689

ine infection is strongly suspected, viral culture of the urine for CMV and examination of the spinal fluid for protein and cells may be helpful.

Because the infant is small and often hypoxic, heat loss and heat production may be impaired and temperature control defective. Careful attention should be paid to thermal environment, particularly when the infant is wet or exposed for examination or procedures.

Metabolic complications such as hypocalcemia and hypoglycemia should be watched for and treated.

Some infants with chronic in utero hypoxia have a high hematocrit level, and blood flow to various organs may be diminished because of increased blood viscosity. These infants are particularly susceptible to hypoglycemia. Plasma reduction exchange transfusion may be useful in infants with hematocrits in central venous samples of over 65 per cent, especially if clinical manifestations suggest hyperviscosity syndrome.

Early postnatal weight gain and early head growth may be indicators that an infant will do well. The ultimate prognosis for infants with extreme intrauterine growth retardation must be guarded, particularly when the cause is unknown. The infant need not be kept in the hospital until a particular weight is achieved. When he is gaining well, feeding well, and can obtain heat balance, he may be discharged home.

BIRTH INJURIES

WILLIAM D. COCHRAN, M.D.

In the realm of neonatology, there are malformations (defects of embryogenesis resulting in congenital anomalies), deformations (resulting from alteration during fetal life of a previously normal part and usually representing a spontaneously correcting "congenital anomaly"), and birth injuries, the last occurring almost exclusively because of a hard or prolonged labor, a malpresentation, an obstetrical manipulation, or a combination of these. Such birth injuries are often associated with some deformation. The increasing number of cesarean sections for most breech presentations and for "failure to progress" in cephalic presentations has certainly decreased the number and severity of birth injuries now seen. However, because they are less common, one must guard against failing to consider them a possibility.

HEAD INJURIES

Head injuries are hematologic, bony, neurologic, or a combination thereof. Besides the almost ubiquitous caput, the most common is a *cephalhematoma,* usually overlying the left parietal bone and associated with an undisplaced simple fracture of the underlying parietal bone some 20 per cent of the time. Maturing to its full size by the time the neonate is 3 days of age, the subperiosteal swelling should be left alone and never aspirated. Some cephalhematomas calcify and take up to a year to resolve, while others are at least partially, if not completely, gone by 10 to 14 days. A *deviated*

nasal septum occasionally is found with a nose that has been held deviated in utero for some time, probably both during and prior to labor. In the great majority of instances, by 2 weeks or so, one will see that all deviation is resolving and that no surgical manipulation is necessary. Lower *cranial nerve VII* injuries, with and without the prior use of forceps, are still seen and are largely unilateral. Though on very rare occasions the cause is absence of the nerve (or its nucleus, as in Möbius syndrome), the usual weakness or paralysis is due to peripheral pressure, with resulting edema or hemorrhage, rarely avulsion. All resolves in the great majority of instances over days, occasionally weeks. There is no definitive treatment. *Forceps marks* or lacerations are now much less common, but *scalp punctures* secondary to internal monitors are being seen more and more frequently. Forceps marks, no matter how alarming, are best left alone in the hope that no fat necrosis or nerve injury has occurred. Secondary infection is only a most unusual sequela. Actual forceps lacerations are extremely rare these days and need individualized attention, possibly stitches. Scalp punctures are best left alone and kept clean and uncovered, so observation for possible infection can more easily be done. *Skull fractures* are now extremely uncommon, save for those found under cephalhematomas. Depressed skull fractures (usually of the parietal bone) are usually elevated neurosurgically, even in the absence of clinical symptoms.

Internal hemorrhage (epidural, subdural, subarachnoid, intracerebral, or intraventricular) secondary to head trauma following labor of more than an average length (or hard labor) is less frequent now but more important to consider, since, especially with computed tomographic scan (but also ultrasonography), more definitive lesions can be identified and hence treated. In the term infant, all but intracerebral lesions have shown some association with a history of labor or anoxia or both. Subarachnoid and intracerebral sites, if not accompanied by other bleeding sites or extremely life-threatening symptoms, are best left alone to resolve. Evacuation of epidural and subdural lesions is lifesaving more than occasionally. Symptoms are most often seizures and apnea, but irritability, persistent hypotonia, and occasionally even deep, irregular respirations are seen. These warrant, as a minimum, a lumbar puncture and, with a history of trauma, probably a prompt computed tomographic scan. Since hypoglycemia and even hyponatremia are common side effects, these possible deviations should also be investigated. The common intraventricular hemorrhage now being reported in the very small premature (<1500 gm birth weight) does not seem to be associated with birth trauma and luckily is usually of minimal degree.

INJURIES TO LONG BONES AND JOINTS

Significant trauma to long bones is becoming exceedingly rare. By far, the most common fracture is that of the *clavicle.* The diagnosis of these fractures is commonly still missed. However, since permanent nonunion is almost unheard of, even in our present litigious society. The old saw that "so long as you put both ends in the same room, they'll heal" still holds for the great majority of such simple fractures. If the fracture seems especially painful, pinning the arm in its shirt against the thorax is usually helpful. Very occasionally, an infant needs the affected arm taped to his or her side. Though figure-of-eight dressings have also been resorted to, they are largely unnecessary. If there is accompanying evidence of brachial nerve injury, greater immobilization should be used.

Dislocated hips are still common, reportedly three to five times more common in female babies. Though reported otherwise, almost invariably the dislocation is posterosuperior. Found more often after breech presentation (and especially after a vaginal delivery), these dislocations are often transient, with the head of the femur staying firmly in the acetabulum after only a day or two of a treatment as simple as using triple diapers. A continued finding of a dislocatable hip necessitates more stringent therapy, possibly a harness or even casting. Even ideal care, however, is not always successful.

Long-bone fractures (usually the humerus but occasionally the femur) are so extremely rare these days they should be treated carefully and conservatively. However, on occasion, a simple humeral fracture will heal optimally with just the arm taped to the infant's side. Epiphyseal fractures (of the humerus and femur) are reported. *Hyperextended knees* are still occasionally seen. Although they are dramatic in their presentation and cause the unexperienced to diagnose an absent patella, using simple flexion immediately after birth and then holding the joint flexed for a day with something as simple as small sand bags is usually all that is necessary to prevent future re-extension. A radiograph reveals little, since the epiphyses involved are not well visualized and the patella is not calcified at all.

INJURIES TO SKIN

Dramatic *ecchymoses* in the absence of bleeding disorders are still seen, especially with face or breech presentations. Almost without exception they should be left untreated and uncovered, as air is a great healer (as is "tincture of time"). Hemorrhages in the sclerae are even more common and are, by themselves, universally benign. Even fundal hemorrhages tend to heal completely without sequelae in the great majority of instances. *Fat necrosis*, probably from some extrinsic pressure, occurs occasionally and rarely is extensive. Seen largely on the face (mostly the cheeks) or on the back, the lesion appears reddened, hot, and lumpy. Again, time—a matter of days or occasionally weeks—brings about resolution.

NEUROLOGIC INJURIES

See also head injuries, discussed previously, regarding cranial nerve VII injuries. By far, the most common injury to the brachial plexus, and usually the most benign, is *Erb's palsy*. Believed to be due to edema in or around the upper brachial plexus, most of the time the weakness or paralysis begins clearing within days, if not hours. Historically, there has usually been some physical pulling on the head to deliver the infant's body. Strapping the arm and physiotherapy are largely unnecessary

treatments, unless the abnormality is accompanied by pain or is very persistent. Checking for accompanying fractures of the clavicle is wise. *Klumpke's paralysis* or palsy is far less common (or at least far less appreciated as being present). However, it seems more apt to be persistent and permanent. Therapy is necessary only in those extremely rare long-term cases and usually consists of some splinting device for positioning. *Diaphragmatic paralysis* (phrenic nerve injury) probably is secondary, again to some strong manipulative delivery process. It is rarely recognized unless it represents a severe nerve involvement, and then it is often a permanent paralysis.

THORACOABDOMINAL INJURIES

Today, thoracoabdominal injuries are rare—indeed, have almost vanished. Traumatic pneumothorax, chylothorax, subcapsular hematomas of the liver, and ruptured hollow viscera or spleen are mentioned in past textbooks. Some have never been seen by this author in years of practicing neonatology. Often what is found after birth to be chylothorax is diagnosed before labor. Treatment depends on the lesion and its impact on the infant's condition.

MANAGEMENT OF THE NEWBORN AT DELIVERY

KATHLEEN S. CARLSON, M.D.

The goal of delivery room resuscitation is to assist the infant in his or her transition from the intrauterine to the extrauterine environment. Respiratory and circulatory changes must occur within the first several minutes of life for the transition to be successful. Respiratory adaptations to extrauterine life include adequate lung expansion and effective gas exchange. Termination of the right-to-left intracardiac shunts normally present in the fetus is a necessary circulatory adaptation for the neonate.

Antenatal and intrapartum factors may influence the type and extent of resuscitation required. Antenatal factors that may be of significance include maternal toxemia, chorioamnionitis, diabetes or cardiac disease, fetal prematurity, asphyxia, lung immaturity, hydrops, intrauterine growth retardation, or previously diagnosed congenital anomalies. Significant intrapartum factors include meconium-stained amniotic fluid, cord prolapse, bleeding, nuchal cord, precipitous descent, or fetal bradycardia. Despite attention to antenatal or intrapartum factors (or both) that may increase an infant's likelihood of requiring resuscitation, the absence of these factors does not ensure that resuscitation will not be required.

PERSONNEL

At least two experienced persons are needed to resuscitate an infant in the delivery room. In the case of a severely asphyxiated infant, three experienced persons may be required. One member of the resuscitation team should be an individual skilled in airway management and ventilation. This person should coordinate the resuscitative efforts of the team. The second person should be responsible for monitoring the infant's heart rate by auscultation or palpation and performing cardiac massage if the heart rate is less than 60 beats per minute. A third person may be needed if administration of medications, umbilical catheterization, or volume resuscitation is required. Of critical importance is the experience or skill of the individuals carrying out the resuscitation. Therefore, the most experienced persons, be they physicians, nurses, or respiratory therapists, should assume responsibility.

EQUIPMENT

Equipment needed for neonatal resuscitation should be readily available in every delivery room. This equipment should include a radiant warming table; an oxygen source with an adjustable flow meter; a sterile bulb syringe and wall suction with adjustable vacuum and suction catheters; face masks of appropriate sizes; a flow-through anesthesia bag capable of delivering 100 per cent oxygen with an adjustable pressure valve; a laryngoscope with Miller 0 and Miller 1 blades; flanged and unflanged endotracheal tubes of 2.5-, 3.0-, and 3.5-mm diameter; flexible intubation stylets and adaptors for the ventilation bag; a stethoscope; a sterile umbilical catheterization tray and 3.5 and 5 French catheters; drugs, including epinephrine, sodium bicarbonate, 10 per cent dextrose, 10 per cent calcium gluconate, naloxone, and 5 per cent albumin; and syringes, needles, saline flush, tincture of benzoin, and tape. In addition, a transport incubator with a portable oxygen supply and battery-operated heat source should be available to move the infant from the delivery room to the nursery.

When a person is called to attend a delivery, the transport incubator, containing a full tank of oxygen, should be moved into the delivery room and plugged in. The individual coordinating the resuscitation should introduce himself or herself to the parents, obtain a history from the obstetrician, and proceed to prepare the equipment. The radiant warmer should be turned on, and dry, warm blankets should be laid out. The oxygen source should be turned on and the flow adjusted to the ventilation bag. The pop-off valve should be checked. One must ensure that the laryngoscope bulb is bright. Appropriate-sized endotracheal tubes should be set out, and the wall suction should be adjusted.

METHODS

Following delivery, the infant should be placed on the radiant warming table. The airway should be cleared. In most infants, the mouth, oropharynx, and nares can be cleared effectively with a suction bulb. If thick, particulate meconium is present, the infant should be intubated immediately and direct tracheal suctioning performed. In the absence of meconium, the infant should be wiped dry concomitantly with airway clearance. When particulate meconium is present, drying should be deferred until after intubation. Respiratory efforts may be stimulated by drying and may

contribute to further aspiration of meconium. An assessment of heart rate, respiratory effort, muscle tone, reflex irritability, and color—that is, the Apgar score—should be made. An immediate Apgar score (*before 1 minute of age*) should dictate the type and sequence of resuscitative efforts required. Throughout the resuscitation, the infant's condition or Apgar score must be continuously evaluated to modify the intensity of resuscitative efforts appropriately.

More than 90 per cent of all babies will exhibit an initial Apgar score of 8, 9, or 10. In these infants, airway clearance and drying will be all that is required. Nasopharyngeal stimulation by a suction catheter, which may precipitate vagally induced arrhythmias, should be avoided, if possible, until the child is 5 minutes of age. A brief physical assessment should be followed by allowing the parent or parents to bond with the infant.

Infants with Apgar scores of 5, 6, or 7 are mildly depressed at birth and will require stimulation and oxygen in addition to airway clearance and drying. These infants usually have a normal heart rate. One hundred per cent oxygen should be provided by anesthesia bag and mask held by the baby's face. The infant can be stimulated to breathe by gently rubbing the back or slapping the feet or both. Naloxone should be considered if the mother has received a recent narcotic analgesic during labor (this drug is contraindicated if the mother is a known narcotic addict).

If stimulation plus oxygen by mask does not improve respiratory efforts, tone, and color after 1 minute, or if the initial Apgar score is 3 or 4 (i.e., slowing heart rate) after airway clearance and drying, the infant should be ventilated with a bag and mask, with 100 per cent oxygen and pressures sufficient to move the chest wall. Bagging should be continued until the heart rate exceeds 100 beats per minute, the color is pink, and good respiratory effort is maintained. If the heart rate falls to less than 60 beats per minute or the chest is not moving adequately with bag-and-mask ventilation, the infant should be intubated. Cardiac massage (two compressions per second) should be initiated if the heart rate remains less than 60 beats per minute. Sternal compression just below the nipple line with the thumbs over the middle third of the sternum and the fingers wrapped around the back is the preferred technique.

The severely asphyxiated infant has an initial Apgar score of 0, 1, or 2 and appears cyanotic and flaccid and exhibits no respiratory effort or periodic gasps. The heart rate is slow or absent. The airway should be cleared, and the infant should be immediately intubated and bagged with 100 per cent oxygen at 40 to 60 breaths per minute and pressures adequate to move the chest wall. Cardiac massage should be started. If the heart rate does not increase after 1 to 2 minutes of ventilation and cardiac massage, one should ensure that the endotracheal tube is not malpositioned (down the right mainstem bronchus or in the esophagus) or plugged (with mucus, blood, or meconium). One should confirm that the bag is delivering 100 per cent oxygen (i.e., that the connections are appropriate and secure). The vast majority of severely asphyxiated infants can be resuscitated by adequate ventilation, and pharmacologic intervention is rarely necessary. One cannot emphasize enough the importance to a successful resuscitation of a *properly positioned, patent endotracheal tube* as well as bagging with *100 per cent oxygen* and *pressures that move the chest.*

If by 3 to 5 minutes after delivery, the heart rate has not exceeded 100 beats per minute, despite adequate ventilation with 100 per cent oxygen and continued cardiac massage, drug therapy will be needed. Epinephrine, 0.1 to 0.2 ml/kg, 1:10,000 diluted 1:1 with sterile water, should be administered. If the heart rate remains less than 100 beats per minute, an umbilical venous catheter should be inserted as rapidly and aseptically as possible. The catheter should be inserted just far enough to get good blood return, approximately 1 to 2 cm past the abdominal wall. Sodium bicarbonate, 2 to 4 mEq/kg diluted 1:1 with 10 per cent dextrose, should be administered over 2 to 4 minutes through the umbilical vein. This therapy should correct acidosis and provide the myocardium with glucose. The importance of ensuring adequate ventilation prior to bicarbonate administration needs to be emphasized. If bradycardia persists, 0.2 ml/kg (up to 1.0 ml) of a 1:10,000 solution of epinephrine should be given. One to 2 ml/kg of 10 per cent calcium gluconate may then be given as a slow infusion if cardiac output remains poor. Rapid administration of calcium may exacerbate bradycardia. All medications should be flushed through the catheter. Volume expansion with colloid, blood, or other fluids may be lifesaving in the face of significant blood loss from the infant (e.g., abruptio placentae, vasa praevia, fetal-maternal hemorrhage, ruptured viscus, or severe cord compression) or severe anemia secondary to hemolytic disease. If an infant's hypotension and poor perfusion are secondary to asphyxial myocardial damage, volume expansion may precipitate congestive heart failure and make matters worse.

When adequate oxygen delivery and ventilation have been achieved and the heart rate is greater than 100 beats per minute, the infant should be transferred to the neonatal intensive care unit for further evaluation and therapy.

RESPIRATORY DISTRESS SYNDROME

IVAN D. FRANTZ, III, M.D.

To discuss the management of respiratory distress syndrome requires discussion of all aspects of care of the premature infant. It is beyond the scope of this article to cover temperature control, fluid and electrolyte management, nutrition, treatment of patent ductus arteriosus, mechanical ventilation, and the various complications associated with these therapies. It has been 30 years since Avery and Mead first demonstrated that surfactant deficiency was the cause of respiratory distress syndrome, yet specific therapy aimed at surfactant replacement is only now being tested and is several years away from commercial availability. Nonetheless, the original observation that surfactant is lacking in

infants with respiratory distress syndrome, coupled with the observation that symptoms can be relieved with surfactant replacement, justifies renaming the syndrome surfactant deficiency disease (SDD). Such a renaming allows us to consider therapy aimed at a specific underlying problem but should not result in our forgetting about the remainder of problems of prematurity, which will continue to exist even when surfactant deficiency has been corrected or adequately treated.

Although the prevention of SDD is largely in the hands of the obstetrician, pediatricians are frequently involved in the decision-making process. SDD may be prevented through two approaches: prevention of premature labor and acceleration of fetal lung maturation. The pediatrician is frequently asked to provide data on the risk of neonatal mortality to be balanced against the risk of fetal mortality or maternal morbidity. In addition to neonatal mortality, the pediatrician must be aware of the risk of SDD at various gestational ages and the likelihood of other complications. Table 1 indicates neonatal mortality, risk of SDD, and risk for other complications, including necrotizing enterocolitis, intracranial hemorrhage, sepsis, and so on. The data were obtained from St. Margaret's Hospital in Boston for the years 1984 to 1986.

The pediatrician may be asked to render an opinion about whether or not steroids should be given to the mother prenatally for the enhancement of fetal lung maturation. The data are overwhelmingly in favor of steroid use. There are few risks to mother, fetus, or newborn. Beneficial effects have been noted in most circumstances. In those few studies in which little effect has been shown in certain groups, the groups have been too small to have demonstrated statistical significance, or the incidence of SDD within the control groups has been so low as to make demonstration of a reduction impossible. Therefore, if delivery can be safely postponed, a trial of steroids is warranted.

Given the birth of an infant with SDD, respiratory support with oxygen, continuous positive airway pressure (CPAP), or mechanical ventilation becomes the backbone of treatment. In general, the goal of therapy is to maintain oxygen and carbon dioxide tensions in physiologically acceptable ranges. Because of the risks of retinopathy of prematurity and bronchopulmonary dysplasia, one may choose to maintain the PaO_2 some-

TABLE 1. Gestational Age and Morbidity and Mortality of Prematurity

Gestational Age (wk)	Mortality (%)	SDD (%)	Morbidity (%)
35	2	11	14
34	2	14	18
33	2	23	34
32	2	20	34
31	2	41	62
30	7	53	76
29	7	47	72
28	10	61	80
27	15	62	90
26	30	77	100
25	30	81	100
24	73	73	100
23	90	—	100

what lower than normal and the $PaCO_2$ higher than normal. Exact values may vary with the stage of illness as well. One can expect SDD to worsen over the first 24 to 48 hours of life, so that one may wish to leave a margin for error on the high side for PaO_2 and on the low side for $PaCO_2$. The initial treatment for SDD includes provision of adequate inspired oxygen to maintain oxygen saturation greater than 90 per cent. This generally requires that the PaO_2 be kept in the range of 50 to 60 torr. $PaCO_2$ should be maintained in a range that prevents significant acidosis (pH>7.25). In most cases a $PaCO_2$ of 50 to 55 torr can be tolerated.

CPAP has been shown to be beneficial in preserving surfactant function and diminishing the oxygen requirement. Although there are no convincing data demonstrating improved survival with the early use of CPAP, most neonatologists support its early use. To most, this means the institution of CPAP when clinical signs of SDD are present and the FIO_2 requirement approaches 0.40. Administration of CPAP with nasal prongs is effective for most infants and avoids the necessity for tracheal intubation. Mask and headbox CPAP techniques are currently out of favor, although continuous negative pressure applied to the chest wall is in use in some centers.

Mechanical ventilation must be initiated for the infant who develops apnea or severe respiratory distress, who requires an FIO_2 greater than 0.70 to maintain a PaO_2 of 60 torr, or whose $PaCO_2$ exceeds 55 torr.

Because of the inhomogeneous nature of surfactant deficiency, the lung disease is marked by patchy alveolar atelectasis and expansion, resulting in a risk of pneumothorax. This risk varies with the severity of the disease, so that infants who require oxygen have only a 5 per cent risk of pneumothorax, those who are sick enough to require CPAP have a risk of 10 per cent, and those who require mechanical ventilation have a risk of 20 per cent. Physicians who manage infants with SDD must be prepared to diagnose and treat pneumothorax.

High-frequency ventilation and surfactant replacement are relatively new approaches to the treatment of SDD. Studies of high-frequency ventilation suggest that although it is successful in effecting gas exchange, it may not have advantages over conventional ventilation for routine cases of SDD. It does appear to have a role in those infants for whom conventional ventilation is inadequate, particularly if pulmonary air leaks are present.

As indicated in the introduction to this article, surfactant replacement is both the proof of the underlying cause of SDD and its most promising means of therapy. Studies thus far have demonstrated clear, short-term benefits of surfactant replacement, including improved blood gas tensions and decreased requirement for mechanical ventilation. Longer-term benefits, such as decreases in the occurrence of bronchopulmonary dysplasia and mortality, are less dramatic. The exact indications and dosage are not yet established. Exogenous surfactant has been tested both prophylactically for all infants at risk of developing respiratory distress from surfactant deficiency and therapeutically for in-

fants with symptoms. Initial studies utilized a single dose of surfactant, which in some cases appeared to have transitory effects. Studies are currently under way to evaluate the response to multiple doses. If proved safe and effective, surfactant replacement may be a simple approach to reducing morbidity and mortality for large numbers of premature infants.

NEONATAL PNEUMOTHORAX AND PNEUMOMEDIASTINUM

PAUL M. COLOMBANI, M.D.,
and J. ALEX HALLER, M.D.

Approximately 20 per cent of newborn infants with pulmonary disease will develop pneumothorax or pneumomediastinum during the course of their management. Pneumothorax and pneumomediastinum are defined as an escape of alveolar air from the lung into the pleural space and mediastinum, respectively. The overwhelming majority (95 per cent) of these infants are preterm infants with respiratory distress syndrome requiring mechanical ventilatory support. Fewer than 10 per cent of infants are spontaneously breathing when they develop pneumothorax or pneumomediastinum. Other etiologies include those for which infants require assisted ventilation: meconium aspiration, pneumonia, wet lung syndrome, recurrent apnea, and congenital anomalies. Presenting signs and symptoms range in severity from an incidental chest radiograph finding of a small, simple pneumothorax to profound cardiopulmonary collapse from tension pneumothorax or pneumomediastinum.

Optimal management for pneumothorax or pneumomediastinum is determined by the patients' clinical condition and the degree of respiratory compromise. The asymptomatic patient who is spontaneously breathing may be observed for signs of deterioration. Frequent vital sign determinations and careful physical examinations should be performed. Monitoring of the patient using pulse oximetry or arterial blood gas determinations is useful in managing these patients. Transillumination, which has been helpful in the diagnosis of pneumothorax, can also be used. Chest radiographs should be repeated at 4- to 6-hour intervals to determine whether the pneumothorax is increasing in size. If there is evidence of clinical deterioration during observation or if chest radiographs reveal that the pneumothorax is increasing in size, then optimal management would be the placement of an intercostal chest tube to re-expand the lung.

Any infant requiring positive-pressure ventilation for respiratory disease who develops a pneumothorax should have a chest tube placed to reinflate the lung and ensure that the pneumothorax will not increase and contribute to further respiratory compromise. It is likely that continued positive pressure will only increase the size of the pneumothorax, resulting in further respiratory deterioration in these critically ill patients. In the patient with cardiopulmonary collapse from tension pneumothorax, the accumulated air must be evacuated under pressure immediately. It is important to note that congenital malformations, such as lobar emphysema and cystic adenomatoid malformation, or acquired deformities, such as pneumatic lung cyst, may mimic tension pneumothorax. A careful radiographic differentiation is required prior to the definitive treatment of a pneumothorax. When a presumptive diagnosis of tension pneumothorax is made, needle aspiration of the accumulated air pocket is the preferable first step and may be lifesaving. Under sterile conditions and using a closed system (a large syringe, a three-way stopcock, and a butterfly needle or "angiocath"), the needle is placed through the chosen interspace just over the upper rib margin. This placement will avoid the neurovascular bundle that runs under the lower rib margin. Insertion of the needle in the upper half of the chest cavity is preferred, to avoid injuring solid organs such as the liver, spleen, diaphragm, or heart. Our preference is to place the needle at the anterior axillary or midclavicular line, at the second or third interspace. Care must be taken to prevent inserting a long needle too deeply into the pleural cavity. When air is obtained by applying suction to the syringe, the needle may be stabilized using a clamp to prevent further penetration of the needle. When air under tension is aspirated, an immediate improvement in cardiopulmonary function is to be expected. The plastic needle may be left in place until a chest tube is placed. It is frequently necessary to aspirate intermittently ongoing air accumulations while setting up and performing the chest tube insertion.

Surgical placement of a chest tube for symptomatic pneumothorax may be lifesaving and should be in the armamentarium of any physician who cares for infants in a critical care setting. The typical chest tube placement site for a large pneumothorax or tension pneumothorax is the anterior axillary line in the third or fourth interspace. The catheter is directed superiorly and anteriorly into the apex of the pleural cavity. Infants with pneumothorax may often have loculated pockets of air, which may not be optimally drained using this approach. In these situations, close examination of anteroposterior and lateral chest radiographs will localize the position of the pocket of air.

There are a number of methods for chest tube placement. The safest approach is to identify the interspace and location along the rib that will be optimal for the drainage of air. Local anesthetic is infiltrated into the skin and subcutaneous tissue of the area just inferior to the rib and interspace to be utilized. A transverse incision is then made in the skin. With use of a curved clamp, a tunnel is made from the skin site, ascending through the subcutaneous tissue and musculature to the rib above. The clamp is then passed through the intercostal muscles just over that rib, the pleural space is entered, and the clamp is spread to enlarge the tunnel. A catheter is then placed through the tunnel and into the pleural space, using a curved clamp as a guide to place the chest tube in the desired location. The size of the patient dictates the size of tube that is required, usually an 8 or 10 French chest tube. The tube is then connected with a closed drainage system with underwater seal or vacuum suction or both. A rule of thumb regarding the amount of negative pressure to place on the closed drainage system is to utilize the same amount of negative pressure as the size of the chest tube (e.g., 10 French chest tube = 10 cm H_2O negative pressure). The catheter is then sutured to the skin to ensure that accidental dislodgment does not occur. Re-expansion of the affected lung should be immediate following placement of the chest tube to vacuum suction drainage. This re-expansion should be confirmed by chest radiograph. Vacuum suction is continued until the air leak stops. Most pneumothoraces resolve within 48 to 72 hours, but longer periods may be needed in infants requiring prolonged ventilatory support. Following resolution of the leak and full expansion of the lung on the chest radiograph, the chest tube may be connected to underwater seal. If the lung remains inflated after 24 hours of underwater seal, the chest tube then can be safely removed. An occlusive dressing should be placed over the chest tube exit site to prevent reaccumulation of air through the tract made for the chest tube. Those infants whose air leak resolves but who continue on ventilatory support will usually benefit from leaving their chest tube in place until ventilator support is withdrawn and they are spontaneously breathing.

Occasionally, patients with multiple, loculated pneumothoraces may require several chest tubes for optimal management to remove accumulated air pockets for improved ventilation.

Pneumomediastinum is usually well tolerated in patients requiring ventilatory support and is often an incidental radiographic finding during routine monitoring of these patients. Rarely, a tension pneumomediastinum may develop and cause symptoms suggestive of cardiac tamponade with cardiac decompensation. In this situation, needle aspiration is the first step. This may be performed by placing a needle carefully via a subxiphoid approach, using the above-mentioned closed system, with gentle suction as the needle is advanced. From a subxiphoid position, the needle is carefully advanced toward the left shoulder of the patient in a superficial plane of approximately 20° to 30°. The catheter is gently advanced until air is encountered. The air is then evacuated, and the patient is observed for improvement in cardiopulmonary status. In inserting the needle, care must be taken to ensure that the direction of the needle is not changed once it has entered the subxiphoid position. Changing the direction of the needle may create a laceration of the liver, diaphragm, or heart. Most patients will improve with needle aspiration. The patient is then observed over the next few hours for evidence of reaccumulation of air, either by deterioration in vital signs or by chest radiographs. Slow reaccumulation of air may be treated by a second needle aspiration. Rarely, a mediastinal chest tube can be placed through the same xiphoid approach to evacuate accumulated air.

Accelerated air resorption by placing the patient on 100 per cent oxygen and washing out accumulated nitrogen from the extra-alveolar location may be useful in older children. For the sick premature infant or the term infant with respiratory compromise, such an approach should not be utilized because of the considerable risk associated with placing these infants on 100 per cent oxygen.

Complications of needle aspiration and chest tube placement in newborns include laceration of the lung parenchyma, with increased air leak and bleeding from the damaged lung, as well as lacerations of the diaphragm, spleen, kidney, or liver if chest tubes are placed in a caudal position. These complications can be avoided by direct dissection into the pleural space using a hemostat clamp. Blind trocar insertion of a tube is dangerous. Infection of the pleural space or chest tube tract is rarely encountered. Bleeding from an intercostal artery can occur if the chest tube is placed below the rib rather than over the rib. Placement of a chest tube in a patient with lobar emphysema or pulmonary pneumatocele, incorrectly diagnosed as pneumothorax, will complicate the optimal management of these conditions and can be avoided by a careful differential diagnosis of pneumothorax.

Air leak into the pleural space or mediastinum during the course of positive-pressure ventilation for respiratory disease is a common problem in the neonate, especially in the preterm baby with respiratory distress syndrome. Optimal and deliberate management of these problems should be undertaken immediately upon diagnosis. Prompt re-expansion of the lung will allow for improvement in respiratory parameters. Then ongoing efforts to withdraw respiratory support from these patients, as their underlying conditions improve, can continue unimpeded by complicating factors such as pneumothorax and pneumomediastinum.

BRONCHOPULMONARY DYSPLASIA

JOAN E. HODGMAN, M.D.

A syndrome of chronic respiratory distress and oxygen dependency accompanied by changes in the chest radiograph commonly follows assisted ventilation of the infant of very low birth weight.

Sensible management of ventilated infants involves control of oxygen levels and respirator pressures and early weaning from endotracheal tubes. Relative fluid restriction during the first week of intensive care will decrease the incidence of bronchopulmonary dysplasia (BPD) in surviving infants. Physiotherapy and tracheal toilet are particularly important, considering the decrease in cilial function and the increase in mucus secretion characteristic of the condition. Caloric intake should be pushed as soon as tolerated because BPD is accompanied by a 25 per cent increase in metabolic rate, presumably due to increased work of breathing. Growth failure is prominent in the first year, with improvement in pulmonary function occurring with acceleration of physical growth.

There is a compulsion to decrease oxygen levels as rapidly as possible in order to facilitate discharge of the infant. This is probably an error that contributes to increased pulmonary vascular resistance and cor pulmonale. Ambient oxygen should be given to maintain a PaO_2 of 55 mm Hg and a RPEP/RVET below 0.35. These levels can be readily attained in home programs with the use of nasal catheters. Oxygen levels can be readily followed in an outpatient setting using a pulse oximeter. Readings should be obtained during sleep when oxygen levels are lowest.

Diuretics have a beneficial effect on pulmonary mechanics and are recommended to control the increase in interstitial fluid that occurs in BPD. Furosemide is the drug of choice for initiation of treatment in doses of 1 to 2 mg/kg/day. Electrolytes must be monitored to minimize the complications of hyponatremia, hypokalemia, and metabolic acidosis. Renal calcification associated with calciuria has been reported after 12 days of furosemide therapy; this was reversed when treatment was changed to oral diuretics. In infants who respond to furosemide, substitution of chlorothiazide (Diuril) at 20 mg/kg bid should be made as soon as possible.

The characteristic smooth muscle hypertrophy present in BPD suggests that bronchodilators should have a place in therapy. Theophylline in doses recommended for apnea of prematurity improves pulmonary mechanics and may shorten the length of time ventilation is needed when used early in the course of the disease before the development of significant fibrosis. Isoproterenol also decreases airway resistance and increases conductance. Before chest physiotherapy and airway suction, brief inhalation of a 0.1 per cent solution is recommended, especially for infants who wheeze.

The place of steroids in the management of BPD has not been settled. Recent controlled studies have shown good results from short courses of dexamethasone in ventilator-fast infants. Weaning from the ventilator was possible in all treated infants, but long-term outcome was not influenced. Rate of complicating infections was high in one study but not in the most recent. A 2- to 3-week trial of dexamethasone at beginning doses of 2 to 3 mg/kg/day, which are tapered after the first week, is indicated in the ventilator-dependent infant early in the disease course. Although good results using a 42 day course have been reported in one study, the place of long-term treatment has not been established, and the effects of steroids on both susceptibility to infection and growth must be considered.

Although administration of vitamin E showed apparent early promise in prevention of BPD, studies, including one by the original proponents of this therapy, have failed to confirm a protective effect.

Infants do not need to remain hospitalized for their full convalescence. Oxygen therapy and chest physiotherapy are feasible at home, with proper patient selection and a program for parental support. Early discharge will decrease both the expense of intensive care and the emotional deprivation associated with the treatment of the infant with BPD.

NEONATAL ATELECTASIS

RICHARD J. MARTIN, M.D.,
and MICHELE C. WALSH-SUKYS, M.D.

Atelectasis, the collapse of segments or lobes of the lung, is a frequent neonatal problem. Atelectasis may result from extrinsic compression caused by the intrathoracic accumulation of gas or fluid, from thoracic masses, or from adjacent emphysematous lung parenchyma. More commonly, however, atelectasis occurs in infants in association with endotracheal tube misplacement or as a complication of recent extubation. In the former situation, the endotracheal tube enters the right mainstem bronchus, and atelectasis in all or part of the left lung results. There may also be occlusion of the bronchus to the right upper lobe, causing additional right upper lobe collapse. The treatment is to withdraw the endotracheal tube after radiographic confirmation of its position, so that air entry returns to the right lung. This step alone almost always results in complete radiographic resolution of the atelectasis. The orotracheal or nasotracheal tube must then be well secured and the position of the infant's head and neck stabilized.

Postextubation atelectasis is one of the most common complications of weaning very low birth weight infants from assisted ventilation. It may occur from hours to days after extubation and is often recurrent and relatively refractory to treatment. The right upper lobe appears to be most frequently involved. Treatment should be directed toward dislodging or removing thick mucus secretions and increasing the infant's spontaneous respiratory efforts. The latter may be achieved with the use of methylxanthines (theophylline and caffeine). These drugs probably enhance the chances of successful extubation of the smallest, sickest infants by increasing respiratory drive or respiratory muscle contraction and so decreasing the risk for atelectasis.

Persistent lobar atelectasis, particularly that involving the right upper lobe, may indicate the presence of granulation tissue in the superior segmental bronchus. This tissue may form after prolonged or recurrent malposition of the endotracheal tube in the right mainstem bronchus. After confirmation by fiberoptic bronchoscopy, granulation tissue can be excised surgically.

Therapy for atelectasis should be directed at the primary cause. A pneumothorax or pleural effusion can be adequately relieved by thoracostomy tube placement. Atelectasis produced by intrinsic bronchial obstruction should be treated with suctioning, vibration or percussion of the chest wall, and postural drainage or positioning of the infant. Infants with bronchopulmonary dysplasia or other very low birth weight infants should not be manipulated too vigorously. Hypoxemia may occur during prolonged suctioning, and transcutaneous oxygen monitors or pulse oximeters should alert caregivers to this complication. If the secretions appear to have become purulent, pneumonia should be considered a cause of the atelectasis, and appropriate cultures should be obtained. The selection of catheter size during suctioning is determined by the viscosity of the secretions and the endotracheal tube diameter.

Although some authors have recommended the use of large-bore endotracheal tubes to facilitate suctioning, the use of excessively large tubes is associated with subglottic stenosis and therefore cannot be encouraged. The use of bronchodilator agents has also been suggested, but the therapeutic benefit is undocumented. Direct laryngoscopy to permit blind suctioning of the lower airway may lead to "suction biopsy" of the lower airway, with significant bleeding, and therefore is to be discouraged. With persistent unilateral atelectasis, lateral positioning of the infant so that the atelectatic lung is upward (or superior), and so preferentially ventilated, may be beneficial.

The skillful use of fiberoptic bronchoscopy can relieve persistent atelectasis with minimal risk in all but the smallest, sickest infants. Mucous plugs or even bronchial casts sometimes are removed intact, and prompt clinical and roentgenographic improvement may be noted. Unfortunately, the problem may rapidly recur after successful bronchoscopy, and vigorous conservative therapy must be sustained after reinflation has occurred. If gas exchange is severely compromised despite these measures, reintubation may be indicated. Infants with atelectasis occurring (or persisting) during assisted ventilation may benefit from a small increase in positive end-expiratory pressure or continuous positive airway pressure. If atelectasis fails to resolve, ventilator settings should be returned to prior levels to avoid unnecessary barotrauma.

LOBAR EMPHYSEMA

HENRY L. DORKIN, M.D.

Lobar emphysema may be defined as marked overdistention of a lung subunit, usually a segment or lobe, with anatomic and/or physiologic consequences to other intrathoracic structures. This entity may present acutely or subacutely as a cause of neonatal respiratory distress. Acutely, signs and symptoms are usually present in the first days of life and include dyspnea, compression of normal ipsilateral and contralateral lung tissue, ventilation-perfusion mismatch, and vascular compromise. Clearly this is an emergency. Infants with subacute disease have milder but often progressive respiratory distress and are usually diagnosed by 4 months of age. Alternatively, lobar emphysema can present more subtly in older patients with intermittent symptoms of cough, wheeze, tachypnea, or recurrent chest infection.

Both congenital and acquired forms of the disease are seen. Congenital or infantile lobar emphysema is more common in males and usually affects the upper or middle lobes. The etiology is uncertain, but it has been attributed to localized abnormalities of both the bronchi and parenchyma. Bronchial obstruction may occur from various causes, such as bronchomalacia, bronchial stenosis/atresia, extrinsic compression, or intraluminal secretions. Parenchymal involvement may be in the form of either abnormally developed alveoli or a polyalveolar lobe. Acquired lobar emphysema is seen in patients with bronchopulmonary dysplasia or pulmonary interstitial emphysema and is thought to be a consequence of the underlying lung disease or its therapy. The lesion is seen predominantly in the middle and lower lobes, more often involving the right lung. Endobronchial damage from repetitive tracheal suctioning, especially suctioning after the catheter tip has adhered to the mucosa, has been proposed as an iatrogenic factor.

Therapy is in part a function of the presenting clinical scenario and requires an early team approach coordinating the pediatrician, surgeon, radiologist, and anesthesiologist. Clinical and laboratory signs of respiratory failure or vascular compromise require aggressive management. Patients modestly distressed may deteriorate rapidly and, therefore, all should be closely watched by experienced personnel using frequent vital sign checks and cardiorespiratory monitors.

Respiratory care of the distressed neonate includes frequent assessment of respiratory effort and gas exchange efficacy. Nasal flaring, cyanosis, increasing tachypnea, retractions, paradoxical respiratory motion of the lower rib margin or abdominal wall, asymmetric breath sounds or percussion, and shift of the cardiac impulse toward or across the midline are objective signs of increasing respiratory embarrassment. Careful, sequential use of chest roentgenography helps to confirm the diagnosis, illustrates rapidity of progression, and may prevent confusion with tension pneumothorax (which is treated quite differently). An arterial line (umbilical or radial) should be established for frequent blood gas determination and continuous arterial pressure monitoring. Transcutaneous O_2/CO_2 monitors and oximetry complement the arterial line data but will not give direct hemodynamic information.

Medical management should include humidified oxygen sufficient to assure adequate oxygen delivery to vital organs and the periphery. It should be remembered that addition of oxygen will diminish the usefulness of cyanosis as an indicator of respiratory insufficiency. When possible, the patient should be placed in the lateral decubitus position with the affected lobe dependent. Intubation may be necessary for good pulmonary toilet and ventilatory support. Positive-pressure ventilation may be necessary but should be used carefully. Such ventilation, especially when used with positive end-expiratory pressure, may cause increased air trapping with deterioration. Sometimes selective intubation of the nonemphysematous lung may improve gas exchange with concomitant partial deflation of the diseased lobe. This may be more successful with the acquired form.

Nonrespiratory medical management should include the evaluation of electrolytes, glucose, urea nitrogen, and hematologic data. A secure venous line should be placed with fluids appropriate to replete and maintain fluid/electrolyte balance. A peripheral intravenous line is often adequate, although a central line also provides data on central venous pressure. Urine output should reflect good renal perfusion. A nasogastric tube should be placed and the child given nothing by mouth because of feeding-related stress, possible aspiration, and pre-

operative precaution. The significant incidence of associated cardiac defect (patent ductus, ventricular septal defect) warrants preoperative evaluation if time permits.

For neonates with severe distress, definitive therapy is surgical excision of the affected lung tissue. Preoperative blood typing and clotting studies are needed and careful anesthesia induction performed such that the patient does not struggle and develop respiratory deterioration. The surgeon may elect bronchoscopy prior to thoracotomy if it is thought that an obstruction amenable to an airway approach is present. Otherwise, relief of mediastinal compression does not occur until the emphysematous lobe is removed.

Nonoperative management may be appropriate for infants growing well with minimal symptoms, particularly those in whom diagnosis was delayed to beyond 4 months of age. Acute decompensation during viral respiratory tract infection can occur as a result of progressive air trapping during tachypnea. Such patients should be monitored accordingly. If the population for nonoperative management is carefully selected, follow-up comparison between conservatively and surgically treated patients with similar degrees of disease suggests similar results.

MECONIUM ASPIRATION SYNDROME
BRUCE R. BOYNTON, M.D., M.P.H.

The aspiration of meconium-stained amniotic fluid causes a syndrome characterized by respiratory distress and hypoxemia and is often accompanied by multiple air leaks, pulmonary hypertension, and hypoxic damage to multiple organ systems. Symptoms may be limited to mild tachypnea if only a small amount of meconium is aspirated, whereas aspiration of large volumes often results in cardiopulmonary failure and death.

The best treatment for meconium aspiration is prevention. Women at high risk for delivering infants with meconium aspiration (e.g., those who are post-term, hypertensive, or toxemic) should be monitored closely during labor. If the amniotic fluid becomes meconium stained, the fetal heart rate must be monitored continuously, and if it is abnormal, a blood sample from the fetal scalp should be obtained for pH measurement. A scalp pH lower than 7.2 indicates fetal asphyxia and the need for immediate delivery. Finally, a pediatrician must attend all deliveries involving meconium staining.

As soon as the infant's head is delivered, the obstetrician should clear the airway by suctioning the oropharynx and nasopharynx with a DeLee suction catheter and trap. The infant is then delivered and handed immediately to the pediatrician, who clears the mouth of remaining meconium with a bulb syringe or large-diameter suction catheter. If the amniotic fluid is only slightly stained and the child is vigorous, laryngoscopy and intubation are probably not needed. However, infants born through thick, or "pea soup," meconium should be intubated and suctioned, even when no meconium is seen in the oropharynx. The reason for this is that symptomatic meconium aspiration has been reported even when the oropharynx is meconium free.

Previous recommendations called for the operator to place his or her mouth over the endotracheal tube adaptor and suck meconium from the trachea into the endotracheal tube. Because of recent concern over the risk of inhaling human immunodeficiency virus (HIV)–contaminated amniotic fluid, we recommend that meconium not be removed by oral suction. A device is now available that connects the wall suction unit directly with the endotracheal tube adaptor and allows controlled suction to be applied intermittently (Meconium Aspirator, Neotech Products, Chatsworth, California).

Tracheal suction should be continued as long as meconium remains in the airway and the infant is not bradycardic. If the heart rate falls below 60 beats per minute, attempts to suction meconium should stop, and the child should be hand-ventilated using gentle pressure with a prolonged inspiratory time to inflate the lungs. If respiratory distress continues, the infant should be ventilated about 60 times per minute with moderate end-expiratory pressure and whatever peak inspiratory pressure is needed to move the anterior chest wall. We do not recommend saline lavage of the trachea in the delivery room. Large meconium plugs cannot be removed by this method, and particulate meconium may be carried into the peripheral airways. It is important to empty the stomach of meconium as well as the airways because the infant may vomit and aspirate gastric contents.

Suctioning the airway will prevent most cases of meconium aspiration syndrome. However, some infants aspirate before delivery. If the infant has aspirated meconium, he or she should be observed in a special care unit staffed by experienced nurses. Many of these infants will have tachypnea without other symptoms and be ready for transfer to the normal nursery after 8 hours of observation. Others will become progressively ill.

The infant should be placed in a neutral thermal and minimal stress environment with continuous respiratory and heart rate monitoring. Because these infants are at high risk for acute deterioration in oxygenation, they need to be monitored continuously by oximeter or transcutaneous electrode. If the infant requires an FIO_2 of greater than 0.4, an umbilical artery catheter can be inserted for easy arterial access and continuous blood pressure monitoring. If the infant has cardiovascular instability, it is useful to insert an umbilical venous catheter as well. Venous catheters can be inserted quickly, provide venous access during prolonged attempts to insert an arterial catheter, and may be used to measure central venous pressure.

Oral feedings should be delayed for 24 hours, and 10 per cent dextrose should be given by intravenous infusion. Infants with meconium aspiration syndrome are often hypoglycemic or hypocalcemic. The serum glucose level should be estimated by Dextrostix (Ames Laboratories) upon admission and repeated periodically. If the Dextrostix reading is less than 40 mg/dl, a serum glucose level should be obtained for confirmation and intravenous glucose given (6 to 8 mg/kg/min). Calcium gluconate (50 mg/kg intravenously [IV] every 6 hours) can be given if the level of ionized calcium is low.

Polycythemia frequently accompanies meconium aspiration syndrome. If the hematocrit of a venous blood sample exceeds 65 per cent and the infant is symptomatic, he or she needs a partial exchange transfusion with 5 per cent albumin.

Hourly chest percussion, vibration, postural drainage, and suction are useful adjuncts in removing residual meconium from the lungs. The infant is placed in a 20° Trendelenburg position and rotated from side to side to drain all pulmonary segments. However, these treatments are stressful for some infants and must be deferred if they compromise gas exchange.

Although meconium is sterile, it is customary to evaluate these infants for sepsis and treat them with broad-spectrum antibiotics (ampicillin, 100 mg/kg/24 hr, and gentamicin, 5 mg/kg/24 hr) if there are special risk factors, such as chorioamnionitis or prolonged rupture of membranes. If the cultures have not grown pathogens in 72 hours, antibiotics can be discontinued.

Many infants who aspirate meconium will have progressive respiratory distress and will require mechanical ventilation. We use ventilator rates between 60 and 100 per minute, with short inspiratory times (<0.3 second). Moderate end-expiratory pressures (4 to 7 cm H_2O) improve oxygenation in these infants, probably by maintaining the patency of airways that are partially obstructed by meconium. Peak inspiratory pressures should be kept as low as possible to reduce the risk of air leaks. We adjust FIO_2 to maintain the arterial PO_2 at about 100 torr in term infants and about 70 to 80 torr in preterm infants. High-frequency ventilation has not been shown to have any advantage over conventional ventilation in the treatment of meconium aspiration.

About 25 per cent of infants who aspirate meconium develop air leaks, usually pneumothoraces. The incidence is even higher in those who require mechanical ventilation. A chest radiograph should be obtained on admission and after any unexplained hypoxemia. If a pneumothorax is found, it may be treated by placing a chest tube through the third or fourth intercostal space in the anterior axillary line. The tube is then attached to a water trap and continuous suction device.

Persistent pulmonary hypertension is the most serious complication of meconium aspiration and is associated with a high mortality rate. Treatment is controversial, but most practitioners use a combination of hyperventilation, inotropes, and vasodilators. We try to maintain the PO_2 at about 100 torr, the PCO_2 at 25 to 30 torr, and the pH at 7.50 to 7.55. We avoid using paralyzing drugs but find that sedation with fentanyl (2 to 5 μg/kg every 2 hours) prevents agitation and "fighting" the ventilator. If the infant continues to be hypoxemic despite these treatments, it is worthwhile trying a vasodilator. We use tolazoline (1 mg/kg/hr IV) in a continuous infusion and omit any test dose. If the infant remains hypoxemic and is not hypotensive, we increase the infusion rate progressively (up to 5 mg/kg/hr) until oxygenation improves. Some infants who fail to respond to tolazoline will have improved oxygenation after infusion with other vasodilators such as prostaglandin E_1 (0.1 to 0.4 µg/kg/min). Tolazoline and prostaglandin E_1 are systemic as well as pulmonary vasodilators and may cause hypotension. With use of these drugs, dopamine may be needed to maintain systemic blood pressure. There is recent evidence that some infants with meconium aspiration syndrome and severe pulmonary hypertension may be helped by extracorporeal membrane oxygenation.

Meconium aspiration is almost always accompanied by asphyxia, and the infant may suffer hypoxic damage to multiple organ systems, including the heart, brain, and kidneys. If cardiac impairment is suspected, an electrocardiogram and echocardiogram should be obtained immediately. Frequent echocardiographic findings include right ventricular dysfunction and tricuspid regurgitation. A right-to-left shunt across the foramen ovale may also be present. This shunt can be detected on the four-chamber view of the heart by injecting 1 to 2 ml of saline through a peripheral vein and visualizing microbubbles in the right atrium cross the foramen to the left atrium. Serial echocardiograms can also help in assessing the response of a poorly functioning ventricle to inotropic drugs. Hypotensive infants should be given a bolus of colloid suspension, such as 5 per cent albumin (10 ml/kg), to increase intravascular volume. If this is not effective, it can be followed with a continuous infusion of dopamine (5 µg/kg/min).

Infants with hypoxic-ischemic encephalopathy may be hypertonic, hypotonic, or tremulous and often have seizures in the first 12 hours of life. Phenobarbital is the drug of choice, in a loading dose of 20 mg/kg IV, followed by 4 mg/kg/24 hr. Phenytoin can be added if needed (a loading dose of 20 mg/kg IV and a maintenance dose of 5 mg/kg/24 hr). Additional phenobarbital may be given if the seizures continue, but it should be remembered that phenobarbital is a myocardial depressant and must be used with caution in infants with impaired cardiac function.

Infants with meconium aspiration syndrome may be oliguric or anuric from hypoxic damage to their kidneys. Until the infant urinates, he or she should not receive potassium and fluids should be limited to replacement of insensible losses (40 to 60 ml/kg/24 hr). Urine output must be measured carefully; determination of urea nitrogen and serum creatinine levels is also helpful.

DISORDERS OF THE UMBILICUS

JOSEPH L. KENNEDY, Jr., M.D.

The umbilical cord comprises two arteries and a vein embedded in a mucoid gel, Wharton's jelly. (A fine nutrient vessel is rarely visible on the surface of the cord as a thin red line.)

Appearance. Thick cords are associated with healthy premature infants; thin cords are more often found in term infants and are associated with intrauterine growth retardation. The average length of the cord is 55 to 60 cm. The cord is significantly shorter (<35 cm) when there is diminished fetal movement, usually from uterine constraint secondary to oligohydramnios. The cord is stained yellow or green with bilirubin or meconium, respectively, in the amniotic fluid; pink or red cords indicate recent intra-amniotic hemorrhage, usually abruption. Localized areas of yellowish edema are occasionally seen normally.

Involution. After birth, the umbilical cord begins to atrophy and the vessels begin to thrombose and become obliterated. The cord stump will remain for 1 to 2 weeks, rarely for as long as a month. Delayed separation of the cord is associated with local or systemic antibiotic therapy, with cesarean birth, and with certain rare disorders of leukocyte function.

Cord Care. The cord is clamped 2 to 4 cm from the abdominal wall with a clamp providing constant pressure. Prevention of umbilical infection, granuloma, or colonization with pathogens is best achieved by daily treatment of the cord with a topical antimicrobial agent, dispensed from an individual or single-use container. Povidone-iodine ointment, bacitracin ointment USP, chlorhexidine gluconate skin cleanser, or 1 per cent silver sulfadiazine cream is effective. The use of 70 per cent alcohol is effective in promoting drying of the cord but may be associated with increased bacterial colonization; triple dye is efficacious in preventing staphylococcal colonization but is not well accepted by parents or nursery personnel. Routine washing or cleansing of the cord is contraindicated, since dry conditions inhibit bacterial growth.

Infection. Local mild chronic infection of the cord may be associated with the development of an umbilical granuloma. Care must be taken to distinguish this from a patent omphalomesenteric duct or patent urachus. Treatment consists of careful repeated cauterization with topical 75 per cent silver nitrate. More serious infection of the umbilicus, omphalitis, can be caused by group A or B streptococci, or by *Staphylococcus aureus*. Contamination of the umbilicus with soil or feces can result in neonatal tetanus when maternal immunity is lacking. Parenteral antibiotic treatment appropriate to the organism should be undertaken immediately. Complications of omphalitis include hepatic abscess, septicemia, portal vein thrombosis, periumbilical gangrene, and umbilical arteritis.

Injury. Injury to the cord, with hematoma, rupture, avulsion, or blood loss, can occur from maternal abdominal trauma, external version, or amniocentesis or percutaneous umbilical blood sampling or may occur during delivery with a velamentous insertion of the cord or vasa praevia. The cord may be inadvertently incised at episiotomy or at cesarean delivery.

Vascular Problems. Other causes of bleeding are hemorrhagic disease of the newborn and failed ligation after umbilical vessel catheterization or from a slipped clamp; fetal-maternal or twin-twin transfusion or fetal-placental hemorrhage may occur in utero. Exsanguination or severe hemorrhagic shock may ensue. Umbilical artery thrombosis, coarctation, or narrowing can be associated with fetal distress or demise. Constriction of the umbilical cord may also occur with idiopathic in utero torsion or from an amniotic band; such bands may cause disruption of distal extremities in the infant.

Congenital Anomalies. *Single umbilical artery* is associated with some degree of intrauterine growth retardation, with twinning, and with an increased incidence of nonspecific congenital anomalies. Single umbilical artery occurs in 1 per cent of newborns and is almost always found when the infant has trisomy 18. The abdominal skin commonly grows out a short distance along the cord (*umbilicus cutis*); rarely, it is absent around the insertion of the cord (*umbilicus amnioticus*). *Umbilical hernias,* common in blacks, are usually small and often not recognized at birth because of the overlying cord stump. They resolve spontaneously over several years, do not rupture or incarcerate, and do not need surgical repair or strapping. Umbilical hernias may also be found with congenital hypothyroidism.

Omphaloceles, often now diagnosed in utero, are obvious at birth. A search should be made for accompanying congenital anomalies; Beckwith syndrome may manifest at birth, with macrosomia, macroglossia, omphalocele, and symptomatic hypoglycemia. Eventration of the abdominal contents onto the abdomen without an enclosing membrane is almost always gastroschisis rather than a ruptured omphalocele. In this instance, a normal umbilicus will be located lateral to the defect.

Cord *mucoceles* or cord *cysts* are seen uncommonly. They may be mucoid, allantoic, or omphalomesenteric in origin but seldom have any clinical significance. Care should be taken to clamp or ligate the cord proximal to these lesions so as not to cause localized infection or delayed separation of the cord.

Patent urachus or *omphalomesenteric duct* may be associated with drainage of urine, mucus, or stool. The differentiating urinary and gastrointestinal tracts are, during early embryonic life, in close proximity to the umbilicus. Communicating structures may persist; partial patency of these structures may be associated with cystic masses.

Cysts or polyps of the umbilicus itself are usually omphalomesenteric duct remnants and often require surgical removal. A persistent patent omphalomesenteric duct will cause a yellowish secretion and wetness of the cord stump. The diagnosis can be made by inspection or microscopic examination of the cross-section cut surface of the cord or by probing the umbilicus for a fistulous duct. Rarely, the ileum will prolapse through the duct, and surgical repair will be required. Such a prolapse can be associated with a small bowel volvulus.

Aberrant gastric mucosa can be found in the umbilicus, producing an acid mucous secretion.

Patent urachus may cause wetness of the umbilical stump; it may be associated with bladder neck or urethral obstruction and must be managed surgically.

Tumors of the umbilical cord are rare; hemangiomas can bleed or be associated with fetal death.

NEONATAL ASCITES
TIMOS VALAES, M.D.

The emphasis in this article is on the management of isolated neonatal ascites in contrast to generalized edema and fluid accumulation in all the body cavities (hydrops fetalis). Nevertheless, there is considerable overlap in the causes of the two conditions, and often ascites predominates in the clinical picture of hydrops and requires immediate paracentesis to relieve the respiratory embarrassment. In the great majority of the cases the ascites is present at birth; i.e., the onset is in intrauterine life. Ultrasonography has considerably facilitated the etiologic diagnosis of ascites and, even more importantly, has shifted the diagnosis and often the treatment to intrauterine life.

Management of Fetal Ascites

Distention of the fetal abdomen by free fluid is relatively easy to detect and differentiate from dilatation of abdominal hollow organs such as the gastrointestinal tract, the urinary collecting system, the female genital tract, and the bile ducts and the gallbladder. The presence or absence of generalized fetal edema and of hepatosplenomegaly provides key information in the etiologic diagnosis of fetal ascites. Appropriate laboratory investigations should be undertaken whenever the sonographic information does not provide a definite etiology. Because of the frequency of urinary ascites and the possibility of intrauterine intervention to relieve the underlying obstructive uropathy, it is important in the sonographic investigation of fetal ascites to visualize the kidneys, the ureters, and the bladder and to estimate the volume of amniotic fluid as an indicator of renal function. A further refinement involves the real-time assessment of bladder filling after percutaneous urine aspiration. In the absence of a definite cause for early fetal ascites, continuous sonographic monitoring is indicated because spontaneous resolution has been well documented. This is more likely to happen if cryptogenic fetal ascites is associated with polyhydramnios. Following spontaneous resolution of fetal ascites, laxity of abdominal wall with, as an extreme, the "prune belly" appearance is the tell-tale finding at birth. Resolution of fetal ascites accompanied by oligohydramnios indicates progressive renal failure as a result of retrograde pressure from urinary obstruction. In this event renal dysplasia and pulmonary hypoplasia incompatible with survival are already present.

Intrauterine drainage of early fetal ascites either by repeated paracentesis or by placement of a special shunt catheter from the fetal abdomen to the amniotic cavity should be undertaken in order to avoid the effects on pulmonary development of the elevation of the diaphragm and in cases of urinary ascites in order to decompress the obstructed urinary tract, avoid renal dysplasia, and maintain an adequate volume of amniotic fluid, thus preventing the development of Potter's syndrome.

It should be emphasized that both in utero and after birth only a small percentage of the cases with obstructive uropathy are complicated by urinary ascites. In the majority of the cases megacystic megaureters and hydronephrosis are present, and decompression in utero requires the placement of a shunt catheter from the dilated bladder to the amniotic cavity. Theoretically, preterm delivery with extrauterine decompression of the urinary tract offers an alternative solution. Nevertheless, it appears that by 30 to 32 weeks of gestation, when the risks due to prematurity are acceptable, the majority of the fetuses have suffered irreparable renal damage and pulmonary hypoplasia, whereas those that have escaped this fate can safely be left to be delivered spontaneously, provided that they are closely monitored sonographically.

Ascites and, more commonly, hydrops can result from fetal paroxysmal supraventricular tachycardia, which is relatively easily diagnosed with fetal heart monitoring or fetal ECG. Correction of tachycardia and heart failure has followed digitalization by administering digitalis to the mother. Resolution of the tachycardia and of the ascites and hydrops may take 1 to 2 weeks, and digitalization should continue up to the delivery. Whether transplacental digitalization or diuretics will be helpful in the management of fetal ascites or hydrops due to cardiac malformations or congenital heart block has not been well documented but may be worth trying.

Fetal ascites of other than renal or cardiac etiology is not amenable to intrauterine treatment, and fetal paracentesis for diagnostic purposes is rarely justified. (The treatment of immunologic hydrops fetalis with intrauterine transfusion is outside the scope of this discussion.) Occasionally fetal abdominal paracentesis during early labor will be necessary to allow for vaginal delivery and to prevent respiratory difficulties after birth.

Management of Neonatal Ascites

A long list of diseases and conditions is associated with ascites in the newborn and small infant. Obviously, the treatment of the underlying condition, if available, leads to the permanent resolution of ascites. Irrespective of the etiology of ascites, aspiration of the ascitic fluid is often indicated for diagnostic purposes and to relieve the respiratory embarrassment caused by the increased intra-abdominal pressure and the resultant elevation of the diaphragm.

Technique of Abdominal Paracentesis. The newborn is placed in supine position with the extremities restrained. The right or left lower abdominal quadrant is prepared with an antiseptic solution, such as povidone-iodine (Betadine), and draped. A 20- or 22-gauge "Intracath" needle and catheter are introduced just below the umbilicus and outside the lateral border of the rectus muscle. When the peritoneal cavity is entered, as indicated by the feeling of "give," the catheter is advanced and the needle removed while suction is applied with a syringe. Enough fluid is removed to relieve the respiratory embarrassment. Complete removal of the ascitic fluid should be avoided for fear of abrupt shift of intravascular fluid and circulatory collapse. A sterile dressing is placed after withdrawal of the catheter. Some leakage of ascitic fluid through the puncture site is likely to occur. Vital signs should be followed closely after the

paracentesis. The fluid should be sent for laboratory analysis (total protein, electrolytes, urea, creatinine, and triglycerides, if milky in appearance), cell count, Gram's stain, and culture. Laboratory data for the ascitic fluid, particularly in cases of urinary ascites, when high urea and creatinine are expected, can be misleading, as the fluid rapidly equilibrates with the rest of the extracellular fluid and loses its diagnostic characteristics. This is not likely to occur with meconium or infectious peritonitis or with bilious or chylous ascites. In the latter the characteristic appearance and chemistry develop only after milk feedings have been given.

Specific Treatment. The etiology determines the specific medical or surgical treatment of neonatal ascites. Thus, laparotomy and the appropriate surgical closure, anastomosis, or "-ostomy" are the treatments used for bilious ascites and ascites associated with the generalized type of meconium peritonitis. Similarly, relief of the obstruction leads to resolution of the ascites associated with hydrometrocolpos from imperforate hymen or atresia of the vagina.

The treatment of urinary and chylous ascites and the ascites associated with liver disease will be discussed separately.

Management of Neonatal Urinary Ascites

Whether present at birth or developing in the first few days of life, the leakage of urine into the peritoneal cavity is the result of obstructive uropathy, and the principles of treatment are the same irrespective of the level of obstruction. The site of leakage or perforation is not always apparent, and its localization is not essential for treatment. Decompression of the urinary tract, initially by catheterization, should be attempted. If the cause of obstructive uropathy is posterior urethral valves or bladder neck obstruction, catheter drainage is often sufficient. Prolonged adequate drainage, necessary for recovery of renal function, is achieved by suprapubic vesicostomy. This achieves adequate drainage and allows for the recovery of renal function. If the initial ultrasonographic assessment and the cystourethrogram demonstrate unilateral or bilateral obstruction proximal to the bladder, nephrostomy or ureterostomy is necessary. Nephrostomy is also necessary when, in spite of vesicostomy, urinary ascites persists and the upper urinary tract remains dilated. Very rarely will it be necessary to localize the site of perforation and close it surgically. Even when urinary ascites results from transection of a persistent urachus during umbilical artery cut-down, catheter drainage of the bladder proves sufficient to seal the perforation.

In spite of its dramatic clinical presentation, urinary ascites from obstructive uropathy has good prognosis. Ascites indicates that there is good urine production and renal function. The initial impression of severe renal failure is misleading. Anuria or oliguria is due to the escape of urine into the peritoneal cavity, whereas the grossly elevated BUN, creatinine, and often potassium reflect not the functional status of the kidneys but the fact that the urine in the peritoneal cavity equilibrates with the plasma—reverse peritoneal dialysis. Occasionally, life-threatening hyperkalemia will need to be

INFANTS OF DRUG-DEPENDENT MOTHERS **703**

treated with Kayexalate retention enema (1 gm of resin per kg of body weight every 2 to 6 hours) and/or glucose-insulin infusion (1 unit of insulin per 3 gm of glucose). Initially fluid administration should be restricted to insensible water loss (400 ml per square meter of body surface per day) and liberalized as soon as adequate drainage and decreasing ascites are demonstrated. The effectiveness of the treatment is monitored by following closely the changes in body weight, abdominal girth, and sonographic appearance of the urinary tract and by the improvement in urine output, blood electrolytes, BUN, and serum creatinine.

The surgical techniques used to correct the various types of urinary tract obstruction are beyond the scope of this discussion.

Management of Neonatal Chylous Ascites

A variety of malformations of the intestinal lymphatics have been described in isolated congenital chylous ascites as well as in chylous ascites associated with sporadic or hereditary congenital lymphedema. Chylothorax often coexists. The diagnosis is based on the characteristic milky appearance and high triglyceride content and lymphocyte count of the fluid after milk feeding has been started. Chylous ascites associated with lymphedema is often complicated by protein-losing enteropathy with severe malnutrition as an additional problem. Surgical exploration, in an effort to localize the site of the leakage of lymph, is seldom rewarding. Success has been reported with formulas containing only medium-chain triglycerides (e.g., Portagen), which are transported directly by the portal system without chylomicron formation, which increases the intestinal lymph flow. When this fails, a trial of complete bowel rest, achieved by total parenteral nutrition—including lipid infusion—for a period of several weeks, has resulted in permanent sealing of the leaking lymphatics.

Surgical efforts to excise the malformed cisterna chyli, resection of the loops with the most extensive lymphangiectasia, and finally, peritoneovenous shunts should be considered in intractable chylous ascites but offer few chances of success.

Management of Neonatal Ascites Due to Liver Failure

The treatment of ascites due to liver failure and cirrhosis is similar in all pediatric age groups and, with few exceptions, independent of the primary cause of liver failure. The predominant liver diseases of early infancy, extrahepatic biliary atresia and cryptogenic "neonatal hepatitis," do not produce liver failure and ascites early in the neonatal period. Fetal and neonatal ascites or hydrops has been described as an early manifestation of several hereditary storage diseases, such as Wolman's and Gaucher's, gangliosidoses, mucopolysaccharidoses, and sialadenosis. Other metabolic diseases that can result in a rapidly evolving liver failure and ascites include galactosemia and fructose intolerance. The latter is unlikely to manifest in the neonatal period, as modern infant formulas do not contain cane sugar, and fruit juices are not introduced in the diet of infants before several weeks of age. Early recognition and

special diets lacking the offending monosaccharide result in reversal of the liver failure and ascites.

Of the transplacentally transmitted agents, *Toxoplasma*, *Treponema*, and the cytomegalovirus can cause fulminant hepatic failure. The hepatitis B virus is usually transmitted perinatally, and the rare acute yellow atrophy develops after the first month of life. Similarly, cholestasis and ascites in sick, very low birth weight infants on parenteral nutrition develop slowly and after at least 3 weeks of total parenteral nutrition.

The ill-defined familial fatal neonatal hepatitis offers the most dramatic example of acute liver failure and ascites in early life. Cholestatic jaundice, coagulopathy, and hyperammonemia with convulsions and coma develop within the first week of life, leading rapidly to death in spite of supportive treatment. The histology of the liver is that of "giant cell hepatitis" with extensive hepatocellular necrosis. The search for an infectious agent or metabolic disorder has been unrewarding. Specifically, extensive search for the markers of hepatitis viruses, including the non-A, non-B virus(es), in both the patients and their mothers has been negative. The author has treated two infants in two families with exchange transfusions to correct the coagulopathy and ameliorate the hyperammonemia. Immediate improvement of the general status followed the procedure, with gradual resolution of jaundice, hepatosplenomegaly, and ascites in the next several months. At follow-up at 7 and 12 years of age there was no evidence of liver or other metabolic disease, and growth and development were normal. It is difficult to explain this experience and to argue that exchange transfusion is the specific treatment for this condition. Nevertheless, with the excuse of using an effective method to correct the coagulopathy, exchange transfusion should be tried in neonatal acute liver failure of unknown etiology and should be used definitely in familial cases.

The symptomatic management of ascites accompanying liver disease includes (a) sodium restriction to 1 to 2 mEq/kg/day and (b) diuretics. Spironolactone, 3 to 5 mg/kg/day with a maximum dose of 10 mg/kg/day, is the agent of choice, since ascites from liver disease is associated with secondary hyperaldosteronism. If there is no response after treatment with increasing doses for 6 to 8 days, furosemide (1 to 2 mg/kg/day) is added. Electrolytes should be closely monitored and deviations corrected. (c) Correction of hypoproteinemia and reduced intravascular volume is carried out by administration of either 1 gm/kg salt-poor human albumin or 10 ml/kg of fresh frozen plasma over 2 to 3 hours followed by furosemide or ethacrynic acid. Success with this symptomatic treatment will be transient if the underlying process is irreversible.

INFANTS OF DRUG-DEPENDENT MOTHERS

ROSITA S. PILDES, M.D.,
and GOPAL SRINIVASAN, M.D.

Drug withdrawal is only one of the problems in the neonate who has been exposed in utero to pharmacologic agents that may adversely affect total development as well as development of individual organ systems. Treatment, therefore, should be instituted as early in pregnancy as possible.

INTRAPARTUM CARE

A detailed history of drug intake should be taken on all pregnant women at the time of admission, keeping in mind that not all neonatal withdrawal syndromes are due to narcotics and not all women taking drugs are drug dependent. This information must then be relayed to the pediatrician to facilitate therapeutic intervention in the neonate without excessive investigation because of inadequate information. Drugs that have been reported to cause neonatal withdrawal symptoms are listed in Table 1.

Cocaine abuse increases the risk of placental abruption, premature labor, and fetal distress secondary to decreased uterine blood flow and to increased oxygen requirement by the fetus. The intrapartum period is the most inopportune time for withdrawal of drugs from the mother, who is already undergoing the additional stress from labor and delivery. Methadone and meperidine are commonly used to prevent intrapartum withdrawal. Excessive fetal movements and increased oxygen requirements secondary to withdrawal may cause fetal distress; fetal monitoring is therefore essential, and a physician well versed in resuscitation should be present in the delivery room. Respiratory depression at birth may result from excessive use of drugs prior to delivery but can usually be overcome by prompt attention to the airway. Naloxone (Narcan) is not recommended because the drug may precipitate acute withdrawal symptoms, including seizures.

Most drug-dependent mothers do not take a single drug, and the presence of other drugs may alter or potentiate the withdrawal response of the infant. Cocaine alone or in conjunction with other drugs acounts for 70 to 80 per cent of the drugs found in maternal or neonatal urine. A very careful history of additional drugs must be obtained, and a toxicology screening of cord blood and urine collected during the first day of postnatal life should be performed.

NEONATAL CARE

Treatment in the neonatal period is directed not only at therapy of the withdrawal syndrome but also at problems secondary to prematurity and intrauterine growth retardation. Supportive therapy includes correction of hypoxemia, hypoglycemia, and polycythemia and provision of adequate fluid and calories. Respiratory alkalosis secondary to tachypnea rarely requires therapy. The increased incidence of syphilis, gonorrhea, and hepatitis in drug-dependent mothers must be kept in mind and the infant checked accordingly.

Therapeutic intervention is not always necessary, since symptoms, when present, are often self-limited. A quiet, comforting environment with gentle handling, swaddling, and frequent feedings may be sufficient. Therapy is indicated when the symptoms interfere with adequate weight gain and well being. These include

TABLE 1. Drugs Associated with Neonatal Withdrawal Syndrome

Cocaine
Narcotics
  Heroin
  Methadone
  Codeine
Barbiturates
Analgesics
  Pentazocine (Talwin)
  Propoxyphene hydrochloride (Darvon)
Tranquilizers and sedatives
  Bromides
  Chlordiazepoxide (Librium)
  Desipramine hydrochloride (Pertofrane)
  Diazepam (Valium)
  Ethchlorvynol (Placidyl)
  Glutethimide (Doriden)
  Hydroxyzine hydrochloride (Atarax)
Combination of drugs
  Ts and blues [Talwin and tripelennamine (Pyribenzamine)]
Alcohol
Sympathomimetics
  Amphetamines
Phencyclidine (PCP)

vomiting or diarrhea, marked irritability and tremors that interfere with sleep or feeding, and seizures.

Therapeutic regimens vary considerably among centers, and a number of scoring systems have been developed in an attempt to standardize evaluation of symptoms and treatment responses. Most of the pharmacologic agents used have been successful in controlling the acute withdrawal syndrome. Although narcotic withdrawal symptoms are relieved most specifically by use of a narcotic, most pediatricians are reluctant to use a narcotic in the infant for fear of promoting drug dependence.

The various pharmacologic agents that have been used for therapy of drug withdrawal are outlined in Table 2. The choice of drugs is arbitrary; we prefer phenobarbital or chlorpromazine, but paregoric is often used in infants with diarrhea. In general, the drug is titrated starting with the smallest recommended dose until the desired effect is achieved. Once the infant is asymptomatic for 2 to 3 days, the drug is tapered until it is completely discontinued. Infants whose symptoms are controlled for only short periods of time may need more frequent administration. Tapering should be started by first gradually lowering the dose and then increasing the length of time between administrations. The tapering process may proceed every 48 hours as long as withdrawal symptoms do not reappear. Tremors, however, may persist for months.

Phenobarbital has been used extensively since 1947 and appears to provide adequate control of symptoms. Suppression of withdrawal signs is accomplished by a generalized, nonspecific central nervous system depres-

TABLE 2. Drugs Used for Treatment of Neonatal Withdrawal Syndrome

	Dose/kg	Route	Interval Between Doses
Phenobarbital	1–2 mg	IM or PO	q6h
Chlorpromazine	0.5–0.7 mg	IM or PO	q6h
Paregoric	0.05–0.1 ml	PO	q4–6h
Diazepam	0.3–0.5 mg	IM or PO	q8h

sion. Side effects include excessive sedation, which may lead to inadequate fluid and caloric intake. Diarrhea may remain uncontrolled. The duration of phenobarbital therapy ranges from 4 to 14 days in our nursery. The potential for withdrawal symptoms from phenobarbital therapy must be kept in mind; usually, infants requiring treatment for 2 weeks or less have not shown signs of barbiturate dependence.

Chlorpromazine was introduced in 1959 and is effective in controlling symptoms within hours after it has been initiated. The drug may be given orally or intramuscularly if vomiting or diarrhea is present. Side effects include extrapyramidal signs in infants who have received more than 2.8 mg/kg/24 hr. In our nursery, the mean duration of therapy with chlorpromazine has been 9 days, with a range of 3 to 17 days.

Paregoric (camphorated tincture of opium) has been used since the nineteenth century. Paregoric appears to control symptoms, with restoration of normal central nervous system function as measured by sucking behavior, whereas central nervous system depression may be observed with phenobarbital or diazepam therapy. The usual dose of paregoric is 0.05 to 0.1 ml/kg every 4 hours before feeding. If at the end of the 4-hour period symptoms have not decreased, the dose may be increased. Once the symptoms are controlled for at least 48 hours, tapering may begin. One of the drawbacks in the use of paregoric is the prolonged period often required for the tapering process (20 to 45 days). In addition, paregoric contains camphor, a known central nervous system stimulant. Camphor is absorbed rapidly and excreted slowly in the urine because it is lipid soluble and requires glucuronide conjugation. For this reason, tincture of opium (laudanum) is preferable whenever a narcotic is used. Care must be exercised in using the correct dilution, since laudanum comes in a 10 per cent solution equivalent to 1 per cent morphine, whereas paregoric contains 0.04 per cent morphine. Laudanum must be diluted 25-fold to obtain the same dilution and can then be used similarly to paregoric.

Diazepam is effective in suppressing withdrawal signs but does not appear to offer any advantages over the other drugs. Diazepam is usually given intramuscularly at the onset but may be continued orally. Once symptoms are controlled, the initial dose is cut in half; the time interval between doses is then increased to 12 hours, then the dose is cut in half again. The drug is usually administered for only a few days, since it is poorly metabolized and excreted and has a prolonged half-life. Moreover, the parenteral preparation contains sodium benzoate, which competes with bilirubin for albumin-binding sites.

Methadone has been introduced more recently because of its wide use in the therapy of heroin addiction in adults. Theoretically, methadone is the drug of choice in infants of methadone-dependent mothers.* However, methadone is not easily available, the dose is not standardized, and there is greater difficulty in weaning the infant. Moreover, withdrawal symptoms from methadone respond to the same drugs used for heroin withdrawal.

*The use of methadone in infants is not listed by the manufacturer.

The variety in therapeutic approaches indicates that the optimal regimen has yet to be demonstrated. Further studies based on clinical as well as biochemical observations are necessary to compare the effects of the various drugs. Unfortunately, long-term effects are difficult to obtain, since follow-up of infants of addicted mothers is fraught with numerous problems.

Cocaine abuse is different from other drug addictions and therefore deserves special attention. It is unclear whether cocaine withdrawal produces clear-cut abstinence syndrome. Infants exposed to cocaine in utero have significant depression of interactive behavior and poor organizational response to environmental stimuli by Brazelton neonatal behavior scale assessment. In addition to prematurity and IUGR, fetal and neonatal hypertension, tachycardia, stroke, hemorrhagic cerebral infarctions in "neonatally silent areas of brain," and abnormal EEGs have been reported. The etiology and incidence of teratogenic effects are unclear; they include genitourinary anomalies, skull defects, and exencephaly.

Management of the neonate also requires sensitivity toward the needs of the mother. Support, encouragement, and teaching are necessary to improve the mother's self-esteem. The infant should not be transferred to the high-risk nursery except when therapeutic intervention is necessary. Since the mother will frequently be discharged prior to the infant, these hours of early contact may be the most important in promoting maternal-infant bonding and possibly preventing the high incidence of child abuse.

Breast feeding by drug-addicted mothers should be undertaken cautiously, with careful monitoring of the infant. The advantage of promoting maternal-infant bonding must be weighed against the potential risk to the neonate. For example, methadone is excreted in breast milk; yet, breast feeding should be encouraged in mothers enrolled in methadone programs, and the dose of methadone cut down to minimum levels. Drugs such as heroin have been known for years to be excreted in breast milk, and at one time withdrawal symptoms were treated by breast feeding with gradual weaning. Breast feeding is contraindicated during cocaine abuse, since the drug is excreted up to 60 hours after maternal use. Hypertension, tachycardia, sweating, mydriasis, apnea, and seizures have been observed in infants intoxicated with cocaine through breastfeeding. Almost all analgesics (meperidine, propoxyphene hydrochloride, pentazocine, diazepam, and barbiturates) appear in breast milk in low levels but may accumulate in the neonate. Individual variation in drug excretion will determine whether the neonate will be sleepy, hypotonic, or depressed or have poor sucking. Thus, breast feeding recommendations must be individualized and should be based on the risk-to-benefit ratio to the infant.

POSTNEONATAL CARE

Exacerbation or recurrence of withdrawal symptoms may be present for 3 to 6 months after birth and include restlessness, agitation, tremors, and brief periods of sleep. Medication should be avoided if at all possible. Additional problems that arise after discharge are thrombocytosis and an increased incidence of sudden infant death syndrome.

DISCHARGE PLANNING

The social service department should be involved with the family, and the infant can be discharged to the mother if there are adequate support systems in the home. Reporting of an infant with positive urine screen is mandatory in some states. Many addicted mothers appear anxious to keep their babies but do not have a realistic view of their own ability to care for the infant. Good prognostic signs include a stable marital relationship, successful raising of other children, addiction to a single drug, enrollment in a drug program, and a short duration of addiction. The caretakers should be aware of the expected behavior of the infant, such as increased sensitivity to auditory stimuli, decreased visual orientation, excessive crying, and increased sucking needs. The infants often respond to a soft soothing voice, gentle rocking, holding, and use of a pacifier. Follow-up visits by a visiting nurse, social worker, or ex-addict counselor may be helpful. A great deal of time and energy is invested in each case to ensure supervision of the child's care, but despite all efforts, approximately 15 to 20 per cent of the infants require placement in foster homes.

LONG-TERM PROGNOSIS

Early withdrawal symptoms of irritability, hyperactivity, sleep, feeding problems, and hypertonicity may persist for several months. Longitudinal studies are scarce because a large percentage of the patients are lost to follow-up. Postnatal environmental conditions such as inconsistent care, poor living conditions, and perinatal HIV infections also influence the outcome. In one study, behavioral disturbances, brief attention span, and temper tantrums were identified in 7 of 14 infants of mothers addicted to heroin. Children of mothers maintained on methadone who were followed up to 18 months of age were noted to have a higher incidence of otitis media, head circumference below the third percentile, neurologic findings of tone discrepancies, developmental delays, poor fine motor coordination, and lower scores on Bayley mental and motor developmental indices. Striking deficits in free play situations that require self-organization, self-initiation, and follow-through have been observed. This lack of creativity in toddlers may be a better predictor of long-term outcome than the performance on structured developmental tests. High correlation has been reported between the hyperexcitable state in the neonate and neurologic and behavioral dysfunction at 1.5 to 4 years of age.

Acquired immune deficiency syndrome (AIDS) has been reported in infants born primarily to intravenous drug-addicted mothers or those who are sexually promiscuous. Intrauterine growth retardation, failure to thrive, lymphadenopathy, hepatosplenomegaly, parotitis, interstitial pneumonia, profound cell-mediated immunodeficiency with reversed T4/T8 ratios, and hypergammaglobulinemia have been observed in children with AIDS. Although the mode of transmission is unclear, clinical histories strongly suggest vertical transmission.

MATERNAL ALCOHOL INGESTION: EFFECTS ON THE DEVELOPING FETUS

STERLING K. CLARREN, M.D.

Because the effects of prenatal exposure to alcohol are not reversible postnatally, management is confined to prevention and remediation.

PREVENTION

Primary Prevention. It is clear that maternal alcohol consumption during pregnancy can adversely affect the developing embryo or fetus. Frequent high-dose exposures may produce the fetal alcohol syndrome (FAS). Frequent moderate-dose exposures or infrequent high-dose exposures have not generally been associated with FAS but may be linked to increased rates of major malformations, decreased infant size, and decreased intellectual performance. Unfortunately, the words "frequent," "infrequent," "high dose," and "moderate dose" cannot be precisely defined in terms of maternal alcohol consumption. Blood alcohol concentration is not determined solely by the number of drinks consumed but is also related to maternal size, rate of alcohol absorption and metabolism, duration of the period of consumption, and types of food consumed with the alcoholic beverage. Other maternal factors, such as the number of years during which alcohol has been consumed, smoking, and nutritional deficiencies, and individual fetal resistance to teratogenesis may be other important determinants of embryo-fetal outcome. Therefore, the *safest* recommendation for alcohol use in pregnancy remains the following: Women who are pregnant or even considering pregnancy should avoid alcohol altogether. Given our society's general attitude, however, more realistic (albeit highly arbitrary) advice would be that pregnant women and those considering pregnancy should avoid intoxication at all times and should use alcohol only in low doses (less than the amount in two standard drinks per occasion) on an intermittent basis (7 days between occasions). Women who are pregnant and acknowledge abusive drinking behaviors should be encouraged to stop drinking. Although early gestational exposure is probably the most dangerous period for teratogenicity, middle and third trimester exposure may adversely affect overall growth and brain development. There are some data to suggest that growth deficiency and some intellectual deficits may be at least partially ameliorated through the discontinuation of alcohol consumption in later pregnancy.

The women most likely to produce infants with FAS or other alcohol-related birth defects are alcoholics or heavy intermittent binge drinkers who are unlikely to alter their drinking behavior simply because they have heard a cautionary tale. If our society is serious about preventing FAS, a condition that may account for 10 per cent of the mental retardation in this country, we will need to develop alcohol treatment programs specifically designed for pregnant alcoholics and effective outreach methods for identifying and attracting these high-risk individuals into therapy.

Secondary Prevention. No prenatal test has yet been shown to be capable of diagnosing FAS in the fetus. Some fetuses with FAS are very small or have severe malformations of the heart, kidney, or brain that may be detected by ultrasonography. No pattern of drinking has been linked to the production of FAS at a rate of more than 30 to 40 per cent. Consequently, termination of pregnancy cannot generally be decided strictly on the basis of early gestational alcohol exposure history or diagnostic imaging results.

REMEDIATION

Neonatal Assessment. The diagnosis of FAS is made correctly in only about one third to one half of affected newborns. This fact is not surprising, since the diagnosis is based in part on brain dysfunction, which may not be apparent until later in childhood, and on facial features, which can be subtle in the neonate. Early diagnosis is especially relevant, however, when the infant is to be placed for adoption. Potential adoptive parents of infants gestationally exposed to any multiple pattern of intoxicating amounts of alcohol should be warned of the potential dangers of future medical and educational problems, even when the newborn's physical examination is normal.

If a woman is intoxicated at the time of delivery, the newborn will have about the same blood alcohol concentration as the mother at parturition. Although alcohol is slowly metabolized by newborns, supportive treatment is generally all that is required. Irritability, jitters, and poor feeding are often observed in FAS infants. Neonatal seizures are occasionally reported and should be considered in any infant with FAS. When the neurologic irritability is not due to seizures, the baby may be calmed by reducing environmental stimuli, such as dimming the lights and tight swaddling.

Medical Management. Growth failure is the most consistent health problem in children with FAS. No treatable explanation for growth deficiency has yet been found. Children with FAS should be screened for occult renal anomalies and should be carefully followed for commonly associated problems like visual refractive errors, strabismus, middle ear disease, cardiac anomalies, and scoliosis. Occlusal problems are very common in older children with FAS, who frequently develop a Class III occlusion (prognathism). Nearly every major malformation has been reported in some child with FAS.

Educational Management. No specific level or pattern of cognitive disability is found in children with FAS, and consequently, individual assessments are needed. Infant stimulation programs, physical therapy, occupational therapy, speech therapy, and educational remediation may all be required.

A large number of children with FAS show signs of marked distractibility. This may be manifested as jitteriness in the infant, hyperactivity in the preschool child, and an inability to concentrate on academic topics in the schoolchild. The usual medications prescribed for hyperactivity, like methylphenidate, have not been particularly helpful in children with FAS. Behavioral modification may be of use.

Family Management. Long-term follow-up studies of children with FAS reveal that a large percentage of their mothers are missing or dead 5 years after the birth of the children. Mothers of children with FAS are often far-advanced alcoholics, and every effort should be expended in bringing them into treatment.

Mothers and fathers of children with FAS generally feel tremendous guilt and anger. They generally benefit from psychological support and family counseling in addition to the other services mentioned previously.

PREPARATION OF THE NEONATE FOR TRANSFER
JEFFREY B. GOULD, M.D., M.P.H.

Successful infant *transport* is dependent upon (1) anticipating the need for transport before the infant critically deteriorates, (2) stabilizing the infant to minimize stress and hypoxemia, and (3) preparing the parents.

When to Transport

The decision to transfer an infant to a more specialized facility is ideally made when the patient's diagnostic and therapeutic requirements are expected to exceed those available in the hospital of birth. The key to success is to initiate transfer before the patient's condition seriously deteriorates, thus avoiding many possible complications and greatly improving the outcome. Lists of conditions "requiring transport" usually include such categories as very low birth weight (<1500 gm), severe asphyxia, respiratory distress, sepsis/meningitis, metabolic abnormality, multiple congenital anomalies, and surgical emergencies. As hospitals become more experienced members of perinatal transport networks, there has been local refinement of these lists by multidisciplinary newborn committees consisting of physicians, nurses, and administration and technical staff. This local refinement based on an assessment of the local facilities, medical, nursing, and support capabilities; past experience caring for "transport infants"; and past experience with the time and difficulties of transports serves to "fine tune" the transport decision. It is often difficult to decide if an infant really needs transport or should be observed for "a few more hours." When in doubt, consultation with the senior transport physician on call will be useful.

The Initial Transport Call

The initial transport call sets into motion a course of collaborative care that begins in the local hospital (stabilization phase), continues in the tertiary care center (intensive care phase), and often terminates with transport of the infant back to the local hospital (growth and preparation for discharge to home phase). This initial call must contain information that will identify the patient's immediate and projected needs. Such factors as perinatal history, condition at birth, subsequent course, and current status are critical, as they allow the transport consultant to evaluate the working diagnosis, assess the ongoing treatment, and suggest steps to further stabilize the infant. The initial call also helps the team set their operational priorities; establish the composition of the transport team (need for respiratory therapist, senior neonatologist, etc.); assess the need for special or extra equipment (e.g., extra heat devices for a very small premature, extra supplies of saline for a large gastroschisis), and in some cases recommend the tertiary care facility that can best meet the infant's specific needs.

Another important aspect is the determination not to transport an infant. Such decisions are usually reserved for moribund infants whose likelihood for survival would not be improved by transport to a more specialized facility. It is often helpful to make this decision in consultation with the "transport neonatologist."

Stabilization Prior to Transport

Regardless of the illness, the more stable the infant at the time of transport, the greater is the likelihood of a favorable outcome. The stabilized infant has (1) a normal temperature (37°C rectal, 36.3° to 36.5°C skin); (2) an arterial oxygen level that is neither brain damaging (<40 mm Hg) or eye damaging (>80 mm Hg); (3) a pH that is not severely acidotic (<7.3); (4) a hematocrit and blood volume that provide for good tissue perfusion; (5) fluid status that avoids dehydration and water intoxication; and (6) no metabolic derangement such as hypoglycemia or hypocalcemia.

Temperature. Infants who are hypothermic have increased oxygen consumption, a tendency toward acidosis and hypoglycemia, and tolerate stress poorly. One of the most important aspects of stabilization is to keep the patient from getting hypothermic. The typical transport infant is a premature who has required extensive resuscitation in the delivery room. These infants are usually cold when they reach the nursery. While their physiologic needs are being attended to (e.g., intubation, starting intravenous line, placing catheters) their temperature and chances for intact survival will continue to fall unless special equipment (such as radiant warmers) is used and special precautions are taken. Even though a small premature is on a radiant heat bed, a prolonged period under sterile drapes while a catheter is being placed can lead to a serious drop in temperature. Also, an infant will rapidly cool when removed from a warm incubator for emergency intubation. An adequate number of devices to supply heat to exposed infants is a sound investment for even the smallest nursery. A hypothermic infant's temperature should be checked every 15 minutes until normal.

Oxygenation. The use of a continuous pulse oximeter is often helpful in supporting clinical assessment between blood gas determinations. Oxygen saturations of 88 to 92 per cent for the less than 1000 gm, 92 to 93 per cent for the 1000 to 1500 gm, and 92 to 95 per cent for the greater than 1500 gm infant usually indicate a safe level of PaO_2. Central cyanosis, and an oxygen level below 50 to 60 mm Hg should be treated by increasing the per cent oxygen. The persistence of poor color, low oxygen levels, and high levels of CO_2 (>60

mm Hg) suggests that ventilation is inadequate, especially when the cardiac rate falls to less than 100. The patient should be treated with artificial ventilation by bag and mask or bag and endotracheal tube. The adequacy of ventilation and the specific treatment of a persistently low heart rate may be established using the guidelines for neonatal resuscitation (see section on Resuscitation).

Acidosis. The pH may be determined from a warmed heel stick or even a venous sample. When the pH is <7.28 to 7.30, acidosis should be treated. If the CO_2 is >50, this respiratory acidosis should be treated by increasing the depth (watch the chest for adequate movement) or rate of ventilation. If the base deficit is greater than 5, correct this metabolic acidosis by giving a slow infusion of sodium bicarbonate (as described in section on Resuscitation).

Hypovolemic Shock. Shock due to low blood volume may present as pallor, cool skin, poor capillary filling, poor urine output, and persistence of low oxygen and a metabolic acidosis. This should be treated with whole blood or blood products as described in section on Resuscitation.

Dehydration. The signs of dehydration are similar to those of hypovolemic shock. While the hematocrit is usually low in hypovolemia, it is often high in dehydration. Treatment involves expansion of the blood volume with 10 ml/kg of 5 per cent albumin or normal saline followed by the infusion of D5W.

Metabolic Considerations. The blood sugar should be followed with dextrostix. Hypoglycemia may be treated with 2 ml/kg of D10W IV over 2 to 3 minutes, repeated once if necessary, and followed by a continuous infusion of D10W at 6 to 8 mg/kg/min. Be sure to continue following with Dextrostix.

In addition to the major steps to stabilize infants, some acute processes will require medical intervention prior to the arrival of the transport team. Suspected sepsis as evidenced by hypo- or hyperthermia, lethargy or irritability, vomiting, unexplained deterioration, or pneumonia, especially in an infant born to a mother with prolonged rupture of membranes or a temperature, must be immediately treated using standard guidelines. A gastric aspirate for smear and culture, blood culture, lumbar puncture, suprapubic tap, one surface culture, and a culture of the placenta should be obtained. In many instances these specimens are sent with the infant to the tertiary center.

Seizures will also require immediate treatment following standard guidelines.

A pneumothorax is often diagnosed following sudden and unexplained pulmonary deterioration. This must be immediately aspirated if symptomatic. However, one need not use a chest tube, as the introduction of an "Intracath" type needle at the anterior axillary line at the level of the nipple will often suffice as a temporary measure. The needle should be attached to a syringe or vacuum and water trap set up for continuous evacuation.

Intestinal obstruction at esophageal, duodenal, or lower levels should always be treated with an indwelling catheter attached to an intermittent suction device.

Intermittent suctioning by staff using a syringe is usually not very effective and poses a serious risk of aspiration.

Certain surgical conditions also require immediate therapy. Myelomeningocele, gastroschisis, and omphaloceles should be kept moist and clean by covering with moist, warm saline packs. The infant must be positioned to take the stress off the mass, and evaporative heat loss must be avoided.

There are two common pitfalls to be avoided in caring for a critically ill infant prior to transport: (1) not giving standard neonatal care such as eye prophylaxis, vitamin K, or identification prints, and (2) not recording the time and quantity of all medications and fluids given the infant and all urine and stool output.

While it is impossible to discuss all the problems and their immediate treatments here, this is precisely the goal of the initial transport call—to assess the patient's needs and to develop therapies to be followed prior to the arrival of the transport team.

Preparation of Parents

To most parents transport of their infant is devastating. The period of maternal-infant separation increases their anxiety and despair. It is helpful to explain to both parents the reason for transport and the greatly improved outlook for the majority of transported infants. Prior to transport, the transport physician should also speak with the parents. The father or another central family member should be encouraged to visit the infant as soon after admission as possible. Firsthand experience with the neonatal intensive care unit (NICU) and its staff can then be carried back and serve as a source of support to the mother. The NICU should contact the referring hospital several hours after admission so that a report of the infant's current status and prognosis can be relayed to the mother.

Although a great deal of time may have been spent with the mother or parents prior to transport, during this initial shock period it is unlikely that many of the details will be remembered. It is helpful to meet with the mother or parents 12 hours after transport. I have found the question, "Things were pretty hectic after the birth of your baby. I wonder if you could tell me what you understand about his/her condition and its treatment?" to be extremely useful.

Final Preparation for Transport

Prior to the arrival of the transport team one should collect copies of the mother's and infant's charts, 10 ml of clotted maternal blood, 10 ml of clotted cord blood, copies of x-rays and ECGs, culture specimens, and the placenta. With the arrival of the transport team, the status of the patient's stabilization will be re-evaluated, as will the need to institute further therapy prior to transport. Attempts will be made to ensure optimal stabilization and decisions will be made as to whether the infant should have a more stable peripheral intravenous line, an umbilical artery catheter, or perhaps intubation for marginal respiratory status, if these were not already required during the period of pretransport stabilization; as a last step the team will contact the tertiary center for a final consultation. The patient's course, needs, and expected time of arrival will be discussed. At this point it is important that the route from nursery to ambulance be cleared by holding elevators, clearing corridors, and positioning the vehicle.

BREAST FEEDING

MARIANNE R. NEIFERT, M.D., *and*
K. MICHAEL HAMBIDGE, F.R.C.P. (Ed.), Sc.D.

Infant feeding experts universally agree that breast milk represents optimal nutrition during the early months of life. Breast feeding confers protection against gastrointestinal and upper respiratory infections, which has profound significance in underdeveloped countries and lesser but real importance in more developed areas. In addition, allergic disease is less prevalent among infants who have been breast fed. The relationship developed through breast feeding can be an important part of early maternal-infant interaction and provides a source of security and comfort for the infant, apart from the provision of nutrients.

PREPARATION FOR BREAST FEEDING

The Decision. When feasible, the pediatrician should inquire prenatally about the intended feeding method. If bottle feeding has been selected, one should ask in a nonjudgmental manner how the decision was made, as many women decline to breast feed because of misinformation rather than a true preference for bottle feeding. If breast feeding is planned, the physician should support the decision, reiterate the advantages, and encourage the parents to attend a prenatal breast-feeding class.

Breast Examination. A clinician should perform a prenatal breast examination to assess physical factors potentially having an impact on lactation performance. Breast enlargement during pregnancy is a favorable prognostic sign, implying adequate glandular development. The presence of scars should prompt an inquiry about previous breast surgery potentially affecting lactation, particularly reduction mammoplasty and procedures involving periareolar incisions that might have severed ducts. Abnormal breast appearance, including hypoplasia or marked asymmetry, may be associated with compromised lactation potential.

The nipple should be inspected for inversion by being compressed between the thumb and forefinger. The normal nipple will protrude with stimulation, while the inverted nipple retracts inward. To improve nipple protractility, Hoffman's exercises can be performed several times daily in the last trimester. The woman should place her index fingers at opposite areolar margins and gently stretch the tissues outward, moving circumferentially around the areola. Breast shells, also known as milk cups or breast shields, can be worn over inverted nipples during the latter months of pregnancy to help draw them out.

Nipple Preparation. Because manipulating the nipples prenatally may produce uterine contractions, approval from the woman's obstetrician should be obtained before instituting regular prenatal nipple preparation. The axiom "first do no harm" should be respected, since overvigorous nipple manipulation may be traumatic and actually predispose to nipple pain once breast feeding commences. Gently rolling or pulling the nipples may enhance elasticity, but no proof exists that prenatal nipple manipulation actually minimizes postpartum nipple tenderness or fosters success in breast feeding. A positive attitude and confidence, acquired through discussions with health care providers, reading materials, and classes, probably do more to guarantee success than physical preparation of the breasts.

INITIATION OF BREAST FEEDING

Breast feeding can begin as soon after delivery as both mother and baby are stable. Correct positioning and proper breast-feeding technique are necessary to ensure effective nipple stimulation and optimal breast emptying, with minimal nipple discomfort.

Technique. To nurse while the mother is sitting, the infant should be elevated to the height of the breast and turned completely to face the mother so that their abdomens are touching. The mother's arm supporting the infant should be held tight at her side, bringing the baby's head in line with her breast. The breast should be supported by the lower fingers of her free hand, while the nipple is compressed between the thumb and index finger to make it more protractile. The infant's initial licking and mouthing of the nipple help make it more erect. When the infant opens his or her mouth *widely*, the mother should rapidly insert as much nipple and areola as possible favoring the inferior area.

Rigid time restrictions should not be imposed, but sensible guidelines are 5 minutes per breast at each feeding the first day, 10 minutes on each side at each feeding the second day, and 15 minutes or more per side thereafter. To maximize milk intake and optimally stimulate and empty both breasts, it is preferable to nurse at both breasts at each feeding. In the presence of a well-conditioned let-down, or milk ejection, reflex, a vigorous infant can obtain most of the available milk in 5 to 7 minutes, but additional sucking time ensures breast emptying and ongoing milk production, as well as satisfies the infant's sucking urge. The mother should alternate the side on which she begins feedings, so that the breast last suckled is the one first nursed at the next feeding. To prevent nipple trauma, the mother should break suction gently after nursings by inserting her finger between the baby's gums.

Hospital Routines. The successful initiation of breast feeding is fostered by unrestricted rooming-in, access to bedside instruction from knowledgeable nurses, "demand" rather than scheduled feedings, and early follow-up after discharge. Supplemental water or formula should not be offered routinely to breast-fed infants, nor should appropriate supplement be withheld when medically indicated. Individualized assessment of lactation risk factors and infant nursing technique should determine before discharge those mother-baby pairs needing additional intervention.

Lactogenesis. Lactogenesis, or the onset of copious milk secretion, usually occurs on the second to fourth postpartum day and is associated with engorgement, or swelling, of the breasts. Engorgement can cause the nipple-areola junction to be tense and convex, making it difficult for the infant to grasp correctly. Hand or pump expression of milk prior to nursing will soften the areola and facilitate the infant's latch-on.

Failure to relieve breast engorgement promptly by effective infant nursing or by pumping is probably the leading preventable cause of subsequent insufficient lactation. The pressure of unrelieved engorgement causes involution of mammary glandular tissue and rapidly diminishes milk supply. Thus, maternal-infant separation, infants with latch-on or sucking problems, and reluctant nursers should be viewed as posing risks for the successful onset of lactation.

When an infant is not nursing effectively for any reason by the time the milk has come in, it is important that the mother commence emptying her breasts at regular feeding intervals, preferably with one of the efficient piston electric breast pumps equipped with a double collection system (Medela or Egnell). Only regular and effective breast emptying will preserve her milk supply while she is trying to establish breast feeding. Meanwhile, her expressed milk can be used to supplement the infant.

Common Problems in the Initiation of Breast Feeding

Sore Nipples. Many women experience transient, mild nipple tenderness during the early days of breast feeding. Tenderness usually begins to resolve once milk is in and the oxytocin-mediated, let-down reflex is conditioned. Ensuring proper positioning of the infant and correct latch-on is paramount in managing sore nipples. Nursing for shorter periods more frequently, beginning feeds on the least sore side, air drying the nipples well after nursings, and applying lanolin cream are ancillary measures to help minimize tenderness.

Severe nipple pain almost always indicates improper attachment by the infant, with associated poor breast emptying and diminished milk supply. If nipples are severely cracked or denuded, breast feeding may need to be disrupted temporarily to permit healing. In the interim, milk supply can be increased and maintained by regular milk expression. Even when breast feeding produces exquisite pain, women typically report no discomfort using the piston electric breast pump. Once the nipples have healed, breast feeding can be reinstituted, with particular emphasis on correct positioning of the infant.

Nipple Confusion. Despite abbreviated postpartum confinement and enlightened hospital protocols, many infants still receive bottle supplements during their nursery stay. Routine supplements may cause an infant to prefer bottle feeding, with its different tongue-and-mouth action and the rapid, easy flow of fluid. A "nipple-confused" infant may refuse to grasp the maternal nipple, having become accustomed to a stiff rubber nipple and prompt milk flow. Prevention of nipple confusion should be emphasized, by introducing breast feeding promptly after delivery and by avoiding elective bottle feeding until the infant is nursing well.

Infant Jaundice. Hyperbilirubinemia occurs more often among breast-fed than formula-fed infants, but the mechanism for jaundice is often misinterpreted.

In a small percentage of breast-fed infants, an unidentified property of the milk inhibits the conjugation of bilirubin and leads to persistent indirect hyperbilirubinemia, which peaks in the second week of life and may persist for several weeks. *Breast milk jaundice* should not be diagnosed unless other causes of hyperbilirubinemia have been ruled out, a normal conjugated bilirubin level has been documented, and the infant is exhibiting a normal rate of weight gain with breast feeding. If the severity of jaundice warrants intervention, a 24- to 36-hour trial of formula feeding usually results in a dramatic decline in bilirubin level. While breast feeding is interrupted, it is important to instruct the mother how to maintain her milk supply by emptying her breasts with a piston electric breast pump on a regular nursing schedule.

Breast-feeding jaundice is much more prevalent among breast-fed infants than breast milk jaundice, but the latter is often misdiagnosed to explain exaggerated or persistent jaundice in an underweight breast-fed infant. Breast-feeding jaundice, perhaps more accurately described as "lack of breast milk jaundice," is exaggerated physiologic jaundice associated with inadequate intake of breast milk, infrequent stools, and unsatisfactory weight gain. Actually, nonhemolytic, unconjugated hyperbilirubinemia in the first week of life is a common marker for poor nursing and inadequate milk intake. Rather than undermine breast feeding further by disrupting nursing, one should attempt to facilitate breast emptying and to increase the infant's milk consumption by enhancing breast-feeding technique, increasing the frequency of nursing, and augmenting the infant's suckling stimulus with regular breast pumping. If supplemental feedings are indicated, expressed milk or formula or both can be given.

Breast Feeding the Premature or Sick Newborn. When an infant's illness, prematurity, or a birth defect precludes direct nursing at the breast, specialized information and equipment are necessary for the mother to establish and maintain lactation successfully until breast feeding can occur. The mother should have access to a piston electric breast pump and double collection system to empty her breasts simultaneously at regular intervals, thereby preserving an adequate milk supply. Although milk can be expressed using a variety of methods, including hand expression, manual pumps, battery-operated pumps, and small electric pumps, the vast majority of women find the piston-type electric breast pumps, rented from surgical supply outlets and pharmacies, to be the most effective, efficient, and physiologic means of initiating and maintaining full lactation. As soon as the infant is stable, he or she should be introduced to the breast so that nutritive nursing can eventually be accomplished. Mothers should continue to pump their breasts after feedings until it is documented that the infant obtains appropriate milk volumes with nursing and is gaining well with breast feeding. Because subjective evaluations of the quality of a breast feed may be highly misleading, infant test weights with an accurate scale should be used to verify intake at the breast.

MANAGEMENT OF BREAST FEEDING

Normal Routines. An important role of the physician is to establish for new mothers the norms for breast-fed infants. A mother should expect her infant to nurse as often as every 2 to 3 hours for the first several weeks. During this period, it is critical that the mother be allowed sufficient rest. Guidelines for minimizing outside activities, household chores, and other duties in order to nurse every few hours will prove more helpful than using pacifiers, water, or formula supplements to prolong the normal feeding interval. Breast-fed infants usually pass a yellow, seedy stool with every feeding during the early weeks. Infrequency of stools during the first month is a sensitive indicator of inadequate milk intake. After the first or second month, the stool frequency usually diminishes, and the older breast-fed infant may normally pass a stool once every several days. Night nursings are both normal and necessary to the maintenance of a generous milk supply. Many parents have found that taking the infant into their own bed to nurse at night is a harmless method of making the night-time feedings less disruptive to their sleep.

Nutrient Composition of Breast Milk. The protein content of mature human milk (9 gm/L) is adequate for the normal infant without imposing unnecessary demands on maternal resources. Protein deficiency occurs in the occasional breast-fed infant with cystic fibrosis who has some impairment of protein absorption. The relatively low concentration of phenylalanine in human milk has led to the increasing use of some breast milk in the dietary management of infants with phenylketonuria. More than 50 per cent of the calories in breast milk are supplied by fat; a high fat intake is important for the young, rapidly growing infant. The percentage of polyunsaturated fatty acids varies with the maternal diet but is always adequate to meet essential fatty acid requirements. The calcium content of breast milk is 13 mEq/L with a calcium (mg)-phosphorus (mg) ratio of 2:1. Neither the calcium nor the phosphorus supplied in breast milk is sufficient to meet the requirements of the very low birth weight infant, who also requires a protein supplement. The exceptionally low sodium concentration of human milk (7 mmol/L) is noteworthy, and there is increasing evidence that this is a favorable feature.

The content of vitamins A, C, E, and most B vitamins is adequate in breast milk. Breast milk of alcoholic mothers may be deficient in thiamin, malnourished mothers may have deficient levels of folate in their milk, and vitamin B-12 deficiency has been described in breast-fed infants of vegan mothers who have neglected to take B-12 supplements. Vitamin K levels are relatively low in breast milk, and it is especially important to ensure that the standard vitamin K prophylaxis is administered intramuscularly to all neonates who will be breast fed. Breast-fed infants whose bodies are exposed to sunlight for 30 minutes per week or whose heads are exposed to sunlight for 2 hours per week will synthesize adequate vitamin D, or 1, 25(OH)$_2$D$_3$. Dark-skinned infants need more prolonged exposure. Sufficient vitamin D will also be provided in breast milk if the mother's vitamin D status is very good. However, if the mother's vitamin D status is only fair or marginal and the infant is not exposed to sunlight, vitamin D supplements are advised for the breast-fed infant.

The fluoride content of breast milk is low, even in areas where the water supply is fluoridated. Although the incidence of caries in fully breast-fed infants is relatively low, standard fluoride supplements (0.25 mg/day) are recommended for fully breast-fed infants, especially if breast feeding continues to be the only source of nutrients after the age of 6 months. Breast milk contains adequate iron to meet the needs of fully breast-fed infants for 4 to 6 months and provides an optimal source of zinc and copper during the same interval.

Inadequate Infant Weight Gain. Poor weight gain among breast-fed infants is a common, frustrating problem that is best prevented by appropriate anticipatory guidance and early follow-up. An initial visit at 5 to 7 days is suggested for all breast-fed infants, particularly for infants of primiparous women, to establish that the infant is nursing with appropriate technique at frequent intervals and is voiding and producing stools normally. Once the mother's milk has come in, the breast-fed infant should commence regular weight gain, approximating an ounce per day. Thus, most infants will be above their birth weight by 2 weeks of age. If an infant loses greater than 8 per cent from the birth weight, has not established appropriate weight gain by the end of the first week, or is not above birth weight by 10 to 14 days, a detailed evaluation of breast feeding should be elicited. The infant feeding and elimination pattern should be obtained, maternal and infant lactation risk factors should be explored, breast feeding should be observed, and the maternal breasts should be examined.

Temporarily augmenting the infant's suckling by pumping the breasts with a piston electric breast pump after each nursing has proved effective in maximizing milk yield, increasing the infant's intake during nursing, and obtaining expressed milk for supplemental feedings. Pumping is especially important if the infant is receiving necessary bottle supplements and consequently is nursing less vigorously.

Often, a formula supplement is indicated to ensure the nutritional well-being of an underweight infant. Formula can be offered by bottle, or if the mother prefers, the Supplemental Nutrition System (SNS) (Medela, Inc.) can be used to provide supplement simultaneously while the baby is breast feeding. With the SNS device, the baby suckles both the maternal nipple and a thin tube connected to a plastic bottle filled with formula and suspended around the mother's neck.

Modest declines in growth percentiles after 3 to 4 months may signal the need for introduction of beikost. Solids should be offered after nursings to complement, not displace, breast milk in the infant's diet.

Weaning. Infant weaning has evolved from the predominantly mother-led process observed during the past several decades to the baby-led process now being witnessed with increased frequency. Although contemporary women are nursing their infants longer, late nursing is not yet a societal norm. Apart from the nutritional role of breast feeding, clinicians need to recognize the legitimate psychological needs of infants and toddlers that can be met by nursing. Weaning gradually, by allowing the baby to outgrow the need to nurse, is preferable to abrupt, imposed weaning. In addition, the maternal engorgement associated with abrupt weaning can be physically uncomfortable and can predispose the mother to mastitis.

MATERNAL ISSUES

Diet. Nursing mothers should eat a well-balanced, nutritious diet with increased protein, calcium, and fluids. Dieting to reduce weight is contraindicated during lactation. Prepregnancy weight will usually be attained by 6 months post partum without dieting. No dietary restrictions are necessary for the nursing mother unless she observes reactions in the infant following ingestion of specific foods. Typical offenders are cow's milk, eggs, peanut butter, chocolate, citrus, corn, and other common allergens. Infantile "colic" among breast-fed babies can sometimes be traced to a specific food antigen in the maternal diet.

Mastitis. A small percentage of nursing mothers experience mastitis during the course of breast feeding. Predisposing factors include cracked nipples, incomplete breast emptying, and breast trauma. Weaning is not necessary with mastitis; in fact, failure to empty the affected breast regularly does predispose to abscess formation. Mastitis should be suspected whenever a nursing mother complains of a "flulike" illness with local breast tenderness. Associated symptoms include malaise, chills, fever, headache, and erythema and pain in the affected breast. Antibiotic therapy offering adequate coverage against beta-lactamase–producing organisms should be initiated promptly and continued for 10 days. Analgesics may be necessary for several days to control discomfort.

The mother may find it more comfortable to initiate nursing on the unaffected side and then move the infant to the affected breast once let-down has been triggered. Synthetic oxytocin, as Syntocinon Nasal Spray, can be prescribed to enhance the let-down reflex. A piston electric breast pump is another helpful adjunctive therapy to facilitate milk expression.

Working and Nursing. Specific recommendations are necessary for the large population of women who elect to breast feed but who, out of necessity or choice, return to work before the infant is weaned. Working and nursing need not be mutually exclusive, but special effort is required for a woman to maintain lactation while separated from her infant during the work day.

If the mother wishes to maintain her milk supply and obtain milk for her baby's feedings, she should arrange regular "lactation breaks" at her workplace to express milk privately. The frequency of milk expression might range from one to three times during the work day, depending on the age of her infant. Expressed milk can be refrigerated for approximately 24 hours and frozen for approximately 3 months in a freezer with a separate door or for 6 months or longer in a deep freezer at $-20°C$ ($-4°F$). Some workplaces provide "pumping lounges" with electric pump facilities for lactating employees. Other options include nearby or on-site childcare so that the mother might nurse her baby on her lunch break.

Maternal Drug Therapy. Many factors play a role in determining the effect of maternal drug therapy on the nursing infant, including the route of administration, the dosage, the molecular weight of the drug, as well as its ionization, fat solubility, pH, and protein binding. Fortunately, the dosage of most drugs delivered to the nursing infant via breast milk is subtherapeutic. In general, any drug prescribed therapeutically for newborns can be consumed via breast milk without ill effect. Drugs delivered to the infant via breast milk should always be viewed with a risk-benefit assessment. For example, it is probably preferable to nurse while taking low-dose birth control pills than to forego breast feeding altogether or to experience an unplanned pregnancy during lactation.

Very few drugs are absolutely contraindicated; these include radioactive compounds, antimetabolites, and lithium. The knowledge base about drugs in breast milk is rapidly changing, and many drugs contraindicated in the past have subsequently been shown not to pose a real hazard to the breast-fed infant. The *Physician's Desk Reference (PDR)* offers a paucity of information about drug excretion in breast milk and is typically overly conservative in its recommendations for lactating women. A regional drug center, such as the Rocky Mountain Drug Consultation Center (303–893–DRUG), can serve as a reliable source of knowledge about drugs in breast milk.

CONCLUSION

An important role for pediatricians is to promote optimal infant nutrition through breast feeding and to help nursing mothers accomplish the full course of lactation by offering accurate information about breast feeding, professional support, and appropriate anticipatory guidance. When a woman achieves her breast-feeding goal, she not only contributes immeasurably to her infant's health but also experiences competence in an important aspect of early mothering, which may set the tone for her subsequent parenting.

FEEDING THE LOW BIRTH WEIGHT INFANT

EKHARD E. ZIEGLER, M.D.

In recent years there has been a much expanded use of parenteral nutrition in low birth weight infants. This has been associated with increased sophistication in the formulation of parenteral regimens. A major impetus for the expanded use of parenteral nutrition has been the tendency to delay introduction of enteral feedings in the belief that this will reduce the risk of necrotizing enterocolitis. Feeding protocols in use today call for withholding of enteral feedings for up to 4 weeks in infants considered at high risk of necrotizing enterocolitis. This approach is feasible only because safe methods of parenteral nutrition using central and peripheral veins are available.

Nutritional support of low birth weight infants typically proceeds in three phases: a *parenteral phase*, during which enteral feedings are not provided at all; a *transition phase*, during which enteral feedings are gradually introduced and parenteral nutrition is reduced; and a final *enteral phase*, during which all feedings are enteral. Typically, infants do not grow during the parenteral phase but begin to grow during the transition phase and grow rapidly (catch-up growth) during the enteral phase.

THE PARENTERAL PHASE

Administration of fluids intravenously is begun shortly after birth, providing energy in the form of glucose. Electrolytes are frequently omitted for the first 24 hours. A decision to provide amino acids and minerals as well as glucose—referred to subsequently as parenteral nutrition—should be made as early as possible and not later than 48 hours of age. Factors entering into the decision include birth weight, perinatal risk factors with regard to necrotizing enterocolitis, the severity of postnatal illness, and any other factors that may delay introduction of enteral feedings. As a general rule, infants with birth weights less than 1500 gm should receive parenteral nutritional support, unless they are among the unusual infants who have no major medical problems and who are considered likely to tolerate enteral feedings by 3 days of age. Larger infants may tolerate somewhat longer periods with only glucose and electrolytes, but even term infants should usually be given parenteral nutrition if enteral feedings cannot be initiated by 4 days of age.

The immediate postnatal period is often quite stormy, and it is unlikely that true growth will occur even if sufficient nutrients are provided. Therefore, nutritional support should be based on the limited objective of preventing nutritional depletion by replacement of ongoing losses, including expenditures of energy. A variety of parenteral nutrition regimens for high-risk infants are currently employed in nurseries across the country, testifying to a certain lack of consensus regarding optimal composition. The composition of the peripheral venous nutrition (PVN) solution used at the author's institution is indicated in Table 1.

The solution is designed to provide adequate, but not excessive, intakes of amino acids, minerals, and vitamins when used as the primary source of intravenous fluids. It has the advantage of providing flexibility with regard to concentrations of glucose and potassium. It is available at two amino acid concentrations (1.4 and 2.1 gm/dl) and, on a special request basis, sodium concentrations other than those specified are available. In order to avoid administration of excessive amounts of amino acids and, perhaps, of other nutrients, the PVN solutions are not administered in amounts exceeding 200 ml/kg/day. In the occasional premature infant requiring fluid intake greater than 200 ml/kg/day, the additional

TABLE 1. Peripheral Venous Nutrition Solution for Low
Birth Weight Infants*

Nutrient	Amount per 100 ml
Amino acids	1.4 or 2.1 gm
Glucose	2.5–15.0† gm
Acetate	1.7 mEq
Sodium	3.0 mEq
Potassium	0.0–3.0† mEq
Chloride	1.0‡ mEq
Calcium	40 mg
Phosphorus	31 mg
Magnesium	3.6 mg
Zinc	0.2 mg
Copper	40 μg
Manganese	20 μg
Chromium	0.4 μg
Selenium	0.1

*1.5 ml of M.V.I. Pediatric (Multi-Vitamin Infusion) (Armour Pharmaceutical Co.) are added to each 24-hour supply.

†Desired concentration to be specified by prescribing physician; K > 3.0 mEq/100 ml available on request.

‡Cl will vary depending on concentration of K+, which is added as KCl.

fluids are generally administered as a 5 per cent glucose solution. It must be emphasized that the amino acid concentration of 1.4 gm/dl is intended for the immediate postnatal period and is not sufficient for growing infants. Therefore, if and when energy intakes exceed 80 kcal/kg/day, it is advisable to increase the amino acid concentration to 2.1 gm/dl.

Because biochemical evidence of essential fatty acid deficiency may develop in small premature infants within a few days of birth, parenteral administration of lipid emulsions should be initiated between 4 and 6 days of age unless enteral feedings have been initiated. The dose of lipid required to prevent essential fatty acid deficiency is about 0.5 gm/kg/day. When infused slowly (0.05 gm/kg/hr), intravenous lipid emulsions at this dosage rarely give rise to hyperlipidemia and are probably safe even in the presence of moderate hyperbilirubinemia. Monitoring for hyperlipidemia is mandatory, however, and should be performed by determination of serum triglyceride concentration at the end of the daily infusion period. Triglyceride concentrations should be kept below 150 mg/dl. To avoid exceeding this value, it may be necessary to reduce the rate of infusion or the total amount infused. Inspection of a spun hematocrit tube for serum lactescence is frequently used instead of triglyceride determination, but it must be cautioned that this method does not reliably detect hyperlipidemia of a mild to moderate degree. If the amount of intravenous lipids is increased beyond 0.5 gm/kg/day in order to increase energy intake, monitoring of serum triglyceride concentrations is particularly important. Most neonatologists prefer not to exceed doses of 2.5 to 3.0 gm/kg/day.

THE TRANSITION PHASE

An important initial role of enteral feedings is to test the functional maturity of the gastrointestinal tract and to provide a stimulus for morphologic, functional, and endocrine maturation of the gut. Thus, there may be major beneficial effects of enteral feedings even during the period in which most of the intake of energy and specific nutrients is provided by the parenteral route.

There are two decisions to be made: what to feed and by what method. Expressed milk from the infant's own mother is the feeding of choice. It is important that the milk collected by the mother is fed in the order in which it was collected. In this way the infant receives initially colostrum, followed by transitional milk, and eventually mature milk. Donated breast milk, when available, is the second choice, especially when it is mature milk. Since some form of heat treatment is required to prevent transmission of infectious agents, cellular elements of the milk are lost and some loss of protective factors is inevitable. If formula is to be used, it should be one of the premature infant formulas (see the section Feedings). Most neonatologists prefer to start milk or formula at energy concentrations less than 67 kcal/dl. However, the scientific basis for this practice is not established.

The second decision is whether to feed by continuous intragastric infusion or by bolus. Continuous infusion is associated with fewer cardiovascular and pulmonary effects and is the preferred method for very small infants. At the author's institution a regimen of cycles consisting of 3 hours of infusion followed by 1 hour without infusion has been used for years and has worked satisfactorily. Gastric contents are aspirated before the next cycle, and the physician is notified if the volume aspirated exceeds 20 per cent of the volume infused.

Transpyloric feeding, i.e., introduction of feedings into the duodenum or jejunum, has the advantage that the often sluggish rate of gastric emptying does not limit the volume of milk or formula that can be administered. However, many neonatologists believe that the disadvantages (e.g., impaired nutrient absorption) and risks (e.g., intestinal perforation) outweigh the advantages, and transpyloric feeding is not widely used today.

THE ENTERAL PHASE

During the transition phase just described the objective of nutritional management was the replacement of ongoing losses. Now that the infant is growing, greater intakes of energy and nutrients are needed for the formation of new body tissues. If energy or protein intake are inadequate, growth rate will be limited. When sufficient energy and protein but too little calcium and phosphorus are provided, the infant will develop rickets. It is apparent that nutritional management of the growing premature infant must be based on an understanding of nutrient requirements.

Nutrient Requirements. Until requirements can be established for all nutrients by appropriately designed feeding studies, estimates of nutrient requirements obtained by the factorial method serve as interim guidelines. These estimates represent for each nutrient the sum of tissue accretion plus losses via feces, urine, and skin. Use of the fetus as a model for the growing premature infant has the major advantage that body composition of the human fetus is known. No more satisfactory model is available.

Estimates of nutrient requirements obtained by the factorial method form the basis for the advisable intakes presented in Table 2. Because of variability among infants, the requirement, which is based on average values, has been increased by 10 per cent to give an advisable intake. A margin of only 10 per cent above requirements has been used because premature infants have very limited tolerance to excessive intakes. Advisable intakes of nutrients have been stated in relation to energy requirements (i.e., are expressed per 100 kcal) because for most nutrients it is more important that they be provided in the correct proportions to each other rather than in relation to body weight.

It is evident from the values presented in Table 2 that advisable intakes of nutrients decrease somewhat with increasing body weight. At still higher body weights (not shown) they gradually approach those of the full-term infant.

Feedings. As mentioned previously, the feeding of choice is milk from the infant's own mother. The mother should be encouraged to attempt lactation and every effort should be made to aid her in this effort. The success rate is likely to be a direct function of the support provided. Milk should be placed in suitably small containers that should be dated so as to enable subsequent use of the milk in sequence. Usually, milk will need to be frozen, although refrigeration is adequate if storage is required for only a few days. By feeding the milk in sequence the infant receives initially colostrum, with its high concentration of anti-infectious substances, followed by transitional and eventually mature milk. Because of the small volumes of milk consumed, the time scale is expanded compared with the time over which the milk was collected.

Even preterm milk, with its somewhat higher protein content compared with term milk, provides a number of nutrients in inadequate amounts, i.e., amounts that do not meet the needs of the growing low birth weight infant. From a comparison of advisable intakes of the low birth weight infant with the nutrient content of preterm milk (Table 2), it is evident that per unit of energy lesser amounts of protein and of most minerals are provided than are presumed to be advisable.

In essentially every feeding study of preterm infants in which human milk has been compared with formulas designed for low birth weight infants, weight gain has been found to be less rapid with human milk than with formula. The difference is greatest when pooled donor milk is used, but even with milk from the infant's own mother there is slower growth than with formula. In addition, undermineralization of the skeleton is more pronounced with human milk than with formula. There seems to be little dispute about these facts. There is dispute, however, about what should be done about the problem. One school of thought holds that somewhat slower growth is of no particular consequence and is therefore an acceptable price for the benefits mother's milk confers on the infant. Similarly, undermineralization of the skeleton may have no long-term consequences. The opposing view, to which the author subscribes, holds that from a physiological point of view a diet that permits less than full realization of the subject's growth potential cannot be considered optimal. In addition, slowed growth exposes the infant to the risks of extra days or weeks of hospitalization. Although skeletal undermineralization does not generally progress to such an extent, in some infants spontaneous fractures occur.

We therefore recommend the supplementation of human milk with protein and minerals. Such supplementation corrects the nutritional inadequacies without diminishing the advantages of human milk. Supplementation should be initiated when the infant begins to gain weight. Supplements specifically designed for the purpose are preferable to use of concentrated infant formula. Table 3 indicates the composition of such a supplement. The Enfamil Human Milk Fortifier is supplied in packets containing 0.95 gm and is added to 25 ml of human milk. Protein and minerals are the main ingredients and are supplied in amounts calculated to raise intakes of these nutrients to levels that approximately meet requirements.

When the infant's mother does not provide milk, and there is no other source of human milk available, three formulas specifically designed to meet the nutritional needs of low birth weight infants are available. As may be seen in Table 2, these formulas vary somewhat in the amounts of nutrients provided (relative to energy). On the whole these formulas meet nutrient requirements of the low birth weight infant more closely than formulas designed for term infants. All three formulas contain as their source of protein a blend of bovine whey proteins and casein in a ratio of 60:40. All three formulas provide half the amount of carbohydrate in the form of lactose. The fat blend of each formula contains at least some medium-chain triglycerides to capitalize on the ease and efficiency with which this fat is absorbed. The content of polyunsaturated fatty acids

TABLE 2. Advisable Nutrient Intakes and Composition of Human Milk and of Formulas for Low Birth Weight Infants (per 100 kcal)

Nutrient	Advisable Intake 700–1000 gm	Advisable Intake 1000–1500 gm	Human Milk*	Similac Special Care	Enfamil Premature	"Preemie" SMA Ready-to-Feed
Protein (gm)	3.60	3.30	2.30	2.70	3.00	2.50
Calcium (mg)	175.00	154.00	36.00	178.00	165.00	93.00
Phosphorus (mg)	120.00	107.00	19.00	89.00	83.00	49.00
Magnesium (mg)	6.60	5.90	4.80	12.30	7.60	8.60
Sodium (mEq)	3.28	2.73	1.70	2.20	1.70	1.70
Potassium (mEq)	2.28	2.00	2.10	3.60	2.80	2.40
Chloride (mEq)	2.90	2.40	1.90	2.50	2.40	1.80
Iron (mg)	2.40	2.20	0.20	0.37†	0.25†	0.37
Zinc (mg)	1.50	1.30	0.50	1.50	1.56	1.00
Copper (mg)	0.18	0.16	0.08	0.25	0.13	0.09

*Preterm, 14 days post partum.
†Also available with 1.8 mg/100 kcal.

TABLE 3. Composition of Human Milk Fortifier
(amounts added to each 100 ml of milk)

Nutrient	Enfamil Human Milk Fortifier
Energy (kcal)	14.00
Protein (gm)	0.70
Carbohydrate (gm)	2.70
Sodium (mEq)	0.30
Potassium (mEq)	0.40
Chloride (mEq)	0.50
Calcium (mg)	90.00
Phosphorus (mg)	45.00
Magnesium (mg)	4.00
Zinc (mg)	0.71
Copper (mg)	0.08

(PUFA) is higher in the formulas than in human milk, but sufficient vitamin E is present to provide a satisfactory E:PUFA ratio. It should be noted that all formulas are low in iron content (Table 2), reflecting the widely held belief that iron has adverse effects on small preterm infants and should therefore be withheld, despite the recognized need for an exogenous source of iron. Two of the formulas are also available fortified with iron (1.8 mg/100 kcal) and are routinely used at the author's institution.

Although there is no consensus regarding optimal intakes of each vitamin, formulas for preterm infants and the available human milk fortifiers provide ample amounts of all vitamins.

NEONATAL INTESTINAL OBSTRUCTION

ROBERT M. FILLER, M.D.

Neonates with bilious vomiting, abdominal distention, and failure to pass meconium within 24 hours have intestinal obstruction until proved otherwise. The four most common causes include intestinal atresia, malrotation, meconium ileus, and Hirschsprung's disease. The diagnosis of intestinal obstruction is usually made on flat and upright radiographs of the abdomen. Barium enema is used to better define the specific type of obstruction and to rule out an unsuspected colonic atresia.

To prevent aspiration and progressive intestinal distention, nasogastric intubation and suction should be instituted in all patients prior to diagnostic studies and transport of the patient. In most cases, a No. 10 French nasogastric catheter can be used. Smaller tubes often fail to achieve the desired result. Infants should be nursed in a thermoneutral environment, and care must be taken to avoid hypothermia during radiologic studies. Correction of fluid and electrolyte abnormalities may be necessary before surgery when the diagnosis is delayed; but when the diagnosis is made early, dehydration and electrolyte imbalance are not usually problems. Ampicillin (200 mg/kg/day) and gentamicin (5 to 7.5 mg/kg/day) are given intravenously just prior to surgery and continued for 24 hours in uncomplicated cases. In patients with significant peritoneal contami-

nation antibiotics are continued for 1 week and clindamycin (50 mg/kg/day) is added to the regimen.

Intestinal Atresia

The principle of surgical treatment for intestinal atresia is to excise the atretic area of intestine and join the ends to establish continuity. However, for atresias at certain sites, resection and end-to-end anastomosis are technically dangerous or not feasible, and alternative measures are necessary. For example, it is often easier to bypass an atresia in the second portion of the duodenum by means of a duodenojejunostomy than to excise an atretic segment near the common bile duct. Similarly, an end-to-end anastomosis may be technically impossible in those with high jejunal atresia because of the marked discrepancy in size between the dilated proximal bowel and the ribbon-like distal bowel. In these cases, a side-to-side jejunostomy becomes the best solution even though a small percentage of patients develop a blind loop syndrome that needs later correction. It has been known for many years that a grossly dilated intestine just proximal to an atresia has ineffective peristalsis even after the obstruction has been relieved. This may result in partial intestinal obstruction. In addition, the overdistended loop tends to become a stagnant pool of intestinal fluid, with bacterial overgrowth that can produce a blind loop syndrome. To prevent this problem, enormously dilated intestine is excised with the atretic segment. However, when this is not feasible because of overall short intestinal length or duodenal involvement, the diameter of the dilated segment is narrowed by plication or tapering.

Intestinal Malrotation

Malrotation of the intestine is associated with intestinal obstruction when the duodenum is compressed by bands that run from the cecum to the posterior parietes (Ladd's bands) or when midgut volvulus occurs. The latter event is an extreme emergency, since the viability of all of the small intestine and half of the colon is in jeopardy. When midgut volvulus is suspected, immediate operation is necessary even if fluid and electrolyte resuscitation is incomplete. At surgery, the intestines are eviscerated, and volvulus is corrected by counterclockwise rotation of bowel around the axis of the superior mesenteric artery. Ladd's bands are divided in all cases, and the duodenum is freed so that it descends in a straight line into the abdomen to the right of the spine. The cecum ends up in the left upper quadrant. If the bowel is viable, an incidental appendectomy is performed. Intestinal resection for localized areas of bowel necrosis is necessary. When the viability of the entire midgut is in doubt after reduction of a volvulus, the intestines are replaced in the abdomen, and the wound is closed. The abdomen is re-explored 24 hours later and intestine that is definitely necrotic is excised. In general, it is wiser to exteriorize the cut ends of potentially ischemic intestine than to perform an end-to-end anastomosis.

Meconium Ileus

Meconium ileus is caused by inspissated meconium in the lumen of the distal small bowel and almost always is associated with cystic fibrosis. In 50 per cent of cases meconium ileus is complicated by intestinal atresia, volvulus, intestinal infarction, and meconium peritonitis.

In cases of simple meconium ileus attempts at disimpacting the obstructing meconium by enema techniques are preferable to immediate surgical therapy. Various enema preparations have been used. Gastrografin, a hypertonic iodine solution combined with a wetting agent, has received the most attention in the literature. Its high osmolarity draws fluid into the bowel lumen and separates the meconium from the intestinal wall. However, because of this high osmolarity, Gastrografin can produce hypovolemic shock when large fluid shifts into the intestine occur. Therefore, we prefer to employ an enema solution of 25 per cent diatrizoate sodium (Hypaque) with 5 per cent acetylcysteine (Mucomyst), which has an osmolarity less than half that of Gastrografin and yet appears to be as effective. Intravenous fluid therapy during the Hypaque enema is not necessary in the well-hydrated neonate. Care must be taken to avoid intestinal perforation during the procedure, which usually requires several instillations of irrigating fluid until it passes into the dilated intestine above the obstruction.

Operative treatment is required for all infants with complicated meconium ileus as well as for those in whom enema therapy has failed. Many surgical methods have been used to relieve the obstruction. We prefer to relieve the obstruction by enterotomy and irrigations with 5 per cent acetylcysteine. If irrigation fails to relieve the obstruction (less than 10 per cent of cases), an intestinal stoma is created proximal to the point of obstruction.

In infants with complicated meconium ileus, the atretic, infarcted, or perforated intestine is excised. It is usually unwise to attempt intraoperative irrigations and end-to-end anastomoses in these patients because of the likelihood of anastomotic complications. Creation of a double-barreled ileostomy is preferable.

Hirschsprung's Disease

When radiographic evaluation suggests that intestinal obstruction is due to Hirschsprung's disease, a punch biopsy of the rectal mucosa 1.5 cm above the dentate line is performed at the bedside. If this indicates the absence of ganglion cells, a right transverse loop colostomy is performed. The colostomy is also biopsied to confirm the presence of ganglion cells at the stoma. A definitive operation to correct Hirschsprung's disease is performed when the child is 6 to 12 months of age.

The postoperative management of infants who require surgery for intestinal obstruction is similar regardless of the type of corrective procedure employed. Nasogastric suction is maintained until bowel movements begin and nasogastric tube output is minimal. Oral feedings are then started with breast feeding or with infant formula except in those patients with cystic fibrosis in whom Pregestimil, a protein hydrolysate formula with medium chain triglycerides and added amino acids, is used. Postoperative antibiotic therapy is maintained as previously noted.

A significant number of infants with short intestinal length or complicated surgical problems have prolonged malabsorption after surgery. Often they do not tolerate a full diet for several weeks (or even years) after surgery. Nutrition must be maintained intravenously in these infants while dietary manipulations and intestinal regeneration are proceeding.

HEMOLYTIC DISEASE OF THE NEWBORN
HEBER C. NIELSEN, M.D.

Fortunately, advances in obstetric and perinatal medicine have significantly reduced the frequency of hemolytic disease of the newborn. A side effect of this medical triumph has been that pediatricians are now less experienced in the diagnosis and management of those few infants who manifest hemolysis and hyperbilirubinemia.

Some of the treatment options now available to the pediatrician have been developed during this era of reduced incidence of disease and therefore have not had the large-scale rigorous clinical testing that allows one to choose with complete assurance the correct option and the optimal time to intervene in all varieties of hemolytic disease. Other treatments were tested in term infants suffering from Rh disease of the newborn; the guidelines developed for this clinical situation are frequently adapted to other causes of hemolysis without formal testing. This practice may lead to the establishment of "rules" for treatment that have been set on a somewhat arbitrary basis. This article will try to avoid such an approach and will, rather, develop general guidelines by which an approach to caring for an individual infant can be formulated.

It is of primary importance in working with any infant who presents with hyperbilirubinemia to establish the cause of the elevated bilirubin level. Hemolysis is only one of several important considerations. For the purpose of this discussion, it is assumed that a diagnosis of hemolytic disease has been appropriately arrived at. The guidelines proposed in this article may not be applicable to other causes of neonatal hyperbilirubinemia.

Infants who present with hemolytic disease may suffer from one or more of three problems directly related to the hemolytic process. Most frequently, there is hyperbilirubinemia, which either is at a level that presents a high risk for neurologic damage or is rising at such a rate that it is predicted that it will reach a potentially neurotoxic level. In addition, there may be significant anemia as a result of the ongoing hemolysis. Finally, there is the process that is causing the hemolysis. All three of these problems may present a real danger to the infant, and therapy for each individual factor should be considered.

TREATMENT
Hematocrit

A tolerable hematocrit is not easy to define. Such variables as gestational age, weight, and respiratory status need to be taken into consideration. Infants will exhibit tachycardia and signs of congestive heart failure in response to severe anemia. However, one should not wait for these symptoms before beginning treatment. In general, a hematocrit less than 30 per cent or a hemoglobin less than 10 gm/dl in a term, otherwise healthy infant warrants treatment. These values may be higher in premature infants, infants with respiratory distress, or infants with severe hemolytic disease resulting in evidence of hydrops fetalis.

All infants suspected of having hemolysis should have their central hemoglobin and hematocrit measured as part of the initial evaluation. This should be done immediately after birth (the sample should be obtained while the baby is in the delivery room following resuscitation) in newborns in whom significant in utero hemolysis is suspected. Treatment is directed at elevating the hematocrit. This goal is best accomplished by a partial exchange transfusion with packed red blood cells (PRBC) that have not been reconstituted. Only enough volume is replaced to raise the hematocrit (Hct) to the desired level. One formula for calculating this volume is the following:

$$\text{Volume PRBC} = (\text{body weight}) \times 120 \times (\text{desired Hct} - \text{actual Hct})$$

PRBC represents the packed red blood cell volume to be administered during the partial exchange; 120 is a constant taking into account the average infant's blood volume of 80 ml per kilogram of body weight and an expected hematocrit of 67 per cent of the PRBC. In general, a desired hematocrit of 40 per cent is appropriate. This treatment should not be expected to alter the serum bilirubin level significantly.

Infants with hemolytic disease may develop a late (after 1 week of age) fall in hematocrit. This decrease may appear as late as 1 month of age. These infants should receive careful follow-up with a hemoglobin and hematocrit measurement to determine the possible need for a booster transfusion.

Bilirubin

An elevated bilirubin level is the abnormality in hemolytic disease of the newborn that most frequently requires treatment. In general, hyperbilirubinemia and jaundice are the presenting complaints that lead to a work-up and diagnosis of hemolytic disease. Treatment of the hyperbilirubinemia may be instituted before the diagnosis is established, but a diagnosis must still be vigorously pursued. The major consideration is which of the various types of treatment to begin.

Phototherapy. Phototherapy is an effective therapy for lowering the serum indirect bilirubin level, but its use does not remove the necessity of determining the cause of hyperbilirubinemia. It may reduce the likelihood of needing an exchange transfusion or may reduce the total number of exchanges performed, but it should not be regarded as an alternative to exchange transfusion if the exchange transfusion is required.

The level of serum bilirubin at which phototherapy should be started has not been clearly established. Since the bilirubin level rises normally over the first several postnatal days, and since the premature brain appears to be more sensitive to the effects of bilirubin, the level requiring treatment would be dependent on gestational and postnatal age. Other factors such as poor hydration, poor feeding, acidosis or other metabolic abnormalities, or the presence of hemolysis should prompt one to begin phototherapy earlier. All infants with hemolytic disease who are jaundiced on the first day of life should immediately be started on phototherapy. Many clinicians further use the general guideline of beginning phototherapy when the bilirubin level is rising at a rate of greater than 0.25 mg/dl/hr, or when the indirect bilirubin has reached one half of the predetermined level at which an exchange transfusion would be performed. Hemolysis caused by Rh isoimmunization may be rapid and severe. Infants with this hemolytic process should be started on phototherapy as soon as the diagnosis is made rather than waiting for the indirect bilirubin level to rise to a predetermined, arbitrary value.

The effectiveness of phototherapy is directly related to the dose of radiant energy absorbed through the skin. This dose is maximized by using high-energy output lights in the blue wavelengths and by exposing the greatest amount of body surface area to the lights. Phototherapy units should be given routine maintenance to ensure proper working order. The use of many phototherapy units simultaneously on one infant may significantly increase the energy delivery to the skin, but this should be documented in any particular case.

Phototherapy may cause increased free water loss. Hydration status should thus be carefully monitored during its use.

Exchange Transfusion. Double-volume exchange transfusion is the most effective therapy for lowering the bilirubin level rapidly. It should be performed when the indirect bilirubin fraction has reached a level that has a high risk of being neurotoxic or when the indirect bilirubin is rising at such a rate that reaching a potentially neurotoxic level is very likely.

Recommendations about what constitutes a potentially neurotoxic level of indirect serum bilirubin have been developed from experience with term infants with Rh disease. On the basis of this experience, an exchange level of 20 mg/dl is accepted as the standard for term infants with hemolytic disease. Recommendations for premature infants are less clear. Infants with birth weights between 1500 and 2000 gm might be exchanged for an indirect serum bilirubin of 18; infants with birth weights between 1000 and 1500 gm should be exchanged for an indirect serum bilirubin of no greater than 15; and infants with birth weights below 1000 gm should be exchanged for an indirect serum bilirubin of no greater than 12. These levels should be lowered in infants who, as mentioned, are acidotic or have a low serum albumin, other metabolic abnormality, or neurologic abnormality.

The rate of rise of the serum bilirubin level may prove to be a more useful index of the need for exchange transfusion in some infants, as an early exchange will not only clear bilirubin but also will clear some of the antigen and the abnormal red blood cells. This practice may lead to fewer exchanges in some severely affected infants. A rate of rise in the serum indirect bilirubin that is greater than 0.5 mg/dl/hr over a period of 4 hours or more indicates that the bilirubin will likely reach an exchange level and that an exchange transfusion should be now undertaken. If it is early in the course of hemolytic disease not due to Rh incompatibility, especially if the serum bilirubin level is still much lower than the projected exchange level, it may be reasonable to begin with phototherapy in an effort to slow the rate of rise. In many cases, particularly of hemolytic disease arising from ABO incompatibility, the early use of phototherapy may cause the rate of rise to slow significantly and prevent the bilirubin from reaching the exchange level.

Exchange transfusion is not a benign procedure. It is associated with a low but real risk of significant morbidity and mortality in the most experienced hands. With the improvements in prenatal care previously mentioned, fewer and fewer physicians have the opportunity to become expert in this procedure. It is best that infants who require or are likely to soon require exchange transfusions be transferred to a tertiary care center. Infants require close cardiorespiratory monitoring during and immediately after exchange transfusions. Serum electrolyte status, glucose and calcium levels, and blood counts need to be closely followed. Facilities for emergency cardiorespiratory resuscitation and support, as well as individuals who are appropriately trained and experienced in this area, need to be on hand at all times.

Type O, Rh-negative blood is generally the best blood to use for an exchange transfusion. Blood may be obtained as fresh or banked. Fresh heparinized blood is metabolically superior. However, it is extremely difficult to obtain for an exchange transfusion because the time required for obtaining, screening, and preparing the blood for use is so long that waiting for the blood generally presents an unacceptable risk to the infant requiring the exchange. If heparinized blood is used, the infant should be given protamine at the end of the transfusion to reverse the anticoagulation of the heparin.

Banked blood is generally stored as packed cells in the anticoagulant citrate-phosphate-dextrose (CPD). The anticoagulant acid-citrate-dextrose (ACD) is now rarely used. Recently, some blood banks have added Adsol to the stored blood to prolong its stability during storage. Cells stored in Adsol must be washed by the blood bank before use to remove the Adsol. CPD and ACD bind calcium; infants receiving these may have problems with calcium metabolism during the exchange. ACD contains a high acid load and is the least preferable anticoagulant for neonatal purposes. All packed cells should be restored to a hematocrit of approximately 50 per cent with plasma. It is best to use blood that has been stored for the shortest period, as the stored red blood cells release significant quantities of potassium over time. Storage in Adsol lessens but does not eliminate this problem. In general, blood that is older than 5 days should not be used for neonatal transfusions.

Phenobarbital. Phenobarbital may be a useful adjunct to therapy. It will induce the hepatic glucuronyl transferase enzyme system to conjugate more efficiently indirect bilirubin into the safer direct bilirubin product. Phenobarbital is most effective in lowering neonatal bilirubin levels when it is administered to the pregnant mother for 2 weeks before delivery and continues to be administered in the newborn. In cases of severe hemolysis, phenobarbital may be added to other therapies early on, with the expectation of ameliorating the long-term course. Since the effect of phenobarbital is not apparent for 2 to 3 days, it should not be thought of as an alternative to exchange transfusion or to phototherapy. The dose used is similar to the anticonvulsant dose in newborns. Infants receive a loading dose of 10 mg per kilogram of body weight if the mother was not already treated and thereafter a maintenance dose of 3 to 5 mg/kg every 12 hours. The respiratory status must be closely monitored because of the well-known depressant effects of phenobarbital. Phenobarbital is more effective with advancing gestational age. It is not beneficial in infants with a gestational age of less than 32 weeks.

Experimental Therapies. Other therapies to help lower the indirect bilirubin fraction of the newborn have been proposed. Binding agar has been shown to be effective in reducing the serum bilirubin. It binds bilirubin, which has been secreted via the biliary system into the small bowel, thus preventing the re-uptake of bilirubin. Tin-protoporphyrin has recently received attention in early animal and human clinical trials. It competes with natural protoporphyrin for enzymatic conversion, thus reducing the rate of bilirubin formation. Both of these therapies must be considered experimental and are not recommended at this time for general clinical application.

Removal of the Cause of Hemolysis

If hemolysis is not reduced or stopped, bilirubin production will remain elevated, and the serum bilirubin level will be difficult to control. In addition, the cause of hemolysis occasionally is itself a threat to the health of the infant. Exchange transfusion removes antibody and antibody-coated cells, or cells with unstable membranes that are rapidly breaking down (as in hereditary spherocytosis). Severe infections, such as sepsis, may occasionally be the source of hemolysis. This possibility should always be considered and evaluated whenever an infant presents with an unexpected onset of hemolysis postnatally. Environmental toxins rarely may be the cause of hemolysis in such problems as glucose-6-phosphate dehydrogenase deficiency. Eliminating exposure to the toxin will stop the hemolytic process and allow a more rapid recovery.

FOLLOW-UP

Infants who have hemolysis on the basis of blood type incompatibilities or red blood cell abnormalities require particular attention beyond the period of acutely elevated bilirubin levels. As mentioned before, the hematocrit will continue to fall for up to several weeks postnatally, even though bilirubin production is no longer a problem. Infants with Rh disease, severe ABO disease, and red blood cell abnormalities should have their hemoglobin and hematocrit checked at 1 month of age to determine if they are inappropriately anemic. A booster transfusion may be required.

Infants who have had a prolonged course of hemolysis may have chronic elevation of conjugated bilirubin, presumably as a result of acquired defects in bile excretion. These problems are generally self-limiting, but the total and direct bilirubin levels should be monitored until it is clear that the problem has resolved. In severe cases, treatment with phenobarbital will assist in stimulating the excretory mechanisms and aid in resolution.

Many of the causes of severe hemolytic disease involve hereditary elements. A full knowledge of the diagnosis and course of disease in any infant should be made available to the obstetrician, who may be caring for a future pregnancy.

NEONATAL POLYCYTHEMIA AND HYPERVISCOSITY

WILLIAM OH, M.D.

Neonatal polycythemia, defined as a venous hematocrit exceeding 65 per cent, is a common condition in the newborn. Hyperviscosity, defined as blood viscosity exceeding 2 SD (standard deviations) of the normal newborn population, is commonly associated with polycythemia. However, there are infants whose venous hematocrit is below 65 per cent and yet who may have hyperviscosity. Since blood viscosity measurement is rarely available in most clinical laboratories and the association of hyperviscosity and polycythemia is very close, the diagnosis of hyperviscosity is often inferred when polycythemia is present.

The management of polycythemia and hyperviscosity consists of prevention and therapeutic reduction of venous hematocrit. Since the pathogenesis of polycythemia and hyperviscosity is closely connected with high-risk obstetrical events that lead to fetal and/or perinatal hypoxia, appropriate management to minimize these high-risk events is highly desirable to prevent the development of neonatal polycythemia and hyperviscosity. Postnatal placental transfusion is also an important factor in the pathogenesis of polycythemia and hyperviscosity. It has been demonstrated that an approximately 20 to 25 per cent increase in blood volume can occur if placental transfusion is allowed to take place in the infant (delivered vaginally) because of a delayed cord clamping of about 2 to 3 minutes after the delivery. This acute expansion of blood volume results in hemoconcentration during the first 6 hours of life, leading to the development of polycythemia and hyperviscosity. Therefore, one approach to minimizing the incidence of polycythemia and hyperviscosity is to clamp the cord within 15 to 30 seconds to avoid excessive placental transfusion. This approach is particularly important in high-risk infants who have perinatal hypoxia.

The therapeutic reduction of red blood cell mass can

be achieved by partial exchange transfusion. This is a procedure that is generally accomplished by inserting an umbilical venous catheter under aseptic conditions to perform the exchange transfusion. Ideally, the catheter should be placed in the inferior vena cava just above the diaphragm and through the ductus venosus. This placement can be accomplished in many cases if the procedure is done during the first 6 hours of life. However, in the older infant, because of the collapse of the ductus venosus, it is often difficult (sometimes impossible) to pass the umbilical venous catheter beyond this structure to gain entry into the inferior vena cava. Under this circumstance, the umbilical venous catheter can be placed in the portal sinus for performance of the partial exchange transfusion. The actual procedure involved in the partial exchange transfusion is similar to that described for the exchange transfusion used in treating hyperbilirubinemia. The difference is that rather than replacing the removed blood volume with an equal volume of blood, we replace it with an equal volume of Plasmanate. The aim of this procedure is to reduce the hematocrit (Hct) from the polycythemic to a normal range. The following formula can be used to calculate the amount of blood to be removed and replaced with Plasmanate:

Amount of blood (ml) =

$$\frac{\text{observed Hct } (\%) - \text{desired Hct } (55\%) \times 85 \text{ ml/kg}}{\text{observed Hct } (\%) \times \text{ body weight (kg)}}$$

The desired hematocrit of 55 per cent is the normal value for term newborns, and the reason for not attempting to reduce the hematocrit lower than this value is to prevent the development of anemia at a future date. A figure of 85 ml/kg is the estimated blood volume in normal term newborns.

Venous hematocrit should be monitored at 4 to 6 hours following the procedure; if the venous hematocrit exceeds 65 per cent again, another partial exchange transfusion may be considered. If the formula previously shown is utilized to derive the volume to be exchanged, infants rarely require a repeat partial exchange transfusion. The infant should be fasted for 3 to 6 hours before and after the partial exchange transfusion procedure. Since the amount of blood removed is small (ranging between 10 and 20 per cent of the infant's estimated blood volume), acid-base or calcium imbalance is rarely encountered. Therefore, it is not necessary to monitor these parameters unless one is dealing with a sick newborn and there are indications for monitoring these biochemical measurements. If the procedure is done under strict aseptic technique, prophylactic or therapeutic antibiotics are also unnecessary. Gastrointestinal complications, including feeding intolerance and necrotizing enterocolitis, have been reported in infants with polycythemia and hyperviscosity who were treated with partial exchange transfusion. Therefore, these infants should be monitored very closely for these potential complications.

The long-term neurodevelopmental outcome of infants with polycythemia and hyperviscosity (many of whom were symptomatic) who were treated with partial exchange transfusion was found to be more favorable than that of those who were not treated. This finding argues for treating these infants with the partial exchange transfusion, particularly if they are symptomatic. A controversial issue concerns the indication for treating infants who have polycythemia (and probably hyperviscosity) but who are asymptomatic. The reason for this controversy is that long-term outcome data to evaluate the role of treating asymptomatic polycythemia and hyperviscosity in the newborn are lacking. Furthermore, the procedure itself (partial exchange transfusion) is not without potential risk and complications. Most clinicians make decisions for treating asymptomatic infants with polycythemia and hyperviscosity on an individual basis. If the infant's hematocrit exceeds 70 per cent, if there are subtle questions about whether or not the infant is indeed asymptomatic, and if the infant is young (less than 6 hours of age), most clinicians would elect to use the partial exchange transfusion. Another argument for the treatment is that the procedure will reduce the red blood cell mass and eliminate the possibility of hyperbilirubinemia later in life, which requires therapeutic intervention. If the hematocrit is between 65 and 70 per cent and the infant is truly asymptomatic, a more conservative approach—that is, not treating the infant with partial exchange transfusion—may be considered.

23

Special Problems in the Adolescent

CHILDREN OF DIVORCING PARENTS

MICHAEL JELLINEK, M.D.

Over the past 30 years divorce has become increasingly common. Currently one third of the nation's children have experienced a separation or divorce. The rate since the 1950's has tripled, and over 1 million children each year endure the divorce process. Since the average length of marriage is between 6 and 7 years, many of these children are young and especially vulnerable.

How do pediatricians first learn of the separation or divorce? Unless a parent volunteers the information or asks directly about their child's related emotional difficulties, most pediatricians do not know acutely about the divorce because they do not routinely ask about marital status or parental discord. Instead, pediatricians often learn of a divorce indirectly and late in the process through a change of address, a request to send records to another pediatrician, or problems in collecting bills as family finances are frozen in negotiations or in hostility.

Once aware that a divorce is in process or has taken place, the pediatrician must consider a number of issues in addressing the development and psychosocial needs of the child or children in the family. Inevitably divorce is a loss and must be mourned. However, the nature of this loss is not like a death, which is involuntary, irreversible, relatively unambiguous, and elicits a broad-based, supportive response from the community. Divorce is voluntary, one or both parents separating of their own accord, and the consequent explanations, hostile behaviors, and community reaction may make little sense to the child. The losses are multiple. During the divorce, the initial level of contact between the child and parents is less than when the family was intact, and even this level decreases further, especially for the noncustodial parent (the father in 90 per cent of divorces). In addition to the absolute decrease in time

with the parents, there is also a change in the quality of the time spent. Both parents are frequently preoccupied by their own form of mourning the marriage, trying to manage the rage they feel toward their former spouse, and dealing with the many details of the divorce process. The child must also face the loss of the family unit—a complex social structure that until now had supported a view of the world that was safe, predictable, filled with expectations, and encouraging of hope.

The financial impact frequently is crushing. Setting up two households and paying for the divorce are frequently overwhelming. The financial consequences for mothers are especially severe. Following divorce, mothers on average have suffered a 50 per cent drop in disposable income; in direct contrast, fathers no longer in the home have a relatively modest 15 per cent decrease in disposable income. Child support payments are frequently erratic and, like visitation, tend to decrease over time. Only recently has legislation been in effect that encourages court action to enforce financial agreements.

If the parents need to work harder or more hours, then again the amount and quality of time available to the child diminishes. If the family's home has to be sold, the losses secondary to the divorce are compounded by the loss of the child's room, neighborhood friends, local school, and the community supports (religious groups, sports teams, familiar routines, etc.).

Whether leading to divorce, following divorce, or a constant source of tension within a marriage that remains intact, ongoing parental discord is probably the single most damaging feature to the child's well-being and functioning. The child's sadness, anxiety, self-blame, private tension, and loneliness are daily realities. Children exposed to chronic, ongoing discord are more likely to be depressed, angry, and dysfunctional in school, with peers, and in extracurricular activities.

DEVELOPMENTAL CONSIDERATIONS

The expectable reactions to divorce depend upon the child's developmental level and the quality of the child's

722

relationship to the custodial parent or parents (joint custody).

In one of few prospective studies, Wallerstein and Kelly reported on children of various ages who were followed after divorce. Infants' and toddlers' reactions were most sensitive to the mother's ability to function. Many reacted to the divorce stresses by regression in toilet training, increased irritability, and greater dependency. Children whose homes were characterized by maternal depression and ongoing parental discord had more severe symptoms lasting over a year.

The preschool or young school-aged child is particularly vulnerable because the child's frame of reference has gone beyond the mother to include the entire family. At this cognitive level the child is confused by the events and length of the divorce process and uses an egocentric explanation of causation. Emotionally, the child is developing a conscience and is thus very ready to accept responsibility and blame for family events. Guilt-ridden fantasies are substantiated in part by arguments about "the children" overheard, often unbeknownst to the parents, prior to the separation and divorce. In addition, the child feels helpless as events beyond the child's understanding and control (especially lawyers and courts) dictate new realities.

School-aged children are more sophisticated and less likely to feel solely responsible for the divorce. Their reactions to divorce are more diverse and indirect. Children of this age feel sad, lonely, and powerless. They present with depression, psychosomatic disorders, problems in peer relationships, and a decrease in school performance. In addition, there is a higher incidence of aggressive behavior in boys who live with their mothers. These boys cope with missing their fathers by taking his place and behaving "just like his father," which quickly provokes the mother's anger and worst fears. School-aged children frequently consider changing homes to see what life would be like with the other parent and, possibly, as an effort to reunite the family. These real or imagined efforts may not end until one parent remarries.

The adolescent's developmental task is to separate from the family unit and establish an adult identity. Divorce disrupts this developmental process. Home is no longer a place for daily contact and identification with both parents. A frequent defensive reaction is the 10- to 11-year-old's early entry into adolescent behavior or the adolescent's premature closure of identity formation, i.e., uncritical adoption of the absent parent's characteristics. The pseudomature adolescent appears aloof, overly controlled, and overly controlling. Peer groups may become a major source of nurturance, and experimentation with drugs and alcohol may become a daily attempt to hide feelings of shame, suppress anxiety, dull depression, and test the limits in the newly structured family. The evolution of the adolescent's sexual identity may be accelerated in an effort to find temporary companionship.

CLINICAL ASSESSMENT AND MANAGEMENT

How should the pediatrician approach the child and family facing divorce? What questions should be asked of all families? Which children are at special risk?

Given the high prevalence of divorce and the serious impact of ongoing discord, the pediatrician should ask about the quality of family life as a routine part of primary care. If it is early in the course of marital problems, then the pediatrician may be able to take a preventive stance and refer the couple for counseling. If a separation or divorce has already been implemented, then the pediatrician should (1) focus on a brief review of the child's functioning in the major areas of daily life (family, friends, school, play, and the child's mood), (2) assess how the child is reacting to the divorce, and (3) determine if the child is at special risk. Children at special risk are more likely to have serious ongoing dysfunctions that include (1) predisposing vulnerabilities—children with a chronic disease or previous psychiatric disorder, a family history of psychiatric disorder (e.g., depression), children having suffered previous losses (especially as a preschooler or earlier). (2) chronic family discord before the divorce—divorce often serves as a marker for a disintegration process that has been active for many years. The child may have been used by one parent against the other, a process that takes a terrible toll on the child's emotional development. (3) ongoing discord after the divorce—includes parents who cannot communicate about childrearing or financial matters, use of visitation to provoke the former spouse, and repeated court actions. Court-ordered joint custody is a growing trend and potentially very supportive to the child's long-term development. However, joint custody also requires frequent contact and cooperation between parents—the same adults who could not communicate or achieve harmony in their marriage. If joint custody is agreed to by the parents only grudgingly or ordered by the court as an expedient to avoid a bitter trial, then the risks of damaging, ongoing discord are very high. Children who have to walk through a "demilitarized" zone from the car to one or another of their parents' front door are clearly at special risk. (4) emotional status of parent(s) after the divorce—Is the mother or father seriously depressed, agitated, abusing substances, or dysfunctional in meeting the child's physical and emotional needs? If the parents have been or continue to be overwhelmed by their marital difficulties, then it is quite possible that the child was used by one or both parents as an emotional support rather than treated as a child deserving of appropriate attention and nurturance.

After assessing the child's daily functioning and the presence of any risk factors, the pediatrician can decide whether follow-up appointments are necessary to reassess the child's well-being or if an immediate referral is indicated. In general, pediatricians can be of real help by remembering that parents are under great stress during a divorce. Simple, nonjudgmental listening and emotional understanding can be very supportive and can give the pediatrician some sense of how well the parent is functioning. Options for referral depend upon the circumstances. Some parents may benefit from a referral to a local self-help group, others by suggestions concerning daycare. A seriously depressed mother may require a psychiatric referral, ongoing discord about parenting issues may need to be referred to a psychologically sophisticated mediator, and the individual child's dysfunctional reaction may need to be evaluated by a child psychologist or psychiatrist.

Pediatricians themselves may get caught up in the ongoing battles between the parents. One parent, commonly the mother, may have a closer relationship with the pediatrician than the other. Consequently, the pediatrician may be more sympathetic to that parent's perspective and try to be supportive by agreeing with that parent's views on visitation or educational decisions to the point of writing letters to the court. If the child has a medical illness such as diabetes or asthma, the pediatrician may be used as part of one parent's legal plan to make the other parent appear unfit to care for the child. Unless the need to take sides is quite clear, the pediatrician probably will be of maximum help to the family by focusing on the child's well-being from a long-term and generally neutral perspective.

Although divorce issues are often complex and personally stressful, being available for 10 or 15 minutes to listen, assess, and, if necessary, intervene is a satisfying and increasingly vital aspect of pediatric practice.

OBESITY*

ADRIANE S. KOZLOVSKY, M.S., R.D., L.D.
and FELIX P. HEALD, M.D.

Obesity, an enlargement of the adipose tissue organ, is multifactorial in origin. As a result of limited understanding of the etiology of obesity, it is not surprising that the results of treatment are disappointing. In children and adolescents recent evidence strongly suggests genetics as a significant factor in obesity. This fact, combined with the influence of family lifestyle, results in a high prevalence of obesity among children and adolescents. The lack of success in treating obesity has resulted in more than 2000 different diets and a multiplicity of commercial weight-control programs.

Each obese child or adolescent presents a unique problem in management. Factors such as age, sex, fat distribution, eating and activity patterns, and motivation need to be considered when designing a therapeutic program. Regardless of external pressures, the teen must have significant personal motivation to make the lifestyle changes necessary to be successful in the weight loss attempt. These motivators may be physical (limited mobility) or psychological (poor body image, difficulty in buying clothes). Of particular importance is the determination of family history of obesity. If there is a strong family history of obesity, the therapist, adolescent, and family need to establish realistic therapeutic goals. The difference between treating children and adolescents versus adults is their growth and development. In physiologic terms, weight loss occurs when a state of catabolism is created and the body burns fat while sparing lean body mass. The issue of how this can be accomplished in children, and particularly in adolescents, has not been resolved. Finally, the physician must always be on the alert for excessive preoccupation with weight loss as a prelude to anorexia nervosa.

TREATMENT

The primary goal of most treatments for obesity is the reduction of caloric intake with the concurrent increase of caloric expenditure. Caution is advised against implementing fasting or very low calorie regimens to achieve weight loss during an adolescent's developing years. The most widely recommended treatment for obesity includes a triad approach of dietary monitoring, behavior modification, and exercise on a regular basis.

To achieve compliance with the various aspects of treatment, the prescribed regimen should be compatible with the teenager's lifestyle and daily routine. A 24-hour or typical dietary recall, coupled with inquiries of food preferences, can be indicative of the most frequently chosen foods and eating patterns. The Diabetic Food Exchange system, which divides food into six general categories, allows for selection and flexibility, while exposing the teenager to nutrient-dense food choices and reasonable portion sizes. Initially, specific aspects of the teenager's eating habits reflected in the food recall should be addressed. Issues such as excessive consumption of sugar-sweetened beverages, frequent snacking, and consumption of fast foods should be addressed, with one specific modification at a time. While encouraging gradual weight loss, weekly weigh-in sessions are important, both as indicators of motivation and as positive reinforcement for the teenager when weight loss does occur. Food records may be helpful in identifying significant environmental stimuli, although in the teenage population, records cannot always be relied upon for accurate information. Goal-setting should be concrete and short-term in nature, attempting 1 to 2 pounds weight loss each week. It is helpful to specify the goals by writing them down to represent a formal commitment.

Once treatment is initiated and preliminary weight loss is achieved, relapse prevention is designed for anticipation and coping with future high-risk situations. The ultimate intent is for teenagers to manage the behaviors on their own when the counselor is not available on a daily basis. Finally, teenagers should learn to identify problems unique to their own situation and feel comfortable with their decision-making process.

An exercise program compatible with the teenager's lifestyle should be included in a comprehensive weight-reduction plan. Activities such as television watching or sleeping, which are routinely engaged in after school hours, should be discouraged. Exercises including brisk walking, stair climbing, and low-impact aerobics, which do not require a great deal of prior planning and time allocation or expensive equipment, should be prescribed, on a daily basis if possible.

Currently, treatment plans have not been overwhelmingly successful in their attempts to produce effective weight loss results and even less successful in achieving weight maintenance (especially in the adolescent popu-

*Supported in part by Maternal and Child Health Grant MCJ 000980.

lation). Research has shown that modest losses are possible at the end of 1 year, but 5-year results are no better than no treatment at all. It is hoped that further research will uncover more effective techniques to ensure both phases of active weight loss and weight stabilization.

HOMOSEXUAL BEHAVIOR

LAWRENCE S. NEINSTEIN, M.D.

DEFINITION

Homosexuality is one of the most emotionally charged issues for the adolescent and his or her family and physician. A homosexual can be defined as a person with a persistent, erotic attraction as an adult to members of the same sex, and who usually, but not always, engages in sexual relationships with them. In 1974, the American Psychiatric Association ended its classification of homosexuality as a mental disorder and labeled it as an alternative choice of sexual expression. Several points are important in applying the above definition to an individual, and in particular to teenagers.

1. Sexuality is a continuum—Kinsey developed a seven-point scale (0–6) for rating sexual behavior based on psychological reactions and overt sexual practices. A "0" is a person who is exclusively heterosexual, while a "6" is a person who is exclusively homosexual. The other numbers represent people on a continuum of degrees of homosexual and heterosexual fantasy and behavior.

2. Some homosexual experimental behavior is common for many adolescents. For most adolescents, this genital play appears to be part of a developmental process leading to a heterosexual identity. However, this type of incident can lead to confusion and panic in many teenagers.

3. Sexual behavior during early adolescence may or may not parallel the direction of adult sexual expression. Some adolescents, particularly young girls, may display mainly same-sex sexual behavior (petting and kissing) but have predominantly heterosexual orientation. On the other hand, some adolescents may hide their "true" homosexual tendencies with heterosexual activity.

4. Some heterosexual adolescents will engage in homosexual behavior under certain circumstances. This may include noncoed boarding schools, the armed services, or prison settings. Most of these individuals have heterosexual behavior after leaving such an environment.

In distinction from homosexuals, a transvestite is an individual who derives pleasure by dressing in the clothing of the opposite sex. A transsexual is an individual who believes that the body he or she was born with does not match the sex he or she prefers to be. Neither the transvestite nor the transsexual teenager should be assumed to be homosexual.

PREVALENCE

As many as 30 to 50 per cent of males and 30 per cent of females engage in some homosexual experimentation during adolescence. Approximately 10 per cent of males are exclusively homosexual during at least 3 years of their lives, and 5 per cent of males for their entire lives. The prevalence in females has been more difficult to obtain but is about half that of males.

ETIOLOGY

While there is controversy over the factors involved in homosexual and heterosexual identity, the cause is unknown. The influence of genetics, of prenatal hormone levels, and of environment have all been postulated. While compelling evidence for any one of these factors is lacking, it seems likely that sexual identity is well-formed during childhood—even before adolescence. Several myths exist regarding homosexuality:

1. Homosexuality is a mental disorder. Homosexuality is *not* a mental disorder but a sexual preference. Homosexual adolescents may have problems identifying or adjusting to their sexual preference, leading to other fears and anxieties. The exposure of most homosexual adolescents to a societal environment of negative attitudes, lack of positive role models, and lack of family contacts can lead to problems with self-esteem and sexual behavior.

2. Homosexuals are child molesters. Most child molestation acts are committed by heterosexual males, not homosexual males.

3. Homosexual males are effeminate and wish to be female. The majority of homosexual males cannot be differentiated from heterosexual males and have no desire to be female.

Four stages of acquisition of homosexual sexual identity have been described. Stage I is sensitization. In this stage, the child feels a sense of being different with no understanding of the reason for these feelings. During the second stage, dessociation and signification, the individual may use various defenses to try to ignore any homosexual impulses and activity or regard them as a passing phase. There may be same-sex arousal and limited same-sex sexual experiences followed by periods of guilt and withdrawal. Stage III is the coming out phase. In this stage, which may not come until adulthood (if ever), individuals identify themselves as homosexual. Stage IV, commitment, is the last stage. At this point, the individual experiences satisfaction, self-acceptance, and an unwillingness to alter sexual identity.

The average ages for typical events in the coming out process are as follows:

	Male (age)	Female (age)
Same-sex interest	13	14–16
First same-sex activity	15	20
First same-sex love relationship	21–24	22–23
Disclosure to nonhomosexuals	23–28	28

In a study of gay adolescent males, it was found that 31 per cent were attracted to men during childhood and the rest were aware of their attraction to men in mid-adolescence. The mean age of gay self-identification was 14.

COUNSELING

Physicians should be able to deal with the anxieties of adolescents with strong homosexual tendencies and the fears of heterosexual adolescents involved with homosexual experimentation. If the physician finds it impossible, because of moral or religious convictions, to be objective in counseling and in taking care of a teenager with homosexual behavior, it is important to offer the teenager a referral to another professional.

The goals of the physician in counseling a young person or parent concerned about homosexuality should be to understand the feelings of all involved, to identify what their concerns are, to provide factual information, and to provide practical suggestions to help reduce the concerns and/or frictions.

To achieve any of these goals the concern of homosexuality must be discovered. Most adolescents are reluctant to discuss sexual issues, let alone homosexual concerns. In helping teenagers to discuss sexuality, it is helpful to first build rapport by asking less threatening questions about their medical concerns, school, hobbies, and friends. It is also essential to ensure confidentiality regarding sexual issues. There are different approaches in finding out about sexual identity or concerns. The physician can ask questions about dating and sexual activity and then later ask about sexual preference. It is often helpful to preface this with a reason for the inquiry (e.g., special medical problems). Alternatively, one can ask if there are any concerns or questions regarding the body, sexual activity, or sexual identity. Another approach is to state that many teenagers have concerns or questions about homosexuality and ask if there is anything that the individual would like to ask.

If a concern is raised, it is helpful to explore several areas. What is the teenager actually concerned about? If a homosexual encounter occurred, what actually happened? Is this a single encounter or one of many? Has the teen had sexual experiences with other people? Is there an interest in heterosexual sex? What are the teen's sexual fantasies? What does it mean to the teenager to be homosexual? What makes the teen think he or she is homosexual? What does it mean to the parent to have a homosexual son or daughter?

After these areas are explored, it is important to provide the teen and/or parents with factual information. This includes the prevalence of adolescent homosexual experimentation, the continuum of sexual behavior, and the fact that many teenagers worry about their sexual identity. The adolescent and his or her family must be aware that it is often difficult to assess and predict adult sexual behavior based on adolescent sexual behavior. However, the physician can help clarify the issues and keep the teen integrated into his or her family and social system regardless of sexual preference. The physician should encourage family ties, as acceptance from the family is extremely important to the adolescent. The physician should discourage blame and guilt if homosexuality is discovered. The sexual aspects

should be de-emphasized. The adolescent is a son or daughter who is homosexual, and not a homosexual who is a son or daughter.

Psychosocial areas need to be explored, as the social consequences of homosexual behavior can include peer rejection, family rejection, and harassment at school and job. For those adolescents who have a homosexual orientation, the evaluation should also include an assessment of their desire to remain homosexual or to try and alter their current sexual preference. However, adolescents should not be forced into therapy to change their sexual identity.

MEDICAL CONCERNS

The major medical concerns for physicians caring for adolescents with homosexual behavior include sexually transmitted diseases, gay bowel syndrome, and acquired immune deficiency syndrome (AIDS). Because of multiple partners, the high prevalence of asymptomatic carriers, and anonymity among patients, there is an epidemic of sexually transmitted diseases among the homosexual population. These problems are predominantly in homosexual males.

When evaluating for medical problems among gay adolescents, the physician must first be able to get correct information regarding the teen's sexual practices. Helpful approaches in eliciting this "sensitive" part of the history include establishing confidentiality, establishing a "need to know," and asking questions in a nonjudgmental fashion. Let the adolescent know that some personal questions will be asked and, although they do not have to be answered, honest answers will help the practitioner give the best care possible.

The physician will need to know if the teen has begun to have sexual relations and whether those relations are with members of the same sex, opposite sex, or both. The physician should also inquire into specific sexual practices. This may help to determine the adolescent's risk for sexually transmitted diseases and also furnish an opportunity to provide appropriate education regarding prevention of sexually transmitted diseases. Specifically the physician should ask about fellatio, anal intercourse (inserter or insertee), anilingus (rim or "scat"), number of sexual partners, frequency of sexual contact, use of condoms, prior history of sexually transmitted diseases, and HIV status (if known).

Documentation of this information must be considered carefully. The granting of access to the adolescent's chart by health professionals, allied health care workers, insurance companies, the courts, and parents carries both legal and ethical ramifications. The physician needs to consider him- or herself as a patient advocate protecting confidentiality. The practitioner must also be aware of the local state laws governing documentation, particularly in regard to HIV infection.

In the gay adolescent male who is either not sexually active or sexually active with one partner and is using appropriate barrier methods, a simple routine physical examination and syphilis serology would be adequate. If the gay adolescent male is having sex with multiple partners or is not using a barrier method, a more thorough screening is needed. The physical examination should include close inspection for lymphadenopathy, skin rashes, oral lesions, and anal trauma. The laboratory evaluation should include a gonorrhea culture and Chlamydia DFA or culture. These should be done on all appropriate sites of sexual contact. Additional screening tests include syphilis serology and hepatitis-B surface antigen and antibody. Discussion of HIV screening is appropriate. If HIV screening is ordered, pre- and post-test counseling is mandatory.

Anorectal and pharyngeal gonorrhea are fairly common in homosexual males. The majority of infections are asymptomatic. Symptoms include rectal burning, tenesmus, and mucopurulent discharge. Complications include fissures, abscesses, fistulas, and strictures. The preferred therapy for rectal and pharyngeal gonorrhea is ceftriaxone 250 mg diluted in 1 per cent xylocaine given intramuscularly plus doxycycline 100 mg orally twice a day for seven days. Spectinomycin can be used for rectal gonorrhea in patients allergic to penicillin but is not recommended for pharyngeal gonorrhea. Patients with pharyngeal gonorrhea who cannot be treated with ceftriaxone can be treated with ciprofloxacin 500 mg orally as a single dose. However, ciprofloxacin is contraindicated in growing individuals. Sulfamethoxazoletrimethoprim, 9 tablets daily as a single dose for 5 days, can also be used in pharyngeal gonorrhea as an alternative to ceftriaxone. Gonorrhea cultures from the rectum, urethra, and pharynx are recommended every 3 to 6 months in homosexual males with multiple partners.

Before the AIDS era, syphilis in gay males accounted for approximately 50 per cent of cases among males. In the AIDS era, when condom use has increased substantially among homosexual males, current epidemiologic data show an increase in the percentage of syphilis cases among heterosexual males. The primary lesion may be missed if present in the rectum. Syphilitic lesions are generally painless. However, rectal syphilis can cause pain, and the lesion can appear atypical, resembling a carcinoma with shaggy borders. A syphilis serology is recommended every 3 to 6 months for homosexual males with multiple sex partners.

There is evidence that HIV infections may alter infections with syphilis. This has led to cases of HIV-positive individuals either not responding to traditional therapy or having an accelerated course of syphilis. Cases have also been reported of HIV-infected individuals with evidence of syphilis but with negative syphilis serology. HIV-positive adolescents with syphilis require careful evaluation for late and unusual manifestations of syphilis, including cerebrospinal fluid evaluation. These individuals may also need more aggressive penicillin therapy.

Hepatitis B infections are prevalent in homosexual males, occurring in 37 to 51 per cent of these individuals. A successful vaccine is now available for hepatitis B and should be used in homosexual males with multiple partners.

Up to 80 per cent of homosexual males who are engaging in sexual activity with multiple partners will acquire cytomegalovirus screening each year. While this infection is largely asymptomatic, it may lead to a severe infectious mononucleosis type of illness, particularly in the immune-suppressed HIV-positive teen.

The gay bowel syndrome can include proctitis, colitis, and gastroenteritis. Infecting agents include *Neisseria gonorrhoeae, Treponema pallidum, Chlamydia trachomatis,* herpes simplex virus, human papilloma virus (condylomata acuminata), *Entamoeba histolytica, Giardia lamblia, Shigella, Salmonella,* and *Campylobacter jejuni/fetus.* Anal problems can include anorectal trauma secondary to anal intercourse or use of foreign objects for anal intercourse; proctitis and inflammation or perianal area secondary to allergies caused by contactants such as lubricants and infectious agents; pruritus ani secondary to oil-based lubricants and blockage of anal pores leading to inflammation; anal condylomata; hematochezia secondary to anal lacerations caused by anal intercourse, "fisting," or use of sex toys; anal ulcers secondary to herpes (painful; usually seen in clusters) or syphilis (painless; a single lesion); and anal discharge secondary to bacterial sexually transmitted diseases. The evaluation of the rectum and anus in a symptomatic teen should include proctoscopy, gonorrhea and Chlamydia cultures, stool for routine culture and ova and parasites, and syphilis serology. Treatment is directed at the etiologic agent.

Venereal warts are common in the rectal area in individuals having rectal intercourse. External warts are best treated with podophyllin or trichloracetic acid or a combination of both. Internal warts can be treated with electrocautery or lasers. However, patients with internal warts are best referred to physicians familiar with their treatment, as overly aggressive therapy can lead to strictures. Examining serology for syphilis is essential.

The acquired immune deficiency syndrome (AIDS) is the disease causing the most concern among homosexual males. The cause is the human immunodeficiency virus, a retrovirus. Because of the long incubation period, most cases occur outside the adolescent age group. However, HIV infections are becoming more common among the adolescent population. While all teens need to be informed about AIDS, it is especially important in the homosexually active adolescent. A discussion should take place between the physician and the homosexual adolescent about HIV testing. Use of a condom for all forms of intercourse should be encouraged among all sexually active teens, but particularly in the homosexually active male. The adolescent should understand safer sexual practices, which include limiting sexual partners (abstinence or monogamy); avoiding sexual practices that involve the exchange of body fluids such as blood or semen; avoiding the use, or if used, the sharing of needles; using latex condoms and not those made from natural lamb skin; and using water-based lubricants because oil-soluble ones can damage latex.

SEX EDUCATION

JOHN W. KULIG, M.D.

Sex education should be incorporated into anticipatory guidance provided from birth through late adolescence. Health providers have a unique opportunity to facilitate communication about sexuality between parents and their children as well as to provide specific factual information. Although comprehensive sex education should ideally occur within the home, most teenagers report receiving such information from peers. Parents often believe that sex education is being taught at school, yet only about one third of all schools provide specific courses in sex education, and only 10 per cent are truly comprehensive in nature. Teenagers in particular are often eager to discuss sexuality-related concerns with both parents and health providers yet are often inhibited by the obvious discomfort generated by their questioning. In addition, parents of teenagers still commonly believe the myth that withholding information about sexuality may delay the onset of sexual activity.

Health providers can encourage and support parents in their role as sex educators in the family, provide age-appropriate guidance during the course of primary care visits, and assume an advocacy role on behalf of formal sex education programs in the community. Even in the absence of formal discussions about sexuality at home, children learn much from observing parental attitudes, vocabulary, and interactions. Parents of infants and toddlers should be advised to use proper terms when referring to body parts and to react calmly to the genital manipulation that commonly occurs with increased body awareness. Questions from preschoolers should be answered accurately in a simple, straightforward manner and in language appropriate to age. The concept of privacy should be reinforced at this time, and proper names should continue to be used for both body parts and functions.

An important component of sex education at this age is the introduction of specific warnings aimed at reducing the risk of sexual misuse by an older child or adult. School-age children who have not requested information on their own may be provided with specific data during "teachable moments," such as the birth of a sibling, the experience of "playing doctor," or the chance exposure to sexually explicit magazines or films. A parent's reaction to each of these events in a calm, nonpunitive manner will do much to avert feelings of guilt or discomfort on the part of the child. When explicit questions are posed, the parent should respond promptly with a simple factual answer rather than deferring the question to a later age or to the other parent.

With the onset of puberty, body image and physical development assume paramount importance to the young teenager. At this point it is essential that the adolescent be provided an opportunity for a confidential interview with the health provider as well as privacy during the physical examination. Emphasis on the normalcy of the examination can do much to alleviate the anxieties of an early adolescent faced with a rapidly changing body. At this stage, females should be provided with specific information about breast asymmetry, menarche, menstrual hygiene, and the management of menstrual cramps, while males should be advised about pubertal gynecomastia, erections, and nocturnal emissions. Masturbation should be acknowledged as a nor-

mal means of sexual expression in both sexes. The teaching of both breast self-examination and testicular self-examination should be considered an integral component of primary care for the early adolescent. In addition, adolescent females should be carefully prepared for their first pelvic examination, which should always be conducted in a gentle, sensitive manner.

Sexual history-taking in adolescence is best accomplished through the use of "informative questions," which provide normative data and solicit a broader response than "yes or no" questions. Questioning should vary according to developmental stage, level of anxiety, presenting concern, and mode of sexual expression. Discussion may also be facilitated by asking about the patient's relationship with a best friend, which in a dating relationship may lead to explicit information about sexual activity. A history of sexual activity in an adolescent should lead both to careful questioning about the character of the relationship and to a contraceptive history and the provision of contraceptive counseling, as appropriate. Contraceptive counseling should include specific advice regarding use of barrier methods that reduce the risk of sexually transmitted infection. Questioning with use of "reality testing" may counter the magical thinking and feelings of invulnerability and denial that often characterize adolescent sexual behavior. For example, one might point out that a teenager who is sexually active without the use of contraception has, in fact, made a decision either to become pregnant or to father a child. Few teenagers have considered their response to an unplanned pregnancy. Health professionals who choose not to provide contraceptive counseling services should become aware of community agencies that serve adolescents.

Parents should be encouraged to maintain a dialogue with their adolescents and to express their beliefs openly and honestly. Parents should be cautioned, however, that teenagers do not need their approval to become sexually active and that the provision of contraceptive advice and services may reduce the risk of consequences of this activity. There is no evidence that such information stimulates sexual activity but rather may do just the opposite by satisfying curiosity without the need for experimentation. Numerous contemporary pamphlets, texts, and audiovisual materials on the topic of sex education are available for use by health providers, educators, and parents. A bibliography of low-cost resources on sex education for adolescents is published annually by the Committee on Adolescence of the American Academy of Pediatrics (Publications Department, American Academy of Pediatrics, P.O. Box 927, Elk Grove Village, Illinois 60009-0927).

ADOLESCENT SEXUALITY, CONTRACEPTION, PREGNANCY, AND ABORTION

JOHN W. KULIG, M.D.

Adolescents' health concerns about sexuality include a broad range of issues ranging from questions about the normalcy of their pubertal growth and development to dealing with the consequences of early sexual activity. Sexual expression among teenagers often reflects a developmental sequence that begins with self-exploration during puberty, followed by group dating, and then individual dating, which may initially be exploitative in nature. By high school graduation, approximately two thirds of all American teenagers have experienced at least one episode of sexual intercourse. Health providers must recognize both the medical and social consequences of early sexual activity, including not only sexually transmitted disease and pregnancy but also anxiety, depression, and multiple somatic complaints. Sexual history-taking should include the asking of "informative questions" in a nonjudgmental fashion, with an assurance of confidentiality. Counseling should deal not only with the anatomy and physiology of reproduction and contraception but should also address decision making, positive options, and the denial of consequences that is so commonly seen in midadolescence.

The health provider must assure the adolescent that he or she is comfortable in addressing these concerns in a forthright manner. Questions should be age-appropriate, should not presume sexual preference, and should explicitly address the possibility of sexual abuse if suspected. Physical assessment during adolescence should include specific statements about the normalcy of pubertal development, and health education during this period should incorporate the teaching of breast and testicular self-examination. An annual pelvic examination with Papanicolaou smear and endocervical cultures is indicated in all sexually active adolescent females in order to detect cervical dysplasia and asymptomatic gonococcal and chlamydial infection. Pelvic examination is also indicated in the evaluation of menstrual disorders, lower abdominal pain, vaginal discharge, DES exposure in utero, and in the confirmation of pregnancy and the prescription of contraception.

CONTRACEPTION

Contraceptive counseling is an essential component of health education for the adolescent and may be conducted by the health provider or ancillary personnel and reinforced with the use of free or low-cost handouts and films. Surveys have consistently shown that maintenance of confidentiality is the most important factor in the provision of contraceptive care for teenagers. Counseling should be individualized, should be provided in a nonjudgmental manner for both males and females, and should address choices regarding sexual activity as well as the specific contraceptive methods available. Adolescents who choose to remain abstinent should be supported in this decision and encouraged to resist peer pressure.

Contraceptive Pill. The oral contraceptive pill remains the most popular choice among adolescent females. If indicated, the pill may be started as early as 6 to 12 months postmenarche after ovulatory cycles have been established. Among the medical contraindications to oral contraception, those that are most likely to affect adolescents include pregnancy, migraine headaches, hypertension, congenital heart disease, active liver disease, collagen vascular disease, diabetes mellitus, lipid disorders, severe depression, and a history of thromboembolic disease. Counseling should emphasize the noncontraceptive benefits of the pill, such as the resolution of dysmenorrhea and the reduced risk of pelvic inflammatory disease, iron deficiency anemia, benign breast disease, and certain forms of cancer. Serious complications of pill usage are exceedingly uncommon among teenagers; however, smoking should be discouraged in hopes of further reducing this risk.

A fixed-dose combination pill containing 1 mg of norethindrone and 35 μg of ethinyl estradiol is a low-dose formulation suitable for the vast majority of adolescent women. Recently marketed triphasic formulations may prove equally effective, with an overall reduction in total hormonal dosage per cycle. Lower dose pills and those containing progestin only should be avoided owing to an unacceptable incidence of breakthrough bleeding, which is likely to markedly reduce compliance. A 28-day pill packet is preferred to a 21-day packet, since the patient can simply be advised to take one pill each day at the same time of day, rather than remembering to stop for 1 week prior to beginning a new packet. A complete physical examination including breast and pelvic examination with Papanicolaou smear and cultures should first be performed. The pill should be started on the fifth day of menses or on the Sunday after menses in order to avoid administration during an unsuspected pregnancy. Patients should be scheduled to return to the physician 6 weeks after starting the pill, then at 3-month intervals for the first year and at 6-month intervals thereafter. Weight, blood pressure, and side effects are monitored at the interval visits, and the complete physical examination is repeated annually. Minor side effects such as breast tenderness, weight gain, and spotting often resolve after two or three cycles of use; thus, a change in pill formulation should generally not be instituted until after the 3-month follow-up visit. Drug interactions, particularly with anticonvulsants, may require an adjustment in dosage of both medications. The pill should be discontinued prior to surgery or orthopedic immobilization, but periodic "pill holidays" are not recommended. Concomitant use of a barrier method should be advised to reduce the risk of sexually transmitted infection.

Intrauterine Device. The intrauterine device (IUD) is not commonly used among nulliparous adolescents owing to a relatively high expulsion rate, increased cramping, and an increased risk of pelvic inflammatory disease, with potential for subsequent infertility. The IUD might be considered in patients with a history of prior pregnancy or failure with oral contraception or barrier methods due to poor compliance and in sexually active adolescents with mild mental retardation. Copper- or progesterone-containing devices should be inserted during menses in selected adolescents with no prior history of pelvic infection or multiple sexual partners.

Barrier Methods. Barrier methods would be ideal for adolescents if compliance could be assured. These methods are reversible, have few side effects, and reduce the risk of sexually transmitted infection. Condom use is the only method that allows the male to share directly in the responsibility for contraception. Condoms are available over the counter to minors, do not require a prescription, and do not require visits to a health provider later. Latex condoms with a spermicidal lubricant and reservoir tip are advocated for use by adolescent males, and explicit instructions on proper storage and use should be provided. Natural-membrane condoms should not be recommended, since microscopic pores may permit transmission of viral infection. The newly developed "female condom," which consists of a polyurethane sheath that fits into the vagina and covers the labia, may prove to be an effective alternative. Spermicidal foams and creams are also available over the counter for adolescent females and, when used with condoms, provide a very high level of efficacy. Spermicidal suppositories may be less acceptable owing to the need to wait for dissolution, which may produce an unpleasant burning sensation in the vagina. The vaginal contraceptive sponge is another inexpensive, nonprescription method that acts to absorb semen, block the cervical os, and release a spermicide. The sponge is effective for 24 hours after insertion but must be left in place for 6 hours after intercourse. Some patients have experienced difficulty with removal of the sponge. The diaphragm has been successfully used by motivated older adolescents, especially those who are comfortable with tampon insertion. The diaphragm is used in conjunction with a spermicidal cream or jelly and must initially be fitted by a health provider. Patients are asked to return in 1 week with the diaphragm in place to assure proper size and insertion. Diaphragms should be replaced annually or earlier if a significant change in weight occurs. The cervical cap, recently approved by the FDA, is comparable in function and efficacy to the diaphragm, but is more costly, less available, and has been associated with cervical abnormalities and vaginal odor with prolonged use.

Other Methods. Postcoital contraception has been demonstrated to be highly effective with the administration of only four Ovral oral contraceptive pills. Two pills are taken at each dose, 12 hours apart, within 48 to 72 hours of intercourse. The emetic doses of estrogen prescribed in the past for 5 days are no longer necessary for this indication.

Depo-medroxyprogesterone acetate given in a dose of 150 mg IM every 3 months will induce a secondary amenorrhea in a majority of patients. While not FDA approved for use as a contraceptive, this drug appears to be safe and effective for use in patients with moderate to severe mental retardation or mental illness as well as in selected patients with conditions such as sickle cell disease or severe congenital heart disease, in whom alternate methods are contraindicated yet the risk of pregnancy may be life threatening. The most troublesome side effects include irregular menstrual spotting or bleeding and weight gain.

"Natural family planning" is of limited usefulness among adolescents owing to unpredictable ovulation, the prolonged period of abstinence required each month, and the need to monitor the calendar, basal body temperature, and cervical mucus for optimal results. Withdrawal or coitus interruptus is also ineffective owing to poor control on the part of the adolescent male and the possible presence of sperm in the preejaculate fluid. Despite the lack of efficacy, either of these two methods is preferable to no attempt at contraception. Except in the event of a life-threatening emergency, surgical sterilization is not an option in an adolescent without involvement of the courts. Finally, abstinence should be emphasized as a positive choice, without risks, side effects, or cost.

PREGNANCY

Health providers caring for adolescents are very likely to face the issue of pregnancy diagnosis and referral, since approximately one million teenage pregnancies occur each year. Common presentations include physical symptoms such as amenorrhea, nausea, breast tenderness, back pain, and urinary tract symptoms; behavioral presentations may include personality changes, truancy, and decline in school performance and general signs of anxiety, depression, or even suicidal behavior. A high index of suspicion will result in the correct diagnosis even in the absence of a confirmatory menstrual history. A 2-minute urinary slide pregnancy test is usually positive within 2 to 4 weeks after conception or 4 to 6 weeks since the last normal menstrual period. A negative test should be followed by contraceptive counseling and a repeat urinary pregnancy test in 1 to 2 weeks if menses have not resumed. Positive tests should be confirmed by pelvic examination to estimate uterine size and determine length of gestation. Serum pregnancy testing and pelvic ultrasonography may be helpful in cases of suspected ectopic pregnancy and in confirming gestational age.

Pregnancy counseling should then be conducted to assess the patient's response to the diagnosis and to discuss all options. With the patient's permission, parents and partners should be involved in helping the patient reach a decision. Although patients often express fear of parental reaction to pregnancy, most younger teenagers eventually consent to parental involvement, and their response is usually quite supportive. Options include terminating the pregnancy by therapeutic abortion or continuing the pregnancy, with subsequent adoption of the infant or raising the infant alone or with the assistance of a parent or partner. Early referral for therapeutic abortion or prenatal care is indicated in either case, preferably to a local agency that provides special services for pregnant adolescents and their partners. The medical complications of adolescent pregnancy are most common in patients younger than age 16, but the social consequences impact throughout adolescence. Prenatal programs that attempt to keep the pregnant adolescent in school and to teach parenting skills are aimed at averting serious psychosocial sequelae, including a high risk of repeat pregnancy, child abuse, and neglect.

ABORTION

Since laws governing therapeutic abortion in minors vary by state, each health provider should become familiar with local law as well as area resources. Early referral is indicated to reduce the risk of medical complications. First trimester abortions are performed by suction curettage on an outpatient basis, while second trimester abortions often require an inpatient stay for induction of labor with hypertonic saline or prostaglandin instillation. Medical complications of therapeutic abortion are rare, and future child-bearing is not compromised. Follow-up should include the selection of an appropriate method of contraception.

MANAGEMENT OF A DRUG-USING ADOLESCENT

RICHARD H. SCHWARTZ, M.D.

Adolescents of any socioeconomic group anywhere may be affected by the disease of alcohol/drug (chemical) dependency, the symptoms or social consequences of which include adolescent turmoil, unpredictable explosive temper, conduct disorder (chronic lying, thievery, aggression, and/or promiscuity), bizarre behavior, venereal disease, truancy, serious academic underachievement, depression, involvement in motor vehicle accidents, running away, personality disorders, chronic argumentativeness and disrespect for others, amotivation, low sense of goal direction, and suicidal tendencies. It appears that drug use is the Great Imitator during adolescence and must be considered as a primary cause of, and not merely a secondary effect of, such mood disturbances and behaviors. Because endogenous depression, serious non–drug-related mental illness, and life with a physically or sexually abusive parent may lead to some of the same symptoms as found with drug abuse, pediatricians or their consultants must carefully evaluate each adolescent who exhibits these symptoms in order to reach the correct diagnosis. However, drug use should be a primary consideration.

EVALUATION

The first step in evaluating a teenage patient with any of the above symptoms is to obtain a comprehensive history, preferably during a counseling session. To elicit information about possible drug abuse the physician should ask the patient a few nonthreatening questions about school, family relationships, jobs, friends, and recreational activities, academic performance subject by subject, vocational aspirations, frequency of conflicts with parents, attendance at hard rock concerts, if any close friends are hassled by their parents for drinking a little beer, participation in drinking games at parties, if any close friend has ever been drunk or high, how many cans of beer the adolescent who drinks alcohol may consume before he or she "catches a buzz."

Drug-using adolescents often become proficient in techniques of denial or minimization of their own role, blaming others, selective muteness, and overt hostility when threatened by references to drug use. Therefore, a more thorough drug and alcohol assessment, if the pediatrician's suspicions are aroused, should be done by a professional with expertise and experience in the field of substance abuse, rather than by a well-meaning but naive pediatrician who may easily be manipulated and misled ("conned") by a drug-using adolescent.

The physical examination is unlikely to provide any hard evidence regarding drug use, although some indications of the adolescent's sympathy with the drug culture may be provided by his or her attitude toward the physician and attire. Lack of sustained eye contact, lack of spontaneity, a flattened affect, and an attitude of hostility, secretiveness, or persistent evasiveness should alert the physician to the possibility of drug use, especially when combined with a preference for the hairstyles and clothing favored by drug users. These are "soft signs" and require correlation with the history and laboratory findings as in the diagnosis of any other disease. It is usually more fruitful to concentrate on the adverse social consequences of drug use and avoid threatening direct questions about such use. Intoxicated behavior or concrete evidence of drug use is not often witnessed by parents of a drug-using adolescent until fairly late in the progressive stages of the drug use syndrome.

LABORATORY DIAGNOSIS

Because it is so difficult to diagnose drug use, any array of factors in the history combined with any of the attitudes just described should raise the suspicion that an adolescent has this disorder. And because of the potentially life-threatening consequences of continued drug use, the physician should order laboratory tests to assist in further evaluation of such a patient.

Marijuana Use. Metabolites of marijuana (cannabis) and phencyclidine persist in the body for several days after last use of those drugs and may be detected by laboratory analysis of a urine specimen. The half-life of marijuana is 72 hours, and if the adolescent is using cannabis every day, evidence will be detectable in the urine up to several weeks after the beginning of a period of complete abstinence. Casual or infrequent users of marijuana will have a negative (clean) urine by immunoassay methods after 48 to 72 hours of abstinence.

A urine specimen collected for analysis of these substances should be obtained from a first voiding on a Monday morning (because most adolescents use drugs on Friday and Saturday evenings), preferably under direct surveillance to avoid possible deliberate substitution or adulteration of the urine specimen by the adolescent. Most frequent users of illicit drugs are well aware of procedures for adulterating a specimen for laboratory analysis of such use, including substituting urine of a non–drug-using friend, diluting the specimen with tap water, drinking large quantities of water before voiding, and purposely adding blood, household bleach, salt, or an acidic substance. Thus, when direct observation is not possible, the urine specimen should be checked for color, pH, specific gravity, and freshness (warmth of the specimen when obtained in the physician's office or at home).

Testing urine specimens serially (consecutive Monday morning urine specimens) for the presence of cannabinoids is more informative than a single test for such substances. If cannabinoids are present in two mid-week urine specimens obtained several days apart, or if three weekly spot-checked Monday-morning specimens are positive, it is likely that the adolescent is using marijuana frequently enough to warrant a more complete drug evaluation. Such an adolescent may well need immediate intervention and treatment of his or her drug abuse disorder.

Alcohol Use. Frequent use of alcohol is more difficult to detect than marijuana use, but the patient should be questioned carefully about citations for driving while intoxicated, what he or she does with friends for relaxation, and how often the adolescent or his or her close friends have been incapacitated by alcohol. If alcohol use has been heavy, damage to the parenchyma of the liver may be present and detected as elevation of the hepatic enzyme gamma glutamyl transpeptidase. This test, however, is relatively nonsensitive and nonspecific for adolescent alcoholism.

Acute alcohol ingestion may be detected by administration of a Breathalyzer test or immunoassay of a urine specimen obtained within 6 hours of ingestion. Such use may also be detected, even as late as 12 hours postingestion, by sophisticated urine toxicology methods such as gas chromatography, but such means are much more expensive and the results are not available for some time after the sample is drawn.

CHEMICAL DEPENDENCY

Chemical dependency is the increasingly preferred term for compulsive drug use. Either persistent, frequent use of mood-altering, pleasure-producing drugs or indulgence in prolonged binges of such drug use characterize the adolescent who has lost control of his or her use of drugs. Such an individual has a preoccupation with a self-perceived need to obtain a euphoric "high" not reached by other means, usually in the company of peers who have the same mind-set. These adolescents may develop a tolerance to their drug(s) of choice, so that they require ever increasing quantities of the drug to achieve the same degree of euphoria. Because the chemically dependent young person obtains much of his or her pleasure in life from the social use of drugs, he or she cannot or will not stop using these substances. Thus, even though the adolescent may have tried one or more times to remain abstinent, and despite being apprised of the many adverse consequences of drug use (academic underachievement, family conflicts, internalized shame and guilt, legal complications, acute toxic reactions), it must be recognized that the chemically dependent adolescent usually cannot break free of his or her disease without intensive and prolonged professional help.

Outpatient Management. After the adolescent has been evaluated by a pediatrician or consultant who is an expert in chemical dependency, a time must be chosen when the patient is not under the influence of drugs to bring the entire family together (excluding young children) for treatment. At this initial session the goal is for every family member present to agree to a drug-free lifestyle for him- or herself and for the parents to state unequivocally that they are prepared to do anything and everything to accomplish that goal. Behavioral changes that will be necessary for the drug user include (1) total abstinence from all drugs (including alcohol), (2) complete and immediate dissociation from drug-using friends, (3) co-operation in the provision of periodic urine specimens to monitor compliance with the plan, and (4) participation in family meetings each week.

Other activities in which the drug user must participate include attendance at a peer-support group such as Alcoholics Anonymous or Narcotics Anonymous two or three times a week for the first month, two times a week for the second month, and once weekly for the next 3 months. A sponsor from the support group should be assigned to act as role model for the drug-using adolescent and to monitor attendance and participation at meetings. The adolescent and family may need psychotherapeutic or pastoral counseling, which should be done by someone expert in managing individuals with alcohol- or drug-related problems.

It is important for the adolescent and professionals who are helping him or her to manage the drug problem to communicate on a regular basis with school guidance counselors, teachers, the pediatrician, group therapy sponsor, and interested others. Further, the teenager must comply with a mutually agreed upon list of house rules, the breaking of which will have fair but definite and clear consequences. The adolescent's parents would do well to attend a parent support group such as Al-Anon or Toughlove. Parents of drug-using teenagers often feel embarrassed, guilty, insecure, and alienated from parents of "successful" teenagers. Lastly, if the drug which the adolescent has heavily abused is alcohol, a medically supervised trial of disulfiram (Antabuse) (250 mg/day in a single dose for 2 to 3 months) should be considered. Antabuse requires an intensive education as to the reasons for use and its effects if alcohol is ingested, and it should not be prescribed unless it is part of a comprehensive plan of management including regular attendance at AA meetings.

If this necessarily authoritarian plan of therapy is unsuccessful, the young person dependent on drugs (including alcohol) should be admitted to an adolescent-oriented drug rehabilitation program or therapeutic community with or without his or her consent unless the age of majority has been reached.

In-patient Management. The basic principles of managing drug abuse are the same, regardless of which of the following drugs is abused: alcohol, marijuana, cocaine, stimulants, depressants, hallucinogens, PCP, or inhalants. Methadone may be included in the regimen for management of opiate abuse, Antabuse has been found to be helpful in the treatment of some alcoholics, and phenothiazine or trifluoperazine may be required to treat subacute or chronic drug-related PCP or LSD psychosis as part of the overall treatment plan. Antidepressant medication may be a necessary adjunct in the management of selected severely endogenously depressed and chemically dependent adolescents.

Detoxification is almost always unnecessary for adolescent drug users unless the dependence is on an opiate, barbiturate, or diazepam, or unless the patient had attempted to withdraw from alcohol dependence previously and had shown severe acute symptoms. When necessary, such detoxification can usually be accomplished in 3 to 7 days (unless the drug is diazepam).

Drug rehabilitation programs for adolescent drug users should meet six criteria. (1) No drugs whatever should be permitted in the program, including alcohol, mood-altering drugs, and tranquilizers. (2) Peer-group support should be encouraged. (3) Some staff members should be ex–drug users or alcoholics. (4) Intense family participation should be manadatory. (5) The chemically dependent patient should be separated from friends and/or parents for a minimum of 1 to 2 months. (6) The program must have an aftercare program that includes a large enough group of graduates close enough geographically to the patient that they form an easily accessible peer group of drug-free supporters.

Pediatricians play a crucial role in the identification and treatment of drug-dependent adolescents. By familiarizing themselves with the symptoms of chemical dependency, the techniques of the assessment of a drug-using adolescent, and the resources in their areas to help rehabilitate drug users, they will be much better able to serve their adolescent patients and their families.

24

Miscellaneous

THE IMMUNODEFICIENCIES, INCLUDING HIV-1 INFECTION

GWENDOLYN B. SCOTT, M.D.,
and BRIAN L. HAMILTON, M.D., Ph.D.

GENERAL MANAGEMENT CONSIDERATIONS

Antibiotic Use

The routine use of prophylactic antibiotics for prevention of infection has been found to be beneficial in conditions such as chronic granulomatous disease of childhood (CGD). However, the benefits of such treatment must be carefully weighed against the risks of predisposing to infections with resistant bacteria or fungi. In general, routine prophylaxis of B-cell, T-cell, or combined T- and B-cell immunodeficiencies is not recommended.

Fever in a patient with immunodeficiency should be evaluated promptly. Cultures from appropriate sites should be taken and inoculated onto media for isolation of aerobic and anaerobic bacteria as well as fungi and mycobacteria. Broad-spectrum antibiotics should be begun promptly pending culture results. Knowledge of the specific immune defect may guide initial therapy; i.e., in patients with granulocyte deficiencies, anti-staphylococcal coverage should be included; in patients with complement deficiency or antibody deficiencies, initial therapy should include antibiotics effective against *Streptococcus pneumoniae*, *Haemophilus influenzae* type b, and *Neisseria meningitidis*. When an organism has been identified and its sensitivity pattern to antibiotics is determined, antibiotics should be changed to a more specific therapy.

Prophylaxis for *Pneumocystis carinii* pneumonia is indicated in many of the immune deficiencies discussed in this chapter. The treatment of choice is oral trimethaprim-sulfamethoxazole (TMP-S), 75 mg/M^2 of TMP and 375 mg/M^2 of sulfamethoxazole given every 12 hours on Monday, Tuesday, and Wednesday. Leukocyte counts should be monitored and the medication discontinued if neutropenia occurs. Children with HIV infec-

tion who have an absolute T-helper cell number of 400 cells/mm^3 or less or who have already had an episode of *P. carinii* pneumonia should receive prophylaxis. There are no studies done to date to determine the most effective dosage schedule for prophylaxis in children with HIV infection. The recommended adult dose is 160 mg TMP and 800 mg sulfamethoxazole given twice daily with 5 mg of leukovorin once daily.

The use of aerosolized pentamidine as prophylaxis in adults with HIV infection is well established. For older adolescents and adults, aerosolized pentamidine can be given as 300 mg every 4 weeks using a Respirgard II jet nebulizer. Some patients on this treatment may develop bronchospasm (cough or wheezing), and these patients should be pretreated with a bronchodilator prior to their next treatment. However, there is little information at present on the use of aerosolized pentamidine in children, particularly infants. Long-term effects of this drug are not known. Prophylaxis using aerosolized pentamidine does not protect against extrapulmonary pneumocystosis. None of the above regimens has been shown to be completely protective against *P. carinii* pneumonia, and patients should be monitored closely for this infection.

Immune Serum Globulin, Human (HSIG, Gamma Globulin)

The gamma globulin fraction prepared by cold alcohol precipitation of human serum (Cohn fraction II) is used to treat patients with defective humoral immunity. These preparations contain only the IgG fraction and are not used to replace IgA or IgM. IgG is prepared from large lots of pooled human serum or plasma. Antibodies to most of the common viral and bacterial pathogens are present, but the titers of antibody vary from lot to lot. It should be recognized that these preparations may not include antibody to pathogens that are not commonly present in the donor population (e.g., Dengue) or to pathogens that present a changing serotype each year (e.g., influenza A and B). The standard preparation procedures for gamma globulin destroy known pathogens such as hepatitis B and HIV-1. The original preparations contained sufficient aggregated material to cause severe reactions when given intravenously and thus had to be given intramuscularly. The amount of IgG given by the intramuscular route is limited by the volume required and by the pain associated with the injection. Only modest elevations of the serum IgG levels can be obtained using these preparations. Intravenous gamma globulin (IVIG) is prepared by various treatments that stabilize the material and prevent aggregate formation. Most of the preparations currently available contain normal ratios of the four IgG subclasses and retain biologic activity of the IgG (e.g., complement fixation, transplacental transfer). IVIG is preferred by most immunologists because higher serum levels can be readily achieved, it is less painful, and it is more efficacious in preventing chronic pulmonary disease in patients with hypogammaglobulinemia. In addition, high-dose IVIG appears to suppress endogenous immunoglobulin production. This attribute is the basis for using IVIG to treat autoimmune disorders such as idiopathic thrombocytopenia. The disadvantages of using IVIG are the expense (about $100/gm infused as compared to about $30/dose injected for IMIG) and the inconvenience of intravenous access. The latter has typically required monthly clinic visits, but home therapy is now available through several home health care agencies.

Dosages for the different gamma globulin preparations are as follows:

Intramuscular Immune Globulin (IMIG). A loading dose of 1.5 ml/kg is given followed by maintenance doses of 0.6 to 0.75 ml/kg, usually given every 4 weeks. In general, a maximum of 40 ml/dose is given. The dose is divided between multiple intramuscular sites, usually in 5- to 10-ml volumes. Serum IgG levels are a poor guide to therapy because these preparations do not cause significant elevations. Therapy can be monitored by measuring antibody titers to common antigens such as tetanus toxoid and by clinical response.

Intravenous Immune Globulin (IVIG). For patients with severe hypogammaglobulinemia/agammaglobulinemia, treatment can be initiated with 400 mg/kg given daily for 4 to 5 days. For mild hypogammaglobulinemia, patients may be started on 200 mg/kg/dose given every 4 weeks. The dose is adjusted to maintain trough levels of IgG above 500 mg/dl. The standard maintenance dose is 400 mg/kg, usually given every 4 weeks. Some patients require doses greater than 400 mg/kg to maintain adequate trough levels. Other patients require dosing as frequently as every 2 to 3 weeks to maintain adequate IgG levels and a good clinical response.

Bone Marrow Transplantation

Bone marrow transplantation (BMT) remains the only definitive therapy for congenital disorders of the immune system. All patients with cellular immunodeficiencies (T-cell deficiency), severe combined immunodeficiency (SCID), and severe neutrophil disorders should be considered potential candidates for BMT. The optimal donor is an HLA A, B, and DR matched sibling. Recent advances in the field include the use of HLA-identical but unrelated donors or haploidentical transplants from HLA-mismatched siblings or parents. Allogeneic BMT has proved to be successful in the treatment of a wide spectrum of disorders, including DiGeorge syndrome, Wiskott-Aldrich syndrome, SCID, chronic granulomatous disease of childhood, and Kostman's agranulocytosis.

Enzyme/Growth Factor Replacement

The treatment of congenital immunodeficiencies with appropriate enzymes and growth factors is a promising new approach. This field will grow as additional factors become available through biotechnology for use in the clinic. Replacement therapy should be considered as an alternative to allogeneic bone marrow transplantation.

Some forms of immunodeficiency may respond to enzyme replacement therapy. Patients with severe combined immunodeficiency resulting from adenosine deaminase (ADA) deficiency have been treated in the past with red blood cell transfusions as a source of normal enzyme with some success. The use of bovine ADA that has been modified with polyethylene glycol (PEG-ADA) is currently under investigation and should be considered in these patients.

The use of recombinant granulocyte colony stimulating factor (G-CSF) is currently under investigation in the treatment of congenital agranulocytosis and cyclic neutropenia with promising results.

Vaccines

Patients with immunodeficiency may be safely given denatured protein, carbohydrate, and killed viral vaccines. However, immunodeficient patients may not always produce an adequate humoral response to standard antigens. Patients should receive routine immunization with diphtheria-pertussis-tetanus vaccine (DPT), killed polio vaccine (IPV), and the newer *Haemophilus influenzae* type *b* (HIB)–protein conjugate vaccine. Patients over the age of 24 months should receive polyvalent pneumococcal vaccine (PPS). Patients with deficiencies of the terminal complement components (C5, C6, C7, C8, C9) are more susceptible to infection with *Neisseria* species and may be protected by vaccination with meningococcal vaccine.

These patients should not be given live viral or bacterial vaccines (oral polio, measles, mumps, rubella, yellow fever, or bacillus Calmette-Guerin [BCG]) because they are at risk of developing clinical disease from the attenuated virus or bacteria. This applies to patients with complement deficiencies and neutrophil disorders as well as those with B- and T-cell disorders. Patients with X-linked agammaglobulinemia cannot make antibody and should not be vaccinated. Immunologically normal siblings and household contacts of patients with immune deficiencies should not receive live oral polio vaccine because of the potential for shedding the virus and transmission to immunodeficient siblings. However, siblings and household contacts may receive MMR vaccine, since transmission of these vaccine viruses does not occur.

The major exception to these guidelines involves patients with HIV infection. Currently available data suggest that routine childhood immunizations do not cause serious adverse reactions in either asymptomatic or symptomatic children with HIV infection. However, the efficacy of the various vaccines in this population is unknown, and there are reports of lower rates of seroconversion to some antigens. The current recommendation is to give inactivated polio vaccine (IPV) to all patients. MMR vaccine should be considered for use in all HIV-infected children regardless of symptoms and administered according to the usual schedule. This recommendation is based on the fact that children with HIV infection immunized with MMR have not had adverse effects and the reports of severe and fatal measles occurring in symptomatic infected children. The authors believe that the use of live viral vaccines in this population should be individualized and that patients with severe immune dysfunction should not receive live vaccines.

Passive Immunization

Immunocompromised children exposed to measles should be given immune globulin. This also applies to children with HIV infection regardless of immunization status. The dose of intramuscular gamma globulin is 0.5ml/kg (maximum dose 15 ml) given within 6 days of exposure. If a child has been receiving regular therapy with intravenous gamma globulin, additional gamma globulin may not be necessary if the exposure occurred within 3 weeks of the last treatment. Immunocompromised susceptible children exposed to varicella should receive varicella-zoster immune globulin (VZIG) within 96 hours of exposure.

HUMORAL IMMUNE DEFICIENCIES

Patients with these disorders tend to develop pyogenic infections, particularly of the lungs and sinuses. These infections are frequently chronic and require aggressive long-term, broad-spectrum antibiotic therapy to suppress infection. Older children and adolescents should have pulmonary function studies done yearly and their therapy adjusted if function is decreasing. Good pulmonary toilet and postural drainage are important for children with sinopulmonary involvement. The goal of therapy is to prevent recurrent bacterial and viral infections.

X-Linked Agammaglobulinemia

Patients with X-linked gammaglobulinemia or severe hypogammaglobulinemia require life-long replacement therapy. Replacement therapy can be accomplished with intravenous or intramuscular gamma globulin. Intravenous gamma globulin is recommended, since it is less painful and achieves higher serum levels. It is believed that the use of the intravenous dose may prevent complications such as the chronic lung disease, which is common in this entity. Serum IgG trough levels of at least 500 mg/dl should be maintained to achieve a good response. The actual dose required varies with each patient and may range from 200 to 800 mg/kg. The frequency of infusion may also vary from every 2 to 6 weeks and should be adjusted according to the clinical response of the patient. If a serious infection occurs, then additional gamma globulin may be required. Exposure to varicella or hepatitis B necessitates administration of the appropriate hyperimmune globulin. Immunization with live viral vaccines is contraindicated. These patients are at risk for development of vaccine-associated poliomyelitis.

Common Variable Immunodeficiencies

These patients have a late-onset hypogammaglobulinemia and present as a spectrum of clinical disease because some make normal amounts of antibody to specific antigens, whereas others do not. Patients with borderline or low levels of IgG should have quantitation of IgG subclasses and antibody production. Replacement therapy with IVIG must be individualized by the severity of clinical symptoms. Those with severe recurrent infections should receive immunoglobulin replacement therapy. The dose of IVIG is adjusted to control symptoms and to maintain trough levels greater than 500 mg/dl. The patient with hypogammaglobulinemia should be closely monitored for the development of autoimmune disease.

Transient Hypogammaglobulinemia of Infancy

Transient hypogammaglobulinemia of infancy is a self-limited condition that can be diagnosed only after the deficiency has corrected. Infants with low serum immunoglobulin levels and normal B-cell number who are asymptomatic do not necessarily require treatment. These children should be followed closely and serum immunoglobulins repeated at 3- to 6-month intervals. One would anticipate that normal levels might be achieved by 3 years of age. However, some children require a longer period of time to normalize. Those infants with severe recurrent infections should receive immunoglobulin replacement therapy. Therefore, serum immunoglobulin levels should be checked routinely at 3-month intervals on all infants receiving IVIG, if normal levels are attained, the infusions may be discontinued and serum IgG levels monitored. In some cases, prolonged therapy may be required. Because immunoglobulin replacement may suppress the ability to synthesize one's own IgG, young children treated with IVIG for mild hypogammaglobulinemia should be reassessed between 4 and 6 years of age by stopping the IVIG treatments and monitoring monthly serum IgG levels and clinical symptoms.

IgG Subclass Deficiencies

The patient with an IgG subclass deficiency is usually missing one or two of the subclasses but has normal or increased levels of others. Symptomatic patients should be treated with immunoglobulin injections or infusions, as indicated in the general management section.

IgA Deficiencies

At present, there is no specific treatment available for IgA deficiency. These patients have a higher incidence of *Giardia lamblia* infection; patients with chronic diarrhea or malabsorption syndrome should be thoroughly investigated for this organism. In a small group of patients, autoimmune disease has been a complication. Some children also have associated IgG sublass deficiencies. In most cases of complete IgA deficiency, immunoglobulin replacement or blood transfusions are contraindicated. Since the patient has no immunoglobulin A, there is the possibility that the patient may become sensitized and develop anti-IgA antibodies. However, in some patients with IgA deficiency and associated IgG subclass deficiency, intravenous or intramuscular gamma globulin can be well tolerated and beneficial. In such circumstances, patients should be monitored for the development of antibodies to IgA and should be carefully observed during infusions. Intravenous administration of gamma globulin is preferred over intramuscular injection, since the infusion can be terminated immediately if a reaction occurs. IVIG preparations low in IgA are preferred. A patient with IgA deficiency should be aware that the transfusion of whole blood or blood products may be harmful. If a transfusion is necessary, blood obtained from another IgA-deficient donor or washed red blood cells should be given. A Medic-Alert bracelet is advised to alert physicians to the fact that a transfusion could be harmful.

IgM Deficiency

This disorder is rare and is associated with an increased susceptibility to meningococcal disease. Since immunoglobulin preparations do not contain significant amounts of IgM, immunoglobulin therapy is not generally helpful. Penicillin prophylaxis may be used as an alternative therapy in these patients.

CELLULAR IMMUNE DEFICIENCIES

Patients with T-cell deficiencies frequently have associated B-cell defects. These patients are susceptible to intracellular bacterial infections, viral diseases, and opportunistic infection. The goal of therapy is to correct the deficiency and prevent complications.

T-Cell Deficiencies

Isolated T-cell deficiencies involving thymic hypoplasia can be reconstituted by transplantation of fetal thymic tissue. Fetal thymus fragments implanted in the muscle or injected intraperitoneally have resulted in successful reconstitution of T-cell immunity. Thymic tissue is obtained from a 10- to 14-week human fetus removed by hysterotomy. The thymus is removed, cut into small fragments, and placed into sterile tissue culture medium. Transplantation should be done within 1 or 2 hours by intraperitoneal injection using a sterile 18-gauge peritoneal catheter that is removed after the injection. Cultured thymic epithelial cells have also been transplanted, and partial immune reconstitution has resulted, although more experience with this therapy is needed. Enhanced T-cell immunity may also be achieved using immunomodulators such as thymosin, thymopoietin, and other thymic factors. Bone marrow transplantation from a histocompatible sibling has also been successful in reconstitution of T-cell function.

Patients with complete DiGeorge syndrome initially require treatment for their hypoparathyroidism. Hypocalcemic seizures need to be controlled and prevented with the use of intravenous calcium gluconate. Calcium supplementation, a low phosphorus diet, and large doses of vitamin D are important in the treatment of the hypoparathyroidism. Parathyroid hormone injec-

tions may also be necessary for control of this complication. Since this is a T-cell deficiency, live virus vaccines should not be administered. Blood for transfusion should be irradiated (3000 rad) to prevent graft-versus-host disease, and *P. carinii* prophylaxis should be provided. Over 90 per cent of patients with the DiGeorge syndrome have associated congenital heart defects such as truncus arteriosus, interrupted aortic arch, double aortic arch, and aberrant right subclavian artery. Surgical correction and supportive measures should be provided for the congenital heart defects that often accompany this syndrome. Since the incidence of T-cell deficiency (complete DiGeorge syndrome) in patients with aortic arch abnormalities is not known, all patients with congenital heart defects should receive only irradiated blood products.

Chronic Mucocutaneous Candidiasis

This is a T-cell immunodeficiency characterized by chronic and recurrent infection of the mucous membranes, scalp, skin, and nails with *Candida albicans*. There is a broad spectrum of clinical disease, and some patients have associated endocrinopathies.

The goal of therapy is to prevent and control fungal infection. The type of therapy required depends on the extent and location of the infection. For mild infection, topical therapy with mycostatin or clotrimazole may be adequate. Treatment of lesions of the oral mucosa has been facilitated by the development of troches or pastilles containing the above medications and has proved to be an effective therapy for the older child. For more extensive involvement or esophagitis, oral therapy with ketoconazole or intravenous therapy with amphotericin B or miconazole is indicated. Iron therapy has proved beneficial in some cases. The child with CMC should be evaluated at least yearly for the presence of endocrinopathy and appropriate therapy given if documented. Various measures have been used as treatment for this disorder. Transfer factor, levamisole, and thymosin have produced variable results.

Wiskott-Aldrich Syndrome

These patients have thrombocytopenia, eczema, and abnormal T-cell function that results in an inability to make antibody responses to carbohydrate antigens. These patients, however, may make antibody to carbohydrate antigens that have been conjugated to protein carriers, such as the newer *H. influenzae* type *b* (HIB) conjugate vaccines. Patients with recurrent bacterial infections may respond to monthly infusions of intravenous gamma globulin. Intramuscular gamma globulin is contraindicated because of the low platelet count and the potential for bleeding.

Life-threatening episodes of bleeding should be treated with fresh platelet transfusions irradiated at 3000 rads to prevent graft-versus-host reaction. In most cases, episodes of bleeding decrease with advancing age. Splenectomy usually results in normalization of the platelet count and should be considered for patients who have significant thrombocytopenia and bleeding. Following splenectomy, children should be placed on prophylactic antibiotics to prevent overwhelming infection.

There is an increased incidence of malignancy, particularly lymphoma, in this group of patients. Patients with Wiskott-Aldrich syndrome should be considered for bone marrow transplantation, which has been shown to successfully correct both the platelet and T-cell abnormalities.

SEVERE COMBINED IMMUNODEFICIENCY

These patients have absent T- and B-cell immunity and represent a variety of underlying defects. An evaluation should be done to determine whether an enzyme deficiency such as adenosine deaminase (ADA) or purine nucleoside phosphorylase (PNP) is the cause. In the past, monthly red blood cell infusions have resulted in partial immune reconstitution in some patients with ADA deficiency. Replacement therapy by weekly intramuscular injections of bovine ADA conjugated with polyethylene glycol (PEG-ADA) is currently under investigation. Such therapy has resulted in clinical improvement in a limited number of patients. Bone marrow transplantation, however, remains the treatment of choice for most forms of severe combined immunodeficiency. With this technique, some children have shown full reconstitution of both T-cell and B-cell function, whereas others have had persistence of B-cell deficiency. These patients then require full replacement therapy with intravenous immunoglobulin.

Other therapies have been attempted, such as transplantation of fetal liver, fetal thymus, and cultured thymic epithelial cells. A few patients have shown partial reconstitution, but the majority have failed. These patients should be placed in strict reverse isolation until appropriate diagnostic testing has been completed and treatment arranged.

Other therapeutic considerations include the use of irradiated (3000 rads) blood to prevent a graft-versus-host reaction. Donor blood seronegative for cytomegalovirus (CMV) should be used if possible. These children should not receive live viral vaccines. If they are exposed to varicella, they should be given zoster immune globulin (ZIG). P carinii prophylaxis should be given. Intravenous immunoglobulin therapy should be given until immune reconstitution is accomplished. Fever should be evaluated with aggressive diagnosis and broad-spectrum antibiotics used until culture results are available. Treatment of CMV with a combination of gancyclovir and alternate-day IVIG therapy is under investigation.

COMPLEMENT DEFICIENCIES

In general there are only a few specific therapies available for disorders of the complement system. However, knowledge of the deficiency is important, since it can alert the physician to information important in management of the patient. Patients with C3, C5, C6, C7, and C8 deficiencies are susceptible to infection, and if fever occurs, aggressive diagnosis and treatment should be given. Pneumococcal and meningococcal disease are common with these deficiencies. Immunization with pneumococcal, meningococcal, and H. influenzae

type b (HIB) conjugate vaccine is recommended for these patients. The use of prophylactic penicillin should also be considered. Patients with C3 deficiency present with severe, recurrent pyogenic infections in a pattern similar to that of severe neutropenia.

Patients with complement deficiencies make poor antibody responses to standard antigens. Thus, patients with recurrent infections should be evaluated for their ability to make antibody. Treatment with IVIG may decrease the incidence of infections in some patients. Patients with absence of an early-acting complement component (Clq, Clr, C2, and C4) may develop autoimmune and collagen-vascular disease and should be closely followed for evidence of these disorders.

Hereditary angioneurotic edema results from an absence of C1 esterase inhibitor. These patients can be treated by avoidance of factors such as trauma that might precipitate an event. Knowledge of the presence of this deficiency can prevent unnecessary surgery with unexplained episodes of abdominal pain. Semisynthetic androgens, danazol and stanazolol, have been useful in the prevention of acute episodes of swelling. The mechanism of action of this drug is not known, and it is not generally recommended for use in children. Epsilon-aminocaproic acid (EACA) has also been used prophylactically but has associated side effects. Preoperative administration of EACA has prevented postoperative edema. Patients should be instructed to seek medical help immediately if laryngeal swelling occurs. Tracheostomy should be performed if needed in patients with laryngeal obstruction.

PHAGOCYTIC DISORDERS

Phagocytic dysfunction is associated with an increased susceptibility to severe, recurrent bacterial infections with a poor response to antibiotic therapy. A spectrum of disorders has been described including (1) congenital agranulocytosis (Kostman's syndrome), (2) cyclic neutropenia, (3) adherence glycoprotein defects (LFA-1, Mac-1, Mac-11, C_3bi receptor, CR_3, and p 150,95 deficiency), (4) chemotactic defects, and (5) defects of intracellular killing (chronic granulomatous disease, myeloperoxidase deficiency).

Symptomatic treatment of these patients includes good skin care with antiseptic soaps and chronic prophylaxis with TMP-S (10 mg/kg/day of the trimethoprim component) to decrease the number of infections. Children with fever should be evaluated with appropriate diagnostic tests and treated promptly and aggressively with intravenous antibiotics that include anti-staphylococcal coverage. Granulocyte transfusions are helpful in patients with severe neutropenia (Kostman's) or with adherence glycoprotein defects. Intravenous gamma globulin treatment is usually not necessary because these patients typically have normal humoral immunity. Patients with Chediak-Higashi syndrome should be monitored for neoplastic transformation.

Bone marrow transplantation has the potential to provide definitive therapy for these disorders and should be considered. Marrow transplants from HLA-matched siblings have been used successfully to treat Kostman's syndrome and chronic granulomatous disease. Therapy of neutropenia with recombinant granulocyte/monocyte colony stimulating factor (G/M CSF) or granulocyte colony stimulating factor (G-CSF) is currently under investigation for patients with congenital agranulocytosis or cyclic neutropenia and has shown some success in both conditions. Some patients with Chediak-Higashi syndrome may respond to high doses of ascorbic acid, resulting in normalization of bactericidal activity and decrease in infections while on this therapy.

PEDIATRIC HIV-1 INFECTION

Children with HIV infection have chronic multisystem disease and require a comprehensive care system that includes medical, social service, psychosocial, and community support. This care is best accomplished by a multidisciplinary team that includes both inpatient and outpatient hospital-based and community-based services. This is a family unit disease as well as a chronic disease for children with perinatally acquired infection. Thus, services and counseling should be family oriented. Physicians and medical staff should be aware of issues of confidentiality and testing for HIV in their patients.

Antiretroviral Therapy

At the present time there is not a definitive cure for HIV-1 infection. A number of antiretroviral drugs are being tested in children, but as of this writing, none is licensed for use in the child under 13 years of age. Azidothymidine (Retrovir) has been used under protocol in children with AIDS and symptomatic clinical disease. For the adolescent patient, Retrovir is available as a 100- or 200-mg tablet. Recently in adults, doses of 600 mg/day have been found to be as effective as larger doses. Retrovir syrup (10 mg/cc) is available for children and is used in a dose of 180 mg/M^2/dose given every 6 hours. The drug is well tolerated and is associated with the same adverse reactions as in adults, i.e., bone marrow depression, particularly anemia and neutropenia. These effects are reversible with dose reduction or discontinuation of the drug.

Other new drugs in clinical trials include dideoxycytidine (ddC), dideoxyinosine (ddI), and soluble CD$_4$. Results of these trials are not yet available. For the latest information on drugs available and being tested in both adults and children with HIV infection, call the hotline at 1-800-Trials-A, Monday through Friday, 9 AM to 7 PM Eastern time.

Intravenous Gamma Globulin

The use of intravenous gamma globulin in children with HIV-1 infection is controversial. Some centers give gamma globulin to all children with symptomatic disease. There are at least two clear-cut indications for the use of gamma globulin in these children: (1) the presence of hypogammaglobulinemia, and (2) documented antibody deficiency and recurrent bacterial infections. Our own preference is to limit IVIG therapy to children who meet one or both of these criteria. The initial dose given is 200 mg/kg with increase to 400 mg/kg given

intravenously once every 4 weeks. Other institutions give this same dose at 2- or 3-week intervals.

Therapy for HIV-Associated Conditions

Children should be monitored for developmental delay and neurologic abnormalities. In the presence of hypotonia, hypertonia, microcephaly, or other neurologic abnormalities, a computed tomography brain scan with contrast and a spinal tap should be performed to rule out infection. Children with HIV encephalopathy have brain atrophy, frequently resulting in a secondary microcephaly. Basal ganglion calcification may be present in some children. Infections such as cytomegalovirus, herpes, and toxoplasmosis should be ruled out. Children with severe encephalopathy should have a retinal examination to exclude other infection. A program of physical therapy should be instituted to maintain as much function as possible. Data from studies using azidothymidine in children suggest that central nervous system function may be improved on this therapy.

Children with lymphoid interstitial pneumonitis (LIP) may have a stable or progressive course. In our experience, this condition can radiographically resemble miliary tuberculosis, *P. carinii* pneumonitis, cytomegalovirus, or other viral pneumonias. Opportunistic infection should be ruled out in these patients. Glucocorticoid therapy may improve arterial oxygen saturation in children with LIP. For children with a PaO$_2$ of less than 65 mm Hg, we recommend oral prednisone, 2 mg/kg/day given in divided doses for 2 weeks and then tapering to 1 mg/kg/day. This is continued over several weeks with monitoring of the arterial blood gases. The use of a pulse oximeter to measure transcutaneous oxygen saturations is less traumatic for the patient. In our experience, children usually show improvement in oxygen saturation within the first few weeks of therapy; however, a few have required prolonged treatment over several months. Some children with severe chronic lung disease are refractory to steroid treatment. In those children responsive to steroids, treatment should be tapered slowly, with monitoring of the blood gases. Some children with LIP become oxygen-dependent. We have enlisted the help of visiting nurses to place these children on home oxygen therapy. Pneumonia is common in children with LIP, and episodes of fever and elevated respiratory rate should be aggressively evaluated. These children should have blood gas determinations and blood and sputum cultures as appropriate and should be placed on broad-spectrum antibiotics pending culture results. *P. carinii* pneumonia is found only rarely in association with LIP.

A portion of children develop nephropathy. The majority of these children present with proteinuria as an early finding, although not all children with proteinuria progress to frank nephrosis. Clinical presentation usually includes edema, proteinuria, and elevation of the blood urea nitrogen and creatinine, usually without hypertension. These patients are treated symptomatically with fluid restriction, a low-salt diet, and diuretics. A renal biopsy is indicated in this condition. The majority of patients biopsied have focal segmental sclerosis.

In our experience, steroid therapy has not been useful in this condition. In a few cases, glomerulonephritis has been present and in these cases a trial of steroids could be given with close monitoring.

Cardiomyopathy is a common finding in children with HIV infection. This may present as an acute or subacute infection. Treatment is usually symptomatic, with fluid restriction, diuretics, and digoxin. This is not usually a fatal disease but may become chronic.

Treatment of Opportunistic Infection

P. carinii pneumonia is the most frequent opportunistic infection in children with HIV infection. In perinatal disease it frequently occurs early in life and should be suspected in the child with fever and tachypnea, with or without pulmonary infiltrates. Bronchoscopy is the preferred method of diagnosis. If a diagnostic procedure cannot be done on admission and *P. carinii* pneumonia is suspected, therapy should be begun with TMP-S, 20 mg TMP/kg/day and 100 mg sulfamethoxazole/kg/day divided into four doses. Oxygen therapy should be given as needed. If the patient continues to deteriorate after 48 hours on this therapy, the TMP-S is discontinued and pentamidine, 4 mg/kg/day, is begun. Therapy is continued for 14 to 21 days and *P. carinii* pneumonia secondary prophylaxis is given, usually with TMP-S. In our experience, patients who require intubation and respiratory support have a poor chance of survival. Other modalities of therapy such as aerosolized pentamidine, trimatrexate, and dapsone have little experience in children. Steroids have been used in the treatment of *P. carinii* pneumonia in adults, but there are no published data using this drug in children. *P. carinii* prophylaxis is discussed in the general management section.

Candida infections of the oral mucosa are common. Mild cases respond to topical mycostatin. Gentian violet is another alternative for therapy. For older children with thrush unresponsive to mycostatin, clotrimazole troches are used. In patients with severe oral *Candida* infection unresponsive to topical therapy, oral ketoconazole is given for approximately 7 to 10 days. We prefer not to use ketoconazole for long-term suppression because of the potential for hepatotoxicity. For *Candida* esophagitis, oral ketoconazole is the drug of choice, used for 14 days. Other alternatives for therapy of invasive *Candida* infection include amphotericin B and miconazole given intravenously.

Recurrent episodes of mucocutaneous herpes simplex infection can be treated with intravenous acyclovir (30 mg/kg/day given as three divided doses).

Other

Other therapeutic measures include maintenance of a good nutritional status. The use of high-calorie supplemental formulas, nasogastric feedings, and parenteral hyperalimentation may be necessary in children with wasting syndrome or failure to thrive.

SUDDEN INFANT DEATH SYNDROME AND RECURRENT APNEA

ABRAHAM B. BERGMAN, M.D.

Sudden infant death syndrome (SIDS), commonly known as crib death, claims about 8000 babies a year in the United States. It is responsible for between two and three deaths of every 1000 live births. After the first week of life, SIDS is the most important single cause of death of infants under 1 year of age; it ranks second only to injuries as the greatest cause of death in children between 7 days and 15 years of age.

Although SIDS has been with us since biblical times (I Kings 3:19-20) masquerading under a variety of names, it did not become generally recognized as a distinct disease entity until the early 1970s. Although we can now describe SIDS and have limited knowledge about the mechanisms that produce the end result, our state of knowledge is still limited. Debate continues about what proportion of infants dying suddenly and unexpectedly represent "classic" SIDS, but it is now generally accepted that the vast majority have common epidemiologic, clinical, and pathologic features. Akin to diseases like leukemia and lupus, the diagnosis of SIDS can be made, but the causes and means of prevention remain unknown.

CHARACTERISTICS OF SIDS

SIDS is more likely to occur in males, in low birth weight babies, in low socioeconomic class families, and during seasons of upper respiratory illness. It is uncommon before 2 weeks and after 6 months of age, with the peak incidence occurring between 2 and 4 months of age. Although a low birth weight child from a poor family who is 2 months old, put to sleep with a cold, is more likely to succumb to SIDS than other infants, these are statistical findings of more interest to the scientist conducting research than to the physician dealing with an individual case. SIDS can also kill fat babies as well as thin; children of rich families as well as poor—just not as frequently.

There are two constant clinical features: Death occurs during sleep and is silent in nature. The death scene is often one of disarray. The infant may be found squeezed into a corner of the bed with a blanket covering the head, which causes many parents to think wrongly that the child suffocated. Blood-tinged froth may emanate from the nose and stain the sheets, giving some parents the erroneous impression that their baby suffered an internal hemorrhage. There is usually evidence of a brief burst of spasmodic motor activity; bladder and bowels are empty and sometimes blanket fibers are found under the fingernails.

In classic SIDS, the lungs are filled with hemorrhagic edema fluid, and minor microscopic evidence of respiratory inflammation is often found. Intrathoracic petechiae dot the surfaces of lungs, pericardium, and thymus; the fact that these petechiae are limited to the thoracic cavity is impressive.

THE EMOTIONAL REACTION OF PARENTS

SIDS parents may be more affected than parents of children who die of a better-known disease or whose death is expected for two reasons: (1) the sudden and unexpected nature of the event, and (2) the aura of mystery surrounding the entity. Characteristic grief patterns have been described for adjusting to the loss of a loved one. With most diseases, the family has the opportunity to prepare and begin the grieving process before death. In SIDS, of course, there is no anticipation, and the entire grieving process must take place after death.

Because of the significant relationship between SIDS and socioeconomic class, a large number of families lack any personal physician and thereby are unlikely to gain sympathetic support at a time of greatest need. Their lack of education and low standard of living compound their feelings of guilt. They tend not to seek help nor to participate in parent self-help groups.

Physicians can play a significant part in alleviating prolonged grief and guilt reactions among survivors of the SIDS victim. Autopsies are important and should be available for all infants, not just those whose families can afford them. SIDS can usually be affirmed after a gross examination; it is not necessary to keep families waiting until all microscopic and laboratory studies are completed. If later findings contradict the provisional diagnosis, a decision must be made about whether the new findings are truly significant to the family (i.e., genetic disease) or useful only in altering vital statistics.

In dealing with families, the physician should be familiar with the basic facts about SIDS and with the characteristic grief reactions. Since parents are in a state of shock at the time of death, an attitude of warm concern and the capacity to listen sympathetically are more important than verbal explanations. The two most important points to convey are (1) "your baby died of a definite disease entity (SIDS)," and (2) "currently SIDS cannot be predicted or prevented; you are in no way responsible for the infant's death."

Children are especially vulnerable to guilt feelings about the death of a sibling. Their reactions are often veiled but may be pervasive and long-lasting unless dealt with promptly. Painful as it is, open discussion of the death among family members should be encouraged. A good indication of parental coping mechanisms with grief is determined in what they tell their children about the infant's death.

Referral or contact with agencies working with SIDS can be most helpful. Many families gain comfort from contact with other families who have lost children to SIDS. Referral to such groups is an individual consideration and should be done at the request of the family. Printed information is helpful in answering the invariable questions of relatives and neighbors. The National SIDS Foundation, with over 70 chapters and a prestigious board of medical advisors, exists to educate health professionals and assist families (10500 Little Patuxent Parkway, #420, Columbia, MD 21044. Phone: 1-800-221-SIDS).

The tragedy of SIDS, unfortunately, does not end with the death of the baby. Pervasive and long-lasting guilt reactions occur among family members; the psychiatric morbidity is enormous. The cause of SIDS itself is not yet known. The cause of the guilt *is* known—ignorance; and prevention *is* possible through informed and compassionate counseling.

RECURRENT APNEA

Concomitant with increasing knowledge about SIDS has come an explosion of interest in a related problem, recurrent apnea. The extent to which recurrent apnea and SIDS are interrelated remains under scientific scrutiny. For practical purposes, a history of apneic episodes can be elicited in less than 3 per cent of SIDS victims. Thus, I abhor the terms "aborted" or "near-miss" SIDS applied to all episodes of apnea. The term "apparent life-threatening event" (ALTE) is coming into more common use. It is defined as an episode that is frightening to the observer and that is characterized by some combination of apnea (central or occasionally obstructive), color change (usually cyanotic or pallid but occasionally erythematous or plethoric), marked change in muscle tone (usually limpness), choking, and gagging.

The major known causes of apnea are immaturity, infections (especially sepsis, meningitis, pertussis, and interstitial pneumonia), anemia, metabolic disturbances, seizure disorders, cardiac rate abnormalities, and gastroesophageal reflux. Careful history and physical examination, including evaluation of neurodevelopmental status, often provide clues that are confirmed by appropriate laboratory studies. If answers are not forthcoming from a traditional "work-up," consultation with a center specializing in evaluation of apnea is advisable. Naturally, appropriate intervention is provided when specific diagnoses are made. More often than not, however, no etiology for the apneic episodes is found.

HOME MONITORS

The emotionally charged question of when to employ a home apnea monitor is never easy to answer. The physician must be content to use his clinical judgment and knowledge of the family until further research provides more definitive guidelines.

I recommend home monitors for two general situations, one medical and the other emotional. The medical indications are best stated in a National Institutes of Health Consensus Development Conference Statement (October 1, 1986).

Cardiorespiratory monitoring or an alternative therapy is medically indicated for certain groups of infants at high risk for sudden death. These groups include infants with one or more severe ALTE's requiring mouth-to-mouth resuscitation or vigorous stimulation, symptomatic preterm infants, siblings of two or more SIDS victims, and infants with certain diseases or conditions such as central hyperventilation. Although no controlled clinical trials have rigorously proved monitoring to be effective in these groups, evidence indicates that these infants are at an extraordinarily high risk for dying and that lives can be saved. Alternative or ancillary treatments such as methylxanthines and/or hospitalization may be considered for specific infants.

I also sometimes recommend the use of a home monitor for certain highly charged emotional situations in which parental anxiety about infant death during sleep is so great that the alternative to monitoring is literally standing vigil at the infant's bedside during every sleeping moment. Most parents to whom this indication applies have previously lost an infant to SIDS, but sometimes other factors have produced this anxiety, such as an observed apnea spell in the infant or an alarming report in the media. In these latter situations, the benefits of an "electronic babysitter" might justify the disruption of life caused by home monitors.

Apnea monitors should be prescribed only by personnel experienced in their use and capable of providing continuous supervision. This means 24-hour-a-day availability and technical support to the family. Parents should be trained in use and care of the monitor, as well as in cardiopulmonary resuscitation. Local emergency medical personnel should be available for back-up services.

THE CHILD AND THE DEATH OF A LOVED ONE

MORRIS GREEN, M.D.

Five per cent of children under the age of 15 experience the death of one or both parents, whereas others lose a sibling, a grandparent, or a friend. The manifestations of grief in children differ in many respects from those in adults.

Children under the age of 3 years do not understand what death means beyond a very traumatic separation experience. Preschool children view death as similar to sleep. Those between the ages of 5 and 9 years begin to recognize death as irreversible but not as something that will happen to anyone they know. After the age of 9, children begin to understand that death is irreversible and could happen to them or their loved ones.

Since children and adolescents tolerate grief and depression poorly, they have a short "sadness span." To avoid being overwhelmed, young children try to deflect the frightening impact of their loss by resuming play, reading comic books, watching television, and acting as if nothing upsetting had happened. Some give no outward sign of grief. Adolescents, who may show little inclination to talk about their loss, may deny that they are depressed. The child or adolescent's behavior may be misinterpreted as inappropriate or uncaring, especially when a young child repeatedly asks when he will get a new father or mother. It is important, therefore, that the physician explain to the surviving spouse and other caregivers how the manifestations of grief in children differ from those in adults.

MANIFESTATIONS OF GRIEF IN CHILDREN

In the young child, the symptoms of grief include regression, sadness, fearfulness, anorexia, failure to thrive, sleep disturbance, social withdrawal, developmental delay, irritability, excessive crying, and increased dependency. The preschool child may demonstrate hyperactivity, constipation, encopresis, enuresis, temper tantrums, "out-of-control" behavior, anger, nightmares, and crying spells. The school-age child's academic performance may decline. Other symptoms may include resistance to attending school, crying spells, lying, stealing, nervousness, and somatic complaints. Adolescents may demonstrate depression, somatic complaints, suicide attempts, and school drop-out.

THE PHYSICIAN'S ROLE

When a parent dies, the physician may express his personal condolences to the surviving parent and offer to be of help to the children. A personal note to each of the children is also meaningful and appreciated.

The child should be told of his parent's death by the surviving spouse or someone else whom the child knows well in a manner attuned to his or her developmental age. The explanation should be simple and repeated as needed. It is best not to use the phrase "went to sleep," as the child may then become afraid of going to bed. Since children may also fear that they or the surviving parent may die and that they were somehow responsible for their parent's death, they should be told explicitly that neither the surviving parent nor they are going to die and that the death was not their fault.

Since children worry about food, housing, and school, they need to be reassured that these needs will be met. Continuity should be stressed. If possible, familiar surroundings and routines should be maintained. So much has changed: The child's future seems uncertain, the surviving parent is preoccupied, the child's schedule is disrupted, and there are many visitors, some total strangers to the child. If possible, children should be kept in their own homes with one familiar primary caregiver to read, talk to, and play with younger children. School-age children need someone with whom to share the news of the day, to answer questions repeatedly, and, as they are ready, to talk about their feelings.

Children may be confused and anxious about the dramatic changes in their surviving parent. Sad, anxious, disorganized, impatient, angry, irritable, and erratic, a grieving parent may simply be unable to cope with the heightened needs of the child. Bereaved parents may be insufficiently aware of their need for someone to talk to and for reassurance. Inappropriate "blurring of the generations" may lead, for example, to a mother clinging to the child, expecting her son to be the "man of the house," discussing money and other personal worries, or overburdening the child with chores.

Since bereaved children are very much affected by the mental health of their surviving parent, continuing symptoms in a child are often linked to the parent's unresolved grief. Problems in bereavement in a parent may be manifested by persistent depression, failure to participate in outside social activities, somatic complaints, increased smoking, and abuse of alcohol or drugs. Referral of the parent to a mental health professional may be an important contribution of the physician.

RISK FACTORS IN CHILDREN

In children, the long-term outcome cannot be predicted on the basis of the bereaved child's initial response. Such sequelae, which may include an increased predisposition to illness, depression, and suicide, may not appear until the adult years. The Institute of Medicine Committee on the Health Consequences of Bereavement identified the following risk factors in bereaved children: parental death under 5 years of age or in early adolescence; maternal death when a girl is under 11 years of age; the death of a boy's father; a history of emotional problems in the child; an ambivalent relationship with the deceased parent or sibling; excessive parental dependency on the child; absence of a support network; inability of the surviving parent to use that support; multiple caregivers; lack of environmental constancy; a poor relationship with a step-parent; and bereavement due to sudden death, homicide, or suicide.

INDICATIONS FOR MENTAL HEALTH HELP

"Red flags" that suggest the need of a bereaved child for mental health help include severe anxiety, fear or hope of dying, persistent depression, suicide gestures or attempts, continued regressive behavior, a verbalized hope for reunion with the deceased, unremitting guilt and self-blame, aggressive and destructive behavior, delinquency, avoidance of talking about the deceased, expression of only positive or negative feelings about the deceased, school underachievement, school avoidance, promiscuity, unwillingness to separate from the surviving parent, failure to demonstrate any manifestation of grief, inability to form new attachments to other children or adults, excessive daydreaming, and persistent somatic complaints.

ATTENDING THE FUNERAL

Generally, children who can understand the cause of a sibling's or parent's death are old enough to attend the funeral if they wish. Children should not be forced to do so if they are afraid, reluctant, or revolted by the idea. Many children under 6 years of age are too young, whereas those over 9 may be helped by attending, especially if the service is conducted with the child's needs in mind. Preparation prior to the funeral should include being told what the setting will look like and what will happen. It is also a good idea for the child to be accompanied by a relative or close family friend so that he may be accompanied out of the room if he wishes to leave.

SEXUAL ABUSE AND RAPE
EBERHARD M. MANN, M.D.

Sexual abuse and rape of children and adolescents are now such frequent complaints that all physicians who care for minors are likely to encounter several cases in their practice every year. In order to deal with the often complex medical, psychological, and legal consequences of sexual abuse, special rape crisis centers have been set up in most metropolitan communities.

Whether or not the physician participates in sexual abuse examinations, he or she needs to be familiar with the proper management techniques in order to provide adequate medicolegal assessment and treatment, meet reporting obligations to child protective or law enforcement agencies where required, and advise on relevant referrals for comprehensive services.

DEFINITION

Sexual abuse can be grouped into three major categories:

1. Sexual Assault. Sexual assault involves vaginal, oral, or anal intercourse with an unconsenting victim. Only the slightest penetration is sufficient to meet criteria for these offenses. Since it is assumed that minors below a certain age are developmentally too immature to consent to sexual relations with older persons, any intercourse with them constitutes "statutory" sexual assault. The age of consent to sexual intercourse varies from state to state.

Criminal penalties for sexual assault differ according to severity of bodily injury, degree of force, and state law.

2. Incest. Traditionally, incest has been defined as sexual relations between blood relatives who are not legally permitted to marry. However, this definition is not practical for clinical purposes. The concern is about protection of children and adolescents from sexual involvement with any family member. Family-related sexual abuse is now integrated into child-abuse–reporting laws nationwide. These laws state that professionals—including physicians—are mandated to report any suspicion of sexual relations between a minor and a household member to the state-designated child protection agency. Household members include parents, stepparents, siblings, other relatives, the parents' live-in partners, or any adult who participates in a child care role.

3. Molestation. Molestation means any touching of the sexual organs or other intimate parts, such as breasts, anus, or buttocks, of a person with the intent to gratify sexual desire.

PREVALENCE

Although true prevalence is not known, several surveys estimate that up to one in four girls and up to one in seven boys are sexually abused before the age of 18 years. Seventy-five per cent of reported victims are girls, 25 per cent are boys; 95 per cent of the sex offenders are male. Half of all reported sexual abuse takes place within families.

With increased public awareness and improved treatment services, rates of reporting have dramatically increased over the last 10 years; however, most children and teenagers still do not disclose sexual abuse immediately after its occurrence, and many never tell. Young victims are reluctant to make sexual abuse known because they are often afraid that they will not be believed or will be blamed. Many fear loss of family or loss of reputation.

IDENTIFICATION

Sexual abuse should be suspected and investigated in the following situations:

1. A child makes a sexual abuse allegation.

2. A child shows injuries or infections likely to be caused through sexual contact (e.g., hymenal tears, loose anal sphincter tone, sexually transmitted disease).

3. A child re-enacts specific adult-like sexual behavior with toys, peers, or other people.

4. A child shows specific fear/avoidance behavior around a particular person.

While the first two situations are highly indicative of sexual abuse, the latter two are less specific. In non-threatening but direct talk with the child, the possibility of sexual abuse should be explored.

Overall, most sexual abuse complaints made by children and teenagers are valid (80 to 90 per cent). Allegations of sexual abuse are usually true if they are reported by the children themselves and if sexual activities are described and/or demonstrated in a specific rather than a vague manner.

Lately there has been increasing concern over false allegations of sexual assault. In three situations the possibility of false reporting is slightly higher:

1. Sexual abuse allegations that arise in the context of a custody or visitation dispute, generally involving young children who cannot yet verbally express themselves.

2. Misinterpretation by an adult of either normal sexual child behavior (for example, occasional masturbation) or caretaking behavior (like washing, bathing, diapering, or cleaning the genital area).

3. Deliberate lies by a teenager. While not common, a few teenagers who are knowledgeable about the powerful impact of a sexual abuse complaint may accuse a caretaker falsely if they wish to be removed from an undesirable environment like a conflicted parental or foster home. Also rare is the teenager who invents a rape story to conceal consented intercourse in order to escape the parents' anticipated wrath.

These "sex stress" situations tend to be highly emotionally charged and require an extended psychosocial assessment.

In any case, it is not the physician's role to determine whether a sexual offense has occurred; this remains the responsibility of the legal authorities or child protective services. The physician can assist these agencies, however, in making their decision by describing and/or testifying whether the results of the child's examination are compatible with the alleged sexual abuse complaint.

MANAGEMENT

The physician's responsibilities in the management of sexual abuse can be summarized as follows:

1. Provide emotional support.
2. Take a detailed sexual abuse history (Table 1).
3. Conduct a focused physical examination.
4. Conduct a genital examination when needed.
5. Collect medicolegal evidence.
6. Treat injuries; give tetanus prophylaxis when indicated.
7. Check for sexually transmitted disease; offer prophylactic treatment.

8. Check for pregnancy; discuss pregnancy prevention methods when indicated.
9. Document findings.
10. Offer follow-up treatment and counseling services.
11. Testify in court when required.

The physician's attitude must be supportive and non-judgmental. Teenagers particularly are prone to self-blame. Questions implying criticism like "why did you stay out late at night" may reinforce guilt and increase emotional distress. A teenager who has been raped while running away from home or while partying in defiance of the parents' wishes does not suffer less from the violent trauma than a teenager who was assaulted while sleeping at home.

EMOTIONAL SUPPORT

All sexual abuse cases are to be considered medical and psychological emergencies. Most victims and their families are upset, confused, and anxious but rarely "hysterical" when they come to the doctor's office or hospital. It is important that the physician take sufficient time to inquire about the child's and family's main concerns regarding the alleged abuse and examination. Teenagers should be interviewed without their parents, as they often feel inhibited in their presence. The purpose and each procedure of the examination should be carefully explained; many teenage girls have not undergone a pelvic examination before and feel frightened and embarrassed. Presence of a female chaperone is mandatory. If the alleged sexual assault occurred within 72 hours, the victim needs to be examined immediately to check for presence of semen as medicolegal evidence.

TAKING A SEXUAL ABUSE HISTORY

In order to determine the extent of a physical/genital examination and assess risk for infection and pregnancy, the physician needs to inquire in detail about the types of sexual acts and physical force used during the assault. In each case it is important to find out which parts of the body were touched by what (penis, finger, mouth, tongue, foreign object). Was there ejaculation and where on the body? When did it happen? Who did it? How often? What were the symptoms, worries, and activities after the assault? Did the person shower or douche, which may have washed medicolegal evidence away?

Relevant medical and obstetric/gynecologic information has to be obtained, including data on menstrual history, birth control usage, sexual activity immediately preceding or following the assault, current medications, and allergies.

It is not necessary to inquire extensively about the circumstances of the assault, identifying characteristics of the alleged perpetrator or other information not required for conducting the medical examination. This more legally relevant information is appropriately collected by law enforcement personnel.

Children, even teenagers, are often sexually naive. Many times they do not understand words like *erection*

TABLE 1. Sex Abuse History

1. When did the abuse occur (date and time)?			
2. Who was the assailant?			
3. Did the assailant use force? (What kind?)			
4. Did the assailant put his penis inside your:			
a. vagina	Yes ☐	No ☐	Don't know ☐
b. mouth	Yes ☐	No ☐	Don't know ☐
c. rectum	Yes ☐	No ☐	Don't know ☐
5. Did the assailant reach a climax?	Yes ☐	No ☐	Don't know ☐
If answer is *YES:*			
a. Did he climax inside you?	Yes ☐	No ☐	Don't know ☐
Specify:	vagina ☐	rectum ☐	mouth ☐
b. Did he climax outside you?	Yes ☐	No ☐	Don't know ☐
(If yes, where on your body?)			
6. Did the assailant wear a condom?	Yes ☐	No ☐	Don't know ☐
7. Did the assailant place his mouth on your genitals?	Yes ☐	No ☐	Don't know ☐
8. Did the assailant insert foreign objects into your vagina?	Yes ☐	No ☐	Don't know ☐
Did the assailant insert foreign objects into your urethra?	Yes ☐	No ☐	Don't know ☐
Did the assailant insert foreign objects into your rectum?	Yes ☐	No ☐	Don't know ☐
9. Did the assailant insert fingers into your vagina?	Yes ☐	No ☐	Don't know ☐
Did the assailant insert fingers into your rectum?	Yes ☐	No ☐	Don't know ☐
10. Did the assailant force you to touch his genitals?	Yes ☐	No ☐	Don't know ☐
11. Did the assailant touch your breasts?	Yes ☐	No ☐	Don't know ☐
12. Were any of these acts performed more than once?	Yes ☐	No ☐	Don't know ☐
13. Have you had intercourse after the attack?	Yes ☐	No ☐	Don't know ☐
14. Did you:			
(a) bathe?	Yes ☐	No ☐	Don't know ☐
(b) douche?	Yes ☐	No ☐	Don't know ☐
(c) change your clothes?	Yes ☐	No ☐	Don't know ☐
(d) rinse your mouth or brush your teeth?	Yes ☐	No ☐	Don't know ☐
15. Medical History			
(a) Major illnesses:	_____		
(b) Allergies:	_____		
16. OB/GYN History			

Menstrual History

Age of onset _____ Irregular _____

Regular _____ Duration _____

Cycle _____

Last menstrual period _____

Current contraception _____

Last coitus prior to incident (date) _____

Venereal disease history during last 6 months _____

Other OB/GYN related symptoms, illnesses, or infections _____

or *ejaculation.* Unfamiliar terms need to be described figuratively. Erection may be understood as "a hard penis sticking out"; ejaculation may be described as "white, sticky stuff coming out of his ding-a-ling."

Before the physician interviews the child, he may ask the parents what terminology the child uses for sexual body parts. Young children may be better able to identify body parts and demonstrate sexual acts on dolls than give verbal descriptions.

In our experience, most children and teenagers prefer to be asked specific questions which allow them to answer "yes" or "no," like "Did he put his penis in your vagina?" General questions like "Tell me what happened" deliver vague answers: "I was raped."

To be complete in the interview, physicians are encouraged to utilize questionnaires that contain relevant questions in checklist form.

PHYSICAL EXAMINATION

Fortunately, serious physical injuries occur in less than 5 per cent of child sexual abuse victims. Up to 40 per cent suffer minor physical trauma like bruises, scratches, abrasions, hymenal erythema or lacerations, anal fissures, or rectal bleeding. More than half of sexually abused children and teenagers do not show signs of physical damage. Therefore, absence of physical findings does not rule out sexual abuse, a fact that is often misunderstood by lay people including families, attorneys, police, and juries in court who tend to rely heavily on "physical evidence" to determine whether sexual abuse took place.

A general physical examination focuses on the detection and documentation of any tenderness or injuries sustained during the assault. Whenever possible, injuries should be photographed. Body surface and clothing are to be checked for dirt, blood, stains, debris, or other signs of physical struggle.

The patient's mental state needs to be observed. Signs of emotional upset, level of alertness and orientation, and areas of greatest concern during the assault and at the time of the examination should be recorded.

GENITAL EXAMINATION

Only areas involved in sexual manipulation need to be checked specifically. If an alert patient reports that the assault involved oral sex only, a genital examination is unnecessary and inappropriate. Victims who have no clear recollection of specific sexual activities should receive a complete examination of all orifices. Under no circumstances should victims be examined against their will.

When indicated, the genital/perineal area is inspected for signs of tenderness, irritation, swelling, or injury. In females, the hymenal ring is checked for injuries and size of opening. If the hymenal opening is too small to permit introduction of even a small speculum and no external injury is evident, no full pelvic examination is required, as chances of injury to the vaginal canal are minimal in such cases.

For the purpose of a rape evaluation, it is irrelevant to determine whether the hymen is "virginal" or "marital." Especially in teenagers, the distinction is not always easy to make because of normal variations of hymenal shape, elasticity of the membrane, size of the opening, or trauma from other causes. Legally, penetration of the labia alone constitutes intercourse, and penetration into the vagina is not required to allege rape.

If the hymenal opening allows introduction of a speculum, a full pelvic examination is conducted. The vaginal canal and cervix are checked for injuries, blood, discharge, or secretions, which tend to pool in the posterior fornix. A bimanual examination to rule out anomalies or tenderness of the adnexae concludes the examination.

Genitalia of males involved in sexual acts are examined for pain, edema, erythema, bruises, or other injuries to the penis, scrotum, or perineum. If foreign objects were introduced into the urethra and if there is bloody discharge or pain on micturition, further exploration is required. The anus is checked for tenderness and/or injuries.

If major lacerations or other serious injuries are found, appropriate consultation must be requested from colleagues in the area of obstetrics/gynecology, urology, or surgery.

In cases of oral sex, the oral cavity is checked closely for signs of injuries.

Most sexual assault centers now use colposcopes to document physical findings of genital examinations. The colposcope's excellent lighting and magnification capacity permits production of high-quality photographs, which help the physician explain his findings during court testimony.

COLLECTION OF MEDICOLEGAL EVIDENCE

Only tests relevant to the given sexual abuse history should be performed. For example, in molestation cases that did not include intercourse, sperm search is unwarranted.

All test materials may become part of legal evidence. They must be collected under the rule of "chain of custody" to be admissible in court. This requires that all specimens be properly labeled with the patient's name and date of collection. Any person who handles the test material (for example physicians, nurses, or laboratory personnel) must document accurately the names of the persons from whom the samples were received and to whom they were released.

Table 2 summarizes the medicolegal specimens that need to be collected by the physician.

1. Seminal Fluid. Two markers indicate the presence of seminal fluid: sperm and acid phosphatase, an enzyme that is found in high concentration in prostatic secretions but in low concentrations in the female urogenital tract.

For practical purposes, sperm and acid phosphatase cannot be detected in the vagina 48 to 72 hours after intercourse, and specimens need not be collected after this period.

Permanent smears to document presence or absence of sperm should be prepared by the laboratory from test materials collected from the vagina, cervix, rectum, and oral cavity if indicated.

Acid phosphatase levels in the vagina can be determined from vaginal wash.

Suspected seminal stains on skin or clothing can be checked qualitatively for acid phosphatase. If dried, enzyme activity is found after much longer periods of time than in the vagina. On clothing it is still detectable after several years. Ultraviolet light (a Wood's lamp) causes seminal fluid stains on skin surfaces to fluoresce in dark green patches. Fluorescent stains should be swabbed with a saline-soaked cotton patch, which is placed in a closed container and forwarded to the laboratory for acid phosphatase assay.

2. Other Legal Evidence. The police may request collection of other evidence that may help to identify the alleged perpetrator. Clothing that was worn during the assault should be retained. The victim's pubic hair should be combed; lost pubic hair of the assailant may be found. To distinguish "foreign" hair from that of the victim, two or three of the victim's pubic hairs should be plucked with the root. Scrapings from under the fingernails may yield skin remnants of the assailant, especially when there is a history of physical struggle. Seminal stains may, on special request, be examined for ABO antigen and/or DNA.

MEDICAL TESTS

Screening for sexually transmitted diseases is indicated in patients who report sexual activities that place them at risk for infection or who report symptoms. Cultures should be obtained from susceptible sites for gonorrhea; screening for *Trichomonas* and *Chlamydia trachomatis* infections is advisable. A baseline serology

TABLE 2. Medicolegal Evidence Collection

1. Semen
   a. Spermatozoa
   b. Acid phosphatase
2. Photographs of visible injuries
3. Pubic hair combings and pluckings
4. Fingernail scrapings
5. Preservation of clothes worn during the assault
6. ABO typing of seminal fluid (on special police request only)
7. DNA typing of seminal fluid/blood (on special police request only)

test for syphilis is recommended only for patients who have been sexually active prior to the assault. Examinations for herpes simplex, venereal warts, unspecific vaginitis, or urethritis depend on presenting symptoms. If the perpetrator is a family member, he may agree to venereal disease testing instead of submitting the child victim to a potentially frightening procedure.

A pregnancy test needs to be requested in all cases in which hormonal pregnancy prevention after the sexual assault is considered.

In case of anal intercourse, stool should be checked for blood (guaiac).

Other medical tests such as CBC and radiographs are ordered as clinically indicated.

DOCUMENTATION

The medical record will become a legal document if prosecution is considered or if a child protective agency requests court intervention. Therefore, the physician must record history, medical findings, tests, and treatments legibly and accurately.

As much as possible, the child's statements should be quoted verbatim. Medical jargon is to be avoided, unless the physician wants to be harrassed by attorneys to explain findings and recommendations in layman's terms.

Diagrams, which graphically show location and indicate type, age, and size of injuries, help the physician greatly to remember results of the examination in court, even if many months have passed by.

Rape, sodomy, sexual abuse, and *incest* are legal terms and cannot be used as diagnostic labels by physicians. A proper assessment states the nature of the complaint and describes physical and psychological findings. An example follows:

Diagnostic Impression:
1. Alleged sexual assault
2. Multiple fresh bruises on neck and breasts
3. Fresh hymenal tear
4. Anxiety reaction

TREATMENT

1. Injuries. Injuries should be treated as indicated. When necessary, consultations with other specialists should be requested. Tetanus prophylaxis should be offered to unprotected patients with high-risk injuries. If a patient fights a necessary procedure in a state of panic, general anesthesia has to be considered. Although in most instances injuries are superficial and not in need of special treatment, children and teenagers often develop irrational fears of bodily damage following the assault. They may worry about undetected internal injuries, slowly rotting organs, abnormal looking genitals, or inability to have children. Therefore, clear explanation of physical findings and reassurance become important aspects of treatment.

2. Pregnancy Prevention. The chance of pregnancy from a sexual assault is fairly low even in susceptible teenagers because sexual dysfunction and ejaculation difficulties are high among sex offenders. Nevertheless, the possibility of pregnancy is of great concern to most teenage girls and their families, and options on how to deal with the risk of pregnancy must be discussed.

Adolescent girls who give a history of vaginal intercourse, are menstruating, were in mid-cycle at the time of the assault, and were not protected by a contraception device are at highest risk for pregnancy. Only few choose to wait and see whether a pregnancy develops. If pregnant, they have the option to keep the pregnancy and infant, give the infant up for adoption, or request an abortion or menstrual extraction. The vast majority of teenage girls prefer pregnancy prevention. If taken within 72 hours after intercourse, two tablets of Ovral taken twice within a 12-hour interval have proven highly effective in pregnancy prevention with only few side effects. Before Ovral is prescribed, a pregnancy test needs to be obtained to rule out unsuspected existing pregnancy. Ovral cannot be given if intercourse took place more than 72 hours before the examination or if the teenager engaged in unprotected vaginal intercourse during the present menstrual cycle. Because of possible teratogenic effects, Ovral should also be withheld if the patient would not permit abortion in case of treatment failure.

Written informed consent for hormonal pregnancy prevention should be obtained from the patient and if possible from her parents.

SEXUALLY TRANSMITTED DISEASE PROPHYLAXIS

Any patient who has had sexual contact with an offender who cannot be checked for sexually transmitted disease should receive prophylactic treatment to prevent gonorrhea, *Chlamydia trachomatis,* and syphilis. However, prophylaxis is not routinely necessary for victims of molestation or incest or children and adolescents whose compliance with treatment and medical follow-up are considered reliable. Only positive infection should be treated in these situations. The treatment schedules are summarized in Table 3. Most children fear needles, and whenever possible, oral medication is preferred.

Pharyngeal gonorrhea is difficult to treat; if a positive diagnosis is made, intramuscular ceftriaxone or aqueous penicillin or a course of tetracycline or erythromycin is most effective.

All patients who receive prophylactic treatment must be recultured for gonorrhea within 2 weeks to detect treatment failures. Reculturing for *Chlamydia trachomatis* is not routinely necessary, however, because of the high cure rate if the treatment regimen was followed.

Syphilis serology should be rechecked 6 to 8 weeks after the alleged assault if no prophylactic treatment was given. Syphilitic infection should be treated according to guidelines set by the Centers for Disease Control.

Increasingly, young sexual abuse victims and their families voice fear about AIDS. While the chance of HIV infection in most sexually abused children is probably low, some minors, including gay male teenagers, intravenous drug abusers, prostitutes, or victims assaulted by a member of a high-risk group may be at higher risk, especially in urban AIDS epicenters. Repeated counseling is often necessary to alleviate unrealistic fears and to discuss the significance, benefits, and risks of future HIV testing.

TABLE 3. Venereal Disease Prophylaxis (Gonorrhea, *Chlamydia trachomatis*, Syphilis)

Gonorrhea and Syphilis
A. Amoxicillin 3 gm or ampicillin 3.5 gm plus probenecid 1 gm by mouth in single dose. For children under 45 kg: Amoxicillin 50 mg/kg plus probenecid 25 mg/kg by mouth in single dose.
Note: Curative for incubating syphilis; probably not effective for oral gonorrhea

or

B. Ceftriaxone 250 mg intramuscularly—single dose
For children under 45 kg: Ceftriaxone 125 mg intramuscularly—single dose
Note: Curative for incubating syphilis; effective for pharyngeal gonorrhea

or

C. In case of penicillin allergy
Spectinomycin 2 gm intramuscularly—single dose
For children under 45 kg: Spectinomycin 40 mg/kg intramuscularly—single dose
Note: Not curative for incubating syphilis

Chlamydia trachomatis
A. Doxycycline 100 mg by mouth twice daily for 7 days
Note: Probably curative for incubating syphilis
Do not treat pregnant women or children under age 8 with tetracyclines.

or

B. If tetracyclines are contraindicated or not tolerated,
Erythromycin stearate 500 mg by mouth four times daily for 7 days.
For children under age 8 (and under 45 kg): Erythromycin oral suspension 50 mg/kg/day divided in four doses for 7 days.
Note: Probably curative for incubating syphilis.

COUNSELING SERVICES

Even the most emotionally controlled sexual abuse victim suffers psychological trauma, often for a prolonged period of time. Therefore, counseling services should be offered to every victim and his or her family. In the emergency room, the physician should assess the severity of emotional upset and quality of the victim's support system in order to make appropriate referrals.

For most victims, sexual assault presents a sudden, unpredicted, often life-threatening event. Their sense of security may be shattered. For previously well-adjusted victims with supportive families, crisis intervention by trained rape counselors can be effective in minimizing emotional trauma. Counseling remains issue-oriented with the goal of re-establishing the previous level of functioning as quickly as possible. Anticipatory guidance for common reactions with emphasis on their normality is helpful.

Family-related sexual abuse cases need to be reported to child protective agencies, who will co-ordinate the family's assessment and treatment. They will determine if legal intervention is needed to protect the victim from further abuse.

Patients with intense anxiety reactions who cannot return to a supportive home may need to be hospitalized. Incest victims who fear further abuse or retaliation by their family may also require hospital protection until the safety of their homes has been assessed or another secure placement has been found.

TESTIFYING IN COURT

If a sexual abuse case is prosecuted, the physician is often called to court to testify about the results of the examination. The court is likely to qualify the physician as an expert so that he or she may render interpretations and opinions about the specific findings and to respond to theoretical questions about medical issues in sexual abuse. The purpose of the testimony is to help the judge and jury make a correct decision about an alleged criminal offense. Therefore, the medical findings must be presented accurately and impartially. Diagrams and photographs may be used to clarify injuries or anatomic features if appropriate.

The best preparation for testifying is a pretrial interview with the attorney who has issued the subpoena. At this time, all aspects of the testimony can be discussed frankly. The attorney can explain the legal process step by step from the time of taking the oath and qualification as an expert witness to his line of questioning and anticipated questions during cross-examination. The physician, on the other hand, can educate the attorney about medical aspects of sexual abuse and help him phrase questions in a relevant manner.

The physician must always remember that his participation in court is an important aspect of the overall treatment of the sexual abuse victim.

PARENTERAL FLUID AND ELECTROLYTE THERAPY

RICHARD E. KRAVATH, M.D.,
and LAURENCE FINBERG, M.D.

GENERAL PRINCIPLES

The administration of water and electrolytes to sick children has become the principal modality for maintenance and repair of physiologic homeostasis. All who aspire to give care to infants and children must become experts if the care is to be optimal.

Water and salts may be ingested orally as in ordinary feeding and in special feedings, or fluids may be administered parenterally through veins into the circulation. Most of this discussion will deal with the parenteral route, although the use of oral fluids *when the patient's condition permits* is understood to be preferable because of the potential additional regulating function of the intestinal mucosa. A few specific circumstances for oral therapy will be described. The only parenteral route considered will be the intravenous one. At least in the United States, there is little or no need to consider hypodermoclysis, intraperitoneal fluid, or other parenteral modalities.

A few important principles of electrolyte physiology and water metabolism underlie all the therapeutic advice and regimens to be suggested. A brief review of these principles will place the recommendations in a usable context and permit rational application. One should have a reasonable grasp of the composition of the body with respect to water and the important solutes. Water constitutes about 70 per cent of the lean body mass (LBM), perhaps slightly higher in the newborn infant. There is little water associated with adipose tissue, so that an estimated correction is in order for obese subjects. Infants are rarely obese, so weight and lean body mass for them are approximately the same.

About 45 per cent of the lean body mass of infants is contained within cells, mostly muscle cells. Intracellular water contains most of its solute in ionic form. The cations in highest concentration are potassium (K^+) and magnesium (Mg^{++}). The Mg^{++} is largely bound to cell protein and changes slowly, so that few clinical conditions reflect disturbances with it. The anionic composition consists of phosphates, sulfates, bicarbonate, and organic molecules, large (such as protein) and small (such as Krebs cycle intermediates). In the muscle cell there is virtually no chloride ion (Cl^-) and although calcium (Ca^{++}) is of major importance, it appears in a concentration an order of magnitude below that of concern to this subject. Sodium (Na^+) is found in low concentration in cell water. The exclusion of Cl^- and virtual exclusion of Na^+ has fundamental importance both to homeostasis and to planning fluid therapy, since this biologic phenomenon causes NaCl content to be the determiner of the partition of body fluids.

Extracellular fluid (ECF) consists of two subcompartments. The first is interstitial fluid, which bathes the cells and accounts for about 19 per cent of the LBM. This is slightly higher in the neonate but reaches the infant proportion within the first week. Plasma, the intravascular portion of ECF, accounts for about 6 per cent of LBM. The electrolyte concentration in the water of plasma and interstitial fluid is similar; the presence of 6 to 7 gm of protein per dl in the plasma exerts a minor Donnan effect on the concentration of the other ions. These last variations are not clinically important.

Na^+ is the principal cation, Cl^- (100 mEq/L in plasma) and bicarbonate, HCO_3^- (22 to 25 mEq/L) the anions. Small amounts of K^+, Ca^{++}, Mg^{++}, and HPO_4^- are also present. The boundary between intracellular fluid (ICF) and ECF is maintained by transport mechanisms that extrude sodium and exclude chloride. The two fluids maintain quite constant composition in health while in close proximity across thin cell membranes, retaining the probable ancestral arrangement of early living cells with the primeval sea.

The plasma retains its volume despite hydrostatic pressure from the heart and permeable capillaries, because of the relatively impermeable protein; the albumin, being smaller than the globulins, exerts more osmotic (oncotic) influence per gram. Discussion of therapy will stress maintaining the proportionate volumes of these compartments or "spaces." Note that in health all of these spaces represent a nearly constant fraction of the lean mass, and therefore their reconstitution when they are deficient can be appropriately expressed as a fraction of the patient's weight.

Water turnover, the daily obligatory expenditure of water, relates not to mass but to heat (caloric) loss or metabolic activity. This in turn is a function of body surface, so that either calories expended or surface area may be used as a reference denominator for daily water requirements. Table 1 shows the important relation-

TABLE 1. Basic Caloric Expenditure for Infants and Children*

Age	Weight (kg)	Surface Area (m²)	Cal/kg
Neonate	2.5–4	0.2–0.23	50
1 week to 6 mo	3–8	0.2–0.35	65–70
6 to 12 mo	8–12	0.35–0.45	50–60
12 to 24 mo	10–15	0.45–0.55	45–50
2 to 5 years	15–20	0.6–0.7	45
6 to 10 years	20–35	0.7–1.1	40–45
11 to 15 years	35–60	1.1–1.7	25–40
Adult	70	1.75	15–20

*Water expenditure equals 1 ml/cal.

ships for infants. We prefer to use calories* for teaching purposes because of the more fundamental relationship. Also, neonates, edematous subjects, and a few others do not quite conform to surface area calculations for water loss.

Since neither heat loss nor surface area is measured in actual practice, Table 1 may be used to express the water requirement in terms of weight and age. A quick glance at the table shows that only about four points need be remembered to make interpolation easy. In this way ongoing water requirement may be related to its appropriate reference point, energy, which is distinct from deficit replacement, which relates directly to weight at all ages. There is no single common denominator that may be used for both at all ages and sizes. These considerations also emphasize the special hazard of dehydration to the small infant, whose daily water turnover is about 10 per cent of its weight while the adult turns over 2 per cent.

Note that the table refers to basal conditions. In this state the water is expended approximately as follows for every 100 calories metabolized:

Insensible water	skin, 30 ml	
	lung, <u>15</u> ml	
Total		45 ml
Urine (at 300 mOsm/kg)		50 ml
Stool		<u>5</u> ml
Total		100 ml/100 calories or 1 ml/cal

The assumption of 300 mOsm/kg used for urine is a clinically useful one since the actual capacity to concentrate may reduce the obligatory urine loss by a factor of 2 in infants or 4 in older children and act as a safety factor. Many sick patients temporarily lose this capacity. Patients may be at a basal state on rare occasions. More often elevation of body temperature, movement, and increased ventilation bring the fasting bed patient to about 1.5 × basal, a usual figure for calculation. The presence of high fever, extreme movement, or marked tachypnea occurring would warrant an estimate of 2 × basal, and all these together, an unlikely coincidence, might at the extreme warrant 3 × basal as a calculated expenditure. These estimates have been found useful and appropriate in clinical experience for short-term estimates in a fasting patient. Over the long term one

---

*The calorie used here is the nutritionist's calorie or kilocalorie, which is 1000 of the physicist's calories. In a few years the terminology will probably shift to the joule.

must take into account requirements for growth, for specific dynamic action, and for the greater renal solute loads that accompany feedings.

Partially offsetting ongoing water requirement is the production of water from metabolism. This amounts to 12 ml/100 cal metabolized, or about 12 per cent of the requirement. For short-term situations in which recovery follows quickly, this amount may be neglected in calculations; for problems of longer duration this water becomes potentially important and will be considered later.

Homeostasis of hydrogen ion (H^+) is closely guarded in body fluids by buffers, by the control of the P_{CO_2} by the lung, and by renal excretion of H^+ and base. The details of these important relationships are beyond the scope of this presentation, but awareness of the major disturbances remains important. Primary changes in P_{CO_2} are termed respiratory, and primary changes in other acids are termed metabolic. Acidemia and alkalemia refer to actual changes in H^+ concentration, the pH system being conventionally used and pH 7.35 to 7.45 being the normal range. Acidosis and alkalosis represent a primary change in one or the other direction with compensation returning the pH toward the normal range.

The availability of accurate measurements of pH and P_{CO_2} in the last few years has made the practical application of quantitative acid-base physiology easier—unfortunately, also easier to abuse. Two very important cautions are warranted. First, when ventilatory, circulatory, and renal systems are intact and functioning, H^+ homeostasis is assured except under the most extreme circumstances. This will be further elaborated a few paragraphs below. Secondly, dissolved CO_2 (which, hydrated, forms an acid, H_2CO_3) traverses cell membranes and the CSF-plasma boundary much faster than HCO_3^-, the base form of the buffer system. Therefore, since:

$$HCO_3^- + H^+ \leftrightarrows H_2CO_3 \leftrightarrows H_2O + CO_2,$$

the administration of HCO_3^- rapidly into the ECF causes CO_2 to enter ICF and CSF disproportionately to the HCO_3^- and drives pH down (H^+ ion up). Therefore rapid change in pH in ECF may produce a "paradoxic" opposite change in cells and CSF, to the patient's disadvantage. Thus, except under very unusual circumstances, a slow rate of HCO_3^- infusion is preferred even for marked distortion of acid-base balance.

A final general principle of therapy states that a systematic approach is far superior to a haphazard one. A system should include points of analysis, preferably the same ones used in diagnosing the physiologic disturbance. We recommend five points of analysis with periodic return to them to assess therapy. They are as follows, in order of importance, together with the most useful measurement for each:

1. Volume. There are three considerations in calculating the volume of fluids required: (a) deviation from normal—usually a deficit, rarely an excess, quantitatively a fraction of weight; (b) ongoing obligatory water requirements or maintenance, a function of energy expended over time; and (c) continuing abnormal losses from pathologic states.

The best measure for clinical purposes for this most important consideration is an *accurate weight of the patient*, repeated as often as condition warrants but never less than daily. Changes in weight over 24 hours or less may be taken to represent water changes. Be careful not to extrapolate the principle over several days when it no longer may be true, as other body components may lose weight. The acute weight loss can be taken as the deficit in water, since in the metric system 1 gm approximates 1 ml. Therefore if 500 gm are lost in weight, then 500 ml are required in the deficit fraction. If acute weight loss cannot be measured, it can be estimated using the standard landmarks of 5, 10, and 15 per cent loss of body weight, with 10 per cent loss showing obvious signs of dehydration and circulatory impairment.

2. Body Water Space Proportions. This depends on considerations of osmolar physiology. The critical determinant for the ECF-ICF partition is the NaCl content of the body, for which the Na^+ concentration in serum serves as a guide. Too low usually means relatively increased ICF and too high means relatively increased ECF. Albumin levels in serum similarly guide understanding of the relative plasma volume with a low albumin level indicating low plasma volume and so on.

3. Hydrogen Ion Metabolism. The principles were touched on earlier. Emphasis should be given to the fact that if total volume and space partitions are essentially restored and if lung and kidney are functioning, the homeostatic mechanisms need only minimal help—perhaps, more accurately, an absence of aggravation, to correct the deviation. Measurements include arterial pH, Pa_{CO_2}, and HCO_3^-. An additional useful consideration is the "base deficit," a number indicating the metabolic H^+ disturbance after mathematically adjusting the P_{CO_2} to 40 mm Hg. The contribution of this derived number of Astrup and Siggaard-Andersen has given clinicians a means of quantifying the metabolic component of complex disturbances in H^+ and CO_2. Metabolic acidosis should be corrected slowly and cautiously because of problems already referred to, because complete buffering is undoubtedly more complex than the assumptions imply, and finally because over time a number of physiologic adjustments are occurring.

4. ICF Ion Deficiencies. The concern here is primarily K^+ loss, which is often considerable and on which there are empiric data for a number of disorders. Mg^{++} and phosphate losses appear usually to have less clinical relevance. The best available measure is the K^+ level in the serum, but this concentration represents the result of a complex steady state and therefore it may be normal or high in the face of considerable deficit. The HCO_3^- concentration after hydration may offer a clue here, indicating deficit of K^+ when an otherwise unexplained alkalosis is present. ECG sometimes helps.

5. Skeletal-ECF Steady States. Ionized calcium levels are sometimes altered during hydration aberrations. Total calcium gives a clue; ionized $[Ca^{++}]$ gives direct information. ECG sometimes helps here also.

MAINTENANCE FLUID THERAPY

One use for fluid therapy is to maintain hydration in a patient who cannot use the oral route, either because of alimentary tract disease or as a perisurgical necessity. If the patient is at bed rest and afebrile, which is usual, the volume of the water should be of the order of 1.5 × basal requirements. The requirement for sodium is very small, perhaps as little as 0.1 mEq/100 cal metabolized, and the tolerance in the healthy child very great, up to 10 mEq/100 cal. An allowance of 2 to 3 mEq/100 cal metabolized therefore falls midway in the range and provides a concentration of electrolyte (together with coupled anions) to prevent osmotic forces from rupturing red cells or damaging vessels. Glucose, usually 5 per cent, also serves this protective purpose and also supplies enough calories to combat ketosis.

Potassium conservation is not so good as for sodium, but high concentrations are not tolerated as well, so that 1.5 to 2 mEq/100 cal metabolized is needed for balance. These calculations will result in fluids with Na^+ concentrations from 30 to 50 mEq/L and K^+ of 15 to 25 mEq/L. The anions should be Cl^- and any of several bases, HCO_3^-, acetate, or lactate. The proportion of Cl^- to base should be optimally similar to that in ECF, about 4:1. Such solutions may be made up easily by adding electrolytes to 5 per cent glucose solutions or by purchasing ready-made maintenance solutions. The first approach offers more flexibility and pedagogic advantages to large institutions with many varied problems and a teaching program; the second offers convenience, and, where the service is small, safety as well.

Should anuria, severe oliguria, or other special problems be present, either plain glucose water or modified mixtures either to offer or to restrict Na^+ or K^+, may be concocted. Similarly appropriate anion modification may be achieved.

When fever, increased muscular activity, or hyperventilation is present, the volume of administered fluid should be increased in accordance with the previous schedule. If an anuric or oliguric patient is to be managed, then the water allowance for urine is eliminated and all K^+ removed from the solution. Sodium salts are usually also removed unless deficits or other avenues of loss coexist. The water allocation should be reduced by another 12 ml/100 cal, representing water of oxidation. To this new low allowance may be added the previous 8 hours' urine volume if oliguria rather than anuria should be present.

When oral electrolyte and fluid ingestion is appropriate, as in the recovery period following infantile diarrheal disease, we have successfully used the following pharmacy-prepared "ion mixture" (Table 2). The

amount of glucose has been currently reduced from 5 to 3 per cent. This minor change, for theoretic considerations, is the only one in the last 30 years. The ingredients are prepared for mixture with a liter (quart) of water and dispensed (for home use) one day at a time as a package of dry powder.

Similar solutions may also be purchased, although the commercial ones tend to have lower sodium concentrations because of the public's tendency to overuse the product. Although oral carbohydrate-electrolyte solutions have been in clinical use in the United States since about 1946, there has been increased attention to and extension of their usage for the past few years following work done with cholera patients in Asia. Because the stool losses in cholera have a very high sodium concentration and are lost in high volume, the oral solution best suited for them contains 90 mEq/L of sodium (120 mEq/L for adults). These high-sodium solutions also have been used on severely undernourished children at a point when there was deficit of sodium and water without significant resultant hypernatremia. Such a solution useful to replace deficits would not be advisable in northern North America or Western Europe for *postdiarrheal* disease hydration management or for prevention of dehydration because stool losses tend to have a lower volume and much lower sodium losses. Furthermore, intake is often a high-solute feeding and, related to this, there is a high proportion of infants with hypernatremic dehydration. A wise precaution in utilizing "ion mixture" is to instruct the mother to give plain water ad lib if thirst persists after the recommended day's allotment is complete.

MANAGEMENT OF DEHYDRATION

In managing a dehydrated patient, first analyze the disturbance in the five ways discussed earlier: *volume,* including deficit, maintenance, and abnormal continuing losses; body space proportion or *osmolal status; H^+ ion status; ICF losses;* and *ECF-skeletal steady states.* The most common pediatric problems with dehydration result from the symptoms of diarrhea and vomiting, which in turn produce loss of water and salts plus denial of intake. Most commonly water and salt are lost in physiologic proportion, so that there is symmetric (proportionate) constriction of body fluid spaces. This has been called isotonic, isonatremic, or classic dehydration or, when unqualified, just dehydration. When advanced in degree, circulatory deficit dominates the clinical picture. Accompanying the water and salt loss is a varying degree of metabolic acidosis (or acidemia), because intestinal losses contain relatively more base than body fluids, starvation leads to ketosis, circulatory insufficiency leads to lactic acid production, and, most importantly, a failing circulation interferes with the renal ability to excrete nonvolatile acids.

Before implementing therapy, consider how much fluid will be given and what the solute content should be. Volume factors have been covered and usually where a deficit is involved, in combination with maintenance requirements, will come to 150 to 200 ml/kg/24 hr when dealing with infants and less for older patients in accordance with the principles already outlined. The

TABLE 2. Components of Ion Mixture

Ingredients	Concentrations when Diluted 38 gm/L
KCl, 1 gm	Na, 49 mEq/L
NaH_2PO_4, 1.42 gm	K, 20 mEq/L
NaCl, 0.6 gm	Cl, 30 mEq/L
Na citrate, 2.93 gm	Citrate, 29 mEq/L
Glucose, 30.9 gm	H_2PO_4, 10 mEq/L
	Glucose, 3 per cent, or 167 mM

electrolyte content of the deficit fraction should be taken to be that of normal ECF when dealing with isotonic dehydration: Na^+, 150 mEq/L; Cl^-, 120 mEq/L; base, 30 mEq/L.

In fact, NaCl losses are probably about two thirds of this because some ICF is also lost. The exaggeration permits one the convenience of neglecting maintenance electrolyte entirely in the face of a significant deficit fraction. Similarly, the dehydrated weight may be used for calculation and the offsetting value of water of oxidation also ignored in practical situations. If little deficit is estimated, then proceed as under consideration for maintenance. Potassium replacement must be accomplished from empiric data, and a regimen is indicated in the following paragraphs. The aim is usually about 3 mEq/kg/24 hr in diarrheal diseases and most of the other common disorders.

The plan for 24-hour management may be best divided into three phases: emergency, repletion, and early recovery. Each phase, overlapping on the other two, has a particular emphasis. The first or emergency phase is to restore as rapidly as possible the vascular volume. It should last from 30 minutes to 1 hour and consist of very rapid pushing of fluid intravenously in amounts from 20 to 40 ml/kg, depending on choice of solution and severity of illness. This fluid may be an albumin-containing solution such as single donor plasma, whole blood, 5 per cent human albumin, or one of the modified plasma preparations. If so, 20 ml/kg given rapidly is usually sufficient and ends the emergency phase. In very small (<3 kg) infants or severely undernourished babies, the albumin solutions are advisable. Alternatively, a 10 per cent glucose in water stock solution to which Na^+, 75 mEq/L, Cl^-, 50 to 60 mEq/L, and base (HCO_3^- or lactate), 15 to 25 mEq/L, have been added may be given at 40 ml/kg over 40 to 60 minutes.

There are also suitable commercial solutions of this sort. Some authors recommend Ringer lactate for this phase. We prefer the glucose-based solution because in our hands urine formation is observed earlier, but published results show few if any differences. The emergency "push" phase should always be employed in infants with any detectable or presumed deficit to ensure circulation, even if the infant is not yet seriously ill.

The second phase lasts for the next 6 to 7 hours, with its primary aim being repletion of the ECF. A 5 per cent glucose based solution is recommended, and the Na concentration is reduced to about 40 mEq/L (range, 35 to 55). K^+ should be added *as soon as urine formation is assured*, at a level of 20 mEq/L, the anions to be distributed proportioned as before unless a special problem coexists. The amount given in this period should total, together with the emergency phase, one half of the projected fluid volume for the first 24 hours. If, as is so commonly the case, the projection had been for 200 ml/kg in the first 24 hours, the first and second periods should have delivered 100 ml/kg in 6 to 8 hours.

The third phase, or early recovery period, continues the second phase at a slower rate, completing the projected volume plus additions for ongoing pathologic

losses in 24 hours. K^+ is an important part of this phase of therapy unless severe oliguria persists and the aim is intracellular repletion. Oral therapy may be substituted here with "ion mixture" or other suitable fluid. Table 3 summarizes the preceding paragraphs and is constructed on the assumption of a 10 per cent weight loss isotonic dehydration projected to receive 200 ml/kg in the first 24 hours. This approach should be used as a guideline and therapy individualized in accordance with more precise diagnosis of the physiologic disturbances.

When hypernatremic dehydration is diagnosed or reasonably suspected ($Na^+ > 150$ mEq/L), some modifications of the therapy are in order. If shock is concomitant, or even early circulatory failure, the emergency phase should be a plasma-like solution at 20 ml/kg lest brain swelling occur if hypotonic fluids are given. If no shock is present, no emergency phase exists and the deficit should be replaced gradually over a 48-hour period. The rate of administration of the total volume per hour should be the same over the full 48 hours, combining the deficit and 2 days' worth of allocation. The stock solution should be 2.5 per cent glucose. The Na^+ concentration should be 20 to 30 mEq/L, and *as soon as urine production is manifest*, the K^+ concentration should be maximal (40 mEq/L). One ampule of 10 per cent calcium gluconate should be added to every 500 ml of administered fluid. Anions distribute as in isotonic dehydration. This regimen has been remarkably successful in minimizing complications.

When hyponatremia accompanies diarrheal disease (10 per cent or less of the time), simply increase the Na^+ concentration in phases 2 and 3 of the isotonic regimen to 100 or 120 mEq/L. Rarely is hypertonic salt necessary.

SPECIAL HYDRATION PROBLEMS

Hyponatremic States with Circulatory Symptoms. These conditions result when salt is being lost with water but only water is being replaced. Fistula drainage, nasogastric drainage, dialytic errors, improper dilution of infant formula, and Addison disease constitute some of the etiologic circumstances. The patients have azotemia, dilute or absent urine, and circulatory insufficiency, although they may have a normal or even supernormal water content. Such situations are best corrected by infusion of hypertonic solutions of sodium salts. Sometimes this is the only way to save life, and promptness is essential. The deficit of sodium salts must be understood as a deficit of osmotically active solute, because maldistribution of body water is the most pressing problem. The distribution for calculating the deficit then becomes the *total body water* or 70 per cent of the lean body mass.

For example: A 10-kg baby following surgery which created an ileal fistula has been maintained in water balance, but sodium concentration in serum is only 100 mEq/L and the SUN is 110 mg/dl. A mild acidosis has occurred.

Water volume = $0.7 \times 10 = 7$ liters
Deficit per liter = $140 - 100 = 40$ mEq
$7 \times 40 = 280$ mEq Na

TABLE 3. Scheme for First 24 Hours of Rehydration in Isotonic Dehydration; Deficit = 10 Per Cent of Weight

	Period 1	Period 2	Period 3
Phase	Emergency	Repletion	Early recovery
Duration	0.5 to 1 hour	6 to 7 hours	16 to 18 hours
Emphasis for restoration	Plasma volume	ECF	ICF
Fluid composition	a. Plasma or 5 per cent albumin or b. 10 per cent glucose with Na^+ 75, Cl^- 55, HCO_3^- 20 mEq/L	5 per cent glucose with Na^+ 40, K^+ 20, Cl^- 40, and base 20 mEq/L	5 per cent glucose with Na^+ 40, K^+ 20, Cl^- 40 to 45, and base 15 to 20 mEq/L
Amount in ml/kg of body weight	a. 20 ml/kg or b. 40 ml/kg	60 to 80 ml/kg	100 ml/kg plus ongoing abnormal losses

Presume a balanced anion proportion of 210 Cl^- and 70 HCO_3^-.

The replacement should be either with molar or 0.5 M solution; 200 ml of molar NaCl mixed with 80 ml of molar $NaHCO_3$ will replace the deficit of electrolyte. Customarily, one half is given over a short interval and the patient rechecked. If improvement is noted and no untoward effects have occurred, the other half may be run in slowly, the whole process taking 4 to 6 hours.

Salt Poisoning. Severe salt poisoning is the reverse of the previous situation and is best treated by peritoneal dialysis using 7.5 or 8 per cent glucose as the dialyzing solution, with removal every 90 minutes for two or three infusions.

Diabetic Ketoacidosis. The fluid disturbance of diabetic ketoacidosis is similar to that encountered in enteric disease plus hyperglycemia. This last often makes the disturbance similar to hypernatremia. With the addition of gradual administration of insulin, the principles of therapy are similar to those for hypernatremic dehydration. In particular, the correction of the acidemia should be gradual. Rapid infusion of hypertonic $NaHCO_3$ is doubly dangerous, once for the sodium and a second time for the bicarbonate. Rapid reduction of hyperglycemia predisposes to cerebral edema, also best avoided.

Ventilatory Insufficiency. In conditions of ventilatory failure, whether RDS or severe status asthmaticus, the base excess is helpful to approximate the metabolic component of acidemia which is secondary to hypoxia. Adequate fluid should be given with an increased portion of base, if necessary, but at the calculated rate and volume.

Surgical Conditions. Several disorders in which joint care with surgeons is indicated present special problems. Pyloric stenosis, a rather common disorder, is one of the few that may commonly give rise to a metabolic alkalosis. This is because there is high obstruction, so that gastric but not intestinal juices are lost in vomitus. Potassium losses are marked in part because too high a blood pH encourages urinary loss of $KHCO_3$ until the K^+ loss brings about paradoxic aciduria. The management of the volume and proportionate space problems is the same as in other hydration problems. The alkalosis should never be worsened by administration of any base, and the K^+ as KCl should be replaced as rapidly as is safe to a maximum concentration of 40 mEq/L both pre- and post-operatively but not intraoperatively because of possible scant urine formation. These are rare occasions for administration of NH_4Cl or even intravenous dilute HCl, but these situations are perhaps best left for experts.

In Hirschsprung's disease, the only special consideration is to remember that the large volume of fluid trapped in the colon is physiologically outside of the patient but included in the weight by the scale. The volume may easily be 5 per cent of the patient's weight.

Patients burned extensively similarly develop an "edema space" which is additive to the weight by as much as 10 per cent when 50 per cent or more of body surface is involved. This fluid, similar to plasma and interstitial fluid, is unavailable to support plasma or interstitium for a period of 5 to 8 days. Allowance should be made for addition initially and delivery of the edema a week or so later.

PARENTERAL NUTRITION

Patients who have lost most of the small intestine secondary to disease or from surgery to relieve an anomaly or a disease process, as well as patients with bowel disease and severe malabsorption in whom removal of enteral feeding may lead to healing of inflammatory lesions, have experienced successful intravenous alimentation, sometimes after extended periods of up to a year. This is done by placing a catheter into a large vein, permitting infusion of concentrated solute loads or by using less concentrated solutions by peripheral vein. The technique, however, is inherently hazardous because of the ease of contamination and of thrombus formation, particularly with central veins. In addition, a variety of toxic-metabolic complications have occurred, varying with the solution selected. These include hyperammonemia, other evidences of liver damage, deficiency disease, and others. One aid to avoidance of deficiency of linolenic acid and trace elements has been a small weekly infusion of plasma from a donor who donates an hour after eating a high-fat meal. To date the procedure remains one of a high-level, tertiary care nature and should be employed only by groups who will treat significant numbers of patients and who will maintain a commitment to monitor each patient very closely while supervising an experienced bedside and laboratory team.

Parenteral preparations of fat have become available, which are clinically useful. The amount of fat should be kept down to approximately 1 gm/kg/24 hr, given preferably in divided doses as a supplement to the continuous concentrated glucose-amino acid-electrolyte solution. Higher doses of lipid have produced reductions in pulmonary surfactant while traversing the pulmonary circulation. This points to special hazards for infants (or others) with respiratory distress. It also makes clear the usefulness of entry of foodstuffs via the abdominal venous (portal) system so that the liver is the first organ perfused. Despite a number of hazards, both total and partial parenteral nutrition occupy a valuable place in our current armamentarium.

MALIGNANT HYPERTHERMIA

KEITH J. KIMBLE, M.D.

Malignant hyperthermia (MH) is a syndrome of uncontrolled skeletal muscle hypermetabolism, usually triggered by exposure to potent inhalational anesthetic agents or succinylcholine in genetically susceptible persons. As with neonatal sepsis, the morbidity of early treatment of suspected cases is sufficiently trivial and the mortality rate in neglected cases sufficiently great that definitive therapy is commonly instituted when the diagnosis is merely suspected.

Occasionally, the pediatrician may be called to the operating room or postanesthesia recovery room to assist in the management of a child diagnosed only minutes earlier. Unless the patient has already sustained cardiovascular collapse, immediate therapy must be directed only toward discontinuation of all anesthetic agents; hyperventilation with 100 per cent oxygen; and rapid intravenous administration of dantrolene, a specific antidote, in an initial dose of 2.5 mg/kg. Although diuresis, cooling measures, bicarbonate therapy of acidosis, and replacement of the anesthesia machine may eventually be desirable, their implementation must not delay the preparation and infusion of dantrolene. The initial dose of dantrolene is usually effective, but additional drug (occasionally to as high as 10 mg/kg) may be required to suppress hypermetabolism and muscle rigidity completely.

More commonly, the pediatrician is consulted after the first crucial minutes have passed. Several life-threatening problems may nonetheless arise early on. Persistent hyperthermia, especially if body temperature is continuing to rise, may necessitate surface cooling, iced intravenous solutions, and iced saline lavage. Additional dantrolene should also be given, of course. Hyperkalemia may be extreme, requiring hyperventilation, bicarbonate administration, and occasionally glucose-insulin infusion for correction. Limited experience also suggests that calcium, which is effective in reversing the cardiac effects of hyperkalemia in other settings, can be used safely in MH despite theoretic concerns that it may worsen hypermetabolism. Acidosis is most effectively treated with hyperventilation, although alkali therapy (preferably with bicarbonate—not with lactate) may also be efficacious. Ventricular arrhythmias may resolve as hypermetabolism and acidosis (with attendant catecholamine release) subside. Should drug therapy be deemed necessary, lidocaine, usually the drug of choice, should be avoided because of the theoretic concern that hypermetabolism may be worsened, and procainamide substituted.

Once the immediate crisis has passed, the child should be cared for in an intensive care setting for the first several days. Most patients, if not all, should have an arterial line and bladder catheter placed; and some may benefit from pulmonary artery catheterization. Several major problems must be anticipated during this time. Intravenous dantrolene should be continued for 24 hours following the suppression of hypermetabolism and rigidity, but recrudescence may still occur. Continuous monitoring of end-tidal CO_2 may give an early indication of breakthrough in children on controlled ventilation. Additional dantrolene should then be given. Hypoxic-ischemic encephalopathy must be addressed in children who have sustained hypoxemia, hypotension, significant acidosis, or high fever. The usual supportive and anti–cerebral edema measures are indicated. Such therapy may be made more complex by the threat of renal failure secondary to myoglobinuria and acute tubular necrosis, necessitating simultaneous brain dehydration, diuretic-induced polyuria, hypocarbia, and urinary alkalinization. Electrolyte (including calcium and phosphate) disturbances are commonplace. Hemolysis, hypotension, and tissue thromboplastin release may trigger disseminated intravascular coagulation.

Because stress may occasionally provoke MH in the absence of exposure to anesthetic triggers, sedation may be appropriate in the intensive care unit. Barbiturates, narcotic analgesics (especially fentanyl), and benzodiazepines (especially diazepam) are generally considered to be safe. Ketamine should be avoided because it may produce tachycardia, hypertension, and pyrexia, which may be confused with signs of hypermetabolism. Phenothiazines and butyrophenones should not be used because of their association with the neuroleptic malignant syndrome, which has some clinical (although probably no etiologic) similarities to MH. If muscle relaxants are necessary, nondepolarizing agents (especially pancuronium) are considered safe. These drugs do not reverse rigidity, however.

Finally, although safe anesthetics for virtually any procedure can be provided for children with known or suspected MH susceptibility, some special arrangements must be made in the operating room. Prompt consultation with the anesthesiologist when surgery is first contemplated for such patients ensures the best possible care. Prophylactic dantrolene, until recently used routinely in susceptible patients, may be unnecessary.

COLIC

MARC WEISSBLUTH, M.D.

Determining whether crying is or is not colic helps determine how much therapeutic intervention is needed. Several published studies have diagnosed colic in otherwise healthy infants who had paroxysms of irritability, fussing, or crying lasting more than 3 hours a day, occurring more than 3 days in any one week, and continuing more than 3 weeks during the first 3 months. The criterion "more than 3 weeks" is important for two reasons. First, during the first few weeks, some infants have explosive outbursts of colicky-like behavior lasting less than 3 weeks. Apparent treatment successes, when this brief storm naturally passes, represent only placebo responses. The best treatment during these 3 weeks is watchful waiting. Most parents will accept this treatment if they know that the waiting period is definitely limited to 3 weeks. Second, infant crying always increases and peaks at about 6 weeks of age followed by a dramatic reduction. At this age, most babies do not cry more than 3 hours/day or more than 3 days/week but those that do, do so for less than 3 weeks. Placebo responses also occur after 6 weeks. Narrative diagnostic criteria tend to label too many babies. The importance of clear diagnostic criteria is that in most instances the crying is not diagnosed as colic, and this fact sustains the parents in their wait for the crying to naturally disappear and in their resolve to avoid unproven remedies. Or, if the crying is determined to be colic, organized plans can be made to deal with a 3- to 5-month ordeal.

No treatment of a colicky infant leads to a symptom-free state as a light turned off leads to darkness. Some symptoms will always persist. Claims of treatment success are meaningless in the absence of clear entry criteria and explicit treatment outcome criteria. Exactly how much was the crying diminished and in what percentage of infants? Only when this information is available can a pediatrician or parent reasonably decide whether it is worthwhile to try a proposed treatment.

Many proposed so-called treatments are so simple that they probably will never be studied. These include hot water bottles, noises from vacuum cleaners or hair dryers, different nipple shapes, heart beat or intrauterine recordings, and lamb's wool pads. There is a subtle problem with encouraging parents to try these seemingly benign items. When parents repeatedly engage in minitreatment trials with initial high hopes for success, the inevitable failure to eliminate colicky crying reinforces the parental perception that something is fundamentally very unhealthy with the child, themselves, or both. This unwarranted perception of unhealthiness might persist long after the colic subsides and lead to beliefs and parenting practices that reinforce this false notion: My child is allergic; my child has a sensitive stomach; my child was ill his entire infancy and now needs special care; I could never calm my baby; I never had enough milk; my baby must have hated me then.

There are two older speculative ideas about causation and treatment of colic that have been supported and popularized by eminent physicians. These two nonempirical notions, "maternal anxiety" and "stimulus overload," are really only guesswork. Maternal anxiety as the cause of colic has been described in a famous pediatric psychiatry book (mother's "anxious overpermissiveness psychotoxically" disturbs the baby) and in a popular trade infant-care book (parents overreact and the tension around the infant builds up). Neither author really addressed the issue of directionality of effects but merely assumed that the dominant causative factor was parental or maternal emotionality.

Treating the mother or parents would be the logical conclusion, but it should be clearly understood: There is no study meeting contemporary standards of clinical behavioral research investigating the effects parents and children have on each other that supports this conclusion. In fact, contemporary research suggests that specific parenting patterns do not result from or cause colic. Also, when parents were observed to be trying many different ways to calm their colicky baby, it was assumed by older psychoanalytically inclined writers that parents were causing the colic in the first place by something called stimulus overload. This notion also has no basis in fact. Sensitivity to external stimulation may be a recognizable trait in some postcolicky infants, but the stimulus overload speculation does not fit well with the fact that paroxysmal colicky spells often occur in dark rooms only in the quiet evening hours. Treatment strategies built around the unsupported and, I think, erroneous notion that parents cause colic usually create unnecessary parental guilt, which lowers their self-esteem. If parents can accept the fact that they have a difficult temporary situation that is not their fault, they are better able to avoid feelings of helplessness or hopelessness. When they stop overintellectualizing or practicing self-analysis, they can better carry out simple treatment strategies. Pediatricians should explicitly and repeatedly address this issue of parental nonculpability as part of the treatment process.

Treatment has progressed when parents know that their pediatrician is an ally, when they know what is meant by colic, when they know not to waste their energy and upset their emotional stability on useless gimmicks, and when they feel that they are unlucky but not guilty. What then can be done to reduce the crying? Three maneuvers tend to calm infants: (1) rhythmic motions, including rocking chairs, swings, cribs with springs attached to the casters, cradles, carriages and strollers, walking, bouncing, water beds, and automobile rides; (2) swaddling, including wrapping in blankets, snuggling, cuddling, and nestling; (3) sucking, including at breast, bottle, wrist, finger, or pacifier.

Parents should use other people to help care for the baby when the crying is most severe. Even if this break is only a few hours or a few days a week, it sustains morale because it is a rest period that the parents can anticipate. Tell parents that it is true no one can care for their baby as well as they can, but during their baby's inconsolable crying spell, their baby is probably unaware of who is doing the holding and rocking. Parents must understand that this break is for their pleasure and relaxation; it is not to do errands, chores, or housework. Parents need to be emphatically told that occasionally getting away from their crying baby is smart, not selfish. Taking care of themselves means that they will be better able to nurture their baby.

Parents inevitably want to know whether the constant attention will spoil the child, that is, create a crying habit. Data are available to support the contrary conclusion that consistent and prompt parental responsiveness in early infancy tends to reduce, not increase, crying at age 1 year. However, a potential complication of constant attention during the first few colicky months is that some parents do not change their strategies for the older postcolic child at bedtime and naptime. Thus, after the colic passes, the older child is never left alone at sleeptimes and is deprived of the opportunity to develop self-soothing skills. These children never learn to fall asleep unassisted. The resultant sleep fragmentation/sleep deprivation in the child, driven by intermittent positive parental reinforcement, leads to fatigue-driven fussiness long after the physiologic factors that had caused colic are resolved.

Therapeutic Educational Effort. Drug treatment is usually not needed when the parents are able to calmly learn about normal infant crying, and this learning process should occur before they leave the maternity hospital. Otherwise, after the delivery, the inevitable infant crying, commotion, excitement, inexperience, and fatigue combine to undermine parents' receptiveness to educational efforts. After the delivery, frequent visits, telephone calls, and lengthy conversations are usually required, and nothing will doom this educational effort faster than trying to limit it to a few glib responses hurriedly presented. There is no substitute for spending extra time with these families, and the pediatrician should be sensitive to his or her own feelings on this issue.

There may be situations when even a patient pediatrician might decide that an educational effort is not worth trying because the chances of success appear so dim. This might occur with some families when the infant crying ignites a fire storm of emotionality, fueled by unrelenting strident demands from parents and grandparents for diagnostic tests or drug treatments. "Colic is a medical problem; my child is sick with this problem. Therefore, doctor, give me the medicine to treat this problem." The pediatrician then has to decide whether to treat the child because of the severity of the parental response. Superficially, it seems unwarranted to consider drug treatment of the infant in order to primarily reduce parental anxiety and frustration over their inability to soothe their baby. But this does indirectly promote the health of the child by reducing the possibility of parental anger toward the child, child abuse, or infanticide. Not prescribing medicine in some instances will predictably lead to switching pediatricians, which, given the pediatrician's attitude toward the family, may or may not be in the child's best interest.

Drug Treatment. Dicyclomine hydrochloride* is the only drug of proven value in reducing colicky crying, but there are no widely accepted indications for initiating treatment. Presumably, a colicky infant should be considered a candidate for drug treatment if the spells of irritability, fussiness, or crying consist primarily of prolonged inconsolable crying or if the pediatrician senses that colic is creating a dangerous rift between child and parents. It should not be assumed that drug treatment is needed to reduce pain in the infant. The presumption that colic is pain makes no more sense than assuming that a presocial smile represents pleasure. Nevertheless, parents find it easier to affectionately love their baby when crying is diminished, and this increased social contact is beneficial for both child and parents.

Dosage instructions are given in Table 1. Treatment with dicyclomine hydrochloride in one study eliminated colic in 63 per cent of infants, and placebo was effective in 25 per cent (corrected $X^2 = 5.42$, $P = 0.02$). Infants who responded to treatment had significantly fewer mean daily hours of crying than did nonresponders (mean $\pm$ 1 SD, 1.1 ± 0.8 versus 3.9 ± 1.4, $P < 0.001$). The mechanism of action is unknown but the assumption that it is effective by reducing gastrointestinal smooth muscle contractions is probably incorrect. Based on physiological studies of sleep-wake control and the drowsiness associated with excessive dicyclomine, it is likely that the reduction in crying and increased amount of calm/wakeful behaviors is due to central effects. Risks of drug treatment include accidental poisoning due to parental error and anticholinergic signs with overdosage. Also, there is a weak association with non–life-threatening apnea. Another risk is that parents might be encouraged to expect and demand prescription medicines for minor self-limiting illnesses when the child is older. In my practice, in which parents are from the middle income groups, I no longer prescribe dicyclomine. In similar practices, drug treatment may usually be avoided when educational efforts succeed.

---

*Manufacturer's warning: Bentyl is contraindicated in infants less than 6 months of age.

TABLE 1. Dosage Instructions and Doses for Dicyclomine Hydrochloride*

Instructions
1. Start at lowest dose listed for age of your infant.
2. Give one dose in the morning, one at noon, and a third in the evening.
3. Increase the dose each day, if needed, to a maximum of ½ tsp. four times daily, at morning, noon, afternoon, and evening.
4. Do not exceed the maximum dose of ½ tsp. four times daily.
5. Reduce the dose to next lower dose if excessive drowsiness or infrequent urination (three or fewer times per 24 hours) develops.
6. The medicine may be mixed with a small amount of juice or formula, which must then be finished by your baby.

Doses
Age less than 8 weeks
¼ tsp. 3 times daily
¼ tsp. 4 times daily
½ tsp. 3 times daily
½ tsp. 4 times daily
Age 8 weeks or older
½ tsp. 3 times daily
½ tsp. 4 times daily

*Manufacturer's warning: Bentyl is contraindicated in infants less than 6 months of age.

GENETIC DISEASES

CAREY L. JOHNSON, M.D.,
and DAVID L. RIMOIN, M.D., Ph.D.

Genetic diseases, as an aggregate, are very common in both hospital and ambulatory settings. Hospital surveys indicate that at least one-third of all pediatric inpatients suffer from disease processes with significant genetic elements. A considerable component of a private pediatric practice is devoted to the care of chronic illness in childhood, much of which is genetic in origin.

Birth defects occur in roughly 4 per cent of all neonates, and these congenital malformations rank as the third most common cause of pediatric mortality. Thus, hereditary conditions represent a considerable fraction of pediatric disease and require a multidisciplinary approach to therapy.

The approach to therapy in genetic diseases is similar to that taken in other disciplines, i.e., prevention, therapy, or cure (Table 1). Most genetic diseases have defects at the DNA level as an etiology for their phenotype. A genetic "cure" would require the removal of the defective DNA sequences and replacement with normally functioning sequences. At the present time this type of "gene surgery" is beyond our technology, but we are coming closer to being able to safely add extra functioning genes without removing their faulty counterparts.

PREVENTION

At the present time, the major impact of genetics on disease therapy is in prevention. Genetic counseling, prenatal diagnosis, and screening programs provide efficacious methods of preventing genetic disorders. These areas all seek to deal with disease by primary prevention.

Genetic counseling is a labor-intensive, family-oriented process that seeks to provide medical and genetic information relevant to the disorder. In this way, the family is given an opportunity to appreciate the genetics of the disorder, disease progression, and options for treatment. The education of the family provides information that permits informed decisions regarding adjustments to the disorder, reproductive options, and appropriate therapy.

The prospective identification of genetic disorders creates an enormous challenge for counseling. The diagnosis of an affected family member has immediate implications to related individuals, especially those in the reproductive years. The explanation of the genetic risks, disease progression, and options can be extremely abstract concepts to a couple with no personal experience with the disease. It is difficult enough to illuminate the nature, course, and prognosis of a disorder to an affected family; these problems are magnified when the disease is predicted rather than experienced.

One of the primary objectives of genetic counseling is the provision of reproductive options for parents facing the risk of an abnormal offspring. Implicit in this objective is the personal evaluation of risk versus benefit for the family. For any particular disease, the risk-benefit ratio is influenced by many personal factors: whereas one family may view a risk of 10 per cent as far too high, another may be willing to accept such odds.

As research in reproductive medicine progresses, there has been a concomitant increase in the reproductive options available. As previously, a couple may decide to continue with their prior reproductive plans or may decide to forego having children. If these options are viewed as unacceptable, the family may opt for donor insemination, in vitro fertilization, or surrogate motherhood. The development of prenatal diagnostic technology has provided additional options that dramatically reduce a family's risk of having an affected child.

Amniocentesis has become a widely accepted method of obtaining prenatal information. Amniotic fluid is obtained at 16 to 20 weeks' gestation, and exfoliated fetal cells are harvested. A viable cell line can be established in 2 to 3 weeks which is adequate for most cytogenetic and molecular studies. In this fashion, most chromosomal defects and a rapidly expanding number of metabolic defects can be detected.

The new molecular technology has now progressed to the point that the presence or absence of abnormal gene markers can aid in diagnosis. This technology is now available for many diseases, including cystic fibro-

TABLE 1. Genetic Therapy

Prevention
1. Counseling for genetic disorders
2. Carrier screening
3. Prenatal diagnosis

Treatment

1. Replace gene product	Hemophilia A and B
	Growth hormone deficiency
	Agammaglobulinemia
2. Dietary elimination	Phenylketonuria
	Galactosemia
	Hyperammonemias
	Organic acidemias
3. Avoid precipitating agents	G-6-PD deficiency
	Porphyrias
	Malignant hyperthermia
4. End-product supplementation	Thyroid synthetic defects
	Congenital adrenal hyperplasia
	Glycogen storage diseases
5. Metabolic suppression	Congenital adrenal hyperplasia
	Acute intermittent porphyria
6. Cofactor supplementation	Methylmalonic acidemia (B_{12})
	Multiple carboxylase deficiency
	B_6-responsive seizures
	Vitamin D–dependent rickets
7. Enzyme induction	Crigler-Najjar syndrome (phenobarbital)
	Methemoglobinemia (methylene blue)
8. Metabolic inhibition	Lesch-Nyhan syndrome (allopurinol)
	Type III hyperlipidemia (clofibrate)
9. Detoxification	Wilson's disease (penicillamine)
	Hypercholesterolemia (cholestyramine)
	Hemochromatosis (desferoxamine)
	Hyperammonemias (benzoate)
10. Surgery	Cleft lip (cosmetic)
	Limb-lengthening (skeletal dysplasia)
	Retinoblastoma (extirpation)
	Spherocytosis (splenectomy)
11. Transplantation	Immunodeficiency syndromes
	Polycystic kidney
	Mucopolysaccharidoses
	Cystic fibrosis
12. Gene therapy (futuristic)	Severe combined immunodeficiency and other disorders to be tested in the future
13. Miscellaneous	Prenatal therapy
	Physiotherapy
	Psychological counseling

sis, sickle cell disease, the thalassemias, adult polycystic kidney disease, and Huntington's disease. This list of disorders is currently expanding at an explosive rate and will be the diagnostic modality of choice in the near future.

The amniotic fluid itself can be tested for the presence of specific enzymes. The quantitation of amniotic fluid alpha-fetoprotein (AFP) and intestinal microvillar enzymes can dramatically alter the risk predictions in neural tube defects and cystic fibrosis, respectively.

Another method of obtaining fetal tissue for diagnostic purposes is chorionic villus sampling (CVS). This technique employs the per cervical insertion of a flexible plastic catheter and aspiration of fetal cells from the developing chorion. Some of the advantages of CVS are that the procedure is done at 9 to 11 weeks' gestation, information is available the same week as the procedure, and decisions regarding an affected fetus can be made prior to the second trimester. In experienced hands, the procedural mortality risk for CVS appears to be only marginally higher than the 0.5 per cent risk quoted for amniocentesis. CVS does not provide alpha-fetoprotein information, but a screening procedure of maternal serum AFP (discussed later) is available at 16 weeks' gestation. Although CVS will not supplant amniocentesis for diagnosis, it certainly will become an important alternative procedure in the future.

Less frequently utilized forms of invasive investigation include fetoscopy, percutaneous umbilical blood sampling (PUBS), and fetal tissue sampling. Some of these techniques may be associated with a significant risk to the pregnancy, and their use is confined to situations in which the benefit of the information obtained outweighs the risk of the procedure.

Other noninvasive procedures are also available for evaluating the fetus at risk. Fetal ultrasonography provides valuable physical information regarding gestational development, biophysical profile, and fetal well-being. Ultrasonography is also valuable in detecting specific anatomic anomalies of the developing organ systems. Standards for fetal bone length at weekly intervals have been developed which allow for the detection of many fetal growth disorders. Although fetal radiography is rarely used today, it can provide important information in specific situations such as the evaluation of skeletal dysplasias or amniographic evaluation of the fetal upper gastrointestinal tract.

Until recently, the investigation of genetic diseases was largely limited to affected individuals. The advent of molecular techniques has changed the focus of research toward "nonaffected" carrier detection. The identification of individuals at risk for bearing affected children is becoming much more common now, and this promises to be an area of major contribution to preventive medicine.

Genetic screening programs are designed to minimize the impact of genetic disease by identifying genetic abnormalities prior to the onset of clinical disease. Early detection of metabolic disease such as phenylketonuria, galactosemia, and hypothyroidism provides examples of successful mass screening programs. To implement such newborn screening, several prerequisites must be available: a simple, inexpensive, and sensitive test; impeccable recording and follow-up; and effective therapy are all mandatory.

The screening of nonaffected carriers is aimed at identifying couples at risk of bearing affected children. The requirements for carrier screening are a sensitive, inexpensive screening test; an at-risk population; prenatal diagnosis; and coupled genetic counseling. Several genetic disorders fulfill these criteria and include successful programs such as Tay-Sachs disease in European Jews, sickle cell disease in African blacks, alpha-thalassemia in Orientals, and beta-thalassemia in Mediterraneans. Recent advances in the molecular biology of cystic fibrosis suggest that this disease will soon join the list of carrier screening programs.

Probably the most rapidly expanding volume of genetic screening is currently observed in the population of advanced maternal age pregnancies. At age 36, the risk for carrying a fetus with a chromosomal abnormality is 1 in 200, and this risk increases to 1 in 40 at 40 years and to 1 in 12 by 45 years. The social tendency to delay pregnancy and the increasing public awareness of the effects of advanced maternal age have made this indication the most common referral for prenatal studies.

Maternal serum screening programs have long been available for the evaluation of Rh sensitization in Rh-negative women. More recently, it has been demonstrated that screening maternal blood for elevated alpha-fetoprotein (AFP) at 16 to 20 weeks' gestation is a sensitive indicator for open neural tube defects such as spina bifida and anencephaly. A fortuitous consequence of this program has been the observation that low maternal serum AFP levels can be indicative of a trisomy condition. In currently operating programs, low levels of maternal serum AFP have been detecting approximately 20 per cent of unsuspected trisomy-21 (Down's syndrome) fetuses and most of these in younger mothers. It must be stressed that maternal serum AFP is a screening test, and positive results must be followed up by a more definitive examination. It is clear that maternal serum AFP screening enables the identification of open neural tube defects and many of the chromosomally abnormal fetuses early in gestation. Maternal serum AFP screening is now provided through a state program in California and will likely become a routine part of prenatal care in North America.

THERAPY

Crucial to the implementation of therapy is accurate diagnosis. The recent explosion in biomedical technology has provided rapid and accurate information for many genetic disorders and is now revolutionizing diagnosis in infectious diseases and forensic medicine. The applications of molecular biology to disease carrier detection and predisposition to common diseases such as coronary artery disease and diabetes may soon allow for extensive premorbid therapy.

Treatment modalities can be considered at four levels: clinical, biochemical, protein, and DNA. Clinical interventions in genetic disorders represent tertiary therapy. Some examples of this mode include cleft lip repair, splenectomy for hereditary spherocytosis, limb-lengthening procedures for skeletal dysplasias, beta-blockers in Marfan's syndrome, and psychological counseling in Huntington's disease. Maneuvers such as intrauterine transfusion for erythroblastosis fetalis and surgical bypassing of cerebrospinal fluid or urinary tract obstruction have been successfully completed in the prenatal period.

Metabolic therapy focuses on those conditions in which an abnormal metabolic process is recognized. In general, the successful therapies in this group result from a clearance of toxic metabolites by dietary elimination, altered enzyme activity, feedback suppression, or detoxification. In some way, each of these methods circumvents the genetic defect and imposes an external regulation of toxic metabolites.

Classic examples of dietary elimination include phenylalanine restriction in phenylketonuria and galactose restriction in galactosemia. Enzyme induction with phenobarbital or methylene blue is recognized treatment for Crigler-Najjar syndrome and methemoglobinemia, respectively. Enzyme inhibition results in decreased toxins in Lesch-Nyhan syndrome (allopurinol) and hyperlipoproteinemia III (clofibrate). The steroid treatment in the adrenogenital syndromes not only corrects the steroid deficiency but also acts to suppress enzymatic pathways that produce masculinizing or feminizing hormones.

Metabolic therapies involve detoxification and excretion, such as Wilson's disease (penicillamine), familial hypercholesterolemia (cholestyramine), and urea cycle defects (benzoate and phenylacetate). The conjugation and excretion of toxic end-products as nontoxic by-products is another method of maintaining external control over homeostasis.

Many genetic diseases result from absent production or function of proteins. Genetic therapy at this level is designed to replace the abnormal protein. Replacement of protein is effective therapy in hemophilia A and B, growth hormone deficiency, and agammaglobulinemia. Some metabolic diseases have enzymatic defects but are amenable to end-product supplementation, and these include the thyroid synthetic disorders (thyroxine) and congenital adrenal hyperplasia (steroids).

A small group of metabolic disorders is amenable to vitamin supplementation. Pharmacologic doses of these cofactors may induce adequate activity of the abnormal enzyme and normalize the pathway. These disorders include vitamin B_6–responsive convulsions, vitamin D–dependent rickets, multiple carboxylase deficiency (biotin), methylmalonic acidemia (vitamin B_{12}), and vitamin B_6–responsive homocystinuria.

CURES

The advances in immunosuppression and the clinical transplant experience have expanded the role of organ transplantation in the therapy of human genetic diseases. In addition to replacing a malfunctioning organ, the surgical implantation of genetically distinct tissue can provide the organism with the ability to manufacture a deficient protein and thus circumvent the sequelae of the genetic defect.

Bone marrow transplantation has been used successfully in many disorders, including many immunodeficiency states, thalassemias, and Gaucher's disease. Liver transplant has been undertaken for familial hypercholesterolemia, tyrosinemia, and glycogen storage diseases. Renal transplant has been used for cystinosis and Fabry's disease. Transplanting other organ systems is currently being considered (pancreas, heart/lung, skin) for specific conditions. These examples show that organ transplantation is rapidly becoming a recognized option for human genetic therapy.

Certainly the most controversial form of genetic therapy at present involves the manipulation of hereditary material to achieve a genetic "cure." So-called gene therapy has arisen from the simultaneous development of methods to stably clone mammalian genes and to introduce these genes into cultured cells. The obvious extension of this technology is to attempt the correction of disease by human gene therapy.

The concept of altering the human hereditary material has spawned a myriad of scientific and ethical controversies. Recent consensus meetings have laid down general guidelines that such experimental therapy must follow. Most importantly, it has been decided that gene therapy will not be applied to germ cells and initially will be limited to somatic cells. In this way the hereditary alterations cannot be transmitted to subsequent generations.

Somatic gene therapy involves the introduction of new genes to the human body in an effort to reconstitute a genetically defective function. The technical difficulties in replacing defective genes for clinical benefit are many. The identification and characterization of the disease gene are the initial steps. One also must be able to manufacture large quantities of the normal gene and have a way to introduce this gene into the patient's genome. Molecular methods have now identified more than 100 disease genes, and cloning technology has facilitated production of usable quantities of normal genes. A variety of methods have been developed to introduce the normal genes into cells, but the most efficient technique at present has been virus-mediated gene transfer.

Retroviral vectors are suitable for gene transfer because human genes can be carried by the virus and efficiently integrated into the chromosomes of infected hosts. The virus itself has been altered and is unable to replicate. Several concerns have been raised with the use of recombinant retroviruses. These viruses may combine with naturally occuring oncogenes, possibly activating malignant potential. The viral integration site may occur within an otherwise normal gene and produce a mutation. The retroviruses themselves may be able to recombine with native viruses and generate potentially dangerous infectious particles. These matters are currently being addressed in animal and human tissue studies.

The most formidable obstacle in gene therapy is placing the corrected gene where it is needed (targeting) and ensuring that the gene functions in a way to alleviate the disease state and not to create a new set of problems. Many disorders are primarily expressed in specific tissues (thalassemias, neurodegenerative disorders, muscle disorders) and would require site-directed gene transfer. Once positioned in the correct tissue, the appropriate regulation of the new gene is crucial. Over or underproduction of the gene product can produce further clinical difficulties.

Despite the many problems associated with gene therapy technology, severe combined immune deficiency (SCID) appears to be a likely candidate for the first human experiments in gene replacement therapy. SCID results from a deficiency of the enzyme adenosine deaminase (ADA), and the target tissue is bone marrow. Only 5 per cent ADA activity is required to produce functional immunity, and the disease is otherwise lethal. Marrow cells would be removed from the patient and a corrected ADA gene inserted. The patient would then undergo an autologous transplant of this marrow aimed at engrafting stem cells that have an active ADA gene.

A considerable number of human genetic disorders are potentially treatable by gene therapy, and it is a reasonable expectation that current technical problems will be circumvented and somatic gene therapy will be a realistic alternative form of treatment.

SUMMARY

The diversity of genetic disease necessitates a broad interpretation of the term "therapy." In many ways, the preventive aspects of genetic counseling, prenatal diagnosis, and screening programs provide stellar examples of primary therapy. This approach to genetic treatment combines communication skills and technical strategies to provide cost-effective intervention in genetic diseases.

Genetic therapy on a clinical level continues to make significant advances. Treatment of hyperlipidemia and growth disturbances has changed dramatically in recent years. The rapid development of transplant technology has given hope to many people afflicted with severe genetic diseases.

The realistic hope for major advances in genetic therapy lies with the "new" genetics. Molecular biologic approaches to disease diagnosis and therapy will influence all fields of medicine in the near future. The bounty of this new technology will not be limited to genetic diseases as currently exemplified by the genetic engineering of hormones and the polymerase chain reaction diagnosis of infectious diseases such as human immunodeficiency virus and malaria. Somatic gene therapy will one day become an option for a select group of genetic disorders, and developments in this area are among the most exciting and controversial.

Options for genetic therapy are rapidly expanding. The preventive aspects of disease screening and counseling are exemplary of primary prevention. Clinical management of genetic disease is becoming widespread throughout all areas of medicine. Genetic "cures" are becoming increasingly practical with advances in surgery, transplant technology, and somatic gene therapy. Management of genetic diseases has become one of the most controversial and exciting areas of medicine today. The future holds promise for all specialties.

Index

Note: Page numbers followed by (t) refer to tables; page numbers in *italics* refer to illustrations.

Epidermal nevi, 452
  in newborn, 430
Epidermolysis bullosa, 456
Epidermolytic hyperkeratosis, 454
Epididymitis, 381
Epidural abscess, 59
Epiglottitis, 112–113, 527
Epilepsy, 75–83, 86
  drugs for, 79–82, 80(t), 83(t), 636(t)
    laboratory monitoring of patients
      treated with, 79, 79(t), 80(t)
    pharmacokinetics of, 78–79, 79(t)
    poisoning by, 635
    rickets in patients treated with, 318
Epimerase deficiency, 332
Epinephrine, for anaphylaxis, 619, 620,
      621, 674, 674(t)
  for angioedema, 435, 610, 616
  for asthma, 607(t), 608
  for cardiac failure, in septic shock, 596
  for croup, 112
  for physical allergy, 617(t)
  for urticaria, 616
  overdose of, phentolamine for, 621
Epiphora, 474
Epiphrenic diverticulum, 174
Episcleritis, 473
Epispadias, 380–381
Epistaxis, 101–102
Epstein-Barr virus, 565–567
Epulis, congenital, 167
Erb's palsy, 96, 691
Ergocalciferol, for hypoparathyroidism, 290
Ergotamine, for migraine headache, 88
Erosive gastritis, acute, 194
Eruption(s), fixed drug, 615
  in diaper region, 431–432
  polymorphous light, 450
Erythema chronicum migrans, tick bites
      and, 568, 677
Erythema multiforme, 438
Erythema nodosum, 436–437
Erythema nodosum leprosum, 547
Erythema toxicum neonatorum, 429
Erythrocyte(s), antibodies to, transfusion of,
      239
  membrane disorders of, 233
  transfusion of, adverse reactions to, 237–
      238
Erythrocyte metabolism, enzyme deficien-
      cies affecting, 233–234
Erythromelalgia, 159
Erythromycin, interaction of, with carbam-
      azepine, 67
Erythropoietic porphyria, 333
Erythropoietic protoporphyria, 333, 450
Erythropoietin, for chronic renal failure
      and anemia, 230
  increased secretion of, and polycythemia,
      308
Escharotomy, for burns, 682
Escherichia coli infection, 511, 512(t), 517–
      519
  and pneumonia, 508, 508(t)
  in newborn, 511, 517
Esophageal atresia, 173
  with tracheoesophageal fistula, 173
Esophageal compression tubes, control of
      variceal hemorrhage with, 209, 212
Esophageal dysfunction, in cerebral palsy,
      175
  in connective tissue disease, 175
  in dystrophic epidermolysis bullosa, 456
Esophageal foreign bodies, 176, 197, 637
Esophageal varices, bleeding, 177, 207,
      209–210, 212

Esophageal varices *(Continued)*
  cystic fibrosis and, 220–221
Esophagitis, 177, 179
  cyclic vomiting syndrome and, 182
  herpetic, 176
Esophagus, chemical injury to, 176–177,
      640
  disorders of, 173–177
Esotropia, 479
Estrogen, for secondary hypogonadism, 280
  for tall stature, 284
Ethambutol, for tuberculosis, 543–544
Ethanol poisoning, 633
Ethchlorvynol, poisoning by, 658, 658(t)
Ethionamide, for leprosy, 546
  for tuberculosis, 544
Ethosuximide, 636(t)
  for seizures, 80(t), 81, 83(t)
  laboratory monitoring of patients treated
      with, 80(t)
  pharmacokinetics of, 79(t)
Ethylene glycol poisoning, 643
Ethylnorepinephrine, for asthma, 607(t)
Etoposide, for acute leukemia, 264(t)
  for leukemia, in acute cases, 264(t)
Evans' staging system, for neuroblastoma,
      267(t)
  treatment based on, 268–269
Evisceration, 195–196
Ewing's sarcoma, 408–409
Exanthematous conjunctivitis, 467
Exanthematous keratitis, 471–472
Exchange transfusion, for disseminated in-
      travascular coagulopathy, 161
  for hyperbilirubinemia, 206
    in hemolytic disease of newborn, 718–
      719
  for polycythemia, 307, 720
Exercise. See also *Physical therapy.*
  as aid to management, of diabetes melli-
      tus, 310–311
  of hypertension, 148–149
Exercise-induced anaphylaxis, 619–620
Exercise-induced asthma, 607–608, 619
Exocrine pancreas, insufficient enzyme pro-
      duction by, 215
  cystic fibrosis and, 219–220, 224
Exotropia, 479
Exstrophy of bladder, 375
External auditory canal, fractures of, 485
External ear, infection of, 484
External hordeolum, 464–465
Extracorporeal shock wave lithotripsy, 371
Extracranial injury, 46
Extradural hematoma, 49–50
Eye(s), disorders of, 462–480, 592
  foreign body impaction in, 475
  irrigation of, after exposure to toxins,
      624
  trauma to, 475–477
Eye drops, 464(t)–466(t), 469(t)
Eye examination, in patients with cerebral
      palsy, 73
  in patients with rheumatoid arthritis, 340
Eye medications, 463, 463(t)–466(t), 469(t)
Eye ointments, 464(t)–466(t), 469(t)
Eyelid(s), disorders of, 464–465
  pediculosis of, 447
  trauma to, 475–476

Fabry disease, 335
Facial burns, 684
Facial clefts, 167–168
Facial dysplasia, lateral, 394–395
Facial malformations, 392–395
Facial nerve, trauma to, 171

Facial tumors, 452–453
Facial wound management, 170
Factitious vomiting, 182
Factor deficiencies, 254, 259–260
  transfusion for, 239, 255, 259, 260
  complications of, 257–259
Factor inhibitors, 257–258
Factor replacement, for disseminated intra-
      vascular coagulopathy, 161, 161(t)
Factor replacement therapy, 255, 259, 260
  complications of, 257–259
Failure to thrive, 1
  degenerative CNS diseases and, 69
Fallopian tube infections, 390
Familial dysautonomia, 94–96
  and corneal drying, 95, 472
Familial hypercholesterolemia, 331
Familial Mediterranean fever, 687
Familial pemphigus, benign, 455–456
Familial polycythemia, benign, 307
Family counseling, about mental retarda-
      tion, 15
Family support, in cases of chronic renal
      failure, 357
  in cases of degenerative CNS disease, 70
Family therapy, 17
Fanconi's syndrome, 318
Fasciitis, eosinophilic, 342
Fat-soluble vitamin(s), deficiencies of, 7–8
  excesses of, 7, 8
  recommended allowances of, 8(t)
  supplemental, for hepatobiliary disease,
      206, 212
    for malabsorption, 215, 224
Febrile convulsions, 83–86
  and status epilepticus, 83
Febrile nonhemolytic transfusion reaction,
      238, 258
Feeding. See also *Diet* and *Nutrition.*
  after pyloromyotomy, 192
  breast milk in. See *Breast feeding* and
      Breast milk.
  enteral, 2. See also *Parenteral nutrition.*
    after treatment of necrotizing enteroco-
      litis, 203
    in burn victims, 684
    in low birth weight infants, 714
    in patients with diarrhea, 187
  formula, in low birth weight infants,
      715(t), 715–716
  of infants, 3, 174
    caries associated with, 166
    familial dysautonomia and, 94
    low birth weight and, 713–716, 715(t)
Feeding problems, in infants of diabetic
      mothers, 306
Feet. See *Foot (feet).*
Femoral shunt, as vascular access in hemo-
      dialysis, 361
Fenoterol, for asthma, 607(t)
Ferrous sulfate, for iron deficiency, 229
Fetal alcohol syndrome, 706–707
Fetal ascites, 701–702
Fetal death, maternal diabetes and, 301
Fetal growth disturbances, 689
Fetal growth retardation, 689
  maternal diabetes and, 301
Fetal macrosomia, maternal diabetes and,
      301
Fetal supraventricular tachycardia, 702
Fetus, asphyxia of, 96
  effects of rubella on, 559
Fever, and convulsions, 83–86
  and status epilepticus, 83
  burns and, 683
  in familial dysautonomia, 94